DAVIS'S
NCLEX-PN REVIEW

DAVIS'S
NCLEX-PN REVIEW
SECOND EDITION

PATRICIA GAUNTLETT BEARE, RN, PhD

Professor
Louisiana State University Medical Center
School of Nursing
New Orleans, Louisiana

F. A. DAVIS COMPANY • Philadelphia

F. A. Davis Company
1915 Arch Street
Philadelphia, PA 19103

Printed in the United States of America

Last digit indicates print number: 10 9 8 7 6 5 4 3 2 1

Acquisitions Editor: Alan Sorkowitz
Developmental Editor: Ann Houska
Production Editor: Jessica Howie Martin
Cover Designer: Alicia Baronsky
Cover Photograph: Doug Rickards

As new scientific information becomes available through basic and clinical research, recommended treatments and drug therapies undergo changes. The author and publisher have done everything possible to make this book accurate, up to date, and in accord with accepted standards at the time of publication. The author, editors, and publisher are not responsible for errors or omissions or for consequences from application of the book, and make no warranty, expressed or implied, in regard to the contents of the book. Any practice described in this book should be applied by the reader in accordance with professional standards of care used in regard to the unique circumstances that may apply in each situation. The reader is advised always to check product information (package inserts) for changes and new information regarding dose and contraindications before administering any drug. Caution is especially urged when using new or infrequently ordered drugs.

Library of Congress Cataloging-in-Publication Data
Davis's NCLEX-PN review / [edited by] Patricia Gauntlett Beare. — 2nd ed.
  p.   cm.
Includes bibliographical references and index.
ISBN 0-8036-0403-3 (paperback)
  1. Practical nursing—Examinations, questions, etc. 2. Practical nursing—Outlines, syllabi, etc. I. Beare, Patricia Gauntlett.
  [DNLM: 1. Nursing, Practical examination questions.   WY 18.2D265 1999]
RT62.D38   1999
610.73'076—dc21
DNLM/DLC
for Library of Congress   98–27802
                                                                                    CIP

PREFACE

The purpose of this book is to provide the candidate for practical/vocational nurse licensure with a concise review of the information necessary to pass the NCLEX-PN licensing examination and assist the candidate to apply this information in simulated clinical situations by using effective test-taking skills. Chapters 1 and 2 (Unit I) provide basic information on the development, administration, and scoring of the NCLEX-PN and how to prepare for and take the examination.

Clinical Specialties Content Reviews and Tests (Unit II)

In Chapters 3 through 6 recognized nursing authors and experts have prepared the nursing content reviews in outline form. These include reviews of maternity nursing, pediatric nursing, medical/surgical nursing, (with a special section on caring for the older adult), and psychiatric-mental health nursing. The nursing content has been organized according to the nursing process to enable the student to study according to client needs. Test questions were formulated to apply this content in typical clinical situations. The test answer section of each chapter includes the correct answer, rationales for the correct and incorrect answers, the relevant step of the nursing process, and the general category of client need, based on the revision of categories in the new NCLEX-PN test plan.

Related Sciences Reviews and Tests (Unit III)

The chapter on procedures for the licensed practical nurse, now Chapter 7, has been updated. Major revisions and additions have been made to the chapters containing pharmacology review tests and nutrition and combined nutrition-pharmacology review tests. These are now Chapters 8 and 9.

Integrated Comprehensive Practice Tests (Unit IV)

Because the NCLEX-PN test is intended to measure ability to practice as a licensed practical/vocational nurse, these three tests are designed to apply nursing knowledge to health-care situations that demand nursing intervention. Test items have been prepared by nurse-clinicians and educators who have written items for the NCLEX-PN examination and who represent schools or hospitals throughout the United States.

Summary

The content as presented in this book will enable the NCLEX-PN candidate to review essential nursing knowledge and apply this knowledge to test questions in the examination. The number of test questions has been expanded to give the student more practice in applying content to simulated clinical practice settings. Through careful review, candidates will no longer fear the unknown as they review and understand the content and skills necessary to pass the examination.

Patricia Gauntlett Beare

ACKNOWLEDGMENTS

Many people have helped make this second edition a reality.

To Alan Sorkowitz, who supervised the labor and delivery of the text, for his patience and support.

To our special contributors who shared their expertise.

To Danielle Trepagnier, who typed and modified the manuscript.

To Bob Butler, who adroitly guided this book through the production process.

To the reviewers, who critiqued the manuscript for accuracy and clarity.

To my friends, who provided support throughout the publishing process.

CONTRIBUTORS

Lizabeth L. Carlson, RNC, MSN
Coordinator: Maternal/Infant Nursing
Copiah-Lincoln Community College
Wesson, Mississippi

Elizabeth Puneky Covington, RN, MN, CCRN
Assistant Professor of Clinical Nursing
Louisiana State University Medical Center School of Nursing
New Orleans, Louisiana

Kathleen R. Culliton, RN, CS, MS, GNP
Assistant Professor
Weber State University
Ogden, Utah

Diane B. Hamilton, RN, PhD
Professor
Western Michigan University
School of Nursing
Kalamazoo, Michigan

Eileen W. Keefe, RN, CNS
Assistant Professor of Clinical Nursing
Louisiana State University Medical Center School of Nursing
New Orleans, Louisiana

Mary Taylor Martof, RN, EdD
Associate Professor of Clinical Nursing
Louisiana State University Medical Center School of Nursing
New Orleans, Louisiana

Jane Ellerbusch Parrish, BS, MN
Director of Recruitment and Staff Development
University Hospital
New Orleans, Louisiana

Demetrius J. Porche, RN, CCRN, DNS
Associate Professor
Nicholls State University
Thibodaux, Louisiana

Larry D. Purnell, RN, PhD
Professor
College of Health and Nursing Sciences
University of Delaware
Newark, Delaware

Susan I. Ray, RN, MS
Nursing Faculty
Copiah-Lincoln Community College
Wesson, Mississippi

Caroline Bunker Rosdahl, RN, MA
Nursing Faculty
Vocational Education Department
University of Minnesota,
Minneapolis, Minnesota

Kara Schmitt, PhD
Director, BOPR—Testing Services
State of Michigan CIS/Office of Health Services
Lansing, Michigan

Lisa Schulmeister, RN
Adjunct Nursing Faculty
Louisiana State University Medical Center School of Nursing
New Orleans, Louisiana

Danny G. Willis, RN, MN
Clinical Nursing Faculty
Doctoral Student
Louisiana State University Medical Center School of Nursing
New Orleans, Louisiana

CONTENTS

UNIT I

What You Need to Know about the NCLEX-PN

CHAPTER 1

Development, Administration, and Scoring of the NCLEX-PN™*

Patricia Gauntlett Beare, RN, PhD

The National Council Licensure Examination for Practical Nurses (NCLEX-PN), prepared by the National Council of State Boards of Nursing (NCSBN), is designed to measure a candidate's knowledge, skills, and abilities essential to the safe and effective practice of practical nursing. The examination is comprehensive in terms of testing a candidate's ability to work as a practical nurse without harming clients. The results determine whether a candidate can react and respond appropriately to various clinical situations typically encountered by a practical nurse. Candidates who pass the examination are viewed by their boards of nursing as being competent to protect the health, safety, and welfare of clients.

Overview of the NCLEX Examination Testing Process

In April 1994, nurse licensure candidates began taking the National Council Licensure Examination (NCLEX) on computers at many conveniently located test centers across the United States and its territories. The change to computerized adaptive testing (CAT) for the nurse licensure examination came about as a result of a decision made in August 1991 by the NCSBN. The Chauncey Group International, LTD, along with Sylvan Prometric, provides test development and administration services.

To sit for the examination, you, as a practical nurse licensure candidate, must first complete an examination application and submit it, along with the appropriate fee(s) and other required documents, such as a certificate of graduation from a school of nursing, to the relevant board of nursing before the deadline date.

Because each state has different procedures and deadlines,

*NCLEX, NCLEX-PN, and NCLEX-RN are trademarks of the National Council of State Boards of Nursing.

you must be thoroughly familiar with the requirements of the jurisdiction in which you wish to be licensed. In most instances, the nursing program that you attended will instruct you regarding the forms that must be completed as well as the procedures to follow. If the school does not provide you with this information, or if you wish to be licensed in another jurisdiction, it is your responsibility to contact the specific board office for information. (All state boards of nursing, their addresses, and their phone numbers are listed in Appendix A.)

Eligibility Requirements

To take the NCLEX, candidates must satisfy these requirements:

- Apply for licensure in the state or territory in which you wish to be licensed.
- Meet all of the board of nursing's eligibility requirements to take the NCLEX.
- Register for the examination with The Chauncey Group.
- Bring the *Authorization to Test* and acceptable forms of identification to the NCLEX administration. Each candidate will receive an Authorization to Test in the mail from The Chauncey Group after the board of nursing declares the candidate eligible to sit for the examination.

When completing the NCLEX-PN application, be certain that you do so legibly and correctly, as this information will be used in printing your admission card, recording results, providing cumulative data to nursing programs, and perhaps even printing the eventual license.

Foreign-trained candidates should recognize that additional documentation of education and proof of English-language proficiency may be required when a licensure application is submitted to a board of nursing office. For this reason, if you were educated outside the United States, you should send your application as early as possible. It is essential that you contact the jurisdiction in which you wish to be licensed to learn what specific documentation or additional examination results, or both, are required. In addition, you should contact the Commission on Graduates of Foreign Nursing Schools (CGFNS) for detailed information about the requirements that you may have to meet, using the following address and phone number:

Commission on Graduates
of Foreign Nursing Schools
3624 Market Street
Philadelphia, PA 19104
215-349-8767

Basis for the Examination Content

The NCLEX-PN administered in October 1990 was the first to use the results of a job analysis completed in 1987.[1] A new job analysis was completed in 1994. The purpose of the job analysis was to determine the frequency with which certain tasks are performed by practical nurses entering the profession, as well as the criticality of these tasks (i.e., which tasks, if performed incorrectly, could do serious or critical harm to a client). Nurses throughout the country and in a variety of clinical settings completed a survey that listed several hundred tasks typically performed by practical nurses. The respondents' answers, in terms of the frequency and criticality of these tasks, formed the basis for the NCLEX-PN.

Components of the Examination

The examination is not designed merely to measure a candidate's ability to recall or recognize certain facts. Rather, the purpose of the examination is to determine how well a candidate can relate learned facts to common nursing situations. Most items in the examination deal with a candidate's ability to (1) apply information or knowledge learned in one situation and correctly transfer it to another situation, or (2) analyze a relationship by breaking it into simpler components, by making comparisons, or by identifying the relationships between and among certain pieces of information. Remember, the examination is designed to determine how well you will respond in typical, real-life clinical situations and not just whether you are able to recognize facts learned in school.

The test plan or specifications for constructing each form of the examination consists of four phases of the nursing process.[2] Each phase of the nursing process is tested by 15–35% of the items. The test plan also includes four general categories of client needs, a 4 × 4 matrix (Table 1–1) into which each of the examination items must be placed.

So that you can better understand the nursing phases and client health needs, a brief description of each follows.

Phases of the Nursing Process

Data Collection (27–33%)

The practical nurse contributes to the development of a database from which to make decisions about clients. This phase includes five steps: (1) observing the physiological, psychosocial, health, and safety needs of clients; (2) collecting information from the client and others; (3) deciding whether more information is needed; (4) communicating information to others; and (5) participating in the formulation of nursing diagnoses.

Planning (17–23%)

The practical nurse contributes to the development of nursing care plans for clients by (1) assisting in the formulation of goals; (2) participating in the identification of clients' needs and nursing measures that may require changes to the plan; and (3) communicating with the client and others in planning the care.

Implementation (27–33%)

In implementing care for clients, the practical nurse (1) performs basic therapeutic and preventive nursing measures by following a prescribed plan to achieve established goals; (2) provides a safe and effective environment; (3) assists clients and others in understanding the client's plan of care; and (4) records client information and reports it to other health team members.

Evaluation (17–23%)

The final phase in the process involves evaluating the extent to which client goals were achieved. Aspects of the practical nurse's work in this phase include (1) participating in evaluating the effectiveness of the client's care; (2) assisting in evaluating the client's response to nursing care and in making appropriate alterations; (3) evaluating the extent to which identified outcomes of the care plan were achieved; and (4) recording and describing the client's responses to therapy or care, or both.

Table 1–1. **NCLEX-PN Test Plan Matrix**				
	Phases of the Nursing Process			
Client Health Needs	Data Collection 27–33%	Planning 17–23%	Implementation 27–33%	Evaluation 17–23%
Safe, effective care environment 16–22%				
Physiological integrity 49–55%				
Psychosocial integrity 8–14%				
Health promotion/maintenance 15–21%				

Client Needs

Four broad categories are identified in considering the health needs of clients. A brief description of these needs follows, along with the percentage of items covering each.

Safe, Effective Care Environment (16–22%)

The practical nurse assists in meeting client needs in this area by providing nursing care in the categories of (1) management of care and (2) safety and infection control.

Health Promotion and Maintenance (15–21%)

The practical nurse participates as a member of the health-care team to assist in promoting fulfillment of the client's (1) growth and development through the life span and (2) prevention and early detection of disease.

Psychosocial Integrity (8–14%)

Practical nursing care is provided to promote achievement of the client's (1) coping and adaptation and (2) psychosocial adaptation.

Physiological Integrity (49–55%)

The practical nurse provides care to promote achievement of the client's needs in the areas of (1) basic care and comfort, (2) pharmacological and parenteral therapies, (3) reduction of risk potential, and (4) physiological adaptation.

Computerized Adaptive Testing

The NCLEX, administered by computer, uses the methodology called computerized adaptive testing (CAT), mentioned on page 3. With CAT, the computer selects the questions you will answer during the examination to give you the best opportunity to demonstrate your competence.

All questions in the NCLEX are multiple-choice. The questions are presented to you one at a time on a computer screen. You can view each question as long as you like, but you cannot go back to previous questions once you have recorded your answer choices, nor can you leave a question unanswered.

Using the Computer

Although the NCLEX is given on a computer, you are not expected to know how to use a computer before you take the examination. Only two keys—the space bar and the enter key—are used to highlight and record your answer. You will be instructed how to record answers at the test center, and you will have an opportunity to practice on three sample questions before the examination begins. Even after the examination starts, you will be able to request help regarding the use of the computer. The computer practice disk that accompanies this book operates using the same combination of keys that you will use on the test itself, giving you more than 600 questions on which to practice using the computer.

Examination Format

The examination typically presents a situation or incident involving a client, family members, or both. Following each situation is a series of multiple-choice questions pertaining to this information. Some items contain new information and ask additional questions. Because this examination is designed to assess a candidate's ability to practice safely in the work setting, the test items generally relate to various real-life situations in which the practical nurse would be involved. Although candidates must possess basic nursing knowledge to answer the questions, the primary focus is on the ability to apply the basic knowledge to a variety of clinical settings.

Each test item consists of an introductory statement or problem known as the *stem*. The stem is followed by four choices or possible responses to the problem. Only one of these choices is correct; the other three choices are known as *distractors*. Distractors are created in such a way that they may seem correct to someone who is unfamiliar with the terminology, procedure, or general practice. The distractors are not designed to "trick" candidates, but rather to discriminate between those candidates who are qualified to enter the profession and those who are not.

Examination Length

Practical/vocational nurse (PN/VN) candidates take a minimum of 85 questions. The maximum number of questions a PN/VN candidate will answer is 205 during the 5-hour maximum testing period. As you take the examination, questions are selected for you based on your responses to previous questions. Once the minimum number of questions have been taken, testing stops when a candidate's performance is estimated as being either above or below the passing standard with a predetermined level of certainty regardless of the number of questions taken or the amount of testing time elapsed. Depending on individual patterns of correct and incorrect responses, different candidates will answer varying numbers of questions and use varying amounts of time. The examination also stops when the maximum number of questions have been answered or the 5-hour time limit has been reached.

It is important to understand that the length of your examination does not indicate a pass-or-fail result. The number of questions answered is not related to a pass-or-fail decision. A candidate with a relatively short examination may pass or fail the same as a candidate with a long examination. Each candidate, no matter what the length of the examination, has ample opportunity to demonstrate true competence and is given an examination that conforms to the NCLEX test plan.

Guessing

You must answer every question even if you are not sure of the right answer. The computer will not allow you to go on to the next question without answering the question on the screen. If you are not sure of the correct answer, make your best guess and move on to the next question.

Reviewing Answers

After you select an answer to a question, you will have a chance to think about your answer and change it as many times as you like. However, once you confirm your answer and go on to the next question, you will not be allowed to go back to any previous question.

The Passing Standard

To ensure a consistent standard of competence in nursing practice, the National Council uses a criterion-referenced standard. This means that passing or failing depends solely on a candidate's level of performance in relation to the established point that represents entry-level competence. There is no fixed percentage of candidates that pass or fail each examination.

Diagnostic Profile

A diagnostic profile is provided to candidates who fail the examination. The diagnostic profile is mailed to candidates by their respective board of nursing, along with the results of the examination. Using this information, failing candidates can determine their areas of relative strength and weakness based on the test plan and design their study accordingly before retaking the NCLEX.

Reporting Results

Although the NCLEX is scored as the candidate completes each question, *no results* are released at the test center. NCLEX results, available *only* from your board of nursing, will be mailed to candidates approximately 1 month after the examination. *Do not call* your board of nursing, The Chauncey Group, or the National Council for NCLEX results.

Retake Policy

The National Council's retake policy states that candidates must wait a minimum of 91 days between examinations. In addition, each board of nursing may establish its own retake policies, with retakes permitted no more frequently than the policy established by the National Council. This is an important policy that allows the National Council to be certain that all candidates receive a valid examination.

Personal Identification and Examination Security

Because of the importance of the NCLEX, numerous security measures are enforced during the administration of the examination. Strict candidate identification (ID) requirements have been established.

Identification Requirements

When you arrive at the test center, you will be required to present two forms of ID and your Authorization to Test. You will not be admitted to the examination without the proper ID and your Authorization to Test.

- Both pieces of ID must be signed and one must bear a recent photograph of you. The name on the ID with the photograph must be the same as the name that appears on your Authorization to Test.

- Candidates wishing to make a legal name change or an address change must contact their board of nursing.

Please note the following examples of acceptable forms of ID. At least one of your forms of ID must be from the list of primary forms of ID. Examples of acceptable forms of primary ID (must include your signature and photograph) are:

- Valid driver's license with photograph
- Employee ID card with photograph
- School ID card with photograph
- State ID card with photograph
- Valid passport

Secondary forms of ID must include your signature. Examples of acceptable forms of secondary ID include your Social Security card, valid credit cards, and bank automated teller machine cards.

Additional Precautions

Additional security measures that will be taken at the test centers include the following:

- Your thumbprint and photograph will be taken. Your photograph will be included on the report of your results. In some cases, your thumbprint may be used to confirm your identity by the board of nursing in the jurisdiction in which you have applied for licensure. You cannot be tested without having your thumbprint and picture taken.
- You will be observed at all times while taking the examination. This observation will include direct observation by test center staff, as well as video and audio recording of your examination session.

Special Testing Circumstances

Testing accommodations for candidates with disabilities will be made only with the authorization of your board of nursing. To ensure that adequate time is available to evaluate any request for an accommodation, contact your board of nursing as early as possible, preferably before submitting your registration to The Chauncey Group.

Procedure for Requesting Special Accommodations

To request special accommodations, you must do the following:

- Request information from your board of nursing concerning its requirements for requesting testing accommodations.
- Make a request for accommodations to your board of nursing. Your request must comply with requirements established by your board of nursing for persons requesting testing accommodations. Typically, boards of nursing require documentation of past accommodations, if any, and a specific diagnosis by an appropriate health-care professional that includes a description of the accommodations appropriate for your condition.
- Send your request to your board of nursing as early as possible so that, if approved by the board of nursing, the special accommodations can be made in a timely manner.

Table 1–2. **Communicating about the NCLEX**	
Questions about:	Answers
• Registering to take the NCLEX • Authorization to Test • Name corrections on your Authorization to Test • Lost Authorization to Test • Acceptable forms of identification • Comments about the test center	**Call:** 1-800-551-1912 Monday through Friday, 8 AM to 8 PM Eastern Time. Candidates with hearing impairments who use a Telecommunications Device for the Deaf (TDD) may call 1-800-692-5395 for information (open Monday through Friday 8 AM to 4:30 PM Eastern Time). **Write:** NCLEX The Chauncey Group International, LTD 506 Carnegie Center Princeton, NJ 08540 **Fax:** NCLEX The Chauncey Group International, LTD Educational Testing Service FAX 609-951-6767
• NCLEX development • General NCLEX information • Unresolved concerns related to examination administration • Name or address changes • Licensure • Endorsement • Interpretation of results • Diagnostic profiles • Scheduling an appointment to test • Rescheduling or canceling your testing appointment • Examination results	**Write:** National Council of State Boards of Nursing 676 N. St. Clair, Suite 550 Chicago, IL 60611 **Call:** 312-787-6555 Write or call your board of nursing. Wait until you receive your Authorization to Test and the bulletin that will accompany it entitled *Scheduling and Taking Your NCLEX.* Follow directions in the bulletin. Examination results are sent to you by your board of nursing. Wait a minimum of 4 weeks after your examination for your results to arrive in the mail.

Overview of the NCLEX Examination Testing Process*

To be licensed as a PN (sometimes referred to as LPN, VN, or LVN), a candidate must take the NCLEX. To take this examination, candidates must generally go through the following steps, listed in chronological order:

1. The candidate applies to the board of nursing for a license, following instructions from that board.
2. The candidate gets an *NCLEX Candidate Bulletin* from the board of nursing.
3. The candidate submits a registration form to The Chauncey Group (the National Council's contracted testing service) or registers by phone. The Chauncey Group will acknowledge the candidate's registration by mail.

   NOTE: Candidates seeking licensure from Florida, Illinois, Massachusetts, and New York do not register directly with The Chauncey Group. They should follow registration instructions provided by the board of nursing of their state.

4. The board of nursing communicates the candidate's eligibility to test to The Chauncey Group.
5. The Chauncey Group sends the candidate an Authorization to Test (ATT) with a booklet called *Scheduling and Taking Your NCLEX* and a list of test centers.
6. The candidate will call a Sylvan Technology Center and schedule an appointment to test.
7. On the appointed day, the candidate takes the test at a Sylvan Technology Center.
8. The Sylvan Technology Center transmits the test results to The Chauncey Group. After verifying the accuracy of the results, The Chauncey Group transmits them to the designated board of nursing.
9. The board of nursing sends results to the candidate.

Table 1–2 lists telephone and fax numbers and addresses where you may request more information about the NCLEX.

REFERENCES
1. Kane, M and Colton, D: Job Analysis of Newly Licensed Practical/Vocational Nurses, 1986–87. National Council of State Boards of Nursing, Chicago, 1988.
2. NCLEX-PN Test Plan for the National Council Licensure Examination for Practical Nurses. National Council of State Boards of Nursing, Chicago, 1989.

*The information in this section is copyright by the National Council of State Boards of Nursing, Inc., Chicago, Illinois, 1998. Available at: http://www.ncsbn.org.

CHAPTER 2

Preparing for and Taking the NCLEX-PN

Kara Schmitt, PhD

While preparing for and taking the NCLEX-PN, you must constantly remember that you have the ability to pass the examination. Although the manner in which you respond to items may be different and although the number of items may be more than in other tests you have taken during your studies, the examination is still just an examination. To do well, you have to be both psychologically and intellectually prepared.

Test Anxiety

Although stress and anxiety are *not* really the same, these terms are used as meaning the same in this chapter. Stress and anxiety are normal reactions to situations such as preparing for and taking the NCLEX-PN. If you were to ask your friends who have already passed the examination if they were anxious before and during the test, the answer would certainly be "yes." In fact, some amount of anxiety is actually *good* for you and has been found to improve test-taking ability. On the other hand, uncontrollable anxiety hurts your ability to do well. It has been said that stress is "the spice of life or the kiss of death—depending on how we cope with it."[1]

By learning how to handle stress effectively, you can use it to your advantage. Stress or anxiety and the manner in which you recognize and respond to it (your ability to react positively) are personal. No one method works for everyone; therefore, the information given in this chapter is merely designed to give you some ideas of ways in which you might be able to reduce large amounts of stress. The best way to deal with stress is to take specific steps to cope with and reduce the stress-producing situation. Studying and preparing for an examination is the *best* way to reduce the stress felt before an examination. An inappropriate approach, which in the end will increase the stress, is to deny the importance of the task (examination) that you must do. Statements such as "The ex-

amination is filled with trick questions anyway, so why bother studying?" or "If I don't do well, I just wasn't lucky" are inappropriate and will not help you. You need to concentrate your efforts in proper study and positive thinking. The information presented in this chapter is generally applicable to paper-and-pencil examinations as well as computerized adaptive testing (CAT). If something is not relevant to CAT, a notation is made in the text.

Some of the characteristics frequently associated with test anxiety include[2]:

1. Feeling insecure about your performance
2. Worrying a great deal about things that are not under your control
3. Thinking about how much brighter or better others are
4. Thinking about what will happen if you fail
5. Feeling that you are not as prepared as you could or should be (assuming that you have prepared)
6. Worrying about not having enough time to finish the test
7. Feeling that you will be letting yourself or others down
8. Feeling that you could and should have done better

These eight feelings can be viewed as constituting four major symptoms of anxiety,[3] which can and must be handled to overcome the problem. Each of these four symptoms is discussed briefly in the following paragraphs.

Anxiety-Producing Mental Activities

Worrying about nonspecific problems or situations and fretting over everything that could go wrong is associated with this symptom. Self-criticism, self-blame, and general negative self-talk lead to low self-confidence and disorganized problem solving. Telling yourself that you cannot do something or that you are stupid leads to failure. Another trait associated with this symptom is false thinking about yourself and the world around you—the "everyone-is-so-much-smarter-than-I" syndrome.

Misdirected Attention

Instead of focusing on the task at hand, such as studying for or taking the examination, you focus on internal and external distractors. These could include watching other people study, looking at the clock, or daydreaming. If you focus on the wrong thing, you are less efficient and may become emotionally upset.

Physiological Distress

When you are anxious, your body reacts both physiologically and psychologically. Some of the physiological symptoms include sweating, increased heart rate, nervous stomach, and headache. If you focus significantly on the physiological symptoms, you will be less able to focus on your studies or the examination.

Inappropriate Behavior

This symptom is exhibited by avoiding the task that needs to be done (procrastination), withdrawing prematurely from the task, or doing something else when you should be focusing on the task at hand (e.g., talking to your roommate instead of studying). Other aspects of inappropriate behavior include rushing through the examination or study material without focusing on the information or, at the opposite extreme, being excessively compulsive and rereading everything more than is necessary. A final element is trying to push yourself to keep going when you are tense rather than taking time to relax.

To reduce stress to a manageable level, you need to determine what symptoms or behaviors you are exhibiting. One way to learn more about your individual expressions of stress is to find a comfortable, relaxing environment, close your eyes, and really imagine and concentrate on how you feel or what you do when you study. How are you going to feel when it is 1 week before the examination? When it is 1 day before the examination? When it is the day of the examination? When you are sitting in the room taking the examination? Try to think carefully about these events and how you *really* will feel. If you are honest in your evaluation of your feelings, you will be better able to change the way you handle stressful situations.

Another activity you can do to learn more about your own coping ability is to make notes of what you do while studying. Do you watch other people? Do you daydream? Do you begin to worry about the test? Do you give up studying because you think it will do no good? You will probably need to keep a log of your behaviors during several study periods so that you have a complete picture of your behaviors. After you have recorded all of your distractors, make a list of what you could do to reduce your level of anxiety. For instance, telling yourself that you can never learn the material is self-defeating; instead, remind yourself that you learned the material in the past and that you have done well in school. After all, you either have graduated or are ready to graduate, so you must have learned what is necessary to reach this point.

Another aid to learning more about yourself and your reaction to stress is to answer the following questions in terms of what *you* do or how *you* respond during periods of stress:

1. Do I bite my nails, fidget with my hair, or tap my fingers constantly?
2. Do I smoke or drink more frequently?
3. Do I tend to eat more or less or to eat less healthy foods?
4. Do I avoid doing what I should be doing, such as studying?
5. Do I feel as though there is too much to do in too little time?
6. Do I worry about everything—the examination, my health, my family, my work, and so on?
7. Do I seem to have more physical or health-related problems?
8. Do I become irritated or lose my temper more quickly over trivial matters?
9. Do I seem to have less energy or to want to sleep more?
10. Do I have trouble falling asleep or sleeping according to a normal schedule?
11. Am I more critical of myself, or do I think of myself as worthless?
12. Do I seem to forget more day-to-day activities or responsibilities, such as forgetting to shop for groceries, forgetting an appointment, or forgetting to return a phone call?
13. Do I have trouble relaxing and enjoying myself even when I am at a social event or with people I like?
14. Do I tend to daydream more?

Questions 1–3 may be viewed as bad habits that simply become more prevalent during times of stress or anxiety. The key to deciding whether any of these are major problems is to determine whether you are doing them *more than usual* during times of anxiety. If the answer is yes, they could negatively influence your effectiveness in preparing for and taking the examination. At the same time, if you try to be perfect and eliminate normal bad habits during a time of stress, you may actually increase your level of stress. Although it may not be necessary to eliminate bad habits at this time, you should keep them under control.

The other questions (4–14) focus more on symptoms of anxiety. If you responded "yes" to most of the questions, it is time to reevaluate your thoughts about yourself and the future examination. You need to focus less on what is going on around you or inside you and more on how to solve the problem that is causing the anxiety. Begin to view the examination as a problem to be solved or a challenge to be met. Do not view it as something that is a punishment or an imaginary catastrophic event.

Begin to view the test realistically. It is not a measure of your self-worth, your ability to succeed, or your future happiness. It is merely a measure of what you know, as well as your ability to take tests.

Develop a positive attitude toward the test. Eliminate the negative thoughts and feelings you have about it and do not think about how well you will or will not do.

Choose to take the test. The examination is not being forced on you; rather, you elected to take it. By viewing the examination as something you want to do, you are in control and the examination is no longer controlling you. Because you have chosen to take the examination, you must also choose to study for it.

Concentrate on what you can and must do *now*. Do not think about what you should have studied yesterday (the past) or what will happen when you take the exam (the future).

Rather, direct your attention on the present task of studying, and expend your energy on that.

As stated previously, some test anxiety is good for you. Too much, however, will hinder your performance, and you will not be able to demonstrate adequately the knowledge you actually have. Some ways test-anxious persons are helped are by[2]:

1. Learning to be less demanding of themselves
2. Revising their expectations about the consequence of failure and viewing the task as less alarming
3. Strengthening their study skills
4. Gaining more self-control over their worry and emotionality

If anxiety is handled in a positive manner, it can assist in "promoting survival, healthy adaptation and development. In its nonadaptive modes, it can promote incompetence and extreme and lasting misery."[2]

In any situation, if you convince yourself that you are going to fail, you will. Instead of being negative about yourself, trying to decide what others will think if you fail, or how poorly you might do on the examination, *think positively*. Negative statements made either to yourself or to others can significantly reduce the effectiveness of the studying you do. Think positively and you'll *feel* positive.

Read the examples of typical negative and positive statements shown in Table 2–1. Are you guilty of making any of the negative statements? If so, begin working at using statements in the positive column.

Avoid "why," "if only," and "what if" types of questions or statements; for example, "Why did I ever think I could be a nurse?" or "If only I had more time, I could do better" or "What if I don't do well on the examination?" These expressions tend to reinforce feelings of helplessness, frustration, and anger. Try to eliminate them from your internal thoughts and external statements.

Stress and anxiety can and will be reduced if you take *positive* action and think *positive* thoughts about yourself and your abilities. At the same time, recognize that you are going to worry about the examination. The statement "Don't worry" is useless advice because we all worry. You must, however, worry in a constructive manner and must have prepared for the examination.

Study Environment

Not only what you study but also the conditions under which you study are important in your ability to learn and remember. Both internal (daydreaming) and external (noise) distractors can lessen your ability to concentrate.

Think about where and how you typically study. Are you studying in an optimal place and manner? You want to be comfortable and relaxed while studying, yet at the same time you need to be able to focus all of your attention on the material you are reading and reviewing.

The following series of questions should assist you in your evaluation of whether the location and way in which you study are most conducive to learning.

1. When I begin studying, do I have all necessary books, paper, pencils and pens, and other study materials with me so that I do not waste time finding them?
2. Do I schedule at least 1–2 hours at a time for studying?
3. Do I take short breaks (10–15 minutes) while studying for long periods of time and then return to work immediately?
4. Do I spread out my studying over a period of time rather than trying to do it all at the last minute?
5. If I study with friends, do they have good study habits?
6. Do I have a plan for studying and, if so, do I stick to it?
7. Do I feel rested when I study?
8. If I begin to feel tense or tired, do I stop studying for a while and try to relax?

Table 2–1. Changing Negative Self-Talk to Positive Self-Talk

Negative Statements	Positive Statements
"I have to get a perfect score."	"I want to do well, but I don't need to get every item right."
"I always get upset during a test."	"If I feel myself getting tense during the test, I know how to relax."
"I'm a failure because I didn't remember."	"Just because I forgot . . . doesn't mean I'm a failure; I remember lots of other material."
"If the test has questions on . . . topic, I'll fail."	"If the test has questions on . . . topic, I had better study it more."
"What if I fail the exam?"	"I don't expect to fail, but if I do, I'll just have to study harder and do better the next time."
"I'll let my family down if I don't pass this test."	"Sure, my family wants me to do well, but they'll still accept me if I don't pass."
"I'm too stupid to be a nurse."	"I made it through school and I can make it through the exam."
"The test is designed to trick candidates, so it doesn't matter if I study or not."	"If I study, I can do well; it's my responsibility to prepare."
"I'll never be able to understand this material."	"Just relax and try rereading this section; I know I can figure it out."
"Thank heavens, I made it through this study session!"	"Wow, I really learned a lot while studying today. Hope tomorrow goes as well."
"I just know I'll be scared during the examination."	"I know I'll do well on the exam because I'm capable and I studied."
"Everyone expects me to do poorly, so why bother trying to do otherwise."	"I don't care what others think about my chance of passing the test; I know I can do it."
"I don't know why I have to take this test. I got good grades in school."	"I want to take this test simply because it will confirm that I really did learn while in school."

9. If I begin daydreaming or worrying, do I take a few minutes' break to daydream or worry rather than let those activities interfere with my studying?
10. Do I concentrate on the material that I am studying rather than thinking about other things?
11. Have I included time in my schedule for social activities and exercise?
12. When I am finished studying for the day, do I feel I have accomplished something?
13. Am I able to remove myself mentally from the environment; that is, can I block out potential distractions?
14. Is the area in which I study relaxing and comfortable, but not so much so that I fall asleep?
15. Is the area in which I study quiet and basically free from interruptions?
16. Is my desk neat and well organized so that I have enough room to study effectively?
17. Is the lighting sufficient and nonglaring?
18. When it is time to study, do I do so immediately and eagerly?
19. Do I reward myself when I feel I have done an exceptionally good job of studying?

Each of these questions should have been answered "yes" if you are studying in an appropriate atmosphere and with the proper frame of mind. If there were some questions to which you answered "no," try to determine what you need to do to improve the conditions. Remember, how, when, and where you study do make a difference in your ability to learn.

Preparing for the NCLEX-PN

One of the first tasks for you to do is learn all you can about the actual test—how it is constructed, what type of questions are included, how long you have to complete the test, and so on. The information provided in Chapters 1 and 2 serves as a good starting point, but you should also read the material provided by the National Council of State Boards of Nursing (NCSBN) and ask your instructors about the test. The better informed you are about the examination, the better you can prepare in a positive manner.

The suggestions in this chapter are provided so that you can learn to study aggressively and actively. Underlining or highlighting key words is a good start, but that is passive learning and is not as effective for long-term memory. You need to develop active learning skills to improve your chances for remembering the material.[4,5]

Relate the material you have just read to other information you have learned in the past. Does knowledge of something new relate to how you would handle a given situation? Is there a relationship between various facts you have learned? If so, what is that relationship? *Think, don't just memorize.*

Ask yourself questions about the material you have read. Predict how the material might be worded in the examination.

Form study groups to review information and ask each other questions. You may wish to develop a list of questions during one study period and respond to them the next time. All members of the study group need to be actively involved in the process and willing to devote sufficient time for the group interaction to be effective.

Make notes of key concepts or facts that are important to remember. Also, take notes on areas in which you feel uncertain, and use these notes as a reminder that you need to continue learning about the topics.

Be interested in the material. Just because you want to be a practical nurse does not mean that everything you study will be personally interesting to you. However, as you prepare for the examination, you need to become interested in the total field so that you can learn better.

Use prepared test questions such as those in this book to help you study. Use the results of the tests to help you determine your own strengths and weaknesses. Take the tests more than once so that you can see improvement. Use other sources of test items to become more familiar with the different ways in which the same information can be presented.

Set specific goals for yourself. A goal of "needing to learn about nursing" is not much help. Rather, you need to establish a definite goal for each study period.

Establish a schedule for each day's studying and reviewing. Remain flexible, however, so that if you wish to go to a party or go out to dinner when you are supposed to be studying, you can do so without feeling guilty. This does not mean, however, that you forfeit that study time; rather, you make it up later.

Write summaries of what you have read. Rephrase information so that you can better understand it. Restating information in your own words will help you remember it better.

If some information is not clear after reading it in one book, read another book to see if the material is explained any better. Do not forget to ask your instructors or peers for clarification.

Visualize the information that you have just read. Try to imagine how what you have read would actually look. Try to visualize a client with certain conditions or symptoms. What would you need to do?

Overlearn the material. Everyone forgets information, so you should not expect to remember everything you read. However, if you continue studying and learning material even after you think you have learned it, you will forget less.

At the end of each study period, take a few minutes to **outline the key material you just learned.** These outlines can then serve as your final review materials just before the examination. Some key elements of a good outline include:
1. Using underlining or symbols to identify key points
2. Using sufficient space to allow for clarification or expansion based on later studying
3. Recording all formulas, equations, and rules exactly
4. Writing legibly on one side of the paper
5. Writing your own ideas or questions as well as facts
6. Using your own words to help reinforce a concept
7. Using personal nursing care experiences to clarify points

Now that you have learned what you should be doing to become a more active learner, you need to put these activities into place. During the next few study periods, do not try to study any differently than you normally do. Instead, at the end of each study period, take the checklist test shown in Table 2–2. Use the questions to evaluate the ways in which you need to change your studying behavior.

Whenever you answered "no," keep those points in mind the next time you study. Do not feel frustrated if you find you have not included all of the steps in your studying; just keep trying to improve. The overused phrase "Rome wasn't built in a day" is applicable in this instance. It will take time

Table 2-2. **Study Approach Checklist**		
	Yes	No
1. Did you note which material you were unsure of so that you can return to it later?		
2. Did you look over the material before beginning to study it?		
3. When you finished the initial reading, reciting, and reviewing, did you look over your notes and check your memory as to the major headings and subpoints under each heading?		
4. Did you select what is important to be learned and determine your time frame for learning it?		
5. Did you take brief notes as you reviewed?		
6. Did you read the material and try to answer your own questions?		
7. After reading the section or chapter, did you look away and try to recite the answers to questions and give examples of patients with similar problems?		
8. Did you vary your speed of reading according to the difficulty and familiarity of the material and according to your purpose in reading?		
9. Did you pause after reading each section to underline the important points and make marginal notes on the material about which you had questions?		
10. Did you go back to the material that you were unsure of and review again?		

and effort for you to learn how to study more effectively and actively.

How to Take a Multiple-Choice Test

There is a right way and a wrong way to answer multiple-choice items. Although you have probably answered thousands of them during your course of study, you may find it advantageous to review the suggestions given in this section. Part of doing well on an examination is being "test wise," that is, knowing how to figure out the correct answer even if you are not certain. You may have a wealth of knowledge and be one of the smartest in your class, but if you do not know how to respond to multiple-choice questions, you will be unable to prove this knowledge. For better or worse, part of the score you receive on any examination depends on your test-taking ability.

Use logic and common sense to figure out the correct response. The items are usually based on situations that a practical nurse entering the field would most likely encounter rather than exotic or unique situations.

Use cues in the stem and distractors to help you figure out the correct response.

Try to figure out the meaning of unfamiliar words in the stem in terms of the sentence context. You might also be able to figure out the meaning of words by dividing them into prefixes and suffixes that you know.

Read each question thoroughly but quickly. Do not keep reading the same question over and over. Select your response and move on. (In CAT, it is even more critical that you read each item thoroughly. Once you decide on an answer, you cannot change your mind later.)

Read all options before selecting the one you think is correct. A well-constructed test has four plausible responses, and it is your responsibility to select the *best*. Too often, candidates read the first and second options and decide that one of them is correct without reading the other options. Later they may discover that their choice was not really the best.

Eliminate the distractors that are obviously incorrect and then choose between or among the remaining ones.

Do not try to make an item any more difficult than it is. Do not read anything into the question and do not waste your time looking for "tricks" or hidden meanings. As a rule, the items are straightforward and basic.

Relate each option to the stem. Make sure that the answer you select fits the intent of the stem and is grammatically correct.

Focus on key words in the stem.

Select the option that is most inclusive. If two options are similar, but one contains more details, select the option that is more complete.

Break down complex stems into smaller, more manageable sections.

Make certain that the response you select is correct for each of the separate components.

Try answering the question before you have read the options given. This process will help you find the correct response and will also save you time even if the answer you give is not one of those provided. At least you will be thinking about what to look for.

Do not stop trying. Even if there are several items in a row that seem unfamiliar to you, do not start worrying about the examination as a whole. Just answer the items to the best of your ability and move forward.

Concentrate on one item at a time. Do not worry about how many more items you need to answer or how much time remains. Focus on the item that is before you.

Focus on whether the question is asking for a positive or negative response. Negative words (e.g., not, except) are usually emphasized in the stem to help you recognize that you must reverse your thought process.

If a question requires calculations, **talk yourself through each step of the process.** Double-check your computations to be certain you have not made some minor mistake. Generally, the options included in computational questions are based on mistakes typically made in calculation. This means you may find the answer as you worked the problem and still be wrong.

Try to relate a situation in the question to something with which you are familiar. Determine whether the same concepts would apply.

Reword a difficult question and see if that helps you better understand the intent of the item. If you are deciding between two reasonable answers, select the one that focuses on the client as being a worthy human being.

Be aware of double negatives. In these instances, the statement becomes positive.

Look for the most common or typical response to the problem. The examination is designed for nurses entering the field; therefore, the test writers do not expect you to have knowledge that would normally be obtained from years of experience.

Never leave an item unanswered. There is no penalty for guessing, and you have a chance of getting the item correct by guessing. In CAT, you must answer all items presented before any other items are shown.

If you must guess, do so logically. Eliminate the options that you know are wrong, and then see if there is any test construction flaw that might help you figure out the intended answer. Given the extensive editing done before assembling the NCLEX-PN, it is doubtful that these "errors" will be found, but you might as well look for them. Some of the more common test construction errors are:

Length: Select the longest response if all others are approximately equal.

Location: The correct response is more likely to be in the middle.

Grammar: Incorrect options may not grammatically fit the stem.

Language: Unusual or highly technical language typically indicates an incorrect option.

Qualification: If one option includes qualifiers such as "generally," "tends to," or "usually" and other options do not, select that option.

Generalizability: The correct option tends to have greater applicability or flexibility.

Specifics: Options that include "always" or "never" are typically not the correct answer.

Reread the question in its entirety as well as each option you select. Does your response still make sense? Usually your first response will be correct if you read the stem and all distractors carefully. There are instances, however, when you reread a question and decide that another option is better. If this is the case, then by all means change your answer. Do so only with sufficient reason and not just because you are uncertain. You need to read each item carefully as it is presented and respond accordingly.

Study Schedule

The following schedule is provided to help you prepare for the NCLEX-PN without trying to learn and remember everything at the last minute. Keep in mind that cramming has no long-term benefit; you may remember the material for a few hours but not for the entire examination. At some point during your education, you probably stayed up all night studying for an examination, took the examination, and returned to your room and slept. How much of the material did you remember later that day? Probably not much. Therefore, if you want to do well on the examination, you will have to begin preparing early and *not* try to cram all the information into a few nights of studying.

Two to Three Months before the Examination

Although it may seem early to start preparing for the examination, it really is not. At this time, you should:
1. Begin organizing your textbooks and lecture notes meaningfully.

2. Begin noting areas about which you feel less comfortable.
3. Begin learning about the format (CAT) and content of the examination.
4. Take a practice test that includes items similar to those likely to be on the actual NCLEX-PN to see how well you do; assess your strengths and weaknesses.
5. Establish a study schedule that includes adequate time to prepare but also recognizes the need for flexibility (4–5 days per week, with 1–3 hours of study per day). Your schedule should be based on how well you did on the practice test, how confident you feel, and how many weeks are left before the examination.

Four to Eight Weeks before the Examination

At this time, you should:
1. Begin reviewing areas of known weakness *first* so that you will have time to review them again before the examination.
2. Develop, organize, and maintain your own notes in each subject for a final review just before the examination.
3. Form a study group that meets at least weekly; prepare specific topics for discussion when the group meets.
4. Take at least one test a week to help you become more familiar with the types of questions that may be asked.
5. After several weeks of studying, take the original pretest to see how well you are doing, assess strengths and weaknesses again, and readjust your study schedule as necessary.
6. Develop your own situational questions as a technique for reviewing.
7. Maintain sufficient time for eating, sleeping, exercising, socializing, and working—do not become a study hermit.

One Week before the Examination

At this time, you should:
1. Begin a concentrated *review* of the material.
2. Take the pretest for the last time and evaluate your performance.
3. Recite key ideas to yourself; make sure all essential formulas or equations are memorized correctly.
4. Rest, eat well, and do not dwell on the test during the nonstudy times.
5. Make sure you have all documents required for admission to the examination. If you have any questions, call the Board of Nursing office or the agency that administers the examination.

One Day before the Examination

1. Do something you enjoy during the day; have a nice quiet dinner; and relax that evening by doing something pleasant that will keep your mind off the examination.
2. If you are with colleagues who are taking the test, refrain from discussing it.
3. If you feel the need to review your notes, do so once and then not again—do not keep returning to them.
4. Get sufficient sleep—you need to be both physically and mentally alert on the next day.

5. Double-check that you have all required documents and materials for the next day.

Actual Examination Administration

The examination day has finally arrived and, although you may be anxious or worried, you know how to maintain a helpful level of anxiety. Be confident as you start the day.

1. Get up early enough to have a good breakfast.
2. Wear comfortable clothes—preferably layered, so that you can be comfortable whether the room is warm or cool.
3. Make certain you have everything you need—admission card, identification, money for lunch or parking, and so on.
4. Arrive at the examination site *on time.* If you are driving, start at least ½–1 hour earlier than you think is necessary in case an unexpected problem occurs.

Most researchers have found that the greatest level of anxiety in a testing situation occurs while waiting for the test to begin or during the first few minutes of the examination. If you find this happening to you at the start of the test or at anytime during the test, some rapid relaxation may be helpful. You should use this technique as soon as you are aware of feelings of anxiety; if you wait, these feelings may become heightened and more difficult to allay.

One recommended procedure is as follows[3]:

1. Close your eyes. As you sit in your seat, tense all of your muscles. Really try to "scrunch up" as many muscles as you can.
2. Once you have tensed the muscles, take a deep breath (inhale through your nostrils) and hold your breath for a count of five, keeping your muscles tensed all of the time.
3. After counting to five, simultaneously exhale rapidly through your lips and quickly let go of your muscle tightness by silently telling yourself to *relax.*
4. With your eyes still closed, go as limp in the chair as you possibly can after relaxing.
5. Now with your muscles relaxed, take a second deep breath through your nostrils. Hold your breath for a couple of seconds. Then *slowly* exhale through your lips.
6. As you exhale, repeat the word *"calm"* to yourself. You

will probably repeat the word 7–10 times while slowly exhaling.
7. Repeat these steps once or twice to achieve greater relaxation. Each time through the steps will take about 30 seconds.

In addition to the foregoing relaxation technique, you should take a number of other steps to remain calm during the examination.

1. Once you are told to begin the test, jot down formulas or ideas that you think you might forget during the examination in the front of your booklet.
2. Develop an *assertive* yet realistic attitude. Approach the test determined that you will do your best, but also accept the limits of what you know. Use everything you know to do well, but do not blame yourself for what you do not know.
3. Remember the guidelines on how to take multiple-choice tests.
4. Do *not* spend too much time thinking about alternative responses, especially after you have selected the one you think is correct.
5. *Pay attention* to the test, not to yourself or others. Do not waste time worrying, doubting yourself, or wondering how others are doing. Do not worry about what you should have done; instead, pay attention to what you are doing now.
6. Do not let lapses of memory produce unhealthy anxiety or fear; such lapses are normal.
7. Do not waste time with emotional reactions to the questions.
8. *Remain confident* and resolve to work at top efficiency throughout the entire examination. At all times, remain positive and convinced that you will be successful on the examination.

REFERENCES

1. Fiore, N and Pescar, SC: Conquering Test Anxiety. Warner Books, New York, 1987.
2. Sarason, IG (ed): Test Anxiety: Theory, Research and Application. Laurence Erlbaum Associates, Hillsdale, NJ, 1980, pp 18,112–113.
3. Ottens, AJ: Coping with Academic Anxiety. Rosen Publishing Group, New York, 1984.
4. Sherman, TM and Wildman, TM: Proven Strategies for Successful Test Taking. Charles E Merrill, Columbus, OH, 1982.
5. Kesselman-Turkel, J and Peterson, F: Test Taking Strategies. Contemporary Books, Chicago, 1981.

Clinical Specialties Content Reviews and Tests

CHAPTER 3

Maternity Nursing: Content Review and Test

Lizabeth L. Carlson, RNC, MSN

The process of childbearing involves exciting changes in the life of a woman and her family. The changes in physical, emotional, and psychosocial factors have an enormous impact on the expectant family. Factors that affect successful adaptation to pregnancy include personal values, family member roles, social support factors, and cultural effects. Maternity nurses have both the opportunity and responsibility to help the expectant family make the necessary transitions to welcome their new baby into the family. The maternity nurse is responsible for incorporating the psychosocial, cultural, and physiological aspects of pregnancy in the educational, emotional, and physical needs of the childbearing woman and her family.

Antepartal Care

I. Conception
  A. Fertilization
    1. Conception occurs in the upper third of the fallopian tube when egg and sperm unite.
      a. Conception occurs approximately 14 days before the start of the next menstrual cycle.
        1) Each ovum has 23 chromosomes.
        2) Each sperm has 23 chromosomes.
        3) Each fertilized egg is called a *zygote*.
        4) Each zygote has a total of 46 chromosomes (23 from each parent).
          a) A woman has two X chromosomes.
          b) A man has one X and one Y chromosome.
      b. The zygote moves from the fallopian tube to the uterus for implantation.
      c. The fertilized egg is called an *embryo* from implantation until the eighth week of gestation.
      d. From the eighth week of gestation until birth the fertilized egg is called a *fetus*.

  B. Placenta
    1. Structure
      a. Made up of cotyledons
      b. Connects to the fetus via the umbilical cord
      c. Connected to the mother through adherence to the uterine wall
    2. Function
      a. Nutrient and waste exchange between maternal and fetal systems
      b. Gas (oxygen and carbon dioxide) exchange between maternal and fetal systems
      c. Production of pregnancy hormones
        1) Progesterone: stimulates placental growth; decreases uterine contractions, suppresses ovulation, maintains endometrium (decidua) throughout pregnancy
        2) Estrogen: stimulates enlargement of breasts and uterus; stimulates contractions
        3) Human placental lactogen: increases maternal metabolism; aids in preparing breasts for lactation
        4) Human chorionic gonadotropin (HCG): works to develop placenta until about 11 weeks' gestation
  C. Umbilical cord
    1. Structure
      a. Contains two arteries.
      b. Contains one vein.
      c. Arteries and vein are surrounded by Wharton's jelly (for protection).
    2. Function
      a. Attaches placenta to growing fetus at the umbilicus
      b. Carries nutrients, gases, and wastes between mother and fetus
  D. Amniotic membranes

1. Structure
   a. Thin membranous sac surrounding the fetus
   b. Two layers
      1) Amnion
      2) Chorion
   c. Filled with fluid
      1) Saline
      2) Alkaline
   d. Fluid constantly replaced
2. Function
   a. Protects the fetus
   b. Allows free fetal movement
   c. Maintains a stable temperature
   d. Prevents amnion from adhering to the fetus
   e. Allows for fetal respiration
   f. Provides fluid for fetal swallowing
E. Maternal circulation
   1. Blood that is under pressure from the maternal heart is circulated to the aorta, common iliac vessels, and hypogastric and uterine arteries through the uteroplacental shunt, to the cotyledons of the placenta. Three transfers take place:
      a. Oxygen: simple diffusion
      b. Glucose: facilitated diffusion
      c. Proteins: active transport
F. Fetal circulation
   1. The umbilical vein carries oxygen and nutrients to the fetus.
   2. Umbilical arteries carry carbon dioxide and waste to the placenta.
   3. The ductus venosus bypasses digestive tract and liver; shunts blood directly to the inferior vena cava.
   4. The foramen ovale shunts blood from right to left atria, bypassing lungs and ventricles.
   5. The ductus arteriosus shunts blood from pulmonary artery to the aorta, bypassing the lungs.
G. Normal fetal heart rate: 110–160 bpm.
H. Liver and lungs: little function in fetal life
   1. Liver is major source of oxyhemoglobin.
   2. Fetus "practices" breathing amniotic fluid in and out (fetal respiration).
II. Disorders related to conception and implantation
A. Abortion: termination of pregnancy before 20 weeks' gestation
   1. Types
      a. Spontaneous
         1) Threatened: possible loss of pregnancy evidenced by vaginal bleeding
         2) Incomplete: part but not all of pregnancy tissue expelled
         3) Habitual: spontaneous loss of three or more pregnancies
         4) Complete: all pregnancy tissue expelled
         5) Inevitable: cervical dilatation
      b. Induced
         1) Therapeutic: an abortion performed to save the woman's life
         2) Voluntary: occurs up to 24 weeks with medical intervention at the woman's request

3) Criminal: an illegal termination of pregnancy
B. Ectopic pregnancy: implantation of a fertilized ovum outside the uterus, usually in the fallopian tube
   1. Signs and symptoms
      a. Sharp localized pain in the lower abdomen
      b. Painless irregular vaginal bleeding
      c. Syncope
      d. Hypovolemic shock, pallor, anxiety, air hunger, increased thirst, palpitations
C. Hydatidiform mole: a disorder in placental development that causes the ovum to deteriorate and grapelike vesicles to form; may become malignant (choriocarcinoma)
   1. Signs and symptoms
      a. Vaginal bleeding around the 12th week of pregnancy
      b. Hyperemesis
      c. Larger fundal height than expected for dates
      d. Extremely high HCG levels
      e. No fetal heart tones
      f. Symptoms of pregnancy-induced hypertension (PIH) before 20 weeks of pregnancy
   2. Avoidance of pregnancy and follow-up for 2 years is essential to ensure that HCG levels return to normal and to rule out malignancy.
III. Therapeutic management; nursing interventions
A. Data collection
   1. Physical
      a. Vaginal bleeding
         1) Amount
         2) Color
         3) Consistency
         4) Presence of clots
      b. Pain
         1) Type
            a) Sharp
            b) Crampy
            c) Dull
         2) Location
            a) Abdominal
            b) Pelvic
            c) Lower quadrants
            d) Shoulder
      c. Vital signs, especially blood pressure
      d. Tissue passed from vagina
      e. Level of consciousness
   2. Psychological
      a. Fear of death
      b. Anxiety
      c. Guilt
      d. Grief
      e. Disappointment
      f. Denial
      g. Uncooperativeness
   3. Laboratory tests
      a. HCG
         1) Lower for abortion and tubal pregnancies
         2) Elevated for hydatidiform mole
      b. Complete blood cell (CBC) count

1) Values normally decreased during pregnancy
   a) Hemoglobin (Hgb)
   b) Hematocrit (Hct)
2) Values normally increased during pregnancy
   a) White blood cells (WBCs)
   b) Red blood cells (RBCs)
   c. Other specialized evaluations
      1) Ultrasound
      2) Culdocentesis
      3) Pelvic examination
B. Medical and surgical intervention; planning and nursing implementation
   1. Provide information regarding treatment plan.
   2. Prepare for surgery.
      a. Dilatation and curettage (D&C)
         1) Incomplete abortion
         2) Hydatidiform mole
      b. Laparoscopy
         1) Ectopic pregnancy
         2) Possible removal of tube or ovary or both
   3. Provide opportunity for support and counseling.
   4. Prepare for recovery and self-care.
   5. Perform nursing interventions.
      a. Emphasize importance of bedrest.
      b. Save all expelled tissue and clots.
      c. Observe vaginal bleeding.
         1) Count perineal pads.
         2) Estimate blood loss with the cm/ml method (5-cm diameter on peripad equals approximately 10 ml of blood loss).
         3) Monitor vital signs every 5 minutes to 4 hours, depending on the woman's condition.
         4) Institute treatment for shock as needed.
         5) Observe for postsurgery hemorrhage or infection.
         6) Administer drug therapies:
            a) Oral contraceptives
               i) For 1 year post-hydatidiform mole
               ii) For 3 months after ectopic pregnancy
            b. Anticancer drugs for hydatidiform mole
   6. Evaluate nursing interventions.
      a. The woman participates in decisions.
      b. The woman has normal vital signs according to her baseline and pain is controlled.
      c. Woman demonstrates physical and psychological recovery.
      d. Woman identifies support systems.
IV. Maternal adaptations to pregnancy
   A. Physiological
      1. Cardiovascular
         a. Pulse rate increases by 10 bpm.
         b. Blood volume increases by 50%.
         c. WBCs increase to an average of 15,000 mm^3.
         d. Clotting factors increase.
         e. Systolic and diastolic blood pressures are lower by 5–10 mm Hg in the first and second

trimesters; they return to prepregnancy levels in the third trimester.
   2. Respiratory
      a. Rate does not change; depth changes with enlarging uterus.
      b. Oxygen consumption increases during the last half of pregnancy.
   3. Gastrointestinal
      a. Gums swell and bleed easily.
      b. Nausea and vomiting are common in the first trimester.
      c. Gastric emptying is delayed and intestinal motility decreased (caused by effects of progesterone).
      d. Hemorrhoids and constipation are common.
   4. Urinary tract
      a. Frequency is common in first and third trimester; it is caused by pressure on the bladder from the uterus.
      b. Dilation of kidneys and ureters is caused by progesterone.
      c. Glycosuria is caused by increased glomerular filtration.
   5. Reproductive
      a. Uterus
         1) Hypertrophy of myometrial cells results in uterine enlargement.
         2) Number of blood vessels to the uterus increases.
         3) Gentle, rhythmic (Braxton Hicks) contractions start in the first trimester.
      b. Cervix
         1) Goodell's sign: softening of the cervix
         2) Hegar's sign: softening of the lower uterine segment
         3) McDonald's sign: easy flexion of the uterus against the cervix
         4) Chadwick's sign: dark blue-purple coloration of the cervix (color change can extend to the vagina and labia)
         5) Development of a thick mucus plug
      c. Ovaries
         1) Cease egg production
         2) Produce corpus luteum for first 12 weeks of pregnancy
      d. Vagina
         1) Vaginal secretions increase.
         2) Color changes (Chadwick's sign) may be present.
      e. Breasts
         1) Size and tenderness increase.
         2) Nipples become more erectile.
         3) Areola darkens and enlarges.
         4) Montgomery's tubercles develop.
         5) Leakage of colostrum occurs in third trimester.
   6. Skin
      a. Darkening of areola, nipples, vulva, and linea nigra occurs.
      b. Mask of pregnancy (chloasma) may develop.
      c. Stretch marks (striae gravidarum) are possible.

1) Breasts
2) Abdomen
3) Hips
4) Thighs
   d. Spider nevi may develop.
    1) Face
    2) Chest
    3) Arms
7. Skeletal
  a. Relaxation of pelvic joints, caused by influence of relaxin and progesterone
  b. Postural changes (lordosis) as pregnancy advances
8. Metabolism
  a. Average weight gain: 25–30 lb
  b. Increased water retention (caused by influence of estrogen)
  c. Physiological anemia caused by hemodilution
  d. Increased iron demand
9. Psychological
  a. Accomplishment of developmental tasks depends on:
   1) Woman's emotional makeup
   2) Woman's support systems
   3) Acceptance of the pregnancy
   4) Cultural beliefs
  b. Common responses
   1) Ambivalence in early pregnancy very common, even with planned pregnancies
   2) Acceptance
    a) Happy
    b) Fewer physical discomforts
   3) Introversion
    a) Focus on self and fetus
    b) Occurs in the second trimester
   4) Mood swings
    a) Common throughout pregnancy
    b) Caused by increased hormonal production
   5) Body image
    a) Woman's view of herself
    b) Woman's perception of others' views (about her)

V. Care in the first trimester
  A. Data collection
   1. History: present obstetric (OB) experience
    a. Determine first day of last menstrual period (LMP).
    b. Assess for bleeding or cramping since LMP.
    c. Determine if this pregnancy was planned or unplanned.
   2. History: past OB experiences
    a. Number of pregnancies, abortions, stillbirths, premature births, and living children
    b. Difficulties with other pregnancies
    c. Blood type and Rh factor
   3. History: past medical
    a. Childhood diseases
    b. Hospitalizations
    c. Serious illnesses
    d. Handicaps

4. History: current medical
  a. Medications
  b. Usual weight and height
  c. Use of drugs, alcohol, tobacco
  d. Disease conditions or infections
5. History: family
  a. Genetic diseases
  b. Chronic diseases
   1) Diabetes mellitus
   2) Cardiovascular problems
   3) Pulmonary diseases
   4) PIH
   5) Multiple births
6. Physical
  a. Presumptive signs
   1) Amenorrhea
   2) Breast tenderness and enlargement
   3) Nausea and vomiting
   4) Urinary frequency
   5) Quickening
   6) Chloasma
   7) Linea nigra
  b. Probable signs
   1) Hegar's
   2) Goodell's
   3) Ballottement
   4) Chadwick's
   5) Enlargement of abdomen
   6) Changes in cervix and uterus
   7) Braxton Hicks contractions
  c. Positive (diagnostic) signs
   1) Fetal heartbeat heard
    a) By Doppler at 10–12 weeks
    b) By fetoscope at 18–20 weeks
   2) Ultrasound visualization of gestational sac, fetus, and fetal heartbeat
   3) Fetal movement palpated by a professional individual
   4) Fetal heart rate (FHR) tracing (electrocardiogram)
   5) Uterine souffle
7. Psychological
  a. Emotional lability
  b. Disbelief or shock over pregnancy
  c. Physical symptoms possibly experienced together by both members of the couple (couvade)
  d. Partner possibly protective
  e. View of pregnancy: as illness or as normal life process

B. Planning
  1. Provide education about pregnancy and safety.
  2. Promote maternal and fetal well-being.
  3. Assist with psychosocial adaptation.
C. Implementation
  1. Obtain complete health history.
   a. Gravidity (number of pregnancies)
    1) Primigravida: pregnant for first time
    2) Multigravida: pregnant for at least second time
   b. Parity: number of births past 20 weeks (alive or not)
    1) Nullipara: never delivered after 20 weeks

2) Primipara: one birth after 20 weeks
3) Multipara: several births after 20 weeks
2. Calculate estimated date of delivery (EDD): subtract 3 months from LMP, and add 7 days.
3. Peform data collection.
   a. Measure weight and height.
   b. Assess blood pressure, pulse, and respirations.
   c. Palpate breasts.
   d. Assist with speculum examination.
      1) Pap smear
      2) Gonorrhea culture
   e. Inspect abdomen by palpation and auscultation for FHR at 10–12 weeks.
   f. Obtain urine specimen and check for sugar and protein.
   g. Collect blood for syphilis (Venereal Disease Research Laboratory [VDRL]).
   h. Collect blood for CBC, rubella, blood type, and Rh factor.
   i. Provide nutritional information; encourage a nutritionally sound diet.
4. Provide education about:
   a. Exercise: avoid:
      1) High-impact aerobics
      2) Saunas
      3) Hot tubs
   b. Work: no heavy lifting (>10 lb)
   c. Common discomforts
      1) Urinary frequency
      2) Breast tenderness
      3) Pelvic cramping (without vaginal bleeding)
      4) Backache
      5) Heartburn
      6) Mood swings
      7) Nausea and vomiting
      8) Constipation
      9) Broad ligament pain
   d. Schedule for prenatal visits
   e. Discussion on childbirth education classes
   f. Sexuality
   g. Elimination of harmful substances
      1) Drugs
      2) Tobacco
      3) Alcohol
      4) Caffeine
      5) Artificial sweeteners
   h. Nausea: keeping crackers at bedside
   i. Danger signs and symptoms
      1) Sudden gush of fluid from vagina
      2) Severe headache, blurred vision, seeing spots before eyes
      3) Swelling of face, eyelids, hands, lower legs, feet
      4) Vaginal bleeding
      5) Fever and chills
      6) Lack of fetal movement
      7) Pain in abdomen or chest
      8) Scant or bloody urine
      9) Persistent vomiting
   j. Testing

1) Ultrasound
2) Chorionic villus sampling
3) Amniocentesis
D. Evaluation
   1. The expectant woman participates in decisions.
   2. The expectant woman verbalizes understanding of safety.
   3. The expectant woman and her fetus maintain good health during the first 12 weeks.
   4. The expectant woman asks questions about self-care.
   5. The expectant woman voices acceptance of the pregnancy.
VI. Care in the second trimester
   A. Data collection
      1. Physical
         a. Weight gain: 1 lb/wk
         b. Nausea and vomiting should cease
         c. Gravid uterus moves upward, out of the pelvis; results in decreased urinary frequency
         d. Quickening occurs (fetal movement 18–20 weeks)
         e. Blood pressure decreased compared with prepregnancy levels
         f. FHR auscultated between 110–160 bpm
         g. Fundus at umbilicus by 20 weeks
      2. Psychological
         a. Woman and family verbalize feelings about pregnancy.
         b. Woman wears maternity clothes.
         c. Woman and family verbalize changes they are making in planning for the new baby.
         d. Woman is reflective about maternal role.
   B. Planning
      1. Provide counseling about safety for mother and fetus.
      2. Promote psychosocial adaptation by expectant woman.
         a. Therapeutic communication
         b. Teaching
            1) Family roles
            2) Fetal feedback (activity in response to a stimulus)
      3. Involve woman and family in childbirth education.
   C. Implementation
      1. Document and report any abnormalities to the physician.
      2. Listen to fetal heart tones, allowing woman and family to hear.
      3. Determine fundal height.
      4. Discuss common discomforts and treatment.
         a. Heartburn: benefits of eating small, frequent meals, sitting up for 30 minutes after eating, avoiding fatty foods
         b. Varicose veins: elevating legs, wearing support hose, avoiding crossing legs
         c. Ankle edema: elevating legs, avoiding salty food, wearing support hose
         d. Hemorrhoids: advising client to walk more, increasing fiber in diet, taking warm sitz baths

        e. Constipation: advising client to walk more, increasing fluids and fiber

        f. Backache: helpful to wear low-heeled shoes; practice proper posture; perform pelvic-lift exercises

        g. Leg cramps: benefits of increasing calcium in diet, exercising leg to release cramp, dorsiflexing foot

     5. Review prenatal exercises.

   D. Evaluation

     1. The expectant woman verbalizes self-help therapies for common discomforts.

     2. The expectant woman verbalizes acknowledgment of the pregnancy.

     3. The expectant woman relates plans for incorporating the new baby into the family.

     4. The pregnancy proceeds normally during the fourth through the sixth months.

VII. Care in the third trimester

   A. Data collection

     1. Physical

        a. Weight gain: approximately 16 lb by the beginning of the third trimester

        b. FHR 110–160 bpm

        c. Fetal activity monitored by expectant mother (kick count)

        d. Return of urinary frequency

        e. No sugar or protein in urine

        f. Slight edema in ankles, relieved by elevation

        g. Growth determination by fundal height (each centimeter in height equals weeks of pregnancy)

        h. Vaginal secretions: clear; no bleeding

        i. Blood pressure normally rises somewhat higher than prepregnancy levels (however, if increased to 30 mm Hg systolic or 15 mm Hg diastolic, considered hypertension)

     2. Psychological

        a. Increased anxiety related to:

          1) Labor and birth

          2) Mutilation of her body

          3) Ability to cope

        b. Partner experiencing increased anxiety about:

          1) Healthy baby

          2) Safety of woman

          3) Preparation of home for baby

   B. Planning

     1. Involve couple in childbirth classes.

     2. Involve couple in parenting activities as preparation for baby.

     3. Provide opportunity for tour of the OB unit and hospital.

     4. Discuss fears and labor events.

     5. Provide support.

   C. Implementation

     1. Document and report any abnormalities to the physician.

     2. Determine fundal height.

     3. Auscultate FHR.

     4. Discuss labor and delivery plan with the woman and her partner.

     5. Discuss:

        a. Signs of labor

        b. When to go to the hospital

        c. When to call the physician

        d. Possible sibling reactions

     6. Determine fetal presentation

     7. Provide information about specialized tests

        a. Ultrasound

        b. Amniocentesis for fetal maturity

          1) Lecithin:sphingomyelin (L:S) ratio

          2) Phosphatidyl glycerol (PG)

          3) Creatinine

        c. Nonstress test

          1) Reactive: FHR accelerations with fetal movement last for 15 seconds at least 15 beats above the baseline; must occur at least twice in 20 minutes

          2) Nonreactive: no FHR accelerations with fetal movement

        d. Contraction stress tests

          1) Oxytocin challenge test: use of oxytocin (Pitocin) to produce uterine contractions

          2) Nipple stimulation test: use of nipple self-stimulation to produce uterine contractions spontaneously

          3) Contraction stress test: performed when woman is already having uterine contractions

          4) Results

            a) Negative: no late decelerations with uterine contractions

            b) Positive: presence of two or more late decelerations with uterine contractions

            c) Equivocal: one late deceleration only, with uterine contractions; test must be repeated next day

   D. Evaluation

     1. Woman or couple attend childbirth classes and hospital tour.

     2. Woman is aware of and reports fetal activity patterns.

     3. Couple expresses expectations of the birthing experience and parenthood.

Disorders and Complications of Pregnancy

  I. Placental

   A. Placenta previa

     1. Types

        a. Complete: center of placenta completely covers cervical os

        b. Partial: a portion of placenta covers cervical os

        c. Marginal: lower edge of placenta lies on or near cervical os

     2. Data collection

        a. Physical

          1) Increased incidence with parity, multiple gestation, fetal defects, previous endometritis

2) Painless, unexplained uterine bleeding or spotting, usually in third trimester
3) Intermittent gushes of blood
4) Profuse hemorrhage as cervix dilates
5) Fetal distress possibly present as late decelerations
b. Psychological: apprehension about safety of self and fetus
3. Planning
a. Maintain vital signs within normal limits (WNL).
b. Monitor bleeding and fetal status.
c. Provide support and information about condition.
4. Implementation
a. *No* vaginal examinations are permitted.
b. Do not give enemas.
c. Prepare for ultrasound of abdomen.
d. Manage bleeding:
1) Give nothing by mouth (NPO).
2) Hydrate with intravenous (IV) fluids.
3) Apply external fetal monitor.
4) Perform pad count: weigh pads (1 gm = 1 ml), or estimate vaginal bleeding with the cm/ml method hourly.
5) Monitor vital signs.
6) Obtain type and crossmatch for at least 2 units of blood.
7) Have client maintain bedrest.
8) Prepare client for cesarean delivery if necessary
e. Get informed consent.
f. Allow verbalization of feelings.
g. Provide double setup for delivery (i.e., vaginal and cesarean instruments) if vaginal examination is performed
5. Evaluation
a. Woman is prepared for cesarean birth if bleeding is severe.
b. Self-limited bleeding episodes do not endanger mother or fetus.
c. Woman verbalizes anxiety, fear, and anger.
B. Abruptio placentae
1. Types
a. Concealed: separation occurs centrally, causing uterus to fill with blood
b. Marginal: separation occurs near edge, causing bright-red bleeding from the vagina
2. Data collection
a. Physical
1) Vaginal bleeding
a) Scant
b) Heavy
2) Couvelaire uterus
a) Tender
b) Irritable contractions
c) Rigidity
d) Uneven tone
3) Constant painful, low backache
4) Abdominal pain constant or intermittent
5) Maternal shock
6) Low or absent FHR with late decelerations

7) Extreme fetal activity followed by inactivity
b. Psychological
1) Confusion caused by shock or overwhelming pain
2) Restlessness, weakness, uncooperativeness
3. Planning
a. Monitor maternal vital signs closely.
b. Establish fetal well-being through electronic fetal monitoring (EFM).
c. Reduce apprehension; explain procedures.
4. Implementation
a. Treat shock:
1) Administer O_2 at 6–10 L/min by mask.
2) Administer rapid infusion of IV fluids.
3) Maintain client in Trendelenburg's position.
4) Assess vital signs every 5–10 minutes.
5) Monitor intake and output (I&O).
6) Use external fetal monitor for labor pattern and FHR.
b. Remain at bedside.
c. Prepare for emergency delivery.
d. Prepare to transfuse.
e. Monitor fibrinogen, prothrombin time (PT), partial thromboplastin time (PTT) platelets, Hgb, and Hct.
5. Evaluation
a. Couple verbalizes understanding of treatment plan.
b. Woman should be physically stable: normotensive, with adequate Hgb and Hct.
c. Woman verbalizes relief or gratitude or both once emergency is over.
d. Fetal status stabilizes.
C. Incompetent cervix: painless dilatation of the cervix in the second trimester
1. Causes
a. Previous surgical trauma (cone biopsy)
b. Mechanical defect
2. Surgical treatment
a. Cerclage
b. McDonald's procedure
c. Shirodkar's procedure
3. Data collection
a. Physical
1) Painless dilatation
2) Presence of vaginal bleeding or bloody discharge
3) Recurrent spontaneous second-trimester abortions
4) Fetal membranes visible with pelvic examination
b. Psychological
1) Discouragement about ability to deliver full-term infant
2) Guilt about activity and sexual relations
3) Anxiety about outcome
4. Planning
a. Prepare for surgical procedure.
b. Monitor for preterm labor.
c. Provide opportunities for discussion of feelings.
d. Teach woman warning signs of labor.

5. Implementation
   a. Obtain history of other pregnancies.
   b. Maintain bedrest.
   c. Monitor FHR.
   d. Prepare for surgery.
   e. Observe for complications after surgery.
      1) Spontaneous rupture of membranes
      2) Uterine contractions
      3) Signs of infection
      4) Vaginal bleeding
   f. Discuss discharge teaching.
      1) Notify physician if cramping, bleeding, or gush of fluid is present.
      2) Be aware of fetal activity.
      3) Notify physician if fever >100.4°F (38°C), chills, or dysuria is present.
6. Evaluation
   a. Woman voices understanding of the need for the procedure and what will be or was done.
   b. Labor is delayed until 38–42 weeks' gestation.
   c. The woman verbalizes self-confidence regarding carrying a pregnancy to term.
   d. The woman lists signs and symptoms (S/S) of problems and agrees to notify the physician of the same.
D. Hyperemesis gravidarum: continuous episodes of vomiting caused by hormones or stress or both
   1. Data collection
      a. Physical
         1) Weight loss
         2) Dehydration
         3) Epigastric pain
         4) Uncoordinated movements, jerking
         5) Electrolyte imbalance
      b. Psychological
         1) Excessive stress in the woman's or family's life
         2) Unplanned pregnancy
   2. Planning
      a. Establish normal fluid and electrolyte levels.
      b. Assist with coping strategies.
      c. Teach about nutrition.
      d. Provide therapy to stop vomiting and restore balance.
   3. Implementation
      a. Administer IV fluids, vitamins, and antiemetics.
      b. Weigh daily.
      c. Observe vomitus for amount and consistency.
      d. Assess I&O every shift.
      e. Slowly introduce small, frequent meals high in complex carbohydrates.
      f. Obtain psychiatric consultation if needed.
   4. Evaluation
      a. Attain adequate hydration, as evidenced by:
         1) Good skin turgor
         2) Moist mucous membranes
         3) Electrolytes within normal limits
         4) Urine output averaging at least 30 cc/hr
      b. Establish normal eating patterns.
      c. Promote woman's verbalization of ability to cope.

II. Preexisting conditions
   A. Cardiac
      1. Types
         a. Mitral valve stenosis or prolapse common
         b. Congestive heart failure from increased cardiac demands
      2. Data collection
         a. Physical
            1) Pedal edema
            2) Generalized edema
            3) Moist cough
            4) Fatigue
            5) Tachycardia or irregular pulse
            6) Dyspnea on exertion
            7) Systolic murmurs
            8) Cyanosis of nailbeds and lips
         b. Psychological
            1) Anxiety about death of self or fetus
            2) Frustration over reduced activity
            3) Concern for other family members' functioning
            4) Family role changes
      3. Planning
         a. Promote rest and relaxation; limit activity.
         b. Protect from infection.
         c. Promote acceptance of limitations and the condition.
      4. Implementation
         a. Prevent infection (prophylactic antibiotic therapy) early.
         b. Have client avoid strenuous exercise.
         c. Provide frequent rest periods.
         d. Help client and family identify acceptable methods of accomplishing tasks.
         e. Encourage woman and family to verbalize feelings.
         f. Prepare for vaginal delivery by assisting with administration of regional anesthesia and use of forceps.
         g. Help woman identify ways to avoid or deal with emotional stress.
         h. Administer medications:
            1) Digitalis
            2) Furosemide (Lasix)
            3) Penicillin
         i. Position client for best circulatory perfusion (left lateral postion).
         j. Administer O_2 at 6–10 L/min via mask.
      5. Evaluation
         a) Woman remains free of infection.
         b) Woman follows dietary and activity limitations.
         c) Woman's condition stabilizes during labor and delivery.
   B. Hypertension
      1. Essential
         a. Occurrence in second trimester
         b. Permanent condition
         c. No preeclamptic symptoms
      2. Data collection
         a. Physical

1) Blood pressure elevation above baseline
   a) 140/90 mm Hg or greater
   b) Systolic 30 mm Hg above baseline
   c) Diastolic 15 mm Hg above baseline
2) Retinal changes
  b. Psychological: may be depressed about permanent condition
3. Planning
  a. Monitor blood pressure frequently.
  b. Provide education about self-care.
  c. Assess fetal well-being
4. Implementation
  a. Monitor blood pressure every 2 weeks for first 24 weeks, and then weekly.
  b. Provide low-sodium diet information.
  c. Administer medications; teach self-administration:
   1) Diuretics
    a) Thiazides
    b) Furosemide
   2) Antihypertensives
    a) Calcium channel blockers
    b) Hydralazine
  d. Encourage frequent rest on left side.
  e. Avoid stress.
  f. Discuss disease and associated problems.
5. Evaluation
  a. Woman remains normotensive.
  b. Woman demonstrates knowledge of treatment regimen.
  c. Pregnancy progresses without maternal-fetal complications.

C. PIH (toxemia)
1. Preeclampsia symptoms
  a. Edema
  b. Proteinuria
  c. Hyperreflexia
  d. Elevated blood pressure during pregnancy
2. Eclampsia symptoms
  a. Preeclampsia symptoms
  b. Severe frontal headache
  c. Visual changes
  d. Epigastric discomfort
  e. Convulsions
  f. Decreased urine output
3. Data collection
  a. Physical
   1) Edema in pretibial, facial, hand areas
   2) Proteinuria: 1+ to 4+
   3) Weight gain: 2 lb/wk or more or rapid increase
   4) Elevated blood pressure
    a) 140/90–160/110 mm Hg: preeclampsia
    b) 160/110 mm Hg: eclampsia
   5) Blurred vision, frontal headache
   6) Epigastric pain
   7) Hyperreflexia, twitching, convulsions
   8) Oliguria
  b. Psychological
   1) Anxiety about safety of self and fetus
   2) Frustration about activity restrictions and possible hospitalization

4. Planning
  a. Prevent progression to convulsions.
  b. Promote fetal well-being.
  c. Provide teaching about condition.
5. Implementation
  a. Assess blood pressure, urine for protein, edema, reflexes, and weight gain.
  b. Provide high-protein diet, no added salt.
  c. Encourage client to rest on left side in quiet, shaded atmosphere.
  d. Teach S/S that client should report immediately.
  e. Teach self-administration of medications:
   1) Phenobarbital
   2) Hydralazine
   3) Magnesium gluconate
  f. Prevent convulsions:
   1) Obtain electrolyte, magnesium, and uric acid levels.
   2) Administer magnesium sulfate ($MgSO_4$):
    a) Give loading dose IV piggyback.
    b) Give hourly maintenance dose of 1–2 gm.
    c) Never put $MgSO_4$ in the mainline IV infusion.
    d) Administer by IV controller or pump.
  g. Perform hourly assessment of output, respirations, reflexes, and proteinuria.
  h. Monitor vital signs every 15 minutes if woman is in labor.
  i. Have calcium gluconate available to reverse magnesium effects.
  j. Use fetal monitor to evaluate fetus and labor.
  k. Continue $MgSO_4$ administration for at least 24 hours after delivery.
6. Evaluation
  a. Convulsions are avoided.
  b. Progress to delivery is uncomplicated for mother and fetus.
  c. Woman and family verbalize support and acceptable coping methods.

D. Diabetes mellitus
1. Types
  a. Gestational: carbohydrate intolerance during pregnancy
  b. Insulin-dependent: lack of insulin from pancreas requires external source; can be preexisting or develop in pregnancy.
  c. Non-insulin-dependent: partial insulin is secreted; requires diet control.
2. Data collection
  a. Physical
   1) Hyperemesis during early pregnancy
   2) Sugar and ketones in urine
   3) Elevated results of fasting blood sugar (FBS), resting glucose level, and glucose tolerance test (GTT)
   4) Rapid weight gain
   5) Polyuria, polydipsia, polyphagia
   6) Previous large baby ($\geq$4000 gm)

b. Psychological
  1) Anxiety associated with fetal anomalies or death
  2) Stress in learning to cope with the disease
3. Planning
  a. Test regularly for glucose level.
  b. Obtain periodic hemoglobin A_{1c} (HbA_{1c}).
  c. Implement diet and medication if needed.
  d. Provide teaching about disease and its effects on pregnancy.
  e. Observe for signs of hypoglycemia or hyperglycemia.
  f. Monitor fetal well-being.
4. Implementation
  a. Obtain OB history.
  b. Test urine for sugar, protein, ketones, and bacteria.
  c. Assess for large size of fetus, FHR, weight gain, blood pressure, yeast infections, and polyhydramnios.
  d. Provide diet instruction.
  e. Instruct about insulin injections:
    1) Blood sugar levels dictate dose.
    2) Use blood monitoring device before meals and at bedtime.
    3) Synthetic regular insulin (Humulin) is drug of choice.
    4) Synthetic Hagedorn insulin (NPH) may be used.
    5) No oral agents are permitted during pregnancy or lactation.
  f. Hypoglycemia and ketoacidosis require rapid intervention.
  g. Initiate and maintain fetal surveillance for fetal well-being:
    1) Fetal kick counts
    2) Nonstress test
    3) Biophysical profile
  h. Insulin needs increase during pregnancy, abruptly decrease after delivery.
  i. Encourage breastfeeding (decreases insulin requirements).
  j. Instruct woman to avoid use of oral contraceptives.
5. Evaluation
  a. The woman remains stable with normal blood sugar levels (60–120 mg/dl).
  b. The woman verbalizes her knowledge of reasons for fetal surveillance and blood glucose monitoring throughout her pregnancy.
  c. The woman makes decisions regarding her care whenever possible.
  d. The woman complies with her diet and medication regimen.
E. Acquired immunodeficiency syndrome (AIDS) and human immunodeficiency virus (HIV)
  1. Acquired through blood contact with infected person (usually IV drug user, homosexual, or bisexual man), through a blood transfusion, or possibly from breast milk (newborns)
  2. Data collection
    a. Physical

      1) Detailed history of risk behaviors
      2) Night sweats
      3) Malaise
      4) Weight loss
      5) Fever or diarrhea or both
      6) Lymph node enlargements
      7) Kaposi's sarcoma (reddish-purple lesions)
      8) *Pneumocystis carinii* pneumonia
    b. Psychological
      1) Anxiety about self and transmission to fetus
      2) Fear of worsening condition with pregnancy
  3. Planning
    a. Protect from opportunistic infection.
    b. Prevent transmission to health-care workers:
      1) Instruct about Universal Precautions.
      2) Instruct health-care workers how the virus is and is not transmitted.
      3) Administer ziduvodine (AZT) during the third trimester and during labor and delivery.
    c. Provide counseling.
  4. Implementation
    a. Follow blood and body fluids precautions.
    b. Use aseptic technique to prevent infection.
    c. Test infant or cord blood for HIV antibodies.
    d. Teach woman about asepsis when handling the infant.
    e. Provide counseling about contraception and safe sex.
    f. Encourage bottle-feeding.
  5. Evaluation
    a. Woman verbalizes her feelings about prognosis of the disease for herself and her baby.
    b. Protection from infection should be maintained by use of Universal Precautions.
    c. Woman adheres to blood and body precautions in handling baby.
    d. Woman should probably not breast-feed her infant.

Intrapartal Care

I. Labor
  A. Premonitory signs
    1. Lightening: fetus settles into pelvis (drops)
    2. Bloody show (discharge): pink-tinged vaginal mucus
    3. Diarrhea
    4. Burst of energy
    5. Cervical softening (ripening)
    6. Spontaneous rupture of the amniotic membranes (bag of waters)
    7. Braxton Hicks contractions become uncomfortable and frequent
  B. First stage (stage of dilatation)
    1. Begins with labor contractions
      a. Come at regular intervals
      b. Increase in frequency and duration over time
      c. Are increased in intensity by walking

d. Are typified by discomfort radiating from back to abdomen
2. Ends with complete dilatation of cervix (10 cm)
3. Latent phase (0–3 cm)
   a. Mild to moderate intensity of contractions.
   b. Cervix dilates to 3 cm.
   c. Contraction duration is short (15–30 seconds).
   d. Contraction frequency increased from 15 minutes apart to 3–5 minutes apart.
   e. Mood of excitement.
4. Active phase (4–7 cm)
   a. Moderate-to-strong intensity of contractions.
   b. Cervix dilates to 7 cm.
   c. Contraction duration is 45–60 seconds.
   d. Contraction frequency 2–3½ minutes.
   e. Mood serious.
5. Transition phase (8–10 cm)
   a. Strong intensity of contractions.
   b. Cervix dilates to 10 cm.
   c. Contraction duration 45–90 seconds.
   d. Contraction frequency 1½–2 minutes.
   e. Mood of losing control.
   f. Signs indicating that delivery (second stage) is impending: mustache of perspiration, bulging perineum, nausea and vomiting, anal dilatation, increased restlessness, desire to push, desire to move bowels, cries of "my baby is coming."
C. Second stage: stage of expulsion
   1. Begins with complete cervical dilatation
   2. Ends with birth of baby
   3. Includes a "bearing-down," pushing effort
   4. Variable length of time ranging from one contraction to several hours
   5. Mood serious, with great energy expended
D. Third stage
   1. Begins with birth of baby
   2. Ends with delivery of placenta
   3. Lasts between 5–30 minutes
   4. Mood exhilarated
   5. Beginning of attachment
E. Fourth stage
   1. Begins with delivery of placenta
   2. Ends with stabilization of mother 1–4 hours after delivery
   3. Mood of exhilaration and/or exhaustion
   4. Rest period
   5. Optimal time for interaction with baby
F. Mechanisms of descent (cardinal movements)
   1. Engagement: biparietal diameter of fetal head passes through midpelvis
   2. Descent: fetal head moves down into birth canal
   3. Flexion: fetal chin touching fetal chest
   4. Internal rotation: fetal head turns to pass ischial spines
   5. Extension: fetal head passes under symphysis pubis and raises chin off chest
   6. External rotation: turning of fetal head to allow shoulders to pass through the ischial spines
G. Physiological maternal response
   1. Cardiovascular

a. Supine hypotension: caused by vena cava compression secondary to supine position
   1) Turn woman onto left side (left lateral position).
   2) Increase IV fluids.
   3) Administer O_2 by face mask at 6–10 L/min.
   4) Monitor FHR.
   5) Monitor maternal vital signs.
b. Systolic blood pressure rises during contractions
   1) During labor, cardiac output increases (approximately 500 ml of blood that supplies the uterus is squeezed into the maternal circulation during contractions).
   2) Immediately after delivery, cardiac output surges.
2. Blood components
   a. WBCs increase up to 25,000 mm^3.
   b. Increase in fibrinogen.
3. Respiratory
   a. Respiratory rate and depth increase during contractions.
   b. Oxygen consumption doubles during second stage of labor.
4. Pain: variable
   a. First stage
      1) Felt in lower abdomen and back
      2) Caused by:
         a) Hypoxia of uterine muscle tissue during contractions
         b) Cervical dilatation
         c) Stretching of cervix and lower uterine segment
   b. Second stage
      1) Felt in lower abdomen, thighs, and perineum
      2) Caused by:
         a) Muscle hypoxia during uterine contractions
         b) Pressure and distention of vagina and perineum
   c. Third stage
      1) Caused by:
         a) Uterine contractions *and*
         b) Passage of the placenta
   d. Fourth stage
      1) Felt as:
         a) Contractions
         b) Perineal pain
      2) Caused by:
         a) Uterine involution
         b) Episiotomy repair
H. Fetal response
   1. FHR: 110–160 bpm
      a. Early deceleration
         1) A decrease in the FHR with contractions
            a) Generally starts before or at the peak of the contraction
            b) Ends with the end of the contractions
            c) Caused by fetal head compression during contractions and descent
            d) Has reassuring pattern

b. Variable deceleration
1) Occurs at any time during labor (not always associated with a contraction)
2) Has an abrupt (sharp) onset and end
3) Caused by umbilical cord compression
4) Is nonreassuring if:
a) Deep
b) Prolonged
c) Repetitive
d) Associated with decreased variability of the fetal heart tracing
c. Late deceleration
1) Onset can occur at any time during the contraction.
2) Always continues after the end of the contraction.
3) Caused by uteroplacental insufficiency.
4) Nonreassuring pattern.
d. Acceleration
1) Short increase in heart rate (8–15 bpm) in response to fetal movement or uterine contractions
2) Reassuring pattern
e. Baseline variability
1) Most important parameter to fetal well-being
2) Indicates healthy parasympathetic and sympathetic responses

II. Nursing care during first stage
A. Data collection
1. History
a. Name and age
b. Physician
c. Gravida, para
d. EDD
e. Blood type, Rh factor
f. Characteristics of contractions
g. Status of the amniotic membranes
h. Presence of bloody show
i. Time of last meal
j. Allergies
k. Medications currently used
l. History of substance use or abuse in pregnancy
m. Labor and delivery plan
n. Desires regarding infant feeding
2. Physical
a. Assess FHR:
1) Use Doppler, fetoscope, or electronic fetal monitor.
2) FHR may not be heard during contractions and for 15–30 seconds afterward unless monitor is used.
3) FHR can be heard between contractions.
4) Normal range is 110–160 bpm.
b. Evaluate FHR pattern:
1) Variability: should fluctuate by 8–15 beats
a) Beat-to-beat: only seen with internal scalp electrode
b) Long-term: 3–5 beat fluctuations per minute

c) Monitor externally over 10 minutes
d) Indicates whether fetus can tolerate stress of labor
2) Accelerations
a) Normal response to movement or other stimuli
b) Indicate fetal well-being
c) No intervention needed
3) Early decelerations
a) Indicate compression of fetal head against cervix
b) Have uniform shape
c) Start and end with the contraction
d) Need no intervention
4) Late decelerations
a) Indicate insufficient blood flow from placenta to fetus
b) Have smooth shape
c) Can be 5–30 beat drop
d) Usually start after peak of contraction
e) End after contraction over by 5–60 seconds
f) Indicate fetal distress
g) Interventions
i) Turn woman onto left side.
ii) Start O_2 by mask at 6–10 L/min.
iii) Increase IV fluids.
iv) Turn off oxytocin if running.
v) Notify physician.
5) Variable decelerations
a) Indicate umbilical cord compression, cord problems, and/or fetal disorders
b) Have irregular shape, usually in form of V, W, or U
c) Can occur any time with or without contractions
d) Interventions
i) Change maternal position.
ii) Start O_2 by mask at 6–10 L/min if severe.
iii) Check for prolapsed cord.
iv) Notify physician if persistent.
6) Decreased variability
a) Indicates:
i) Fetal hypoxia
ii) Medications for analgesia
iii) Fetal sleep
b) FHR fluctuations of ≤2 bpm
c) May be ominous if persisting >30 minutes
d) Interventions
i) Turn woman onto left side.
ii) Start O_2 by face mask at 6–10 L/min.
iii) Notify physician.
7) Tachycardia
a) Heart rate >160 bpm
b) Indicates:
i) Fetal response to tocolytics
ii) Maternal fever
iii) Dehydration

iv) Possible infection of amniotic sac
v) Beginning fetal hypoxia
vi) Possible precursor to fetal distress
c) Interventions
i) Increase IV fluids.
ii) Start O$_2$ by face mask at 6–10 L/min.
iii) Check maternal temperature.
iv) Notify physician.
v) Check vital signs.
vi) Determine frequency, duration, and intensity of contractions by palpation or external monitor.
vii) Examine for cervical dilatation and effacement.
viii) Assess fetal presentation and station by Leopold's maneuvers and vaginal examination.
3. Psychosocial
a. Assess anxiety level of woman and coach.
b. Assess coping skills of woman and coach.
c. Observe interactions between woman and coach.
d. Assess support shown woman by coach.
B. Planning
1. Provide explanation and honesty about maternal and fetal well-being in labor.
2. Assist with self-comfort measures in labor.
3. Promote safety and familiarity with the area.
4. Provide emotional support to the couple.
C. Implementation
1. Monitor vital signs (blood pressure, pulse, and respirations):
a. Hourly in early labor
b. Every 30 minutes in active labor
c. Every 15 minutes in transition
d. Every 15 minutes if blood pressure elevated or oxytocin infused
2. Take oral temperature:
a. Every 4 hours if membranes intact
b. Every 2 hours if membranes ruptured
3. Assess FHR:
a. Every 30 minutes in latent stage
b. Every 15 minutes in active stage
4. Evaluate progress of labor:
a. Dilatation, effacement, and descent
b. Uterine contractions
1) Every 30–60 minutes in latent stage
2) Every 15 minutes in transition
5. Support breathing patterns:
a. Slow chest breathing
b. Pant-blow
c. Panting
6. Provide comfort measures:
a. Fluid or ice chips
b. Massage, warm blankets to back, or both
7. Encourage ambulation.
8. Encourage voiding every 1–2 hours.
9. Change position frequently.
10. Provide effleurage.
11. Apply cool cloth to forehead and face.

12. Administer analgesics as ordered or requested:
a. Meperidine (Demerol)
b. Butorphanol tartrate (Stadol)
c. Pentazocine (Talwin)
d. Morphine
13. Assist with regional anesthesia:
a. Give 500-ml bolus of IV fluids.
b. Position with spine "curled" for administration of spinal or epidural.
c. Teach woman sensations to expect, expected results, and side effects.
d. Monitor vital signs every 5 minutes for 30 minutes.
e. Position woman off vena cava, using pillow (usually to left side).
f. Maintain IV fluids.
g. Provide emotional support.
14. Use electronic fetal monitor if:
a. Abnormal FHR pattern
b. Decreased fetal movement
c. Meconium passage
d. Small-for-dates or postdates fetus
e. Maternal complications
f. Oxytocin use
g. Vaginal bleeding
h. Maternal fever or infection
15. Maintain hydration (administer IV fluids carefully—do not overload with fluid).
16. Watch for signs of fetal distress:
a. Late decelerations
b. Severe variable decelerations
c. Loss of variability
d. Lack of fetal activity
e. Tachycardia
f. Bradycardia (<110 bpm baseline)
g. Meconium-stained fluid
D. Evaluation
1. Mother and fetus experience labor and delivery without complications.
2. Couple verbalizes appreciation of nurse's support during labor.
3. Couple verbalizes feeling safe and secure in surroundings.
4. Woman verbalizes effectiveness of comfort measures used in labor.
III. Special procedures during labor
A. Amniotomy: artificial rupture of membranes
1. Purposes
a. To stimulate labor
b. To see color of amniotic fluid
c. To enable application of internal monitor
2. Disadvantages
a. Commits woman to delivery.
b. Increases risk of infection.
c. Poses risk of prolapsed cord if fetal head not well applied to cervix.
3. Implementation
a. Auscultate FHR before and after procedure; record findings.
b. Document color, consistency, and amount of fluid.

c. Instruct woman regarding need for bedrest unless fetal head is well engaged.

d. Change linen frequently to keep woman dry.

B. Application of electronic fetal monitor

1. Purpose
   a. Continuous monitoring of FHR and contraction pattern to detect fetal distress
   b. Medical-legal record

2. Ultrasound transducer (fetal)
   a. Requires belt and aquasonic jelly.
   b. Upper area of graph is FHR recording.
   c. Records FHR by soundwaves.
   d. FHR can be heard through speaker on machine.
   e. FHR baseline, long-term variability, and decelerations can be determined.

3. Toco transducer (uterine)
   a. Requires belt.
   b. Lower area of graph records contractions.
   c. Records contractions by pressure from the muscle tightening during a contraction:
      1) Contractions can still be palpated.
      2) Frequency and duration of contractions are recorded.
      3) Intensity cannot be determined without palpation because placement affects tracing on graph.

4. Implementation
   a. Explain procedure to couple.
   b. Demonstrate how to read contraction pattern and FHR.
   c. Chart important data on graph sheet.
   d. Assist physician with application of internal monitors.
   e. Readjust external monitor as needed to obtain a clear tracing.
   f. Save all tracings, properly labeled, for the medical record.

C. Induction of labor

1. Purpose:
   a. Artificial stimulation of labor
   b. Medical intervention
      1) Postdate pregnancies
      2) PIH
      3) Diabetes mellitus
      4) Fetal death
      5) Premature rupture of membranes (PROM)

2. Procedure
   a. Administration of IV oxytocin (Pitocin)
      1) Use IV piggyback.
      2) Always use with IV controller.
      3) EFM is necessary.
      4) Monitor maternal blood pressure every 15 minutes.
      5) Risks
         a) Uterine hyperstimulation: not enough rest between contractions
         b) Tetanic uterine contractions: lasting >90 seconds
         c) Uterine rupture
         d) Increased blood pressure
         e) Risk of water intoxication if used in combination with D_5W IV fluids
         f) Fetal distress related to uterine hyperstimulation
         g) Contraindications
            i) Previous classic cesarean incision
            ii) Placenta previa or abruptio placentae
            iii) Fetal distress
            iv) Preterm fetus

3. Implementation
   a. Follow established protocols for initial dosage and incremental increases of oxytocin.
   b. Monitor vital signs and FHR at least every 15 minutes.
   c. Increase only after assessing FHR, blood pressure, and contractions.
   d. Do not increase once desired pattern is achieved (contractions 1–3 minutes apart, lasting 45–60 seconds).
   e. Discontinue immediately if fetal distress is present or if contractions <2 minutes apart or last >90 seconds.
      1) Turn woman on left side.
      2) Administer O_2 at 6 L/min by face mask.
      3) Report to physician.
      4) Document.

D. Forceps or vacuum extraction delivery

1. Purpose
   a. Assists with rotation and descent of presenting part
   b. Provides help for exhausted woman
   c. Provides help if regional anesthesia has blocked pushing urge
   d. May decrease need for cesarean delivery

2. Complications
   a. Maternal
      1) Perineal tears
      2) Hematomas
      3) Vaginal lacerations
      4) Postpartum hemorrhage
   b. Newborn
      1) Facial bruising
      2) Facial nerve damage
      3) Forceps marks on cheeks or ears
      4) Severe edema of occiput (Chignon) possible with use of vacuum extractor
      5) Breastfeeding grasping ability difficulty

3. Implementation
   a. Explain procedure and feeling of pressure.
   b. Encourage woman to relax during application.
   c. Encourage woman to push with contractions.
   d. Examine newborn infant for injury.

E. Episiotomy: surgical incision of perineum

1. Types
   a. Midline: straight toward rectum from vaginal orifice
   b. Mediolateral: cut angles from vaginal orifice to the right or left and down

2. Purpose
   a. Increase size of outlet for birth

b. Decrease length of pushing time

c. Lessen trauma to the fetal head

3. Implementation

   a. Apply ice after delivery to reduce swelling in first 24 hours.

   b. Examine for bruising, swelling, hematoma, bleeding, and intact sutures.

   c. Teach proper hygiene.

   d. Use analgesics (as needed) and sitz baths (after the first day) for pain.

F. Cesarean delivery: birth through an abdominal incision

1. Indications

   a. Cardiopulmonary disease

   b. Fetal distress

   c. Dysfunctional labor

   d. Failure of descent

   e. Prolapsed cord

   f. Placenta previa

   g. Abruptio placentae

   h. Active herpes

   i. Breach presentation (in a primipara)

   j. May be performed in women with HIV to prevent transmission to the fetus or newborn

2. Complications

   a. Infection

   b. Hemorrhage

   c. Maternal bladder injury

   d. Transient tachypnea (wet lung) of the newborn

3. Implementation

   a. Obtain signature for consent.

   b. Explain procedure.

   c. Explain need for procedure.

   d. Obtain CBC and urinalysis (UA) if not already done.

   e. Ensure typing, screening, and crossmatching done.

   f. Hydrate with IV fluids.

   g. Explain cesarean preparation procedures before carrying them out:

      1) Insert Foley catheter.

      2) Shave abdominal area.

      3) Reassure woman and partner.

      4) Obtain FHR strip.

      5) Remove fetal monitor when ready to go to surgery.

   h. Recovery

      1) Provide usual postpartum assessments.

      2) Check abdominal dressing for bleeding.

      3) Apply antiembolitic stockings.

      4) Have client turn, cough, and breathe deeply every 2 hours.

      5) Measure I&O every shift.

G. Vaginal birth after cesarean delivery

1. Purpose: to allow normal labor and delivery without surgical intervention in a woman who has had a previous cesarean delivery

2. Advantages

   a. Fewer maternal and fetal complications

   b. Quicker maternal recovery

   c. Facilitation of attachment process

3. Contraindications

   a. Cephalophalic disproportion

   b. Fetal distress

   c. Previous classic cesarean (longitudinal) scar on uterus

   d. Placenta previa

   e. Multiple gestation

4. Implementation

   a. Monitor labor closely.

   b. Check vital signs and FHR every 15 minutes.

   c. Watch for signs of uterine rupture:

      1) Loss of FHR

      2) Shearing pain, followed by comfort

      3) Shock

      4) Fetal parts easily palpated in the abdomen

      5) Occult (in the abdomen) and vaginal bleeding

IV. Nursing care during second stage: delivery

A. Data collection

1. Physical

   a. Labor progress

      1) Complete dilatation and effacement

      2) Station of descent of presenting part

      3) Contractions 2–3 minutes apart, lasting 60–75 seconds, strong intensity

      4) Bloody show increases

      5) Urge to bear down

   b. Fetal status

   c. Maternal vital signs

2. Psychological

   a. Willingness or eagerness to finish labor process

   b. Mood of intense concentration

   c. Possible faltering of coping skills

B. Planning

1. Encourage effort of couple to deliver child.

2. Support comfort measures.

3. Monitor maternal and fetal status.

4. Promote quiet, peaceful environment for delivery.

C. Implementation

1. Monitor FHR every 5 minutes; document.

2. Choose position for pushing that is comfortable and effective:

   a. Side-lying

   b. Squatting

   c. Hands-and-knees

   d. Semi-Fowler's

   e. Lithotomy

3. Observe for impending birth:

   a. Strong urge to push continuously

   b. Perineal bulge

   c. Fetal hair or scalp

4. Provide comfort measures.

5. Prepare for delivery:

   a. Position instrument table.

   b. Place warmer for baby.

   c. Perform perineal scrub.

   d. Assist physician.

   e. Adjust mirror if woman desires to watch.

   f. Record time and position of birth.

D. Evaluation
 1. Woman's comfort maintained
 2. Mother and fetus physiologically stable
 3. Couple able to focus on delivery of baby
 4. Atmosphere supportive of family-newborn interaction and attachment
V. Nursing care during third stage: delivery of placenta
 A. Data collection
  1. Physical
   a. Contractions resume after birth of baby.
   b. Abdomen changes shape.
   c. Gush of blood from vagina.
   d. Cord lengthens.
   e. Placenta delivered 5–30 minutes after baby.
   f. Expulsion:
    1) Schultze's placenta: shiny; fetal side first
    2) Duncan's placenta: rough; red cotyledons appear first; associated with retained placental parts
   g. After delivery of placenta:
    1) Uterus remains firm.
    2) Two fingerbreadths below umbilicus.
    3) Chills and shivering common.
    4) Maternal blood pressure monitored every 15 minutes.
    5) Neonate dried and placed in mother's arms and covered with a warm blanket:
     a) Dry newborn infant with warm blanket.
     b) Assign Apgar score (0–10 points):
      i) Color pink: 2 points
      ii) Heart rate >100: 2 points
      iii) Grimace or cry: 2 points
      iv) Muscle tone; motion: 2 points
      v) Respirations regular, or crying present: 2 points
   h. Examination of newborn infant for:
    1) Gross anomalies
    2) Three-vessel cord
    3) Clear lungs
    4) Heart rate
    5) Temperature
    6) Color
    7) Gestational age
    8) Reflexes
  2. Psychosocial
   a. Readiness to interact with neonate
   b. What is said about and to neonate
   c. Need for support and praise after delivery
 B. Planning
  1. Promote stabilization of the newborn infant.
  2. Provide opportunity for interaction with baby.
  3. Monitor mother's and baby's status.
  4. Provide comfort measures.
 C. Implementation
  1. Record time of delivery of placenta and expulsion style.
  2. Monitor maternal vital signs.
  3. Complete neonatal assessment.
  4. Provide neonatal care.
   a. Warmth
   b. Eye prophylaxis (may be delayed up to 2 hours)

   c. Attachment process
  5. Administer drugs as ordered to mother:
   a. Oxytocins
    1) Pitocin
    2) Methergine
    3) Syntocinon
   b. Analgesics
  6. Massage uterus if required for uterine atony.
  7. Assist physician.
 D. Evaluation
  1. Newborn infant has stable vital signs.
  2. Mother and newborn infant are given the opportunity to interact.
  3. Mother reports feeling comfortable.
  4. Mother and newborn infant are physically stable.
VI. Nursing care during the fourth stage
 A. Data collection
  1. Physical
   a. Blood pressure and pulse return to prepregnant baseline measures.
   b. Fundus is firm, midline, and at the umbilicus or 1–2 fingerbreadths below.
   c. Lochia is red (rubra) and scant to moderate in amount.
   d. Bladder is not distended.
   e. Perineum is slightly swollen, with no bruising; sutures are intact.
   f. Maternal exhaustion.
  2. Psychosocial
   a. Emotions possibly labile
   b. Desire to interact with baby
 B. Planning
  1. Monitor vital signs, lochia, and uterine status.
  2. Provide information on perineal and breast care.
  3. Instruct woman to call for assistance getting up.
  4. Measure first three voids:
   a. Must be at least 100 cc each
   b. If less than 100 cc, continue to measure until 3 voids of ≥100 cc each are obtained
  5. Support maternal-infant attachment.
 C. Implementation
  1. Palpate uterus for consistency and placement.
  2. Observe lochia:
   a. Color
   b. Amount
   c. Clots
    1) Number
    2) Size
   d. Odor
  3. Check vital signs.
   a. Every 15 minutes for 1 hour
   b. Then every 30 minutes for 1 hour
   c. Then hourly for 2 hours
  4. Assist mother to empty bladder if full.
  5. Massage uterus if not fully contracted (boggy).
  6. Provide comfort measures:
   a. Warm blanket
   b. Ice pack to perineum
   c. Clean perineal pads; changed as needed and each time client gets up to go to the bathroom
   d. Shower or tub bath

e. Linen change as needed
f. Drink or food or both
g. Analgesics if needed
h. Bra for support
i. Breast binder if bottle-feeding

D. Evaluation
1. Mother's vital signs remain WNL (based on the prepregnant baseline).
2. Fundus remains firmly contracted and at or just below the umbilicus.
3. Lochia remains scant to moderate.
4. Any clots are smaller than a half dollar.
5. Opportunity for family-newborn interaction is provided.
6. Mother demonstrates perineal and breast care and uterine massage.

Labor and Delivery Complications

I. Fetal death
A. Caused by:
1. Chromosomal abnormality
2. Spontaneous abortion
3. Maternal or fetal illness
4. Unrecognized fetal distress
B. Data collection
1. Physical
a. Vaginal bleeding
b. Uterine cramping
c. Lack of fetal movement and FHR
d. Fundal height small for dates
e. Low weight gain
f. Urine estriol level decreased
g. Confirmation with abdominal or pelvic ultrasound necessary
2. Psychological
a. Stages of grieving
1) Shock (denial)
2) Anger
3) Guilt
4) Acceptance
5) Possibly skipping appointment(s) as means of denial
C. Planning
1. Provide information regarding delivery plan.
2. Provide woman with emotional support; reassure her that she is not to blame.
3. Discuss follow-up testing of woman or products of conception or both.
D. Implementation
1. Obtain prenatal history to date.
a. Review fetal activity with woman.
b. Prepare for diagnostic tests to confirm fetal death.
c. Clarify procedure for induction.
d. Provide time alone for family with fetus.
e. Assist in working through grief.
f. Obtain consents for genetic testing, pathology, and burial of fetus.
E. Evaluation
1. Couple verbalizes understanding of procedure for delivery.

2. Couple voices feelings.
3. Woman demonstrates self-care after delivery.

II. Preterm labor: uterine contractions that cause cervical dilatation before 37 weeks' gestation
A. Causes
1. Preterm, premature rupture of membranes
2. Infection
3. Cocaine use
4. Dehydration
5. Fetal death
6. Unknown
B. Data collection
1. Physical
a. Spontaneous contractions
b. Spontaneous rupture of membranes common
c. Cervical dilatation and thinning (effacement) with contractions
2. Psychological
a. Fear and anxiety
b. Guilt feelings
C. Planning
1. Provide information about treatment.
2. Administer medications to stop contractions (tocolytics).
3. Promote verbalization of feelings.
D. Implementation
1. Maintain woman at bedrest lying on left side.
2. Provide oral or IV hydration.
3. Assist with laboratory and ultrasound procedures.
4. Assist with the initiation of tocolytic therapy to decrease or stop uterine contractions.
5. Draw blood to assess:
a. Electrolytes
b. CBC
c. Type and crossmatch before starting medication
6. Apply external fetal monitor.
7. Monitor vital signs and breath sounds every 5–15 minutes.
8. Administer drugs:
a. Always give as piggyback solution by controller or pump.
b. Observe for tachycardia, hypotension, and arrhythmias.
c. Administer ritodrine, terbutaline, or $MgSO_4$ by protocol.
d. Monitor contraction pattern and FHR.
e. Avoid narcotic administration.
f. Administer steroid (betamethasone) if ordered:
1) Helps mature fetal lungs.
2) Use with caution with tocolytics, as pulmonary edema can occur.
g. Alert nursery to prepare for preterm newborn.
E. Evaluation
1. Uterine contractions slow to 0–4 per hour.
2. Fetus and woman tolerate effects of therapy without serious side effects.
3. Woman verbalizes concerns regarding self and fetus.

4. Woman can verbalize:
    a. Warning signs of preterm labor
    b. Medication regimen
    c. Need for rest and limited activity
    d. When to call physician

III. Ineffective labor
  A. Hypotonic contractions: intensity of regular contractions decreases during active labor
  B. Hypertonic contractions (uterus does not rest sufficiently between contractions): contractions occur frequently, usually during latent phase
  C. Uncoordinated contractions (coupling): two pacing cells active
  D. Data collection
    1. Physical
      a. Cervical dilatation slows or stops.
      b. Fetal descent slows or stops.
      c. Woman is exhausted or dehydrated or both.
      d. Extreme pain occurs with hypertonic and uncoordinated contractions.
        1) Turn woman on her left side.
        2) Provide IV hydration.
        3) Observe for S/S of fetal distress.
        4) Document.
        5) Provide pain relief measures.
    2. Psychological
      a. Feelings of discouragement
      b. Extreme fatigue
      c. Uncooperativeness
  E. Planning
    1. Assess progress of labor.
    2. Promote rest and relaxation.
    3. Prepare for augmentation of labor with oxytocin.
  F. Implementation
    1. Hypotonic
      a. Examine vaginally for:
        1) Descent
        2) Dilatation
        3) Effacement
        4) Position
      b. Assist with ultrasound or pelvimetry to rule out CPD.
      c. Hydrate woman vigorously.
      d. Promote rest and a quiet atmosphere.
      e. Sedate woman for sleep as ordered.
      f. Start IV oxytocin infusion:
        1) Give fluids as ordered, except plain D_5W.
        2) Administer via IV piggyback on infusion controller or pump.
        3) Follow protocol.
    2. Hypertonic
      a. Change woman's position.
      b. Encourage woman to empty bladder.
      c. Teach and support relaxation techniques.
      d. Provide analgesia sedation.
      e. Monitor fetus closely.
      f. Use heavy sedation or $MgSO_4$ to decrease uterine tone.
  G. Evaluation
    1. Woman verbalizes understanding of and agrees with treatment plan.

2. Woman and fetus tolerate treatment without complications.
3. Woman reports comfort measures as effective.

IV. Prolapsed cord
  A. Types
    1. Concealed: between presenting part and amnion
    2. Palpable: protruding through the cervix or vagina or both
  B. Data collection
    1. Physical
      a. Umbilical cord seen or palpated
      b. FHR slow and irregular or absent
      c. Violent fetal activity followed by no activity
      d. Severe variable decelerations on the fetal monitor
      e. Associated factors
        1) Breech or transverse presentation
        2) Multiple gestation
        3) Prematurity
        4) Polyhydramnios
    2. Psychological
      a. Confusion and fear, once woman realizes what has happened
      b. Anxiety over rapid intervention
  C. Planning
    1. Relieve pressure on the cord.
    2. Monitor FHR constantly.
    3. Provide for informed consent for emergency cesarean.
    4. Offer emotional support.
  D. Implementation
    1. Monitor FHR immediately after rupture of membranes.
    2. Relieve cord compression immediately:
      a. Knee-chest position
      b. Trendelenburg position
      c. Pushing the presenting part off the cord through the vagina with a sterile gloved hand
        1) Do not try to push the cord back in.
        2) Do not remove hand until fetus is delivered.
        3) Administer O_2 at 10 L/min by face mask.
        4) Prepare for emergency cesarean delivery.
        5) Witness informed consent.
        6) Monitor FHR continuously
  E. Evaluation
    1. Infant born by cesarean section without S/S of hypoxia.
    2. Couple verbalizes feelings of support after delivery.

V. Ruptured uterus: rupture caused by:
  A. Uterine scars
  B. Use of oxytoxic drugs
  C. Unknown cause
  D. Data collection
    1. Physical
      a. Pain
      b. Shearing or tearing
      c. Diffuse or local
      d. Severe
      e. Contractions cease; labor stops
      f. Loss of FHR or very low FHR (severe bradycardia)

g. Abdominal rigidity

h. Fetal parts palpated easily through abdomen

i. Maternal shock

  2. Psychological

    a. Anxiety, confusion

    b. Restless and combative even though weak

E. Planning

  1. Initiate emergency care.

  2. Deliver infant as soon as possible.

  3. Maintain stable physiological status of mother.

F. Implementation

  1. Discontinue oxytocin if infusion is running.

  2. Initiate treatment for shock:

    a. Trendelenburg position

    b. O$_2$ by face mask at 10 L/min

    c. Open IV fluids for rapid infusion

    d. FHR monitoring

    e. Transfusion preparation

    f. Vital signs checked every 5–15 minutes

  3. Prepare for emergency cesarean section with possible hysterectomy.

  4. Inform family members.

G. Evaluation

  1. Infant is born in stable condition or is successfully resuscitated.

  2. Woman's uterus is repairable or hysterectomy is performed without complications.

  3. Woman's physiological status stabilizes.

  4. Couple verbalizes feelings of support.

Postpartum Complications

I. Hemorrhage

A. Early: loss >500 ml within 24 hours of delivery

B. Late: loss >500 ml after 24 hours postpartum

C. Data collection

  1. Physical

    a. Uterine atony

    b. Lacerations of cervix, vagina, perineum

    c. Retained placental parts

    d. Overdistended uterus that will not clamp down

  2. Psychological

    a. Uncooperativeness because fundal massage is painful

    b. Confusion, restlessness

D. Planning

  1. Assess abnormal bleeding.

  2. Maintain vital signs.

  3. Prevent shock.

E. Implementation

  1. Massage uterus.

  2. Assess amount of bleeding (use cm/ml method).

  3. Monitor vital signs.

  4. Increase IV fluids.

  5. Have woman empty bladder.

  6. Administer oxytoxic medication (methergine).

  7. Evaluate blood loss by Hgb and Hct.

  8. Assist with transfusion as needed.

  9. Assist with D&C if required.

  10. Treat shock.

F. Evaluation

  1. Woman's fundus is firm, midline, and at appropriate level for postpartum day.

  2. Vaginal bleeding is scant to moderate.

  3. Woman's vital signs remain WNL of prepregnant baseline.

  4. Laboratory values stabilize WNL.

  5. Woman verbalizes need to rest and drink fluids.

II. Infection: any infection of reproductive system within 10 days of delivery, excluding the first 24 hours postpartum

A. Data collection

  1. Physical

    a. Fever >100.4°F (38°C) and chills

    b. Urinary frequency, dysuria, and inadequate emptying of bladder

    c. Foul odor and greenish color of lochia

    d. Abdominal tenderness, enlarged lymph nodes

    e. Purulent drainage from incision(s)

    f. Increased WBC count (>25,000 mm^3)

  2. Psychological

    a. Extreme fatigue

    b. Distress over inability to be "back to normal"

    c. Uncooperativeness

    d. Anger

B. Planning

  1. Promote proper hygiene after delivery.

  2. Support woman in expression of feelings.

  3. Administer medications.

C. Implementation

  1. Obtain cultures (blood, urine, cervical, and incisional).

  2. Evaluate area and amount of pain.

  3. Evaluate lochia for color and odor.

  4. Check vital signs every 2–4 hours.

  5. Encourage use of sitz bath, K-pad hot pack, and warm compresses for pain relief.

  6. Provide a private bathroom.

  7. Offer reassurance.

  8. Teach personal hygiene.

D. Evaluation

  1. Woman demonstrates personal hygiene care.

  2. Woman verbalizes adequate pain relief.

  3. Medication should be taken for full course.

III. Mastitis: inflammation of milk ducts in breasts 2–4 weeks postpartum

A. Data collection

  1. Physical

    a. Nipple cracks, fissures, and bleeding

    b. Hot, reddened area on breast

    c. Fever and chills

    d. Engorgement and pain

    e. Causes

      1) Incomplete emptying during breastfeeding

      2) Migration of bacteria through cracked nipples

  2. Psychological

    a. Feelings of inadequacy and guilt

    b. Fatigue, depression

B. Planning

  1. Promote breast hygiene.

  2. Reassure woman about mothering skills.

C. Implementation
   1. Teach woman to take antibiotic and analgesic.
   2. Complete emptying of breast essential (can continue to breast-feed, or use manual pump).
   3. Warm compresses should be applied to area.
   4. Bra should be worn day and night.
   5. Reassure woman that normal lactation will return.
   6. Reinforce breast hygiene care:
      a. Wash with water only.
      b. Apply breast milk to nipples and areola after feeding.
      c. Expose nipples to air.
      d. Change breastfeeding positions frequently:
         1) Cradle hold
         2) Football hold
         3) Side-lying hold
D. Evaluation
   1. S/S of infection are decreased or absent.
   2. Breastfeeding continues.
   3. Woman verbalizes and demonstrates breast hygiene measures.

Postpartal Care

I. Immediate: during hospitalization
   A. Data collection
      1. Physical
         a. Temperature: first 24 hours normal up to 100.4°F (38°C)
         b. Pulse: bradycardia 50–70 bpm common up to 10 days
         c. Blood pressure: should return to prepregnancy baseline
         d. Breasts
            1) Soft for up to 3 days, then may become engorged
            2) Very firm and full when engorged
            3) Nipples may become tender if breastfeeding
         e. Abdomen
            1) Flabby and loose, with possible striae
            2) Possible separation of rectus abdominis muscles, which may feel like a hernia
         f. Gastrointestinal
            1) Extreme hunger and thirst
            2) Constipation common
            3) Hemorrhoids common
         g. Urinary
            1) Large urine output occurs over first 24 hours.
            2) Emptying bladder is sometimes difficult.
               a) Swelling of perineum.
               b) Nerve paralysis is caused by pressure during delivery.
               c) Woman should void within 6 hours after delivery.
         h. Uterus
            1) Fundus should be firm; if boggy, massage.
            2) Height is at level of umbilicus for a couple of days.
               3) Height decreases by 1 fingerbreadth/day.
               4) Uterus is not palpable above symphysis after ninth postpartum day.
               5) Lochia: discharge from uterus:
                  a) Rubra: blood, mucus, and decidua; red; first 2–3 days.
                  b) Serosa: serous, watery; pink to brown; 3–10 days.
                  c) Alba: leukocytes and cellular debris white; starts days 6–10, lasts 1–3 weeks.
                  d) Foul odor is indicative of infection.
                  e) Lochia commonly contains small clots (large clots should not be present).
                  f) Lochia becomes heavier with activity and when getting out of bed after lying supine for a long time.
      2. Psychological
         a. "Taking-in" phase: first 24 hours
            1) Reflective of pregnancy, labor, delivery
            2) Dependent
            3) Sense of wonder about baby
         b. "Taking-hold" phase: up to 2 weeks postpartum
            1) Provides self-care
            2) Impatient with discomfort
            3) Independent
            4) Interested in baby; wants to learn
         c. "Letting-go" phase: 3–4 weeks postpartum
            1) Woman feels loss of pregnancy.
            2) Woman must view infant as separate person.
            3) Woman experiences emotional lability.
            4) Woman experiences exhaustion.
   B. Planning
      1. Provide support and anticipatory guidance for parenting.
      2. Allow quiet time for parent-baby interaction.
      3. Instruct in self-care of perineum, breasts, and bowels.
      4. Promote relaxing atmosphere.
   C. Implementation
      1. Assess at least every 8 hours:
         a. Fundus
         b. Breasts
         c. Abdomen
         d. Perineum
         e. Calves (Homans' sign)
         f. Bowels
         g. Urinary function
         h. Vital signs (every 4 hours)
      2. Maintain bladder and bowel function:
         a. Measure urine to assess emptying.
         b. Catheterize woman if she is unable to void.
      3. Insert Foley catheter if woman is unable to void after third straight catheterization.
      4. Encourage intake of fluids (2000–3000 ml daily), especially water.
      5. Provide stool softener and suppositories as ordered.
      6. Encourage high-fiber foods.
      7. Encourage natural laxative foods.

8. Promote perineal healing:
   a. Provide ice pack, first 24 hours.
   b. Have woman take sitz baths, at least three per day after first 24 hours.
   c. Administer topical medications for pain and hemorrhoids.
   d. Teach importance of front-to-back wiping.
   e. Have woman change perineal pads with each toileting, applied front to back.
   f. Teach signs of infection and when to seek help.
   g. Emphasize proper handwashing techniques.
   h. Instruct in perineal lavage (pericare):
      1) Use plain warm tap water, or warm tap water and a bactericidal.
      2) Apply stream of solution from front to back.
      3) Encourage breast care:
         a) Bra should be worn all the time for support.
         b) Nipples should be washed with plain water only.
         c) Breasts should be massaged to promote the letdown reflex or to relieve discomfort or both.
         d) Topical cream should be applied for sore nipples.
         e) Warm towels may be applied to breast for relief if engorged.
         f) Assist with breastfeeding.
         g) Apply breast binder if woman desires bottle-feeding.
         h) Discuss signs and symptoms of mastitis.
         i) Review postpartum exercises:
            i) Kegel
            ii) Modified situps
            iii) Walking
         j) Provide information about sexual relationships:
            i) Sex is permitted when it feels comfortable (approximately 2 weeks postpartum).
            ii) Barrier method of contraception is preferred.
            iii) Woman may need lubricant until normal vaginal secretions return.

D. Evaluation
   1. Parents are given time to interact with baby.
   2. Woman verbalizes and demonstrates self-care methods.
   3. Anticipatory guidance regarding baby care is discussed.
   4. Mother states that she feels rested before discharge.

II. Hospital care of the newborn infant (term)
A. Data collection
   1. Physical
      a. Vital signs
         1) Tympanic or axillary temperature: 97.6–98.8°F (36.4–37.1°C)
         2) Apical pulse: 110–160 bpm
         3) Respirations: 30–60/min
      b. Measurements
         1) Length: average 19–20.5 inches
         2) Head circumference: average 33–35 cm (13–14 inches)
         3) Chest circumference: average 32 cm (12–13 inches)
         4) Average weight: 7–7½ lb (normal range: 2500–4000 gm)
      c. Head
         1) Molded (caput succedaneum)
         2) Fontanels (soft spots)
            a) Anterior: diamond-shaped
            b) Posterior: triangle-shaped
            c) Should be soft and flat
         3) Face
            a) Puffy
            b) Round
         4) Eyes
            a) Blue-gray
            b) Puffy
            c) White sclera
         5) Ears
            a) One-third above outer canthus of eye
            b) Ear flips back to position when folded over
         6) Nose
            a) Pug
            b) Preferential nose breather
         7) Mouth
            a) Hard and soft palates present and intact
            b) Sucking and rooting reflexes
            c) Symmetrical grimace
            d) Tongue smooth; should not protrude
      d. Neck
         1) Short
         2) Skinfolds present
      e. Chest
         1) Symmetrical
         2) Possible breast engorgement
         3) Possible breast discharge
      f. Abdomen
         1) Cylindrical shape
         2) Umbilical stump
         3) Bowel sounds present
         4) Femoral pulses present and equal
      g. Genitalia
         1) Female
            a) Large labia minora
            b) White milky discharge (may be blood-tinged)
            c) Majora covering minora when legs extended
         2) Male
            a) Small penis
            b) Urinary meatus in midline
            c) Foreskin cannot retract
            d) Testes descended
            e) Full rugae on scrotal sac
            f) Scrotum enlarged
         3) Urination within 24 hours
         4) Meconium stool within 24 hours

h. Back
 1) C-shaped
 2) Dimples over sacrum
i. Extremities
 1) Short
 2) Symmetrical
 3) May have extra digits
j. Skin
 1) Milia: clogged glands on face
 2) Lanugo: fine, downy hair on body
 3) Vernix caseosa: thick white substance found in creases
 4) Acrocyanosis: bluish hands and feet
 5) "Stork bites": flat, red birthmarks on eyes, forehead, neck
 6) Newborn rash: red maculopapular lesions (erythema toxicum)
k. Sleep
 1) Period of 2–4 hours after birth.
 2) Infant awakens with increased secretions.
 3) Infant may choke and gag on feeding.
 2. Psychological
a. Parents accept newborn infant and state that he or she is beautiful.
b. Parents hold infant close and speak to him or her.
c. Eye contact is established between newborn infant and parents.
d. Parents discuss infant's health.
e. Newborn infant is held during feedings.
f. Parents demonstrate tolerance of fussiness.
B. Planning
 1. Monitor newborn infant's physical parameters.
 2. Teach infant care to parents.
 3. Encourage interaction with family.
 4. Provide a safe environment for newborn infant.
C. Implementation
 1. Wearing gloves for unwashed babies
 2. Admission assessment
a. Respiratory
 1) Grunting
 2) Nasal flaring
 3) Sternal and intercostal retractions
 4) Signs of distress
 5) Tachypnea
 6) Breath sounds
  a) May hear crackles, suction with bulb syringe
  b) Is common for respiratory rate to be irregular
b. Gestational age
c. Dextrostick for glucose
d. Blood type if mother is O group or Rh negative
e. Eye prophylaxis
f. Vitamin K administered
g. Body temperature maintained
h. Identification bracelet checked
 3. Ongoing care
a. Complete assessment every 8 hours and as needed
b. Daily weight assessment

c. Infection precautions
 1) Perform 3-minute wash to elbow at beginning of shift.
 2) Perform 20-second wash between infants.
 3) Keep infant's eyes free of discharge.
 4) Apply triple dye or alcohol to umbilical cord stump.
 5) Change diapers frequently.
 6) Remove cord clamp after 24 hours if cord is dried.
d. Feeding
 1) Breast at delivery or within first hour
 2) Glucose water at 4–6 hours for bottle-fed babies
 3) Breastfeeding or bottle-feeding on demand, at least every 4 hours
 4) Anticipation of spitting up mucus
 5) Assistance with infant position for breastfeeding
e. Elimination
 1) Meconium: green or black first 24 hours
 2) Transitional: green or brown
 3) Then yellow
f. Circumcision
 1) Observe for bleeding.
 2) Apply Vaseline or ointment if ordered.
 3) Cleanse gently.
 4) Document voiding after procedure.
 5) Teach as needed regarding use of Plastibel clamp.
 4. Discharge
a. Screen newborn infant for:
 1) Phenylketonuria (PKU)
 2) Galactosemia
 3) Hypothyroidism
 4) Sickle cell depending on state law
b. Remove cord clamp.
c. Give instructions to parents:
 1) What crying means
 2) Methods to help with colic
 3) How to suction baby
 4) How to change diapers
 5) How to take temperature
 6) How to give bath
 7) How to care for umbilical stump until healed
 8) Discussion of infant needs for feeding on demand
 9) Positioning on the right side after feeding to promote gastric emptying
 10) Positions for burping
 11) Positioning the infant supine for sleeping (prevents sudden infant death syndrome [SIDS])
 12) Follow-up care
 13) Safety in the home
d. Complete birth certificate.
D. Evaluation
a. Parents interacting appropriately with infant
b. Newborn infant eating and eliminating normally
 1) Breast: nursing until at least one breast is completely soft and empty

2) Diapers: 6–10 wet diapers a day
3) Stools: yellow; soft, curdy; have a sharp odor
4) Bottle
   a) Taking ½–1 oz at each feeding
   b) Minimal spitting up of formula
   c) Stools: yellow-brown, pasty, have an unpleasant odor
   d) Parents' demonstration of infant care to nurse

Common Newborn Problems

I. Full-term infant
  A. Hypoglycemia: blood sugar <40 mg/dl
    1. Causes
      a. Infant stress from delivery
      b. Large infusion of D_5W to mother during labor
      c. Mother with diabetes
      d. Mother with hypertension
      e. Infant large for gestational age (suspect maternal diabetes)
    2. Data collection
      a. Physical
        1) Jitteriness, twitching, jerking movements
        2) Poor, weak sucking reflex
        3) Skin cool, clammy
        4) Irregular respirations, possible respiratory distress
        5) Poor muscle tone
        6) Low blood sugar, low blood calcium
        7) Weak cry; may be high pitched
      b. Psychological
        1) Parents anxious about physical condition of infant
        2) Guilt feelings if mother diabetic or hypertensive
    3. Planning
      a. Assess for signs of hypoglycemia.
      b. Stabilize and maintain normal blood sugar for infant.
      c. Discuss infant's condition with parents.
    4. Implementation
      a. Monitor vital signs frequently.
      b. Obtain serum glucose level every 30 minutes as needed and before feedings.
      c. Administer 10–15% glucose water PO or IV as ordered.
      d. Schedule frequent feedings to maintain blood sugar levels.
      e. May have to supplement breastfeeding in first 48 hours.
      f. Maintain normal body temperature.
      g. Monitor I&O.
    5. Evaluation
      a. Tremors cease.
      b. Parents verbalize questions and concerns about infant's condition.
      c. Hypoglycemia is readily detected and treated rapidly.
      d. Blood sugar levels stabilize by time of discharge.
  B. Respiratory distress
    1. Causes
      a. Fetal lung immaturity (lack of surfactant)
      b. Aspiration of fluid or meconium during labor and delivery
      c. "Wet lung" due to pulmonary fluid collection caused by absence of "thoracic squeeze"
        1) Usually in cesarean births
        2) Sometimes in precipitous vaginal births
        3) Pneumonia: infection of lungs
    2. Data collection
      a. Physical
        1) Predisposing factors are low Apgar score, cesarean section, and bleeding.
        2) Hypothermia and hypotonia may be present.
        3) Skin may be mottled, pale, or cyanotic.
        4) Respirations
          a) Assessment of rate, rhythm, cyanosis, depth of respiration, type of retraction
          b) Grunting and wheezing
          c) Nasal flaring
          d) Tachypnea (respiratory rate 60 or greater)
          e) Diminished breath sounds
          f) Retractions
          g) Provisions for parent-infant interaction
      b. Psychosocial (parental)
        1) Anxiety presenting as anger, shock, and withdrawal
        2) Fear of having permanently disabled child
    3. Planning
      a. Assess whether infant meets criteria for administration of surfactant.
      b. Assess infant's respiratory status frequently.
      c. Provide opportunity for parents to verbalize questions and concerns.
    4. Implementation
      a. Ensure availability of surfactant.
      b. Administer antibiotics (intramuscularly [IM] or IV).
      c. Administer IV fluids.
      d. Assess IV access site: umbilical or peripheral.
      e. Monitor respiratory function.
      f. Check blood gases every 4 hours:
        1) Pulse oximetry
        2) Oxygen via oxygen hood or ventilator
        3) Warm humidified air
      g. Give bicarbonate if ordered to correct acidosis.
    5. Evaluation
      a. Infant progresses to normal respiratory rate and pattern.
      b. Infant's color is pink.
      c. Infant's tissue perfusion is adequate (capillary refill).
      d. Parents verbalize feelings.
      e. Parents state understanding of medical and nursing care of infant.

C. Hyperbilirubinemia
   1. Causes
      a. Physiological jaundice caused by decreases in conjugation at 3–5 days of age
      b. ABO and Rh incompatibility caused by antigen and antibody breakdown of RBCs
      c. Breast milk, which produces a hormone that can delay excretion of bilirubin
      d. Bruises, cephalhematoma, and petechiae resulting from delivery
      e. Immature liver function
   2. Data collection
      a. Physical
         1) Lethargy, irritability
         2) Poor feeding and sucking ability
         3) Color: ruddy to deep yellow
         4) Abdominal distention, bowel sounds present
         5) Dark urine
         6) Elevated total and direct bilirubin levels
      b. Psychological
         1) Parental anxiety and fear about having permanently disabled child (brain damage due to kernicterus)
         2) Guilt if dehydration occurs or phenol-containing agents are used in cleaning bilirubin
   3. Planning
      a. Recognition of jaundice
      b. Tip of nose yellow
      c. Skin undertones yellow when blanched
      d. "Peach" coloring
      e. Sclera yellow
      f. Maintenance of good hydration of infant
      g. Offering oral fluids every 2 hours (breast milk, water, formula)
      h. IV hydration in severe cases
      i. Provision of teaching and reassurance for parents
   4. Implementation
      a. Provide phototherapy treatment with fluorescent or natural (through the window) light.
      b. Undress infant with genitals only covered.
      c. Shield infant's eyes from lights with protective mask.
      d. Provide stable air temperature and monitor every 2 hours.
      e. Change infant's position every 2 hours.
      f. Monitor total and direct bilirubin every 6–8 hours.
      g. Cleanse skin with water after infant voids or has a bowel movement.
      h. Monitor I&O.
      i. Weigh infant every 12–24 hours.
      j. Encourage parents to visit nursery frequently.
      k. Provide auditory stimulation.
      l. Assist in providing exchange transfusion if needed:
         1) Obtain parental informed consent.
         2) Compare type and crossmatch for compatibility.
         3) Suction trachea if needed before starting.
         4) Place under radiant heater with easy access.
         5) Keep NPO 3 hours before and during procedure.
         6) Restrain if necessary.
         7) Monitor vital signs every 5–15 minutes.
         8) Record amounts of blood withdrawn and replaced.
         9) Assess hydration.
         10) Watch for reaction to transfusion.
         11) Monitor blood glucose and calcium levels.
   5. Evaluation
      a. Infant's jaundice resolves with bilirubin levels returning to normal.
      b. Parents demonstrate infant-care skills.
      c. Parents consent to treatment plan.
D. Infection
   1. Causes
      a. Prolonged labor
      b. PROM
      c. Maternal infection
      d. Multiple procedures on infant
   2. Data collection
      a. Physical
         1) Lethargy, irritability
         2) Abdominal distention
         3) Poor sucking and feeding
         4) Elevated WBC count ($>$10,000 mm^3)
         5) Hypothermia or hyperthermia
         6) Irregular respirations; sometimes periods of apnea
         7) Rapid respiratory rate
      b. Psychological
         1) Parental anxiety related to infant's condition
         2) Guilt if mother had infection
   3. Planning
      a. Monitor for signs of infection.
      b. Provide education for parents about infant's condition.
      c. Provide parents with opportunities to verbalize feelings.
   4. Implementation
      a. Administer antibiotics as ordered.
      b. Maintain Universal Precautions.
      c. Obtain cultures (gastric, urine, blood, stool, cord).
      d. Provide oxygen, warmed and humidified, via hood or ventilator.
      e. Check temperature, pulse, and respirations every 2 hours.
      f. Weigh daily.
      g. Monitor I&O.
      h. Suction as needed.
      i. Reposition every 2 hours.
      j. Assess hydration by checking:
         1) Fontanels
         2) Eyes
         3) Skin turgor
         4) Mucous membranes
      k. Share infant's progress with parents.

5. Evaluation
    a. No S/S of infection within 7–10 days.
    b. Parents verbalize feelings.
II. Preterm infant: delivered at <37 weeks' gestation
  A. Data collection
    1. Physical
      a. Extremities thin
      b. Few creases on soles of feet
      c. Fine lanugo over body
      d. Respirations irregular; spells of apnea common
      e. Undescended testicles
      f. Protruding labia minora
      g. Hypothermia
      h. Skin parchmentlike, with many blood vessels visible
      i. Poor coordination of suck-and-swallow reflex
      j. Sluggish peristalsis; infrequent stools
      k. Position with extremities extended (full-term infant has flexed extremities)
    2. Psychological
      a. Parental fear of attachment to fragile infant
      b. Parental grief over loss of perfect infant
      c. Parental depression caused by long-term care and financial cost required
      d. Parental anxiety over possibly harming the infant by touch
  B. Planning
    1. Assess at frequent intervals.
    2. Avoid excess stimulation.
    3. Stabilize and maintain vital signs.
    4. Provide nutrition as ordered—likely to be parenteral at first.
    5. Promote normal growth and development.
    6. Encourage parent-infant interaction.
    7. Encourage "kangaroo care."
  C. Implementation
    1. Prepare warm, quiet environment.
    2. Monitor (axillary or tympanic) temperature every 2 hours.
    3. Take apical pulse and respirations every 2–4 hours.
    4. Maintain IV access and fluid balance.
    5. Administer medications IV.
    6. Handle infant very gently, turning every 2 hours.
    7. Monitor oxygenation (oxygen hood or ventilator supplied).
    8. Coordinate laboratory, medical imaging, and pulmonary function studies.
    9. Maintain meticulous hygiene and Universal Precautions.
    10. Bathe head and diaper area as needed with small gentle strokes.
    11. Gavage-feed every 2–3 hours when ordered; progress as ordered.
    12. Discuss infant's care with parents.
    13. Involve parents in infant care.
    14. Assist parents with expressing feelings.
    15. Help to set realistic time frame for hospitalization.
    16. Reinforce positive adaptive skills.
    17. Instruct mother in pumping and storing breast milk.
    18. Prepare parents for common problems of preterm infant:
      a. Jaundice
      b. Hypoglycemia
      c. Feeding difficulties
  D. Evaluation
    1. Frequent assessment facilitates early intervention.
    2. Parents verbalize feelings.
    3. Parents participate in infant care.
      a. Touching
      b. Stroking
      c. Holding
      d. Feeding
    4. Infant condition stabilizes.
    5. Infant gains weight appropriately.
    6. Parents demonstrate infant-care skills.

BIBLIOGRAPHY

Abrams, A: Clinical Drug Therapy: Implications for Nursing Practice, ed 4. JB Lippincott, Philadelphia, 1994.
Beare, PG: Davis's NCLEX-RN Review. FA Davis, Philadelphia, 1997.
Burroughs, A: Maternity Nursing: An Introductory Text, ed 6. WB Saunders, Philadelphia, 1992.
Fogel, A: Infancy: Infant, Family, and Society, ed 3. West Publishing Co, St Paul, MN, 1997.
Gorrie, T, McKinney, E, and Murray, S: Foundations of Maternal-Newborn Nursing. WB Saunders, Philadelphia, 1994.
Martin, EJ (ed): Intrapartum Management Modules: A Perinatal Education Program, ed 2. Williams & Wilkins, Baltimore, 1996.

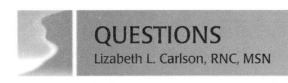
1. A client who is 6 months pregnant comes to the clinic for a routine visit. She asks what she can do to relieve constipation. The nurse should teach the client that the most appropriate measures to alleviate this problem include which of the following recommendations?

   A. Take a mild laxative and use a Fleet enema as needed.
   B. Drink 8 to 10 glasses of water a day and take a daily walk.
   C. Add more protein and fat to the daily diet.
   D. Drink hot coffee or tea each morning at breakfast.

2. A client at 26 weeks' gestation asks why she is having trouble with constipation during her pregnancy. Which of the following explanations by the nurse would be most accurate?

   A. The muscle movement of the intestines slows down, which causes dry, hard stools.
   B. The muscle movement of the intestines speeds up, which causes dry, hard stools.
   C. The intestines are compressed during pregnancy, which causes stool stasis.
   D. The intestines are expanded during pregnancy, which causes stool stasis.

3. A client was admitted to the OB unit on 9/10/97 with c/o labor. The nurse palpated regular uterine contractions of moderate intensity every 5 minutes. A sterile vaginal examination revealed a soft cervix that was 85% effaced and dilated to 2 cm. Which of the following admission information is most important in planning nursing care?

   A. The client's blood type and Rh were A+.
   B. The client's Hgb was 11 gm/dl.
   C. The client's LMP was 2/15/97.
   D. The client's blood pressure was 100/64 mm Hg.

4. A 22-year-old client at 7 weeks' gestation attended the first-trimester class on nutrition. Which of the following statements indicates a need for further teaching?

   A. "I should gain around 30 pounds by my due date."
   B. "Planning meals around the Food Guide Pyramid is best."
   C. "Frozen foods are more nutritious than canned foods."
   D. "My cravings are probably caused by iron deficiency."

5. A client admitted to the OB unit with contractions every 8–10 minutes, with cervical effacement of 100% and dilatation of 3 cm, reported that she and her support person planned to use prepared childbirth techniques. The nurse would expect the couple to use which of the following pain relief methods during this phase of labor?

   A. Slow, deep breathing
   B. Rapid, shallow breathing
   C. Local anesthesia
   D. Narcotic analgesia

6. A 30-year-old gravida 5, para 4 client at 12 weeks' gestation asks the nurse, "Do you think I'm having a boy? If I don't have a boy this time, my husband will probably divorce me." Which of the following explanations by the nurse would be most accurate?

   A. "Girls probably run in your family; there's nothing you can do about it."
   B. "The heartbeat of the baby is fast; that means it's a boy."
   C. "The father's sperm determines if the baby is male or female."
   D. "Don't worry, you are carrying this baby low, that means it's a boy."

7. A client at term states, "I would like to breast-feed, but my mother-in-law told me my breasts are too small and I won't have enough milk for my baby." The best response by the nurse would be which of the following?

   A. "Your breasts are small, but if you don't produce enough milk, you can give the baby some formula."
   B. "The size of the breasts doesn't matter. All women have about the same amount of milk-producing tissue."
   C. "You will produce more milk if you use a breast pump and then give it to your baby in a bottle."
   D. "Milk production is increased by the hormone estrogen. You can ask your doctor for a prescription to take estrogen."

8. A 32-hour-old baby has yellowish skin undertones and a serum bilirubin level of 14 mg/100 ml. The blood type of the baby is B+. The mother's blood type is O+. The infant is being breastfed. The nurse would include which of the following measures in his or her plan of care?

   A. No special measures are necessary; newborns normally get a little jaundiced.
   B. Tell the mother to stop breastfeeding and give the baby formula instead.
   C. Place the infant under the bililights and prepare for an exchange transfusion.
   D. Encourage the mother to increase the frequency of breastfeeding sessions.

9. A primiparous client at 18 weeks' gestation had an ultrasound examination done that showed the fetus in a breech position. The client asked the nurse, "Does this mean I will have to have a C-section?" Which of the following responses by the nurse would be most accurate?

   A. "If a first baby is breech, it must always be delivered by cesarean section."
   B. "The baby will have more room to turn as your delivery date nears."
   C. "You can probably deliver normally; most babies are born breech."
   D. "Many babies are breech at this stage of pregnancy; most turn before delivery."

10. A client in labor has been dilated 9–10 cm for 2 hours. The fetal head has remained at zero station for 45 minutes despite adequate pushing efforts by the client. A sterile vaginal examination reveals a position of occiput

posterior. Which of the following actions by the nurse would be most appropriate?

A. Assist the client to a hands-and-knees position.
B. Assist the client to a supine position.
C. Prepare the client for a forceps rotation.
D. Prepare the client for a cesarean delivery.

11. A client with preterm contractions at 34 weeks' gestation had an amniocentesis for fetal lung maturity. Which of the following laboratory tests should the nurse monitor?

A. HCG
B. PG
C. Alpha-fetoprotein (AFP)
D. PTT

12. A client at 12 weeks' gestation has just been told that she is carrying dizygotic twins. She asks the nurse what the difference is between monozygotic and dizygotic twins. Which of the following explanations by the nurse would be most accurate?

A. "Monozygotic twins come from two different eggs and sperm."
B. "Dizygotic twins come from one fertilized egg that split."
C. "Monozygotic twins come from one egg and two sperm."
D. "Dizygotic twins come from two different eggs and sperm."

13. A 20-year-old client has come to the OB/GYN clinic because her menstrual period is 7 days late. She tells the nurse, "I'm sure I'm pregnant because my period is late and my breasts are tender." Which of the following responses by the nurse would be most accurate?

A. "Missed menses and breast tenderness are positive signs of pregnancy."
B. "Missed menses and breast tenderness are presumptive signs of pregnancy."
C. "Missed menses and breast tenderness are probable signs of pregnancy."
D. "Missed menses and breast tenderness are negative signs of pregnancy."

14. A client is seen in the emergency room (ER) at 16 weeks' gestation with pelvic cramping and bright-red vaginal bleeding. For which of the following signs and symptoms should the nurse observe the client?

A. Increased temperature
B. Increased pulse pressure
C. Increasing heart rate
D. Increased blood pressure

15. The anesthetist has just placed an epidural catheter dosed with marcaine in a client at term in active labor. The nurse should observe the client for which of the following side effects?

A. Hypotension
B. Hypertension
C. Hyperventilation
D. Hypoventilation

16. A client at 12 weeks' gestation has a history of thromboembolitic disease. The client is placed on daily heparin therapy. The nurse should monitor the results of which of the following laboratory tests?

A. PTT
B. PT
C. Bleeding time
D. Coagulation time

17. A postpartum client complains of sharp pain in the calf of her right leg when walking. The nurse notes that the leg has a circumscribed area of redness, warmth, and tenderness. Which of the following nursing actions is most appropriate in this client's nursing care?

A. Instructing the client to massage the affected area to relieve the tenderness
B. Applying cold packs to the affected area to decrease inflammation
C. Encouraging the client to ambulate to increase circulation
D. Elevating the affected extremity to promote venous blood flow

18. A client has just started the third stage of labor. Which of the following nursing actions has priority at this time?

A. Encouraging the client to push
B. Administering an oxytoxic medication
C. Performing physical assessment of the infant
D. Promoting the bonding process

19. A client who delivered 45 minutes ago comes into the transitional nursery to see her infant. She asks the nurse, "My baby's head is shaped like a cone! Will it stay like that?" Which of the following responses by the nurse is most accurate?

A. "That is called a caput. It usually lasts for 3 or 4 days."
B. "That is called molding. It usually lasts for a few days."
C. "That is called a cephalhematoma. It usually lasts for a few weeks."
D. "That is called a nevus. It usually lasts several months."

20. A 20-year-old primiparous client who is breastfeeding is preparing to be discharged home with her newborn son. The nurse has completed discharge instructions on newborn care. Which of the following statements by the client would indicate a need for further teaching?

A. "I should clean the cord stump with alcohol or peroxide every day until it falls off."
B. "If my baby has at least two wet diapers and one bowel movement a day, he is getting enough to eat."
C. "I should dress my baby in clothing I would be comfortable in, plus a light blanket."
D. "I should nurse my baby whenever he acts hungry and for as long as he wants to nurse."

21. The nurse is planning care for a client who had a spontaneous vaginal delivery with epidural anesthesia over an intact perineum. She is currently in the fourth stage of labor. Which of the following nursing goals would be most appropriate for this client?

A. The client will ambulate in the room without assistance.
B. The client will turn, cough, and breathe deeply 10 times every hour.
C. The client's episiotomy will remain clean, dry, and intact.
D. The client will maintain physiological homeostasis.

22. A client delivered a full-term infant 6 hours ago. Which of the following assessment findings indicates normal postpartum progression?

A. Firm fundus at the umbilicus and midline with moderate lochia rubra
B. Firm fundus 1–2 fingerbreadths above the umbilicus and midline with moderate lochia rubra
C. Firm fundus 1–2 fingerbreadths above the umbilicus and deviated to the right side with moderate lochia rubra
D. Firm fundus 3–4 fingerbreadths below the umbilicus and midline with moderate lochia rubra

23. A client is pregnant at 12 weeks' gestation. Which of the following laboratory tests would the nurse need to interpret that would indicate a need for change in the client's plan of care?

A. WBC level = 70 mm^3
B. Hct = 32%
C. Hgb = 10 g/dl
D. Serum glucose level = 105 mg/dl

24. A client in labor received epidural anesthesia with marcaine for contraction pain 1 hour ago. Considering the effects of epidural anesthesia, which of the following nursing measures is important in her care?

A. Assessing the client hourly for respiratory depression
B. Assessing the client hourly for bladder distention
C. Assessing the client hourly for uterine atony
D. Assessing the client hourly for hypertension

25. A client arrived on the OB unit at term with mild irregular contractions. Findings from a sterile vaginal examination were as follows: cervical dilatation of 3 cm, membranes intact, and the presenting part at −1 station. An external fetal monitor was placed and the fetal heart tracing revealed a baseline of 130 bpm with accelerations to the 150s during contractions. Which of the following nursing actions would be most appropriate considering the client's situation?

A. Prepare the client for an immediate operative delivery.
B. Turn the client to her left side and administer oxygen.
C. Notify the registered nurse to start an IV infusion stat.
D. Send the client home and encourage her to ambulate.

26. A postpartum client who is breastfeeding asks for information on birth control methods that do not affect breast-milk production. Which of the following statements would indicate the client needs further instruction?

A. "Using condoms would be a good choice for me."
B. "I can use Depo-Provera and breastfeed without problems."

C. "Breastfeeding itself is effective at preventing pregnancy."
D. "I can use the contraceptive sponge for birth control."

27. An antepartum client at 16 weeks' gestation has tested positive for gonorrhea. All the tests for sexually transmitted diseases had negative results. Which of the following information is most important in planning her nursing care?

A. Client drug allergies
B. Fishy-smelling discharge
C. Presence of a chancre
D. Presence of vesicles

28. A client with non-insulin-dependent diabetes has just found out that she is pregnant. She asks the clinic nurse what she should do about her diabetes. The most appropriate response by the nurse would be which of the following?

A. "You can control your blood sugar with oral hypoglycemic agents."
B. "You can control your blood sugar with insulin injections."
C. "You can control your blood sugar with dietary changes."
D. "You can control your blood sugar by exercising more."

29. A client at 18 weeks' gestation with insulin-dependent diabetes has arrived for AFP testing. She asks the nurse why this test is being performed. Which of the following explanations by the nurse would be most accurate?

A. "This test is to determine the sex of your baby."
B. "This test is for fetal lung maturity."
C. "This test is for neural tube defects."
D. "This test is to determine glycemic control."

30. A postpartum client had a spontaneous vaginal delivery 30 minutes ago. During the postpartum assessment, the nurse notes that there is constant trickling of bright-red vaginal blood in the presence of a contracted uterus at midline. Which action by the nurse would be most appropriate in this situation?

A. Massage the fundus.
B. Call the health-care provider.
C. Have the client empty her bladder.
D. Increase the oxytocin infusion.

31. The nurse enters the room of a breastfeeding client who delivered 3 hours ago and who is in tears. "I just don't know what I'm doing wrong!" she sobs. "I can't get my baby to take the nipple!" Which of the following nursing diagnoses would be most appropriate in this case?

A. Altered parenting related to difficulty in breastfeeding
B. Altered comfort related to sore nipples
C. Altered bonding process related to maternal frustration
D. Knowledge deficit related to breastfeeding techniques

32. A client delivered her first infant 1 day ago at term. Which of the following actions by the nurse would be most likely to promote the attachment process?

A. Take pictures of the baby for the mother to see.
B. Tell the mother what her baby looks like.
C. Take the mother to the nursery window to see her baby.
D. Give the baby to his mother and point out his features.

33. A 20-year-old multipara at 18 weeks' gestation reports symptoms of thick white vaginal discharge and intense itching. A wet mount specimen reveals budding yeast cells and a diagnosis of infection with *Candida albicans*. The client asks how to prevent future infections. Which of the following responses by the nurse is most accurate?

A. "Eat a serving of live-culture yogurt daily."
B. "Douche after intercourse with vinegar and water."
C. "Douche with live-culture yogurt daily."
D. "Take antibiotics as ordered until all yeast cells are gone."

34. A 24-year-old primipara at 32 weeks' gestation comes into the clinic with complaints of nasal stuffiness, nosebleeds, and bilateral hearing loss. She asks why she is having these symptoms. Which of the following explanations by the nurse is most accurate?

A. "This sounds like a bad cold; you need to take a decongestant."
B. "These symptoms are common in pregnancy because pregnancy hormones cause increased blood flow, which causes head congestion."
C. "These are symptoms of a major problem. You need to be referred to a specialist."
D. "This sounds like a sinus infection. It is caused by exposure to allergens, such as cat dander or pollen. You need to take antibiotics and an antihistamine."

35. A client in the second trimester of pregnancy has blood drawn for routine 12-week laboratory work. Which of the following results would be considered normal for this stage of pregnancy?

A. Hgb of 11 g/ml
B. Hgb of 18 g/ml
C. Serum glucose level of 80 mg/dl
D. RBC count of 4.0×10^6 cells/μl

36. A nurse educator teaching a prenatal class asked for feedback from the class on the topic "Breast Changes during Pregnancy." Which of the following statements from one of the attendees would indicate that further instruction is needed?

A. "My areola will get smaller and lighter in color."
B. "My breasts will be tender and swollen."
C. "The nipples will get darker and more erect."
D. "My breasts will enlarge and may feel lumpy."

37. A 36-year-old professional woman who is pregnant for the first time at 10 weeks' gestation tells the nurse that her pregnancy was planned but that "I'm feeling like maybe this wasn't such a good idea." Which of the following responses by the nurse would be most appropriate?

A. "These are unnatural feelings. You should be happy to be pregnant."

B. "Maybe you should consider abortion since you feel this way."
C. "Don't worry, you'll feel differently once the baby is born."
D. "Many women have mixed emotions when they are first pregnant."

38. A 20-year-old client comes in for her first prenatal appointment at 10 weeks' gestation. Blood is drawn for routine prenatal screening. Which of the following laboratory results would indicate a risk to the fetus for erythroblastosis fetalis?

A. Low AFP
B. B−, antibody+
C. L:S ratio of 2:1
D. O+, antibody−

39. A client is in active labor at term with cervical findings of 5 cm dilated, effacement of 90%, and station −1. The FHR baseline is in the 120s with long-term variability. Three late decelerations were noted within the last hour with a quick return to the 150s and then baseline. Which of the following nursing actions would be most appropriate?

A. Position the client on her back so that the monitor strip is more accurate.
B. Prepare for a stat cesarean section.
C. Turn the client to her left side.
D. Encourage the client to ambulate.

40. A client in the 26th week of gestation has been admitted to the OB unit with a diagnosis of PIH. Which of the following symptoms would indicate worsening of the disease?

A. Epigastric discomfort
B. Blood pressure of 140/90 mm Hg
C. Deep tendon reflexes of 2+
D. Dependent edema of 2+

41. A client at 32 weeks' gestation was admitted to the OB ward 3 days ago with preterm labor. Oral terbutaline 2.5 mg every 3 hours was ordered. Which of the following nursing measures would have the *highest* priority in her antepartum care?

A. Check the pulse before each dose of terbutaline.
B. Maintain continuous fetal monitoring.
C. Place the client on strict bedrest.
D. Monitor closely for respiratory depression.

42. An Asian client in labor with her first child has a cervical dilatation of 7 cm, effacement of 100%, and the presenting part is at zero station. Contractions are every 3 minutes, strong in intensity, and lasting 90 seconds. She smiles each time the nurse enters the room. She stiffens her body during contractions but does not otherwise indicate that she is feeling any pain. She has not asked for any pain medication. Which of the following interpretations of the client's behavior would be most accurate?

A. The client is not experiencing acute pain.
B. The client is in control of her pain.
C. The client is demonstrating a moral value.
D. The client is demonstrating a cultural value.

43. A client who delivered a healthy term infant 1 day ago is talking on the telephone when the nurse enters her room to do her postpartum check. Which response by the nurse would be most appropriate?

    A. Instruct the client to hang up the phone immediately so that she can be checked.
    B. Ask the client if doing the check now or in a few minutes would be better.
    C. Ask the client about her vaginal bleeding instead of doing a check.
    D. Postpone the postpartum check until later in the shift.

44. A client at 28 weeks' gestation has been admitted to the OB unit for preeclampsia. Her blood pressures have been ranging from 140s/100s to 160s/110s. She has proteinuria of 3+, generalized edema, and has been complaining of a headache. Which care environment would be most appropriate for this client?

    A. Semiprivate room, up ad lib, vital signs every shift with fetal heart tones, 2-gm sodium diet
    B. Private room, bedrest with bathroom privileges, vital signs with fetal heart tones every 4 hours, regular diet
    C. Three-bed ward, ambulation three times a day, vital signs twice daily with fetal heart tones, low-protein diet
    D. Labor room, strict bedrest, vital signs every 15 minutes with continuous fetal monitoring, NPO

45. A client at 24 weeks' gestation comes into the OB clinic for a routine visit and a CBC. Results of the CBC include a WBC count of 10,000 mm³, RBC count of 5.0 mm³, Hgb of 9 gm/dl, and Hct of 32 PCV%. The client asks what these results mean. Which of the following explanations by the nurse would be most accurate?

    A. "Your lab results are normal for this stage of pregnancy."
    B. "Your white count is high; you may have an infection."
    C. "Your Hgb and Hct are on the low side of normal for pregnancy."
    D. "Your Hgb and Hct are low. It looks like you are a little anemic."

46. A client with severe preeclampsia is being treated with IV MgSO₄. The nurse checks the deep tendon reflexes and they are absent. Which of the following nursing actions has priority?

    A. Notify the RN and continue to monitor the client.
    B. Notify the RN to decrease the rate of infusion.
    C. Notify the RN to increase the rate of infusion.
    D. Notify the RN to stop the infusion.

47. A 22-year-old nulliparous client at 16 weeks' gestation asks the nurse how she can help her husband "get more excited about this pregnancy." Which of the following actions by the nurse would be most appropriate in assisting the father to bond with the fetus and validate the reality of the pregnancy?

    A. Allow the father to listen to fetal heart tones.
    B. Show the father a model of a fetus at the same developmental stage as his fetus.
    C. Give the father a typed handout on fetal development.
    D. Encourage the father to attend an ultrasound of his fetus.

48. A client at 36 weeks' gestation is admitted to the OB unit for severe PIH. The health-care provider performs an amniocentesis for fetal lung maturity to determine the risks of delivery. Which of the following nursing actions has priority after this procedure?

    A. Monitor the puncture wound for S/S of infection.
    B. Monitor fetal heart tones and assess for uterine contractions.
    C. Explain the purpose of the procedure to the client.
    D. Encourage the client to verbalize her concerns.

49. A client with PIH at 32 weeks has been admitted to the OB unit. Her S/S indicate mild PIH. The nurse should monitor which of the following laboratory tests that would signal progression of the disease?

    A. Liver function tests
    B. Serum glucose levels
    C. Serum magnesium levels
    D. Erythrocyte sedimentation rate

50. A 30-year-old client at term has had normal progression of her labor and is now completely dilated and pushing. The fetal presentation is vertex, with the presenting part occipitoposterior (OP) and at 1+ station. Which of the following procedures would the nurse expect to prepare the client for?

    A. Assistance to a lithotomy position and pushing with the breath held
    B. Simpson forceps rotation and delivery with a mediolateral episiotomy
    C. Nurse-administered fundal pressure and midline episiotomy
    D. Piper forceps rotation and delivery with a midline episiotomy

51. A 25-year-old client at term has been admitted to the labor and delivery unit for induction of labor. Sterile vaginal examination reveals cervical dilatation of one fingertip, effacement of 90%, and presenting part floating. Before the induction of labor starts, the client calls the nurse and says, "I felt a gush; I think my water broke." Which of the following nursing actions has the highest priority?

    A. Check for cervical dilatation.
    B. Check maternal vital signs.
    C. Check fetal heart tones.
    D. Check for vaginal bleeding.

52. A breastfeeding client is discharged home with her 24-hour-old infant. Which of the following statements would indicate that the client needs further instruction about nipple care?

    A. "I should clean my nipples with soap and water daily."
    B. "I should leave the flaps of my bra down between feedings."
    C. "I should run a little colostrum on my nipples after nursing."
    D. "I should change the position of the baby with each feeding."

53. A formula-feeding client has been discharged home with her term infant. She calls the nursery after 1 day at

home. She is concerned because the infant is taking only ½ oz at each feeding. Which of the following explanations by the nurse would be most accurate?

A. "The baby needs to take at least an ounce at each feeding no matter what you have to do to get it down."
B. "Maybe the baby is allergic to that formula. You should switch to a soy formula."
C. "If the baby is having at least four wet diapers a day, she or he is getting enough."
D. "½ oz is all the stomach of a newborn can hold. The baby will take more in a few days."

54. A 16-year-old client in the 35th week of gestation has attended childbirth preparation classes at the local hospital. Which of the following statements made by the client to the nurse educator indicates a need for further instruction?

A. "My boyfriend will be my coach and help me relax during contractions."
B. "If I practice these techniques, I won't need any pain medication."
C. "These techniques help control labor pain, but I can ask for pain meds if I need them."
D. "I should practice Kegel exercises several times a day."

55. A newborn boy was just delivered. Which of the following nursing actions has the highest priority?

A. Completely dry the infant.
B. Suction the nose and mouth.
C. Put on ID bands.
D. Check the heart rate.

56. A 24-year-old client delivered a term infant boy 30 minutes ago over a midline episiotomy after normal progression of labor. Vital signs are currently stable. Oxytocin 10 mg is infusing in 500 ml of D_5 lactated Ringer's solution at 125 ml/h. The current postpartum check revealed firm fundus 1 fingerbreadth below the umbilicus, moderate lochia rubra, and two nickel-sized clots. The newborn is in the father's arms. The mother makes the following statement to the nurse. "We were hoping for a little girl, but it's OK as long as the baby is healthy." Which of the following nursing diagnoses would be most appropriate for this situation?

A. Risk for injury related to uterine atony and hemorrhage
B. Altered family processes, potential for growth
C. Potential for infection related to altered skin integrity
D. Anxiety related to the new role of parenting

57. A primigravida with blood type O and −Rh factor has just delivered the placenta. She plans to bottle-feed. Pitocin 20 units is added to 1000 ml of LR solution and hung. The client asks the nurse why she needs this medication. The most accurate explanation by the nurse would be which of the following?

A. "This medication is to dry up your breast milk."
B. "This medication reduces blood clotting."
C. "This medication is to prevent Rh antibodies from forming."
D. "This medication is to make your uterus clamp down."

58. A client at 28 weeks' gestation admitted to the OB unit with symptoms of mild PIH complains of epigastric pain. Which of the following nursing actions would be most appropriate?

A. Pad the siderails and position the client on her left side.
B. Place the client on continuous fetal heart monitoring.
C. Check the medication administration record to see when the client last received an antacid.
D. Notify the RN to start an IV line stat.

59. A client who has just found out she is pregnant tells the nurse, "I'm a vegan. What diet modifications should I follow?" The best reply by the nurse is which of the following responses?

A. "You will have to eat meat during your pregnancy. Babies need complete proteins."
B. "If you drink soy milk and combine grains and legumes, your protein intake will be sufficient."
C. "You need to eat lots of dark-yellow fruits and dark-green leafy vegetables as protein substitutes."
D. "You need to add cheese and eggs to your daily diet. These are high-quality protein sources."

60. A 14-year-old client at 24 weeks' gestation has come into the prenatal clinic for her first visit. She is underweight for her height and pregnancy stage. The nurse asked her for a 24-hour diet recall, which revealed a fast-food diet. Which of the following meal suggestions by the nurse would be both nutritious and acceptable to this client?

A. Baked chicken, baked potato, broccoli, and milk
B. Fried steak fingers, mashed potatoes, fried vegetable sticks, and iced tea
C. Double-cheese pizza with green and red peppers and ham and a strawberry shake
D. Cheeseburger, french fries, fried apple pie, and a soft drink

61. A healthy term infant whose mother plans to breast-feed was admitted to the transitional nursery 30 minutes ago. The infant is under a radiant warmer. The nurse caring for the infant noted that he or she had an axillary temperature of 97°F (36.1°C), a respiratory rate of 60/min, and a heel-stick glucose of 45 mg/dl. Which of the following actions by the nurse would be most appropriate?

A. Wrap the baby warmly and take to the mother for breastfeeding
B. Give the baby an oral glucose feeding of $D_{10}W$.
C. Increase the temperature setting on the radiant warmer.
D. Call the health-care provider regarding an order for a chest x-ray.

62. A cold-stressed infant was warmed to 99°F (37.2°C) (core temperature) over a period of 2 hours. The infant has maintained his or her temperature WNL for the last 24 hours and has been breastfeeding well every 3–4 hours (per mother's report). The nurse should monitor which of the following laboratory results?

A. Serum calcium level
B. Serum glucose level
C. Serum sodium level
D. Serum bilirubin level

63. A 1-day-old infant has just been fed ½ oz of formula and burped. He is placed in his crib in the nursery. To prevent aspiration, in which position should the nurse place the infant?
    A. Right lateral with the crib mattress flat
    B. Left lateral with the crib mattress flat
    C. Prone with the crib mattress flat
    D. Prone with the foot of the crib mattress elevated

64. A pregestational client with diabetes attending a prenatal class on breastfeeding reported to the nurse educator that "I want to breast-feed, but my friend told me that because I'm a diabetic, my milk will be too high in sugar and will make my baby diabetic also." Which of the following responses by the nurse would be most accurate?
    A. "That information is correct. Diabetic women shouldn't breast-feed because of high-sugar content in the breast milk."
    B. "You should definitely breast-feed. It has major health advantages for you and your baby."
    C. "You can breast-feed. The insulin you take will control sugar levels in your milk."
    D. "Your breast milk won't have too much sugar in it, but you would have to add 500 calories to your diet. That is too many calories for a diabetic woman."

65. A routine postpartum assessment on a breastfeeding client reveals bilaterally reddened nipples. No cracking or blisters are noted. The client reported nipple soreness and asked what she could do to decrease the soreness. The best response by the nurse would be which of the following suggestions?
    A. Limit nursing time to 5 minutes on each breast. Then increase nursing time by 1 minute at each subsequent feeding.
    B. Dry the nipples with a soft cloth and then rub them with Massé cream after each feeding.
    C. Make sure the infant's mouth is wide open before latching on and that most of the areola is taken into the mouth.
    D. Breast-feed only every other feeding to rest the nipples. Pump the breast milk into a bottle for other feedings.

66. A client at 8 weeks' gestation called the OB clinic at 10 AM to report streaking of blood on the toilet tissue when she used the bathroom that morning. She also reported having intercourse the night before. She denied any further bleeding or spotting. She asked, "What is causing this bleeding?" Which of the following responses by the nurse would be most accurate?
    A. "You are probably having a miscarriage. You need to go to the emergency room right away."
    B. "What you are experiencing is bleeding caused by implantation of the embryo. It is nothing to be concerned about."
    C. "Some women continue to have a small period each month. Just take it easy during the time you would normally be having your period."
    D. "Penile penetration can cause slight bleeding. It is usually nothing to be concerned about, but call us if the bleeding gets heavier or if you start cramping."

67. A 26-year-old primigravida at 8 weeks' gestation is admitted to the OB unit for severe vomiting. She has been treated in the ER with IV fluids three times in the last week. She reports, "I can't keep anything down, even water." IV fluids are started and promethazine (Phenergan) 25 mg IM/PO q4h is ordered. The client asks the nurse, "Why am I getting that medicine?" The most accurate reply by the nurse is which of the following answers?
    A. "Hyperemesis is connected to emotional disorders. Phenergan reduces anxiety."
    B. "Hyperemesis is caused by exhaustion. Phenergan will help you rest."
    C. "Hyperemesis causes electrolyte imbalances. Phenergan is an electrolyte replacement."
    D. "Hyperemesis is uncontrolled vomiting. Phenergan controls vomiting."

68. A client who has just arrived on the OB unit for a nonstress test brings her clinic records with her. She looks at the records and asks the nurse the meaning of the following notation: G4 T2 P1 A0 L3. Which of the following explanations by the nurse would be most accurate?
    A. "This means you have been scheduled for four prenatal visits; you have been on time for two, canceled one, were a no-show for one, and were late for three."
    B. "This means you have four children; two were born when they were due, one was early, and three were overdue."
    C. "This means you have had four pregnancies; two babies were born when they were due, you had one baby born early, no miscarriages, and you have three living children."
    D. "This means you have four children; two were born early, you miscarried one time, and three children were born when they were due."

69. A primigravida in the sixth week of gestation attends a prenatal class on self-care in the first trimester. In conversing with the nurse educator, she reviews potential hazards to pregnancy. Which of the following statements would indicate a need for further teaching?
    A. "I can clean out the cat box if I wear gloves."
    B. "I shouldn't take any medicine without checking with my doctor first."
    C. "It is better for me if I eat five small meals a day."
    D. "I shouldn't use my hot tub while I'm pregnant."

70. A 15-year-old athlete who weighs 110 lbs and is 66 inches tall is seen in the OB/GYN clinic because her periods have stopped. She told the nurse she didn't understand why this had happened because she was a virgin. Which of the following explanations by the nurse would be most accurate?
    A. "It could be caused by abnormal uterine tissue growth that causes scarring of the ovaries and stops ovulation."
    B. "It could be caused by strenuous exercise that has resulted in low percentage of body fat."
    C. "It could be caused by monthly hormone changes that also cause headaches, irritability, and depression."
    D. "It could be caused by a bacterial infection that has spread to the pelvic organs."

71. A client at 24 weeks' gestation had her Hgb checked at her routine prenatal visit. The Hgb level was 11 gm/dl. She asked the nurse why the level was so low. The most accurate explanation by the nurse is which of the following statements?

    A. "You are not getting enough iron in your diet."
    B. "The hemoglobin is diluted by the fluid in your blood."
    C. "The fetus is building up iron stores by taking it from you."
    D. "During pregnancy, there is decreased production of red blood cells."

72. A client noticed that her health-care provider wrote "positive Chadwick's sign" on her prenatal record. She asked the nurse what this meant. The most accurate response by the nurse would be which of the following?

    A. "It means that your cervix is a bluish color."
    B. "It means that your cervix is getting softer."
    C. "It means that your uterus can flex against the cervix."
    D. "It means that your cervix is dilating."

73. A client at 20 weeks' gestation comes to the clinic for a routine prenatal visit. The nurse measures the fundal height and finds that it is at the umbilicus. The correct interpretation of this finding is which of the following?

    A. The fundal height is lower than expected for gestational age.
    B. The fundal height is higher than expected for gestational age.
    C. The fundal height is appropriate for gestational age.
    D. The fundal height is irrelevant to gestational age.

74. A client at 35 weeks' gestation is seen at the OB clinic. Which of the following complaints by the client would require further nursing assessment?

    A. Shortness of breath when doing housework
    B. Swollen ankles at the end of the day
    C. Sharp, intermittent groin pain
    D. Increase in vaginal discharge

75. An Asian client delivered a full-term infant 2 hours ago. While teaching the client pericare, the nurse noted that she would not make eye contact. The correct interpretation of this behavior is which of the following?

    A. The client is embarrassed.
    B. The client does not understand English.
    C. The client is excessively modest.
    D. The client is demonstrating cultural beliefs.

76. A client in the first trimester of pregnancy is attending a prenatal class on nutrition for pregnancy. She tells the nurse educator that she is lactose-intolerant and asks if there are any other food sources of calcium. The nurse should teach the client that her diet should include which of the following foods?

    A. Sardines, peanuts, broccoli.
    B. Poultry, whole grains, tomatoes.
    C. Liver, dark yellow vegetables, green peppers.
    D. There are no food sources of calcium.

77. A client at 28 weeks' gestation has gained 16 lb. She expresses concern to the nurse about her weight gain. Which of the following responses by the nurse is most appropriate?

    A. "You have gained too much weight for this stage of pregnancy."
    B. "You have not gained enough weight for this stage of pregnancy."
    C. "Your weight gain is appropriate for this stage of pregnancy."
    D. "Weight gain does not matter at this stage of pregnancy."

78. A client at 34 weeks' gestation is seen at the clinic for a nonstress test. She asks the nurse the purpose of the test. Which of the following explanations by the nurse would be most accurate?

    A. "This test determines fetal well-being by assessing the FHR, body tone, and amniotic fluid."
    B. "This test determines fetal well-being by assessing the response of the FHR to fetal movement."
    C. "This test determines fetal well-being by assessing fetal movement several times each day."
    D. "This test determines fetal well-being by assessing the response of the FHR to contractions."

79. A client at 41 weeks' gestation has undergone a nonstress test for fetal well-being. The results of the nonstress test were three FHR accelerations of 18 bpm that lasted for 15 seconds over a 15-minute period. The nurse knows that these results would be considered which of the following?

    A. Positive
    B. Negative
    C. Reactive
    D. Nonreactive

80. A client at 18 weeks' gestation preparing to undergo amniocentesis for fetal anomalies made the following remark to the nurse, "My husband insisted that I have this test." Which of the following responses by the nurse would be most appropriate?

    A. "Don't worry, everything will be fine."
    B. "Make up your mind if you're having the test."
    C. "I'll call the doctor to cancel the test."
    D. "You seem to have some concerns about this test."

81. A client in active labor at term has been using prepared childbirth techniques effectively. She asks the nurse, "Why do contractions hurt so much?" The most accurate reply by the nurse is which of the following responses?

    A. "It hurts because of stretching of uterine muscles."
    B. "It hurts because of irritation to the nerves in the vagina."
    C. "It hurts because the nerves in the uterus are inflamed."
    D. "It hurts because of decreased oxygen to the uterine muscle."

82. A client at term has just been admitted to the OB unit in active labor. The admitting nurse noted the client had a

prepregnancy history of IV drug use and is positive for hepatitis B virus (HBV+). Considering this client's history, which of the following substances would require the nurse to wear personal protective equipment?

  A. All body fluids
  B. Saliva
  C. Feces
  D. Amniotic fluid

83. A client at 24 weeks' gestation has gained 5 lb since becoming pregnant. The nursing diagnosis—Nutrition: altered, less than body requirements, related to diet choices inadequate to meet the nutrient requirements of pregnancy—was developed. Which of the following goals would be most appropriate for this client?

  A. The client will develop a nutritious daily menu plan.
  B. The client will gain 30 lb by term.
  C. The client will take prenatal vitamins and iron daily.
  D. The client will eliminate all snack foods.

84. The spouse of a laboring woman tells the nurse that he does not think he wants to be present for the birth of his child. "I feel like I should be there for my wife, but all that blood and everything is disgusting. Besides, newborn babies are ugly." Which of the following nursing diagnoses would be most appropriate for this situation?

  A. Impaired parenting related to negative perceptions of childbirth and newborns
  B. Role conflict related to unrealistic expectations of the childbearing process
  C. Decisional conflict related to ambivalence toward the anticipated role in childbirth
  D. Impaired family function related to father's nonsupportive attitude toward his wife

85. A client in early labor is complaining of back pain during contractions. Which of the following nursing interventions would be most effective for this type of pain?

  A. Light massage over the abdomen
  B. Massage of the upper back
  C. Firm pressure over the sacrum
  D. Encouraging pant-blow breathing

86. A client in the second trimester is seen in the OB clinic for a urinary tract infection (UTI). She asks the nurse what actions she can take to prevent recurrences. Which of the following responses by the nurse would be most accurate?

  A. "Hold your urine for as long as you can before voiding."
  B. "Empty your bladder before and after intercourse."
  C. "Drink lots of cranberry juice to acidify your urine."
  D. "Eat live-culture yogurt every day to prevent infection."

87. A client dilated to 8 cm with the presenting part at zero station and FHR ranging from 110–120 bpm is complaining of facial numbness and tingling of her hands and feet. Which of the following nursing interventions would be most appropriate for this situation?

  A. Encourage deep-breathing techniques.
  B. Initiate oxygen therapy via face mask.

  C. Turn the client to a lateral position.
  D. Have the client blow into a paper bag.

88. A client attending a prenatal class on labor and delivery asks the nurse what factors can slow or stop descent of the presenting part during labor. Which of the following explanations by the nurse is most accurate?

  A. "During labor, peristalsis decreases and slows fetal descent."
  B. "If the uterus decreases in size during contractions, descent slows."
  C. "If the urinary bladder is full, fetal descent slows."
  D. "Ruptured membranes slow down descent of the fetus."

89. A client has been admitted to the OB unit for observation of labor. The admitting nurse auscultates fetal heart tones with a fetoscope for 1 minute. The FHR was 76 bpm. Which of the following nursing actions would be most appropriate?

  A. Prepare for an emergency cesarean section.
  B. Prepare to assist with internal fetal monitoring.
  C. Report the finding to the RN in charge.
  D. Assess the maternal pulse.

90. A client who delivered an infant boy 24 hours ago had her 2-year-old daughter in the room. The newborn was brought into the room. The 2-year-old girl turned her head away and stated, "I hate that baby; send him back." The mother asked the nurse to return the infant to the nursery. Which of the following nursing diagnoses would be most appropriate for this situation?

  A. Altered parenting related to depression
  B. Altered role performance related to postpartum psychosis
  C. Low self-esteem related to lack of confidence in ability to care for two children
  D. Altered family processes related to sibling rivalry

91. A breastfeeding client has put the infant to the breast for the first time. To facilitate latch-on, the nurse should teach the mother which of the following techniques?

  A. Using a finger to depress the breast tissue so the infant can breathe while nursing
  B. Placing the forefinger and middle finger around the nipple in a "scissors" position
  C. Ensuring that only the nipple is taken into the infant's mouth
  D. Placing the infant in a "belly-to-belly" position with the mother

92. A new mother is preparing for discharge with her full-term infant boy. In discussing infant safety concerns, which of the following statements by the client to the nurse would indicate a need for further instruction?

  A. "We put the car seat in the back seat facing backwards."
  B. "We bought a backpack to carry the baby in."
  C. "We stripped my old crib and painted it with lead-free paint."
  D. "We will put the baby to sleep on his back or side."

93. A 15-year-old client at 28 weeks' gestation tells the school nurse that she has decided to put her baby up for adoption. Which of the following responses by the nurse would be most appropriate?

   A. Tell her it is too soon to make such an important decision.
   B. Support her decision and acknowledge her maturity in making it.
   C. Ask her if she is being pressured into making this decision.
   D. Question her reasons for giving up her baby for adoption.

94. A primigravida at term is admitted to the OB unit in early labor. Contractions are 5 minutes apart and moderate in intensity, and cervical changes are dilatation at 4 cm, effacement at 100%, and presenting part at −1 station. Which of the following changes would indicate the nurse would need to prepare for imminent delivery?

   A. Cervical dilatation of 8–9, presenting part at 1+ station
   B. Client stating, "I feel like I have to have a BM."
   C. Contractions every 3 minutes, hard intensity
   D. The client vomiting and stating, "I can't do this any more."

95. A client in preterm labor was treated with IV magnesium sulfate for 6 hours and is now on subcutaneous (SQ) terbutaline. IV hydration was given with several 500-cc boluses of crystalloid solution since admission. The IV is now infusing at 125 cc/hr. Which of the following symptoms would indicate that the client has developed a fluid overload?

   A. Pulse 120 bpm, heart palpitations
   B. Intake of 3000 cc, output of 3500 cc
   C. 2+ pedal edema
   D. Fine crackles in the base of the lungs

96. A client who abused cocaine while pregnant is getting ready to be discharged home with her infant boy. The infant has a rigid body posture and is difficult to console. The nurse discusses with the client appropriate methods of play for the infant. Which of the following nurse recommendations is appropriate for this situation?

   A. "You need to get a musical mobile for his crib."
   B. "A wind-up swing will quiet him when he cries."
   C. "Tell your friends that rattles are a good toy for him."
   D. "Get a tape player and play soft music in his room."

97. The nurse in the transitional nursery suspects that a newly delivered infant was born to a mother addicted to narcotics. Which of the following physical manifestations would the nurse expect to find in this newborn?

   A. Rigid muscle tone, seizures, poor suck-and-swallow reflex
   B. Flat midface, low-set ears, small for gestational age
   C. Small for gestational age, decreased head circumference, developmental delays
   D. Poor muscle tone, flat midface, epicanthal folds near the bridge of the face

98. A well-dressed client at 24 weeks' gestation presents to the ER with facial and abdominal bruises. She reported, "I walked into a door." Physical assessment reveals numerous bruises in various stages of healing. The nurse suspects intimate partner abuse. Which of the following nursing actions would be most appropriate in this situation?

   A. Encourage the client to leave her partner.
   B. Accept the story. Abuse does not occur in middle-class families.
   C. Refer the client for psychiatric counseling.
   D. Ask the client "Did someone hurt you?"

99. A client is admitted to the OB unit at 34 weeks' gestation with vaginal bleeding. Which of the following symptoms would indicate placenta previa?

   A. Decreased fundal height
   B. Hard, boardlike abdomen
   C. FHR of 180
   D. Painless vaginal bleeding

100. A client whose newborn tested positive for PKU has received teaching from the nurse about the special dietary needs of her infant. Which of the following client statements indicates that teaching has been effective?

   A. "I'll continue breastfeeding."
   B. "I'll have to change to regular formula."
   C. "I'll have to use a soy formula."
   D. "I'll have to get a low-phenylalanine formula."

1. **(B)** Nursing process phase: implementation; client need: prevention and early detection of disease; content area: maternity nursing.

   RATIONALE

   (A) Laxatives and enemas stimulate the intestinal tract, but also can initiate uterine contractions. Intestinal motility is slowed in pregnancy because of the influence of progesterone. **(B)** Increasing fluid intake and exercise stimulates peristalsis. **(C)** High-fat and protein foods contribute to constipation. **(D)** Caffeine can cause tachycardia in the fetus, and its use during pregnancy is discouraged.

2. **(A)** Nursing process phase: implementation; client need: prevention and early detection of disease; content area: maternity nursing.

   RATIONALE

   (A) Progesterone causes peristalsis to slow so that more nutrients can be absorbed. **(B)** An increase in intestinal motility causes diarrhea. **(C)** Compression of the intestines during pregnancy does not contribute to constipation. **(D)** The intestines do not increase in diameter because of pregnancy.

3. **(C)** Nursing process phase: planning; client need: reduction of risk potential; content area: maternity nursing.

   RATIONALE

   (A) Blood type A with Rh positive factor does not present any problems in client care. Maternal blood type O and/or Rh-negative blood types can cause severe jaundice in the newborn because of maternal antibodies that destroy fetal RBCs. **(B)** RBCs are diluted by the increase in plasma volume in pregnancy. A hemoglobin of 11 gm/dl is physiological anemia, as opposed to true anemia. **(C)** According to Nagle's rule, an LMP of 2/15/97 would give an EDD of 11/29/97. This client is in preterm labor at 28⁵⁄₇ weeks' gestation. **(D)** During the first two trimesters of pregnancy, maternal blood pressure normally decreases by 5–10 mm Hg in both systolic and diastolic pressures. This decrease is a result of peripheral vasodilation caused by pregnancy hormones.

4. **(D)** Nursing process phase: evaluation; client need: prevention and early detection of disease; content area: maternity nursing.

   RATIONALE

   (A) Appropriate weight gain for pregnancy is between 25 and 35 lb. **(B)** Intrauterine growth retardation can be caused by poor maternal diets. The Food and Drug Administration recommends following the Food Guide Pyramid recommendations for improved dietary intake. **(C)** Canned foods lose some nutrients in processing. Foods that are frozen are processed less and are more nutritious. **(D)** Pica (cravings for unusual foods or nonfood items) relates more to cultural values and beliefs than to dietary deficiencies. Pica is more likely to cause iron deficiency than to be caused by it.

5. **(A)** Nursing process phase: planning; client need: basic care and comfort; content area: maternity nursing.

   RATIONALE

   (A) This client is in the early phase of labor; slow, deep breathing and relaxation techniques are usually effective in relieving contraction pain during this phase. **(B)** Rapid, shallow breathing, or hyperventilation, is inappropriate for any phase of labor. **(C)** Local anesthesia is used for numbing of the perineum immediately before performance of an episiotomy and delivery of the fetus during the last phase of the first stage of labor. **(D)** Narcotic analgesia is not appropriate for use during early phases of labor.

   It can slow or stop labor if given before 5-cm dilatation. In addition, minimizing use of narcotics is preferred when prepared childbirth techniques are used.

6. **(C)** Nursing process phase: implementation; client need: growth and development through the life span; content area: maternity nursing.

   RATIONALE

   (A) The male sex chromosome is XY; the female sex chromosome is XX. The mother contributes one X chromosome to the future child; the father contributes either an X or a Y chromosome. **(B)** The heart rate of the fetus is neither faster nor slower according to fetal gender. The range for the FHR is 110–160 bpm regardless of gender. **(C)** Meiosis results in the X and Y chromosomes of the man splitting so that each sperm carries either an X or a Y chromosome, thus determining the gender of the fetus. **(D)** How a fetus is carried relates to maternal uterine and abdominal muscle tone. The gender of the fetus does not determine how high or low it is carried.

7. **(B)** Nursing process phase: implementation; client need: growth and development through the life span; content area: maternity nursing.

   RATIONALE

   (A) The volume of breast milk produced relates to how often the breasts are emptied of milk. Formula supplementation decreases breast-milk production because the infant nurses less often. **(B)** The amount of milk-producing glandular tissue in all women is approximately the same. Large breast size is caused by increased fatty tissue. **(C)** An infant is more efficient at emptying a breast than a breast pump. In addition, oral stimulation of the nipples by the infant stimulates the release of oxytocin, which triggers the letdown reflex. **(D)** Estrogen does not stimulate milk production. Oxytocin and prolactin are the hormones responsible for breast-milk production and breastfeeding success.

8. **(D)** Nursing process phase: implementation; client need: reduction of risk potential; content area: maternity nursing.

   RATIONALE

   (A) Bilirubin levels in excess of 12 mg/100 ml may indicate the presence of a pathological process. This jaundice is most likely caused by an ABO incompatibility. Breastfeeding jaundice occurs around the third day of age. Encouraging early and frequent breastfeeding lowers neonatal bilirubin levels. **(B)** Light therapy requires an order from the physician. **(C)** Exchange transfusions for ABO incompatibilities are seldom necessary. **(D)** Early and frequent breastfeeding tends to lower serum bilirubin levels.

9. **(D)** Nursing process phase: implementation; client need: growth and development through the life span; content area: maternity nursing.

   RATIONALE

   (A) If the fetus remains in a breech position, external version may be attempted at around 37 weeks' gestation to change the position of the fetus. If version is unsuccessful in the nulliparous woman with a fetus in a breech position, cesarean delivery is *almost* always certain. **(B)** The uterus becomes more crowded, not less, as pregnancy progresses. **(C)** Few fetuses (3–4%) are in a breech position by delivery; even fewer fetuses in breech positions are delivered vaginally. **(D)** Approximately 96% of fetuses in a breech position turn to a cephalic position by delivery.

10. **(A)** Nursing process phase: implementation; client need: physiological adaptation; content area: maternity nursing.

RATIONALE

(A) Maternal position changes such as sitting, kneeling, lateral, or hands and knees can assist fetal head rotation to an occiput anterior position. (B) The gravid uterus compresses the pelvic blood vessels and compromises uteroplacental blood flow. This position not only has no effect on rotation of the fetal head but can cause fetal compromise. (C) Use of forceps at zero station is considered a high-forceps classification and is not acceptable practice according to the American College of Obstetricians and Gynecologists. (D) Cesarean delivery should be considered only if adequate pushing efforts of ≥2 hours do not result in descent of the fetal head.

11. (B) Nursing process phase: data collection; client need: reduction of risk potential; content area: maternity nursing.

RATIONALE

(A) HCG is a hormone produced by the placenta that stimulates the corpus luteum to persist and secrete estrogen and progesterone, which maintain the pregnancy for the first 20 weeks of gestation. It is found in maternal blood and urine. (B) PG is a major phospholipid of surfactant. Presence of PG in amniotic fluid indicates fetal lung maturity. (C) AFP is a plasma protein that is produced by the fetus. Abnormally high or low levels can indicate fetal anomalies. AFP levels are drawn from maternal blood. (D) PTT levels are drawn to determine if sodium warfarin levels are at therapeutic levels in women with thromboembolitic disease.

12. (D) Nursing process phase: implementation; client need: growth and development through the life span; content area: maternity nursing.

RATIONALE

(A) Monozygotic twins (identical twins) develop from one fertilized egg that splits into identical halves early in embryonic development. (B) Dizygotic twins develop from two different ova fertilized by two different sperm. (C) Once an egg has been penetrated by a single sperm, chemical changes take place that prevent multiple sperm fertilization. (D) See rationale B.

13. (B) Nursing process phase: implementation; client need: growth and development through the life span; content area: maternity nursing.

RATIONALE

(A) The only positive signs of pregnancy are auscultation of fetal heart tones, visualization of the fetus by ultrasound, and fetal movement felt by the health-care provider. (B) Presumptive signs of pregnancy are amenorrhea, fatigue, breast tenderness and enlargement, morning sickness, and quickening. (C) Probable signs of pregnancy are Hegar's sign, ballottement, positive pregnancy test, and Goodell's sign. (D) Amenorrhea and breast tenderness are presumptive, not negative, signs of pregnancy.

14. (C) Nursing process phase: data collection; client need: reduction of risk potential; content area: maternity nursing.

RATIONALE

(A) Increased temperature may be a sign of infection; however, the risk of infection is greatest during the first 72 hours after spontaneous abortion or operative procedures. (B) The client is at risk for excessive blood loss. The pulse pressure decreases with hemorrhage. (C) An increased pulse in the presence of visible bleeding indicates excessive blood loss. (D) Decreased blood pressure is a symptom of excessive blood loss in spontaneous abortion. Increased blood pressure at this stage of pregnancy would be a symptom of hydatidiform mole.

15. (A) Nursing process phase: data collection; client need: reduction of risk potential; content area: maternity nursing.

RATIONALE

(A) Hypotension is common with epidural anesthesia because the sympathetic nerves are also blocked by the medication, which results in vasodilation. (B) Hypertension is not a side effect of epidural anesthesia. (C) Hyperventilation is not a side effect of epidural anesthesia. A client is more likely to hyperventilate during painful contractions. Epidural anesthesia relieves contraction pain. (D) Hypoventilation is possible if epidural narcotics are used. An epidural narcotic (such as fentanyl) was not used in this case.

16. (B) Nursing process phase: data collection; client need: safety and infection control; content area: maternity nursing.

RATIONALE

(A) The PTT is assessed to maintain correct dosages of warfarin (Coumadin). Warfarin crosses the placental barrier and is contraindicated in pregnancy. (B) The PT is evaluated to determine the effectiveness of heparin therapy. (C) A bleeding time is obtained preoperatively to determine how quickly blood clots to maintain homeostasis. It is not routinely performed on pregnant women and is unnecessary for a pregnant woman on heparin therapy. (D) Clotting time is a fictional test.

17. (D) Nursing process phase: implementation; client need: reduction of risk potential; content area: maternity nursing.

RATIONALE

(A) These are symptoms of thrombophlebitis; massage of the area can break the thrombus from the venous wall and cause an embolus. (B) Local application of heat is one of the treatments for superficial thrombosis. (C) The client with symptoms of thrombophlebitis should not ambulate and should be placed on bedrest. (D) Administration of analgesics, local application of heat, bedrest for 5–7 days, and elevation of the affected extremity are often all that is needed to treat superficial thrombophlebitis.

18. (C) Nursing process phase: implementation; client need: basic care and comfort; content area: maternity nursing.

RATIONALE

(A) The third stage of labor is the stage of delivery of the placenta. The placenta will spontaneously separate from the uterine wall and be expelled by uterine contractions. Maternal pushing is unnecessary. (B) Oxytocin should not be administered until after the placenta is delivered, which usually occurs 5–7 minutes after delivery of the infant. (C) The infant's physical condition is a priority at 1 and 5 minutes after delivery. The physical assessment done at this time is known as Apgar scoring. (D) Initiation of the bonding process as soon as possible after birth is important, but the physical stability of the newborn is most important at this time.

19. (B) Nursing process phase: implementation; client need: growth and development through the life span; content area: maternity nursing.

RATIONALE

(A) *Caput succedaneum* is an area of generalized edema of the scalp that was present at birth. (B) *Molding* is an overlapping of the skull bones at the occiput of the skull. It causes the infant skull to have a cone-shaped appearance. (C) A *cephalhematoma* is a collection of blood between the skull bone and its periosteum. It is one-sided (does not cross suture lines) and appears within the first 2 days after delivery. (D) *Nevi* (also known as stork bites) are pink areas on the upper eyelids, nose, upper lip, lower occiput, and nape of the neck.

20. (B) Nursing process phase: evaluation; client need: prevention and early detection of disease; content area: maternity nursing.

RATIONALE

(A) The cord stump should be cleaned with the solution ordered by the health-care provider daily until it falls off. Cord care helps the cord to dry and prevents infection. (B) A breastfeeding infant should have at least six wet diapers daily. Adequate urinary output is a reliable indicator of adequate intake of breast milk. **(C)** The infant should be dressed as parents would dress themselves. Overdressing can cause prickly heat rash. Wrapping the infant in a light blanket maintains body temperature and makes the infant feel secure. **(D)** Breast milk is more completely and quickly digested than formula. Breastfed infants should be fed on demand. It is important for the infant to completely empty the breast, so infant sucking time at the breast should also not be limited.

21. **(D)** Nursing process phase: planning; client need: reduction of risk potential; content area: maternity nursing.

    RATIONALE
    (A) The fourth stage of labor is the immediate (approximately 1 hour) postpartum period. Epidural anesthesia takes approximately an hour to wear off. The client will be unable to ambulate during this time. In addition, *all* postpartum clients should be assisted with ambulation the first few times out of bed. **(B)** Pulmonary hygiene is important in clients with a respiratory condition, or those who have undergone an operative procedure. **(C)** The client does not have an episiotomy. **(D)** The most common complication of the fourth stage of labor is uterine atony and hemorrhage.

22. **(B)** Nursing process phase: evaluation; client need: physiological adaptation; content area: maternity nursing.

    RATIONALE
    (A) The fundal height is approximately 2 fingerbreadths below the umbilicus immediately after delivery. The fundal height increases to 1 fingerbreadth above the umbilicus within 12 hours. The fundal height decreases approximately 1–2 fingerbreadths a day afterward. Lochia rubra is present for 3–4 days after delivery. **(B)** Fundal height increases to 1 fingerbreadth above the umbilicus within 12 hours after delivery. **(C)** Fundal deviation to one side or the other indicates a full bladder and risk for hemorrhage. **(D)** The fundal height is 3–4 fingerbreadths below the umbilicus by the fourth to fifth postpartum day.

23. **(C)** Nursing process phase: data collection; client need: reduction of risk potential; content area: maternity nursing.

    RATIONALE
    (A) WBC counts indicate the presence or absence of infection. The normal range for WBCs in pregnancy is 50–70. There is no evidence of infection. **(B)** The normal Hct in pregnancy ranges from 32–46. **(C)** The normal Hgb in pregnancy ranges from 11–12. This client is slightly anemic. **(D)** The normal serum glucose level in pregnancy is 105.

24. **(B)** Nursing process phase: planning; client need: pharmacological and parenteral therapies; content area: maternity nursing.

    RATIONALE
    (A) Respiratory depression is associated with epidural narcotics. Marcaine is an anesthetic agent. **(B)** The woman may not sense the urge to void because of decreased sensation to the area. Pain caused by bladder distention can last for long periods. **(C)** Uterine atony is associated with administration of oxytoxic drugs. It is not an effect of epidural anesthesia. **(D)** Maternal hypertension is not an adverse effect of epidural anesthesia.

25. **(D)** Nursing process phase: data collection; client need: basic care and comfort; content area: maternity nursing.

    RATIONALE
    (A) This is a reassuring fetal heart pattern; no immediate nursing actions other than comfort measures are necessary. **(B)** There is no fetal distress. **(C)** The client does not need fluid-volume expansion; neither she nor the fetus is in distress. **(D)** This client is in very early labor. The fetal heart pattern is reassuring. Ambu-

lation at home would stimulate labor and descent of the presenting part and decrease hospitalization time.

26. **(C)** Nursing process phase: evaluation; client need: prevention and early detection of disease; content area: maternity nursing.

    RATIONALE
    (A) Condoms are a mechanical barrier method of contraception with an effectiveness rate of 88%. Condom usage does not interfere with breastfeeding. **(B)** Depo-Provera is an injectable form of progestin, with an effectiveness rate of 99.7%. Pregnancy is prevented for 3 months. It is safe for use during lactation. **(C)** High prolactin levels with exclusive breastfeeding can delay ovulation for up to 6 months. However, it is an unpredictable method of birth control. **(D)** The effectiveness of the contraceptive sponge ranges from 72–82%. It has no hormones to affect lactation and is safe for use during the postpartum period.

27. **(A)** Nursing process phase: data collection; client need: pharmacological and parenteral therapies; content area: maternity nursing.

    RATIONALE
    (A) Gonorrhea is usually treated with penicillin. Drug allergies to penicillin are common and can result in an anaphylactic reaction. **(B)** A malodorous vaginal discharge is caused by *Gardnerella vaginalis*. **(C)** A chancre is seen with syphilis. **(D)** Vesicles are seen with herpes.

28. **(B)** Nursing process phase: implementation; client need: pharmacological and parenteral therapies; content area: maternity nursing.

    RATIONALE
    (A) Oral hypoglycemic agents cross the placenta and can cause fetal anomalies. **(B)** Insulin does not cross the placenta and is safe for use in pregnancy. **(C)** Only gestational diabetes can be treated with diet during pregnancy. **(D)** Only gestational diabetes can be treated with exercise during pregnancy.

29. **(C)** Nursing process phase: implementation; client need: prevention and early detection of disease; content area: maternity nursing.

    RATIONALE
    (A) Analysis of amniotic fluid from amniocentesis allows determination of fetal gender. **(B)** The presence of PG and the L:S ratio determine fetal lung maturity. It is obtained from amniotic fluid. **(C)** AFP is a maternal blood test that can detect neural tube defects (the most common anomaly) in fetuses of women with diabetes. It can also indicate the presence of Down's syndrome. **(D)** Glycemic control is determined by HbA_{1c}, a maternal blood test.

30. **(B)** Nursing process phase: data collection; client need: reduction of risk potential; content area: maternity nursing.

    RATIONALE
    (A) Uterine atony would reveal a constant trickle of bright-red blood in the presence of a boggy uterus. **(B)** Excessive lochia in the presence of a contracted uterus suggests lacerations of the birth canal. The health-care provider must be notified so that the laceration can be repaired. **(C)** Excessive bleeding caused by a full bladder would reveal a uterus that was high and deviated to one side. **(D)** Increasing the rate of an infusion of oxytocin would not correct the problem of a lacerated birth canal.

31. **(D)** Nursing process phase: planning; client need: basic care and comfort; content area: maternity nursing.

    RATIONALE
    (A) One session of breastfeeding problems does not result in altered parenting. **(B)** The difficulty is in infant latch-on, not sore nipples. **(C)** Success in breastfeeding has little to do with bond-

ing and attachment. (**D**) Instruction and assistance from the nurse would most likely result in successful latch-on and breast-feeding.

32. (**D**) Nursing process phase: implementation; client need: psychosocial adaptation; content area: maternity nursing.

    RATIONALE

    (**A**) Giving a mother pictures of her baby is appropriate only when an infant is too ill for physical contact. (**B**) Descriptions of the infant do not replace physical contact between mother and baby. (**C**) Direct physical contact between mother and baby is most likely to promote attachment. (**D**) The combination of direct physical contact between mother and baby and discussion of the child's physical and personality attributes assists the mother in recognizing her infant as a distinct individual who is yet a part of her. This process is the beginning of attachment.

33. (**A**) Nursing process phase: implementation; client need: prevention and early detection of disease; content area: maternity nursing.

    RATIONALE

    (**A**) Evidence indicates that ingestion of live-culture yogurt decreases the incidence of vaginal yeast infections. (**B**) Vinegar and water douches decrease vaginal pH and inhibit the growth of yeast cells. However, douching is not recommended in pregnancy. (**C**) Douching with live-culture yogurt decreases vaginal pH. However, douching is not recommended in pregnancy. (**D**) All antimicrobials cross the placenta, and many can cause fetal organ damage. In addition, antibiotic therapy can increase the incidence of vaginal yeast infections.

34. (**B**) Nursing process phase: implementation; client need: growth and development through the life span; content area: maternity nursing.

    RATIONALE

    (**A**) Increased estrogen levels cause congestion, swelling, and hyperemia of the capillaries in the upper respiratory tract. These symptoms are not relieved by antihistamines. (**B**) The elevated levels of estrogen during pregnancy cause increased blood flow in the upper respiratory tract. Nasal stuffiness, earaches, hearing loss, and nosebleeds are common. (**C**) Referral to a specialist is not necessary because these are normal pregnancy symptoms. (**D**) These are normal pregnancy symptoms. Many antibiotics cross the placenta and are contraindicated in pregnancy. Antihistamines are also generally not recommended in pregnancy.

35. (**A**) Nursing process phase: evaluation; client need: physiological adaptation; content area: maternity nursing.

    RATIONALE

    (**A**) Blood volume increases by 30–50% in pregnancy. This causes hemodilution of RBCs and physiological anemia. Normal Hgb levels in pregnancy range from 11–12 gm/dl. (**B**) Plethora is not a normal finding in pregnancy. (**C**) The normal serum glucose level in pregnancy is 105. (**D**) This is a normal RBC count for nonpregnant persons. Normal RBC counts in pregnancy range from $11–12 \times 10^6$ cells/µl.

36. (**A**) Nursing process phase: evaluation; client need: prevention and early detection of disease; content area: maternity nursing.

    RATIONALE

    (**A**) Pregnancy causes the areola to darken and enlarge. (**B**) Breast tenderness and swelling are almost universal findings in pregnancy. (**C**) Pregnancy causes darkening of the pigment in the nipples and causes the nipples to become more erectile. (**D**) Breast enlargement is caused by the influence of progesterone and estrogen. Nodularity is caused by an increase in the size of the mammary glands during the second trimester.

37. (**D**) Nursing process phase: implementation; client need: coping and adaptation; content area: maternity nursing.

    RATIONALE

    (**A**) Ambivalent feelings about pregnancy are common in all women. Response A respresents a block to therapeutic communication. The nurse is telling the client how she "should" feel. (**B**) Even women with a desired pregnancy have ambivalent feelings. Such feelings do not necessarily mean the woman desires an abortion. (**C**) "Mother love" does not necessarily appear right after birth, especially in a first pregnancy. It may take time for such feelings to grow. (**D**) Ambivalence is a normal response experienced by any person preparing for a new role.

38. (**B**) Nursing process phase: data collection; client need: safety and infection control; content area: maternity nursing.

    RATIONALE

    (**A**) AFP is drawn in the second trimester, around 18 weeks of gestation. Low AFP may indicate Down's syndrome. (**B**) Antibodies formed by a mother because of an ABO or Rh incompatibility cause erythroblastosis fetalis. Blood and Rh typing and antibody screening can alert the health-care provider to the possible development of this condition. (**C**) An L:S ratio is obtained from amniotic fluid analysis and indicates fetal lung maturity. (**D**) There is a possibility of ABO incompatibility that could result in erythroblastosis fetalis; however, the antibody screen is negative.

39. (**C**) Nursing process phase: implementation; client need: management of care; content area: maternity nursing.

    RATIONALE

    (**A**) Compression of the major vessels of the pelvis occurs with a supine position. This position will compromise placental perfusion and contribute to fetal distress. (**B**) Fetal reserves are still present as evidenced by long-term variability, "shoulders," and a return to baseline. An operative delivery is not yet required. (**C**) Late decelerations are caused by decreased uteroplacental perfusion. Positioning a woman on her left side promotes fetal well-being by increasing placental perfusion and subsequent fetal oxygenation. This position change may stop the late decelerations. (**D**) Ambulation stimulates uterine contractions and promotes fetal descent. Increased frequency and/or intensity of contractions impairs uterine perfusion.

40. (**A**) Nursing process phase: data collection; client need: reduction of risk potential; content area: maternity nursing.

    RATIONALE

    (**A**) Epigastric pain or discomfort is a sign of impending seizure in the client with severe PIH. (**B**) A blood pressure reading of 140/90 indicates hypertension. Hypertension is considered severe when diastolic blood pressures exceed 110. (**C**) Normal deep tendon reflexes are 2+. (**D**) Dependent edema is a normal finding of pregnancy. Edema of the hands or face or pitting edema indicate a worsening of the disease.

41. (**A**) Nursing process phase: implementation; client need: reduction of risk potential; content area: maternity nursing.

    RATIONALE

    (**A**) Terbutaline can cause maternal tachycardia (>120 bpm). Maternal tachycardia can reduce cardiac output and oxygenation. The dosage may need to be reduced or discontinued if tachycardia occurs. (**B**) Continuous fetal monitoring is maintained during initial tocolysis and active labor. Fetal heart tones and fetal activity logs are more appropriate for determining fetal well-being at this stage of treatment. (**C**) Bedrest with bathroom privileges is the most common activity restriction for clients with preterm labor after initial stabilization. (**D**) Terbutaline is likely to cause hyperventilation. It does not cause respiratory depression.

42. **(D)** Nursing process phase: data collection; client need: psychosocial adaptation; content area: maternity nursing.

    RATIONALE

    (A) Absence of requests for pain medication and smiling do not mean that a client is not experiencing pain. These responses may reflect personal or cultural values. **(B)** The progress of the client's labor and her tension may indicate that the client needs help with pain control. **(C)** Moral values relate to an individual's sense of right and wrong. Pain-control methods are not associated with morality. **(D)** Asian women usually value stoicism and maintaining harmonious relationships. It is incorrect to assume that pain relief is not needed because of these responses.

43. **(B)** Nursing process phase: implementation; client need: prevention and early detection of disease; content area: maternity nursing.

    RATIONALE

    (A) It is important to collaborate with postpartum clients. Postpartum checks can safely be deferred for a few minutes when a client is stable. **(B)** Allowing postpartum clients choices gives them more of a sense of autonomy. OB nurses should foster independence as much as possible. **(C)** Important physical information can be missed if a thorough check is not done. A client may not know what constitutes normal lochia flow, cannot evaluate the episiotomy, and cannot describe the consistency of the fundus. **(D)** The nurse needs a baseline database to evaluate changes in the condition of the client later in the shift.

44. **(B)** Nursing process phase: implementation; client need: management of care; content area: maternity nursing.

    RATIONALE

    (A) A semiprivate room would not afford the client the quiet environment she needs. Routine vital signs are not frequent enough to detect early changes in maternal or fetal condition. Salt restriction has no effect on the edema and is not necessary. **(B)** Loud noises and bright lights can trigger seizures in a preeclamptic client; these stimuli can be minimized in a private room. The client needs to rest as much as possible and avoid stress. Vital signs and fetal heart tones should be monitored a minimum of every 4 hours. There are no dietary restrictions for a client with PIH or preeclampsia. **(C)** This client needs to be in a quiet environment and on bedrest. The vital signs and fetal heart tones are not frequent enough to detect early changes in maternal or fetal condition. A low-protein diet is prescribed for clients with renal conditions. Pregnant clients need adequate amounts of protein to support the pregnancy. **(D)** Unless the condition of the client worsens or she starts to labor, there is no reason for her to be in a labor room. Continuous fetal monitoring and vital signs every 15 minutes do not promote rest. NPO status is not necessary.

45. **(D)** Nursing process phase: implementation; client need: growth and development through the life span; content area: maternity nursing.

    RATIONALE

    (A) Normal laboratory values for pregnancy are as follows: WBCs = 5,000–10,000, RBCs = 4.2–5.4, Hgb = 12–16, and Hct = 37–47. This client is anemic. **(B)** The WBC count is within the normal range for pregnancy. **(C)** The Hgb and Hct are below the normal ranges for pregnancy. **(D)** Most cases of iron deficiency develop after the 20th week of pregnancy because of expanding blood volume and fetal demands. Hgb values below 10 g/dl and/or Hct below 35 PCV% are considered to constitute a true anemia.

46. **(D)** Nursing process phase: implementation; client need: pharmacological and parenteral therapies; content area: maternity nursing.

    RATIONALE

    (A) Absence of deep tendon reflexes is an early indication of magnesium toxicity. The infusion should be stopped immediately. **(B)** Excessive magnesium depresses the entire central nervous system. Magnesium toxicity can culminate in respiratory arrest. **(C)** The infusion of magnesium should never exceed a rate of 150 mg/min. Administration of additional magnesium will make the condition worse. **(D)** Magnesium should be discontinued if the respiratory rate is 12/min or if deep tendon reflexes are absent.

47. **(D)** Nursing process phase: implementation; client need: coping and adaptation; content area: maternity nursing.

    RATIONALE

    (A) Listening to the fetal heart tones helps validate the reality of the pregnancy, but does not help; allowing the father to visualize the new family member best facilitates paternal-fetal attachment. **(B)** Fetal models are good teaching tools for explaining physical development and size of the fetus but are not the best way of encouraging paternal attachment to the fetus. **(C)** Typed handouts are too abstract to be helpful in encouraging paternal-fetal attachment. **(D)** Having a father present at the ultrasound of his fetus promotes paternal-fetal bonding by allowing him to see the features of the fetus. This visualization makes the pregnancy and new role more real.

48. **(B)** Nursing process phase: implementation; client need: safety and infection control; content area: maternity nursing.

    RATIONALE

    (A) Amniocentesis is performed under sterile conditions. In addition, S/S of infection usually take 12–24 hours to manifest after an invasive procedure. **(B)** Amniocentesis involves inserting a long needle through the uterus and into the amniotic sac. There is a risk for stimulation of uterine contractions and of fetal injury. **(C)** Informed consent is required before any invasive procedure. Explanations should take place before the procedure. **(D)** Although encouraging a client to verbalize concerns is always a good nursing intervention, physical needs have priority over psychosocial needs in this instance.

49. **(A)** Nursing process phase: data collection; client need: reduction of risk potential; content area: maternity nursing.

    RATIONALE

    (A) Liver function tests can indicate the development of hemolysis, elevated liver enzymes, low platelets (HELLP) syndrome. HELLP syndrome develops as PIH worsens. **(B)** Expectant mothers with diabetes are at higher risk for developing PIH, but the serum glucose is not a diagnostic test for PIH. **(C)** $MgSO_4$ is administered to prevent convulsions in severe PIH (eclampsia). Magnesium levels indicate a therapeutic level of the medication. This client has mild PIH and is not on magnesium. **(D)** The erythrocyte sedimentation rate is not associated with PIH.

50. **(B)** Nursing process phase: implementation; client need: management of care; content area: maternity nursing.

    RATIONALE

    (A) An OP position will result in prolonged pushing and maternal exhaustion because a larger diameter is presenting to the pelvis and birth canal. Fetal compromise can also result from prolonged pushing. **(B)** The occipitoanterior position is desired for vaginal delivery. The occiput has the smallest fetal diameter and passes through the birth canal easier. Forceps rotation is the quickest way of rotating the fetus to an OP position. Simpson forceps are most commonly used for vertex presentations. A mediolateral episiotomy gives the health-care provider more room for application of the forceps, with decreased risk of episiotomy extension into the anus. **(C)** In a face (OP) position, a midline episiotomy would very likely extend into the anus. Fundal pressure is always contraindicated because of the risk of uterine prolapse. Any assistive pressure by the nurse should be suprapubic. **(D)** Piper forceps are used in breech deliveries to deliver the head.

51. **(C)** Nursing process phase: implementation; client need: prevention and early detection of disease; content area: maternity nursing.

    RATIONALE

    (A) A vaginal examination on a woman with ruptured membranes who is not in labor will increase the risk of infection. **(B)** Maternal vital signs are important to establish a baseline for comparison. However, they are not a priority at this time. **(C)** If the fetal presenting part is not well engaged before rupture of membranes, there is a high risk for a prolapsed fetal umbilical cord. A prolapsed cord can become trapped between the fetal presenting part and the maternal pelvis. The fetal oxygen supply will then be compromised. The presence of fetal heart tones can be a reassuring sign of adequate oxygen delivery to the fetus. **(D)** Vaginal bleeding is a sign of either cervical dilatation or of placenta previa; it is not associated with ruptured membranes unless the client is in active labor.

52. **(A)** Nursing process phase: evaluation; client need: prevention and early detection of disease; content area: maternity nursing.

    RATIONALE

    (A) Soap removes protective oils and dries out the nipples. This can lead to cracking, soreness, and infection. **(B)** Increased air circulation around the nipples prevents maceration. **(C)** Colostrum, or breast milk, contains healing properties, such as lysozymes. **(D)** The area of the nipple directly in line with the infant's nose and chin is most stressed during feedings. Varying the position of the infant can prevent overstress of any one area.

53. **(D)** Nursing process phase: implementation; client need: basic care and comfort; content area: maternity nursing.

    RATIONALE

    (A) The stomach capacity of a newborn is approximately 15 ml. This lasts for the first few days of life. **(B)** Cow's milk allergy manifests in a newborn as vomiting after each feeding. **(C)** A newborn infant should have 6–10 wet diapers a day if the fluid intake is adequate. **(D)** The average capacity of a newborn's stomach increases to 75–90 ml by the age of 7 days.

54. **(B)** Nursing process phase: evaluation; client need: basic care and comfort; content area: maternity nursing.

    RATIONALE

    (A) In the Lamaze method, the labor coach assists the woman by providing feedback during labor and helping her to relax. **(B)** Lamaze techniques are used to increase the ability of the woman to cope with pain through conditioning and relaxation. There are no promises that the methods will completely relieve pain. **(C)** Teachers of prepared childbirth recognize that labor is painful and do not promise that no other methods of pain control will be needed. Pain medications are always available for the laboring woman. **(D)** In the Lamaze method, women learn exercises to condition and tone muscles to prepare for childbirth. The exercises include the pelvic tilt, tailor sit, and Kegel exercises.

55. **(A)** Nursing process phase: implementation; client need: reduction of risk potential; content area: maternity nursing.

    RATIONALE

    (A) Cold stress is extremely dangerous to the newborn. It increases oxygen demands and can cause hypoxia. Drying the infant decreases heat loss through evaporation. **(B)** The physician should suction the oropharynx of the infant while the head is on the perineum. Immediate suctioning after delivery can stimulate the vagus nerve and lower the infant's heart rate. **(C)** Placement of the ID bands can be done any time after the infant is stabilized.

(D) The heart rate should be checked at 1 minute after birth, after the infant is dried and warmed.

56. **(B)** Nursing process phase: planning; client need: coping and adaptation; content area: maternity nursing.

    RATIONALE

    (A) There were normal findings on the postpartum assessment. In addition, actual problems have priority over possible risks. **(B)** This family has entered a new phase of development. The nurse needs to plan and implement measures to promote attachment, so that the parents can start to assume their new roles. This is an actual problem. **(C)** There is a potential for infection of the episiotomy and IV sites; however actual problems have priority over potential ones. **(D)** There is no evidence of anxiety at this time. Altered family processes would be a more appropriate nursing diagnosis.

57. **(D)** Nursing process phase: implementation; client need: pharmacological and parenteral therapies; content area: maternity nursing.

    RATIONALE

    (A) There are currently no approved drugs for lactation suppression. **(B)** Heparin is given to decrease blood clotting ability. **(C)** $Rh_o(D)$ immune globulin (RhoGAM) is given to prevent the formation of anti-Rh antibodies in Rh-negative women who deliver an Rh-positive infant. It is given within 72 hours of delivery. **(D)** Pitocin is an oxytocin that promotes firm contraction of the uterus after birth to control postpartum bleeding.

58. **(A)** Nursing process phase: implementation; client need: safety and infection control; content area: maternity nursing.

    RATIONALE

    (A) Epigastric pain is caused by hepatic edema and hemorrhage in clients with PIH and is a sign of impending seizures. **(B)** Although fetal well-being is a concern, the priority is to ensure the safety of the mother. The FHR can be monitored after seizures have ceased if the fetus did not deliver during the seizures. **(C)** The epigastric area is located in the right upper quadrant of the abdominal area as opposed to just below the xyphoid process, where "heartburn," or acid reflux, a burning sensation, occurs. **(D)** It is unlikely there will be time to start an IV before the onset of seizures. The client needs to be protected from injury first.

59. **(B)** Nursing process phase: implementation; client need: prevention and early detection of disease; content area: maternity nursing.

    RATIONALE

    (A) Meat is not the only source of complete protein. **(B)** Soy is a good protein source. Combining legumes and grains results in proteins with all the essential amino acids. **(C)** Dark-yellow fruits and dark-green leafy vegetables are good sources of iron and vitamin C. They are not good sources of protein. **(D)** This client does not eat any animal product. This includes meats, eggs, and milk products.

60. **(C)** Nursing process phase: implementation; client need: prevention and early detection of disease; content area: maternity nursing.

    RATIONALE

    (A) Although this is a nutritionally well-balanced meal, it is likely too drastic a dietary change for this client. **(B)** Occasional fried foods are all right, but this meal has too much fat. In addition, it is recommended that caffeine be avoided. **(C)** This diet is both nutritious and likely to be accepted by the client. The double-cheese pizza and milkshake help to meet calcium and protein needs. Ham is usually the leanest meat available for pizza. The peppers are a good source of fiber and vitamin C. **(D)** This fast-food meal is likely to be highly acceptable to the client, but it is high in fat and poor in nutrition.

61. **(A)** Nursing process phase: implementation; client need: basic care and comfort; content area: maternity nursing.

    RATIONALE

    (A) Cold stress increases an infant's need for oxygen and can upset the acid-base balance. The infant reacts by increasing its respiratory rate. The infant needs to be wrapped in double blankets and a cap placed on his or her head. Cold stress also increases the metabolic rate and glucose stores are rapidly used up. A protein feeding is preferred because it increases blood glucose levels and maintains them. **(B)** $D_{10}W$ rapidly increases blood glucose levels but does not sustain them. If glucose water is used, it should be followed with a protein feeding 1 hour later. In addition, the cause of the low glucose level is not addressed. **(C)** Too-rapid warming can cause apnea. **(D)** The infant is not in respiratory distress. There are no retractions or grunting. The normal range for respirations in a newborn is 30–60/minute.

62. **(D)** Nursing process phase: data collection; client need: prevention and early detection of disease; content area: maternity nursing.

    RATIONALE

    (A) Hypocalcemia is strongly associated with newborns of mothers with such risk factors as diabetes, perinatal asphyxia, trauma, low birth weight, and preterm birth. **(B)** Glucose levels normally fall in the newborn over the first few hours of life. Infants with risk factors (large or small for gestational age, low birth weight, ongoing cold stress, or neonatal asphyxia) may require frequent glucose monitoring for the first few hours of life. Feeding the infant treats hypoglycemia. **(C)** Water intoxication results in hyponatremia and is associated with excessive feeding of water to infants. Diluting formula with water is another cause of water intoxication. This infant is breastfed and not at risk for hyponatremia. **(D)** Cold stress of the newborn can result in acidosis and raise the levels of free fatty acids. In the presence of acidosis, albumin binding of bilirubin is weakened and bilirubin is freed, resulting in hyperbilirubinemia.

63. **(A)** Nursing process phase: implementation; client need: safety and infection control; content area: maternity nursing.

    RATIONALE

    (A) Turning the infant to the right side promotes emptying of the stomach into the small intestine. A side-lying position also facilitates drainage from the oropharynx. **(B)** The infant should be turned from one side to the other to help develop even contours of the head and to ease pressure on other parts of the body. The left lateral side, however, does not promote stomach emptying. **(C)** The prone position has been associated with an increased incidence of SIDS. **(D)** The prone position has been associated with SIDS. Elevating the foot of the crib increases the risk of aspiration.

64. **(B)** Nursing process phase: implementation; client need: prevention and early detection of disease; content area: maternity nursing.

    RATIONALE

    (A) Blood glucose levels do not affect the amount of lactose in breast milk. **(B)** Breastfeeding is encouraged in mothers with diabetes because it decreases insulin requirements. In addition, breastfed infants have a decreased risk of developing insulin diabetes than those who are formula fed. **(C)** Neither glucose nor insulin enters breast milk from the bloodstream of the lactating woman. **(D)** Adding calories for breastfeeding will not affect dietary control for the woman with diabetes. The caloric demands of breastfeeding easily use up the extra 500 calories needed per day.

65. **(C)** Nursing process phase: implementation; client need: basic care and comfort; content area: maternity nursing.

RATIONALE

(A) Limiting time at the breast does not prevent sore nipples and can create a fussy, unsatisfied infant. The infant has to nurse at least 10 minutes to get the "hind milk," or the higher fat portion of breast milk. **(B)** Any technique that involves friction increases nipple soreness. Nipples should be air-dried. Massé cream is made from lanolin and can create more problems if the woman is allergic to wool (a common allergy). **(C)** If the infant has his or her mouth open wide before latching on, it is more likely that most of the areola will be taken into the mouth. When the infant is positioned with the nipple and most of the areola in his or her mouth, there should not be any tissue damage or pain. **(D)** Use of a breast pump contributes to nipple soreness because of its mechanical action and friction.

66. **(D)** Nursing process phase: implementation; client need: basic care and comfort; content area: maternity nursing.

    RATIONALE

    (A) Signs of a miscarriage are bleeding with cramps, severe pain with or without vaginal bleeding, vaginal bleeding as heavy as menses, or light staining that continues for more than 3 days. **(B)** Implantation occurs from 7–10 days after conception. **(C)** Slight bleeding at the time a period would have been expected is common. No special precautions are necessary. **(D)** The cervix becomes very soft and vascular during pregnancy. Deep penetration of the penis may cause bleeding if the cervix is bumped.

67. **(D)** Nursing process phase: implementation; client need: pharmacological and parenteral therapies; content area: maternity nursing.

    RATIONALE

    (A) Promethazine can decrease anxiety; however, it is no longer believed that women experiencing hyperemesis are attempting to "throw up" the pregnancy. **(B)** Promethazine can have the side effect of sleepiness; however, hyperemesis is not associated with maternal exhaustion. **(C)** Hyperemesis can cause fluid and electrolyte imbalances; however, promethazine is not an electrolyte solution. **(D)** Promethazine is used as an antiemetic in pregnancies when nausea and vomiting are uncontrolled by other means.

68. **(C)** Nursing process phase: implementation; client need: growth and development through the life span; content area: maternity nursing.

    RATIONALE

    (A) GTPAL stands for *gravida* (number of times pregnant, including the current pregnancy), *term* (number of babies delivered after 36 weeks' gestation), *preterm* (number of babies delivered before 36 weeks' gestation), *aborta* (number of pregnancies miscarried or therapeutically aborted), and *living* (number of living children). **(B)** The client had four pregnancies; two were term deliveries, one preterm; she had no abortions, and she has three living children. **(C)** See rationale B. **(D)** See rationale B.

69. **(A)** Nursing process phase: evaluation; client need: prevention and early detection of disease; content area: maternity nursing.

    RATIONALE

    (A) Cats can carry *Toxoplasma gondii* in their stools. This organism can cause fetal anomalies. The organism can be inhaled from litter box dust as well as be transferred on the hands. **(B)** Many medications, including over-the-counter (OTC) medicines, cross the placenta to the fetus. The greatest risk for teratogenic effects is during the first 12 weeks of gestation. **(C)** Gastrointestinal motility is decreased in pregnancy because of the influence of estrogen. The hormone HCG may also affect morning sickness. Pregnant women should avoid overloaded and/or empty stomachs. Five to six small meals a day accomplish this goal. **(D)** Any activity or condition that increases the body temperature to more than 102°F (38.8°C) for more than 10 minutes can cause fetal central nervous system damage.

70. **(B)** Nursing process phase: implementation; client need: growth and development through the life span; content area: maternity nursing.

    RATIONALE

    (A) Endometriosis is endometrial tissue that is found outside the uterus on other pelvic organs. This tissue bleeds at the time of the menses and causes scarring. This scarring can lead to infertility. Endometriosis does not cause cessation of menses. **(B)** Menstrual regularity requires maintenance of body weight and fat above a certain level. A woman who weighs <115 lb or has lost 10 or more pounds through strenuous exercise often experiences cessation of menses. This condition is known as *hypogonadotropic amenorrhea.* **(C)** These are symptoms of premenstrual syndrome (PMS), which include edema, emotional instability, panic attacks, irritability, impaired ability to concentrate, headache, fatigue, and backache. The cause of PMS is unknown. PMS does not affect menses. **(D)** A generalized infection of the female pelvic organs (pelvic inflammatory disease [PID]) is a significant cause of infertility. It is most commonly caused by sexually transmitted organisms. It causes severe lower abdominal pain and tenderness. Cessation of menses is not a symptom of PID.

71. **(B)** Nursing process phase: implementation; client need: growth and development through the life span; content area: maternity nursing.

    RATIONALE

    (A) Normal Hgb levels for pregnancy are 11–12 gm/dl. If the hemoglobin level falls below 11, a true anemia exists. **(B)** Physiological anemia is the result of dilution of hemoglobin concentration by blood-volume expansion. **(C)** The fetus does not rob the maternal body of iron. **(D)** RBC production is increased during pregnancy.

72. **(A)** Nursing process phase: implementation; client need: growth and development through the life span; content area: maternity nursing.

    RATIONALE

    (A) The increased vascularity of the cervix during pregnancy results in congestion of blood and a resulting bluish color. This is known as *Chadwick's sign.* **(B)** The cervix becomes softer as a result of pelvic vasocongestion. This is known as *Goodell's sign.* **(C)** Starting at about the sixth week of pregnancy, the lower uterine segment is so soft that it can be compressed against the cervix. This is called *McDonald's sign.* **(D)** Dilation of the cervix occurs when uterine contractions thin and open the cervix. This is called *cervical dilatation.*

73. **(C)** Nursing process phase: data collection; client need: growth and development through the life span; content area: maternity nursing.

    RATIONALE

    (A) Fundal height in centimeters is correlated to gestational age. The umbilicus is approximately 20 cm from the symphysis pubis. The fundal height is at the appropriate level for a gestational age of 20 weeks. **(B)** See rationale A. **(C)** See rationale A. **(D)** See rationale A.

74. **(D)** Nursing process phase: planning; client need: reduction of risk potential; content area: maternity nursing.

    RATIONALE

    (A) Shortness of breath even at rest is a common complaint of late pregnancy. It is caused by abdominal organ pressure on the diaphragm. **(B)** Dependent edema is a common finding in pregnancy. **(C)** Sharp, intermittent groin pain is caused by stretching of the round ligaments as the uterus enlarges. **(D)** A change in vaginal discharge can indicate preterm labor or a vaginal infection. The health-care provider should be notified.

75. **(D)** Nursing process phase: planning; client need: psychosocial adaptation; content area: maternity nursing.

    RATIONALE

    (A) Making eye contact means different things in different cultures. It does not necessarily mean the client is embarrassed. **(B)** The lack of eye contact does not mean a lack of understanding. **(C)** Asian women are extremely modest; however, this modesty is not manifested in eye contact. **(D)** It is a sign of disrespect in the Asian culture to make eye contact with one considered to be in authority. This client is exhibiting a cultural belief.

76. **(A)** Nursing process phase: implementation; client need: prevention and early detection of disease; content area: maternity nursing.

    RATIONALE

    (A) Dietary calcium can be found in fish with the bones left in (e.g., sardines and salmon), legumes, nuts, dried fruits, and dark green leafy vegetables (except spinach or Swiss chard). **(B)** Poultry is a good source of protein, whole grains of fiber and phosphorus, and tomatoes of vitamin C. **(C)** Liver is high in iron and vitamin E, yellow vegetables contain riboflavin and vitamin A, and peppers are a good source of vitamin C. **(D)** See rationale A.

77. **(C)** Nursing process phase: implementation; client need: growth and development through the life span; content area: maternity nursing.

    RATIONALE

    (A) The recommended rate of gain is approximately 3.5 lb during the first 12 weeks of pregnancy and 0.8 lb each week thereafter. Total weight gained at 28 weeks' gestation should average between 16–20 lb. **(B)** For a woman of normal prepregnant weight, 16 lb is appropriate for this stage of pregnancy. **(C)** This weight gain is within the expected range for 28 weeks of gestation. **(D)** Weight gain in pregnancy, especially after the first trimester, is an important factor in fetal growth. Insufficient weight gain causes increased fetal mortality and morbidity, and excessive weight gain is associated with birth trauma and operative deliveries.

78. **(B)** Nursing process phase: implementation; client need: basic care and comfort; content area: maternity nursing.

    RATIONALE

    (A) This response describes three of the five parameters of a biophysical profile. The other two parameters are fetal breathing and body movements. **(B)** A nonstress test evaluates the ability of the fetal heart to accelerate either spontaneously or in association with fetal movement. **(C)** A fetal kick count is a maternal assessment of the fetus. Fetal movement is associated with fetal condition. **(D)** A contraction stress test is another method of evaluating fetal well-being. Uterine contractions are initiated with either nipple stimulation or IV administration of oxytocin. The fetal response on an external monitor strip is then evaluated once three contractions are obtained in 10 minutes. The test indicates how well a fetus will tolerate labor.

79. **(C)** Nursing process phase: evaluation; client need: prevention and early detection of disease; content area: maternity nursing.

    RATIONALE

    (A) Nonstress test results are either reactive or nonreactive. Contraction stress test results are either positive or negative. **(B)** See rationale A. **(C)** A reactive nonstress test result is normal (reactive) when there are two or more FHR accelerations of at least 15 bpm with a duration of at least 15 seconds in a 20-minute period. **(D)** A nonreactive nonstress test result would be less than two FHR accelerations, or there was an increase of <15 seconds in the two accelerations, or the duration of the accelerations lasted <15 seconds, or the accelerations did not occur within a 20-minute time period.

80. **(D)** Nursing process phase: implementation; client need: coping and adaptation; content area: maternity nursing.

    RATIONALE

    (A) False reassurances are a block to communication. (B) Impatience is a block to communication. (C) The client has not indicated that she wishes to have the test canceled. This is also a block to communication. (D) Open-ended comments or questions that reflect the meaning of the statement by the client are most likely to lead to therapeutic communication.

81. **(D)** Nursing process phase: implementation; client need: physiological adaptation; content area: maternity nursing.

    RATIONALE

    (A) Uterine muscle contracts during labor. (B) There are few nerve endings in the vaginal walls. (C) Nerve inflammation is painful, but it does not cause contraction pain. (D) When the uterus contracts, blood flow is reduced to uterine muscle, resulting in ischemia and pain.

82. **(D)** Nursing process phase: planning; client need: safety and infection control; content area: maternity nursing.

    RATIONALE

    (A) Universal Precautions do not always apply to certain body fluids. Body fluids such as feces, nasal secretion, saliva, sputum, and sweat do not require the use of personal protective equipment unless they are visibly contaminated with blood. (B) Universal Precautions do not apply to saliva except in dental settings. (C) Universal Precautions do not apply to feces unless they are contaminated with visible blood. (D) Universal Precautions apply to blood, amniotic fluids, pericardial fluid, peritoneal fluid, pleural fluid, synovial fluid, cerebrospinal fluid, semen, vaginal secretions, and any body fluid visibly contaminated with blood.

83. **(A)** Nursing process phase: planning; client need: prevention and early detection of disease; content area: maternity nursing.

    RATIONALE

    (A) Involving the client in developing menus that incorporate her food preferences will result in better adherence to a nutritional plan. (B) Weight gain is important in pregnancy, but the nutrient value of the calories ingested is even more important. (C) Dietary sources of nutrients are preferable to supplements because they are absorbed better. In addition, many times foods have other beneficial nutrients that are not contained in vitamin and mineral supplements. (D) It is unrealistic to expect elimination of all snack foods. This goal will almost ensure nonadherence to a nutritional plan.

84. **(C)** Nursing process phase: planning; client need: coping and adaptation; content area: maternity nursing.

    RATIONALE

    (A) Perceptions of the childbirth process do not impact parenting abilities. (B) These are not unrealistic expectations. (C) Ambivalence is manifested by mixed emotions about the impact of an event on one's life. This father feels he "should" be present for the birth but is uncertain about the process. Ambivalent feelings are common during pregnancy and childbirth for both mother and father. (D) Factors that interfere with family function are low socioeconomic status, inadequate family support, the birth of a child with special needs, unhealthy habits, and the inability to make mature decisions.

85. **(C)** Nursing process phase: implementation; client need: basic care and comfort; content area: maternity nursing.

    RATIONALE

    (A) Effleurage is massage of the abdomen performed during contractions. Light-pressure effleurage stimulates small-diameter nerve fibers and may actually increase pain. (B) Massage of the shoulders may help women relax that area; however, this pain is in the lower back. (C) Firm sacral pressure is effective when a woman is experiencing most of the contraction pain in her back. This technique can be combined with thermal stimulation to increase effectiveness. (D) Patterned paced breathing is used when slow-paced and modified-paced breathing are no longer effective. It is commonly used during transition (8–10 cm dilatation).

86. **(B)** Nursing process phase: implementation; client need: prevention and early detection of disease; content area: maternity nursing.

    RATIONALE

    (A) The bladder should be emptied frequently to prevent urine stasis and growth of bacteria. (B) Emptying the bladder before and after intercourse helps wash out any microorganisms that may be introduced onto the urinary meatus and urethra. (C) Cranberry juice does not acidify the urine; it prevents adherence of bacteria to the bladder wall. (D) Ingestion of live-culture yogurt helps prevent vaginal yeast infections, not bladder infections.

87. **(D)** Nursing process phase: implementation; client need: physiological adaptation; content area: maternity nursing.

    RATIONALE

    (A) This client is hyperventilating during an extremely difficult period of labor. The maternal focus is inward. Deep breathing will not reverse the effects of hyperventilation rapidly enough to reverse the respiratory alkalosis this client is developing. (B) The client has already blown off too much carbon dioxide. (C) A position change to lateral is done to increase uteroplacental oxygenation. The fetus is not in distress. (D) Rapid, deep respirations cause the laboring woman to lose carbon dioxide during exhalation, producing respiratory alkalosis. Rebreathing exhaled carbon dioxide in the paper bag will help reverse this condition.

88. **(C)** Nursing process phase: implementation; client need: prevention and early detection of disease; content area: maternity nursing.

    RATIONALE

    (A) Slowed peristalsis can cause vomiting during labor and a higher risk for aspiration of gastric contents. It does not affect fetal descent. (B) The uterine muscle shortens during labor contractions. This results in decreased uterine size, which facilitates fetal descent. (C) A full urinary bladder inhibits fetal descent because it occupies space in the pelvic cavity. (D) Ruptured membranes decrease the duration of labor by an average of 30 minutes.

89. **(D)** Nursing process phase: planning; client need: management of care; content area: maternity nursing.

    RATIONALE

    (A) Auscultation of an FHR of <100 does not indicate operative delivery. If fetal bradycardia is verified, then noninvasive measures should be attempted first and their effectiveness evaluated. (B) Internal fetal monitoring is an invasive procedure that requires rupture of membranes. In the absence of verified fetal bradycardia, this intervention is not warranted. (C) Fetal bradycardia should be verified before any other action is taken. (D) The fetoscope may be placed over the placental or uterine blood vessels and may reflect the maternal pulse rather than fetal bradycardia.

90. **(D)** Nursing process phase: planning; client need: psychosocial adaptation; content area: maternity nursing.

    RATIONALE

    (A) Postpartum depression is characterized by the woman showing less interest in her surroundings and a loss of the usual emotional responses toward her family. She is unable to feel pleasure in her new baby and often has strong feelings of guilt and shame.

(B) Postpartum psychosis is characterized by tearfulness, guilt feelings, sleep and appetite disturbances, and thoughts of harming the infant or self. **(C)** There is no evidence that this client has low self-esteem or is feeling unable to care for both of her children. **(D)** Sibling rivalry is characterized by the older child experiencing feelings of jealously and fear that she will be replaced in the parent's affections by the newcomer. Parental reassurance of love and time spent alone with the older child can help her to cope with these feelings.

91. **(D)** Nursing process phase: implementation; client need: growth and development through the life span; content area: maternity nursing.

    RATIONALE

    (A) Infants' noses are made so that they can breathe while nursing. Depressing breast tissue at the nose can pull the nipple and areola out of the correct position in the infant's mouth. **(B)** Using the scissors position of the fingers can prevent the infant from taking in enough of the areola for effective breastfeeding. **(C)** The lactiferous ducts are found underneath the areola. Proper latch-on includes the nipple and as much of the areola as can be gotten into the infant's mouth. **(D)** Positioning the infant at nipple level prevents nipple trauma. Keeping the body of the infant in a straight line with the head allows the infant to swallow while nursing.

92. **(B)** Nursing process phase: evaluation; client need: growth and development through the life span; content area: maternity nursing.

    RATIONALE

    (A) The back seat is the safest place in a car. The car seat should face the back of the car until the infant weighs at least 20 lb. **(B)** Backpacks should be used only for infants old enough to hold their heads up alone. **(C)** An infant may chew the crib during teething. Lead paint causes brain damage. **(D)** SIDS is associated with the prone position in young infants.

93. **(B)** Nursing process phase: implementation; client need: coping and adaptation; content area: maternity nursing.

    RATIONALE

    (A) A pregnant adolescent must decide what course of action she is going to take. Putting up a child for adoption can be a painful process. Making a decision earlier in the pregnancy allows painful feelings to be resolved before the birth of the baby. **(B)** The autonomous decision by an adolescent to give up her baby for adoption can be considered an important step toward maturity. **(C)** Adolescents who place their infants for adoption because of external pressure frequently feel anger at those who placed the pressure on them. **(D)** The choice of adoption leaves the adolescent with mixed messages from society regarding her pregnancy. She needs affirmation that this decision is a significant event and help in dealing with her feelings.

94. **(B)** Nursing process phase: data collection; client need: management of care; content area: maternity nursing.

    RATIONALE

    (A) These are the findings of transition, which is cervical dilatation from 8–10 cm. Delivery will take place in approximately 2 hours. **(B)** Pressure of the presenting part as it progresses through the birth stimulates the sensation of needing to have a bowel movement. A vaginal examination needs to be done stat as delivery may occur very quickly. **(C)** Contractions can increase in frequency and intensity without much change in the cervix. A judgment about delivery cannot be made from this information. **(D)** Vomiting and a sense of "having enough" are signs of transition.

95. **(D)** Nursing process phase: data collection; client need: prevention and early detection of disease; content area: maternity nursing.

    RATIONALE

    (A) A pulse rate up to 120 and palpitations are normal side effects of terbutaline. **(B)** This output exceeds the intake, which decreases the risk of fluid overload. **(C)** Pedal edema is not uncommon in pregnant women; 3+ edema could indicate PIH, not pulmonary edema. **(D)** Fluid overload would result in pulmonary edema. The lower bases of the lungs are the first to fill with fluid.

96. **(D)** Nursing process phase: implementation; client need: growth and development through the life span; content area: maternity nursing.

    RATIONALE

    (A) Visual and auditory stimulation should not be presented to the infant at the same time. Drug-exposed infants are easily stressed. **(B)** Wind-up swings make a clicking noise and also stimulate the visual system. **(C)** Rattles provide both visual and auditory stimulation. **(D)** Drug-exposed infants need physical contact and soft auditory stimulation.

97. **(A)** Nursing process phase: data collection; client need: growth and development through the life span; content area: maternity nursing.

    RATIONALE

    (A) Hypertonicity and poor coordination of the suck-and-swallow reflex are characteristic of the narcotic-exposed infant. Seizures may also be present. **(B)** These are the typical features of the infant with fetal alcohol syndrome. **(C)** These are the typical features of the tobacco-exposed newborn. **(D)** These are the typical features of the infant with Down's syndrome.

98. **(D)** Nursing process phase: implementation; client need: prevention and early detection of disease; content area: maternity nursing.

    RATIONALE

    (A) Many women fear that disclosure of abuse will result in their being told that they must leave their partners to receive treatment. Pregnant women or those with a newborn are least likely to leave a relationship. **(B)** One in three women is a victim of partner abuse regardless of socioeconomic status. **(C)** The client does not have a psychiatric problem. Sensitivity, acceptance, and guidance on where she can receive help when ready are needed. **(D)** The most significant intervention for partner abuse is being asked about being hurt or frightened by a partner. Studies show that victims of partner abuse frequently go to a health-care provider with obvious injuries and wait for the provider to ask about their injuries because they are too ashamed to volunteer the information.

99. **(D)** Nursing process phase: data collection; client need: reduction of risk potential; content area: maternity nursing.

    RATIONALE

    (A) Decreased fundal height is associated with "lightening" or engagement of the fetal presenting part in the pelvis. **(B)** Abruptio placentae is the separation of the placenta from the uterine wall. If the separation is in the middle of the placenta, bleeding is concealed. **(C)** Fetal tachycardia can occur with tocolysis or maternal infection. **(D)** Painless, bright red vaginal bleeding is symptomatic of placenta previa.

100. **(D)** Nursing process phase: evaluation; client need: growth and development through the life span; content area: maternity nursing.

    RATIONALE

    (A) Breast milk contains the amino acid phenylalanine, which cannot be metabolized by the infant with PKU. Moderate to high levels of phenylalanine can result in mental retardation. **(B)** Formula is modified cow's milk, which contains phenylalanine. **(C)** Soy milk contains phenylalanine. **(D)** PKU is treated with a special low-phenylalanine diet. A special formula is used for infants.

CHAPTER 4

Pediatric Nursing: Content Review and Test

Susan I. Ray, RN, MS

The Ill or Hospitalized Child

Nursing Care of the Ill Child

Meaning of Illness to Child

I. Infant
   A. Change in familiar routine and own bedroom
   B. Separation from favorite toy or blanket
II. Toddler
   A. Fear of separation, being left alone; separation anxiety highest in this age group
   B. Blames self for illness
III. Preschool
   A. Fear of being hurt or fear of mutilation
   B. Afraid of pain and bleeding
   C. Separation anxiety less than for toddler
   D. Often considers illness punishment for wrongdoing
IV. School-age
   A. Fear of physical nature of illness
   B. Concern regarding separation from peers and ability to maintain position in group
   C. Thinks there is an external cause for illness, although located in body
V. Adolescent
   A. Anxiety regarding loss of independence, control, identity
   B. Concern about privacy
   C. Able to explain illness

Response to Separation

I. Greatest impact between ages 1 and 3 years
II. Three phases identified:
   A. Protest: cries for parents; refuses attention of anyone else
   B. Despair: ceases crying; shows evidence of depression; "settles in"
   C. Detachment (denial): superficially appears to adjust; ignores parent in effort to escape emotional pain

Signs and Symptoms of Separation Anxiety

I. Protest: lasts from hours to days
   A. Cries and screams
   B. Searches with eyes for parent
   C. Clings to parent when present
   D. Avoids and rejects contact with strangers
   E. Verbally and physically attacks strangers
   F. Attempts to physically prevent parent from leaving
II. Despair: length of time variable
   A. Inactive
   B. Withdrawn
   C. Depressed, sad
   D. Uninterested in environment
   E. Noncommunicative
   F. Regresses to earlier behaviors (e.g., thumbsucking, bedwetting, use of bottle)
   G. Often refuses to eat
III. Detachment: rarely seen
   A. Shows increased interest in surroundings
   B. Interacts with strangers or familiar caregivers
   C. Forms new but superficial relationships
   D. Appears happy
   E. Shows only passive or superficial interest in parents

Response to Pain

I. Young infant (0–1 years old)
   A. Generalized body response: sometimes local reflex withdrawal on stimulation

B. Movements may be increased: squirming, jerking, and flailing
C. Crying becoming more intense
D. Facial expression reflecting pain
E. Skin changes: pale or flushed
F. Vital sign (VS) fluctuations
G. Irregular eating and sleeping patterns

II. Older infant or toddler (1–3 years old)
A. Localized body response: deliberate withdrawal on stimulation
B. Loud crying
C. Facial expression reflects pain
D. Physical resistance; attempt to push stimulus away when applied

III. Young child or preschooler (3–6 years old)
A. Loud crying, screaming
B. Verbal expressions
C. Thrashing of extremities
D. Physical resistance before and during application of stimulus
E. Requires physical restraint for painful procedures
F. Clings to parent; solicits emotional support
G. Restless and irritable with continuing pain
H. May see these behaviors if child anticipates painful experience

IV. School-age child (6–11 years old)
A. Same behaviors observed in young child
B. Stalling behavior in anticipation of painful procedure
C. Muscular rigidity in anticipation

V. Adolescent (12–18 years old)
A. Less vocal protest and motor activity
B. More verbal complaints such as "It hurts"
C. Increased muscle tension and body control

Fear and Anxiety Reduction

Reducing Response of Fear from Separation, Anxiety, and Pain

I. Infants
A. Promote interaction between infant and primary caregiver.
B. Role-model comfort activities such as cuddling and talking to infant.
C. Provide appropriate activities and toys for age, such as swing, bath toys, mobiles.
D. Be calm and gentle during procedures.
E. Allow caregivers time to comfort infant after procedure.
F. Provide consistent staff.
G. Avoid performing procedures in crib.

II. Toddler
A. Promote visitation from primary caregiver.
B. Provide consistent staff.
C. Play games of disappearance such as hide-and-seek, peek-a-boo.
D. Encourage parents to bring items from home, such as toy, blanket, pictures, and tape recording of bedtime story.
E. Discourage parental departure when child is asleep.
F. Comfort and cuddle child when crying.

G. Continue home habits such as bottle, pacifier, potty chair if trained, diapers if not.
H. Explain unpleasant procedures to child just before procedure. Be honest.
I. Provide distraction: blowing bubbles, kaleidoscope, and pop-up toys.
J. Allow child to play with hospital supplies and equipment that are safe for age: bandages, tongue blade, and stethoscope.
K. Avoid performing painful procedures in crib or bed.

III. Preschool child
A. Prepare child for hospitalization.
B. Reassure child that he or she is not responsible for the hospitalization.
C. When parents or primary caregivers leave, they should relate their return to time frame the child can understand, such as breakfast, lunch, dinner, bedtime. Do not give false return times.
D. Prepare child for procedures by explaining or illustrating the body part that will be involved and what the part will look like after the procedure.
E. Answer child's questions in age-appropriate terms.
F. Allow child to play with hospital supplies and equipment that are safe for age.

IV. School-age child
A. Encourage parents or primary caregiver to avoid extended absences from hospitalized child.
B. Allow child to talk and ask questions. Listen and respond to questions.
C. Promote play through competitive table games.
D. Be familiar with child's home routine and incorporate it into hospital routine as much as possible.
E. Provide positive reinforcement for behavior. Avoid negative feedback.
F. Encourage continuation of school work if child's condition permits.
G. Provide a familiar face (consistent nurse) during procedures when possible.
H. Allow children to express feelings regarding procedure through drawing and talking, or acting-out procedure with doll or stuffed animal.

V. Adolescent
A. Allow adolescent to participate in decisions related to treatment and care. Give information on the rules and policies of the hospital unit.
B. Promote support and visitation from peers and family.
C. Promote positive perception of illness.
D. Explain procedures and what can be expected after a procedure. Allow a question-and-answer period. Be honest.
E. Provide privacy as much as possible.

Nursing Care of the Hospitalized Child

Data Collection

I. Assist in obtaining health history and history of hospitalization.
II. Assist with diagnostic procedures.

Planning

I. Safe, effective care environment
  A. Reduce or eliminate environmental hazards.
  B. Transport, restrain, and position child safely.
  C. Ensure safety during procedures, including surgery.
II. Physiological integrity
  A. Carry out procedures with minimum distress to child.
  B. Prevent or minimize bodily injury or pain or both.
III. Psychosocial integrity
  A. Prevent or minimize effects of separation.
  B. Support and educate child and family.
  C. Help child to maintain control.
  D. Prepare child and family for procedures, surgery as needed.
  E. Use play as diversion and for stress reduction.
IV. Health promotion and maintenance
  A. Promote optimum health.
  B. Promote nutrition and hydration.
  C. Prepare family for home care.

Implementation

I. Keep harmful items out of reach of child.
II. Keep siderails up for infants and young children.
III. Allow freedom on unit within defined and enforced limits.
IV. Restrain child if necessary for safety, but limit use of restraints.
V. Explain hospital routines, items, procedures, and events in language appropriate for child's age.
VI. Use terms familiar to the child (e.g., those for bodily functions).
VII. Maintain a routine similar to that of child at home whenever possible.
VIII. Provide consistency of personnel as much as possible.
IX. Promote family interaction; encourage child and family contact and rooming-in whenever possible.
X. Allow parents to participate in care.
XI. Maintain contact with family: talk to child about home.
XII. Allow sibling visitation if possible.
XIII. Provide an atmosphere that allows free expression of feelings.
XIV. Allow child choices whenever possible.
XV. Explain procedures to the child, what child will experience, and what he or she can do to help: explain at the child's level of understanding; relate unfamiliar things and events to those familiar to the child; clarify terms; explain just before performing procedure.
XVI. Convey an attitude of confidence and indicate that cooperation is expected.
XVII. Allow child to see and handle strange and potentially frightening items, if possible.
XVIII. Be honest with child.
XIX. Be consistent in behaviors toward child.
XX. Communicate disapproval of undesired behavior—not disapproval of child.
XXI. Accept regressive behaviors.
XXII. Praise child for cooperation.
XXIII. Allow ample time for play.
XXIV. Encourage play activities and diversions appropriate to child's age, condition, and interests.
XXV. Use play as a way of explaining procedures.
XXVI. Encourage interaction with other children, when appropriate.
XXVII. Help family support child and refer to agencies providing family support.
XXVIII. Use services as available in neighborhood or region (e.g., Cystic Fibrosis Foundation, Easter Seals, Spina Bifida Association, American Cancer Society).
XXIX. Refer for home health nursing as indicated with discharge planning.

Evaluation

I. Child has consistent caregivers.
II. Child exhibits no evidence of discomfort.
III. Child verbalizes or plays out feelings and concerns.
IV. Child discusses home and family.
V. Child exhibits an understanding of information presented.
VI. Child cooperates in care and participates in care activities.
VII. Parents visit frequently or constantly.
VIII. Parents cooperate in care.
IX. Family demonstrates an understanding of child's behavior and becomes familiar with therapies.
X. Family demonstrates the ability to provide home care.
XI. Family demonstrates an understanding of the child's behavior.
XII. Family uses community resources appropriately.

Nursing Care of the Chronically Ill or Disabled Child

Data Collection

I. Observe for signs of suspected or determined diagnosis.
II. Assist with diagnostic procedures.
III. Be alert for evidence of overprotection or neglect.
IV. Determine family routines and abilities related to special care needs at home.

Planning

See also Nursing Care of the Ill Child.
I. Safe, effective care environment
  A. Promote safe environment according to needs of individual child.
II. Physiological integrity
  A. Follow plan of care.
  B. Prevent complications.
III. Psychosocial integrity
  A. Teach child and family as needed.
  B. Prepare child and family for procedures, surgery as needed.
IV. Health promotion and maintenance
  A. Promote optimum health.
  B. Prepare family for home care.

Implementation

I. Support child and family at time of diagnosis.
  A. Project an attitude that shows acceptance of child and family.

B. Allow expression of feelings and concerns.
II. Explain or reinforce explanation of condition or disease and treatment.
III. Help family develop a thorough plan of care.
IV. Encourage participation in care of hospitalized child.
V. Be available to family as listener or a resource.
VI. Encourage social activity for both child and family.
VII. Emphasize child's abilities.
VIII. Assist with improving appearance and grooming.
IX. Encourage self-care appropriate to capabilities and as much independence as condition allows.
X. Teach family skills and procedures needed for home care.
XI. Encourage sibling participation when possible.

Evaluation

I. Child exhibits no evidence of overprotection or neglect.
II. Child appears clean, well groomed, and attractively dressed.
III. Child and family (when appropriate) demonstrate an understanding of the disease or condition and the ability to provide home care.
IV. Child and family verbalize feelings and concerns.
V. Child and family develop realistic short- and long-term plans.
VI. Child and family comply with plan of care.
VII. Family displays an attitude of confidence in ability to cope.

Newborn Disorders

The Preterm Infant

Description

Infant born before completion of 37 weeks' gestation, regardless of birth weight.
I. Low-birth-weight infant: infant whose birth weight is <2500 gm regardless of gestational age
II. Very-low-birth-weight infant: infant whose birth weight is <1500 gm.
III. Small-for-date or small-for-gestational-age infant: infant whose rate of intrauterine growth was slowed and who was delivered at or later than term; the infant's birth weight falls below the 10th percentile on intrauterine growth curves
IV. Intrauterine growth retardation: infant whose prenatal growth is retarded or below 10th percentile on standardized growth curves

Pathophysiology

I. Factors related to prematurity (more than one often involved)
A. Multiple pregnancies
B. Maternal disease
C. Heavy smoking
D. Poor maternal nutrition
E. Teenage pregnancy
F. Illegal drug use or abuse

G. Low income or socioeconomic status
II. Intensive care nursery necessary

Signs and Symptoms

I. Very small, wrinkled
II. Skin: red to pink with visible veins
III. Fine, feathery hair; lanugo on back and face
IV. Little or no evidence of fat
V. Head large in relation to body
VI. Limbs extended
VII. Lax, easily manipulated joints
VIII. Absent, weak, or ineffectual grasping, sucking, and swallowing reflexes
IX. Inability to maintain body temperature
X. Small thorax
XI. Breathing irregular
XII. Vernix caseosa after 24 weeks of gestation
XIII. Bottom of feet smooth: absence of creases
XIV. Undescended testes in male infant

Therapeutic Management

I. Determination by status of infant, especially in relation to:
A. Respiratory support
B. Body temperature regulation
C. Ability to suck
D. Susceptibility to infection
E. Activity intolerance
II. Prevention of complications

Nursing Care

DATA COLLECTION

I. Perform routine newborn assessment.
II. Assist with diagnostic procedures.
III. Perform ongoing systematic assessment of functioning:
A. Weigh twice daily.
B. Provide respiratory assessment:
1. Rate and regularity
2. Presence of retractions, nasal flaring
3. Breath sounds, secretions
C. Assess cardiovascular system:
1. Heart rate, rhythm
2. Heart sounds, including suspected murmurs
D. Make gastrointestinal (GI) assessment:
1. Feeding behavior
2. Regurgitation or emesis
3. Stool patterns: color, amount, odor, consistency
4. Abdominal distention
5. Bowel sounds
E. Make genitourinary assessment:
1. Abnormalities, if any
2. Urinary output: amount, color, consistency
3. Hydration
F. Assess neurological and musculoskeletal systems:
1. Movements: random, jittery, twitching, spontaneous, elicited
2. Position at rest
3. Changes in head circumference
4. Reflexes: level of response

G. Assess temperature:
   1. Axillary
   2. Rectal
H. Assess skin:
   1. Color: cyanosis or jaundice
   2. Discolored areas
   3. Texture, turgor, characteristics (dry, flaky, peeling)
   4. Skin lesion, rash

PLANNING

I. Safe, effective care environment
   A. See Hospital Care of the Newborn Infant under Postpartal Care in Chapter 3.
   B. Provide external warmth.
   C. Protect from infection.
II. Physiological integrity
   A. Facilitate respiratory efforts.
   B. Conserve energy.
   C. Prevent complications.
III. Psychosocial integrity
   A. Promote parent-infant relationships.
   B. Support and educate family.
   C. Prepare family for procedures.
IV. Health promotion and maintenance
   A. Promote optimum health.
   B. Achieve and maintain optimum hydration and nutrition.
   C. Prepare family for home care.

IMPLEMENTATION

I. Position for maximum respiration: head of crib slightly elevated.
II. Provide supplemental oxygen.
III. Provide external warmth according to infant's condition and tolerance:
   A. Keep well wrapped if placed in open crib.
   B. Use Isolette.
   C. Use overhead warming unit.
   D. Position away from windows or drafts to prevent heat loss.
   E. Provide humidified atmosphere to reduce evaporative heat loss.
   F. Provide infant with knitted cap.
IV. Reduce energy expenditure.
   A. Ease respiratory effort.
   B. Maintain neutral thermal environment.
   C. Implement gavage feeding if infant becomes tired with conventional feeding methods to promote growth and conserve energy.
   D. Organize nursing activities and assessments to minimize disturbance.
   E. Promote rest: reduce environmental distractions (e.g., dim lights or cover crib with blanket, eliminate or reduce noise).
V. Implement institutional policies to prevent spread of infection; teach precautions to family.
VI. Provide nutrition:
   A. Nipple-feed with soft nipple that supplies nourishment without exertion (expressed mother's milk, banked breast milk, special formula).
   B. Assist with breastfeeding (with families who indicate desire).
   C. Gavage-feed.
VII. Prevent skin breakdown.
   A. Clean with clear water or mild, nonalkaline cleanser two to three times a week.
   B. Avoid damage to delicate skin (e.g., removing tape, careful use of scissors for removal of bandages).
   C. Change position of infant every 1–2 hours.
VIII. Encourage family to become involved in infant's care.
IX. Teach family skills needed for home care.

EVALUATION

I. Infant's breathing is regular, unlabored, and within normal limits.
II. Infant's temperature remains within desirable limits (97.7°F [36.5°C]).
III. Infant exhibits no evidence of dehydration.
IV. Infant consumes appropriate amount of nourishment without difficulty.
V. Infant exhibits a steady weight gain.
VI. Infant remains free of complications.
VII. Infant responds to appropriate stimuli.
VIII. Family becomes involved in infant's care.
IX. Family demonstrates an understanding of the condition and the ability to provide home care.

Hyperbilirubinemia

Description

Hyperbilirubinemia is excessive accumulation of bilirubin in the blood.

Classification

I. Pathological
   A. Before 24 hours of age
   B. With Rh-negative mother
II. Physiological
   A. After 24 hours of age
   B. With a bilirubin level of <12.0 normal (reference value) for full-term infant 2–5 days old; preterm level <16.0

Pathophysiology

I. Breakdown of red blood cells (RBCs)
II. Increased levels of bilirubin in the blood
III. Associated with breastfeeding
   A. Cause: unknown
   B. Early: 3–4 days of age
   C. Late: 4–5 days of age

Signs and Symptoms

I. Jaundice: yellowish discoloration of skin
   A. Bright yellow or orange
   B. Greenish, muddy yellow

Therapeutic Management

I. Observe closely for increase in jaundice.
II. Remove excess bilirubin.

A. Phototherapy to alter bilirubin into a more soluble form
B. Exchange transfusion
C. Prevention of blood incompatibility by administration of Rh_0 immune globulin to all unsensitized Rh-negative mothers after delivery

Nursing Care

DATA COLLECTION

I. Perform routine assessment.
II. Assist with diagnostic procedures: serum bilirubin levels, Coombs' test (infants of Rh-negative mothers).

PLANNING

I. Safe, effective care environment (see Hospital Care of the Newborn Infant under Postpartal Care in Chap. 3)
II. Physiological integrity
    A. Assist with measures to reduce serum bilirubin levels.
    B. Prevent complications from therapy.
III. Psychosocial integrity
    A. Support and educate family.
    B. Prevent complications.
IV. Health promotion and maintenance
    A. Promote optimum health.
    B. Prepare family for home care.

IMPLEMENTATION

I. Explain or reinforce explanation of condition and therapies.
II. Place infant under fluorescent light.
III. Turn frequently to expose all body surface areas to light.
IV. Shield infant's eyes with opaque mask of proper size.
    A. Close eyes before application.
    B. Position to prevent occlusion of nares.
    C. Assess several times per day for evidence of discharge, excessive pressures on lids, corneal irritation.
V. Avoid oily lubricants or lotions on skin.
VI. Promote adequate fluid intake.
VII. Observe for evidence of dehydration and drying skin.
VIII. Assist with exchange transfusion.
    A. Use sterile technique.
    B. Assist with procedure.
    C. Keep accurate records of blood volumes exchanged.
    D. Monitor infant's condition: VSs, temperature.

EVALUATION

I. Infant exhibits no evidence of jaundice.
II. Infant's serum bilirubin is within normal limits.
III. Infant remains well hydrated and free of complications.
IV. Family demonstrates an understanding of the condition.
V. Family demonstrates the ability to care for child.

Respiratory Distress Syndrome (Hyaline Membrane Disease)

Description

Respiratory distress syndrome is a dysfunction in newborns, primarily related to developmental delay in lung maturation.

Pathophysiology

I. Decreased surfactant production
II. Diminished oxygen to tissues and inability to excrete excess carbon dioxide
III. With each breath, increased energy expenditure to re-inflate
IV. Decreased lung expansion, with fewer inflated alveoli

Signs and Symptoms

I. Dyspnea
II. Tachypnea (up to 80–120 breaths/min)
III. Pronounced retractions
IV. Audible expiratory grunt
V. Flaring of external nares
VI. Cyanosis

Therapeutic Management

I. Provide oxygen.
    A. Increased oxygen concentration provided in Isolette or by oxygen hood
    B. Assisted ventilation instituted: continuous positive airway pressure (CPAP)
II. Maintain acid-base status.
III. Maintain thermal environment to conserve energy and oxygen use.
IV. Conserve energy by minimal handling and use of gavage feeding.

Nursing Care

DATA COLLECTION

I. Perform routine assessment of premature infant.
II. Perform thorough respiratory assessment.
    A. Determine respiratory rate and regularity.
    B. Describe retractions and nasal flaring.
    C. Describe breath sounds: wet diminished sounds, areas of absence of sound, grunting.
    D. Describe secretions.
    E. Determine whether suctioning is needed.
    F. Describe cry.
    G. Describe oxygen and method of delivery; if infant is intubated, describe size of tube, type of ventilator, and settings.
III. Assist with diagnostic procedures: x-ray, blood gas measurements.

PLANNING

I. Safe, effective care environment
    A. Protect from injury and infection.
    B. Provide warmth.
II. Physiological integrity
    A. Promote respiratory effort.
    B. Conserve energy.
    C. Prepare family for procedures.
III. Psychosocial integrity
    A. See Hospital Care of the Newborn Infant under Postpartal Care in Chapter 3.
    B. Support and educate family.
    C. Prepare family for procedures.

IV. Health promotion and maintenance
  A. Promote optimum health.
  B. Achieve and maintain optimum hydration and nutrition.
  C. Prepare family for home care.

IMPLEMENTATION

  I. Place infant in Isolette or crib with overhead warmer.
  II. Maintain a thermal environment.
  III. Maintain oxygen as prescribed.
  IV. Remove secretions from airway as needed.
  V. Monitor oxygen administration, including ventilator if used.
  VI. Provide nutrition by one of the following:
    A. Gavage-feed to conserve energy and provide sufficient calories.
    B. Nipple-feed with soft nipple, allowing sufficient time for rest.
  VII. Employ careful skin care to prevent breakdown or injury.
  VIII. Teach family skills needed for home care.

EVALUATION

  I. Infant breathes without effort.
  II. Infant maintains optimum blood gas measurements without ventilatory assistance.
  III. Infant remains free of complications.
  IV. Family demonstrates an understanding of the condition and the ability to provide home care.

Neonatal Sepsis (Septicemia)

Description

Neonatal sepsis is generalized bacterial disease in the bloodstream.

Pathophysiology

  I. Acquired
  II. Prenatal: infected amniotic fluid, across placenta from maternal bloodstream
  III. Birth: contact with maternal tissues
  IV. Postnatal: cross-contamination from other infants, personnel, or objects in environment
  V. Occurs more frequently in high-risk infants: preterm infants and those born after a difficult or traumatic delivery

Signs and Symptoms

  I. Respiratory distress
    A. Apnea
    B. Irregular, grunting respirations
    C. Retractions
  II. Gastric distress
    A. Vomiting
    B. Diarrhea
    C. Abdominal distention
    D. Absent stools (from paralytic ileus)
    E. Poor sucking and feeding

  III. Skin manifestations
    A. Cyanosis
    B. Pallor
    C. Jaundice
  IV. Central nervous system (CNS) involvement
    A. Irritability
    B. Apathy
    C. Seizures
  V. Temperature instability

Therapeutic Management

  I. Administration of antibiotics
  II. Oxygen administration
  III. Careful regulation of fluid and electrolytes

Nursing Care

DATA COLLECTION

  I. Perform routine physical assessment.
  II. Assist with diagnostic procedures: cultures of blood, spinal fluid, urine, stool, and any skin lesion examinations.
  III. Observe for side effects of antibiotics.

PLANNING

  I. Safe, effective care environment
    A. See Hospital Care of the Newborn Infant under Postpartal Care in Chapter 3.
    B. Prevent spread of infection.
  II. Physiological integrity
    A. Help to eradicate organisms.
    B. Prevent complications.
  III. Psychosocial integrity
    A. Support family.
  IV. Health promotion and maintenance
    A. Promote optimum health.
    B. Achieve and maintain optimum hydration and nutrition.

IMPLEMENTATION

  I. Provide external warmth (see Nursing Care under The Preterm Infant).
  II. Reduce energy expenditure (see Nursing Care under The Preterm Infant).
  III. Maintain and implement institutional policies to prevent spread of infection.
  IV. Monitor intravenous (IV) infusion.
  V. Administer antibiotics as prescribed.
  VI. Explain or reinforce explanation of condition and therapies.
  VII. Teach family skills needed for home care.

EVALUATION

  I. Infant exhibits no evidence of infection.
  II. Infant remains free of complications.
  III. Family demonstrates an understanding of the condition and the ability to provide home care.

Respiratory Disorders

Croup (Laryngotracheobronchitis)

Description

Croup is an inflammation of the larynx, trachea, and bronchi.

Pathophysiology

I. Narrowing of the air passages produced by edema of respiratory mucosa, causing variable degrees of airway obstruction
II. Condition usually follows 1–3-day cold
III. Most common in children aged 3 months to 3 years
IV. Usually viral in origin.

Signs and Symptoms

I. Restlessness
II. Hoarseness
III. "Brassy" or "barking" cough
IV. Inspiratory stridor
V. Respiratory distress
VI. Fever: low grade
VII. Condition usually occurs suddenly during night

Therapeutic Management

I. Mild disease; can be treated at home
  A. Careful observation for symptoms of respiratory obstruction
  B. Bedrest
  C. Cool, humidified environment
  D. Encouragement of fluid intake
  E. Temperature reduction (if elevated)
II. Severe disease; hospitalization
  A. As previously listed
  B. High-humidity environment
  C. Oxygen
  D. IV fluids
  E. Corticosteroid therapy
  F. Epinephrine for transient relief
  G. Availability of endotracheal intubation equipment

Nursing Care

DATA COLLECTION

I. Perform routine physical assessment.
II. Perform in-depth assessment for:
  A. Rate, depth, and rhythm of respirations
  B. Presence of flaring nares, grunting, and retractions
  C. Pallor, cyanosis
  D. Dyspnea
  E. Stridor
  F. Type, frequency, and intensity of cough
  G. Sputum
  H. Oxygen saturation
III. Assist with diagnostic procedures: chest x-ray, serum electrolytes, blood gas measurements, pH.

PLANNING

I. Safe, effective care environment
  A. See Nursing Care of the Ill Child.
  B. Prevent spread of infection.
II. Physiological integrity
  A. Assist respiratory efforts.
  B. Promote rest.
  C. Promote comfort.
  D. Reduce temperature (for significant elevation).
III. Psychosocial integrity
  A. Support child and family.
IV. Health promotion and maintenance
  A. Prevent dehydration.
  B. Provide nourishment.
  C. Prevent complications.
  D. Prepare family for home care.

IMPLEMENTATION

I. Administer humidified oxygen as prescribed (mist tent, nasal).
II. Position for optimum breathing, with head of bed elevated.
III. Monitor respiratory status regularly.
IV. Administer nose drops and suction nasal passages to facilitate breathing.
V. Administer medication as prescribed.
VI. Support child and family (see Nursing Care of the Ill Child or Nursing Care of the Hospitalized Child).
VII. Encourage presence of family.
VIII. Provide constant attendance during acute illness.
IX. Encourage intake of cool fluids such as fruit juices, soft drinks, and gelatin.
X. Monitor parenteral fluid administration, if prescribed.
XI. Have emergency endotracheal or tracheostomy equipment available.
XII. Implement measures to prevent spread of infection to others.
XIII. Administer antibiotics as prescribed.
XIV. Administer chest physiotherapy, if prescribed.
XV. Teach family procedures needed for home care, including expected results of medication and their possible side effects.

EVALUATION

I. Child remains free of respiratory distress.
II. Child rests comfortably and plays quietly.
III. Child demonstrates adequate nutrition.
IV. Child and family comply with therapeutic regimen.

Epiglottitis

Description

Epiglottitis is an inflammation of the glottitis.

Pathophysiology

I. Edema of tissues above the vocal cords (supraglottic swelling)
II. Narrowing of airway inlet that can result in total obstruction

III. Usually caused by *Haemophilus influenzae* type B
IV. Most common in children 2–5 years old
V. Possible precursor: sore throat

Signs and Symptoms

I. Abrupt onset
II. Rapid progression to severe respiratory distress
III. Elevated temperature
IV. Toxic appearance
V. Characteristic posture with client insisting on sitting upright, leaning forward with chin thrust out, mouth open, and tongue protruding
VI. Irritability
VII. Anxious, apprehensive, frightened expression
VIII. Thick, muffled voice and "croaking, froglike" sound on inspiration
IX. Red, inflamed throat with distinctive large, cherry-red edematous epiglottitis (seldom observed except by qualified examiner, as described earlier)
X. Predictive symptoms: absence of spontaneous cough, drooling, and agitation.

Therapeutic Management

I. Throat examined with extreme care, where facilities are available for emergency endotracheal intubation or tracheostomy
II. Antibiotics to eradicate organisms
III. Corticosteroids to reduce edema

Nursing Care

DATA COLLECTION

I. Assessment is same as for laryngotracheobronchitis.
II. Perform routine physical assessment.
III. Collect data for:
   A. Rate, depth, and rhythm of respirations
   B. Presence of flaring nares, grunting, and retractions
   C. Pallor, cyanosis
   D. Dyspnea
   E. Stridor
   F. Type, frequency, and intensity of cough
   G. Sputum
   H. Oxygen saturation
IV. Assist with diagnostic procedures: chest x-ray, serum electrolytes, blood gas measurements, pH.

PLANNING

I. Prevention of respiratory obstruction
II. Safe, effective care environment
   A. See Nursing Care of the Ill Child.
   B. Prevent spread of infection.
III. Physiological integrity
   A. Assist respiratory efforts.
   B. Promote rest.
   C. Promote comfort.
   D. Reduce temperature (significant elevation).
IV. Psychosocial integrity
   A. Support child and family.
V. Health promotion and maintenance
   A. Prevent dehydration.

B. Provide nourishment.
C. Prevent complications.
D. Prepare family for home care.

IMPLEMENTATION

I. Refer to physician immediately.
II. Administer humidified oxygen as prescribed (mist tent, nasal).
III. Position for optimum breathing with head of bed elevated.
IV. Monitor respiratory status regularly.
V. Administer nose drops and suction nasal passages to facilitate breathing.
VI. Administer medication as prescribed.
VII. Support child and family (see Nursing Care of the Ill Child or Nursing Care of the Hospitalized Child).
VIII. Encourage presence of family.
IX. Provide constant attendance during acute illness.
X. Encourage intake of cool fluids such as fruit juices, soft drinks, and gelatin.
XI. Monitor parenteral fluid administration, if prescribed.
XII. Have emergency endotracheal or tracheostomy equipment available.
XIII. Implement measures to prevent spread of infection to others.
XIV. Administer antibiotics and corticosteroids as prescribed.
XV. Administer chest physiotherapy, if prescribed.
XVI. Teach family procedures needed for care, including expected results of medication and their possible side effects.

EVALUATION

I. Child remains free of respiratory distress.
II. Child rests comfortably and plays quietly.
III. Child has adequate nutritional intake.
IV. Child and family comply with therapeutic regimen.

Pneumonia

Description

Inflammation in the lungs resulting in the alveoli becoming filled with exudate. It can be primary illness or secondary to another infection or surgery.

Pathophysiology

Cause of the pneumonia is usually viral in children but can be from bacteria, mycoplasma, or aspiration. Less often caused by histomycosis, coccidioidomycosis, or fungi.

Signs and Symptoms

I. Dry cough, progressing to productive cough.
II. Fever (103–104°F [39.3–40.0°C]).
III. Shallow, rapid respirations.
IV. Sternal retractions and nasal flaring can occur.
V. Listlessness.
VI. Poor appetite.
VII. Preference for positioning on affected side.
VIII. Onset could be sudden or preceded by upper respiratory infection (URI).

Therapeutic Management

I. Chest x-rays to confirm diagnosis.
II. Elevated white blood cell (WBC) count.
III. Cultures from sputum, nose, and throat may be taken.
IV. Bacterial pneumonia is treated with antibiotics.
V. Viral pneumonia treatment is supportive; if respiratory synctial virus is present, may treat with riboviran via inhalation.
VI. Antipyretics for fever.
VII. Oxygen for cyanosis and dyspnea.
VIII. Oxygen administration with cool mist, chest physiotherapy and postural drainage in some cases.

Nursing Care

DATA COLLECTION

I. Perform routine physical assessment.
II. Collect data for:
   A. Rate, depth, and rhythm of respirations.
   B. Presence of nasal flaring, grunting, and retractions.
   C. Pallor, cyanosis.
   D. Dyspnea.
   E. Stridor.
   F. Cough, nonproductive or productive. Note characteristics of productive cough.
   G. Oxygen saturation.
   H. Alertness of child.
   I. Vital signs.
   J. Fluid status.

PLANNING

I. Safe, effective care environment.
   A. Avoid exposure to infectious agents.
   B. Provide environment appropriate for age.
   C. Routine safety precautions with oxygen.
II. Physiological integrity
   A. Relieve symptoms.
   B. Adhere to therapeutic regimen.
III. Psychosocial integrity
   A. Promote growth and development.
   B. Promote family involvement.
IV. Health promotion and maintenance
   A. Maintain optimum health, good nutrition, and adequate rest.
   B. Prepare child and family for home care.
   C. Promote self-care management.

IMPLEMENTATION

I. Position for optimum ventilation.
II. Provide humidified oxygen as prescribed.
III. Antipyretics for fever.
IV. Administer medications as ordered.
V. Assist in chest physiotherapy and postural drainage.
VI. Monitor intake and output (I&O); prevent dehydration through adequate hydration.

EVALUATION

I. Child exhibits normal respiratory rate, rhythm, and quality.
II. Child exhibits appropriate nutritional intake for age.
III. Child and family adhere to prescribed regimen.

Tonsillitis

Description

Tonsillitis is an inflammation of the tonsillar structures in the oropharynx.

Pathophysiology

I. Bacterial or viral invasion of tonsillar tissues with inflammation, swelling, and erythema (sometimes exudate)
II. Usually occurs in association with pharyngitis
III. Tonsillar enlargement, which causes discomfort and difficulty in swallowing

Signs and Symptoms

I. Difficulty swallowing and breathing
II. Nasal, muffled voice
III. Persistent cough common
IV. Condition often associated with otitis media and hearing difficulty
V. Enlargement of tonsils causing discomfort and difficulty in swallowing
VI. Elevated body temperature possible

Therapeutic Management

I. Medical
   A. Symptomatic treatment
   B. Antibiotics (for throat culture positive for group A β-hemolytic streptococcus)
II. Surgical
   A. Tonsillectomy (removal of the palatine tonsils)
   B. Usually with adenoidectomy (removal of adenoids)

Nursing Care (Tonsillectomy)

DATA COLLECTION

I. Preoperatively
   A. Perform routine assessment.
   B. Assist with diagnostic procedures: bleeding and clotting times.
   C. Prepare child in advance for procedure using simple explanation of procedure. Include what child can expect when he or she awakes.
II. Postoperatively
   A. Take pulse and respirations frequently.
   B. Observe for signs of bleeding:
      1. Rapid pulse
      2. Restlessness
      3. Frequent swallowing, clearing of throat
      4. Nausea and vomiting
   C. Inspect throat for evidence of oozing or hemorrhage.
   D. Inspect vomitus for evidence of fresh bleeding.

PLANNING

I. Safe, effective care environment
   A. See Nursing Care of the Ill Child.
II. Physiological integrity
   A. Promote hydration and nutrition.
   B. Relieve discomfort.
   C. Facilitate drainage.

D. Prevent complications.
III. Psychosocial integrity
  A. Support child and family.
IV. Health promotion and maintenance
  A. Prepare family for home care.

IMPLEMENTATION

I. Offer cool fluids and liquid diet when child is fully alert and there is no evidence of bleeding.
II. Apply ice collar.
III. Offer soft diet after 24 hours; then advance to regular diet for age. Avoid red or brown popsicles to distinguish any bleeding.
IV. Administer analgesics the first 24 hours for discomfort and then as needed for discomfort.
V. Position on side or stomach while child is sleeping and when he or she is awake.
VI. Discourage child from swallowing mucous secretions.
VII. Discourage child from coughing frequently, clearing throat, or blowing nose.
VIII. Avoid acidic fluids or foods (e.g., orange or tomato juice) until healing takes place; do not use straw.
IX. Reassure child and family about what to expect (e.g., expectoration of blood-tinged mucus, temporary alteration in voice).
X. Support child and family.
XI. Teach skills needed for home care.

EVALUATION

I. Child recovers from surgery uneventfully:
  A. No evidence of bleeding
  B. No difficulty with nutritional intake

Acute Otitis Media

Description

Acute otitis media is an infection of the middle ear.

Pathophysiology

I. Usually following an upper respiratory infection
II. Primarily the result of a blocked eustachian tube
III. Impaired drainage, which prevents normal drainage of middle-ear secretions
IV. Rapid growth of organisms in this warm, fertile environment
V. Usual cause: *Streptococcus pneumoniae, Haemophilus influenzae,* and *Moraxella catarrhalis*

Signs and Symptoms

I. General
  A. Earache
  B. Fever
  C. Possible purulent drainage
  D. Loss of appetite
  E. Irritability
  F. Complaints of pain (older children)
  G. Evidence of hearing loss in affected ear
II. In infants
  A. Crying

B. Restless and difficult to comfort
C. Rolling of head from side to side
D. Tendency to rub, hold, or pull affected ear
III. Otoscopic examination reveals:
  A. Bright-red or opaque, bulging or retracting tympanic membrane with diminished mobility
  B. Possibly no visible bony landmarks or light reflex

Therapeutic Management

I. Medical
  A. Antibiotics to eradicate organisms
  B. Analgesics to control discomfort
  C. Acetaminophen for high fever
  D. Decongestants (of questionable value)
II. Surgical
  A. May require myringotomy (surgical incision of eardrum)

Nursing Care

DATA COLLECTION

I. Perform routine assessment.
II. Assess for evidence of generalized infection.
III. Examine external auditory canal for evidence of inflammation.
IV. Assess child for evidence of hearing loss in affected ear.
V. Perform or assist with diagnostic procedures: audiography, tympanometry, pneumatic otoscopy, acoustic reflectometry.

PLANNING

I. Safe, effective care environment
  A. See Nursing Care of the Ill Child.
II. Physiological integrity
  A. Assist in eradication of organism.
  B. Relieve discomfort.
III. Psychosocial integrity
  A. Support child and family.
  B. See Nursing Care of the Ill Child.
IV. Health promotion and maintenance
  A. Prevent complications.
  B. Prepare family for home care.

IMPLEMENTATION

I. Administer antibiotics as prescribed.
II. Administer analgesics as prescribed.
III. Administer decongestants, if prescribed.
IV. Apply local heat; have child lie (affected ear down) on a heating pad wrapped in a towel.
V. Cleanse external ear with sterile cotton swabs or pledgets soaked in saline; then keep ear dry to prevent excoriation.
VI. Cleanse any drainage from ear and keep area dry to prevent excoriation.
VII. Encourage fluid intake.
VIII. Prepare family for surgical intervention, if appropriate:
  A. Myringotomy
  B. Placement of pressure-equalizing tubes
IX. Emphasize the importance of following a full course of antibiotics.
X. Emphasize the importance of follow-up care.

XI. Teach primary caregiver measures to reduce occurrence of otitis media.
XII. Teach family skills needed for home care, including expected results of medications and their possible side effects.

EVALUATION

I. Child appears comfortable.
II. Child's ear canal and surrounding skin are free of drainage and irritation.
III. Child remains free of complications.
IV. Family complies with therapeutic regimen.

Bronchial Asthma

Description

Bronchial asthma is a lower-airway disorder characterized by smooth muscle constriction (bronchospasm), increased thick mucus secretions, and mucosal edema—usually in response to an allergen.

Pathophysiology

I. Symptoms possibly precipitated by allergic response to an allergen (pollens, dust, animal dander), exercise, certain foods, smoke or other irritants, rapid changes in environmental temperature, upper respiratory infection, or emotional stress
II. Bronchospasm
III. Increased mucus secretion
IV. Edema
V. Reduced diameter of air passage

Signs and Symptoms

I. Hacking, paroxysmal, irritative, nonproductive cough
II. Shortness of breath; flaring nares
III. Elevated pulse
IV. Prolonged expiratory phase of respiration
V. Audible wheeze
VI. Restlessness and apprehension, accompanied by an anxious facial expression
VII. In children, speaking with short, panting, broken phrases common
VIII. In older children sitting upright, hunched over, with hands on bed or chair and arms braced common
IX. Chest auscultation revealing coarse, loud breath sounds; sonorous rales; coarse rhonchi; and generalized expiratory wheezing, which becomes increasingly high pitched
X. With repeated episodes, common for children to develop barrel chest, elevated shoulder, and use of accessory muscles of respiration

Therapeutic Management

I. Eliminate or avoid proved or suspected irritants and allergens.
II. Prevent attacks: avoid precipitating factors; administer cromolyn sodium.
III. Relieve or minimize symptoms:
   A. Bronchodilators to relax bronchiole musculature

   1. Rapid-acting β-adrenergic agonists and methylxanthines
   B. Corticosteroids to reduce edema
IV. Treat acute attacks promptly.
V. Educate child and family regarding short- and long-range management.

Status Asthmaticus

I. Hospitalization with intensive nursing care
II. IV fluids
III. Continuous respiratory and cardiac monitoring
IV. Bronchodilators
   A. Short, rapid-acting sympathomimetics: epinephrine, Sus-Phrine, terbutaline
V. Corticosteroids
VI. Humidified oxygen therapy

Nursing Care

DATA COLLECTION

I. See Assessment under Respiratory Distress Syndrome.
II. Obtain history to determine possible precipitating factors.
III. Gather data on environment for presence of possible allergens.
IV. Assist with diagnostic procedures: chest x-ray, sputum examination, immunologic blood tests, skin tests, pulmonary function tests, challenge tests.
V. Assess family interpersonal relationships for evidence of dissension, overprotection, or manipulation.
VI. Provide acute care:
   A. Monitor IV fluids and output.
   B. Monitor VSs frequently.

PLANNING

I. Safe, effective care environment
   A. Remove allergenic materials from environment.
   B. Avoid exposure to infection.
   C. Prevent situations that precipitate an attack (e.g., extremes of weather; air pollutants, especially smoke; and infections).
II. Physiological integrity
   A. Relieve symptoms (e.g., bronchospasm).
   B. Adhere to therapeutic regimen (e.g., medications, breathing exercises).
III. Psychosocial integrity
   A. Promote normal activities.
   B. Discourage overprotection by family.
   C. Promote short- and long-term adaptation to the disease.
IV. Health promotion and maintenance
   A. Maintain optimum health with good nutrition, adequate rest, and appropriate exercise.
   B. Avoid exposure to infections.
   C. Manage minor illnesses at onset.
   D. Prepare child and family for home care.
   E. Promote self-care management.

IMPLEMENTATION

I. Acute attack
   A. Administer bronchodilators, corticosteroids, and antibiotics as prescribed.

B. Position in high-Fowler's position for optimum ventilation.
C. Provide humidified oxygen as prescribed.
D. Administer mucolytic agents as prescribed.

II. Long-term supervision and support
  A. Teach preventive management, avoidance of precipitating factors, appropriate exercise, sound health maintenance.
  B. Explain expected results of medications and their possible side effects.

EVALUATION

I. Child exhibits normal respiratory rate, rhythm, and quality.
II. Child engages in activities appropriate to age and interests.
III. Child and family comply with therapeutic regimen.
IV. Child and family maintain optimum health practices.
V. Child and family cope with life stresses appropriately.

Cystic Fibrosis

Description

Cystic fibrosis is a multisystem disorder primarily affecting the exocrine (mucus-producing) glands.

Pathophysiology

I. Instead of thin, freely flowing secretions, mucous glands produce a thick mucus.
II. Mucus accumulates, dilating and eventually obstructing small ducts and passages.
III. Pancreatic ducts become blocked:
  A. Prevents enzymes from reaching the duodenum
  B. Results in marked impairment in the digestion and absorption of nutrients
  C. Also results in cystic dilatation, degeneration, and eventual fibrosis of the acini (small gland lobes)
IV. Respiratory tract bronchioles and bronchi become blocked:
  A. Manifests as patchy atelectasis and hyperinflation
V. Males usually do not produce sperm.
VI. Sweat glands fail to reabsorb sodium.
VII. Abnormally high levels of sodium and chloride are present in the sweat.
VIII. Sodium depletion may occur.
IX. Disease is inherited as an autosomal recessive trait.

Signs and Symptoms

I. Meconium ileus in newborn period (earliest sign)
  A. Abdominal distention
  B. Vomiting
  C. Failure to pass stools
II. Gastrointestinal
  A. Large, bulky, loose, frothy, extremely foul-smelling stools
  B. Weight loss
  C. Marked tissue wasting
  D. Failure to grow
  E. Abdominal distention

F. Thin extremities
G. Decreased or absent pancreatic enzymes, especially trypsin, in stools
III. Pulmonary
  A. Frequent upper respiratory infections
  B. Chronic cough, which becomes paroxysmal
  C. Thick, tenacious mucus
  D. Eventual barrel chest, dyspnea, clubbing of fingers and toes
  E. Radiographic evidence of patchy areas of atelectasis and obstructive emphysema
IV. Biochemical
  A. Diagnosis by sweat chloride concentrations > 60 mEq/L
  B. Salty taste to sweat (often reported by parents)
V. Delayed puberty

Therapeutic Management

I. Remove obstruction (meconium ileus).
II. Facilitate lung clearance.
III. Prevent and treat pulmonary infections.
IV. Replace pancreatic enzymes.
V. Facilitate growth.
VI. Prevent complications.

Nursing Care

DATA COLLECTION

I. See Data Collection under Respiratory Distress Syndrome.
II. See Data Collection under The Preterm Infant.
III. Perform or assist with diagnostic tests: chest x-ray, sweat electrolytes, pulmonary function, tests for pancreatic enzymes, fat-absorption tests.
IV. Assess family's interpersonal relationships with child and response to the disease.

PLANNING

I. Safe, effective care environment
  A. See Nursing Care of the Ill Child.
  B. Avoid exposure to infections.
II. Physiological integrity
  A. Improve breathing.
  B. Facilitate bronchial clearance.
  C. Promote growth.
III. Psychosocial integrity
  A. Explore feelings regarding an inherited disease.
  B. Explore family's feelings regarding a child with a potentially terminal illness.
  C. Encourage genetic counseling.
  D. Provide long-term support and follow-up care.
IV. Health promotion and maintenance
  A. Maintain optimum health.
  B. Prevent complications.
  C. Prepare family for home care.
  D. Encourage as normal a lifestyle as possible.

IMPLEMENTATION

I. Assist with diagnostic procedures (perform sweat chloride test as prescribed).

II. Provide and/or supervise respiratory therapy as prescribed:
  A. Nebulization
  B. Chest physiotherapy
  C. Breathing exercises
III. Administer antibiotics, mucolytics, and expectorants as prescribed.
IV. Provide nutritious and attractive meals and snacks. Diet should have increased protein and moderate amount of fat.
V. Encourage extra intake of fluids.
VI. Monitor IV infusion, if prescribed.
VII. Administer pancreatic enzymes as prescribed.
VIII. Provide conscientious skin care (salt accumulation may be irritating).
IX. Implement and maintain appropriate infection-control measures.
X. Teach family administration of medications, including expected results and possible side effects.
XI. Teach family about use of equipment and about respiratory management.
XII. Promote compliance with prescribed therapies.
XIII. Encourage and promote self-care.
XIV. Promote as normal a lifestyle as possible (e.g., engaging in activities within capabilities, attending school, developing peer relationships).
XV. Support child and family.
XVI. Refer to genetic counseling services.

EVALUATION

I. Child breathes easily.
II. Child manages bronchial secretions with minimal stress.
III. Child appears well nourished and gains weight appropriate for developmental stage.
IV. Child remains free of complications, especially URIs.
V. Child engages in activities appropriate to developmental level, capabilities, and interests.
VI. Family complies with therapeutic regimen.
VII. Family seeks appropriate counseling.

Gastrointestinal Disorders

Cleft Lip and/or Cleft Palate

Description

Cleft lip is a congenital malformation consisting of one or more clefts in the upper lip. Cleft palate is a congenital defect consisting of a fissure in the midline of the palate.

Pathophysiology

I. Cleft lip: failure of the maxillary and median nasal processes to fuse during prenatal development
  A. May range from a notch in the vermilion border of lip to complete separation extending to the floor of the nose
II. Cleft palate: failure of the two sides of the palate to fuse during prenatal development
  A. May occur as an isolated defect or in association with cleft lip

Signs and Symptoms

These defects are readily apparent at birth.

Therapeutic Management

I. Surgically close the defects at the optimum age.
II. Prevent complications.
III. Facilitate normal growth and development of the child.
IV. Rehabilitate for optimum speech and hearing within limitation of residual impairment, if any.

Nursing Care

DATA COLLECTION

I. Assess for palatal defects by placing examining fingers directly on palate.
II. Assess infant's or child's ability to suck and take nourishment.
III. Assess nutritional status of the child.

PLANNING

I. Safe, effective care environment
  A. See Hospital Care of the Newborn Infant under Postpartal Care in Chapter 3.
  B. Provide an environment appropriate for age.
  C. Promote the involvement of the primary caregiver.
II. Physiological integrity
  A. Facilitate healing of operative site.
  B. Prevent complications.
  C. Facilitate nutritional intake.
III. Psychosocial integrity
  A. Facilitate family's adjustment to a child with a facial defect.
  B. Promote normal lifestyle for child.
IV. Health promotion and maintenance
  A. Implement a feeding method appropriate to extent of the defect, parental preference, and ease of management.
  B. Prepare family for home care.

IMPLEMENTATION

I. Use special nipple or appliance when feeding (e.g., lamb's nipple, flanged nipple, gravity-flow nipple, rubber-tipped syringe, or specially designed feeding appliance); modify standard nipple with small single slit or cross-cut at end.
II. Feed with infant's head held upright to prevent aspiration.
III. Provide soft diet postoperatively for older children until healing takes place.
IV. Breastfeeding mothers are taught positioning of infant as for formula feeding and placing nipple well back in the infant's mouth for more efficient compression.
V. Bubble (burp) frequently during feeding.
VI. Convey an attitude of acceptance of infant and family; indicate by behavior that infant is a valuable human being.
VII. Protect operative site (cleft lip):
  A. Avoid positioning on stomach.
  B. Apply elbow restraints.
  C. Maintain metal appliance (if applied in the operating room).

D. Cleanse operative site, as prescribed, after feeding and as indicated.
E. Prevent excessive crying.
VIII. Protect operative site (cleft palate):
A. Avoid placing objects in child's mouth (e.g., standard spoon: use only wide-bowled spoon, tongue depressor, thermometer).
B. Restrain arms.
IX. Support and educate family regarding home care.
X. Teach family to observe for signs of speech or hearing impairment.

EVALUATION

I. Infant takes feedings well and displays appropriate weight gain.
II. Surgical site remains clean and free of trauma and infection.
III. Child develops normal patterns of speech articulation and intonation.
IV. Child hears without difficulty.
V. Family uses community resources appropriately.
VI. Family exhibits evidence that the child is an accepted and loved member of the household.

Tracheoesophageal Fistula, Esophageal Atresia

Description

Tracheoesophageal fistula is a congenital malformation resulting from failure of the esophagus to develop a continuous passage; the esophagus may or may not form a connection to the trachea.

Pathophysiology

The anomaly appears in one of the following ways:
I. Proximal esophageal segment terminating in a blind pouch; distal segment connected to the trachea or primary bronchus by a short fistula at or near the bifurcation (most common anomaly)
II. Blind pouches at end of the proximal and the distal esophagus, which are widely separated and have no communication to the trachea
III. Otherwise normal trachea and esophagus connected by a common fistula
IV. Fistula from the trachea to the upper esophageal segment or to both the upper and lower segments (rare)

Signs and Symptoms

I. Excessive salivation and drooling
II. Coughing
III. Choking
IV. Cyanosis
V. Ceasing breathing possible
VI. Possibility of catheter gently passed into the esophagus meeting with resistance if the lumen is blocked
VII. Diagnosis established by radiographic demonstration of anomaly

Therapeutic Management

I. Patent airway
II. Prevention of pneumonia

A. Feed by gastrostomy.
B. Drain oral secretions via tube inserted into proximal blind pouch or cervical esophagostomy.
III. Surgical repair of defect (time of repair depends on the type of defect and condition of the infant)

Nursing Care

DATA COLLECTION

I. Perform routine assessment. (Does mother have a history of polyhydramnios?)
II. Observe for evidence of anomaly, primarily the 3 Cs: coughing, choking, and cyanosis (especially following ingestion of fluid). Also excessive salivation.
III. Assist with diagnostic procedures: gastric lavage, chest x-ray.

PLANNING

I. Safe, effective care environment
A. Prevent complications.
B. Provide safe environment according to the needs of the child.
II. Physiological integrity
A. Prevent aspiration of fluid and secretions into trachea.
B. Feed via gastrostomy as prescribed.
C. Provide conscientious postoperative care at time of surgical correction.
III. Psychosocial integrity
A. Meet oral needs of infant.
B. Facilitate family's adjustment to an infant with a physical defect.
IV. Health promotion and maintenance
A. Provide health supervision as appropriate.
B. Prepare family for home care.

IMPLEMENTATION

I. Recognize defect as soon after birth as evident.
II. Position for optimum drainage of secretions—usually supine, with head elevated at least 30 degrees.
III. Suction oropharynx as needed.
IV. Aspirate secretions from proximal blind pouch, manually or by intermittent or continuous suction.
V. Feed prescribed formula via gastrostomy tube.
VI. Provide for infant's sucking needs with pacifier, especially during gastrostomy feedings.
VII. Observe postoperatively for ability to swallow without choking and for satisfactory eating behavior.
VIII. Prepare family for appearance of child (e.g., presence of chest tubes).
IX. Assist family in coping with the infant's needs and therapies.
X. Provide for maternal and infant bonding.
XI. Teach family skills needed for home care.

EVALUATION

I. Infant remains free of respiratory distress.
II. Infant's lungs remain clear.
III. Infant retains feedings and exhibits appropriate weight gain.
IV. Family exhibits appropriate behavior with infant.
V. Family demonstrates an understanding of the condition and the ability to provide home care.

Pyloric Stenosis

Description

Pyloric stenosis is a narrowing of the opening at exit of the stomach.

Pathophysiology

I. Enlargement (hypertrophy) of the pyloric musculature causing obstruction at the stomach exit (may be genetic)

Signs and Symptoms

I. Vomiting
   A. Is forceful to projectile
   B. Occurs shortly after a feeding
   C. May follow each meal or appear intermittently
II. Infant hungry and irritable, accepts second feeding after vomiting
III. No evidence of pain or discomfort
IV. Weight loss
V. Signs of dehydration
VI. Hard, olive-shaped tumor possibly palpable

Therapeutic Management

I. Correct any dehydration and electrolyte imbalance.
II. Provide surgical relief of obstruction by pyloromyotomy (Fredet-Ramstedt procedure).

Nursing Care

DATA COLLECTION

I. Perform routine assessment.
II. Observe infant's eating behaviors, especially vomiting pattern.
III. Assess for dehydration. Monitor electrolytes.
IV. Assist with diagnostic procedures: upper GI series, ultrasound, laboratory assessment of electrolyte status.

PLANNING

I. Safe, effective care environment
   A. See Nursing Care of the Ill Child.
   B. Promote an environment that is appropriate for the age of the child.
II. Physiological integrity
   A. Provide nutrition.
   B. Prevent vomiting.
   C. Prevent complications.
III. Psychosocial integrity
   A. Meet infant's sucking needs.
   B. Support family and prepare for surgery.
   C. Promote healthy parent-child relationships.
IV. Health promotion and maintenance
   A. Provide health supervision.
   B. Prepare family for home care.

IMPLEMENTATION

I. Obtain baseline weight and monitor daily.
II. Monitor IV infusion as prescribed.
III. Monitor I&O.
IV. Monitor electrolytes.

V. Monitor nasogastric suction, if present.
VI. If feeding, minimize vomiting by:
   A. Feeding slowly
   B. Holding infant in semiupright position
   C. Bubbling frequently (before, during, and after feeding)
   D. Placing on right side after feeding
   E. Handling minimally after feeding
VII. Teach family skills needed for home care.

EVALUATION

I. Infant takes and retains feedings.
II. Infant exhibits a satisfactory weight gain.
III. Parents demonstrate an understanding of the condition and the ability to provide home care.

Imperforate Anus

Description

Imperforate anus is a congenital malformation in which the rectum has no outside opening.

Pathophysiology

I. Rectum ends as a closed or blind pouch.
II. End may connect to the vagina by a fistula.

Signs and Symptoms

I. Absence of an anus; dimple present
II. Failure to pass meconium stool
III. Passage of stool through inappropriate opening

Therapeutic Management

I. Perform surgery to construct opening.
II. Sometimes a temporary colostomy may be necessary.
III. In vaginal fistula, surgery may be delayed 4–6 months.

Nursing Care

DATA COLLECTION

I. Perform routine assessment.
II. Observe for meconium stool.
III. Assist with diagnostic procedures: endoscopy, x-ray, renal ultrasound.

PLANNING

I. Safe, effective care environment
   A. See Hospital Care of the Newborn Infant under Postpartal Care in Chapter 3.
   B. Promote environment appropriate for age.
II. Physiological integrity
   A. Promote wound healing.
   B. Promote normal bowel function.
   C. Prevent infection and trauma.
III. Psychosocial integrity
   A. See Hospital Care of the Newborn Infant under Postpartal Care in Chapter 3.
   B. Support family.
   C. Prepare family for surgical procedure.

D. Promote involvement of primary caregiver in the care.
IV. Health promotion and maintenance
  A. Provide appropriate hydration and nutrition.
  B. Prepare family for home care.

IMPLEMENTATION

I. Avoid taking temperature rectally.
II. Monitor IV fluids as prescribed.
III. Monitor I&O; weigh daily.
IV. Maintain nasogastric suction, if prescribed.
V. Offer pacifier to satisfy nonnutritive sucking needs.
VI. Observe stool pattern.
VII. Support family and teach skills needed for home care.

EVALUATION

I. Infant is well hydrated and well nourished.
II. Infant displays normal stool pattern.
III. Operative site remains free of infection.
IV. Family demonstrates an understanding of the condition and the ability to provide home care.

Hirschsprung's Disease (Megacolon)

Description

Hirschsprung's disease is a lack of normal peristalsis.

Pathophysiology

I. Lack of peristaltic movements due to absence of autonomic parasympathetic ganglion cells
II. Retention of stool
III. Distention of the bowel

Signs and Symptoms

I. Absence or small amount of stool in the newborn period
II. Anorexia
III. Abdominal distention and vomiting
IV. Constipation
V. Ribbonlike stool
VI. Inadequate weight gain in infancy

Therapeutic Management

I. Temporary colostomy
II. Bowel reconstruction (usually at 1 year of age)

Nursing Care (Operative)

DATA COLLECTION

I. Perform routine assessment.
II. Observe bowel pattern.
III. Assess general hydration and nutritional status.
IV. Assist with diagnostic procedures: x-ray, rectal biopsy, anorectal manometry.

PLANNING

I. Safe, effective care environment
  A. See Nursing Care of the Ill Child.

II. Physiological integrity
  A. Provide nutrition and hydration.
  B. Facilitate bowel movements.
III. Psychosocial integrity
  A. Foster healthy parent-child relationships.
  B. Prepare child and family for surgical procedure and postoperative colostomy care.
IV. Health promotion and maintenance
  A. Prevent complications.
  B. Prepare family for home care, including postoperative colostomy care.

IMPLEMENTATION

I. Preoperative
  A. Maintain nasogastric suction.
  B. Keep client on nothing by mouth (NPO) regimen.
  C. Monitor IV therapy.
  D. Administer enemas and laxatives as prescribed.
  E. Administer antibiotics as prescribed.
II. Postoperative
  A. Maintain nasogastric suction.
  B. Avoid rectal temperatures.
  C. Monitor IV therapy.
  D. Provide colostomy care as prescribed.
  E. Provide diet as prescribed.
  F. Support family and teach colostomy or wound care or both as indicated.

EVALUATION

I. Child exhibits a normal bowel elimination pattern.
II. Child remains well nourished and well hydrated.
III. Child exhibits no evidence of infection.
IV. Family demonstrates an understanding of the disease and the ability to provide home care.

Celiac Disease

Description

Celiac disease is a malabsorption disease characterized by hypersensitivity to gluten.

Pathophysiology

I. Inability to digest wheat, barley, rye, and oats (gluten)
II. Accumulation of toxic substances in the gut
III. Inflammation and ulceration of intestinal mucosa

Signs and Symptoms

I. Age of onset: 1–5 years
II. Failure to thrive: malnutrition and hypocalcemia
III. Muscle wasting, especially of buttocks and extremities
IV. Diarrhea, acute or insidious; stools often pale and watery with odor
V. Some cases of vomiting and constipation
VI. Anemia; easy bruising and bleeding
VII. Irritability, uncooperativeness, apathy
VIII. Celiac crisis
  A. Precipitated by infection

B. Prolonged fluid and electrolyte depletion
C. Emotional disturbance

Therapeutic Management

I. Dietary elimination of wheat, barley, rye, and oats
II. Supplemental vitamins and minerals

Nursing Care

DATA COLLECTION

I. Perform routine assessment.
II. Pay particular attention to bowel elimination patterns, amount, color, and character.
III. Assist with diagnostic procedures (such as stool collection, intestinal biopsy, gluten challenge).

PLANNING

I. Safe, effective care environment
   A. See Nursing Care of the Ill Child.
   B. Promote an appropriate environment for age.
II. Physiological integrity
   A. Implement and maintain gluten-free diet.
III. Psychosocial integrity
   A. See Nursing Care of the Ill Child.
   B. Promote healthy parent-child relationship.
   C. Promote normal lifestyle and peer relationships.
IV. Health promotion and maintenance
   A. Promote good health practices.
   B. Prepare family for home care.

IMPLEMENTATION

I. Provide special gluten-free diet: eliminate barley, wheat, oats, and rye.
II. Substitute offending grains with other grains: corn, rice, or soybean.
III. Administer vitamin and mineral supplements as prescribed.
IV. Teach family about the disease and its management.
V. Teach family diet planning:
   A. Appropriate grain products
   B. Reading food labels for hidden presence of gluten, including gravies, hydrogenated vegetable protein, and vegetable protein added
   C. Introducing recipes that promote adherence to diet
VI. Teach family signs of celiac crisis.
VII. Reinforce explanations of the disease and therapies.
VIII. Encourage child to assume responsibility for diet adherence as early as possible.
IX. Stress that gluten restriction is usually a lifelong necessity.

EVALUATION

I. Child achieves age-appropriate weight and height.
II. Child engages in activities appropriate to age.
III. Family complies with prescribed diet.

Intussusception

Description

Intussusception is telescoping of a portion of the intestine into an adjacent portion.

Pathophysiology

I. Most common site for telescoping is the ileocecal valve.
II. Stopping passage of intestinal contents beyond the defect.
III. Inflammation, edema, and decreased blood flow.
IV. Stool contains primarily blood and mucus: the characteristic "currant-jelly" stool.
V. Condition usually affects males between 3–6 months old.

Signs and Symptoms

I. Sudden, intermittent, severe abdominal pain.
   A. Child screams and draws knees up to chest.
   B. Child appears comfortable between pain episodes.
II. Vomitus is bile stained or contains stool.
III. Loose, scant stools.
IV. Passage of red currant-jelly-like stools, usually 12 hours after the onset of pain.
V. Tender, distended, boardlike abdomen.

Therapeutic Management

I. Nonsurgical: reduction by barium enema
II. Surgical: reduction or resection

Nursing Care

DATA COLLECTION

I. Perform routine assessment.
II. Listen carefully to family's description of symptoms.
III. Assess vomitus.
IV. Assess stools.
V. Assess patterns of pain and relief.
VI. Assist with diagnostic procedure: x-ray.

PLANNING

I. Safe, effective care environment
   A. See Nursing Care of the Ill Child.
II. Physiological integrity
   A. Prepare child for emergency therapeutic procedures.
   B. Observe child for complications (e.g., fever, dehydration, peritonitis).
III. Psychosocial integrity
   A. Support child and family.
   B. Prepare child and family for procedures.
IV. Health promotion and maintenance
   A. Promote and maintain optimum hydration and nutrition.
   B. Promote elimination.
   C. Prepare family for home care.

IMPLEMENTATION

I. Monitor stooling pattern.
II. Monitor vital signs and IV infusion.
III. Maintain nasogastric suction, if used.

EVALUATION

I. Child exhibits normal stooling pattern.
II. Child is free of discomfort.

III. Family demonstrates an understanding of the condition and the ability to provide home care.

Diarrhea

Description

I. A noticeable or sudden increase in the number of or change in consistency of stools
II. Watery stools

Pathophysiology

I. Infection
II. Malabsorption syndromes
III. Loss of fluid and electrolytes

Signs and Symptoms

I. Mild diarrhea: few loose stools daily but no other symptoms
II. Moderate diarrhea: several loose or watery stools daily
III. Severe diarrhea: numerous stools to continuous stooling
IV. Accompanying signs
   A. Weight loss
   B. Dry skin and mucous membranes
   C. Decreased urine

Therapeutic Management

I. IV fluid therapy
II. Correction of electrolyte and acid-base imbalances
III. Elimination and/or correction of cause of diarrhea
IV. Prevention of spread of infection
V. Prevention of complications

Nursing Care

DATA COLLECTION

I. Perform routine assessment.
II. Observe stool pattern and consistency.
III. Assess (on admission and throughout care) weight and state of hydration.
IV. Assist with diagnostic procedures: laboratory tests of fluid and electrolyte status, acid-base balance; stool examination.
V. Test stools for pH, glucose, and blood, if prescribed.

PLANNING

I. Safe, effective care environment
   A. See Nursing Care of the Hospitalized Child.
   B. Prevent spread of diarrhea to others.
II. Physiological integrity
   A. Promote rehydration and maintain adequate hydration.
   B. Re-establish nutrition appropriate to age and condition.
   C. Prevent complications.
III. Psychosocial integrity
   A. See Nursing Care of the Hospitalized Child.
   B. Support and educate child and family.
   C. Prepare child and family for procedures.

IV. Health promotion and maintenance
   A. Promote optimum health.
   B. Prepare family for home care.

IMPLEMENTATION

I. Monitor IV fluid administration, if prescribed.
II. Feed oral rehydration fluids as prescribed.
III. Gradually reintroduce diet for age as indicated.
IV. Implement appropriate isolation precautions. Instruct family and others in their use.
V. Record color, consistency, and appearance of stool.
VI. Keep accurate I&O records.
VII. Measure and record weight.
VIII. Avoid rectal temperature measurements.
IX. Provide skin care, especially of anal, perineal, and buttock areas.
X. Provide for sucking needs with pacifier if NPO or if receiving limited oral fluids.
XI. Promote parent-child interaction.
XII. Teach family skills and procedures needed for home care.

EVALUATION

I. Child takes and retains prescribed oral fluids.
II. Child exhibits evidence of good hydration and satisfactory weight for age.
III. VSs remain within normal range for age.
IV. Child consumes adequate diet for age.
V. Child's skin exhibits no evidence of discoloration or irritation.
VI. Mucous membranes remain moist and clean.
VII. Family demonstrates an understanding of the condition and the ability to provide home care.

Pinworms

Description

Pinworms are an intestinal infestation with *Enterobius vermicularis*, the common pinworm.

Pathophysiology

I. Infection begins when eggs are inhaled or swallowed.
II. Eggs hatch in intestine and mature.
III. Female worms proceed to anal area and lay eggs.
IV. Movement of worms on skin and mucous membrane surfaces causes intense itching.
V. Eggs are deposited on hands and under fingernails during scratching, and child puts fingers in mouth, causing reinfection.

Signs and Symptoms

I. Intense perianal itching
II. Evidence of itching in young children
   A. General restlessness and irritability
   B. Sleep disturbances
   C. Bedwetting

Therapeutic Management

I. Administration of mebendazole (Vermox) or pyrantel pamoate (Antiminth)

Nursing Care

DATA COLLECTION

I. Perform routine assessment.
II. Assist with diagnostic procedures: identify parasite. Specimens must be sent to laboratory while still warm.

PLANNING

I. Safe, effective care environment
   A. Prevent spread of infestation.
II. Physiological integrity
   A. Help to eradicate organisms.
III. Psychosocial integrity
   A. Support and educate child and family.
   B. Prepare child and family for collection of specimens and administration of medication.
IV. Health promotion and maintenance
   A. Promote optimum health.

IMPLEMENTATION

I. Explain or reinforce explanation of condition and therapies.
II. Collect specimens for examination.
   A. Construct loop of transparent tape, sticky side out, and place around the end of a tongue depressor.
   B. Apply to perianal region in morning as soon as child awakens and before a bowel movement or bath.
   C. Place in jar or plastic bag loosely.
III. Teach family to administer medication: single dose, followed in 2 weeks by second dose.
IV. Teach child and family preventive measures:
   A. Wash hands after toileting and before eating.
   B. Keep child's fingernails short.
   C. Bathe or shower daily.
   D. Discourage child from biting nails, placing fingers in mouth, and scratching anal area.
   E. Wash linen in hot water.
   F. Sanitize linen, underpants, and diapers in hot water.
V. Prevent spread by keeping toys separate and avoid shaking linen.

EVALUATION

I. Child exhibits no evidence of infestation.
II. Family demonstrates an understanding of the condition and the ability to perform home care.
III. Others exhibit no evidence of infestation.

Cardiovascular Disorders

Congenital Heart Disease

Description

Congenital heart disease is a defect in the heart resulting from developmental arrest or deviation during the prenatal period.

Pathophysiology

I. Acyanotic defects
   A. A narrowing of the pulmonary artery
   B. An opening that moves arterial blood into the venous system (left to right shunting)

II. Cyanotic defects
   A. Unoxygenated blood mixed with oxygenated blood in the systemic circulation
   B. Usually right-to-left shunting of blood through an abnormal opening and/or vessel configuration
III. Characteristics of major acyanotic defects
   A. Patent ductus arteriosus: failure of fetal ductus arteriosus to completely close after birth, increasing pulmonary circulation
   B. Coarctation of aorta: narrowing of the aorta, causing decreased circulation
   C. Atrial septal defect: abnormal opening between the right and left atria
   D. Ventricular septal defect: abnormal opening between the right and left ventricles (defect can vary in size from pinhole to complete absence of septum)
   E. Pulmonary stenosis: narrowing or stricture at the entrance to the pulmonary artery
   F. Aortic stenosis: narrowing or stricture of the aortic valve or the entrance to the aorta
IV. Characteristics of major cyanotic defects
   A. Tetralogy of Fallot: classic form consists of four defects:
      1. Ventricular septal defect
      2. Pulmonic stenosis
      3. Overriding aorta
      4. Right ventricular hypertrophy
   B. Transposition of the great vessels (arteries) (pulmonary artery leaves the left ventricle and the aorta exits from the right ventricle, with no blood flow between systemic and pulmonary circulations)

Signs and Symptoms

I. Infants
   A. Generalized cyanosis
   B. Cyanosis during exertion, especially crying, feeding, straining
   C. Dyspnea, especially following physical effort
   D. Fatigue (with eating)
   E. Failure to thrive
   F. Tachypnea
II. Older children
   A. Small for age
   B. Delicate, frail body
   C. Fatigue
   D. Dyspnea with exercise
   E. Clubbed fingers (cyanotic defects)
   F. Squatting for relief of dyspnea (cyanotic defects)
III. Other possible observations
   A. Bounding pulse
   B. Murmur
   C. Thrill
   D. Tachycardia
   E. Difference in pulse between upper and lower extremities (coarctation of the aorta)

Therapeutic Management

I. Medical
   A. Improve circulatory effort:
      1. Digitalis administration

B. Remove and prevent excess fluid retention:
1. Low-sodium diet (formula)
2. Diuretic administration
C. Prevent complications:
1. Supplemental vitamin administration
2. Supplemental iron administration
3. Potassium chloride administration
II. Surgical
A. Cardiac catheterization to establish diagnosis
B. Surgical correction appropriate to the specific defect
C. Relief of symptoms until surgical correction can be accomplished

Nursing Care

DATA COLLECTION

I. Perform routine assessment, with particular attention to the following:
A. Assess rate and quality of pulses.
B. Measure blood pressure.
C. Observe for cyanosis, dyspnea, and clubbing of fingers.
D. Listen for murmurs.
II. Take careful health history, especially relative to:
A. Weight gain
B. Feeding behavior
C. Exercise intolerance
D. Frequency of infection
E. Unusual posturing (squatting, assuming knee-chest position)
III. Assist with diagnostic procedures: electrocardiography (ECG), x-ray, sonography, echocardiography, cardiac catheterization.

PLANNING

I. Safe, effective care environment
A. See Nursing Care of the Ill Child.
B. Promote environment appropriate for age.
II. Physiological integrity
A. Decrease energy output.
B. Improve circulatory effort.
C. Prevent complications (e.g., excess fluid retention, congestive heart failure [CHF], URI).
III. Psychosocial integrity
A. See Nursing Care of the Ill Child.
B. Assist child and family to cope with the condition.
C. Support and educate child and family.
D. Prepare child and family for procedures or surgery.
E. Promote as normal a lifestyle as possible.
IV. Health promotion and maintenance
A. Promote optimum health.
B. Maintain optimum fluid and nutrition.
C. Prepare family for home care.

IMPLEMENTATION

I. Limit physical activity.
II. Feed slowly.
III. Allow for frequent rest periods; schedule nursing activities to minimize disturbance of rest.
IV. Help child and family select activities appropriate to the condition.

V. Monitor I&O.
VI. Avoid extremes of temperature.
VII. Administer drugs as prescribed: digoxin (Lanoxin), iron preparation, diuretic, potassium chloride.
VIII. Administer oxygen as prescribed.
IX. Administer oral and IV fluids as prescribed.
X. Feed low-salt formula, if prescribed.
XI. Protect child from contact with persons with infections.
XII. Explain or reinforce explanation of condition and therapies.
XIII. Teach family skills and procedures needed for home care, including expected results of medications and their possible side effects.
XIV. See Nursing Care of the Ill Child.

EVALUATION

I. Child rests quietly and breathes easily.
II. Child's VSs are within acceptable limits.
III. Child consumes enough fluid and food for age.
IV. Child achieves normal growth for age.
V. Child exhibits no evidence of infection.
VI. Family demonstrates an understanding of the condition and therapies and the ability to provide home care.

Rheumatic Fever

Description

Rheumatic fever is an inflammatory disease affecting the heart, joints, CNS, and subcutaneous tissue.

Pathophysiology

I. Occurs after an infection with group A β-hemolytic streptococcus
II. Believed to occur as an autoimmune response
III. Characterized by inflammatory reaction of heart, joints, and skin
IV. Characterized by edema of involved tissues

Signs and Symptoms

I. Diagnosis based on Jones' criteria
II. Major manifestations
A. Carditis: tachycardia, cardiomegaly, murmur
B. Polyarthritis: migratory swollen, hot, red, painful joints
C. Chorea: sudden aimless, irregular movements of extremities, involuntary facial grimaces, speech disturbances
D. Subcutaneous nodes: nontender swelling located over bony parts
E. Erythema marginatum: transitory, nonitching rash
III. Minor manifestations
A. Fever: low-grade
B. Arthralgia without arthritic changes
C. History of previous rheumatic fever or rheumatic heart disease
D. Increased erythrocyte sedimentation rate (ESR)
E. C-reactive protein (CRP)
F. Leukocytosis
G. Anemia

H. Prolonged PR interval on ECG
I. Elevated antistreptolysin-O titer

Therapeutic Management

I. Treatment of group A β-hemolytic streptococci with penicillin
II. Prevention of permanent cardiac damage
   A. Bedrest during acute phase
   B. Corticosteroids to decrease inflammation
III. Supportive care for other symptoms
   A. Anti-inflammatory agents to suppress joint inflammation
   B. Mild sedation to decrease anxiety and restlessness caused by chorea
   C. Acetaminophen to relieve discomfort
IV. Prevention of further infections with long-term penicillin

Nursing Care

DATA COLLECTION

I. Perform routine assessment.
II. Take history of infections in the last 2 weeks.
III. Assist with diagnostic procedures: ECG, laboratory tests.

PLANNING

I. Safe, effective care environment
   A. See Nursing Care of the Ill Child.
   B. Provide appropriate environment for age.
II. Physiological integrity
   A. Help to eradicate organism.
   B. Alleviate symptoms.
   C. Prevent complications.
III. Psychosocial integrity
   A. See Nursing Care of the Ill Child.
   B. Support and educate child and family.
   C. Prepare child and family for procedures, surgery as needed.
   D. Promote child and primary caregiver interaction.
IV. Health promotion and maintenance
   A. Maintain and promote optimum health.
   B. Prepare family for home care.

IMPLEMENTATION

I. Administer penicillin or other antibiotic as prescribed.
II. Administer corticosteroids, anti-inflammatory drugs, analgesics, and sedatives as prescribed.
III. Help family cope with child's enforced limited activity, if prescribed.
IV. Teach family skills and procedures needed for home care, including expected results of medications and their possible side effects.
V. Teach the importance of long-term penicillin therapy.

EVALUATION

I. Child exhibits no evidence of cardiac problems.
II. Child exhibits no rash or swollen nodes and moves joints without pain.
III. Child displays no evidence of streptococcal infection.
IV. Child is able to exercise without fatigue.

Kawasaki Disease

Description

Kawasaki disease (KD) is a systemic vasculitis that usually affects children younger than 5 years of age. The cause is unknown.

Pathophysiology

I. Inflammation develops in small vessels (capillaries, venules, arterioles), progressing to medium-size blood vessels.
II. Pericarditis.
III. Aneurysms may develop because of damage to vascular wall.
IV. Vessel walls can be damaged, resulting in scarring, calcification, and stenosis.
V. Thrombus formation can occur.

Signs and Symptoms

I. Acute phase
   A. Irritable, inconsolable child with high fever unresponsive to antipyretics.
   B. Conjunctiva becomes reddened and eyes are dry.
   C. Inflammation of pharynx and oral mucosa.
   D. Strawberry tongue with dryness of lips.
   E. Rash is variable, often affecting perineum.
   F. Lymphadenopathy.
   G. Edematous extremities with erythema of palms of hands and soles of feet.
   H. Decrease in left ventricle function, and ECG changes associated with myositis.
   I. Symptoms of congested heart failure.
II. Subacute phase
   A. Fever subsided, but irritability present.
   B. Clinical symptoms resolving.
   C. Changes in echocardiogram.
   D. Periungual desquamation.
   E. Arthritis can persist into this phase.
   F. Chances of thrombocytosis increase.
   G. Cardiac involvement indicating myocardial infarction (abdominal pain, vomiting, restlessness, inconsolable crying, pallor, and shock).
III. Convalescent phase
   A. Clinical symptoms subsided.
   B. Sedimentation rate increases.
   C. Thrombocytosis may be apparent, and coronary complications are still of concern.
   D. Arthritis can still be present.

Therapeutic Management

I. High dose of IV gamma globulin
II. Salicylate therapy
III. Coumadin when large aneurysms are present.

Nursing Care

DATA COLLECTION

I. Perform routine assessment.
II. Monitor cardiac status (CHF, tachycardia, and respiratory distress).

III. I&O with daily weights. Watch for dehydration.
IV. Assist with ECG and echocardiogram.

PLANNING

I. Safe, effective care environment
  A. Provide environment appropriate for age.
  B. Provide environment for convalescence.
II. Physiological integrity
  A. Promote hydration status.
  B. Prevent complications (CHF, respiratory distress, dehydration, myocardial infarction).
III. Psychosocial integrity
  A. Promote child-parent bonding.
  B. Support and educate the family.
  C. Prepare the child and family for procedures.
IV. Health promotion and maintenance
  A. Promote optimum health.
  B. Prepare family for home care.

IMPLEMENTATION

I. Monitor cardiac status.
II. Monitor I&O along with daily weights.
III. Monitor IV fluids carefully because of the increased chances of CHF.
IV. Monitor infusion of gamma globulin.
V. Advise to dress in cool, loose clothing.
VI. Administer acetaminophen for fever.
VII. Provide good oral hygiene with lubricant for lips.
VIII. Perform range-of-motion (ROM) exercises to prevent stiffness of joints with arthritis. Bath time is an appropriate time for this.
IX. Provide quiet environment to help console child.
X. Teach family skills needed for home care.

EVALUATION

I. Child exhibits no evidence of cardiac problems.
II. Family understands signs and symptoms that require medical attention.
III. Family demonstrates an understanding of the disease and the ability to provide home care.

Hematopoietic Disorders

Leukemia

Description

Leukemia is cancer of the blood-forming tissues.

Pathophysiology

I. Abnormal increase of immature WBCs prevents production and development of normal blood cells in bone marrow.
II. Abnormal WBCs invade tissue and cause symptoms.
III. Symptoms depend on the area of the body invaded by leukemia cells.

Signs and Symptoms

I. Pallor, easy fatigability
II. Susceptibility to infections
III. Easy bruising and bleeding
IV. Bone pain and fractures
V. Enlarged liver, spleen, lymph glands
VI. Headache
VII. Nausea and vomiting
VIII. Irritability
IX. Anorexia and weight loss

Therapeutic Management

I. Achieve and maintain remission.
II. Administer antimetabolites and immunosuppressants.
III. Prevent complications of chemotherapy.
  A. Prevent infection with protective isolation or other appropriate precautions.
IV. Replace blood elements.
V. Relieve pain.

Nursing Care

DATA COLLECTION

I. Perform routine assessment.
II. Assist with diagnostic tests (e.g., blood counts, lumbar puncture, bone marrow aspiration, biopsy).
III. Observe for signs of complications (e.g., bleeding, ulceration, CNS symptoms).
IV. Assess family's coping capabilities and support systems.

PLANNING

I. Safe, effective care environment
  A. See Nursing Care of the Ill Child.
  B. Prevent transfer of infection to the child.
  C. Prevent trauma that might cause bleeding.
II. Physiological integrity
  A. Help to achieve a remission.
  B. Relieve pain.
  C. Alleviate symptoms.
III. Psychosocial integrity
  A. See Nursing Care of the Ill Child.
  B. Educate child and family.
  C. Help child and family to cope with effects of the disease and its therapies.
  D. Prepare child and family for procedures and therapies.
IV. Health promotion and maintenance
  A. Promote optimum health.
  B. Achieve and maintain optimum fluid and nutrition.
  C. Prepare family for home care.

IMPLEMENTATION

I. Implement and maintain protective isolation.
II. Administer antimetabolites and immunosuppressive agents as prescribed.
III. Administer blood products as prescribed.
IV. Administer analgesics as prescribed.
V. Provide frequent oral hygiene with soft toothbrushes or swabs.
VI. Use minimal and gentle physical manipulation.
VII. Avoid taking rectal temperatures.
VIII. Administer antiemetic for nausea as prescribed.
IX. Provide meticulous, nontraumatic skin care.

X. Change position frequently.

XI. Promote rest; encourage frequent rest periods.

XII. Stimulate appetite with attractive meals and foods of child's choice; provide nutritious supplements.

XIII. Encourage family to be with the child at meal times.

XIV. Teach family skills and procedures needed for home care.

EVALUATION

I. Child attains and maintains a remission.

II. Child appears comfortable and verbalizes no complaints of pain.

III. Child eats an adequate amount of appropriate foods.

IV. Child exhibits no evidence of infection, bleeding, or other complications.

V. Child appears rested and engages in appropriate activities.

VI. Child and family cope with effects of therapies.

VII. Family demonstrates an understanding of the disease, the consequences of therapies, and the ability to provide home care.

Sickle Cell Disease

Description

Sickle cell disease is a genetically transmitted disease in which normal adult hemoglobin (HbA) is partly or completely replaced by hemoglobin S (HbS).

Pathophysiology

I. HbS transmitted as an autosomal dominant gene but displaying an autosomal recessive inheritance pattern

II. Disease occurring primarily in blacks or persons of Mediterranean ancestry

III. Rigid crescent or sickle shape assumed by RBCs when oxygen released to tissues (HbS has decreased oxygen-carrying capacity and short life span or increased destruction rate)

Signs and Symptoms

I. Growth retardation and delayed puberty

II. Chronic anemia

III. Marked susceptibility to infection

IV. Vaso-occlusive crisis (sickle cell crisis)

    A. Pain in involved areas

    B. Extremities: painful swelling of hands, feet, joints; ulceration

    C. Abdomen: severe abdominal pain

    D. Chest: pain, pulmonary disease

    E. Liver: jaundice, hepatomegaly

    F. Kidney: hematuria

V. Laboratory evidence of disease

    A. Presence of HbS in blood

    B. Hemoglobin electrophoresis identifies type and extent of abnormal hemoglobin

Therapeutic Management

I. Identify presence of HbS.

II. Prevent sickling phenomenon: promote adequate oxygenation and maintain hemodilution.

III. Treat sickle cell crisis:

    A. Bedrest to minimize oxygen use

    B. Oral or IV fluids

    C. Electrolyte replacement

    D. Administration of analgesics for pain relief

    E. Blood replacement for anemia; exchange transfusion in selected cases

    F. Antibiotics to treat existing infections

    G. Short-term oxygen therapy for severe anoxia

IV. Perform splenectomy for recurrent pooling of blood in the organ (sequestration).

Nursing Care

DATA COLLECTION

I. Perform routine assessment.

II. Assist with screening or diagnostic tests or both: Sickledex, electrophoresis, blood count.

III. Assist in diagnostic testing to assess effects of complications: x-ray, tomography, renal function tests, liver function tests.

PLANNING

I. Safe, effective care environment

    A. See Nursing Care of the Ill Child.

II. Physiological integrity

    A. Relieve pain (crisis).

    B. Promote adequate fluid intake.

    C. Prevent complications.

III. Psychosocial integrity

    A. See Nursing Care of the Ill Child.

    B. Support and educate child and family.

    C. Prepare child and family for procedures, surgery as needed.

IV. Health promotion and maintenance

    A. Prevent sickling crisis.

    B. Promote optimum health.

    C. Prepare family for home care.

IMPLEMENTATION

I. Administer oxygen, if ordered.

II. Administer analgesics as prescribed for pain.

III. Provide warmth to affected areas.

IV. Encourage ample oral fluids; force fluids, if needed; monitor IV infusion, if present.

V. Teach family skills and procedures needed for home care.

VI. Emphasize need for medical attention for infections.

EVALUATION

I. Child does not suffer a sickle cell crisis (i.e., should be free of pain or other symptoms).

II. Child is well hydrated.

III. Child exhibits no evidence of infection.

IV. Family demonstrates an understanding of the disease and the ability to provide home care.

V. Family seeks genetic counseling.

Hemophilia

Description

Hemophilia comprises a group of bleeding disorders in which one of the factors needed for clotting of blood is deficient.

I. Hemophilia A: deficiency of factor VIII (antihemophilic factor; antihemophilic globulin)
II. Hemophilia B (Christmas disease): deficiency of factor IX

Pathophysiology

I. Transmitted by X-linked recessive inheritance pattern
II. Inability of blood to clot
III. Bleeding into tissues possible anywhere

Signs and Symptoms

I. Prolonged bleeding anywhere from or in the body
II. Prolonged bleeding from trauma (e.g., umbilical cord, circumcision, cuts, loss of teeth, nosebleed, injection, surgery)
III. Excessive bruising, even from slight injury

Therapeutic Management

I. Replace missing blood factor with one of the following:
   A. Factor VIII concentrate
   B. Cryoprecipitate
   C. Fresh frozen plasma
II. Prevent chronic crippling effects of joint bleeding:
   A. Corticosteroids or nonsteroid anti-inflammatory agents (or both), to reduce inflammation
   B. Cold compresses applied to joint
III. Administer ibuprofen for discomfort as prescribed.
IV. Identify persons at risk for the disorder.

Nursing Care

DATA COLLECTION

I. Perform routine assessment.
II. Take careful histories:
   A. Health history for evidence of previous bleeding episodes, and present problem
   B. Family history for evidence of other affected members

PLANNING

I. Safe, effective care environment
   A. See Nursing Care of the Ill Child.
   B. Prevent trauma.
II. Physiological integrity
   A. Relieve discomfort.
   B. Prevent and control bleeding episodes.
   C. Prevent crippling effects of bleeding into joints.
III. Psychosocial integrity
   A. See Nursing Care of the Ill Child.
   B. Support and educate child and family.
   C. Prepare child and family for procedures, surgery as needed.
IV. Health promotion and maintenance
   A. Maintain and promote optimum health.
   B. Prepare family for home care.
   C. Promote self-management of therapies.

IMPLEMENTATION

I. Administer clotting factor as prescribed.
II. Administer ibuprofen as prescribed for pain.

III. Prevent trauma.
   A. Prevent falling and impact injuries.
   B. Alter environment to reduce injury, especially in toddlers (carpeted floors, padded furniture).
   C. Encourage use of soft toothbrush.
IV. Control or decrease local bleeding.
   A. Immobilize and elevate affected part.
   B. Apply pressure for 10–15 minutes.
   C. Apply cold to promote vasoconstriction.
V. Prevent crippling effects.
   A. Apply splints as prescribed.
   B. Encourage or perform passive ROM exercises.
VI. Teach family (including the child) skills and procedures needed for home care, especially administration of clotting factor.
VII. Encourage child to assume responsibility for own care.

EVALUATION

I. Child exhibits no evidence of bleeding.
II. Child exhibits no evidence of tissue damage.
III. Family demonstrates an understanding of the disease and the ability to provide home care.
IV. Family seeks genetic counseling.

Idiopathic Thrombocytopenic Purpura

Description

Idiopathic thrombocytopenic purpura (ITP) is an acquired hemorrhagic disorder characterized by a marked decrease in the number of platelets.

Pathophysiology

I. Involves excessive destruction of platelets
II. Interferes with blood clotting
III. Causes easy bleeding, particularly noted beneath the skin

Signs and Symptoms

I. Occurs in children 2–8 years of age
II. Most commonly seen after upper respiratory infections or childhood communicable diseases
III. Makes child prone to easy bruising: evidenced as petechiae, ecchymoses
IV. Results in bleeding from mucous membranes
   A. Epistaxis
   B. Bleeding gums
   C. Hematuria
   D. Hematemesis

Therapeutic Management

I. Restriction of child's activity at onset and if bleeding is active
II. Administration of corticosteroids for children at highest risk for serious bleeding
III. Administration of packed red cells for blood loss
IV. Administration of gamma globulin to increase platelet count (in chronic ITP)
V. Splenectomy in selected cases

Nursing Care

DATA COLLECTION

I. Perform routine assessment.
II. Assist with diagnostic tests.

PLANNING

I. Safe, effective care environment
   A. See Nursing Care of the Ill Child.
II. Physiological integrity
   A. Prevent and/or control bleeding.
   B. Prevent complications.
III. Psychosocial integrity
   A. See Nursing Care of the Ill Child.
   B. Support and educate child and family.
   C. Prepare child and family for procedures, surgery as needed.
IV. Health promotion and maintenance
   A. Promote optimum health.
   B. Prepare family for home care.

IMPLEMENTATION

I. Administer corticosteroids as prescribed.
II. Implement measures to prevent bleeding (see Hemophilia).
III. Administer nonsalicylate preparations for discomfort.
IV. Teach family skills and procedures needed for home care.

EVALUATION

I. Child exhibits no evidence of bleeding.
II. Family demonstrates an understanding of the condition and the ability to provide home care.

Endocrine Disorders

Diabetes Mellitus

Description

Diabetes mellitus is a disease of metabolism characterized by a deficiency of the hormone insulin.
   I. Insulin-dependent diabetes mellitus or type I diabetes: onset typically in childhood and adolescence
   II. Maturity-onset diabetes of youth or type II diabetes: decrease in the amount of needed insulin

Pathophysiology

I. Inadequate insulin for metabolism of carbohydrates, fats, and proteins
II. Inadequate glucose to fuel body needs; proteins and fats broken down
III. Blood glucose concentration increased, spilling over in urine
IV. Increased fluid and electrolytes lost in diuresis

Signs and Symptoms

I. Three "polys"
   A. Polyphagia
   B. Polyuria
   C. Polydipsia
II. Weight loss
III. Fatigue
IV. Hyperglycemia
V. Possible diabetic ketoacidosis
   A. Ketones as well as glucose in urine
   B. Dehydration
   C. Vomiting
   D. Electrolyte imbalance
   E. Metabolic acidosis
   F. Abdominal pain
   G. Fruity acetone breath
   H. Drowsiness progressing to coma

Therapeutic Management

I. Insulin replacement
II. Exercise
III. Nutritional intake that:
   A. Provides sufficient calories to balance daily expenditure of energy
   B. Satisfies requirements for growth and development
   C. Contains no concentrated sugars
IV. Management of hypoglycemia, illness, ketoacidosis
V. Promotion of adherence to regimen and self-management of disease

Nursing Care

DATA COLLECTION

I. Perform routine assessment.
II. Assist with diagnostic tests (e.g., fasting blood sugar, chemical strips, ketones, glucose tolerance).

PLANNING

I. Safe, effective care environment
   A. See Nursing Care of the Ill Child.
   B. Monitor blood sugar regularly.
II. Physiological integrity
   A. Promote regular monitoring of blood sugar and insulin intake.
   B. Promote careful balancing of nutrition and exercise.
   C. Prevent complications.
III. Psychosocial integrity
   A. Support and educate family and child.
   B. Encourage regular activities to prevent child from becoming emotionally crippled.
IV. Health promotion and maintenance
   A. Promote optimum health.
   B. Prepare family for home care.

IMPLEMENTATION

I. Monitor blood sugar regularly.
II. Keep accurate records of food intake and exercise.
III. Monitor for signs of hypoglycemia and hyperglycemia.
IV. Administer insulin as prescribed.
V. Teach family and child to check blood sugar and monitor food intake and exercise.
VI. Teach family and child to give injections.
VII. Teach family and child to regulate insulin intake according to food intake and exercise.

EVALUATION

I. Child has no episodes of hyperglycemia or hypoglycemia.
II. Child participates in normal childhood activities.
III. Family and child demonstrate ability to prepare medications and to give injections safely.
IV. Family and child demonstrate the ability to regulate diet.
V. Family and child demonstrate ability to modify insulin intake to match food and exercise.

Hypothyroidism (Congenital)

Description

Congenital hypothyroidism is a deficiency in secretion of thyroid hormones.

Pathophysiology

I. Deficiency of thyroid hormones causing retardation in growth and development

Signs and Symptoms

I. Infancy
   A. Cool, dry, mottled skin
   B. Coarse, sparse hair
   C. Enlarged tongue
   D. Hoarse cry
   E. Diminished activity
   F. Difficulty feeding
II. Childhood
   A. Continuous constipation
   B. Growth retardation
   C. Mental retardation

Therapeutic Management

I. Administer thyroid hormone.

Nursing Care

DATA COLLECTION

I. Perform routine assessment.
II. Assist with diagnostic procedures: thyroid hormone tests.

PLANNING

I. Safe, effective care environment
   A. See Nursing Care of the Ill Child.
II. Physiological integrity
   A. Prevent complications.
III. Psychosocial integrity
   A. See Nursing Care of the Ill Child.
   B. Support and educate child and family.
   C. Prepare child and family for procedures or surgery, if needed.
IV. Health promotion and maintenance
   A. Promote optimum health.
   B. Prepare family for home care.

IMPLEMENTATION

I. Explain or reinforce explanation of disease and therapies.
II. Teach family administration of thyroid hormone.

EVALUATION

I. Child displays normal growth and development.
II. Family demonstrates an understanding of the disease and the ability to provide home care.

Genitourinary Disorders

Urinary Tract Infection

Description

Urinary tract infection is an infection of any portion of the urinary tract and includes urethritis, cystitis, ureteritis, pyelonephritis.

Pathophysiology

I. Bacterial invasion of urinary structures, usually confined to the bladder but possibly ascending to upper collecting system and kidney, where it produces inflammatory changes, with scarring and loss of renal tissue

Signs and Symptoms

I. Children <2 years old
   A. Fever of abrupt onset
   B. Poor feeding
   C. Vomiting
   D. Diarrhea
   E. Abdominal distention
   F. Frequent or infrequent voiding
   G. Constant squirming
   H. Strong-smelling urine
   I. Diaper rash
II. Children >2 years old
   A. Bedwetting
   B. Daytime incontinence (toilet-trained child)
   C. Fever and chills
   D. Strong or foul-smelling urine
   E. Increased frequency of urination
   F. Localized sharp or dull pain
   G. Urgency
   H. Abdominal pain
   I. Flank pain
   J. Bloody urine
   K. Vomiting (in preschool children)

Therapeutic Management

I. Treat with antibacterial preparations (systemic penicillins, sulfonamides).
II. Detect or correct anatomic abnormalities.
III. Prevent recurrences.
IV. Preserve renal function.

Nursing Care

DATA COLLECTION

I. Perform routine assessment.
II. Observe elimination behaviors, including amount and character of urine output.
III. Assist with diagnostic procedures: urinalysis, IV pyelography, cystoscopy, cystourethrography, ultrasonography.

PLANNING

I. Safe, effective care environment
   A. See Nursing Care of the Ill Child.
II. Physiological integrity
   A. Help to eradicate organisms.
   B. Prevent complications.
III. Psychosocial integrity
   A. See Nursing Care of the Ill Child.
   B. Support and educate child and family.
   C. Prepare child and family for procedures.
IV. Health promotion and maintenance
   A. Promote optimum health.
   B. Achieve and maintain optimum hydration.
   C. Prevent recurrence.
   D. Prepare family for home care.

IMPLEMENTATION

I. Administer antibacterial medications as prescribed.
II. Teach child and family preventive hygiene habits (e.g., wipe genitals from front to back, avoid tight-fitting clothing in genital area).
III. Encourage adequate fluid intake.
IV. Explain procedures needed for diagnosis and evaluation.
V. Teach family skills and procedures needed for home care, including expected results of medication and possible side effects.

EVALUATION

I. Child exhibits no evidence of infection.
II. Child and family demonstrate good hygienic practices.
III. Family demonstrates an understanding of the disease and the ability to provide home care.

Nephrotic Syndrome

Description

Nephrotic syndrome is a chronic renal disease.

Pathophysiology

I. Protein leakage into urine (proteinuria)
II. Fluid accumulation in tissues
III. Reduced renal blood flow

Signs and Symptoms

I. Weight gain
II. Edema
   A. Puffiness around eyes
   B. Abdominal swelling
III. Diarrhea
IV. Anorexia
V. Normal or slightly decreased blood pressure
VI. Increased susceptibility to infection
VII. Easy fatigability
VIII. Urine
   A. Decreased
   B. Frothy
   C. Darkly opalescent

Therapeutic Management

I. Activity as tolerated
II. Salt restriction (during edematous stage)
III. Fluid restriction, if severe edema present
IV. Corticosteroids (prednisone)
V. Immunosuppressive agents in severe cases (cyclophosphamide)
VI. Prevention of infection with prophylactic antibiotics, sometimes

Nursing Care

DATA COLLECTION

I. Perform routine assessment.
II. Observe amount and character of urine.
III. Assess edema: measure I&O, specific gravity of urine; weight; abdominal girth.
IV. Assess pulse and blood pressure.
V. Assist with diagnostic procedures: urinalysis, serum protein measurements, renal biopsy (sometimes).

PLANNING

I. Safe, effective care environment
   A. See Nursing Care of the Ill Child.
   B. Prevent infection.
II. Physiological integrity
   A. Decrease urinary protein output.
   B. Prevent complications.
   C. Conserve energy.
III. Psychosocial integrity
   A. See Nursing Care of the Ill Child.
   B. Support and educate child and family.
   C. Prepare child and family for procedures, surgery as needed.
IV. Health promotion and maintenance
   A. Promote optimum health.
   B. Achieve and maintain optimum fluid and nutrition.
   C. Prepare family for home care.

IMPLEMENTATION

I. Practice careful medical asepsis.
II. Avoid contact with infected persons or items.
III. Administer corticosteroids, immunosuppressive agents, and antibiotics as prescribed.
IV. Administer drugs orally or IV, but never intramuscularly or subcutaneously.
V. Provide good skin care, especially in skinfolds of edematous areas (powder).
VI. Change child's position frequently.
VII. Promote quiet activities.
VIII. Provide high-protein diet, appropriate for age, and snacks to encourage eating.

A. Use no added salt and discourage salty foods (e.g., potato chips).

B. Fluids may be restricted to control edema.

IX. Weigh daily, with same clothes and at same time of day.

X. Accurately record I&O.

XI. Teach family skills and procedures needed for home care, including expected results of medication and possible side effects.

EVALUATION

I. Child exhibits no evidence of edema.

II. Child achieves normal urinary output.

III. Child exhibits no evidence of infection or skin breakdown.

IV. Child engages in activities appropriate to age and condition.

V. Family demonstrates an understanding of the disease and the ability to provide home care.

Acute Poststreptococcal Glomerulonephritis

Description

Acute poststreptococcal glomerulonephritis is an inflammation of the renal glomeruli after a streptococcal infection.

Pathophysiology

I. Reaction of renal tissues to group A β-hemolytic streptococci

II. Retention of water and sodium

Signs and Symptoms

I. Edema, especially periorbital

II. Anorexia

III. Hematuria

IV. Pallor

V. Irritability

VI. Lethargy

VII. Ill appearance

VIII. Headache

IX. Abdominal or flank pain

X. Dysuria

XI. Vomiting

XII. Mild to moderately elevated blood pressure

XIII. Urine
A. Severely reduced volume
B. Cloudy appearance
C. Smoky brown color

XIV. Hematological tests
A. Elevated antistreptolysin-O titer, ESR, CRP

Therapeutic Management

I. Restricted activity during acute phase

II. Regular diet with sodium restricted according to severity of symptoms

III. Dietary potassium restricted during periods of decreased urinary output

IV. Antibiotics

V. Antihypertensives

Nursing Care

DATA COLLECTION

I. Perform routine assessment.

II. Take health history for evidence of recent streptococcal infection.

III. Monitor vital signs and weight.

IV. Assess for signs of cerebral edema.

V. Carefully measure I&O.

VI. Observe character of urine.

VII. Assist with diagnostic procedures: urinalysis, blood count, throat culture, serological tests (e.g., ESR, CRP), streptozyme titer test, and antistreptolysin titer test.

PLANNING

I. Safe, effective care environment
A. See Nursing Care of the Ill Child.
B. Promote rest.

II. Physiological integrity
A. Provide appropriate diet and promote appetite.
B. Prevent and observe for complications.

III. Psychosocial integrity
A. See Nursing Care of the Ill Child.
B. Support and educate child and family.
C. Prepare child and family for procedures, surgery as needed.

IV. Health promotion and maintenance
A. Promote optimum health.
B. Prepare family for home care.

IMPLEMENTATION

I. Encourage frequent rest periods.

II. Provide and encourage quiet activities.

III. Administer antibiotics and antihypertensives as prescribed.

IV. Use no added salt at meals; discourage highly salted foods (e.g., potato chips, salted nuts).

V. Provide low-potassium diet, if prescribed.

VI. Separate from other children with infections.

VII. Teach home care, including expected results of medication and possible side effects.

EVALUATION

I. Child plays quietly and rests as needed.

II. Child eats appropriate diet.

III. Child remains free of complications.

IV. Family demonstrates an understanding of the condition and the ability to provide home care.

Cryptorchism

Description

Cryptorchism is a failure of one or both testes to descend normally into the scrotum.

Pathophysiology

I. Descent can be arrested at any point along the inguinal canal.

II. Condition is usually unilateral and associated with inguinal hernia.

III. Usual course is spontaneous descent within a year.

Signs and Symptoms

  I. Rarely a cause of discomfort
 II. Empty scrotum: unilateral or bilateral
III. Testes palpable if within the inguinal canal

Therapeutic Management

  I. Medical: human gonadotropin administration after 1 year of age
 II. Surgical: orchiopexy before 3 years of age

Nursing Care

DATA COLLECTION

  I. Perform routine assessment.

PLANNING

  I. Safe, effective care environment
     A. See Nursing Care of the Ill Child.
 II. Physiological integrity
     A. Prevent complications.
III. Psychosocial integrity
     A. See Nursing Care of the Ill Child.
     B. Promote a positive body image.
     C. Support and educate child and family.
     D. Prepare child and family for surgery.
IV. Health promotion and maintenance
     A. Promote optimum health.
     B. Prepare family for home care.

IMPLEMENTATION

  I. Provide clean wound care.
 II. Present positive feedback to child and family.
III. Teach family skills and procedures needed for home care.

EVALUATION

  I. Family seeks early evaluation and therapy.
 II. Family demonstrates an understanding of the condition and the ability to provide home care.
III. Child exhibits no evidence of infection.
IV. Child displays a positive body image.

Wilms' Tumor

Description

Wilms' tumor is a malignant neoplasm of the kidney.

Pathophysiology

  I. Develops from abnormal embryonic tissue usually by age 3 years
 II. Starts in renal capsule and grows into the surrounding tissues

Signs and Symptoms

  I. Abdomen that becomes large
 II. Firm, nontender abdominal mass
III. Symptoms related to pressure of tumor on tissues

  A. Constipation
  B. Vomiting
  C. Difficult breathing

Therapeutic Management

  I. Surgical removal of tumor
 II. Chemotherapy and sometimes radiation to treat disease and to minimize metastasis

Nursing Care

DATA COLLECTION

  I. Perform routine assessment.
 II. Assist with diagnostic procedures (e.g., tomography, IV pyelography, ultrasound, biochemical and hematological studies, urinalysis).

PLANNING

  I. Safe, effective care environment
     A. See Nursing Care of the Ill Child.
     B. Avoid touching abdomen and tumor before surgery.
 II. Physiological integrity
     A. Prevent complications.
     B. Assist with chemotherapy and radiation.
III. Psychosocial integrity
     A. See Nursing Care of the Ill Child.
     B. Support and educate child and family.
     C. Prepare child and family for procedures, surgery as needed.
IV. Health promotion and maintenance
     A. Promote optimum health.

IMPLEMENTATION

  I. Avoid palpating abdomen after diagnosis is suspected or confirmed.
 II. Administer antimetabolites as prescribed.
III. Provide support to family and encourage expression of feelings regarding a child with a life-threatening disorder.
IV. Educate family regarding observations for symptoms of side effects of chemotherapy or radiotherapy.
 V. Teach family skills and procedures needed for home care.

EVALUATION

  I. Child displays no ill effects of therapies.
 II. Child does not exhibit signs of metastasis.
III. Caregiver ensures that child has uneventful recovery from surgery.
IV. Family members express their feelings and concerns.
 V. Family demonstrates an understanding of the condition and the ability to provide home care.

Neurological Disorders

Myelomeningocele (Infant)

Description

  I. Spina bifida: defect in closure of vertebral column, with varying degrees of tissue protrusion through vertebral opening

II. Spina bifida occulta: failure of complete closure of the vertebral column with no outpouching
III. Meningocele: hernial protrusion of saclike cyst of meninges containing spinal fluid
IV. Myelomeningocele: hernial protrusion of a saclike cyst containing meninges, spinal fluid, and a portion of the spinal cord with its nerves

Pathophysiology

I. Degree of neurological damage dependent on extent and location of the outpouching.
II. Sensory disturbances match the motor dysfunction (see Signs and Symptoms).

Signs and Symptoms

I. Hernia evident with myelomeningocele and meningocele
II. If lesion is high, severe paralysis
III. If lesion is low, in sacral spine only, minimal weakness of legs
IV. Incontinence
V. Lack of bowel control
VI. Loss of feeling below the lesion

Therapeutic Management

I. Surgically cover skin and close lesion.
II. Treat complications: infections, hydrocephalus, renal problems.
III. Correct any associated orthopedic deformities.
IV. Provide mobility.

Nursing Care

DATA COLLECTION

I. Perform routine assessment.
II. Assess neurological status.
III. Assist with diagnostic procedures: transillumination, x-ray.
IV. Observe pressure areas for signs of skin breakdown.
V. Assess for evidence of complications (e.g., enlarging head, dislocated hip, meningitis).

PLANNING

I. Safe, effective care environment
   A. See Nursing Care of the Ill Child.
II. Physiological integrity
   A. Prevent injury to the sac (preoperative).
   B. Prevent complications.
III. Psychosocial integrity
   A. See Nursing Care of the Ill Child.
   B. Support and educate child and family.
   C. Prepare child and family for procedures, surgery as needed.
IV. Health promotion and maintenance
   A. Promote optimum health.
   B. Achieve and maintain optimum fluid and nutrition.
   C. Prepare family for home care.

IMPLEMENTATION

I. Apply sterile, moist dressing over sac and moisten with saline or antimicrobial solution as prescribed.
II. Use care in cleaning soiled sac.
III. Position infant on stomach or side.
IV. Place infant on fleece pad to reduce pressure on knees and ankles.
V. Maintain legs in abduction with pad between knees and roll beneath ankles.
VI. Avoid diapering; place infant on diaper or pad and change as needed.
VII. Employ meticulous skin care, especially in genital area, because of leaking urine and stool.
VIII. Provide gentle ROM exercises to paralyzed extremities as prescribed.
IX. Observe sac for any change in size.
X. Observe for any leaking fluid.
XI. Teach family skills needed for home care, including signs of increased intracranial pressure (hydrocephalus is frequent complication of myelomeningocele).

EVALUATION

I. Infant's skin remains clean and intact, with no evidence of infection or breakdown.
II. Infant exhibits no evidence of infection.
III. Signs of complications are detected early and appropriate interventions implemented.
IV. Family demonstrates an understanding of the condition and the ability to provide home care.

Hydrocephalus

Description

Hydrocephalus is a condition caused by an increase in the amount of cerebrospinal fluid (CSF) within the cranium.
   I. Communicating: CSF flows freely through the ventricular system to the subarachnoid space.
   II. Noncommunicating: flow of CSF in the ventricular system is obstructed.

Pathophysiology

I. Increased accumulation of CSF in the ventricles
II. Ventricles enlarging
III. Pressure on the brain against the skull
IV. Damage to brain tissue

Signs and Symptoms

I. Infancy
   A. Irritability and vomiting
   B. Bulging fontanels
   C. Crying when picked up; yawning, quiet when set down
   D. Display of changes in level of consciousness possible
   E. Feeding difficulties
   F. Brief, shrill, high-pitched cry
II. Early infancy
   A. Abnormal rapid head growth
   B. Bulging, tense, nonpulsating fontanels

   C. Separated cranial sutures
   D. High-pitched cry
III. Later infancy
   A. Enlarging frontal bones ("bossing")
   B. Depressed eyes
   C. Sclera visible above iris ("setting sun" sign)
IV. Childhood
   A. Headache
   B. Deviation of the eyes
   C. Irritability
   D. Lethargy
   E. Apathy
   F. Confusion

Therapeutic Management

   I. Surgical
   A. Remove obstruction (e.g., tumor, cyst).
   B. Relieve intracranial pressure via ventricular tap during preoperative period.
   C. Shunt CSF from ventricle to extracranial compartment (usually the peritoneum), to relieve intracranial pressure.
   D. Revise shunt as needed during growth.
   II. Medical
   A. Treat complications (infection, shunt malfunction).

Nursing Care

DATA COLLECTION

   I. Perform routine assessment.
   II. Measure head circumference routinely.
   III. Perform neurological examination; observe for signs of increasing intracranial pressure.
   IV. Observe for signs of infection preoperatively and postoperatively.
   V. Assist with diagnostic procedures: echoencephalography, tomography.

PLANNING

   I. Safe, effective care environment
   A. See Nursing Care of the Ill Child.
   II. Physiological integrity
   A. Prevent complications of the disorder or the corrective surgery.
   III. Psychosocial integrity
   A. See Nursing Care of the Ill Child.
   B. Support and educate child and family.
   C. Prepare child and family for procedures, surgery as needed.
   IV. Health promotion and maintenance
   A. Promote optimum health.
   B. Prepare family for home care.

IMPLEMENTATION

   I. Preoperatively, support head to prevent strain on neck; turn frequently to avoid pressure injury.
   II. Position on back or on operated side to prevent pressure on shunt valve.
   III. Keep flat to prevent too-rapid reduction of intracranial fluid, if ordered.

   IV. Place on sheepskin.
   V. Pump valve mechanism as prescribed.
   VI. Monitor I&O, including IV infusion, to prevent fluid overload.
   VII. Check pupil equality.
   VIII. Measure head circumference daily.
   IX. Teach family skills needed for home care.

EVALUATION

   I. Child exhibits no evidence of infection or increased intracranial pressure.
   II. Family demonstrates understanding of the condition and the ability to provide home care.

Bacterial Meningitis

Description

Bacterial meningitis is an infection of the meninges.

Pathophysiology

   I. Usual organisms: *Haemophilus influenzae* (type B), *Streptococcus pneumoniae,* meningococci
   II. Most commonly a result of infection elsewhere in the body

Signs and Symptoms

   I. Fever
   II. Vomiting
   III. Irritability
   IV. Seizures
   V. Rigidity of neck, possibly progressing to opisthotonos
   VI. Infants and young children
   A. Bulging fontanel (infants)
   VII. Children and adolescents
   A. Headache
   B. Changes in ability to feel sensations
   C. Positive Kernig's and Brudzinski's signs
   D. Possible development of delirium, coma

Therapeutic Management

   I. Prevent spread of infection.
   II. Administer antimicrobials.
   III. Maintain optimum fluids.
   IV. Maintain breathing.
   V. Reduce intracranial pressure.
   VI. Manage shock.
   VII. Control seizure.
   VIII. Control extremes of body temperature.
   IX. Treat complications.

Nursing Care

DATA COLLECTION

   I. Perform routine assessment.
   II. Perform regular neurological assessment.
   III. Observe for signs of increased intracranial pressure, shock, respiratory distress.

94 Clinical Specialties Content Reviews and Tests

IV. Assist with diagnostic procedures: lumbar puncture, cultures (CSF, blood), complete blood count (CBC), other laboratory tests.

PLANNING

I. Safe, effective care environment
  A. See Nursing Care of the Ill Child.
  B. Prevent or reduce environmental stimulation.
  C. Prevent transmission of disease to others.
II. Physiological integrity
  A. Help to treat organisms.
  B. Prevent complications.
III. Psychosocial integrity
  A. See Nursing Care of the Ill Child.
  B. Support and educate child and family.
  C. Prepare child and family for procedures, surgery as needed.
IV. Health promotion and maintenance
  A. Promote optimum health.
  B. Achieve and maintain optimum hydration and nutrition.
  C. Prepare family for home care.

IMPLEMENTATION

I. Implement appropriate isolation precautions and maintain as needed.
II. Teach family proper protective procedures.
III. Administer antimicrobials as prescribed.
IV. Monitor and maintain IV infusion.
V. Keep environmental stimuli at minimum (e.g., quiet, dimly lit room); avoid noisy activities and excessive handling of child.
VI. Implement seizure precautions.
VII. Position for comfort: head of bed slightly elevated, side-lying position; no pillow to reduce neck stretching.
VIII. Observe and record any seizure activity.
IX. Administer anticonvulsive medication, if ordered.
X. Teach family skills needed for home care, including expected results of medication and possible side effects.

EVALUATION

I. Child appears comfortable and alert and interacts with family.
II. Child remains free of seizures.
III. Signs of complications are detected early and appropriate interventions implemented.
IV. Family demonstrates an understanding of the disease and the ability to provide home care.
V. Others remain free of infection.

Epilepsy (Generalized, Tonic-Clonic, Grand Mal Seizures)

Description

Epilepsy consists of recurrent convulsive seizures of unknown cause.

I. Petit mal seizure (also known as absence seizure)
  A. Moments of blank staring
  B. Breaks in speech and thinking
  C. Minor tremors
  D. No loss of consciousness

II. Grand mal seizure
  A. Involuntary muscular contractions of the large muscles (tonic-clonic type)

Pathophysiology

I. Spontaneous electric discharge.
II. Partial seizures: discharges limited to a more or less specific region of the cerebral cortex.
III. Generalized seizures: discharges arise in the brain and involve both hemispheres of brain.

Signs and Symptoms

I. Absence seizures
  A. Brief loss of consciousness
  B. Abrupt onset; 20 or more attacks per day
  C. Minor tremors
  D. Often mistaken for inattentiveness or daydreaming
II. Tonic-clonic seizures
  A. Occurrence without warning
  B. Tonic phase lasting about 10–20 seconds
    1. Immediate loss of consciousness
    2. Falling to floor, if standing
    3. Eyes rolling upward
    4. Stiffening in generalized, symmetrical tonic contraction of entire body
    5. Arms usually flexed
    6. Legs, head, and neck extended
    7. Increased salivation
    8. Possibly a peculiar piercing cry
    9. Apneic, possibly becoming cyanotic
  C. Clonic phase lasting about 30 seconds
    1. Violent jerking movements as the trunk and extremities undergo rhythmic contraction and relaxation
    2. Foaming at the mouth possible
    3. Incontinence of urine and feces possible
  D. As attack ends, movements becoming less intense, occurring at longer intervals, then ceasing entirely

Therapeutic Management

I. Control seizures or reduce their frequency with anticonvulsants.
II. Discover and correct cause when possible.
III. Promote as normal a lifestyle as possible.

Nursing Care

DATA COLLECTION

I. Perform routine assessment.
II. Take family history for evidence of seizures.
III. Take careful history of the seizure:
  A. Age at onset of seizures
  B. Time of day when seizures occur
  C. Detailed description of seizure
  D. Any factors causing seizure: environmental, physical
  E. Sensory warning associated with seizure (aura)
  F. Length and progression of seizure
  G. Feelings and behavior after seizure

IV. Observe seizure:
  A. Behavior at onset of seizure
    1. Change in facial expression
    2. Cry or other sound
    3. Involuntary movements
    4. Random activity
    5. Position of head, body, extremities
    6. Time of onset
  B. Movement
    1. Change of position, if any
    2. Description of place movement began
    3. Tonic phase: length, parts of body involved
    4. Clonic phase: twitching or jerking, parts of body involved, sequence of parts involved, any change in movements
    5. Face
     a. Color change: pallor, cyanosis, flushing
     b. Perspiration
     c. Mouth position, teeth clenching, frothing, tongue biting
    6. Eyes
     a. Position: straight ahead, deviation
     b. Pupils (if able to assess): change in size, equality
    7. Respiratory effort
     a. Presence and length of apnea
     b. Any cyanosis
    8. Other: involuntary urination or defecation
  C. Behavior after seizure
    1. State of consciousness
    2. Orientation
    3. Motor ability
    4. Speech
    5. Sensations
V. Assist with diagnostic procedures: electroencephalogram (EEG), skull x-ray, tomography, blood studies.

PLANNING

I. Safe, effective care environment
  A. See Nursing Care of the Ill Child.
  B. Prevent injury to child during seizure.
  C. Provide an environment with seizure precautions.
II. Physiological integrity
  A. Prevent seizures if possible.
III. Psychosocial integrity
  A. See Nursing Care of the Ill Child.
  B. Support child and family.
  C. Educate child and family.
  D. Prepare child and family for procedures.
  E. Promote positive self-image in child.
IV. Health promotion and maintenance
  A. Promote optimum health.
  B. Prepare family for home care.

IMPLEMENTATION

I. Administer anticonvulsants as prescribed.
II. Protect child from injury during seizure:
  A. Do not attempt to restrain child or use force.
  B. If child is standing or sitting, ease child down to prevent falling.
  C. Avoid placing anything in child's mouth.
  D. Loosen restrictive clothing.
  E. Prevent child from hitting hard or sharp objects during uncontrolled movements.
  F. Move furniture or other objects out of way.
  G. Do not attempt to move child, unless he or she is in danger.
III. Promote use of protective helmet for child subject to frequent seizures.
IV. Maintain siderails on bed.
V. Pad bumpers or add padding to the siderail.
VI. Discourage a child subject to daily seizures from engaging in activities in which injury might occur.
VII. Provide comfort after seizure as the child may feel tired and sore.
VIII. Help child and family deal with problems related to the disorder.
IX. Emphasize need for adherence to medical regimen.
X. Help child and family determine activities appropriate to child's condition, interests, and developmental level: avoid contact sports, climbing trees, or apparatus from which child might fall.
XI. Teach family skills needed for home care, including expected results of medication and possible side effects.

EVALUATION

I. Child remains seizure-free.
II. Child exhibits no evidence of physical injury.
III. Child expresses feelings and concerns regarding his or her disease and its ramifications.
IV. Family follows instructions.
V. Family treats child as any other child in the family.
VI. Family demonstrates an understanding of the disease and the ability to provide home care.

Musculoskeletal Disorders

Clubfoot

Description

Clubfoot is a deformity in which the foot is twisted out of its normal shape or position.
I. Talipes: deformity involving the heel
II. Pes: deformity involving the foot

Pathophysiology

I. Cause unknown
II. Some distortions caused by prenatal positioning, not structural problem

Signs and Symptoms

I. Some positional deformities are:
  A. Inversion, or bending inward
  B. Eversion, or bending outward
  C. Plantar flexion (in which toes are lower than heel)
  D. Dorsiflexion (in which toes are higher than heel)
II. Most common deformity is:
  A. Talipes equinovarus: foot points downward and inward in various degrees of deformity

Therapeutic Management

I. Correct deformity by application of successive casts or by surgery.
II. Maintain correction until normal muscle balance is attained.
III. Observe as a follow-up to prevent possible recurrence.

Nursing Care

DATA COLLECTION

I. Perform routine assessment.

PLANNING

I. Safe, effective care environment
   A. See Nursing Care of the Ill Child.
   B. Promote safety for age.
II. Physiological integrity
   A. Promote correction of deformity.
   B. Prevent complications.
III. Psychosocial integrity
   A. See Nursing Care of the Ill Child.
   B. Support family.
   C. Prepare family for casting.
IV. Health promotion and maintenance
   A. Promote optimum health.
   B. Prepare family for home care.

IMPLEMENTATION

I. Implement cast care.
II. Implement stretching or strapping as directed.
III. Teach family skills needed for home care.

EVALUATION

I. Cast remains clean and intact.
II. Family is able to do stretching exercises or to handle straps if that method is prescribed.

Congenital Hip Dysplasia

Description

Congenital hip dysplasia is imperfect development of the hip or dislocation of the hip.

Pathophysiology

I. Subluxation: incomplete dislocation of hip
   A. Femoral head staying in contact with acetabulum
   B. Relaxed ligaments
II. Dislocation
   A. Femoral head out of contact with acetabulum
   B. Displacement posteriorly and superiorly over the rim
   C. Click heard as femur slips out of acetabulum

Signs and Symptoms

I. Infant
   A. Shortening of limb on affected side
   B. Restricted movement of hip on affected side
   C. Unequal thigh folds

Therapeutic Management

Varies with age of child and extent of dislocation
   I. 0–6 months old
      A. Application of external device (Pavlik harness) that maintains femur centered in the acetabulum in the attitude of flexion
   II. 6–18 months
      A. Traction followed by plaster cast immobilization
   III. Older child (>18 months old)
      A. Surgical reduction

Nursing Care

DATA COLLECTION

I. Perform routine assessment.
II. Assess corrective device for proper application and/or maintenance.
III. Assist with diagnostic procedures: x-ray, sonography.

PLANNING

I. Safe, effective care environment
   A. See Nursing Care of the Ill Child.
   B. Promote an appropriate environment for age.
II. Physiological integrity
   A. Maintain correct position of hip in acetabulum.
   B. Prevent complications related to wearing corrective device.
III. Psychosocial integrity
   A. See Nursing Care of the Ill Child.
   B. Support and educate child and family.
   C. Prepare child and family for procedures, surgery as needed.
IV. Health promotion and maintenance
   A. Promote optimum health.
   B. Prepare family for home care.

IMPLEMENTATION

I. Teach family the purpose, function, application, and maintenance of the Pavlik harness, cast, or traction.
II. Help family to adapt routine nurturing activities and equipment to accommodate corrective device or cast: feeding, sleeping, playing, safety measures (e.g., car seat).
III. Avoid lifting child by legs to diaper.

EVALUATION

I. Child is properly maintained in corrective device.
II. Child engages in activities appropriate to age or plays as much as possible.
III. Family demonstrates understanding of the condition and its therapy and the ability to provide home care.

Coxa Plana (Legg-Calvé-Perthes Disease)

Description

Coxa plana is a progressive destruction of the femoral head, producing varying degrees of deformity.

Pathophysiology

I. Lack of circulation to the femoral head
II. Degeneration by bone absorption

III. Regeneration of the bone
IV. Process taking about 4 years

Signs and Symptoms

I. Limp on affected side
II. Pain: soreness or aching
    A. In hip, entire length of thigh, or knee
    B. Worse on rising or at end of a long day
    C. Tenderness over hip capsule
III. Joint dysfunction and limited ROM
IV. Stiffness
V. External hip rotation (late sign)

Therapeutic Management

I. Rest, initially, to reduce inflammation and restore motion
II. Traction to stretch tight adductor muscles (sometimes)
III. Containment of femoral head in acetabulum by non-weight-bearing device (abduction brace, leg cast, leather harness)
IV. Surgical correction (sometimes)

Nursing Care

DATA COLLECTION

I. Perform routine assessment.
II. Assess corrective device for proper application and signs of irritation.
III. Assist with diagnostic procedure: x-ray.

PLANNING

I. Safe, effective care environment
    A. Alter physical environment as necessary to accommodate corrective device.
II. Physiological integrity
    A. Maintain corrective device.
    B. Prevent complications.
III. Psychosocial integrity
    A. Support and educate child and family.
    B. Prepare child and family for procedures.
IV. Health promotion and maintenance
    A. Promote optimum health.
    B. Prepare family for home care.

IMPLEMENTATION

I. Encourage child to maintain usual activities within limitations imposed by the disease and its therapy.
II. Teach family purpose, function, application, and maintenance of corrective device.

EVALUATION

I. Child engages in usual activities.
II. Family complies with therapeutic regimen.
III. Family demonstrates an understanding of the disease and the ability to provide home care.

Scoliosis

Description

Scoliosis is lateral curative of the spine. Usually consists of two curves: the original curve and a compensatory curve in the opposite direction.

I. Functional: caused by another deformity (e.g., unequal leg length)
II. Structural: caused by changes in the spine and its supporting structures

Pathophysiology

I. Structural scoliosis
    A. Spinal and support structure changes
    B. Loss of flexibility

Signs and Symptoms

I. Undressed subject viewed from back:
    A. Primary curvature with a compensatory curvature that places head in alignment
    B. Head and hips out of alignment
    C. Rib hump and asymmetry when child bends forward from waist
II. Dressed subject
    A. In girls wearing dresses, hems that do not hang straight

Therapeutic Management

I. Spinal strengthening and realignment
    A. Medical
        1. External bracing (Milwaukee)
        2. Casting
        3. Skeletal traction techniques
            a. Halo: femoral
            b. Halo: pelvic
        4. Electrical stimulation
    B. Surgical: internal fixation
        1. Harrington rod
        2. Spinal fusion

Nursing Care

DATA COLLECTION

I. Perform routine assessment.
II. Inspect corrective appliance and skin regularly for possible problems (e.g., skin irritation), and assess for correct application and fit.
III. Assist with diagnostic procedure: x-ray.

PLANNING

I. Safe, effective care environment
    A. Prevent injury.
II. Physiological integrity
    A. Nonsurgical treatment: Maintain prescribed appliance.
    B. Surgical treatment: Provide competent postoperative care.
    C. Prevent complications.
III. Psychosocial integrity
    A. Prepare child and family for long-term therapy.
    B. Support and educate child and family.
    C. Prepare child and family for procedures, surgery as needed.
    D. Help child adjust to appliance.

E. Promote a positive self-image.
IV. Health promotion and maintenance
  A. Promote optimum health.
  B. Prepare child and family for home care.

IMPLEMENTATION

I. Explain or reinforce explanation of condition, including:
  A. How appliance corrects defect
  B. Reason for lengthy treatment
  C. Anticipated results of therapy
  D. How client can help achieve desired goals
  E. Maintenance of therapeutic devices
II. Help child adjust to restricted movement.
III. Provide guidance regarding selection of appropriate exercises and anticipated problems (e.g., selection of clothing, reactions of peers).
IV. Discuss freedoms and restraints imposed by brace or rod.
V. Encourage independence and self-care when appropriate.
VI. Emphasize positive long-term outcome.
VII. Provide feedback and praise for positive behavior and compliance.

EVALUATION

I. Child engages in activities appropriate to age and capabilities.
II. Child displays evidence of positive self-image.
III. Child and family comply with therapeutic regimen.
IV. Child and family demonstrate an understanding of the condition and the ability to provide home care.

Fractures

Description

Fractures are traumatic injuries to bone in which the bone is broken.

Pathophysiology

I. Complete: bone fragments separated
II. Incomplete: bone fragments attached
III. Simple, or closed: no break in skin
IV. Open, or compound: bone protruding through break in skin
V. Greenstick: incomplete fracture because soft bone bends
VI. Comminuted: multiple breaks in one spot
VII. In children, at fracture site the periosteum remains intact and remarkably stable

Signs and Symptoms

I. Pain or tenderness at site of break
II. Generalized swelling
III. Diminished functional use of affected part
IV. Possible bruising, severe muscular rigidity
V. Because of attached periosteum at fracture site, child possibly able to use affected part

Therapeutic Management

I. Reduce fracture; regain alignment of bony fragments.
  A. Closed or open reduction

II. Retain alignment and length of part through immobilization.
III. Restore function of injured parts.

Nursing Care

DATA COLLECTION

I. Perform routine assessment.
II. Obtain history of trauma.
III. Assist with diagnostic procedure: x-ray.
IV. Assess casted extremity regularly for pain, swelling, discoloration (pallor or cyanosis), ability to move part, paresthesia, pulse, odor.
V. Assess extremity in traction for maintenance of desired pull, body alignment, correct functioning of apparatus.
VI. For open reduction, assess bleeding over operative site; outline edges of stain to assess increase.

PLANNING

I. Safe, effective care environment
  A. See Nursing Care of the Ill Child.
  B. Prevent injury.
  C. Provide an environment that facilitates healing.
II. Physiological integrity
  A. Maintain bone immobility.
  B. Promote bone healing.
  C. Prevent complications.
III. Psychosocial integrity
  A. See Nursing Care of the Ill Child.
  B. Support and educate child and family.
  C. Prepare child and family for procedures.
IV. Health promotion and maintenance
  A. Prepare family for home care.

IMPLEMENTATION

I. Keep casted extremity elevated on pillows or other support for first day, or as directed.
II. Apply "petaling" moleskin to rough edges of cast.
III. Maintain integrity of cast; keep clean and dry, avoiding damage to cast.
IV. Prevent child from placing crumbs or small items inside cast.
V. For open reduction, administer pain medication as needed.
VI. Teach crutch walking to child with lower-extremity injury.
VII. Teach family skills needed for home care: care of cast, signs of complications.

EVALUATION

I. Cast remains dry and intact.
II. Child exhibits no evidence of circulatory or neurological impairment.
III. Family demonstrates an understanding of the condition and the ability to provide home care.

Cerebral Palsy

Description

Cerebral palsy is impaired muscular control resulting from brain injury or occurring during a period of early brain growth.

Pathophysiology

I. Injury to the brain from pressure or oxygen deprivation before birth
II. Infection or toxicity after birth

Signs and Symptoms

I. Disorder of motor development
II. Possibly abnormal motor performance—slight to severe impairment
   A. Inability to stand or sit
   B. Increased stiffness of muscles
   C. Difficulty in chewing and swallowing
   D. Drooling and impaired speech articulation
   E. Spastic movements—especially scissors gait
   F. Nonspastic: athetoid or atoxic
   G. Seizures
   H. Constipation
   I. Respiratory problems
   J. Orthopedic complications
   K. Dental problems
III. Behavior problems
IV. Vision and hearing problems
V. Learning disabilities
VI. Attention-deficit hyperactivity disorder

Therapeutic Management

I. Establish movement, communication, and self-help with braces, mobilizing devices, speech therapy.
II. Gain optimum appearance and use of motor abilities:
   A. Skeletal muscle relaxants (some older children)
   B. Antianxiety agents to relieve excessive motion
   C. Anticonvulsants for seizures
   D. Dextroamphetamine or methylphenidate (Ritalin) for hyperactivity
III. Correct any associated defects with orthopedic surgery when possible.
IV. Provide educational opportunities adapted to the individual child's needs and capabilities.

Nursing Care

DATA COLLECTION

I. Perform routine assessment.
II. Obtain history of child's behavior and attainment of developmental milestones.
III. Assist with diagnostic procedures: EEG, tomography, screening for metabolic defects, serum electrolytes.

PLANNING

I. Safe, effective care environment
   A. Help modify environment to conform to needs of child.
   B. Promote age-appropriate safety precautions.
II. Physiological integrity
   A. Promote relaxation.
   B. Establish movement and communication.
   C. Prevent complications.
   D. Promote adequate nutritional intake for age.
   E. Promote normal elimination.
III. Psychosocial integrity
   A. Assist with educational program.
   B. Promote positive self-image.
IV. Health promotion and maintenance
   A. Promote optimum health.
   B. Support family in its efforts to meet the needs of the child.

IMPLEMENTATION

I. Provide safe environment with padded furniture, siderails on beds, and sturdy furniture that does not slip; avoid scatter rugs and polished floors.
II. Restrain child when in chair or wheelchair.
III. Provide helmet for child who is prone to falls.
IV. Apply and correctly use braces.
V. Carry out and teach family to perform stretching exercises.
VI. Encourage sitting, crawling, and walking at appropriate ages.
VII. Use play that encourages desired behavior.
VIII. Use special devices that allow child independent motion.
IX. Maintain a well-regulated schedule that allows for adequate rest and sleep.
X. Help family modify equipment and activities to meet needs of child.
XI. Provide extra calories to meet extra energy demands of increased muscle activity.
XII. Encourage child to assist in care.
XIII. Enlist efforts of speech therapist.
XIV. Employ nonverbal communication methods.
XV. Promote and assist bowel elimination.
XVI. Teach family skills needed for care, including expected results of medication and possible side effects.
XVII. See Nursing Care of the Chronically Ill or Disabled Child.

EVALUATION

I. Child is sufficiently rested.
II. Child eats a balanced diet with sufficient calories for needs.
III. Child has normal bowel elimination.
IV. Child is able to communicate his or her needs to caregivers.
V. Family provides a safe environment for the child.
VI. Family demonstrates an understanding of the condition and the ability to provide home care.

Juvenile Rheumatoid Arthritis

Description

Juvenile rheumatoid arthritis is an inflammatory disease of the joints and connective tissues.

Pathophysiology

I. Similar to adult arthritis
II. Chronic inflammation of the joints
III. Joint swelling
IV. Limited motion caused by muscle spasm and inflammation
V. Eventual erosion, destruction, and fibrosis of articular cartilage

Signs and Symptoms

I. Joint characteristics
   A. Stiffness and swelling
   B. Tenderness
   C. Possibly painful to touch or relatively painless
   D. Warm to touch (seldom red)
   E. Loss of motion
   F. Characteristic morning stiffness or "gelling" on arising in the morning or after inactivity
II. Systemic
   A. Fever, higher in evening
   B. Enlarged liver, spleen, and lymph nodes
   C. Anemia
   D. Pallor
   E. Rash
   F. Pericarditis, myocarditis, and uveitis
   G. Aggravated by stress and fatigue

Therapeutic Management

I. Suppress inflammatory process with:
   A. Nonsteroidal anti-inflammatory drugs
   B. Cytotoxic drugs
   C. Corticosteroids
II. Preserve function or prevent deformity (or both) with physical therapy, occupational therapy, splinting, and positioning.
III. Reduce pain with analgesia and heat application.

Nursing Care

DATA COLLECTION

I. Perform routine assessment.
II. Observe for joint discomfort and movement.
III. Assist with diagnostic tests: x-ray, WBC count, rheumatoid factors, ESR, antinuclear antibodies; result of latex fixation test to detect disease in adults is negative in most children.

PLANNING

I. Safe, effective care environment
   A. See Nursing Care of the Ill Child.
   B. Modify environment as needed to facilitate child's mobility.
   C. Promote safe environment appropriate for age.
II. Physiological integrity
   A. Relieve discomfort.
   B. Prevent physical deformity and preserve joint function.
   C. Promote positive self-image and good self-esteem.
III. Psychosocial integrity
   A. See Nursing Care of the Ill Child.
IV. Health promotion and maintenance
   A. Promote good health practices.
   B. Promote self-care.
   C. Prepare family for home care.

IMPLEMENTATION

I. Administer anti-inflammatory preparations as prescribed.
II. Carry out or assist with physical therapy plan.

III. Provide heat to affected joints via bath, hot compresses, paraffin baths.
IV. Carry out ROM activities in appropriate locations (e.g., bath, pool, playroom).
V. Encourage activity appropriate to capabilities.
VI. Apply splints and support equipment (e.g., bolsters, sandbags, pillows) as prescribed.
VII. Help modify environment for safety and utensils to facilitate self-help.
VIII. Use child's natural affinity for play to encourage motion and activity.
IX. Teach family skills needed for home care:
   A. Administration of medications, including possible side effects
   B. Purpose and correct application of splints or appliances
   C. Modification of environment, clothing, and utensils to facilitate self-help

EVALUATION

I. Child moves with minimal or no discomfort.
II. Child engages in suitable play and self-help activities.
III. Child and family demonstrate an understanding of the disease and therapies and the ability to provide home care.

Cognitive and Sensory Disorders

Strabismus and Amblyopia

Description

Strabismus and amblyopia are disorders of vision: respectively, a malalignment of the eyes and a weakness of eye muscle.

Pathophysiology

I. Image viewed does not fall on corresponding parts of retina in both eyes.
II. Double vision (diplopia) occurs.
III. Child suppresses image in deviating eye to avoid double vision.
IV. Disuse causes impaired vision in involved eye.

Signs and Symptoms

I. Deviation apparent on inspection
II. Squinting in attempt to produce clearer vision

Therapeutic Management

I. Uninvolved-eye patching to force child to use and strengthen involved eye
II. Corrective lenses to help focus object on retina
III. Surgical correction

Nursing Care

DATA COLLECTION

I. Perform routine assessment.
II. Assist with diagnostic procedure: ophthalmologic examination.

PLANNING

   I. Safe, effective care environment
     A. Provide safe environment for child with both eyes patched.
   II. Physiological integrity
     A. Provide postoperative care after surgical correction.
     B. Promote compliance in nonsurgical therapies.
   III. Psychosocial integrity
     A. Support and educate child and family.
     B. Prepare child and family for procedures, surgery as needed.
   IV. Health promotion and maintenance
     A. Promote optimum health.

IMPLEMENTATION

   I. Implement safety precautions as for blind adult.
   II. Provide safe postoperative care.
   III. Apply sterile dressing changes.
   IV. Teach child and family proper use of patching or glasses.

EVALUATION

   I. Child exhibits desired oculomotor movements and eye alignment.
   II. Child and family comply with therapeutic regimen.
   III. Family demonstrates an understanding of the condition and the ability to provide home care.

Mental Retardation

Description

Mental retardation is defined as significantly subaverage general intellectual functioning: an IQ of 70 or below on an individually administered IQ test.

Pathophysiology

   I. Inherited disease (e.g., phenylketonuria, galactosemia)
   II. Infection (e.g., rubella)
   III. Drugs (e.g., excessive alcohol, chronic lead ingestion)
   IV. Down's syndrome
   V. Congenital malformations (e.g., microcephaly, hydrocephaly)
   VI. Birth injuries
   VII. Inadequate nutrition
   VIII. Failure to thrive

Signs and Symptoms

   I. Motor delay
   II. Intellectual delay: slower than normal rate of learning new skills
     A. Basic patterns of development maintained
     B. Time scale prolonged
   III. Delayed vision and hearing development
   IV. Delayed language
   V. Neurobehavioral disturbances

Therapeutic Management

   I. Infant stimulation
   II. Special education

   III. Appropriate protective care (home, institution)
   IV. General health supervision
   V. Correction of associated anomalies (e.g., heart defects, facial defects, impaired mobility)

Nursing Care

DATA COLLECTION

   I. Perform routine assessment.
   II. Obtain history of possible etiologic factors.
   III. Obtain developmental history.
   IV. Perform or assist with diagnostic procedures: developmental screening tests, IQ test, specific diagnostic tests (e.g., chromosome analysis, metabolic studies).

PLANNING

   I. Safe, effective care environment
     A. Ensure protected environment.
     B. Ensure safety for age.
   II. Physiological integrity
     A. Promote development.
   III. Psychosocial integrity
     A. Support and educate family.
     B. Promote acceptance by family.
     C. Promote special education for the child.
     D. Promote positive self-esteem in child and family.
   IV. Health promotion and maintenance
     A. Promote optimum health.
     B. Help family adjust to future care.

IMPLEMENTATION

   I. Help family to identify both short- and long-term goals.
   II. Teach family skills needed for home care:
     A. Set realistic goals for child to learn new activities.
     B. Promote self-help skills and independence.
     C. Provide play materials that stimulate development and promote self-help.
     D. Promote development of interpersonal skills.
   III. Help family to investigate and obtain special help for the child:
     A. Infant stimulation programs
     B. Special education
     C. Appropriate institutional care
   IV. Help to identify activities that promote self-esteem.

EVALUATION

   I. Child attains developmental milestones commensurate with cognitive level.
   II. Child develops optimum self-help within the limits of his or her capabilities.
   III. Family demonstrates an understanding of the condition and the ability to provide home care.

Down's Syndrome

Description

Down's syndrome, also called trisomy 21, is a genetic disorder characterized by varying degrees of mental retardation and multiple defects.

Pathophysiology

I. Increased incidence in children whose mothers were >35 years of age at the time of birth
II. In 92–95% of the cases, attributed to an extra chromosome 21

Signs and Symptoms

I. Physical characteristics
   A. Small rounded skull with a flattened appearance
   B. Inner epicanthal folds and eyes slant upward and outward
   C. Small nose with depressed bridge ("saddle nose")
   D. Protruding tongue
   E. Short hands and fingers
   F. Floppy infant
   G. Simian line (transverse palmar crease)
II. Associated characteristics
   A. Cardiac anomalies (most common congenital defects)
   B. Delayed eruption of teeth
   C. Fissured tongue
   D. High susceptibility to URI
   E. Umbilical hernia
   F. Affectionate, placid personality

Therapeutic Management

I. See Mental Retardation.
II. Correct physical defects.
III. Treat infections.

Nursing Care

DATA COLLECTION

I. Perform routine assessment.
II. Assist with diagnostic procedures: chromosome analysis, tests to diagnose suspected anomalies.

PLANNING

I. Safe, effective care environment
   A. See Mental Retardation.
   B. Prevent infection.
II. Physiological integrity
   A. See Mental Retardation.
III. Psychosocial integrity
   A. See Mental Retardation.
IV. Health promotion and maintenance
   A. See Mental Retardation.
   B. Prevent infections.
   C. Prevent additional children with Down's syndrome.

IMPLEMENTATION

I. See Mental Retardation.
II. Avoid exposure to persons with URIs.
III. Encourage genetic counseling when disorder is caused by a translocation.
IV. Prenatal: Encourage amniocentesis for pregnant women >35 years of age.
V. Encourage exercise (e.g., Special Olympics).

EVALUATION

I. See Mental Retardation.
II. Child exhibits no evidence of infection.

Skin Disorders

Scabies

Description

Scabies is a superficial infestation produced by the scabies mite, *Sarcoptes scabies.*

Pathophysiology

I. Impregnated female mite burrows under the skin and lays eggs.
II. Child is sensitized to mite.
III. Inflammatory response occurs 30–60 days after initial contact. If child is sensitized to mite, inflammatory response occurs in 48 hours.

Signs and Symptoms

I. Itching
II. Lesions: minute grayish-brown, threadlike lesion (burrow) with black dot at end
III. Distribution: primarily between fingers and toes, and in axillae, groin, and abdominal areas

Therapeutic Management

I. Treat mite with scabicide, usually 1% lindane (Kwell).
II. Relieve itching with soothing ointments or lotions.

Nursing Care

DATA COLLECTION

I. Perform routine assessment.
II. Assist with diagnostic procedure: skin scrapings observed under microscope for evidence of mite.

PLANNING

I. Safe, effective care environment
   A. Prevent spread of mite to others.
II. Physiological integrity
   A. Eliminate scabies mite.
   B. Relieve discomfort.
   C. Prevent or minimize scratching.
III. Psychosocial integrity
   A. Support and educate child and family.
IV. Health promotion and maintenance
   A. Promote optimum health.

IMPLEMENTATION

I. Explain or reinforce explanation of condition and therapies.
II. Teach family application of scabicide; follow directions accurately:
   A. Apply on cool, dry skin (not after a bath).

B. Leave on for prescribed time.

C. Treat all members of household.

III. Apply lotion or ointment to affected areas.

IV. Employ methods to prevent scratching.

  A. Keep fingernails short and clean.

  B. Keep child in T-shirt or other soft clothing to cover itching area.

  C. Wrap hands in soft cotton gloves or stockings, if needed; pin gloves to shirt sleeves.

EVALUATION

I. Child's skin remains clean and dry with no evidence of scratching.

II. Child rests and plays with no evidence of discomfort.

III. Child and family exhibit no evidence of infestation.

IV. Family demonstrates an understanding of the condition and the ability to provide home care.

Pediculosis Capitis

Description

Pediculosis capitis is an infestation of the head by *Pediculus humanus capitis* (head louse).

Pathophysiology

I. Female louse lays eggs at night on a hair shaft close to junction with skin.

II. Eggs hatch in approximately 7–10 days.

III. Crawling insect and insect saliva on skin produce itching and irritation.

Signs and Symptoms

I. Itching.

II. Nits and nit cases observable on hair shaft.

III. Distribution: usually found in hair at occipital area, nape of neck, behind ears. Has been found in eyebrows and eyelashes.

Therapeutic Management

I. Elimination of lice and nits with pediculocidal shampoos (Kwell, RID, Nix)

II. Manual removal of nit cases

Nursing Care

DATA COLLECTION

I. Perform routine assessment.

II. Inspect scalp for evidence of nits or nit cases at base of hair shaft:

  A. Systematically spread hair with two tongue depressors or popsicle sticks.

  B. Observe for:

   1. Any movement that indicates a louse

   2. Nits (whitish oval specks adhering to hair shaft)

   3. Empty nit cases (translucent oval specks)

  C. Condition is distinguished from dandruff by adherent nature; dandruff falls off hair readily.

PLANNING

I. Safe, effective care environment

  A. Prevent spread to others.

II. Physiological integrity

  A. Eliminate lice and nits.

III. Psychosocial integrity

  A. Support and educate child and family.

IV. Health promotion and maintenance

  A. Promote optimum health.

IMPLEMENTATION

I. Caution children against sharing combs, hats, caps, scarves, coats, and other items used on or near the hair.

II. Reassure family that anyone can get pediculosis, regardless of age, cleanliness, or socioeconomic level.

III. Teach family application of shampoo:

  A. Follow directions described on label of pediculocide:

   1. Read directions several times in quiet environment before application.

  B. Make child as comfortable as possible.

  C. Avoid getting preparation in eyes.

   1. If irritation occurs, flush well with tepid water.

  D. Remove nits with tweezers or between the fingernails.

IV. Launder washable items of clothing and linens in hot water and dry in dryer.

V. Soak combs, brushes, and so on, in pediculocide or lotion and very hot water for 5–10 minutes.

VI. Vacuum mattresses and upholstered furniture carefully.

VII. Support child to prevent feelings of shame or embarrassment.

VIII. Caution family against cutting child's hair or shaving head.

EVALUATION

I. Child and family exhibit no evidence of reinfestation.

II. Family demonstrates an understanding of the condition and the ability to provide home care.

Dermatophytosis (Ringworm)

Description

Infections are caused by a group of closely related fungi.

I. Tinea capitis: ringworm of the scalp

II. Tinea corporis: ringworm of the body

III. Tinea pedis: athlete's foot

Pathophysiology

I. Fungus that invades the skin

II. Production of an enzyme that causes hair to break off at roots

Signs and Symptoms

I. Tinea capitis

  A. Scaly, round patches

  B. Patch, scaling areas of baldness

  C. Itching

II. Tinea corporis
  A. Round or oval red scaling patches that spread outward and heal centrally
III. Tinea pedis
  A. Most frequent in adolescents; rare in young children
  B. Blisters and fissuring between toes
  C. Patches with pinhead-sized vesicles on plantar surface
  D. Itching

Therapeutic Management

I. Eliminate fungus.
  A. Administration of oral griseofulvin
  B. Topical applications of antifungal preparations

Nursing Care

DATA COLLECTION

I. Perform routine assessment.
II. Assist with diagnostic procedure: direct microscopic examination of scales from skin scrapings.

PLANNING

I. Safe, effective care environment
  A. Prevent spread to others.
II. Physiological integrity
  A. Help eliminate fungus.
III. Psychosocial integrity
  A. Support and educate child and family.
IV. Health promotion and maintenance
  A. Promote optimum health.
  B. Prepare family for home care.

IMPLEMENTATION

I. Suggest examination of animals in child's environment for evidence of infection (tinea corporis).
II. Teach family how to administer oral medication and apply topical ointments.
III. Teach family desired effects of medications and possible side effects.
IV. Teach family to improve the ventilation of the feet.

EVALUATION

I. Child exhibits no evidence of infection.
II. Family complies with therapeutic regimen.
III. Family demonstrates an understanding of the condition and the ability to provide home care.

Diaper Dermatitis

Description

Diaper dermatitis is an acute inflammatory disorder caused directly or indirectly by the wearing of diapers.

Pathophysiology; Signs and Symptoms

I. Various types of lesions observed, depending on cause of irritation and inflammation
II. Primary causes
  A. Allergy

B. Poorly washed diapers
C. Infrequent diaper change
D. Ammonia formation urine

Therapeutic Management

I. Promote skin healing.
II. Apply corticosteroids for stubborn inflammations.
III. Apply antifungal ointments or powders for candidiasis.
IV. Prevent recurrence.

Nursing Care

DATA COLLECTION

I. Perform routine assessment.

PLANNING

I. Safe, effective care environment
  A. Promote cleanliness.
II. Physiological integrity
  A. Minimize skin wetness.
  B. Promote normal skin pH.
  C. Prevent secondary infection.
III. Psychosocial integrity
  A. Support and educate family.
IV. Health promotion and maintenance
  A. Promote optimum health.

IMPLEMENTATION

I. Change diaper as soon as wet; change at least once during night.
II. Clean, rinse, and dry area before diapering.
III. Apply ointment (petrolatum, zinc oxide) over clean, dry, *noninflamed* skin to prevent moistness from reaching skin.
IV. Encourage use of diapers that reduce wetness next to skin (e.g., those with absorbent gel).
V. Avoid diaper covering (plastic pants, some elasticized disposable diapers).
VI. Teach diaper care to families who prefer cloth diapers.
  A. Encourage commercial diaper laundries.
  B. Home care: Soak diapers in quaternary ammonium compound:
    1. Wash in hot water with simple laundry soap (e.g., Ivory).
    2. Run through rinse cycle twice.
    3. A dryer enhances softness.
VII. Teach families application of any prescribed medication.

EVALUATION

I. Child remains free of dermatitis in the diaper area.
II. Family demonstrates an understanding of the condition, treatment, and prevention and the ability to provide home care.

Atopic Dermatitis (Eczema)

Description

Atopic dermatitis is a superficial inflammatory process involving primarily the skin.

Pathophysiology

I. Affected individuals have a lower threshold for itching.
II. Characteristic lesions appear after irritation (scratching, rubbing).
III. Appearance and distribution of lesions vary with age of child.
IV. Frequently a family history of sensitivity exists.

Signs and Symptoms

I. Intense itching
II. Unaffected skin dry and rough
III. Infantile form
  A. Generalized distribution, especially cheeks, scalp, trunk, extremities
  B. Erythema
  C. Vesicles and papules
  D. Weeping and oozing
  E. Crusting and scaling

Therapeutic Management

I. Prevent itching with antihistamines, mild baths, detergents, and soaps.
II. Hydrate the skin with emollients and limit bathing.
III. Reduce inflammation with topical corticosteroids.
IV. Prevent or control secondary infection.
V. Modify diet, if indicated.

Nursing Care

DATA COLLECTION

I. Perform routine assessment.
II. Assist with elimination diet, if indicated.

PLANNING

I. Safe, effective care environment
  A. Protect from known irritants.
II. Physiological integrity
  A. Prevent or minimize scratching.
  B. Prevent complications.
III. Psychosocial integrity
  A. Support and educate child and family.
IV. Health promotion and maintenance
  A. Promote optimum health.

IMPLEMENTATION

I. Keep fingernails and toenails short and clean.
II. Wrap hands in soft cotton gloves or stockings and pin gloves to shirt sleeves as needed to prevent scratching.
III. Avoid overheating child.
IV. Provide soothing and emollient tepid water baths or compresses as prescribed.
V. Administer antihistamines, sedatives, topical corticosteroids, and/or antibiotics as prescribed.
VI. Teach family diet planning (if food sensitivity is implicated).
VII. Teach family skills needed for care, including expected results of medications and their possible side effects.
VIII. Provide psychological and supportive care to promote a positive self-image.

IX. Teach parents to keep child protected from people who have infections.

EVALUATION

I. Child's skin remains intact without redness.
II. Child exhibits no evidence of secondary infection or trauma.
III. Family demonstrates an understanding of the condition and the ability to provide care.

Seborrheic Dermatitis

Description

Seborrheic dermatitis is a chronic, recurrent inflammatory condition of the skin.

Pathophysiology

I. Occurs most commonly on scalp ("cradle cap"), eyebrows, external ear canal (otitis externa), inguinal region
II. Related to excessive secretion from sebaceous glands
III. Cause unknown

Signs and Symptoms

I. Characteristic thick, adherent, yellowish, scaly, oily patches
II. May or may not include mild itching

Therapeutic Management

I. Symptomatic treatment
II. Corticosteroid ointment for persistent rash
III. Antibiotics for infected rash

Nursing Care

DATA COLLECTION

I. Perform routine assessment.

PLANNING

I. Safe, effective care environment
  A. Maintain cleanliness.
II. Physiological integrity
  A. Remove lesions.
  B. Prevent complications.
III. Psychosocial integrity
  A. Support and educate family.
IV. Health promotion and maintenance
  A. Promote optimum health.
  B. Prepare family for home care.

IMPLEMENTATION

I. Clean scalp (or other affected area).
II. Shampoo three to four times weekly with mild soap or shampoo.
III. Apply oil to lesion; massage into scalp; allow to penetrate and soften crusts; thoroughly wash out.
IV. Remove loosened crusts from hair strands with fine-toothed comb.
V. Apply any prescribed topical preparation.

VI. Explain or reinforce explanation of condition and therapies, especially regarding fear of damaging infant's soft spot.

VII. Teach family skills needed for care.

EVALUATION

I. Child's skin remains free of lesions.

II. Family demonstrates an understanding of the condition and the ability to provide care.

Acne Vulgaris

Description

Acne vulgaris is an inflammatory disease of the skin.

Pathophysiology; Signs and Symptoms

I. Hormones implicated in production of lesions

II. Distribution: face, neck, shoulders, back, and upper chest

III. Noninflamed lesions: comedones
   A. Compact masses of keratin, lipids, fatty acids, and bacteria
   B. Dilated follicular duct, which may be closed (whitehead) or open (blackhead); open lesions discolored as fatty acids oxidized by air

IV. Inflamed lesions
   A. Dilated follicular wall rupturing to produce papules, pustules, nodules, and cysts
   B. Description and possibility of scarring.

V. Lesions potentially complicated by secondary infection by *Staphylococcus albus*

Therapeutic Management

I. Prevent or reduce formation of new lesions with topical applications of retinoic acid, benzoyl peroxide, or a combination of these.

II. Reduce lesion formation in older adolescent females with cyclic estrogen-progesterone therapy.

III. Reduce inflammatory process and scarring with antibiotics and intralesional steroids.

Nursing Care

DATA COLLECTION

I. Perform routine assessment.

PLANNING

I. Safe, effective care environment
   A. Promote cleanliness.

II. Physiological integrity
   A. Remove comedones.
   B. Reduce number of lesions.
   C. Prevent inflammation and scarring.
   D. Prevent secondary infection.

III. Psychosocial integrity
   A. Support and educate child and family.
   B. Prepare child and family for procedures.
   C. Promote a positive self-image.

IV. Health promotion and maintenance
   A. Promote optimum health.
   B. Prepare child and family for home care.

IMPLEMENTATION

I. Encourage child to assume responsibility for own care.

II. Teach child how to carry out prescribed regimen:
   A. Skin cleansing and hair shampooing
   B. Application of topical preparations
   C. Administration of prescribed medications, including desired effects and possible side effects

III. Teach measures to reduce lesion formation:
   A. Hair styling (off forehead)
   B. Selection and application of makeup (water-based preparations)
   C. Avoidance of excessive scrubbing or pinching, squeezing, or otherwise manipulating lesions
   D. Avoidance of oily substances

IV. Caution against self-medication with over-the-counter preparations.

V. Emphasize importance of clean skin, hair, hands, and implements coming in contact with lesions.

VI. Dispel myths related to cause and treatment of acne.

VII. Allow child to express feelings.

VIII. Provide positive reinforcement for compliance.

IX. Emphasize improved appearance, self-limited nature of disorder.

X. Caution family against nagging or blaming or both.

EVALUATION

I. Child assumes responsibility for care.

II. Acne lesions diminish in number and severity.

III. Acne lesions do not become secondarily infected.

IV. Family displays a supportive attitude.

V. Child and family comply with therapeutic regimen.

VI. Child and family demonstrate an understanding of the condition and the ability to provide home care.

Impetigo Contagiosa

Description

Impetigo contagiosa is a superficial bacterial infection of the skin.

Pathophysiology

I. Caused by staphylococci, streptococci, or both

II. Begins as discolored spots

III. Followed by appearance of vesicles or bullae

IV. Rupture of vesicles or bullae, leaving superficial, moist erosion

V. Spread of germ-laden fluid to surrounding skin

VI. Drying of exudate forms heavy, honey-colored crusts and scabs

VII. Tends to spread outwardly

Signs and Symptoms

I. Vesicles, bullae, and weeping crusts as just described

II. Most often observed on face, hands, or perineum

III. Pruritus common

Therapeutic Management

I. Topical application of bactericidal ointment
II. Systemic administration of antibiotics in severe cases

Nursing Care

DATA COLLECTION

I. Describe lesion accurately; examine skin for evidence of spread to other areas.
II. Assist with diagnostic procedures: exudate culture.

PLANNING

I. Safe, effective care environment
   A. Prevent spread of infection.
II. Physiological integrity
   A. Help to eliminate lesions.
   B. Prevent complications.
III. Psychosocial integrity
   A. Support and educate child and family.
IV. Health promotion and maintenance
   A. Promote optimum health.
   B. Prepare family for home care.

IMPLEMENTATION

I. Practice and teach child and family careful handwashing.
II. Caution child against touching lesions to prevent spread.
III. Treat lesions:
   A. Soak crusts with warm-water compresses.
   B. Carefully remove crusts.
   C. Apply antibiotic ointment to affected areas.
IV. Administer antibiotics, if prescribed.
V. Teach family management of lesions and administration of medications.

EVALUATION

I. Child's skin remains free of lesions.
II. Family demonstrates an understanding of the disease and the ability to provide home care.
III. Others do not contract disease.

Thermal Burns

Description

A thermal burn is an injury to tissues caused by application of excessive heat to skin.

Pathophysiology

I. Physiological response directly related to amount of tissue destroyed
II. Extent of injury: expressed as percentage of body surface area involved; varies according to size of child
III. Depth of injury
   A. Superficial (first-degree): involves epidermis; heals without scarring
   B. Partial-thickness (second-degree): involves epidermis and variable portion of dermis (superficial or deep)
      1. Superficial: heals uneventfully
      2. Deep: may convert to full-thickness injury
   C. Full-thickness (third-degree): involves all layers of the skin
      1. Usually combined with extensive partial-thickness damage
      2. Scarring
   D. Full-thickness (fourth-degree): involves all layers of skin, subcutaneous tissue, and muscle
IV. Severity of injury
   A. Minor burns
      1. Partial-thickness burns over <15% of body surface
      2. Full-thickness burns over <2% of body surface
   B. Moderate burns
      1. Partial-thickness burns over <15–25% of body surface
      2. Full-thickness burns over <10% of body surface, except in small children or when burns involve critical areas (e.g., face, hands, feet, genitalia)
   C. Severe burns
      1. Burns complicated by respiratory tract injury
      2. Partial-thickness burns over 25% or more of body surface
      3. Burns of face, hands, feet, or genitalia
      4. Full-thickness burns over 10% or more of body surface
      5. Any child <2 years of age, unless burn is very small and very superficial
      6. Electrical burns that penetrate
      7. Deep chemical burns
      8. Burns complicated by fractures or soft-tissue injury
      9. Burns complicated by concurrent illness (e.g., obesity, diabetes, epilepsy, cardiac or renal disorders)
V. Local responses
   A. Edema formation
   B. Fluid electrolyte and protein loss
   C. Circulatory stasis
VI. Systemic responses
   A. Circulatory
   B. Anemia from heat-damaged RBCs at burn site
VII. Healing
   A. Superficial burns: damaged epithelium peeling off in small scales or sheets, in 5–10 days, leaving no scarring
   B. Partial-thickness burns: crust forming in 3–5 days; healing occurring from underneath
   C. Deep dermal burns (deep partial-thickness, full-thickness burns): healing slow; thin epithelial covering forming in 25–35 days; scarring common
VIII. Systemic effects of severe burns
   A. Asphyxia from irritation and edema of lungs and respiratory passages
   B. Shock from fluid and protein loss from denuded skin, edema from increased capillary permeability and vasodilation at burn site, diminished intravascular colloidal osmotic pressure (greatest hazard first 48–72 hours)
   C. Renal shutdown from shock

Signs and Symptoms

I. Superficial (first-degree) burns
   A. Dry, red surface
   B. Blanches on pressure, then refills
   C. Painful
II. Partial-thickness (second-degree) burns
   A. Blistered, moist
   B. Mottled pink or red
   C. Red; blanches on pressure, then refills
   D. Very painful
III. Full-thickness (third-degree) burns
   A. Tough, leathery
   B. Dull, dry surface
   C. Brown, tan, red, or black
   D. Does not blanch on pressure
   E. Little pain, but surrounded by painful partial-thickness burns

Therapeutic Management

I. Minor burns
   A. Cleanse and debride wound.
   B. Cover with dry or medicated dressing.
II. Major burns: general care
   A. Hospitalize client.
   B. Establish adequate airway.
   C. Replace and maintain IV fluids and electrolytes.
   D. Feed a high-calorie, increased-protein diet or regular diet.
   E. Administer morphine sulfate for pain on scheduled basis.
   F. Administer zinc and vitamin A preparations to promote epithelial growth.
   G. Use prophylactic antibiotics (controversial).
   H. Administer tetanus toxoid (based on immunization history).
III. Wound management
   A. Debridement of devitalized tissue: hydrotherapy
   B. Topical antimicrobial therapy
   C. Cover: temporary dressing (gauze, biological, synthetic, allograft, and autographs)
   D. Graft
      1. Permanent cover (partial-thickness, full-thickness burns)
      2. Full-cover, postage-stamp, mesh, lace, or slit
   E. Primary excision
IV. Prevention of deformity using splinting and compression garments

Nursing Care

DATA COLLECTION

I. Assess respiratory status.
II. Help to assess burn injury.
III. Obtain a history of burn injury—especially time of injury, nature of burning agent, duration of contact, whether in enclosed area, any medication given.
IV. Obtain pertinent history—especially preburn weight, preexisting illness, allergies.
V. Assess pain.
VI. Check eyes for evidence of injury or irritation.
VII. Observe for signs of respiratory distress.
VIII. Check nasopharynx for edema or redness.
IX. Monitor vital signs frequently.
X. Weigh on admission and daily, or as prescribed.
XI. Measure I&O.
XII. Assess circulation to areas peripheral or distal to burns.
XIII. Assess level of consciousness.
XIV. Observe for signs of altered behavior.
XV. Observe for signs of impending overhydration.
XVI. Observe wound for evidence of healing, stability of temporary cover or graft, and infection.
XVII. Assist with diagnostic tests: CBC, urinalysis, wound cultures, hematocrit.

PLANNING

I. Safe, effective care environment
   A. See Nursing Care of the Ill Child.
   B. Prevent heat loss.
   C. Prevent infection and trauma.
II. Physiological integrity
   A. Relieve pain.
   B. Facilitate wound healing.
   C. Preserve graft site.
   D. Provide nutrition.
   E. Prevent complications.
III. Psychosocial integrity
   A. See Nursing Care of the Ill Child.
   B. Promote positive self-image.
IV. Health promotion and maintenance
   A. Promote optimum health.
   B. Prepare family for home care.

IMPLEMENTATION

I. Place in protective environment according to unit policy:
   A. Prevent contact with infected persons or objects.
   B. Administer good oral hygiene.
II. Maintain environmental temperature to prevent heat loss or place under heat source.
III. Administer analgesics for pain as prescribed.
IV. Administer antibiotics as prescribed.
V. Administer tetanus toxoid (or antitoxin), if prescribed.
VI. Maintain meticulous medical and surgical asepsis.
VII. Carry out wound care as prescribed.
   A. Avoid injury to crusts and eschar.
   B. Keep child from scratching and picking at wound.
   C. Provide distraction (young child) and reasoning (older child).
   D. Restrain infant or younger child as needed.
   E. Position for minimal disturbance of grafted area.
VIII. Provide highly nutritious meals and snacks.
   A. Provide extra calories and protein.
   B. Promote appetite by providing attractive meals, preferred foods, and companionship during meals.
   C. Encourage self-help.
   D. Encourage oral feedings, but feed via other means, if necessary: nasogastric tube.
   E. Administer supplementary vitamins and minerals as prescribed.
IX. Administer antacids as prescribed.
X. Carry out active or passive ROM exercises.

XI. Encourage mobility of affected (if it does not disturb graft) and unaffected areas.
XII. Ambulate as soon as feasible.
XIII. Encourage and promote self-help activities appropriate to abilities and developmental level.
XIV. Position in functional attitude for minimum deformity.
XV. Apply splints as ordered and designed.
XVI. Wrap healing tissue with elastic bandage or dress in elastic garments as ordered.
XVII. Convey a positive attitude to child.
XVIII. Provide reinforcement for positive aspects of appearance and capabilities.
XIX. Explore child's feeling regarding altered physical appearance.
   A. Discuss aids that hide any disfigurement.
XX. Promote positive thinking in child.
XXI. Encourage continuing schooling.
XXII. Encourage peer contact.
XXIII. Help family members to set realistic goals for themselves and the child.
XXIV. Teach family skills needed for home care, including wound care, rehabilitation, diet planning, administration of medication (if needed), and diet supplements.

EVALUATION

I. Child exhibits little or no evidence of pain.
II. Child's wound heals with minimal disfigurement.
III. Child recovers uneventfully.
IV. Child exhibits a positive body image.
V. Child and family comply with rehabilitative efforts.

Communicable Diseases

Chickenpox

Description

Chickenpox is a disease characterized by crops of itching, vesicular skin eruptions, with few systemic symptoms.

Pathophysiology

I. Highly contagious infection with varicella-zoster virus
II. Source of infection: respiratory tract secretions
III. Transmission by direct contact, droplet spread, and contaminated objects
IV. Incubation period: usually 13–17 days
V. Period of communicability: Probably 1 day before eruption of lesions to 6 days after vesicles erupt when crust begins to form.

Signs and Symptoms

I. Slight fever
II. Malaise
III. Anorexia
IV. Highly itchy rash
   A. Lesions: papules, vesicles, and crusts present in varying degrees at any time
   B. Distribution: torso, spreading to face and extremities

Therapeutic Management

I. Symptomatic
II. Aspirin administration contraindicated because of association with Reye's syndrome

Nursing Care

DATA COLLECTION

I. Perform routine assessment.
II. Pay particular attention to type and configuration of lesions.

PLANNING

I. Safe, effective care environment
   A. See Nursing Care of the Ill Child.
   B. Prevent spread of infection to other children.
II. Physiological integrity
   A. Prevent development of secondary infection of lesions.
III. Psychosocial integrity
   A. See Nursing Care of the Ill Child.
   B. Reduce scarring.
IV. Health promotion and maintenance
   A. Promote optimum health.

IMPLEMENTATION

I. Isolate infected child and his or her secretions from others.
II. Implement hospital policy for hospitalized child.
III. Administer soothing lotion (e.g., calamine) to itchy areas.
IV. Prevent scratching:
   A. Keep skin clean.
   B. Keep child's fingernails short.
   C. Apply mittens or elbow restraints, if necessary.
   D. Explain the danger of secondary infection and scarring to older children.
   E. Suggest applying pressure to areas to relieve discomfort.
V. Keep child occupied with diversional activities.
VI. Teach family skills needed for home care, including preventing spread of infection

EVALUATION

I. Child recovers uneventfully, with minimal or no scarring.
II. Others remain free of infection.

Diphtheria

Description

Diphtheria is an infectious disease characterized by respiratory infection and membrane on pharynx.

Pathophysiology

I. Infection with the bacterium *Corynebacterium diphtheriae.*
II. Toxins produced may affect nervous system and heart.

III. Sources of infection: nasopharyngeal secretions, skin, eye, and lesions of affected person.
IV. Incubation period: 2–5 days or longer.
V. Period of communicability: until bacilli are no longer present—usually 2 weeks, but can extend to 4 weeks.

Signs and Symptoms

I. Nasal: resembles common cold
II. Pharyngeal
  A. Anorexia
  B. Malaise
  C. Fever
  D. Smooth, adherent white or gray membrane on mucous membrane
III. Laryngeal
  A. Fever
  B. Hoarseness
  C. Cough
  D. Signs of airway obstruction possible

Therapeutic Management

I. Administer antitoxin.
II. Administer antibiotics.
III. Allow complete bedrest.
IV. Perform tracheostomy or intubation for airway obstruction.
V. Provide symptomatic treatment of shock.
VI. Treat infected contacts and carriers.

Nursing Care

DATA COLLECTION

I. Perform routine assessment.
II. Observe for evidence of respiratory obstruction.
III. Assist with diagnostic procedures: nose and throat culture, sensitivity testing.

PLANNING

I. Safe, effective care environment
  A. See Nursing Care of the Ill Child.
  B. Prevent spread of infection.
II. Physiological integrity
  A. Help to eradicate organisms.
  B. Prevent complications.
III. Psychosocial integrity
  A. See Nursing Care of the Ill Child.
IV. Health promotion and maintenance
  A. Promote optimum health.
  B. Immunize susceptible individuals.

IMPLEMENTATION

I. Maintain strict isolation according to hospital policy and strict bedrest.
II. Immunize susceptible individuals.
III. Administer antibiotics and antitoxin as prescribed.
  A. Participate in sensitivity testing; have emergency equipment (tracheostomy set, epinephrine) readily available in the event of a reaction.
IV. Provide total care to promote rest and prevent cardiac complications.

V. Administer oxygen, humidity, and so on, as prescribed.
VI. Teach family skills needed for home care, including preventing spread of infection.

EVALUATION

I. Child recovers uneventfully.
II. Child remains free of complications.
III. Others remain free of infection.

Infectious Mononucleosis

Description

Infectious mononucleosis is an acute, self-limiting, contagious disease presumed to be of viral origin.

Pathophysiology

I. Mildly contagious disease caused by Epstein-Barr virus
II. Source: oral secretions
III. Transmitted by direct intimate contact with oral secretions
IV. Incubation period approximately 2–8 weeks

Signs and Symptoms

I. Headache
II. Malaise
III. Fatigue
IV. Fever
V. Loss of appetite
VI. Enlarged lymph nodes
VII. Enlarged spleen
VIII. Some liver involvement with jaundice

Therapeutic Management

I. Supportive treatment:
  A. Analgesic (acetaminophen) for headache, fever, malaise
  B. Gargles, hot drinks, analgesic lozenges for sore throat
II. Bedrest for fatigue.
III. Regulate activities according to tolerance.

Nursing Care

DATA COLLECTION

I. Perform routine assessment.
II. Assist with diagnostic procedures: CBC, heterophil antibody test, enzyme immunoassay test, Monospot.

PLANNING

I. Safe, effective care environment
  A. See Nursing Care of the Ill Child.
II. Physiological integrity
  A. Provide comfort.
  B. Prevent secondary infection.
III. Psychosocial integrity
  A. See Nursing Care of the Ill Child.
  B. Support and educate child and family.
IV. Health promotion and maintenance
  A. Promote optimum health.
  B. Prepare family for home care.

IMPLEMENTATION

   I. Provide comfort measures (e.g., analgesics, gargles).
  II. Help child and family to determine appropriate activities according to symptoms and interests.
 III. Allow child to express feelings of depression and resentment related to lengthy convalescence, fatigue, and restriction of activities.

EVALUATION

   I. Child verbalizes feelings and concerns.
  II. Child and family comply with therapeutic regimen.
 III. Family demonstrates an understanding of the disease and the ability to provide home care.

Measles (Rubeola)

Description

Measles is an acute, highly contagious disease involving the respiratory tract and characterized by a blotchy, macular rash.

Pathophysiology

   I. Highly contagious infection with the measles virus
  II. Source of infection: respiratory tract secretions
 III. Transmission by direct contact with infectious droplets
  IV. Incubation period: 10–20 days; 14 days to appearance of rash
   V. Period of communicability: from 4 days before to 5 days after appearance of rash
  VI. Complications: otitis media, bronchopneumonia, or encephalitis

Signs and Symptoms

   I. Onset
      A. Fever and malaise
      B. Cough, conjunctivitis, runny nose
      C. Small, irregular red (Koplik's) spots on mucous membrane of mouth
  II. Rash: appears 3–4 days after onset
      A. Begins as red, round, raised rash on face
      B. Gradually spreads downward
 III. Photophobia (often)
  IV. Anorexia
   V. Enlarged lymph nodes

Therapeutic Management

   I. Supportive
  II. Acetaminophen for fever and discomfort
 III. Prophylactic antibiotics

Nursing Care

DATA COLLECTION

   I. Perform routine assessment.

PLANNING

   I. Safe, effective care environment
      A. See Nursing Care of the Ill Child.
      B. Reduce irritating environmental stimuli.
      C. Prevent spread of infection to others.
  II. Physiological integrity
      A. Promote comfort.
      B. Prevent complications.
 III. Psychosocial integrity
      A. See Nursing Care of the Ill Child.
  IV. Health promotion and maintenance
      A. Promote optimum health.
      B. Prepare family for home care.

IMPLEMENTATION

    I. Isolate as appropriate and according to hospital policy.
   II. Immunize susceptible individuals.
  III. Maintain bedrest and provide quiet activity.
   IV. Dim light in room if child is photophobic.
    V. Administer acetaminophen as prescribed.
   VI. Avoid chilling.
  VII. Cleanse eyelids with warm saline to remove secretions and crusts.
 VIII. Teach family skills needed for home care, including preventing spread of infection.

EVALUATION

   I. Child exhibits no evidence of discomfort.
  II. Child recovers uneventfully.
 III. Child remains free of complications
  IV. Others do not contract the disease.

Mumps

Description

Mumps is an acute infectious disease characterized by swelling of the parotid glands.

Pathophysiology

   I. Highly contagious infection with paramyxovirus
  II. Sources of infection: direct contact and droplet
 III. Incubation period: 14–21 days
  IV. Period of communicability: immediately before and after swelling begins.
   V. Unilateral or bilateral involvement of the parotid glands chiefly
  VI. Frequently extends to include testes in adult men

Signs and Symptoms

   I. Onset: 24 hours
      A. Fever
      B. Headache
      C. Malaise
      D. Anorexia
  II. Parotid gland enlarging to maximum size in 1–3 days
 III. Accompanied by pain and tenderness

Therapeutic Management

   I. Primarily supportive
  II. Respiratory isolation advised

Nursing Care

DATA COLLECTION

  I. Perform routine assessment.
 II. Assist with diagnostic tests: culture from throat washings, urine, or spinal fluid; viral studies.

PLANNING

  I. Safe, effective care environment
    A. See Nursing Care of the Ill Child.
    B. Prevent spread of infection.
 II. Physiological integrity
    A. Promote comfort.
    B. Prevent complications.
III. Psychosocial integrity
    A. See Nursing Care of the Ill Child.
 IV. Health promotion and maintenance
    A. Promote optimum health.
    B. Prepare family for home care.

IMPLEMENTATION

  I. Use respiratory isolation precautions during hospitalization.
 II. Avoid contact with individuals who have not had mumps.
III. Offer easily swallowed bland foods.
 IV. Administer analgesics for discomfort as prescribed.
  V. Apply warm or cool compresses to area of neck swelling.
 VI. Encourage quiet play and nonstrenuous activity.
VII. Teach family skills needed for home care, including preventing spread of infection.

EVALUATION

  I. Child recovers uneventfully.
 II. Child remains free of complications.
III. Others do not contract the disease.

Pertussis (Whooping Cough)

Description

Pertussis is an acute, highly contagious respiratory disease characterized by a paroxysmal cough that ends with a loud "whooping" inspiration.

Pathophysiology

  I. Highly contagious infection with the bacillus *Bordetella pertussis*
 II. Source of infection: respiratory tract
III. Transmission by direct contact, droplet spread, freshly contaminated articles
 IV. Incubation period: 3–21 days, usually 10 days
  V. Period of communicability: highest during runny nose stage; risk diminishing rapidly but lasting up to 3 weeks

Signs and Symptoms

  I. Catarrhal stage
    A. Runny nose
    B. Sneezing
    C. Teary eyes
    D. Cough
    E. Low-grade fever
 II. Paroxysmal stage
    A. Frequent attacks
    B. Cough becoming paroxysmal after 1–2 weeks
      I. Series of short, rapid bursts during exhalation
      II. Followed by characteristic "whoop"
    C. Large amounts of mucus being expelled during or after paroxysm
    D. Vomiting frequently after coughing attacks

Therapeutic Management

  I. Hospitalization of infants and children with potentially severe disease
 II. Supportive care
III. Antimicrobials

Nursing Care

DATA COLLECTION

  I. Perform routine assessment.
 II. Observe coughing.
III. Observe for signs of airway obstruction.
 IV. Assist with diagnostic procedures: throat culture, WBC, direct immunofluorescence to nasal secretions.

PLANNING

  I. Safe, effective care environment
    A. See Nursing Care of the Ill Child.
    B. Reduce or eliminate factors that cause coughing.
    C. Prevent spread of infection.
 II. Physiological integrity
    A. Reduce coughing.
    B. Ease upper respiratory symptoms.
III. Psychosocial integrity
    A. See Nursing Care of the Ill Child.
    B. Reassure child and family during coughing episodes.
 IV. Health promotion and maintenance
    A. Promote optimum health.
    B. Prepare family for home care.

IMPLEMENTATION

   I. Isolate hospitalized child according to hospital policy.
  II. Avoid contact with nonimmunized children.
 III. Immunize susceptible individuals.
  IV. Administer antibiotics as prescribed.
   V. Reduce factors that cause coughing:
    A. Keep room well ventilated.
    B. Keep environment smoke- and dust-free.
    C. Avoid extremes of temperature or chilling.
    D. Keep child playing quietly.
  VI. Provide comfort measures to prevent distress.
 VII. Maintain child in mist tent with high humidity.
VIII. Encourage fluid intake.
  IX. Refeed if child vomits.
   X. Teach family skills needed for home care, including preventing spread of infection.

EVALUATION

I. Child exhibits minimal coughing.
II. Child recovers uneventfully.
III. Child remains free of complications.
IV. Others remain free of infection.

Rubella (German Measles)

Description

Rubella is a mild contagious disease characterized by red, raised rash; swollen lymph nodes; and slight fever.

Pathophysiology

I. Contagious infection with rubella virus
II. Source of infection: nasogastric secretions
III. Transmission by direct contact
IV. Incubation period: 14–21 days, usually 16–18 days
V. Period of communicability: 7 days before to 5 days after appearance of rash

Signs and Symptoms

I. Postnatal
  A. Low-grade fever, malaise, headache
  B. Swollen lymph nodes
  C. Rash
    1. Pinkish-red, round, raised
    2. On face initially
    3. Spreading downward to neck, trunk, and extremities
    4. Disappearing in 3 days in same order as it began
II. Congenital rubella syndrome
  A. Various deformities in infant if contracted during the first trimester of pregnancy
  B. Growth retardation of infant

Therapeutic Management

I. Supportive care

Nursing Care

DATA COLLECTION

I. Perform routine assessment.
II. Assist with diagnostic tests: serological tests; throat, blood, urine, or spinal fluid culture; specific IgM antibody titer.

PLANNING

I. Safe, effective care environment
  A. See Nursing Care of the Ill Child.
  B. Prevent spread of disease.
  C. Prevent prenatal disease.
II. Physiological integrity
  A. Provide comfort measures.
III. Psychosocial integrity
  A. See Nursing Care of the Ill Child.
IV. Health promotion and maintenance
  A. Promote optimum health.
  B. Prepare family for home care.

IMPLEMENTATION

I. Immunize susceptible individuals.
II. Prevent contact with pregnant women.
III. Administer acetaminophen for discomfort.
IV. Teach family skills needed for home care, including preventing spread of infection.

EVALUATION

I. Child recovers uneventfully.
II. Child remains free of complications.
III. Others do not contract the disease.

Streptococcal Infection (Scarlet Fever)

Description

Streptococcal infection, or scarlet fever, is an acute infectious disease of childhood characterized by sore throat, fever, and enlarged lymph nodes and rash.

Pathophysiology

I. Contagious infection with group A β-hemolytic streptococci
II. Source of infection: nasopharyngeal secretions
III. Transmission by direct contact or droplet spread, freshly contaminated articles
IV. Incubation period: 2–4 days
V. Period of communicability: 7 days before to about 5 days after appearance of rash
VI. Complications: otitis media, tonsillar abscess, sinusitis, rheumatic fever, nephritis, or carditis

Signs and Symptoms

I. Onset
  A. Abrupt high fever
  B. Pulse increased out of proportion to fever
  C. Chills, malaise, headache
  D. Vomiting, abdominal pain
II. Sore throat
  A. Tonsils: red, enlarged
  B. Tongue: red, swollen, coated with white ("red strawberry tongue")
III. Skin
  A. Red, pinhead-sized rash (occurs in 12–36 hours)
  B. Rash generalized, seldom seen on face
  C. Face flushed
  D. Desquamation begins at end of first week; usually complete by 3 weeks

Therapeutic Management

I. Full course of penicillin
II. Supportive measures during fever phase

Nursing Care

DATA COLLECTION

I. Perform routine assessment.
II. Assist with diagnostic test: throat culture.

PLANNING

    I. Safe, effective care environment
        A. See Nursing Care of the Ill Child.
        B. Prevent spread of infection.
    II. Physiological integrity
        A. Promote comfort.
        B. Prevent complications.
    III. Psychosocial integrity
        A. See Nursing Care of the Ill Child.
    IV. Health promotion and maintenance
        A. Promote optimum health.
        B. Prepare family for home care.

IMPLEMENTATION

    I. Administer penicillin as prescribed.
    II. Promote bedrest during fever phase.
    III. Administer acetaminophen for sore throat.
    IV. Emphasize importance of adherence to penicillin regimen.
    V. Teach family skills needed for home care, including preventing spread of infection.

EVALUATION

    I. Child recovers uneventfully.
    II. Child remains free of complications.
    III. Others do not contract the disease.

Psychosocial Disorders

Failure to Thrive

Description

Failure to thrive (FTT) is a deviation from the established growth pattern in child <3 years of age.
    I. Organic FTT: growth failure due to major illness
    II. Nonorganic FTT: presence of growth retardation in the absence of organic dysfunction

Pathophysiology

    I. Organic FTT causes: principally neurological, GI, or endocrine dysfunction
    II. Nonorganic FTT causes: neglect, poverty

Signs and Symptoms

    I. Growth failure
        A. Weight 20% or more below the ideal weight for an infant's height
    II. Nonorganic
        A. Apathy
        B. Withdrawal behavior
        C. Feeding or eating dysfunction
        D. No fear of strangers (at age when stranger anxiety expected)
        E. Avoidance of eye contact
        F. Wide-eyed gaze, continual scan of the environment
        G. Muscles stiff and unyielding or flaccid and unresponsive
        H. Minimum amount of smiling

Therapeutic Management

    I. Organic: determination and treatment of cause
    II. Nonorganic: hospitalization for feeding trial and observation
        A. Home treatment
            1. Implement feeding program.
            2. Provide infant stimulation program.
            3. Refer to community resources that provide services to reduce family stress.
            4. Provide mental health services (individual or group).
            5. Perform conscientious medical follow-up.
        B. Recommendation of termination of parental rights, if necessary

Nursing Care

DATA COLLECTION

    I. Perform routine assessment.
    II. Assess feeding behaviors, parent-child interaction.
    III. Obtain detailed history.
    IV. Assist with diagnostic procedures.

PLANNING

    I. Safe, effective care environment
        A. See Nursing Care of the Ill Child.
        B. Provide a nurturing environment for child.
        C. Promote trusting environment between caregiver and child.
    II. Physiological integrity
        A. Plan feeding program that encourages an adequate caloric intake.
        B. Implement care plan for specific organic disorder (if identified).
    III. Psychosocial integrity
        A. See Nursing Care of the Ill Child.
        B. Promote a trusting relationship.
        C. Provide appropriate infant stimulation.
        D. Provide nurturing environment for family.
        E. Foster parental self-esteem.
    IV. Health promotion and maintenance
        A. Promote optimum health.
        B. Achieve and maintain optimum nutrition.
        C. Prepare family for home care.

IMPLEMENTATION

    I. Maintain structured routine in care.
    II. Provide continuity of nursing personnel for care.
    III. Implement feeding program:
        A. Provide unlimited feeding of diet for age.
        B. Avoid interruptions of feedings (e.g., laboratory studies, radiology, examinations).
        C. Remain calm and relaxed during feeding.
        D. Follow child's rhythm during feeding.
        E. Continue feeding even when child tries to refuse food.
    IV. Provide eye contact during care.
    V. Praise child for desired behavior.
    VI. Provide sensory stimulation—tactile, visual, and auditory—appropriate to child's developmental level.
    VII. Provide nurturing environment for family.

VIII. Teach family about child's physical care, developmental skills, and emotional needs.
IX. Serve as role model in child's care.
X. Afford family the opportunity to discuss feelings and concerns.
XI. Provide emotional nurturance without encouraging dependency.
XII. Build family's self-esteem with praise for positive behaviors and achievements.
XIII. Teach skills needed for home care:
    A. Continue teaching skills needed for care.
    B. Provide for continued infant stimulation program.
    C. Provide for a consistent contact system.
    D. Refer to community resources that provide ongoing care and services to reduce family stress.

EVALUATION

I. Infant attains and maintains desired weight.
II. Infant accomplishes expected developmental tasks.
III. Family demonstrates an understanding of the condition and the ability to provide home care.
IV. Family demonstrates nurturing behaviors toward infant.

Child Maltreatment

Description

Child maltreatment is intentional physical abuse or neglect, emotional abuse, or sexual abuse of children.

Pathophysiology

I. Possible characteristics of child
    A. Viewed as difficult or different
    B. Reminds caregiver of an unliked person in life
    C. Often born prematurely
    D. Born to unmarried parents or from an unwanted pregnancy
    E. Seriously or chronically ill
II. Possible parental characteristics
    A. Victim of abuse as a child
    B. Emotionally immature
    C. Violent behavior
    D. Low self-esteem
    E. Inadequate understanding of normal growth and development; expectations beyond capabilities of the child
    F. Role reversal: parent expects child to be nurturer
    G. Living in social isolation
    H. Not seeking support or assistance from others
III. Situational characteristics
    A. Environment of chronic stress: interpersonal relationships, financial, unemployment, alcoholism, drug addiction, poor housing
    B. Lack of adequate support systems

Signs and Symptoms

I. Physical evidence of abuse or neglect or both
    A. Soft-tissue injuries: abrasions, lacerations, bruises
    B. Traumatic bruises in varying stages of healing
    C. Burns, especially symmetrical burns of buttocks, genitalia, legs or hands; round "dug-out" craters (cigarette burns)
    D. Bites, hair loss
    E. Fractures
    F. Drug intoxication
II. Neglect
    A. Evidence of noncare: dirty, ill-fed, and ill-clothed
    B. Evidence of lack of stimulation
    C. FTT
    D. Medical neglect
III. Emotional abuse: extremely varied; difficult to define and identify
    A. Self-destructive behavior
    B. Antisocial behavior
    C. Child humiliated, labeled, put down
    D. Child as family scapegoat
    E. Family with unrealistic expectations of child
    F. Suicide attempts
IV. Sexual abuse
    A. Injuries in genital area
    B. Torn, stained, or bloody underclothing

Therapeutic Management

I. Protect from further abuse.
II. Treat injuries.
III. Provide nurturing environment.

Nursing Care

DATA COLLECTION

I. Perform routine assessment.
II. Describe any physical injury.
III. Observe parent-child interaction.
IV. Identify family strengths and possible support systems.
V. Assist with diagnostic procedures.

PLANNING

I. Safe, effective care environment
    A. Remove child from abusive situation.
II. Physiological integrity
    A. Promote healing of physical injuries.
    B. Prevent complications.
III. Psychosocial integrity
    A. See Nursing Care of the Ill Child.
    B. Promote nonthreatening, nurturing environment.
    C. Support and educate family.
IV. Health promotion and maintenance
    A. Promote optimum health.
    B. Prepare family for home care.

IMPLEMENTATION

I. Establish protective measures for child as indicated.
II. Report suspected abuse to proper authorities.
III. Keep factual, objective records.
IV. Teach family about normal growth and developmental patterns and appropriate expectations for age.
V. Help family accept its parenting role.
VI. Provide anticipatory guidance.

VII. Refer to community resources that provide services to reduce family stresses.

VIII. Reinforce family strengths.

EVALUATION

I. Child remains free of injury.

II. Child exhibits appropriate behavior for developmental level.

III. Child exhibits minimal or no evidence of distress.

IV. Child accepts foster family, when necessary.

V. Family demonstrates an understanding of the condition and the ability to provide safe home care.

Poisoning

General Concepts of Poisoning

Description

Poisoning consists of eating, drinking, or inhaling toxic amounts of drugs, household products, or any item.

Pathophysiology

I. Depends on poison

Signs and Symptoms

I. Increased respirations

II. Severe acidosis

III. Electrolyte imbalance

IV. Restlessness

V. Thirst

VI. Fever

VII. Sweating

VIII. Oliguria

IX. Tinnitus

X. Tremors

XI. Convulsions

XII. Coma

Therapeutic Management

I. Identify toxic substance and antidote.

II. Stabilize cardiovascular and respiratory systems.

III. Remove remaining poison from body.

IV. Increase excretion of toxin.

V. Prevent and/or correct effects of absorbed toxin.

VI. Prevent complications.

Nursing Care

DATA COLLECTION

I. Acquire careful and detailed history regarding what, when, and how much of toxic substance has entered the body.

II. Collect assessment data on area exposed to poison and VSs.

III. Assist with diagnostic procedures: blood and urine examination for presence of specific substances.

IV. Save all evidence of poison (container, plant, vomitus, urine).

V. Observe client for latent symptoms of poisoning.

PLANNING

I. Safe, effective care environment
   A. Protect from injury.

II. Physiological integrity
   A. Dilute poisonous substance.
   B. Remove substance from stomach.
   C. Prevent aspiration of vomitus.
   D. Absorb remaining substance.
   E. Prevent complications.

III. Psychosocial integrity:
   A. Support and educate child and family.
   B. Prepare child and family for procedures.

IV. Health promotion and maintenance
   A. Prevent recurrence.
   B. Prepare family for home care.

IMPLEMENTATION

I. Contact physician for immediate advice regarding treatment, local poison control center, or emergency facility.

II. Implement measures to eliminate or reduce effects of poison.

III. Ingested poison:
   A. Remove pills, plant parts, or other materials from mouth.
   B. Administer water to dilute substance unless contraindicated.
   C. Administer ipecac syrup to induce vomiting (unless client swallowed hydrocarbons or corrosives or is comatose).
   D. Position to prevent aspiration.
   E. Prepare for and assist with gastric lavage, if prescribed.
   F. Administer activated charcoal after vomiting has occurred, to absorb remaining poison, following hospital protocol.

IV. Carry out orders for management of specific poisons (e.g., IV infusion, artificial ventilation), and administer specific antidotes (e.g., chelating agents, antivenom) and anticonvulsants.

V. Provide comfort and reassurance to child and family.

VI. Teach poison prevention.

EVALUATION

I. Child eliminates poison from body.

II. Child remains free of complications.

III. Child does not have a repeated episode of poisoning.

IV. Family demonstrates an understanding of the condition and the ability to provide home care.

QUESTIONS

Susan I. Ray, RN, MS

1. A baby born today at 38 weeks' gestation weighs 5 lb 2 oz (2335 g). The nurse would describe the baby as:

   A. A normal newborn
   B. Chronically ill
   C. Low birth weight
   D. Very low birth weight

2. A baby is a low-birth-weight infant born at 36 weeks' gestation. The nurse planning care for this infant would focus on:

   A. Conservation of energy and warmth
   B. Bathing infant every shift in warm water
   C. Prevention of cradle cap by daily shampooing
   D. Stimulation of senses

3. The nurse knows that pain responses in a low-birth-weight neonate:

   A. Are easy to assess in neonates
   B. Do not exist because of an immature neurological system
   C. Produce crying and flexing of extremities
   D. Require measurement through vital sign (VS) variation

4. In a neonate at 36 weeks' gestation, the nurse would anticipate implementation of nursing care for which disorder?

   A. Acne
   B. Chickenpox
   C. Jaundice
   D. Scoliosis

5. The nurse would clean a neonate with clear water or mild nonalkaline cleanser two or three times per week because:

   A. Cleaning stimulates circulation
   B. Growth of bacteria is minimized
   C. Oils provide nourishment to tissues
   D. Thorough cleansing prevents irritation

6. If a neonate develops respiratory distress syndrome, the nurse should include as an evaluation outcome:

   A. Neonate breathes without effort.
   B. Neonate recovers from surgery uneventfully.
   C. Family seeks genetic counseling.
   D. Others do not contract disease.

7. A 2-year-old infant is given a diagnosis of severe croup (laryngotracheobronchitis). The nurse caring for this child identifies essential therapeutic measures as being hospitalization and:

   A. Corticosteroids
   B. Cool humidification
   C. Intubation
   D. Whirlpool baths

8. The nurse is planning for an admission of a preschooler. The nurse knows that a preschooler thinks about illness in terms of:

   A. Concerns about privacy
   B. External causes for body illnesses
   C. Punishment for wrongdoing
   D. Separation from a favorite toy or blanket

9. A 3-year-old child is being admitted to the pediatric unit. Phases of separation anxiety that the nurse would observe for are:

   A. Crying, withdrawal, and attachment
   B. Depression, detachment, and acceptance
   C. Protest, despair, and acceptance
   D. Protest, despair, and detachment

10. When providing care for a toddler, the nurse knows that the following nursing measures would promote hospital adjustment:

    A. Minimize parental involvement in care.
    B. Provide detailed, professional explanations of routines.
    C. Use siderails when child is sleeping.
    D. Institute visitation provisions for siblings.

11. A toddler is in respiratory distress, but he refuses to stay in his mist tent. The mother wants you to help. The best intervention by the nurse would be to:

    A. Give the child a favorite toy to play with under the tent
    B. Have the mother read to the child as she sits under the tent with him
    C. Administer strong sedation to put the child to sleep
    D. Tell the child that the tent is a spaceship that will take off if he cries

12. A school-age child is being discharged home from the hospital after being treated for respiratory distress from an asthma attack. Criteria for evaluating nursing care would include outcome objectives such as:

    A. Family instead of nursing staff assumes all care.
    B. Family demonstrates ability to provide home care.
    C. Child accepts all care without responding.
    D. Child rejects family as providers of care.

13. The mother of a toddler tells you that her child has been attending day care for 3 weeks. Today, when she picked up the child, she noticed that she had been scratching her chest, which had red bumps on it. The nurse would suspect which condition?

    A. Chickenpox
    B. Diphtheria
    C. Measles
    D. Mumps

14. Which of the following would be the most important nursing intervention for a child with chickenpox?

    A. Administering aspirin to control elevated temperature
    B. Avoiding the use of calamine lotion because of chances of secondary infection
    C. Keeping the child's fingernails short

D. Encouraging siblings to visit to prevent isolation and promote adaptation to illness

15. An infant is admitted to the pediatric unit with a diagnosis of failure to thrive (FTT). The infant is apathetic and withdrawn, avoids eye-to-eye contact with a wide-eyed gaze, and continually watches the environment. On the basis of the signs and symptoms, the nurse would suspect the infant of presenting with:

    A. Endocrine dysfunction
    B. GI dysfunction
    C. Neurological dysfunction
    D. Nonorganic FTT

16. When a nurse observes signs and symptoms of child neglect, appropriate action includes which of the following?

    A. Ensure involvement of a variety of caregivers.
    B. Oppose parental decision making.
    C. Promote a trusting relationship.
    D. Provide extra stimulation.

17. The nurse would consider which objective appropriate to evaluate the outcome of care for an infant with nonorganic FTT?

    A. Family demonstrates dependence on nursing staff for care.
    B. Family demonstrates nurturing behaviors toward infant.
    C. Infant maintains admission weight.
    D. Infant makes slow progress toward developmental milestones.

18. A 4-year-old child has swallowed the contents of one bottle of baby aspirin. The physician has ordered administration of ipecac. The clinic nurse understands that the rationale for this medication is to:

    A. Absorb remaining substance
    B. Dilute poisonous substance
    C. Prevent aspiration of vomitus
    D. Remove substance from stomach

19. A 6-year-old child is admitted to the pediatric unit with partial- and full-thickness third-degree burns. From this information, the nurse can plan burn care that affects:

    A. Dermis only
    B. Epidermis only
    C. All layers of skin
    D. All layers of skin, subcutaneous tissues, and muscle

20. Nursing care for a child with a third-degree burn on the body would focus on:

    A. Encouraging mobility
    B. Helping child to scratch wound
    C. Limiting fluid intake
    D. Removing crusts and eschar

21. Morphine sulfate is prescribed every 4 hours for a burned school-age child. When the nurse arrives to give the medicine, the child's eyes are closed and the child appears to be sleeping. The most appropriate initial response by the nurse is to:

    A. Assess nonverbal pain cues
    B. Give the shot quickly and leave
    C. Leave and go back in 30 minutes
    D. Report the problem to the doctor

22. You are the nurse who takes a burned client to the playroom for the first time. The client has bandages on both arms. The other children are playing and ignore the client. Your response should be to:

    A. Act as a role model, bringing the child in and playing with him at a table
    B. Leave him alone in the room and hope it gets better
    C. Take the child back to his room so he can watch television
    D. Tell the child to find a game and ask someone to play with him

23. A 10-year-old child broke her left leg, and the whole end of the bone protrudes through the skin. The nurse understands this fracture to be:

    A. Compound
    B. Greenstick
    C. Incomplete
    D. Simple

24. A school-age child is in traction. When the nurse enters the room, the child is twisted in bed. She says she's trying to reach her radio. The nurse should:

    A. Arrange games, toys, snacks, and call signal within reach
    B. Take the radio out of the room
    C. Tell her parents that they need to stay with her all the time
    D. Tell the child to call whenever she needs anything

25. A new cast is applied to a school-age child's leg in preparation for discharge. Nursing care of the newly applied cast would include:

    A. Lower the extremity until the cast dries.
    B. Keep the cast moist and clean.
    C. Provide ROM exercises to fractured joint.
    D. Tell the child not to put anything inside the cast.

26. A 14-year-old adolescent has a new diagnosis of diabetes. The nurse would expect this to be:

    A. Glucose intolerance
    B. Insulin-dependent diabetes
    C. Maturity-onset diabetes
    D. Plain diabetes

27. An adolescent with a new diagnosis of diabetes is learning to administer her own medication by injection. The adolescent has drawn up the correct dose, but she cannot give herself a shot. The nurse should:

    A. Give the shot and let her get more practice with an orange
    B. Assist her by guiding her hand, then insert the needle for her
    C. Tell her that she does not need the shot as long as she follows her diet
    D. Tell her that this is a problem that the physician should be made aware of

28. The nurse understands that planning care for an adolescent with diabetes would include:

    A. Balancing diet, exercise, and insulin
    B. Increasing exercise and activity to lower blood glucose
    C. Limiting dietary intake to lower the blood glucose
    D. Limiting exercise and activity to decrease insulin needs

29. Signs and symptoms of ketoacidosis that the nurse would teach a diabetic with a new diagnosis of diabetes would include:

    A. Glucose in urine
    B. Headache
    C. Low blood sugar
    D. Thirst

30. A toddler had an upper respiratory infection (URI) last week. Today the toddler is crying and pulling at his left ear. The nurse would expect a diagnosis of:

    A. Otitis media
    B. Diphtheria
    C. Pertussis
    D. Tonsillitis

31. With a diagnosis of otitis media, the nurse would not anticipate which of the following in nursing care for the child?

    A. Antibiotic administration
    B. Analgesic administration
    C. Oxygen therapy
    D. Surgical intervention

32. The nurse would identify which outcome when evaluating care of the child with otitis media?

    A. Comfort and ear canal status
    B. Completion of antibiotics
    C. Family's ability to give injections
    D. Prevention of secondary infection

33. A teenage girl is admitted to the adolescent unit with a diagnosis of cystic fibrosis. The nurse determines that the adolescent has a typical sign of this disease when which of the following is noted?

    A. Cool, dry skin
    B. Frequent urination
    C. Large, bulky, foul-smelling stools
    D. Poor appetite

34. The nurse knows that the primary cause of the serious pulmonary problems that children with cystic fibrosis can develop is:

    A. Bronchial constriction
    B. Inadequate surfactant
    C. Pulmonic stenosis
    D. Thick, tenacious mucus

35. If pancreatic enzymes are prescribed for a child with cystic fibrosis, the nurse should administer these by which route?

    A. Intramuscularly
    B. IV
    C. Orally
    D. Intradermally

36. The nurse promotes exercise in an adolescent with cystic fibrosis because it is therapeutically important to help promote a sense of well-being and to:

    A. Aid digestion and absorption of nutrients
    B. Enhance heart muscle and vascular tone
    C. Promote mobilization of lung secretions
    D. Stimulate exocrine gland secretions

37. A child with cystic fibrosis may be treated with a mist tent at home. The nurse would want the family to identify the reason for the mist is to help:

    A. Dilate alveoli
    B. Minimize secretions
    C. Prevent dehydration
    D. Relieve dyspnea

38. Postural drainage is prescribed for home care. The family and child need to learn about the therapy and all positions for treatments. The nurse would teach the family and child which position to help move secretions from the right lower lobes?

    A. Lying on back with head lowered
    B. Lying on left side with head lowered
    C. Lying on left side with head raised
    D. Sitting with left knee bent

39. As a nurse, you know that a child with cystic fibrosis must learn to avoid:

    A. Dog and cat hair
    B. Bacterial infections
    C. Sodium chloride
    D. Ultraviolet light

40. A 6-year-old child is admitted to the pediatric unit with a diagnosis of rheumatic fever (RF). The nurse associates the probable cause of the child's recent sore throat with:

    A. Pneumococci
    B. Staphylococci
    C. Streptococci
    D. Influenza B

41. An initial nursing intervention for a child with RF would include:

    A. Administering corticosteroids
    B. Assisting child into squatting position
    C. Encouraging visits by school friends
    D. Protecting from sunlight

42. The mother of a child with a diagnosis of RF is concerned that the physician ordered aspirin for her 6-year-old child. The nurse would explain to the mother that aspirin is important to reduce:

    A. Carditis
    B. Itching
    C. Headaches
    D. Joint tenderness

43. Evaluation of care for a child with RF would include assessing family knowledge of:

    A. Coughing and deep breathing
    B. Fluid and diet restrictions
    C. Long-term penicillin administration
    D. Oxygen therapy

44. A 2-year-old child had a tonsillectomy yesterday. The nurse would be least concerned about:

    A. Halitosis
    B. Increased pulse
    C. Nausea
    D. Restlessness

45. The second day after a tonsillectomy, a child is receiving a full-liquid diet. Which of the following should be discouraged?

    A. Chocolate milk
    B. Ice cream
    C. Orange juice
    D. Popsicles

46. A child is admitted with bronchial asthma. The respiratory signs that the nurse would expect to see include:

    A. Sleep apnea
    B. Inspiratory stridor
    C. Productive cough
    D. Prolonged expirations

47. In the management of an episode of acute asthma, the nurse would not expect to include:

    A. Antibiotics
    B. Antiemetics
    C. Corticosteroids
    D. Bronchodilators

48. An infant was given a diagnosis of a lumbar myelomeningocele at birth. The nurse knows that this is a:

    A. Defect in closure of spinal vertebral column with varying degrees of tissue protrusion through the opening
    B. Failure of complete closure of the vertebral column with no outpouching
    C. Hernial protrusion of saclike cyst of meninges containing spinal fluid
    D. Hernial protrusion of saclike cyst of meninges containing spinal fluid and a portion of the spinal cord with nerves

49. For an infant with myelomeningocele, nursing care before surgery to close the defect would include:

    A. Meticulous skin care, especially in the area of sac
    B. Supine positioning whenever possible
    C. Securing a diaper firmly over buttocks to avoid contamination
    D. Taping a dry dressing over the sac

50. The nurse knows that which of the following is frequently associated with myelomeningoceles?

    A. Hydrocephalus
    B. Intussusception
    C. Mental retardation
    D. Pneumonia

51. A mother brings her 2-year-old child to the clinic. The child is drooling, agitated, and appears to be in respiratory distress. The pediatrician suspects epiglottitis. Which action by the nurse is best?

    A. Allow the mother to hold the child.
    B. Insist that the mother leave the examination room.
    C. Give the child cool fruit juice to drink.
    D. Obtain a throat culture.

52. The nurse explains to the mother that the usual cause of epiglottitis is:

    A. β-Hemolytic streptococcus
    B. *Haemophilus influenzae*
    C. Respiratory syncytial virus
    D. *Staphylococcus aureus*

53. A toddler is being admitted to the pediatric unit with epiglottitis. Which intervention would be the most important for the nurse?

    A. Have tracheostomy equipment available.
    B. Notify the respiratory therapist of the admission.
    C. Have the antibiotics prepared when the child arrives on the unit.
    D. Make the child NPO.

54. An infant is being admitted for a cleft lip repair tomorrow morning. The nurse collecting data from the mother will expect to obtain information about:

    A. Drooling
    B. Noisy respirations
    C. Sucking problems
    D. Swallowing difficulty

55. During the first 24 hours postoperatively after a cleft lip repair, the nurse would:

    A. Apply elbow restraints to the infant
    B. Position the infant prone
    C. Keep the infant upright in an infant seat
    D. Use a mist tent to facilitate the infant's breathing

56. An 18-year-old adolescent is being admitted to the pediatric unit with a low platelet count. The nurse planning care would:

    A. Assess temperature with rectal thermometers
    B. Encourage brushing teeth after each meal and at bedtime
    C. Reduce aspirin intake to once daily
    D. Teach the adolescent the importance of using creams to remove hair on legs

57. When planning care for a child with neutropenia, the nurse would:

    A. Include raw vegetables and fruit in meal plans
    B. Maintain bedrest
    C. Report any temperature elevation to the physician
    D. Restrict visitors

58. A toddler with a diagnosis of sickle cell disease is being discharged home with his parents. Which nursing intervention should take priority?

    A. Assessing the parents' knowledge of pain management

B. Consulting home health care for follow-up
C. Identifying a support group for the family
D. Teaching measures to prevent sickle cell crisis

59. The nurse planning care for a preschooler postoperatively would identify which behavior as characteristic of pain response in this age group?

    A. Demanding explanations
    B. Stoic behavior
    C. Clinging to parents
    D. Stalling behaviors

60. The nurse planning care for a postoperative child receiving meperidine (Demerol) would:

    A. Not administer meperidine longer than 48 hours
    B. Give meperidine on the second postoperative day
    C. Prefer meperidine to morphine because it has fewer side effects
    D. Use naloxone (Narcan) to reverse any side effects of meperidine

61. The nurse planning care for a school-age child immobilized with traction would:

    A. Avoid isometric exercises
    B. Force fluids
    C. Limit peer visitation
    D. Offer detailed description of procedures

62. A child is 12 hours postoperative after repair of a compound fracture of the arm. The nurse would identify which data as requiring immediate attention?

    A. Bruising of the fingers
    B. Capillary refill of 2 seconds
    C. Pallor at the nailbeds
    D. Edema of the extremity

63. The nurse would be concerned that a child could develop compartment syndrome if pain is:

    A. Radiating distally
    B. Responsive to repeated oral medication
    C. Unresponsive to oral medication and responsive to narcotics
    D. Unresponsive to narcotics

64. The nurse is teaching parents cast care. The nurse would identify which of the following as a sign of infection?

    A. Increased pain in the extremity
    B. Temperature of 100°F (37.7°C) orally
    C. Hot areas felt on the cast
    D. Blood-tinged drainage on the cast

65. An adolescent is less than 24 hours postoperative from reduction of a compound fracture. The nurse would be most concerned with:

    A. Blood pressure (BP) 100/60 mm Hg
    B. Petechia noted on the chest
    C. Moderate amount of pain relief from narcotic
    D. Urine output of 600 cc

66. Which action by the nurse is the most important in maintaining Buck's traction on a 4-year-old child?

A. Assessing the weights to ensure that they are hanging freely
B. Conducting neurovascular checks every 4 hours
C. Monitoring the effectiveness of a muscle relaxant
D. Readjusting the fit of the bandage daily to promote countertraction

67. Evaluation of care for a child with a diagnosis of juvenile rheumatoid arthritis would include objectives related to:

    A. Preserving joint function
    B. Preventing side effects of corticosteroid therapy
    C. Minimizing growth to prevent deformities
    D. Promoting home schooling

68. Evaluation of care for a child with lupus would include assessing the family's knowledge of:

    A. High protein and fat diet
    B. Restricting sun exposure
    C. Reducing exercise
    D. Yearly eye examinations

69. The nurse knows that ritualistic behavior provides security for which age group?

    A. Infant
    B. Toddler
    C. Preschool
    D. Adolescent

70. The nurse is aware that which of the following age groups fears body mutilation?

    A. Toddler
    B. Preschool
    C. School-age
    D. Adolescent

71. As the nurse planning care for a school-age child, which activity would be the most appropriate for this age?

    A. Reading stories to the child
    B. Giving the child hospital supplies to collect
    C. Playing a card game
    D. Listening to a tape from peers

72. A child with a history of allergic rhinitis is scheduled for skin testing today. What measure by the nurse would promote the accuracy of the results?

    A. Making sure that the child has no nasal congestion
    B. Making sure that the child has not taken antihistamines in the last several days
    C. Testing for food allergens
    D. Using the posterior legs for testing

73. The nurse would recognize which early sign of anaphylactic shock in a client who received an allergy shot?

    A. Abdominal cramping
    B. Bradycardia
    C. Elevated BP
    D. Sense of doom

74. Which measure would the nurse teach the mother to limit dust mite exposure for her child?

A. Disinfecting the bath area daily
B. Limiting the child's exposure to animals
C. No smoking in the home
D. Restricting the child from playing on the carpet

75. A child with lupus has been placed on corticosteroids for an indefinite period. Which diet would the nurse teach the family to follow?

A. Bland
B. High-protein, high-fiber
C. Low-sodium
D. Reduced fat

76. The nurse knows that which symptom is associated with disease activity in a child with lupus?

A. Abdominal cramping
B. Chest congestion
C. Excessive fatigue
D. Sore throat

77. The nurse would teach a mother to avoid giving which food to a child who is allergic to wheat?

A. Instant drink mixes
B. Chocolate-covered peanuts
C. Salad dressings
D. Wieners

78. A child has been given a diagnosis of allergy to eggs. The nurse would teach the child to avoid which food?

A. Cola
B. Gravy
C. Instant breakfast drinks
D. Mayonnaise

79. The nurse would teach the mother to introduce cereal into the infant's diet at what age?

A. 2 months
B. 4 months
C. 9 months
D. 12 months

80. A mother brought her 6-month-old infant to the well-baby clinic. The mother is interested in starting her infant on cereal. Which cereal would the nurse instruct the mother to introduce first in the infant's diet?

A. Barley
B. Oat
C. Rice
D. Wheat

81. A mother began her 14-month-old child on cow's milk 4 weeks ago. Which symptom would the nurse identify as a possible allergy to cow's milk?

A. Chronic runny nose
B. Excessive urination
C. Irritability
D. Refusal to drink milk

82. A child admitted with a respiratory infection has been placed on continuous pulse oximetry. The nurse would identify which following situation as best for obtaining an accurate pulse oximetry reading?

A. Normal hemoglobin level
B. Room with a cool temperature
C. Very active child
D. A child with a capillary refill of 3 seconds or more

83. An infant is admitted to the pediatric unit with a respiratory infection. Which of the following could indicate to the nurse that the infant might be developing respiratory distress?

A. Heart rate = 100 bpm
B. Grunting on expiration
C. Capillary refill of 2 seconds
D. Urine output of 80 cc for last 4 hours

84. A 4-year-old child is receiving a blood transfusion. Which sign would indicate to the nurse that the child might be having a reaction to the blood?

A. BP = 90/50 mm Hg
B. Heart rate = 90 bpm
C. Oral temperature = 100°F (37.7°C)
D. Respiratory rate = 26/min

85. The order for a 4-year-old child reads gentamycin 1 drop OS qid. Which action by the nurse is appropriate to administer the medicine?

A. Pull the left lower eyelid down, instill drop, and repeat on other eye.
B. Pull the right pinna back and upward to instill drop.
C. Pull the left lower eyelid down to form a reservoir, then instill drop.
D. Pull the right pinna back and down to instill the drop, then repeat with the left.

86. Which action by the nurse is appropriate when instilling eardrops?

A. Pull the pinna back and upward to instill drops.
B. Hold the child still for 10 minutes after the drops are instilled.
C. Increase the head of the bed to facilitate absorption of the drops.
D. Tape a piece of cotton in the child's ears once the drops have been instilled.

87. The physician orders a saline enema for a 4-year-old child. The nurse knows that the appropriate amount of fluid to administer would be:

A. 100 ml
B. 300 ml
C. 500 ml
D. 700 ml

88. The nurse is making midmorning rounds on a child to whom she administered insulin at 7:30 AM. What symptom would alert the nurse that the child might be hypoglycemic?

A. Confused state
B. Irritability and crying
C. Flushed face
D. Fruity breath

89. A nurse is teaching the child and parents when to administer a combination of regular and NPH insulin injections. The nurse would teach the appropriate time as:
    A. Just before meals
    B. Thirty minutes before meals
    C. Just after meals
    D. In the morning and the evening

90. The nurse knows that repeated vaginal yeast infection in an adolescent girl is a classic sign of:
    A. Diabetes mellitus
    B. Poor hygiene
    C. Sexual activity
    D. Urinary tract dysfunction

91. The nurse knows that full-term infants are at a high risk for developing iron-deficiency anemia at what age?
    A. 6 weeks
    B. 4 months
    C. 6 months
    D. 9 months

92. An 11-month-old infant has been given a diagnosis of iron-deficiency anemia. The nurse would use which of the following criteria to evaluate the outcome of teaching a mother about iron supplements?
    A. The mother acknowledges that the iron should be given with fruit juice.
    B. The mother acknowledges that the iron should be given alone.
    C. The mother acknowledges that the iron should be given with meals.
    D. The mother acknowledges that the iron should be given with milk.

93. The nurse could use which of the following to determine if a mother is administering iron supplements to her infant?
    A. The absence of jaundice in the infant
    B. The observance of a tarry stool in the infant's diaper
    C. The mother saying that she is not having difficulty administering the iron
    D. The mother notifying the nurse that the infant no longer has diarrhea

94. The nurse would instruct the mother of a 6-year-old who is receiving iron to administer the iron:
    A. At bedtime
    B. Early in the morning
    C. By straw
    D. With protein

95. A mother complains that her daughter, who has juvenile rheumatoid arthritis, has stiffness in the morning. The nurse would advise the mother to:
    A. Give her warm baths each morning
    B. Administer a pain medication before the child gets up
    C. Do passive ROM with the child before she gets out of bed
    D. Have the child wake up 1 hour early to allow the stiffness to go away

96. The nurse would identify which criterion to evaluate the outcome of discharge teaching with a mother of a child with a diagnosis of rheumatic fever?
    A. Compliance with monthly penicillin shots
    B. Compliance with monthly throat cultures
    C. Compliance with yearly echocardiograms
    D. Compliance with a regular exercise program

97. The mother of a child with a diagnosis of Kawasaki disease asks the nurse, "Why does my child need aspirin when he no longer has a fever"? The nurse would explain that aspirin:
    A. Is given to reduce inflammation
    B. Is given for its antipyretic effects
    C. Prevents valve damage
    D. Decreases the chances of thrombus formation

98. The nurse would identify which child as being at high risk for developing iron-deficiency anemia?
    A. A 4-month-old child who is breastfeeding
    B. A 2-year-old child who drinks 48 oz of milk a day
    C. An 8-year-old child who refuses to drink milk
    D. A 15-year-old adolescent who refuses to eat chicken

99. The nurse would instruct the mother of a child on long-term steroid therapy to:
    A. Add vitamins to diet
    B. Limit social contacts
    C. Reduce sodium and fat in the diet
    D. Restrict physical activity

100. The nurse would identify a complication of meningitis as being:
    A. Hearing loss
    B. Spinal damage
    C. Urinary incontinence
    D. Memory loss during the acute illness

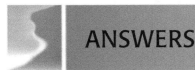

1. **(C)** Nursing process phase: data collection; client need: physiological adaptation; content area: pediatrics.

   RATIONALE
   (A) This infant does not weigh at least 2500 g. **(B)** The data do not give information on an ill child. **(C)** This infant is <2500 g, which describes a low-birth-weight infant. **(D)** A very-low-birth-weight infant is one that is <1500 g.

2. **(A)** Nursing process phase: planning; client need: management of care; content area: pediatrics.

   RATIONALE
   (A) It is very important to conserve warmth and energy in an infant with low birth weight. **(B)** Too much bathing can result in loss of body heat. **(C)** Daily shampooing is not necessary to prevent cradle cap and can cause heat loss. **(D)** Neonates should be placed in an environment with minimal stimulation.

3. **(C)** Nursing process phase: data collection; client need: physiological adaptation; content area: pediatrics.

   RATIONALE
   (A) The nurse must learn to identify behaviors that indicate discomfort in neonates. **(B)** Neonates do respond to painful stimuli. **(C)** Crying and flexing are means of responding to pain in neonates. **(D)** Change in VSs can indicate pain but can also indicate other problems.

4. **(C)** Nursing process phase: planning; client need: physiological adaptation; content area: pediatrics.

   RATIONALE
   (A) Acne does not occur in neonates. **(B)** Chickenpox has an incubation of approximately 2 weeks, and the neonate would be protected by maternal antibodies. **(C)** Jaundice is a common occurrence in newborns and low-birth-weight infants. **(D)** Scoliosis is not common in neonates.

5. **(B)** Nursing process phase: implementation; client need: basic care and comfort; content area: pediatrics.

   RATIONALE
   (A) Bathing can stimulate circulation, but this is not desired in the neonate. **(B)** Bathing two or three times weekly can remove bacteria. **(C)** Oils are not needed because the neonate has natural protection. **(D)** Cleansing is limited because of an increase in temperature loss during bathing.

6. **(A)** Nursing process phase: evaluation; client need: physiological adaptation; content area: pediatrics.

   RATIONALE
   (A) This would indicate that treatment was successful and the problem is resolving. **(B)** Surgery is not a treatment for respiratory distress syndrome. **(C)** Genetics has nothing to do with respiratory distress syndrome. **(D)** This type of respiratory illness is not contagious.

7. **(B)** Nursing process phase: planning; client need: management of care; content area: pediatrics.

   RATIONALE
   (A) Corticosteroids may be used for their anti-inflammatory effect, but they are not among the first measures taken with croup. **(B)** Cool humidification is usually the first measure taken. Cool temperature constricts the edematous blood vessels. Oxygen is supplemented when necessary. **(C)** Prophylactic intubation is no longer a trend. Intubation equipment should be on standby if respiratory failure occurs. **(D)** Whirlpool therapy is not indicated with croup.

8. **(C)** Nursing process phase: data collection; client need: coping and adaptation; content area: pediatrics.

   RATIONALE
   (A) Adolescents are concerned the most with privacy. **(B)** School-age children focus on external causes of illnesses. **(C)** Preschool children focus on illness as punishment for wrongdoing. **(D)** Infants have greater anxiety toward separation.

9. **(D)** Nursing process phase: data collection; client need: coping and adaptation; content area: pediatrics.

   RATIONALE
   (A) Attachment is not a phase of separation anxiety. **(B)** The initial phase is protest, demonstrated by crying. Acceptance is only superficial if this phase is demonstrated. **(C)** Acceptance is not a phase of separation anxiety. **(D)** Protest is demonstrated through crying. Despair is observed in depression of the child. Detachment, which seldom occurs, is demonstrated by an appearance of adjustment.

10. **(D)** Nursing process phase: implementation; client need: psychosocial adaptation; content area: pediatrics.

    RATIONALE
    (A) Parental involvement should be maximized. **(B)** Explanations should be simple and in lay terms. Use of dolls is beneficial. **(C)** Siderails should be used at all times. **(D)** Sibling visitation reduces anxiety and isolation.

11. **(B)** Nursing process phase: implementation; client need: management of care; content area: pediatrics.

    RATIONALE
    (A) A favorite toy is appropriate, but the tent separates him from his mother. The tent might frighten the child. The child in respiratory distress needs the comfort of his mother. **(B)** This choice would provide his mother's comfort while giving him the benefit of humidification. **(C)** Sedation is contraindicated because it could mask some signs of respiratory distress. **(D)** Threatening the child with separation from his mother is inappropriate.

12. **(B)** Nursing process phase: evaluation; client need: prevention and early detection of disease; content area: pediatrics.

    RATIONALE
    (A) Promotion of family involvement is good. Not all families are involved at this level of care. The goal should be family adaptation, not to relieve nurses of responsibility. **(B)** Before discharge, the family should demonstrate the ability to provide care for its child. **(C)** The family should be involved in care. The child is too young to be ultimately responsible for his or her own care. **(D)** Rejection of family indicates an adjustment problem.

13. **(A)** Nursing process phase: data collection; client need: prevention and early detection of disease; content area: pediatrics.

    RATIONALE
    (A) Chickenpox is characterized by itching and vesicular skin eruptions over the body, first on the torso. Incubation is 13–17 days. **(B)** Diphtheria is characterized by respiratory involvement and a membrane on the pharynx. **(C)** Measles is characterized by a macular rash that begins on the face and spreads to the trunk. **(D)** Mumps is characterized by swelling of the parotid glands.

14. **(C)** Nursing process phase: implementation; client need: basic care and comfort; content area: pediatrics.

    RATIONALE
    (A) Aspirin is contraindicated because of the increased chance of

developing Reye's syndrome. (**B**) Using soothing lotions is encouraged to decrease scratching, which can increase chances of secondary infection. (**C**) Keeping the fingernails short decreases the chance of breaking the skin by scratching. (**D**) Child should be isolated for approximately 6 days after the eruptions until crusty patches begin to form. This is a highly contagious disease.

15. (**D**) Nursing process phase: data collection; client need: psychosocial adaptation; content area: pediatrics.

    RATIONALE

    (**A**) Endocrine dysfunction is related to growth failure. (**B**) GI dysfunction indicates an organic FTT. (**C**) Neurological dysfunction is associated with organic FTT. (**D**) These are signs and symptoms of nonorganic FTT associated with neglect.

16. (**C**) Nursing process phase: planning; client need: coping and adaptation; content area: pediatrics.

    RATIONALE

    (**A**) Limiting the number of caregivers promotes consistency and helps to establish trust. (**B**) Parental decisions should be incorporated to promote parental self-esteem. (**C**) Developing the trust of both the child and the family establishes an appropriate environment in which to promote parenting skills. (**D**) Stimulation should be provided in an appropriate manner.

17. (**B**) Nursing process phase: evaluation; client need: psychosocial adaptation; content area: pediatrics.

    RATIONALE

    (**A**) The family demonstrates an ability to care for the child without depending on nursing staff. (**B**) To develop appropriately, the child should be in a family that is able to provide a nurturing environment. (**C**) The infant should be gaining weight. (**D**) Although the nurse wants to see progress toward developmental milestones, it may take longer than this hospital admission. If the family is nurturing and providing for the child appropriately, the milestones will be achieved.

18. (**D**) Nursing process phase: implementation; client need: pharmacological and parenteral therapies; content area: pediatrics.

    RATIONALE

    (**A**) Absorbing the remaining substance would not be recommended, and this is not the action of ipecac. (**B**) Dilution of the poisonous substance would not be recommended. (**C**) Ipecac is not administered to prevent aspiration. (**D**) Ipecac is administered to induce vomiting and remove stomach contents.

19. (**C**) Nursing process phase: planning; client need: basic care and comfort; content area: pediatrics.

    RATIONALE

    (**A**) A superficial burn would heal without scarring. (**B**) The epidermis is the middle layer, and this layer alone could not be burned. (**C**) Partial- and full-thickness burns involve all layers of the skin. (**D**) A fourth-degree full-thickness burn involves all layers of skin, subcutaneous tissue, and muscle.

20. (**A**) Nursing process phase: implementation; client need: reduction of risk potential; content area: pediatrics.

    RATIONALE

    (**A**) The nurse should promote mobility of the area as long as it would not interfere with grafts or healing. (**B**) The nurse should help the child to avoid scratching wound so that injury and delayed healing will not occur. (**C**) The nurse should encourage the child to take fluids and eat nutritious, high-protein meals, not to limit fluids. (**D**) The nurse should keep the wound clean and take care not to damage the crusts and eschar when cleaning.

21. (**A**) Nursing process phase: implementation; client need: physiological adaptation; content area: pediatrics.

    RATIONALE

    (**A**) Children respond to pain differently. One way is sleep or withdrawal. The best response is to assess for increased pulse and respirations, facial grimacing, and restlessness. (**B**) The child should be assessed before administration of the medication. (**C**) This response is acceptable, but the child should be assessed first. (**D**) This response is a nursing judgment that does not require input from a physician.

22. (**A**) Nursing process phase: implementation; client need: psychosocial adaptation; content area: pediatrics.

    RATIONALE

    (**A**) The bandages could be scary and the child may need some help adjusting. The best response is to stay with him until he feels comfortable in asking other children to play. (**B**) This intervention does not promote interaction among the children. (**C**) This response will not help to break the ice and initiate interaction. (**D**) This child may need help in interacting initially because of his different appearance.

23. (**A**) Nursing process phase: data collection; client need: physiological adaptation; content area: pediatrics.

    RATIONALE

    (**A**) A compound fracture occurs when the bone protrudes through the skin. (**B**) A greenstick fracture is an incomplete one in which the bone bends. (**C**) In an incomplete fracture, the bone fragments remain attached. (**D**) A simple fracture does not cause a break in the skin.

24. (**A**) Nursing process phase: implementation; client need: reduction of risk potential; content area: pediatrics.

    RATIONALE

    (**A**) The child's activity needs should be met without jeopardizing her traction. (**B**) The child needs activities appropriate to age. It would be better to assist her to identify how far she can move without assistance, by marking the bed with tape to alert her to a limitation. (**C**) It is not necessary that the parents be present at all times. The parents may not be able to be present all the time. (**D**) Things should be arranged to promote some independence in the child. If needed, she can call.

25. (**D**) Nursing process phase: implementation; client need: reduction of risk potential; content area: pediatrics.

    RATIONALE

    (**A**) Lowering the extremity could cause edema and should be discouraged. (**B**) The cast should stay dry and clean. (**C**) The child should be mobile when the cast is dry, but ROM exercises to the extremity would be dangerous. (**D**) The child should be instructed not to put anything inside the cast. Objects inside the cast could cause pressure points and sores.

26. (**B**) Nursing process phase: data collection; client need: physiological adaptation; content area: pediatrics

    RATIONALE

    (**A**) Glucose intolerance is not recognized as a form of diabetes. (**B**) This type of diabetes usually occurs in childhood. (**C**) This type of diabetes occurs in adult life. (**D**) Plain diabetes not recognized as a form of diabetes.

27. (**A**) Nursing process phase: implementation; client need: coping and adaptation; content area: pediatrics.

    RATIONALE

    (**A**) Give the shot and allow the child to get more practice. It is better to wait until she is comfortable. This would be a time for the nurse to allow the child to express her feelings. (**B**) This could be done when the child is ready to try on her own. (**C**) A balanced diet would help to control the disease, but she will still require medication. (**D**) This is not a physician's problem. The nurse should allow the child more time.

28. (**A**) Nursing process phase: planning; client need: physiological adaptation; content area: pediatrics.

    RATIONALE

    (**A**) Balancing diet, exercise, and insulin is the focus of therapeutic management that promotes optimal functioning. (**B**) Exercise is important in lowering blood glucose, but it must be considered in relation to the overall picture of diet and insulin therapy. (**C**) An adequate amount of nutrition is required to promote growth. (**D**) Exercise, not limiting exercise, decreases insulin needs.

29. (**A**) Nursing process phase: planning; client need: physiological adaptation; content area: pediatrics.

    RATIONALE

    (**A**) Ketoacidosis results if glucose control is not maintained and blood glucose levels rise. Signs and symptoms include ketonuria, glucosuria, dehydration, vomiting, electrolyte imbalance, metabolic acidosis, abdominal pain, fruity acetone breath, and drowsiness progressing to coma. (**B**) Headache is a symptom of low blood glucose. (**C**) Ketoacidosis is the result of high blood glucose levels. (**D**) Thirst does occur in hyperglycemia, but glucose in urine is more specific for ketoacidosis.

30. (**A**) Nursing process phase: data collection; client need: physiological adaptation; content area: pediatrics.

    RATIONALE

    (**A**) It is common for an ear infection to follow a respiratory infection in a toddler. Signs and symptoms include crying, restlessness, rolling head from side to side, and pulling on the affected ear. (**B**) Diphtheria is a respiratory illness that can affect this age group. (**C**) Pertussis is accompanied by a "whooping" cough. (**D**) Tonsillitis is accompanied by difficulty swallowing.

31. (**C**) Nursing process phase: planning; client need: physiological adaptation; content area: pediatrics.

    RATIONALE

    (**A**) Antibiotics are part of the management of otitis media. (**B**) Analgesics may be required. (**C**) Oxygen therapy is usually not a part of management. (**D**) Myringotomy may be required in some children.

32. (**A**) Nursing process phase: evaluation; client need: basic care and comfort; content area: pediatrics.

    RATIONALE

    (**A**) Comfort and absence of drainage would take priority for measuring evaluation of care. (**B**) Completion of antibiotics is an outcome, but it does not indicate status of ear or comfort. (**C**) Family may be required to give medications orally, but usually not injections for ear infections. (**D**) Prevention of secondary infections is also a means of evaluating care, but comfort and absence of infection are more specific.

33. (**C**) Nursing process phase: data collection; client need: physiological adaptation; content area: pediatrics.

    RATIONALE

    (**A**) Cool, dry skin is not a sign of cystic fibrosis. (**B**) Frequent urination is not a sign of cystic fibrosis. (**C**) Large, bulky, foul-smelling stools are a sign of cystic fibrosis. These are attributed to decrease in or absence of pancreatic enzymes, resulting in faulty absorption of nutrients. In addition, salty taste of sweat, weight loss in the presence of a good appetite, distended abdomen, and marked tissue wasting are signs of cystic fibrosis. (**D**) Poor appetite is not a symptom.

34. (**D**) Nursing process phase: data collection; client need: physiological adaptation; content area: pediatrics.

    RATIONALE

    (**A**) Bronchial constriction is not a problem associated with cystic fibrosis. (**B**) Inadequate surfactant is associated with premature infants. (**C**) Pulmonic stenosis is associated with cardiovascular problems that involve a narrowing of heart vessels. (**D**) Thick, tenacious mucus is a classic sign of cystic fibrosis that leads to pulmonary obstruction.

35. (**C**) Nursing process phase: implementation; client need: pharmacological and parenteral therapies; content area: pediatrics.

    RATIONALE

    (**A**) Intramuscular administration is an inappropriate route. (**B**) IV administration is an inappropriate route. (**C**) Pancreatic enzymes are available in capsule form. An adolescent would swallow the capsule. For a child who has difficulty swallowing a capsule, the capsule could be opened and the enzyme sprinkled on the child's food. (**D**) Intradermal administration is inappropriate.

36. (**C**) Nursing process phase: planning; client need: physiological adaptation; content area: pediatrics.

    RATIONALE

    (**A**) Enzymes are given to aid in the digestion and absorption of nutrients. (**B**) Heart muscle and vascular tone are not the focus for medical concerns. (**C**) Exercise promotes mobilization of pulmonary secretions and enhances pulmonary treatments. (**D**) Cystic fibrosis produces secretions; therefore stimulation of secretions is not a goal.

37. (**D**) Nursing process phase: planning; client need: basic care and comfort; content area: pediatrics.

    RATIONALE

    (**A**) Mist does not dilate alveoli. (**B**) Mist does not reduce secretions. (**C**) Mist does not prevent dehydration. (**D**) Mist helps to liquefy the thick secretions, making it easier for the child to bring the secretions up.

38. (**B**) Nursing process phase: planning; client need: reduction of risk potential; content area: pediatrics.

    RATIONALE

    (**A**) This position is not the best for draining the right lower lobe. (**B**) This position is the best for draining the right lower lobe. Postural drainage uses gravity to help move secretions. This position would help secretions move into the larger bronchi toward the mouth. (**C**) This position would not facilitate drainage of the lower lobes into the bronchi. (**D**) This position would not affect the drainage from the lungs.

39. (**B**) Nursing process phase: planning; client need: reduction of risk potential; content area: pediatrics.

    RATIONALE

    (**A**) If the child is allergic to dog and cat hair, then these animals should be avoided. (**B**) Therapeutic management of cystic fibrosis includes prevention and treatment of pulmonary infections. Persons with any kind of infection, bacterial or viral, should be avoided. (**C**) Sodium may become depleted because the sweat glands fail to reabsorb sodium; salt should not be avoided and may need to be supplemented. (**D**) Sunlight is not a problem with cystic fibrosis.

40. (**C**) Nursing process phase: data collection; client need: physiological adaptation; content area: pediatrics.

    RATIONALE

    (**A**) Pneumococcus is not the causative agent for RF. (**B**) Staphylococcus is not the causative agent for RF. (**C**) RF is caused by a group A β-hemolytic streptococcus. (**D**) Influenza B is not the cause of RF.

41. **(A)** Nursing process phase: implementation; client need: pharmacological and parenteral therapies; content area: pediatrics.

    RATIONALE

    (A) Corticosteroids may be administered for pancarditis and valvular involvement. **(B)** Squatting positions are useful in treating certain types of heart defects in children. **(C)** Rest is important for these children. Visits by friends during the acute phase are discouraged. **(D)** Sunlight does not affect this disease process.

42. **(D)** Nursing process phase: planning; client need: pharmacological and parenteral therapies; content area: pediatrics.

    RATIONALE

    (A) Aspirin is not the treatment for carditis in RF. **(B)** The rash associated with RF is nonitching. **(C)** Headaches are not a major complaint of RF. **(D)** Polyarthritis, migratory, swollen, hot, red, painful joints, and fever are symptoms of this disease. Aspirin is prescribed as an anti-inflammatory agent to suppress joint inflammation.

43. **(C)** Nursing process phase: evaluation; client need: pharmacological and parenteral therapies; content area: pediatrics.

    RATIONALE

    (A) Coughing and deep breathing are not home-care interventions. **(B)** There are no diet and fluid restrictions for home care. **(C)** Penicillin therapy is prophylactic to prevent recurrences of RF. **(D)** Oxygen therapy is not a home intervention with RF.

44. **(A)** Nursing process phase: data collection; client need: physiological adaptation; content area: pediatrics.

    RATIONALE

    (A) Halitosis is common for 10–14 days after surgery and can be relieved with oral fluids and mouthwash. This would be the nurse's least concern. **(B)** Increased pulse could be associated with pain or blood loss and requires close observation. **(C)** Nausea can be associated with blood loss and would be of concern. **(D)** Restlessness can be a sign of pain or blood loss, and the child should be observed closely.

45. **(C)** Nursing process phase: implementation; client need: basic care and comfort; content area: pediatrics.

    RATIONALE

    (A) Chocolate milk is appropriate in a full-liquid diet. **(B)** Ice cream is appropriate in a full-liquid diet. **(C)** Acidic fluids and foods such as orange juice should be avoided because they can cause irritation to the throat during healing. **(D)** Popsicles are an appropriate clear liquid. Red or brown popsicles should be avoided because they might mask signs of bleeding.

46. **(D)** Nursing process phase: data collection; client need: physiological adaptation; content area: pediatrics.

    RATIONALE

    (A) Sleep apnea is not a sign of asthma. **(B)** Inspiratory stridor is not a sign of asthma. **(C)** Productive cough is not a sign of asthma. **(D)** A prolonged expiratory phase of respiration with shortness of breath, nasal flaring, audible wheezing, and a hacking, nonproductive cough are signs of asthma.

47. **(B)** Nursing process phase: planning; client need: pharmacological and parenteral therapies; content area: pediatrics.

    RATIONALE

    (A) Antibiotics may be administered if infection is thought to be the cause of the attack or if secondary infection is a concern. **(B)** Nausea and vomiting are not associated with asthma. **(C)** Hypersensitivities and inflammation are a concern with asthma. **(D)** Bronchospasms are of concern with asthma.

48. **(D)** Nursing process phase: data collection; client need: physiological adaptation; content area: pediatrics.

    RATIONALE

    (A) This defect is spina bifida. **(B)** This defect is spina bifida occulta. **(C)** This anomaly is meningocele. **(D)** This anomaly is myelomeningocele.

49. **(A)** Nursing process phase: implementation; client need: safety and infection control; content area: pediatrics.

    RATIONALE

    (A) Meticulous skin care, especially in sac and genital areas, is critical. **(B)** Supine positioning should be avoided because pressure could be placed on the sac. **(C)** The diaper should not be secured around the infant, only placed under him or her. **(D)** A sterile moist dressing should be placed over the sac.

50. **(A)** Nursing process phase: planning; client need: physiological adaptation; content area: pediatrics.

    RATIONALE

    (A) A large number of children with myelomeningocele develop hydrocephalus and require shunting. **(B)** Intussusception is not associated with neural tube defects. **(C)** The majority of children with myelomeningocele have normal IQs. **(D)** Pneumonia can be a potential problem but is not the appropriate choice.

51. **(A)** Nursing process phase: implementation; client need: coping and adaptation; content area: pediatrics.

    RATIONALE

    (A) It is best that the mother hold the child so that the child will not become more upset. Her presence will be a comfort. **(B)** Having the mother leave the examination room could cause the child to become further upset and could further compromise respiratory status. **(C)** Cool fruit juice is appropriate once the immediate distress is over and the inflammation is going down. **(D)** A throat culture could cause complete obstruction in a child with epiglottitis who is in distress. Examination of the throat should take place only if someone is available to intubate the child.

52. **(B)** Nursing process phase: data collection; client need: physiological adaptation; content area: pediatrics.

    RATIONALE

    (A) This organism is not the cause of epiglottitis, but it is the cause of scarlet fever. **(B)** This organism is the usual cause of epiglotittis. **(C)** This virus is frequently associated with laryngitis. **(D)** This organism is the usual cause of bacterial tracheitis.

53. **(A)** Nursing process phase: implementation; client need: reduction of risk potential; content area: pediatrics.

    RATIONALE

    (A) This is the most important intervention. Epiglottitis can cause complete airway obstruction. Emergency equipment would be needed immediately. **(B)** This intervention is appropriate, but the tracheostomy equipment is the most important for a new admission. **(C)** Antibiotics are usually given to the child, but the nurse should wait for the physician's order. **(D)** Initially the child will be NPO, but the tracheostomy equipment is the most important intervention.

54. **(C)** Nursing process phase: data collection; client need: physiological adaptation; content area: pediatrics.

    RATIONALE

    (A) The infant should be able to handle saliva without drooling. **(B)** The infant will more than likely be a mouth breather, but noisy respirations are not expected. **(C)** The infant will have difficulty sucking because of the inability to create a vacuum with the lips. **(D)** The cleft lip should not affect the infant's ability to swallow.

55. **(A)** Nursing process phase: implementation; client need: safety and infection control; content area: pediatrics.

    RATIONALE

    (A) Restraints should be applied to keep the infant from putting fingers in the mouth and causing trauma to the incision. **(B)** The infant should not be placed on the abdomen because the incision site could be traumatized in this position. **(C)** It would be acceptable to position in an infant seat, but the major concern is to avoid trauma to the incision. **(D)** A mist tent is unnecessary.

56. **(D)** Nursing process phase: implementation; client need: basic care and comfort; content area: pediatrics.

    RATIONALE

    (A) Rectal thermometers should be avoided. **(B)** Brushing could cause gums to bleed. **(C)** Aspirin should not be given because aspirin affects platelet function and increases risk of bleeding. **(D)** Using creams is an appropriate means to remove hair, because shaving with a razor could cause bleeding if the skin were cut.

57. **(C)** Nursing process phase: planning; client need: reduction of risk potential; content area: pediatrics.

    RATIONALE

    (A) Raw vegetables and fruit should be avoided because bacteria can be introduced to the child. **(B)** Strict bedrest is unnecessary. **(C)** Temperature elevations should be reported to the physician. **(D)** Visitors should be limited to those without infections, but not restricted.

58. **(D)** Nursing process phase: implementation; client need: prevention and early detection of disease; content area: pediatrics.

    RATIONALE

    (A) It would be important for parents to understand pain management, but preventing sickle cell crisis is the priority. **(B)** Home health care would not be necessary. **(C)** Support groups can be beneficial to the family but would not be the priority intervention. **(D)** Teaching measures to prevent sickle cell crisis is most important to maintain physiological integrity of the child.

59. **(C)** Nursing process phase: planning; client need: coping and adaptation; content area: pediatrics.

    RATIONALE

    (A) The child may be loud and crying, but demanding explanations would be characteristic of an older child. **(B)** The preschooler would be physical, requiring restraint, not stoic. **(C)** Clinging to parents is a typical behavior of the preschooler. **(D)** Stalling behaviors are typical of school-age children.

60. **(A)** Nursing process phase: planning; client need: pharmacological and parenteral therapies; content area: pediatrics.

    RATIONALE

    (A) Meperidine should not be administered for longer than 48 hours because of build-up of a toxic metabolite. **(B)** An oral dose of meperidine would be four times the dose of morphine and might not get the same analgesic effects. **(C)** Morphine can be administered for a longer time than meperidine with fewer side effects. **(D)** Naloxone should not be used with meperidine because it can alter the seizure threshold.

61. **(B)** Nursing process phase: planning; client need: reduction of risk potential; content area: pediatrics.

    RATIONALE

    (A) Isometric exercises should be encouraged. **(B)** Forcing fluids is important to prevent constipation and to promote removal of calcium from the body. **(C)** Peer visitation is important at this age, and engaging in table games is a good activity for this age group. **(D)** An explanation of procedures and their effects on the body is important, but a detailed description is not necessary.

62. **(C)** Nursing process phase: data collection; client need: reduction of risk potential; content area: pediatrics.

    RATIONALE

    (A) Bruising can be expected with compound fracture. The fingers should be observed for further discoloration that would indicate decreased circulation. **(B)** Capillary refill of 2 seconds is normal. **(C)** Pallor suggests a decrease in circulation to the extremity. The surgeon should be notified. **(D)** Edema is expected but should be watched for an increase that might impair circulation.

63. **(D)** Nursing process phase: data; client need: physiological adaptation; content area: pediatrics.

    RATIONALE

    (A) Pain is expected and pressure on nerves can cause pain to radiate. **(B)** Pain responding to oral medication is acceptable. **(C)** Pain responding to a narcotic is acceptable. **(D)** Pain unresponsive to a narcotic indicates deteriorating neuromuscular status. This requires immediate attention.

64. **(C)** Nursing process phase: data collection; client need: safety and infection control; content area: pediatrics.

    RATIONALE

    (A) Increased pain can suggest infection, but other symptoms should be present with pain. **(B)** This temperature should be watched. A low-grade fever can be expected with inflammation. **(C)** Infected areas are hot to touch, and the heat can radiate through the cast. **(D)** Bloody drainage on the cast does not mean infection, but drainage can lead to infection.

65. **(B)** Nursing process phase: data collection; client need: reduction of risk potential; content area: pediatrics.

    RATIONALE

    (A) This is an acceptable BP for an adolescent. **(B)** Petechiae on the chest is a classic symptom of pulmonary fat embolism. This would require immediate attention. **(C)** Pain management is important; additional medication may be required. **(D)** This is an acceptable urinary output.

66. **(A)** Nursing process phase: implementation; client need: reduction of risk potential; content area: pediatrics.

    RATIONALE

    (A) Weights should be hanging freely to get the desired effect. **(B)** Neurovascular checks have no effect on the traction. **(C)** Relaxed muscles will not affect this traction. **(D)** Countertraction is achieved by the body weight, not tightness of the bandage.

67. **(A)** Nursing process phase: evaluation; client need: prevention and early detection of disease; content area: pediatrics.

    RATIONALE

    (A) The disease directly affects joint capsules; therefore, the goal would be directed toward preserving joint functioning. **(B)** Side effects cannot be prevented but can be minimized. **(C)** Normal growth is important. Minimizing growth will not prevent deformities. **(D)** The child should attend school with peers if at all possible.

68. **(B)** Nursing process phase: evaluation; client need: prevention and early detection of disease; content area: pediatrics.

    RATIONALE

    (A) Diet should be low in fat to reduce chances of weight gain. **(B)** Sun exposure should be restricted—especially between 10 AM and 2 PM—by use of sunscreen, hats, and clothing that covers the extremities. **(C)** Exercise should be encouraged, but should not be strenuous. **(D)** Yearly eye examinations are essential if the child is taking hydroxychloroquine sulfate (Plaquenil). Hydroxychloroquine sulfate has been associated with retinal damage.

69. **(B)** Nursing process phase: data collection; client need: growth and development through the life span; content area: pediatrics.

    RATIONALE

    (A) Infants are in the stage of trust versus mistrust, and a consistent primary caregiver is important. **(B)** Toddlers are developing a sense of autonomy, and ritualistic behavior provides a sense of comfort. **(C)** Preschoolers are developing a sense of initiative and exploration. **(D)** Adolescents are interested in peer support and identification.

70. **(B)** Nursing process phase: data collection; client need: growth and development through the life span; content area: pediatrics.

    RATIONALE

    (A) Toddlers fear separation. **(B)** Preschoolers fear body mutilation. **(C)** School-age children fear the physical nature of the illness. **(D)** Adolescents are concerned with loss of independence.

71. **(C)** Nursing process phase: data collection; client need: growth and development through the life span; content area: pediatrics.

    RATIONALE

    (A) School-age children would prefer to be more active. **(B)** Preschool children are interested in collecting. **(C)** School-age children are at an age for competitive games. This would be an appropriate activity. **(D)** Peer relationships are very important to the adolescent.

72. **(B)** Nursing process phase: data collection; client need: pharmacological and parenteral therapies; content area: pediatrics.

    RATIONALE

    (A) This would not affect the testing. **(B)** Antihistamines could alter the results of testing. It is best to wait 48–96 hours after the last dose of antihistamine. **(C)** Only testing for food allergens would limit results for sensitivities to environmental allergens and pollens. **(D)** Forearms and upper back are the best sites for testing.

73. **(D)** Nursing process phase: data collection; client need: physiological adaptation; content area: pediatrics.

    RATIONALE

    (A) Abdominal cramping is a late sign of anaphylaxis. **(B)** Tachycardia is a sign of anaphylaxis. **(C)** Hypotension is seen in anaphylaxis. **(D)** A sense of doom voiced by the client is an early sign of anaphylaxis.

74. **(D)** Nursing process phase: implementation; client need: prevention and early detection of disease; content area: pediatrics.

    RATIONALE

    (A) Disinfecting the bath area reduces exposure to molds. **(B)** Restricting pets does not affect allergies to dust mites. **(C)** Cigarette smoking is an irritant, not an allergen. **(D)** Dust mites are attracted to carpets. Avoiding playing on carpets reduces exposure.

75. **(C)** Nursing process phase: implementation; client need: physiological adaptation; content area: pediatrics.

    RATIONALE

    (A) There are no data to support the need for a bland diet. **(B)** A high-protein, high-fiber diet is not necessary. **(C)** A low-sodium diet would be recommended because of fluid gain with corticosteroids. **(D)** A reduced-fat diet is good, but there is no indication that the child is consuming too much fat.

76. **(C)** Nursing process phase: data collection; client need: physiological adaptation; content area: pediatrics.

    RATIONALE

    (A) Abdominal cramping is usually not associated with disease activity in lupus. **(B)** Chest congestion does not indicate disease activity with lupus. **(C)** Excessive fatigue is a sign of disease activity with lupus. **(D)** Sore throat does not indicate disease activity with lupus.

77. **(D)** Nursing process phase: implementation; client need: prevention and early detection of disease; content area: pediatrics.

    RATIONALE

    (A) Instant drink mixes should not contain wheat products. **(B)** Chocolate-covered peanuts would not affect an allergy to wheat. **(C)** Wheat is usually not contained in salad dressings. **(D)** Wieners do contain wheat.

78. **(D)** Nursing process phase: implementation; client need: prevention and early detection of disease; content area: pediatrics.

    RATIONALE

    (A) Cola should be avoided with allergy to chocolate. **(B)** Gravy should be avoided with wheat allergy. **(C)** Instant breakfast drinks should be avoided with milk allergy. **(D)** Mayonnaise is made with eggs and should be eliminated from the child's diet.

79. **(B)** Nursing process phase: implementation; client need: prevention and early detection of disease; content area: pediatrics.

    RATIONALE

    (A) Two months is too soon. **(B)** Four to six months is an appropriate time to introduce cereal. **(C)** By 9 months of age, fruit, vegetables, and junior foods can be introduced. **(D)** By 12 months of age, cow's milk can be introduced.

80. **(C)** Nursing process phase: implementation; client need: prevention and early detection of disease; content area: pediatrics.

    RATIONALE

    (A) Barley is not the first choice. **(B)** Oat is not the first choice. **(C)** Rice is the first choice because it is easier to digest and has the least potential of allergy than other cereals. Cereals should be introduced one at a time, in case allergies develop. This would make it easier to identify the allergen. **(D)** Wheat should be introduced after rice cereal.

81. **(A)** Nursing process phase: data collection; client need: physiological adaptation; content area: pediatrics.

    RATIONALE

    (A) Chronic runny nose is an allergic response to cow's milk. **(B)** Excessive urination is not indicative of an allergy. **(C)** Irritability can be the result of symptoms of an allergy. **(D)** Refusal to drink milk does not imply an allergy.

82. **(A)** Nursing process phase: data collection; client need: physiological adaptation; content area: pediatrics.

    RATIONALE

    (A) Normal hemoglobin levels give a more accurate pulse oximetry reading. **(B)** Cool temperature can cause vascular constriction, and the reading would not be as accurate. **(C)** Excessive motion can interfere with the reading. **(D)** Poor perfusion can interfere with an accurate reading.

83. **(B)** Nursing process phase: data collection; client need: physiological adaptation; content area: pediatrics.

    RATIONALE

    (A) This is an appropriate heart rate for an infant. **(B)** Expiratory grunting can indicate respiratory distress. **(C)** This is a desirable capillary refill time. **(D)** This is a satisfactory urinary output.

84. **(C)** Nursing process phase: data collection; client need: pharmacological and parenteral therapies; content area: pediatrics.

    RATIONALE

    (A) This is a normal BP. **(B)** This is a normal heart rate. **(C)** This temperature is elevated, which indicates an allergic response to blood. **(D)** This is an acceptable respiratory rate.

85. **(C)** Nursing process phase: implementation; client need: pharmacological and parenteral therapies; content area: pediatrics.
    RATIONALE
    (A) The abbreviation OS means left eye, not both eyes. **(B)** The order is to instill drops in the eye, not the ear. **(C)** The abbreviation OS means left eye, and pulling lower lid down and forming a reservoir are proper actions. **(D)** The order is to instill drops in the eye, not the ear.

86. **(A)** Nursing process phase: implementation; client need: prevention and early detection of disease; content area: pediatrics.
    RATIONALE
    (A) This is the proper way to administer eardrops. **(B)** The child should be held still for a few minutes, but 10 minutes is not necessary. **(C)** It is not necessary to raise the head of the bed. **(D)** This is acceptable, but not required.

87. **(B)** Nursing process phase: implementation; client need: basic care and comfort; content area: pediatrics.
    RATIONALE
    (A) This is too small an amount. Infants are given approximately 200 ml. **(B)** This is the appropriate amount for a 4-year-old child. **(C)** This amount would be in the range for a school-age child. **(D)** This amount is in the range for a school-age child.

88. **(B)** Nursing process phase: data collection; client need: physiological adaptation; content area: pediatrics.
    RATIONALE
    (A) Confusion is a symptom of hyperglycemia. **(B)** An irritable, weepy, and nervous child is consistent with hypoglycemia. **(C)** Flushed face is a symptom of hyperglycemia. **(D)** Fruity breath is a sign of hyperglycemia.

89. **(B)** Nursing process phase: implementation; client need: pharmacological and parenteral therapies; content area: pediatrics.
    RATIONALE
    (A) The insulin should be administered 30 minutes before meals. **(B)** Administering the insulin 30 minutes before meals coordinates the peak of the insulin with the ingestion of food. **(C)** This would be too late; insulin is given before meals. **(D)** Insulin is usually administered to children in the morning and the evening, but this answer does not give information on the time for each of the doses.

90. **(A)** Nursing process phase: data collection; client need: physiological adaptation; content area: pediatrics.
    RATIONALE
    (A) Vaginal yeast infections and urinary tract infections are early signs of diabetes in adolescent girls. **(B)** This is not the cause of yeast infections in girls with diabetes. **(C)** Sexual activity can result in vaginal infections, but a hyperglycemic state contributes to yeast infections in girls with diabetes. **(D)** Urinary tract dysfunction does not cause vaginal yeast infections.

91. **(D)** Nursing process phase: planning; client need: physiological adaptation; content area: pediatrics.
    RATIONALE
    (A) Iron stores are adequate for the first 5–6 months of age in the infant. **(B)** Iron stores from the mother are still adequate when an infant is 4 months old. **(C)** At 6 months, maternal iron stores are depleting, but iron levels are maintained for an additional 120 days, through the life of these RBCs. **(D)** The infant receives iron from the mother in utero that can be stored for up to 6 months. The majority of the iron is stored in the hemoglobin of RBCs, and an additional supply is stored in the liver, spleen, and bone marrow. The life of a normal RBC is 120 days. If the infant is not receiving iron supplements or an adequate amount of iron

in the diet, iron-deficiency anemia will show up at 9 months, after the life of the RBCs stored from the mother.

92. **(A)** Nursing process phase: evaluation; client need: prevention and early detection of disease; content area: pediatrics.
    RATIONALE
    (A) Fruit juice contains vitamin C, which enhances the absorption of iron. **(B)** Iron should be given with juice or a multivitamin to increase its absorption. **(C)** Iron should be administered between meals, because the bulk of a meal can decrease the absorption of the iron in the upper GI tract. **(D)** Milk decreases the absorption of iron.

93. **(B)** Nursing process phase: evaluation; client need: physiological adaptation; content area: pediatrics.
    RATIONALE
    (A) Jaundice does not indicate iron deficiency. **(B)** Iron supplements can cause green, tarry stools. **(C)** It is good for a mother to identify the fact that she is compliant, but evidence of the tarry stool is objective data. **(D)** Iron deficiency does not produce diarrhea. Iron supplements can result in constipation.

94. **(C)** Nursing process phase: implementation; client need: pharmacological and parenteral therapies; content area: pediatrics.
    RATIONALE
    (A) Iron should be administered in divided doses throughout the day to maximize absorption. **(B)** Dividing the dose throughout the day maximizes absorption. **(C)** Iron should be given through a straw or by a dropper or syringe to prevent staining the teeth. **(D)** Iron absorption is enhanced if given with vitamin C, not protein.

95. **(A)** Nursing process phase: implementation; client need: basic care and comfort; content area: pediatrics.
    RATIONALE
    (A) Soaking in warm water decreases stiffness in the joints. **(B)** Pain medication does not reduce stiffness. **(C)** Doing passive ROM reduces stiffness but does not soothe the joint as the warm water does. **(D)** Waking up early does not reduce stiffness.

96. **(A)** Nursing process phase: evaluation; client need: prevention and early detection of disease; content area: pediatrics.
    RATIONALE
    (A) Penicillin shots are usually administered for an indefinite period after the occurrence of RF to prevent reinfection with streptococcus. **(B)** Monthly throat cultures are not necessary. **(C)** Yearly echocardiograms can evaluate the status of the heart but do nothing to prevent reinfection. **(D)** A regular exercise program is good for the child, but the aim of therapy is to prevent reinfection with streptococcus.

97. **(D)** Nursing process phase: implementation; client need: pharmacological and parenteral therapies; content area: pediatrics.
    RATIONALE
    (A) Aspirin controls inflammation, but the reason for aspirin at this time is to decrease thrombus formation. **(B)** Because fever is gone, the aspirin is not needed as an antipyretic. **(C)** Aspirin cannot prevent valve damage, but it can help to control inflammation that contributes to valve damage. **(D)** Aspirin is continued in an antiplatelet dose once fever has subsided to decrease thrombus formation.

98. **(B)** Nursing process phase: data collection; client need: prevention and early detection of disease; content area: pediatrics.
    RATIONALE
    (A) This child is not at high risk because of maternal iron stores. **(B)** A 2-year-old child's diet should be limited to 24 oz of milk per day. **(C)** Refusing to drink milk does not cause iron-defi-

ciency anemia. **(D)** Refusing to eat chicken does not cause iron-deficiency anemia.

99. **(C)** Nursing process phase: implementation; client need: basic care and comfort; content area: pediatrics.

    RATIONALE
    (A) This would not be necessary because of steroid therapy. **(B)** The child needs to be around peers for support and normal development. **(C)** Steroids cause water retention and increase

appetite. Weight gain is common. **(D)** The child still needs to be active, and exercise is encouraged.

100. **(A)** Nursing process phase: data collection; client need: physiological adaptation; content area: pediatrics.

    RATIONALE
    (A) Hearing loss can occur from damage to nerves. **(B)** Spinal damage is not likely. **(C)** Urinary incontinence is not a complication. **(D)** Memory loss is not a complication.

CHAPTER 5

Medical-Surgical Nursing: Content Review and Test

Caroline Bunker Rosdahl, RN, MA
Patricia Beare, RN, PhD

Respiratory System

Basic Information

All body cells depend on adequate oxygen level and carbon dioxide removal. The respiratory system is regulated by the central nervous system (CNS) and depends on the cardiovascular system for its blood supply. Diseases of the respiratory system can be either primary (direct) or secondary (caused by diseases in other body systems). The licensed practical nurse (LPN) needs to make a respiratory assessment of all clients and include this information in the nursing care plan even when secondary to disease in other body systems. In this chapter, "Diagnostic tests and methods" replaces "Planning" step.

I. Basic data collection
 A. Subjective observations (client description)
  1. Cough
  2. Difficulty in breathing
  3. Pain
  4. Weakness, tiredness
  5. Sputum
 B. Client history
  1. Respiratory illness or difficulty
  2. Injuries
  3. Use of extra pillows when sleeping
  4. Smoking
  5. Occupation
  6. Use of medications
 C. Objective observations (LPN description)
  1. Respirations
   a. Rate
   b. Depth
   c. Type
   d. Difficulty in breathing
  2. Symptoms of lack of oxygen
   a. Yawning
   b. Restlessness
   c. Drowsiness
   d. Anxiety
   e. Confusion
   f. Disorientation
  3. Skin
   a. Color
    1) Pale or ruddy (reddened)
    2) Cyanotic (bluish): color of lips, nails, inside of mouth checked
   b. Temperature
   c. Excessive sweating
  4. Cough
   a. Frequency: continuous, sporadic (on and off)
   b. Type: productive, moist, hacking, dry, nonproductive
  5. Sputum
   a. Presence or absence
   b. Type: thick, frothy, watery
   c. Color: white, yellow, rusty, blood-tinged, purulent
   d. Amount: scant, moderate, abundant
   e. Odor
  6. Vital signs
   a. Pulse: rate, quality, type
   b. Blood pressure (BP)
   c. Temperature: rectal, unless ordered otherwise
 D. Recording and reporting of all observations

Major Respiratory Diagnoses

Epistaxis (Nosebleed)

I. Description
 A. Bleeding from the nose

B. Causes
   1. Direct trauma to nose: blow to nose, insertion of foreign object
   2. Nasal polyps
   3. Acute or chronic infections: sinusitis or rhinitis
   4. Systemic diseases such as hypertension
   5. Local irritation: inhalation of chemicals
   6. Varicosities within nasal cavity
   7. Chronic use of aspirin
   8. High altitudes, dry climates
   9. Hodgkin's disease
   10. Scurvy
   11. Vitamin K deficiency
   12. Rheumatic fever
   13. Blood dyscrasias: hemophilia, purpura, leukemia, some anemias
II. Data collection
   A. Subjective symptoms
      1. Bleeding
      2. Pain
      3. Lightheadedness, dizziness
      4. Difficulty in breathing through the nose
   B. Objective symptoms
      1. Observation of bleeding from nose
      2. Trauma around nose
      3. Decrease in BP
      4. Rapid, bounding pulse
      5. Dyspnea
      6. Pallor
      7. Other indications of progressive shock
III. Diagnostic tests and methods
   A. Client history
   B. Physical examination
      1. Examination of nasal cavity
      2. Bruises or bleeding elsewhere
   C. Laboratory tests
      1. Repeated hemoglobin (Hgb) and hematocrit (Hct) tests
      2. Platelet count
      3. Prothrombin time (PT)
IV. Implementation
   A. Check nasal packing.
   B. Keep airway open (have client breathe through mouth).
   C. Control bleeding.
      1. Pinch soft part of nose firmly.
      2. Tilt head slightly forward.
      3. Apply ice collar or cold wet compresses to nose.
   D. Encourage expectoration of blood (swallowing blood causes vomiting).
   E. Monitor skin color.
   F. Monitor vital signs.
      1. Report and record vital signs.
      2. Report any changes in vital signs immediately.
   G. Provide mouth care.
   H. Administer medications as ordered.
   I. Instruct client not to drink hot fluids.
   J. Provide reassurance to client and family.
   K. Explain home care:
      1. Instruct client not to pick nose or insert foreign objects in nose.

   2. Emphasize need for follow-up examinations and periodic blood studies for nosebleeds.
   3. Suggest use of humidifiers if client lives in dry climate or at high elevation, or both, or in home heated with circulating hot air.
V. Evaluation
   A. Client maintains effective airway and breathing pattern.
   B. Bleeding is absent.
   C. Client reports increased comfort.
   D. Vital signs remain stable.
   E. Laboratory blood values remain within normal range.
   F. Pain is decreased or absent.
   G. Client demonstrates an understanding of disease process, treatment, and home care.

Laryngitis

I. Description
   A. Acute or chronic inflammation and swelling of mucous membrane lining of the larynx and vocal cords (enlarged upper end of the trachea)
   B. Acute form possibly occurring as an isolated infection or as part of a generalized bacterial or viral upper respiratory tract infection
   C. Possibly leading to decreased secretion and shrinking of the mucous membrane
   D. Difficulty in breathing if crusts accumulate in laryngeal area and vocal cords, narrowing the breathing area
   E. Possibly becoming chronic because of recurrent irritation after the acute form
   F. Causes
      1. Excessive use of voice
      2. Exposure to cold and wet
      3. Spread of infection from nose and throat
      4. Local irritation caused by smoking
      5. Inhalation of irritating chemicals, dust, fumes
      6. Aspiration of caustic chemicals
      7. Preexisting nose and throat pathology
      8. Association with other diseases such as whooping cough, measles
      9. Alcohol abuse
II. Data collection
   A. Subjective symptoms
      1. Pain on swallowing or speaking
      2. Complaints of hoarseness
      3. Complaints of dry cough
      4. Tickling sensation in throat
      5. Fever
      6. Malaise
      7. Complaints of difficulty in breathing (because of crust formation)
   B. Objective symptoms
      1. Loss of voice
      2. Hoarseness
      3. Dry cough
      4. Increase in temperature
      5. Edema of larynx
      6. Difficulty in breathing (because of crust formation and narrowing of breathing space)

III. Diagnostic tests and methods
   A. Client history
   B. Physical examination
   C. Indirect laryngoscopy (use of mirror visualization to examine the larynx)
      1. Determines presence of red, inflamed, and, occasionally, hemorrhagic vocal cords and exudate (fluid, pus, or serous material)
      2. Checks for swelling
IV. Implementation
   A. Mark intercom to inform other hospital personnel that the client cannot answer.
   B. Explain to client why he or she should not talk.
   C. Provide a "magic slate" or pad and pencil for communication.
   D. Minimize need to talk by anticipating the client's needs.
   E. Provide vaporizer or humidifier.
   F. Administer medications as ordered.
   G. Discourage smoking.
   H. Explain disease process, treatment, and home care:
      1. Use of humidifier during winter
      2. Avoidance of air conditioning during summer (because air conditioning dehumidifies room)
      3. Use of medicated throat lozenges
      4. No smoking
V. Evaluation
   A. Client reports increased comfort.
   B. Laryngitis is absent.
   C. Client demonstrates an understanding of disease process, treatment, and home care.

Carcinoma of the Larynx

   I. Description
      A. Most common form (95%) is squamous cell carcinoma.
      B. Rare forms include adenocarcinoma, sarcoma, and others.
      C. Intrinsic tumors are found on the true vocal cord and do not tend to spread because nearby tissues lack lymph nodes.
      D. Extrinsic tumors are found on the larynx outside of the true vocal cord and tend to spread early.
      E. Cancer of the larynx is nine times more common in men than in women and usually occurs between the ages of 50 and 65 years.
      F. Causes
         1. Major predisposing factors
            a. Smoking (especially heavy)
            b. Alcoholism
            c. Chronic inhalation of noxious fumes
            d. Familial tendency
            e. History of frequent laryngitis and vocal straining
      G. Classification by location
         1. Supraglottis (posterior surface of epiglottis, false vocal cords)
         2. Glottis (true vocal cords)
         3. Subglottis (downward from vocal cords [rare])
   II. Data collection
      A. Subjective symptoms

1. Hoarseness lasting >3 weeks
2. Cough
3. Pain or burning in throat after drinking citrus juice or hot liquid
4. Difficulty in breathing
5. Pain radiating to ear
6. Anxiety
   B. Objective symptoms
      1. Hoarseness
      2. Lump in throat
      3. Dysphagia (difficulty in swallowing)
      4. Cough
      5. Enlarged lymph nodes in neck
III. Diagnostic tests and methods
   A. Client history
   B. Visual examination (indirect laryngoscopy)
   C. Direct laryngoscopy
   D. Biopsy examination
   E. Laryngeal tomography
   F. Chest x-ray to detect metastases
IV. Implementation
   A. Provide emotional support.
   B. Provide general preoperative and postoperative care for:
      1. Laryngectomy (removal of larynx, partial or complete)
      2. Radical neck dissection (excision that includes lymph nodes, epiglottis, muscle tissue, thyroid cartilage)
         a. Permanent tracheostomy
      3. Radiotherapy with surgery
   C. Preoperative care
      1. Before partial or total removal of larynx:
         a. Instruct client to maintain good mouth care.
         b. Instruct bearded male client to shave off beard (helps in giving postoperative care).
         c. Encourage client to talk about concerns and problems in communicating after surgery.
         d. Encourage client to choose method of communication:
            1) Pencil and paper
            2) Magic slate
            3) Sign language
            4) Alphabet board
         e. Explain postoperative procedures:
            1) Suctioning
            2) Nasogastric (NG) feeding
            3) Care of laryngectomy tube
            4) Breathing through neck
            5) Speech alteration
   D. Immediate postoperative care
      1. Maintain open airway (care of tracheostomy, if present).
      2. Place client in Fowler's position.
      3. Check dressing every hour.
      4. Prevent movement of client's head.
      5. Connect wound drain to suction as ordered.
      6. Maintain intravenous (IV) fluids as ordered.
      7. After partial laryngectomy:
         a. Provide tube feedings (first 2 days postoperatively as ordered).

  b. Encourage oral fluids after tube feedings are discontinued.
  c. Keep tracheostomy tube in place until edema subsides:
    1) Encourage client not to use voice until physician orders otherwise.
    2) Caution client to whisper until healing is complete.
8. After total laryngectomy
  a. On return from recovery room, position client on side, elevate head 30–45 degrees.
  b. Monitor vital signs.
  c. Record fluid intake (tube feedings) and fluid output (I&O).
  d. Provide frequent mouth care.
  e. Support back of neck to prevent tension on sutures and possible wound rupture.
  f. Suction gently as ordered; do not use deep suctioning (may damage suture line):
    1) Suction through both tube and nose (client can no longer blow air through nose).
    2) Suction mouth gently.
  g. Give pain medication as ordered.
  h. If tube feeding is ordered, check tube placement and elevate client's head to prevent aspiration:
    1) Have suction available after removal of feeding tube (client may have difficulty swallowing).
  i. Watch for crusting and secretions around stoma (tracheostomy opening).
  j. Provide room humidification (helps prevent crust formation).
  k. Remove crusting (use prescribed ointments, moist gauze).
  l. Check for and report complications:
    1) Redness, swelling, secretions on suture line
    2) Bleeding (may be a ruptured carotid artery: apply pressure to site; *call for help*)
    3) Tracheostomy stenosis (narrowing of opening causing shortness of breath)
    4) Presence of fistula (abnormal opening around tube)
  E. Provide reassurance to client that speech rehabilitation can help him or her speak again.
  F. Support client through grieving process.
  G. Watch for depression.
V. Evaluation
  A. Client reports decreased anxiety.
  B. There are no avoidable complications from surgery.
  C. Client learns alternative forms of communication.
  D. Client uses effective coping strategies regarding altered body image.
  E. Pain is controlled.
  F. Client maintains adequate nutritional intake.

Pneumonia

I. Description
  A. Acute inflammation of lung tissue, with secretions filling the alveolar sacs (air cells of the lungs), allowing bacterial or viral growth

  B. Inflammation spreading to neighboring sacs, resulting in consolidation accompanied by thick exudate in the lung spaces
  C. Sputum having a characteristic rusty color; breathing becoming difficult
  D. Causes
    1. Inhalation of respiratory secretions (droplets) containing infected bacteria or viruses; inhalation of irritating chemicals
    2. Types of bacteria
      a. Pneumococci
      b. *Staphylococcus aureus*
      c. *Haemophilus influenzae*
      d. *Mycoplasma pneumoniae*
    3. Viral infections
    4. Irritating chemicals
      a. Aspiration of chemicals in stomach contents
      b. Inhalation of chemicals (e.g., chlorine)
II. Data collection
  A. Subjective symptoms
    1. Productive cough
    2. Difficulty in breathing
    3. Chills
    4. Pain on inspiration (breathing in)
    5. Weakness
  B. Objective symptoms
    1. Painful, dry cough, changing to a productive cough with green, yellow, or rusty sputum, depending on organism
    2. Marked elevation in temperature
    3. Elevated white blood cell (WBC) count
    4. Positive diagnosis by chest x-ray
    5. Positive sputum culture analysis
    6. Presence of crackles
    7. Hypoxemia (decreased amount of oxygen in blood)
III. Diagnostic tests and methods
  A. Client history
  B. Physical examination with auscultation of chest (listening to chest with a stethoscope)
  C. Chest x-ray and examination
  D. Complete blood count (CBC)
  E. Sputum culture and sensitivity test
IV. Implementation
  A. Keep personal items and call signal within client's easy reach.
  B. Provide mouth care.
  C. Help client conserve energy; schedule rest periods.
  D. Encourage eating small meals and increasing fluid intake.
  E. Place client in semi-Fowler's to high-Fowler's position.
  F. Give oxygen with humidity as prescribed.
  G. Check vital signs every 4 hours, using rectal thermometer.
  H. Check breathing effort.
  I. Check sputum color and thickness.
  J. Collect sputum specimens.
  K. Encourage good handwashing technique.
  L. Isolate as indicated; provide for proper disposal of oral and nasal secretions.
  M. Suction as necessary.

N. Have client turn, cough, and breathe deeply every 2 hours, or as prescribed.

O. Maintain IV fluids and medication schedule as ordered.

P. Administer prescribed antibiotics, antipyretics, analgesics, expectorants, and bronchodilators as ordered.

Q. Document all observations and treatments.

R. Explain disease process, treatment, and home care.

V. Evaluation

A. Client reports increased comfort and decreased anxiety.

B. There are no complications from infection.

C. Client maintains adequate nutritional and fluid intake.

D. Client understands how to take medications as ordered.

E. Client demonstrates an understanding of disease process, treatment, and home care.

Empyema, Suppurative Pleurisy, Pleural Effusion

I. Description of empyema

A. A collection of pus and necrotic (dead) tissue within the pleural space, which normally contains a small amount of extracellular fluid (ECF) that lubricates the surfaces of the pleura

B. Causes
   1. Pneumonia
   2. Lung abscess
   3. Chest trauma or surgery
   4. Liver disease with ascites
   5. Peritoneal dialysis
   6. Fungus infections

II. Description of suppurative pleurisy

A. Purulent inflammation of the pleura, causing pain and a pleural rub

B. Causes
   1. Pneumonia
   2. Lung abscess
   3. Infection
   4. Pulmonary infarction
   5. Chest trauma or surgery
   6. Pulmonary tuberculosis

III. Description of pleural effusion

A. Accumulation of fluid within the pleural space

B. Causes
   1. Pulmonary tuberculosis
   2. Lung cancer
   3. Other infections of lung: pneumonia, lung abscess
   4. Congestive heart failure
   5. Liver disease with ascites
   6. Peritoneal dialysis
   7. Chest trauma

IV. Data collection

A. Subjective symptoms
   1. Chest pain
      a. Empyema
         1) Unilateral (one sided)
      b. Suppurative pleurisy
         1) Sharp pain on inspiration: referred to shoulder, abdomen, or affected side

   2. Malaise
   3. Difficulty in breathing
   4. Cough

B. Objective symptoms
   1. Elevated temperature
   2. Cough
   3. Decreased breath sounds
   4. Chest expansion not symmetrical (one side does not expand to same degree as other side of chest)
   5. Increase in WBC count
   6. Presence of pleural rub (coarse, creaky sound heard during inspiration and early expiration directly over area of inflammation present in pleurisy)
   7. Findings from chest x-ray

V. Diagnostic tests and methods

A. Client history

B. Chest x-ray

C. Physical examination (including listening to lung sounds)

D. Laboratory study of pleural fluid specimen obtained via thoracentesis

VI. Implementation

A. Monitor respirations, breath sounds, and vital signs.

B. Administer antibiotic, anti-inflammatory, and analgesic medications as ordered.

C. Place client in semi-Fowler's or high-Fowler's position to assist in breathing.

D. Provide adequate rest.

E. Demonstrate how to splint chest for coughing.

F. Encourage coughing and deep-breathing exercise.

G. Encourage good handwashing technique.

H. Encourage fluid intake.

I. Prepare client and assist with thoracentesis or chest tube insertion, or both, as ordered for pleural effusion and empyema.

J. Explain disease process, treatment, and home care to client and family.

VII. Evaluation

A. Client reports increased comfort.

B. Client maintains effective breathing pattern.

C. Chest tube systems work correctly.

D. There are no avoidable complications from infection.

E. Client and family demonstrate an understanding of the disease process, treatment, and home care.

Chronic Obstructive Pulmonary Disease

I. Description

A. Chronic obstructive pulmonary disease (COPD) includes a group of lung conditions that are frequently progressive and obstruct pulmonary air flow.

B. COPD affects expiratory (breathing out) air flow.

C. COPD comprises three major conditions: asthma, emphysema, and chronic bronchitis.

ASTHMA

I. Description

A. Sudden narrowing of the trachea (windpipe) and bronchi, obstructing air flow and causing hyperinflation

B. Spasms of the muscle of the bronchi, edema, and swelling of mucous membrane producing thick secretions

C. Air that enters is trapped

D. Characteristic wheeze when client tries to exhale (breathe out) through narrowed bronchi

E. Difficulty in breathing

F. Inability to expectorate in sufficient amounts through coughing

G. Attacks lasting 30–60 minutes with normal breathing between attacks

H. Possibility of status asthmaticus, which is difficult to control

I. Causes
   1. Inhalation of irritating chemicals such as those found in cigarette smoke, polluted air
   2. Recurrent respiratory infections
   3. Allergic reaction
   4. Physical or emotional stress
   5. Family tendency
   6. Seasonal occurrence

II. Data collection
   A. Subjective symptoms
      1. Shortness of breath
      2. Wheezing
      3. Thick, tenacious sputum (after an acute attack)
      4. Chest tightness
      5. Anxiety (feeling of suffocation)
   B. Objective symptoms
      1. Dyspnea
      2. Wheezing on expiration
      3. Thick, tenacious sputum
      4. Flaring nostrils
      5. Use of accessory muscles of respiration
      6. Tachypnea
      7. Tachycardia
      8. Diaphoresis (perspiration)
      9. Flushing

III. Diagnostic tests and methods
   A. Client history
   B. Physical examination
   C. Chest x-ray
   D. Sputum analysis
   E. Arterial blood gases (ABGs)
   F. Electrocardiogram (ECG)
   G. Skin tests for allergies

IV. Implementation
   A. Decrease anxiety; provide time to listen, and do not leave client alone during attack.
   B. Keep environment free from dust and allergens.
   C. Place client in semi- to high-Fowler's position with arms supported by overbed table.
   D. Prevent infection; discourage visits by persons with upper respiratory infections.
   E. Discourage smoking.
   F. Monitor vital signs; assess respirations and skin color frequently.
   G. Administer prescribed medications as ordered.
   H. Give oxygen as ordered.
   I. Note sputum characteristics.
   J. Encourage adequate fluid intake.
   K. Monitor fluid I&O.
   L. Encourage adequate nutritional intake (small, frequent, high-protein, high-caloric meals).
   M. Explain disease process, treatment, prevention, and home care:
      1. Importance of taking medications on time
      2. Breathing exercises
      3. Diet and fluids
      4. Client and family assisting in planning care
      5. Importance of signs and symptoms indicating immediate follow-up.

V. Evaluation
   A. Client reports increased comfort and decreased anxiety.
   B. There are no avoidable complications from infection.
   C. Client maintains effective breathing pattern.
   D. Client maintains open airway and adequate gas exchange.
   E. Client verbalizes feelings regarding disease.
   F. Client discusses intention to stop smoking.
   G. Client discusses intention to check home and work environment.
   H. Client maintains fluid balance.
   I. Client maintains undisturbed sleep pattern.
   J. Client maintains adequate nutritional intake.

EMPHYSEMA

I. Description
   A. Emphysema is a chronic, progressive condition in which the air sacs (alveolar sacs) distend, rupture, and destroy the capillaries.
   B. The alveoli lose elasticity, resulting in trapping of inspired air.
   C. Inspiration (breathing in of air) becomes difficult; expiration (breathing out) is prolonged.
   D. Lung tissue becomes fibrotic (formation of scar tissue).
   E. Exchange of oxygen and carbon dioxide decreases (destruction of alveolar walls decreases surface area for gas exchange).
   F. Causes
      1. Asthma
      2. Recurrent inflammation: pneumonia, air pollution
      3. Cigarette smoking
      4. Pulmonary fibrosis
      5. Family tendency

II. Data collection
   A. Subjective symptoms
      1. Chronic cough
      2. Difficulty in breathing
      3. Anorexia (loss of appetite)
      4. Weight loss
      5. Malaise
   B. Objective symptoms
      1. Chronic cough: productive, purulent sputum
      2. Barrel chest
      3. Use of accessory muscles of respiration
      4. Prolonged expiratory period: grunting, pursed-lips breathing, abnormal rapidity of breathing
      5. Peripheral cyanosis of extremities
      6. Clubbing of fingers

7. Dyspnea on exertion
8. Orthopnea
9. Difficulty in talking: short, jerky sentences
10. Drowsiness, confusion, possible unconsciousness caused by lack of oxygen to brain

III. Diagnostic tests and methods
   A. Client history
   B. Physical examination
   C. Chest x-ray
   D. Pulmonary function tests
   E. ABGs
   F. Sputum analysis
   G. ECG

IV. Implementation
   A. Loosen, liquefy, and remove secretions (clapping, chest physiotherapy, postural drainage) as ordered.
   B. Encourage coughing and deep-breathing exercises to increase respiratory function.
   C. Prevent and control infections.
   D. Discourage smoking.
   E. Avoid air pollution.
   F. Administer antibiotics on time as ordered.
   G. Discourage visits from persons with upper respiratory infections.
   H. Give O_2 in low concentrations (1–2 L):
      1. Higher levels of O_2 are dangerous when CO_2 level is high.
      2. Respiratory center of brain becomes used to low blood O_2 level.
      3. Increases in O_2 level causes respiratory rate to decrease (may lead to unconsciousness and death).
   I. Encourage adequate fluid intake.
   J. Provide humidity.
   K. Use nebulizers and perform intermittent positive-pressure breathing (IPPB) as ordered.
   L. Administer expectorants as ordered.
   M. Provide adequate rest.
   N. Organize care:
      1. Limit exertion.
      2. Assist with turning and getting in and out of bed.
      3. Explain disease process, diagnostic procedures, treatment, and home care.

V. Evaluation
   A. Client reports increased comfort and decreased anxiety.
   B. Client remains free of injury or infection.
   C. Client maintains effective airway clearance and gas exchange.
   D. Client maintains adequate tissue perfusion.
   E. Client maintains adequate nutritional intake.
   F. Client maintains undisturbed sleep pattern.
   G. Client verbalizes feelings regarding disorder and intentions to stop smoking.
   H. Client uses effective coping strategies.
   I. Client demonstrates an understanding of disease process, diagnostic procedures, treatment, and home care.

CHRONIC BRONCHITIS

I. Description
   A. Chronic, progressive condition accompanied by excessive secretions from overactive mucus glands

B. Edema and infection within bronchi obstructing air flow and gas exchange
C. Extension and destruction of alveolar sacs and capillaries possible if acute attacks not prevented or treated
D. Causes
   1. Asthma
   2. Inhalation of irritating chemicals such as those in cigarette smoke
   3. Recurrent respiratory infections
   4. Air pollution
   5. Family tendency

II. Data collection
   A. Subjective symptoms
      1. Cough
      2. Thick, gray, white, yellow, or blood-tinged sputum
      3. Dyspnea on exertion
      4. Weight loss
      5. Swelling of legs
      6. Tachypnea (abnormally rapid breathing)
      7. Wheezing
      8. Anxiety
   B. Objective symptoms
      1. Productive cough with tenacious gray, white, or blood-tinged sputum
      2. Tachypnea
      3. Use of accessory respiratory muscles
      4. Edema
      5. Dyspnea on exertion
      6. Wheezing
      7. Neck vein distention

III. Diagnostic tests and methods
   A. Client history
   B. Physical examination
   C. Chest x-ray
   D. Pulmonary function tests
   E. ABGs

IV. Implementation
   A. Provide safe, effective care environment.
   B. Loosen, liquefy, and remove secretions.
   C. Perform postural drainage, clapping, chest physiotherapy as ordered.
   D. Force fluids as ordered.
   E. Provide adequate rest.
   F. Provide high-protein diet.
   G. Discourage visits from persons with upper respiratory infections.
   H. Administer bronchodilators, antibiotics, corticosteroids as ordered.
   I. Administer ultrasonic or mechanical nebulizer treatments to loosen secretions and aid in mobilization.
   J. Administer diuretics for edema as ordered.
   K. Give oxygen as ordered for relief of hypoxia (reduced oxygen content).
   L. Discourage smoking.
   M. Include client and family in planning care.
   N. Explain disease process, treatment, prevention, and home care to client and family.

V. Evaluation
   A. Client reports increased comfort and decreased anxiety.

B. Client maintains open airway for increased gas exchange.

C. Client has no complications from infection.

D. Client's sleeping pattern improves.

E. Client maintains adequate nutritional and fluid intake.

F. Client verbalizes intention to stop smoking.

G. Client and family demonstrate an understanding of disease process, treatment, prevention, and home care.

Pneumothorax and Hemothorax

I. Description

A. Pneumothorax is an accumulation of air or gas in pleural space causing collapse of the lung.
   1. The amount of air or gas trapped in pleural space determines the degree of lung collapse.
   2. The collapse may be partial or complete.
   3. In tension pneumothorax, air in pleural space is under higher pressure than air in opposite lung and vascular structures.
   4. In an open pneumothorax (usually result of trauma), air flows between pleural space and outside of body.
   5. In a closed pneumothorax, air reaches pleural space directly from the lung.
   6. Prompt treatment is required for tension or large pneumothorax:
      a. Without prompt treatment, fatal pulmonary and circulatory impairment will result.

B. Hemothorax is an accumulation of blood in pleural space.
   1. Blood from intercostal, pleural, mediastinal, and sometimes blood vessels in lung enters the pleural cavity.
   2. Amount of lung collapse and mediastinal shift depends on amount of bleeding and underlying cause.
   3. Pneumothorax often accompanies hemothorax.

C. Causes
   1. Spontaneous (air leakage from congenital blebs next to pleural surface and rupture of emphysematous bulla [large vesicle] after exercise or coughing and tubercular lesions or cancerous lesions that erode into pleural space)
   2. Trauma (knife wound, fractured ribs, venous pressure line insertion, gunshot wound, after thoracentesis)
   3. Postoperative procedure where chest cavity has been entered
   4. Diagnostic and treatment procedures
      a. Thoracentesis
      b. Insertion of CVP line
      c. Closed pleural biopsy

II. Data collection

A. Subjective symptoms
   1. Spontaneous: sudden sharp pleuritic pain increased by breathing and coughing
   2. Anxiety
   3. Dizziness

B. Objective symptoms
   1. Profuse sweating
   2. Shortness of breath
   3. Rapid pulse
   4. Dizziness
   5. Weak, rapid pulse
   6. Pallor
   7. Neck vein distention
   8. Asymmetrical (uneven) chest movements
   9. Crackling under skin
   10. Hypotension
   11. Tachycardia
   12. Decreased vocal fremitus
   13. Decreased or absent breath sounds over collapsed lung
   14. ABG findings: pH <7.35, P_{O_2} <80 mm Hg, P_{CO_2} >45 mm Hg
   15. Respiratory distress
   16. Spontaneous pneumothorax with only a small amount of air in pleural space may cause no or few symptoms

III. Diagnostic tests and methods
   A. Client history
   B. Physical examination
   C. Chest x-ray

IV. Implementation

A. For spontaneous pneumothorax with no signs of increased pleural pressure, lung collapse of <30%, and no signs of dyspnea or other indications of compromise or complications:
   1. Maintain bedrest.
   2. Monitor vital signs hourly for indications of shock.
   3. Give oxygen as prescribed.
   4. Assist in needle aspiration of air, if required.

B. For lung collapse >30%:
   1. Prepare client for thoracostomy and placement of chest tubes.
   2. Prepare client for possible surgical repair.

C. Provide mouth care.

D. Check nutritional status.

E. Watch for pallor, gasping respirations, and sudden chest pain.

F. Check for increased respiratory distress or mediastinal shift.

G. Listen for breath sounds over both lungs.

H. Encourage client to control coughing and gasping during thoracentesis or thoracotomy procedure.

I. Encourage coughing and deep-breathing exercises once chest tubes are in place to facilitate lung expansion.

J. For clients undergoing chest tube drainage:
   1. Watch for air leakage (bubbling), which indicates that lung defect has not closed.
   2. Check around neck or at tube insertion site for crackling beneath the skin, which is a sign of subcutaneous emphysema.

K. Check, record, and report amount and color of drainage.

L. Assist in changing dressings around chest tube insertion site as necessary.
   1. Do not dislodge or reposition tube.
   2. If tube dislodges, place petrolatum gauze dress-

ing over opening immediately to prevent rapid lung collapse; *call for help.*
3. Provide reassurance to client and family.
4. Explain disease process, treatment, and home care.

V. Evaluation
A. Client reports increased comfort and decreased anxiety.
B. Vital signs stabilize.
C. Lungs re-expand.
D. Pain is absent.
E. Respiratory problems are absent.
F. Client maintains effective breathing pattern.
G. Client maintains effective gas exchange (ABGs are normal).
H. Client maintains adequate nutritional intake.
I. Client demonstrates an understanding of disease process, treatment, and home care.

Pulmonary Tuberculosis

I. Description
A. Pulmonary tuberculosis is an acute or chronic infection caused by the tubercle bacillus organism, which leads to inflammation and formation of a permanent nodule containing the tubercle bacillus.
B. The person who has been infected harbors the bacillus for life. It is dormant unless it becomes active during physical or emotional stress.
C. The nodules become fibrosed and the area becomes calcified and can be identified by x-ray.
D. The incidence of tuberculosis is currently increasing, and a drug-resistant strain is becoming a problem. Individuals with acquired immunodeficiency syndrome (AIDS), the homeless, and others living in crowded, poorly ventilated conditions have a higher-than-average incidence of this disease.
E. Transmission of the organism is by airborne droplets.
F. Cause
1. Exposure to airborne droplets containing the tubercle bacillus from infected person
G. Factors contributing to activation of infection
1. Uncontrolled diabetes mellitus
2. Hodgkin's disease
3. Leukemia
4. Treatment with corticosteroids
5. Treatment with immunosuppressive drugs
6. Silicosis

II. Data collection
A. Subjective symptoms
1. Early phase may be asymptomatic
2. Fatigue
3. Weakness
4. Weight loss
5. Anorexia
6. Night sweats
7. Low-grade fever
8. Cough with micropurulent sputum
9. Occasional hemoptysis (coughing up of blood from the lungs)
10. Chest pain
11. Anxiety; fear of public rejection
B. Objective symptoms
1. Productive cough with micropurulent sputum
2. Elevated afternoon temperature
3. Positive chest x-ray
4. Sputum positive for acid-fast bacilli
C. Presence of hemoptysis
D. Positive tuberculin test

III. Diagnostic tests and methods
A. History of tuberculin exposure
B. Physical examination
C. Chest x-ray
D. Tuberculin test
E. Sputum smears and cultures
F. Auscultation of chest
G. Chest percussion

IV. Implementation
A. Isolate client in quiet, well-ventilated room during infective period.
B. Assist with comfort measures.
C. Assess respirations, breath sounds, and vital signs.
D. Instruct client to cough, sneeze, or laugh into tissue.
E. Instruct client to dispose of tissues in receptacle provided for this purpose.
F. Instruct client to wear mask when outside room.
G. Instruct staff and visitors to wear masks.
H. Provide adequate rest.
I. Encourage client to eat well-balanced meals.
J. Encourage him or her to eat small, frequent meals.
K. Record weight weekly.
L. Observe, report, and record hemoptysis.
M. Administer antituberculosis drugs as ordered.
N. Explain need for taking medications (combinations of two or three) as ordered to prevent resistant strains.
O. Watch for drug side effects.
P. Explain disease process, treatment, prevention, and home care to client and family:
1. Report side effects of medications immediately.
2. Emphasize importance of regular follow-up examinations.
3. Report signs and symptoms of recurring tuberculosis.
4. Emphasize need for long-term treatment.
5. Advise persons exposed to infected clients to receive tuberculin tests, and, if ordered, chest x-rays and prophylactic isoniazid.

V. Evaluation
A. Client reports increase in comfort.
B. Hemoptysis is absent.
C. Client maintains adequate nutritional intake.
D. Cough and sputum are absent.
E. Client maintains effective airway clearance.
F. Client and family demonstrate an understanding of disease process; mode of transmission; treatment; including medication and need for long-term treatment; and home care.

Adult Respiratory Distress Syndrome or Shock Lung

I. Description
A. Adult respiratory distress syndrome (ARDS) is res-

piratory failure that occurs as a result of massive trauma to the lungs.

B. ARDS results from increased permeability of alveolar capillary membrane.

C. Fluid accumulates in the tissues of the lung, alveolar spaces, and small airways, causing the lungs to stiffen.

D. Impairment of ventilation occurs, which prohibits adequate oxygenation of pulmonary capillary blood.

E. Condition characterized by hypoxia (low O_2 levels), dyspnea, pulmonary edema, destruction of alveoli, and inflammation, resulting in decreased O_2 and CO_2 exchange.

F. Severe ARDS can cause irreversible and fatal hypoxia; however, clients who recover usually have little or no permanent damage.

G. Contributing factors
   1. Shock
   2. Sepsis
   3. Drug overdose
   4. Blood transfusion reaction
   5. Smoke or chemical inhalation
   6. Pancreatitis, uremia
   7. Near-drowning
   8. Viral, bacterial, or fungal pneumonia
   9. Trauma: lung contusion, head injury, long bone fracture with fat emboli
   10. Disseminated intravascular coagulation (DIC)
   11. Oxygen toxicity
   12. Aspiration of gastric contents
   13. Infection

II. Data collection
   A. Subjective symptoms
      1. Rapid breathing
      2. Dyspnea
      3. Confusion, anxiety
      4. Restlessness, apprehension
      5. Mental sluggishness
      6. Increased heart rate
      7. Decreased urinary output
   B. Objective symptoms
      1. Dyspnea
      2. Cough
      3. Tachypnea
      4. Cyanosis
      5. Elevated temperature
      6. Rapid, shallow breathing
      7. Intercostal and suprasternal retractions
      8. Presence of rales and rhonchi
      9. Restlessness, confusion, and apprehension caused by hypoxia
      10. Motor dysfunction caused by hypoxia
      11. Decreased urinary output
      12. Evidence of initial respiratory alkalosis (decreased PCO_2) and a decrease in PO_2
      13. Evidence of more severe ARDS

III. Diagnostic tests and methods
   A. ABGs
   B. Pulmonary artery catheterization to identify cause of pulmonary edema
   C. Serial chest x-rays
   D. Laboratory tests
      1. Sputum culture and sensitivity
      2. Blood cultures to detect infections
      3. Toxicology screen for drug ingestion
      4. Serum amylase determination if pancreatitis suspected

IV. Implementation
   A. Maintain bedrest in high-Fowler's position.
   B. Administer humidified oxygen via a tight-fitting mask (allows for use of continuous positive airway pressure [CPAP]) as ordered.
   C. Assist with administration of ventilator support as ordered:
      1. Administer sedatives, narcotics, and neuromuscular blocking agents as ordered to minimize restlessness, oxygen consumption, and carbon dioxide production and to facilitate ventilation.
   D. Monitor ventilator, ABGs, and vital signs hourly.
   E. Administer prescribed IV fluids, bronchodilators, and vasodilators to facilitate ventilation.
   F. Maintain open airway; suction as necessary.
   G. Check extremities for color, temperature, and capillary refill hourly.
   H. Restrict fluids as ordered.
   I. Administer diuretics to reduce edema as ordered.
   J. Monitor I&O hourly.
   K. Administer a short course of high-dose steroids as ordered in clients in whom fat emboli or chemical injuries are the cause of ARDS.
   L. Assist with administration of IV fluids and vasopressors as ordered to maintain BP if hypotension occurs.
   M. Administer antimicrobial drugs as ordered for nonviral infections.
   N. Monitor respiratory status at least every 2 hours:
      1. Watch for retractions on inspiration.
      2. Note rate, rhythm, and depth of respirations.
      3. Watch for use of accessory muscles of respiration.
      4. Using stethoscope, listen for abnormal breath sounds.
      5. Check characteristics of sputum (clear, frothy sputum is indicative of pulmonary edema).
   O. Monitor for signs of confusion caused by hypoxia.
   P. Prepare client and assist with insertion of Swan-Ganz catheter.
   Q. Monitor placement and dressing of Swan-Ganz catheter.
   R. Provide emotional support to client and family.
   S. Communicate frequently with client using appropriate communication aids.
   T. Explain condition, treatment, prevention, and home care to client and family.

V. Evaluation
   A. Client reports decreased anxiety.
   B. Client maintains effective gas exchange (oxygen and carbon dioxide).
   C. Client maintains effective breathing pattern.
   D. Client maintains adequate nutritional intake.
   E. Edema is absent.
   F. Client maintains PaO_2 50–60 mm Hg during acute phase.

G. Client maintains normal blood ABGs as condition improves.
H. Client verbalizes feelings regarding condition.
I. Client communicates needs.
J. Client and family demonstrate an understanding of condition, treatment, prevention, and home care.

Respiratory Failure

I. Description
  A. In clients with normal lung tissue, acute respiratory failure usually means PCO_2 >50 mm Hg and PO_2 <50 mm Hg as a result of inadequate ventilation.
  B. Predisposing factors
    1. Pulmonary edema
    2. Chest trauma
    3. Infections: pneumonia, bronchitis
    4. Bronchospasms or accumulating secretions secondary to cough suppression
    5. ARDS
    6. Cancer
    7. Pulmonary emboli
    8. Congestive heart failure
    9. Neuromuscular problems
    10. Extended mechanical ventilation
    11. Head injury
    12. Drug overdose leading to CNS depression
    13. Anesthesia
    14. AIDS
II. Data collection
  A. Subjective symptoms
    1. Headache
    2. Confusion
    3. History of contributing factors
    4. Difficulty in breathing
    5. Increased heart rate
    6. Restlessness
  B. Objective symptoms
    1. ABGs: PaO_2 <50–60 mm Hg, $PaCO_2$ >50 mm Hg, and pH <7.35
    2. Dyspnea
    3. Cyanosis
    4. Hypertension and tachycardia or hypotension and bradycardia
    5. Tachypnea
    6. Arrhythmias
    7. Restlessness
    8. Confusion or irritability
    9. Diaphoresis
    10. Decreased level of consciousness
    11. Alterations in respirations and breath sounds
III. Diagnostic tests and methods
  A. ABGs
  B. Serial chest x-rays
  C. pH blood levels
  D. Tidal volume measurements
  E. Hct and Hgb
  F. Serum electrolyte measurements
IV. Implementation
  A. Maintain bedrest with high-Fowler's position, and turn client every 2 hours.
  B. Monitor vital signs and breath sounds.

C. Monitor ABGs and pH.
D. Give oxygen as prescribed.
E. Monitor for signs of hypoxia.
F. Suction only when secretions are present (preoxygenize before suctioning).
G. Administer prescribed bronchodilators.
H. Prepare client and assist with endotracheal and mechanical ventilation, if necessary:
  1. Administer sedatives, narcotics, and neuromuscular blocking agents as ordered to minimize restlessness, oxygen consumption, and carbon dioxide production and to facilitate ventilation.
  2. Give sedatives to promote relaxation while client is being mechanically ventilated.
  3. Have resuscitation bag with mask available (clients are temporarily pharmacologically paralyzed).
  4. Make sure ventilator alarms are *on*.
  5. Make sure artificial airway is securely stabilized.
  6. Assess client for retained secretions (while temporarily paralyzed, cough reflex is lost).
  7. Keep eyes lubricated to avoid corneal abrasions (temporary loss of corneal reflex).
I. Continuously monitor ECG monitor, indwelling arterial catheter, and pulmonary artery catheter for changes in cardiovascular status.
J. Monitor CNS (level of consciousness, movement, and sensation).
K. Monitor renal status (urine output, blood urea nitrogen [BUN], and serum creatinine levels).
L. Check nutritional status; assist with administration of internal supplementation or total parenteral nutrition (TPN) as ordered:
  1. Provide amount of protein and calories based on client's metabolic state.
  2. Poor gastrointestinal (GI) perfusion and motility interfere with absorption of nutrients.
  3. Avoid gastric distention because it may lead to respiratory insufficiency because of upward pressure against diaphragm.
  4. Check fluid balance and electrolytes (sodium, potassium, chloride, calcium, phosphate, and magnesium blood levels).
M. Give emotional support to client and family.
N. Explain disease process, contributing factors, treatment, and home care to client and family.
V. Evaluation
  A. Client reports increased comfort and decreased anxiety.
  B. Client maintains effective airway clearance.
  C. Client maintains adequate exchange of oxygen and carbon dioxide.
  D. Client maintains effective breathing patterns.
  E. Client maintains improved ABGs and pH.
  F. Client maintains adequate nutritional intake.
  G. Client maintains adequate cardiac output.
  H. Client maintains adequate CNS response.
  I. Client maintains adequate renal status.
  J. Client and family demonstrate an understanding of disease process, contributing factors, treatment, and home care.

Carcinoma of the Lung

I. Description
  A. A primary or secondary (metastatic from a primary site) malignant tumor in the lung or bronchi
  B. Bronchiogenic carcinoma, usually developing within wall or epithelium of the bronchial tree, most common primary tumor
     1. Usually without symptoms until late stages when metastasis has spread to brain, spinal cord, or esophagus
     2. Treatment in late stages usually symptomatic
     3. Prognosis poor unless detected and treated early
  C. Types
     1. Epidermoid (squamous cell) carcinoma
     2. Small cell (oat cell) carcinoma
     3. Adenocarcinoma
     4. Large cell (anaplastic) carcinoma
  D. Precipitating factors for susceptible host
     1. Cigarette smoking
     2. Exposure to asbestos
     3. Exposure to other carcinogens: uranium, arsenic, nickel, iron oxides, chromium, radioactive dust, and coal dust
     4. Familial susceptibility
     5. Primary prevention beginning with cessation or avoidance of cigarette smoking and avoidance of particular industrial and air pollutants

II. Data collection
  A. Subjective symptoms
     1. Asymptomatic in early stages
     2. Depend on location of lesion
     3. Squamous cell and small cell carcinomas
        a. Cough
        b. Wheezing
        c. Dyspnea
        d. Hemoptysis
        e. Chest pain
     4. Adenocarcinoma and large cell carcinomas
        a. Fever
        b. Weakness
        c. Weight loss
        d. Anorexia
     5. Lesions that penetrate into pleural space
        a. Pleural friction rub
        b. Pleural effusion
        c. Clubbing of fingers
     6. Metastasis to distant structures; may involve any part of body: CNS, abdomen, bone, and connective and vascular tissues

III. Diagnostic tests and methods
  A. Chest x-ray
  B. Examination of sputum for cells (requires sputum coughed up from lungs and tracheobronchial tree)
  C. Bronchoscopy
  D. Needle biopsy
  E. Tissue biopsy
  F. Thoracentesis
  G. Chest tomography
  H. Esophagography
  I. Bronchography

  J. Angiocardiography (contrast studies of bronchial tree, esophagus, and cardiovascular tissue)
  K. Tests to detect metastasis
     1. Bone scan
     2. Bone marrow biopsy
     3. Computerized axial tomography (CAT) scan of brain
     4. Liver function tests
     5. Gallium scan (noninvasive nuclear scan) of liver, bone, and spleen
     6. Staging (determines extent of disease and aids in planning treatment)

IV. Implementation
  A. Prevent avoidable complications.
  B. Encourage adequate nutritional intake.
  C. Reduce anxiety.
  D. Assist client and family in coping with fear.
  E. Monitor vital signs, breath sounds, and skin color.
  F. Monitor cough and sputum.
  G. Explain postoperative procedures:
     1. Foley catheter insertion
     2. Endotracheal tube
     3. IV therapy
     4. Dressing changes
     5. Coughing; deep diaphragmatic breathing
     6. Range-of-motion (ROM) exercises
  H. After chest surgery:
     1. Maintain open airway for adequate gas exchange.
     2. Monitor chest tubes.
     3. Prevent postoperative and pulmonary complications.
     4. Check vital signs every 15 minutes for first hour, every 30 minutes for next 4 hours, then every 4 hours.
     5. Observe and report abnormal respirations and other changes immediately.
     6. Suction as necessary; encourage deep breathing and coughing.
     7. Check secretions (initial sputum will be thick and contain dark blood, changing to thin and grayish yellow within 24 hours).
     8. Monitor and record closed chest drainage: watch for air leaks, report immediately.
     9. Position client on surgical side to promote drainage and re-expansion of lung.
     10. Monitor I&O; maintain adequate hydration.
     11. Check for potential infection, shock, hemorrhage, dyspnea, mediastinal shift, atelectasis, and pulmonary embolus.
     12. Use antiembolism stockings and encourage ROM exercises to prevent pulmonary embolus.
     13. Check and report foul-smelling discharge or excessive drainage on dressing.
  I. For clients receiving chemotherapy and radiation:
     1. Encourage client to eat soft, nonirritating foods high in protein.
     2. Explain and watch for possible side effects of chemotherapy and radiation.
     3. Administer antiemetics and antidiarrheals as ordered.
     4. Provide good skin care to decrease skin breakdown.

5. Use reverse isolation technique if bone marrow suppression occurs.
J. Before discharge:
  1. Assist with instruction of client receiving radiotherapy as outclient to avoid sunburn and tight-fitting clothes.
  2. Teach exercises for prevention of shoulder stiffness.
  3. Discourage smoking.
  4. Explain disease process, diagnostic procedures, treatment, and home care.
V. Evaluation
  A. Client reports increased comfort and decreased anxiety.
  B. Client maintains effective airway for gas exchange.
  C. Client uses effective coping mechanisms.
  D. Client verbalizes feelings regarding disease.
  E. Client exhibits acceptable ABGs.
  F. There are no avoidable complications.
  G. Client maintains adequate nutritional intake.
  H. Client demonstrates an understanding of disease process, diagnostic procedures, treatment, and home care.

Chest Injuries

I. Description
  A. Trauma to rib cage, diaphragm, mediastinum, or pleura possibly caused by blunt or penetrating injuries
    1. Blunt chest injuries
      a. Damage to internal structures without chest wall penetration
      b. Commonly caused by vehicular accidents
      c. Types
        1) Myocardial contusion: bruising of heart muscle
        2) Pulmonary contusion: bruising of lung tissue or pleura
        3) Rib and sternal fractures: displacement of ribs and sternum resulting from fractures caused by a powerful impact
        4) Flail chest: asymmetrical (uneven) chest movement during respiration owing to multiple rib or sternal fractures
          a) Possibility that such fractures may cause fatal complications, such as hemorrhagic shock, diaphragmatic rupture, pneumothorax, and hemothorax if not treated correctly
    2. Penetrating chest injuries
      a. Pierce chest wall, causing injury and changes in pressures within chest cavity
      b. Depending on size of injury, may cause varying degrees of damage to soft tissue, bones, nerves, and blood vessels
      c. Commonly caused by knife stabs or gunshot wounds
II. Data collection
  A. Blunt chest injuries
    1. Rib fractures

a. Pain at site of injury, increasing with deep breathing and movement
b. Shallow, splinted respirations that may lead to hypoventilation
c. Evidence of fracture noted on x-ray
    2. Sternal fractures
      a. Paradoxical chest movements
      b. Damage to liver, spleen
    3. Flail chest
      a. Paradoxical chest movements
      b. Damage to liver, spleen
    4. Pulmonary contusion
    5. Myocardial contusion
  B. Penetrating chest injuries
    1. Pneumothorax
      a. Dyspnea
      b. Tachycardia
      c. Absent breath sounds on affected side
      d. Sucking sound with open wound
      e. Cyanosis
      f. Hypotension
      g. Mediastinal shift with tension pneumothorax
      h. Varying levels of consciousness
      i. Weak, thready pulse
      j. Tachycardia
      k. Possible hemothorax (blood in pleural space)
III. Diagnostic tests and methods
  A. Client history
  B. Chest x-ray
  C. Auscultation of chest
  D. ECG
  E. Serial serum glutamic-oxaloacetic transaminase (SGOT), serum glutamic-pyruvic transaminase (SGPT), lactate dehydrogenase (LDH), and creatine phosphokinase (CPK)
  F. Contrast studies and liver and spleen scans to help detect rupture of diaphragm
  G. ABGs
  H. CBC
  I. Palpation and auscultation of abdomen to evaluate damage to nearby organs and structures
IV. Implementation
  A. Assess airway, breathing, and circulation (ABCs).
  B. Place an occlusive dressing over sucking wound.
  C. Check level of consciousness.
  D. Evaluate color and temperature of skin.
  E. Look for distended jugular veins.
  F. Have blood typed and crossmatched.
  G. Check breath sounds and vital signs.
  H. Assist in establishing an open airway and support ventilation as needed.
  I. Monitor for signs of tension pneumothorax.
  J. Stabilize injury:
    1. Assist with insertion of chest tubes or aspiration in pneumothorax.
    2. Support flail chest.
    3. Splint fractured ribs.
  K. Monitor pulses frequently.
  L. Control blood loss (remember to look under client to estimate amount of loss).
  M. Monitor for shock.
  N. Give oxygen as ordered.

O. Place client in Fowler's position unless shock position is required.

P. Monitor telemetry for suspected cardiac damage.

Q. Administer analgesics, antibiotics, and supportive medications as ordered.

R. Provide emotional support.

S. Prepare client for surgical intervention, if required.

T. Follow specific postoperative procedures.

U. Explain condition, treatment, and home care.

V. Evaluation

   A. Client maintains effective open airway for adequate gas exchange and clearance.

   B. Client maintains effective breathing patterns.

   C. Client reports increased comfort and decreased anxiety.

   D. Client resumes prior lung capacity.

   E. Client maintains adequate nutritional intake.

   F. Client demonstrates an understanding of condition, treatment, and home care.

Cardiovascular System

Basic Information

The heart, arteries, veins, and lymphatic system form the cardiovascular system, which serves as the body's transport system. It brings life-supporting oxygen and nutrients to cells, removes metabolic waste products, and carries hormones from one part of the body to another. It is divided into two branches: pulmonary circulation and systemic circulation. Circulation requires normal function of the heart, which pushes blood through the system by continuous rhythmic contractions.

Diseases related to the cardiovascular system constitute the leading cause of death in the United States. Conditions affecting this system occur across the age continuum. Three major strategies to reduce death and disability resulting from disorders of the cardiovascular system include early detection, appropriate treatment to control the progress of the disease, and a reduction of risk factors that predispose individuals to the disease.

I. Basic data collection

   A. Subjective symptoms

      1. Chest pain during periods of physical and emotional stress

      2. Dyspnea on exertion

      3. Dizziness, fainting

      4. Hemoptysis

      5. Easy fatigability

      6. Family history of heart disease and hypertension

   B. Objective symptoms

      1. Irregular pulse

      2. Abnormal respirations

      3. Skin temperature, color (pallor, cyanosis)

      4. Distended neck veins

      5. Abnormal heart sounds

      6. Clubbing of fingers and toes

      7. Presence of edema

      8. Abnormal peripheral pulses

      9. Bruits or thrills over carotid arteries

      10. Pulsations in jugular vein

      11. Pericardial friction rub

Major Cardiovascular Diagnoses

Angina Pectoris

I. Description

   A. Episodes of acute chest pain as a result of an inadequate oxygen supply to the myocardium, owing to a decrease in blood flow from the coronary arteries.

   B. Condition occurs with either gradual or sudden onset; pain usually lasts <15 minutes and not >30 minutes (average 3 minutes).

   C. Chest pain located behind or under sternum, often radiating to back, neck, left arm, jaws, even upper abdomen or fingers.

   D. Mild to moderate pressure, deep sensation; varied pattern of attacks, "tightness," "squeezing," "crushing" sensations.

   E. Predisposing factors

      1. Exercise

      2. Cigarette smoking

      3. Eating a heavy meal

      4. Environmental temperature extremes: cold, hot, or humid weather

      5. Alcohol use

      6. Drugs

   F. Causes

      1. Atherosclerotic plaque within coronary arteries major cause

      2. Thrombus formation within vessel

      3. Vasospasms

      4. Hypotension

      5. Low blood volume

      6. Cardiac arrhythmias

      7. Sustained hypertension

      8. Aortic stenosis

      9. Cardiomyopathy

      10. Mitral valve disease

II. Data collection

   A. Subjective symptoms

      1. Substernal chest pain lasting an average of 3–5 minutes

      2. Report of exertion before episode

      3. Radiation of pain to neck, jaw, left arm

      4. Anxiety

      5. Sensation of heaviness, tightness, suffocation

      6. Indigestion

      7. Desire to void

      8. Belching

      9. Pain alleviated by nitroglycerin or rest

      10. Verbalizing feelings of fear, impending doom, or apprehension

   B. Objective symptoms

      1. Presence of nausea or vomiting

      2. Dyspnea

      3. Potential increase in heart rate

      4. Potential increase in BP

      5. Skin condition: warm and dry or cool and clammy

III. Diagnostic tests and methods

   A. Client history

   B. Physical examination

   C. ECG

   D. Holter monitoring

E. Coronary angiography
F. Treadmill exercise testing
G. Serum lipid and enzyme values
IV. Implementation
  A. Monitor vital signs, especially during attack.
  B. Monitor ECG; record and report any changes.
  C. Provide environment conducive to rest (remove stressors such as noise, bright lights, interruptions).
  D. Give oxygen as ordered.
  E. Decrease activity level.
  F. Monitor weight.
  G. Provide diet (fat- and cholesterol-restricted) as prescribed.
  H. Monitor angina attacks:
    1. Instruct client to notify staff at the onset of an anginal attack.
    2. Record and report onset, duration, location, symptoms, quality, and intensity.
    3. Administer vasodilating medication as prescribed; observe, record, and report results and any side effects.
  I. Give emotional support to client and family.
  J. Explain disease process, predisposing factors, treatment including medication, prevention by avoidance of risk factors, home care including diet and lifestyle modifications to client and family.
V. Evaluation
  A. Client reports increased comfort.
  B. Vital signs remain stable.
  C. ECG remains within normal limits.
  D. Client uses effective coping strategies.
  E. Client and family demonstrate an understanding of disease process, treatment, prevention, and home care.

Hypertension (High Blood Pressure)

I. Description
  A. Intermittent or sustained elevation in diastolic or systolic blood pressure: systolic pressure >140 mm Hg and diastolic pressure >90 mm Hg
  B. Arterioles primarily affected, resulting in an increase in peripheral resistance with rise in blood pressure, which may be caused by responses of the sympathetic nervous system and stimulation of the renin angiotensin mechanism
  C. Damage occurring to organ supplied by these blood vessels over time
  D. Two major types: essential (primary or idiopathic) hypertension, the most common, and secondary hypertension, resulting from renal disease or other identifiable cause
    1. Essential hypertension
      a. Cause unknown
    2. Secondary hypertension
      a. Predisposing factors
        1) Smoking
        2) Obesity
        3) Diet
        4) Occupation
        5) Stress
        6) Familial history
        7) Sex: primarily among men >35 years old and women >45 years old
        8) Race: primarily among blacks: twice the incidence of whites
        9) Birth control pills, estrogen use
      b. Associations with other diseases
        1) Renal disease
        2) Pheochromocytoma
        3) Atherosclerosis
        4) Cushing's syndrome
        5) Thyroid, parathyroid, or pituitary dysfunction
        6) Primary aldosteronism
  E. Malignant hypertension: a severe form of hypertension common to both types
  F. A major cause of cardiac disease, renal failure, decreased supply of blood to coronary arteries, and cerebrovascular accident (CVA)
  G. Prognosis good if condition detected early and treatment begins before the development of complications
  H. Hypertensive crisis (profoundly elevated BP) possibly fatal
II. Data collection
  A. Subjective symptoms
    1. Asymptomatic or vague symptoms; may have condition and not know it
    2. Chest pain
    3. Fatigue
    4. Blurred vision
    5. Morning headache
    6. Irritability
    7. Dizziness
    8. Ringing in ears
    9. Tachycardia and palpitations
    10. Nausea or vomiting
    11. Shortness of breath
    12. Anxiety
  B. Objective symptoms
    1. BP readings >140/90
    2. Epistaxis
    3. Evidence of other associated diseases
    4. Hematuria
    5. Proteinuria
    6. Restlessness
III. Diagnostic tests and methods
  A. Client history
  B. Physical examination
  C. Series of resting BP readings
  D. Tests and examinations to check for other organ involvement
    1. Chest x-ray
    2. ECG
    3. Routine urinalysis and testing of BUN and serum creatinine levels
    4. Serum potassium levels
    5. IV pyelogram
    6. Serum electrolytes
    7. Blood glucose levels
IV. Implementation
  A. Assess, report, and record signs and symptoms and any reaction to treatments.

B. Schedule rest periods.
C. Provide quiet, calm environment.
D. Give emotional support to decrease anxiety.
E. Administer prescribed medications (antihypertensives, sedatives, diuretics).
F. Observe, record, and report side effects of medications.
G. Monitor weight daily to assess results of diuretic therapy.
H. Monitor I&O to evaluate results of diuretic therapy.
I. Monitor vital signs, including BP at same time every day.
J. Provide diet as ordered.
K. Discourage smoking.
L. Explain to client:
  1. Risk factors
  2. Disease process
  3. Monitoring BP
  4. Medications
  5. Weight
  6. Diet restrictions
  7. Planned exercise
  8. Stress management
V. Evaluation
A. Client reports decreased anxiety.
B. BP readings decrease to acceptable limits.
C. Client understands risk factors.
D. Client explains reasons for dietary restriction.
E. Client explains reasons for complying with treatment and medications.
F. Number of existing risk factors decreases.
G. Client states plan for taking BP measurements.
H. Client explains methods to control stress.

Myocardial Infarction (Heart Attack)

I. Description
A. Myocardial infarction (MI) is necrosis (death) of an area of the myocardium as a result of obstruction to blood flow through the coronary artery or one of its branches.
B. The myocardium tissue dies as a result of oxygen deprivation, which causes cell ischemia.
C. The location and size of the necrosed area affect the heart's ability to regain or maintain its function.
D. The leading cause of death in cardiovascular disease; death usually results from cardiac damage or complications of MI.
E. Mortality is high when treatment is delayed.
F. Approximately one-half of sudden deaths caused by MI occur within 1 hour after onset of symptoms and before hospitalization.
G. Prognosis improves if vigorous treatment is started immediately, unless location and size of infarct are profound.
H. Complications
  1. Cardiogenic shock
  2. Arrhythmias
  3. Congestive heart failure
  4. Ventricular aneurysm
  5. Ventricular rupture
  6. Pericarditis
  7. Pulmonary embolism
  8. Postmyocardial infarction
I. Risk factors
  1. Smoking
  2. Positive family history
  3. Hypertension
  4. Elevated serum triglycerides and cholesterol levels
  5. Obesity or excessive intake of saturated fats
  6. Sedentary lifestyle
  7. Aging
  8. Stress
  9. Sex: men more susceptible, although incidence in women is increasing
  10. Diabetes mellitus
J. Causes
  1. Atherosclerosis: approximately 90% of cases
  2. Constriction or spasm of the coronary artery
  3. Coronary artery embolus
  4. Coronary artery thrombus
II. Data collection
A. Subjective symptoms
  1. Chest pain
    a. Tightness, heaviness, squeezing, or crushing sensation in substernal area, which may radiate to other areas such as neck, jaw, left arm, or shoulder
    b. Pain not relieved by rest or drugs and possibly lasting 30 minutes or more
    c. In elderly and those with diabetes, pain possibly absent, mild, potentially confused with indigestion
  2. Precipitating factors
    a. Exertion
    b. Stress
    c. Exercise
  3. Predisposing factors
    a. Respiratory tract infection
    b. Pulmonary emboli
    c. Hypoxemia
    d. Blood loss
  4. Anxiety, fear, apprehension, feeling of doom, denial, depression
B. Objective symptoms
  1. Dyspnea
  2. Nausea and vomiting
  3. Profuse diaphoresis and pallor
  4. Presence of rales
  5. Tachycardia, decreased BP
  6. Rise in temperature after 24–48 hours
  7. Elevation of cardiac enzymes
    a. CPK peaks 1–8 hours after onset.
    b. CPK-MB elevated 2–4 hours after onset.
    c. SGOT peaks 24–36 hours after onset.
    d. LDH peaks 48–72 hours after onset.
    e. LDH_1 and LDH_2 may show a flipped pattern, in which case LDH_1 is greater than LDH_2; present in 48 hours in most infarctions.
III. Diagnostic tests and methods
A. Client history
B. Physical examination
C. Serial 12-lead ECG

D. Cardiac enzyme studies: SGOT, LDH, CPK-MB
E. Serial chest x-rays
F. Erythrocyte sedimentation rate (ESR) and WBC count
G. Scans
IV. Implementation
  A. Provide quiet, calm environment; explain tests, procedures, equipment.
  B. Keep client on bedrest for first 24–48 hours; then allow progressive activity as prescribed:
    1. Turn client every 2 hours, with assistance.
    2. Use antiembolism stockings to prevent venostasis and thrombophlebitis.
    3. Client may be allowed out of bed to use commode (less strain placed on cardiovascular system).
    4. Avoid activities that may strain the cardiovascular system:
      a. Administer stool softeners as prescribed.
      b. Instruct client not to strain during bowel movement.
      c. Monitor pulse during periods of activity.
  C. Administer sedatives as prescribed to decrease anxiety and apprehension.
  D. Administer vasopressor drugs as prescribed.
  E. Perform internal monitoring of BP and pulmonary artery pressure (hemodynamic monitoring).
  F. Keep IV line open as ordered to provide means for IV drug administration.
  G. Relieve chest pain with prescribed medications.
  H. Monitor heart rhythm to detect arrhythmias.
  I. Administer and monitor oxygen as prescribed to relieve respiratory distress.
  J. Administer anticoagulant medications as prescribed.
  K. Record vital signs every hour during acute episode.
  L. Monitor pulmonary artery catheter readings for cardiac function.
  M. Assist with progressive activity when condition stabilizes.
  N. Continue assessment and documentation of symptoms and reactions to treatments.
  O. Monitor for signs of complications:
    1. Pulmonary edema: left ventricle failure resulting in decrease in blood pumped out by the diseased heart to the body per minute
    2. Congestive heart failure
    3. Cardiogenic shock caused by a decrease in cardiac output
  P. Assist with cardiopulmonary resuscitation in event of cardiac arrest.
  Q. Explain disease process, risk factors, treatment including medication compliance, and home care including lifestyle modifications, activity, diet, and stress management to client and family:
    1. Advise client and family to report to the physician any chest pain immediately.
    2. Emphasize need to stop smoking.
V. Evaluation
  A. Client reports increased comfort.
  B. Client reports decrease or absence of chest pain.
  C. Hemodynamic status remains stable.
D. Client shows progress with activity, with decreased fatigue.
E. Client and family demonstrate an understanding of disease process, treatment including medication compliance, and home care including lifestyle modifications, activity, diet, and stress management.

Congestive Heart Failure

I. Description
  A. Congestive heart failure (CHF) is a condition in which the pumping mechanism of the heart is impaired, resulting in an insufficient blood supply to meet the metabolic needs of the body.
  B. A buildup pressure occurs in the vascular beds of the affected side of the heart.
  C. Congestion of systemic venous circulation results in peripheral edema or enlarged liver.
  D. Congestion of pulmonary circulation may result in pulmonary edema.
  E. CHF usually occurs in the left ventricle (left heart failure) but can occur in the right ventricle (right heart failure) primary or secondary to left heart failure or to COPD.
  F. Sometimes left and right heart failure occur at the same time.
  G. CHF is generally considered a chronic disorder with retention of salt and water by the kidneys.
  H. CHF may be acute as a direct result of MI.
  I. Prognosis depends on underlying cause and response to treatment.
  J. Causes
    1. MI
    2. Cardiomyopathy
    3. Myocarditis
    4. Ventricular aneurysm
    5. Aortic or mitral regurgitation or stenosis
    6. Cardiac tamponade
    7. Arrhythmias
    8. Ventricular or atrial septal defects
    9. Condition may become progressively worse from:
      a. Respiratory tract infections
      b. Pulmonary embolism
      c. Added emotional stress
      d. Increased salt or water intake
      e. Failure to comply with prescribed therapy
II. Data collection
  A. Subjective symptoms
    1. Anxiety or restlessness
    2. Fatigue
    3. Dyspnea
    4. Confusion
  B. Objective symptoms
    1. Left-sided heart failure
      a. Dyspnea
      b. Orthopnea
      c. Nonproductive cough: worsens at night
      d. Later, productive cough with frothy, blood-tinged sputum
    2. Right-sided heart failure
      a. Weight gain caused by fluid accumulation in tissues

b. Pitting, dependent edema (ankle and leg edema or sacral edema, or both)

c. Ascites from portal hypertension, resulting in accumulation of fluid in abdominal cavity, which may interfere with respirations owing to pressure against diaphragm

d. Decreased urine output

e. Distended neck veins

f. Nausea, vomiting, and anorexia

III. Diagnostic tests and methods

A. Client history

B. Physical examination

C. Chest x-ray

D. ECG

E. Pulmonary artery monitoring

F. ABGs

G. Renal function tests

H. Liver function tests

IV. Implementation

A. Give and monitor oxygen as ordered.

B. Place client in high-Fowler's position and elevate extremities.

C. Record vital signs every 15 minutes to 2 hours during acute phase.

D. Restrict fluids as ordered.

E. Provide adequate nutritional intake:
   1. Restrict salt intake.

F. Record I&O every hour during acute phase.

G. Provide quiet, calm environment.

H. Provide adequate rest (conserves energy, prevents fatigue).

I. Monitor and record daily weights (report any changes).

J. Monitor mental status.

K. Monitor IV intake as prescribed.

L. Monitor BUN, creatinine, serum potassium, sodium, chloride, and magnesium levels.

M. Assess amount of activity that results in the least discomfort to client.

N. Monitor for pitting dependent edema (ankle, leg, and sacral edema).

O. Assist with use of rotating tourniquets as ordered:
   1. Check radial and pedal pulses often to ensure tourniquets are not too tight.
   2. Remove one tourniquet at a time to prevent sudden upsurge in circulating volume.

P. Assist with ROM exercises to prevent deep vein thrombosis caused by vascular congestion.

Q. Apply antiembolism stockings; watch for calf pain and tenderness.

R. Assist with activities of daily living (ADLs) until client is able to show gradual progress.

S. Administer medications such as digitalis, diuretics, and vasodilators as prescribed:
   1. Check apical-radial pulse when giving digitalis.
   2. Monitor, record, and report response to medications, including any side effects.

T. Monitor digitalis toxicity tests.

U. Assist client to turn, cough, and breathe deeply.

V. Explain disease process, treatment, home care, and follow-up care to client and family:
   1. Advise to avoid foods high in sodium, such as canned prepared foods and dairy products, to reduce fluid overload.
   2. Reinforce information regarding loss of potassium through use of diuretics and replacement with prescribed potassium supplement and eating high-potassium foods.
   3. Emphasize need for regular checkups.
   4. Emphasize importance of taking digitalis exactly as prescribed.
   5. Instruct client to watch for signs of toxicity (anorexia, nausea, vomiting, yellow vision, cardiac arrhythmias).
   6. Emphasize importance of notifying physician immediately for following: irregular pulse or pulse <60 bpm, persistent dry cough, palpitations, increased fatigue, paroxysmal nocturnal dyspnea, swollen ankles, decreased urinary output, or weight gain of 3–5 lb in a week.

V. Evaluation

A. Client reports decreased anxiety.

B. Client displays decreased confusion.

C. Respiratory difficulties are decreased.

D. Client tolerates a progressive activity.

E. Edema is decreased.

F. Client and family demonstrate an understanding of disease process, treatment including medication compliance, home care including need for daily weight monitoring and lifestyle modifications, and follow-up care.

Shock

I. Description

A. Insufficient cardiac output or tissue perfusion

B. Three types
   1. Cardiogenic shock
   2. Hypovolemic shock
      a. Occurs because of reduction in intravascular blood volume resulting in insufficient perfusion of the tissues (loss of fluid within vascular space)
      b. May lead to irreversible cerebral and renal damage, cardiac arrest, and, finally, death
      c. Requires immediate recognition of signs and symptoms and prompt aggressive treatment to improve prognosis
   3. Vasogenic (or neurogenic) shock
      a. Occurs from acute vasodilation of vascular beds with pooling of blood within peripheral blood vessels, resulting in inadequate perfusion of tissues

C. Complications
   1. ARDS
   2. Renal failure
   3. DIC
   4. Cerebral infarction
   5. Liver dysfunction
   6. GI ulcerations

II. Data collection

A. Subjective symptoms
   1. Confusion, lethargy, restlessness

B. Objective symptoms

1. BP: initially normal; then drops
2. Rapid, weak pulse
3. Cold, clammy skin
4. Low urine output
5. Diaphoresis, pallor
6. Increased respiratory rate, dyspnea, cough
7. Decreased level of consciousness
8. Abnormal clotting with DIC
9. Decreased or absent bowel sounds (paralytic ileus)
III. Diagnostic tests and methods
   A. Client history
   B. Physical examination
   C. Cardiogenic shock
      1. ECG
      2. Serum enzyme levels
      3. X-ray to identify internal bleeding sites
   D. Hypovolemic shock
      1. Laboratory tests
      2. Gastroscopy
      3. Aspiration of gastric contents
      4. Coagulation studies
IV. Implementation
   A. Monitor BP and heart rate immediately.
   B. Keep IV line open as ordered for IV drug instillation.
   C. Keep airway open.
   D. Give oxygen as ordered to promote adequate oxygenation of tissues.
   E. Monitor vital signs:
      1. Cardiac arrhythmias or cardiac ischemia may be produced.
      2. Report hypotension immediately.
   F. Monitor ABGs.
   G. Monitor CBC and serum electrolyte levels.
   H. Monitor urinary output.
   I. Administer prescribed vasoactive drugs.
   J. Monitor urinary output (use Foley catheter); notify registered nurse (RN) if output drops to 30 ml/hr.
   K. Administer diuretic as prescribed.
   L. Turn client every 2 hours to prevent skin breakdown.
   M. Monitor for signs of infection.
   N. Provide safe environment for client who is confused and restless.
   O. Provide environment for client to rest; assist in comfort measures.
   P. Provide mouth care.
V. Evaluation
   A. Vital signs remain within normal range.
   B. Client maintains urine output of >30 cc/hr.
   C. Anxiety, confusion, and restlessness are reduced.
   D. Serum electrolyte levels remain within normal range.
   E. BUN and creatinine levels remain within normal range.
   F. Client maintains good skin hygiene.

Acquired Inflammatory Diseases of the Heart

These diseases occur because of an acute or chronic inflammation of the heart, lining of the heart, and heart valves, caused by bacteria, viruses, trauma, or other factors (four types: pericarditis, myocarditis, endocarditis, and rheumatic heart disease).

Pericarditis

I. Description
   A. Inflammation of the pericardium, the fibroserous sac that envelops and protects the heart; can be acute or chronic
   B. Causes
      1. Bacterial, fungal, or viral infections
      2. Neoplasms: primary or secondary from lungs, breasts, and other organs
      3. High-dose radiation to chest
      4. Hypersensitivity or autoimmune disease such as rheumatic fever, systemic lupus erythematosus, and rheumatoid arthritis
      5. Postcardiac injury
      6. Drugs such as procainamide
      7. Idiopathic factors (unknown cause)
      8. Aortic aneurysm with pericardial leakage
      9. Myxedema
II. Data collection
   A. Subjective symptoms
      1. Sharp pain over sternum radiating to neck, shoulders, back, and arms
      2. Pain increases with deep inspiration, decreases when sitting up or leaning forward (pulls heart away from diaphragmatic pleurae of lungs)
      3. Difficulty in breathing
      4. Tachycardia
      5. Feeling of fullness in chest
   B. Objective symptoms
      1. Signs of pericardial effusion
      2. Dyspnea
      3. Orthopnea
      4. Tachycardia
      5. Substernal chest pain
      6. Pallor; cold, clammy skin
      7. Hypotension
      8. Neck vein distention
      9. Hypotension
      10. Signs of constructive pericarditis
      11. Increase in systemic venous pressure
      12. Pericardial friction rub
      13. Symptoms similar to right-sided heart failure: fluid retention, hepatomegaly, ascites
III. Diagnostic tests and methods
   A. Client history
   B. Physical examination
   C. WBC count
   D. ESR
   E. Serum cardiac enzymes
   F. Cardiocentesis
   G. ECG
   H. BUN level
   I. Pericardial fluid culture
   J. Echocardiography to assess valvular disease
IV. Implementation
   A. Assess pain in relation to respiration and body position.

B. Place client in upright position to relieve dyspnea and pain.
C. Provide adequate bedrest.
D. Administer salicylates, antibiotics, and other prescribed medications.
E. Give oxygen as prescribed.
F. Assist with procedures as necessary.
G. Monitor for signs of infection.
H. Explain diagnostic procedures.
I. Monitor BP and venous pressure (decreased BP and increased venous pressure indicate pericardial effusion).
J. Explain surgical procedure, if required.
K. Follow postoperative care procedures.
L. Explain disease process, treatment, home care, and follow-up care.

V. Evaluation
A. Pericardial friction rub is absent.
B. Pericardial effusion and signs of infection are absent.
C. Client reports increased comfort.
D. Pain is absent.
E. Vital signs remain within normal range.
F. Laboratory studies remain within normal range.
G. Client demonstrates an understanding of disease process, treatment, and home care.

Myocarditis

I. Description
A. Inflammation of the cardiac muscle; may be acute or chronic and may occur at any age
B. Resultant impairment of contractility; often does not produce specific symptoms or ECG abnormalities
C. Recovery in these instances often spontaneous without residual effects
D. Complications including congestive heart failure, myocardial ischemia, necrosis, and, rarely, cardiomyopathy
E. Causes
1. Viral infections: influenza, measles, German measles, echoviruses
2. Bacterial infections: diphtheria, tuberculosis, typhoid fever, tetanus, staphylococci, pneumococci, and gonococci
3. Hypersensitive immune reactions: acute rheumatic fever
4. Radiation therapy: large doses to chest for treatment of lung or breast cancer
5. Chemical poisons: chronic alcoholism
6. Parasitic infections

II. Data collection
A. Subjective symptoms
1. Fatigue
2. Difficulty in breathing
3. Feeling of soreness in chest
B. Objective symptoms
1. Dyspnea
2. In severe cases, neck vein distention, tachycardia, fever, arrhythmia

III. Diagnostic tests and methods
A. Client history

B. Physical examination
C. Serum cardiac enzymes
D. WBC count and ESR
E. ECG
F. Throat culture
G. Stool culture

IV. Implementation
A. Assess cardiovascular status frequently.
B. Listen for rales.
C. Take vital signs.
D. Weigh daily.
E. Record I&O.
F. Monitor cardiac rhythm and conduction.
G. Observe for signs of digitalis toxicity.
H. Check serum electrolyte levels.
I. Emphasize importance of bedrest.
J. Assist with activities; schedule rest periods.
K. Provide bedside commode.
L. Instruct client to resume normal activities slowly.
M. Explain disease process, treatment, and home care to client and family.

V. Evaluation
A. Client reports increased comfort.
B. Cardiovascular status remains within normal range.
C. Signs of infection are absent.
D. Client and family demonstrate an understanding of disease process, treatment, and home care.

Endocarditis

I. Description
A. An inflammation of the endocardium, heart valves, or cardiac prosthesis caused by infectious organisms
B. Usually fatal if untreated, but with treatment approximately 70% of affected individuals recover
C. Prognosis worse when severe vascular damage occurs, resulting in insufficiency of blood flow and congestive heart failure, or when a prosthetic valve is involved
D. Causes
1. In acute form, bacteremia after septic thrombophlebitis; open-heart surgery involving prosthetic valves; or skin, bone, and pulmonary infections
2. Group A nonhemolytic *Streptococcus* (rheumatic endocarditis), *Pneumococcus,* and *Staphylococcus* organisms most common
3. Condition caused by organisms such as staphylococci and *Streptococcus viridans* producing vegetative growths on the heart valves, endocardial lining of the heart chambers, or endothelium of blood vessels that may break off and embolize to the CNS, spleen, kidneys, and lungs
E. Occurrence in IV drug users as a result of infections with *Staphylococcus aureus, Pseudomonas* organisms, or *Candida* organisms

II. Data collection
A. Subjective symptoms
1. Anorexia, weight loss
2. Malaise, weakness
3. Chest pain

4. Chills
5. Night sweats
B. Objective symptoms
1. Low-grade fever (99–102°F [37.2–38.8°C]): sub-acute endocarditis
2. High-grade fever (103–104°F [39.4–40°C]): acute infective endocarditis
3. Positive blood cultures
4. Murmurs over valves
5. Clubbing of fingers
6. Petechiae: in 49% of cases
7. Typical symptoms of complications caused by emboli reaching other organs, including spleen, kidney, lungs, peripheral vascular beds; symptoms include hematuria, pleuritic chest pain, upper left quadrant pain
III. Diagnostic tests and methods
A. Blood culture studies
B. WBC count
C. Histocyte studies
D. ESR
E. Rheumatoid factor
F. Echocardiography to identify valvular damage
G. ECG possibly showing artrial fibrillation and other arrhythmias
IV. Implementation
A. Obtain client history of allergies.
B. Administer antibiotics, as ordered, on time to maintain consistent antibiotic blood levels.
C. Monitor for signs of heart failure.
D. Provide mouth care; avoid invasive procedures.
E. Watch for signs of embolization.
F. Monitor renal status (BUN, creatinine levels, and urinary output to check for signs of renal emboli or drug toxicity).
G. Provide reassurance.
H. Explain disease process, treatment, precautions, and home care to client and family:
1. Watch for symptoms of relapse.
2. Instruct on need for prophylactic antibiotics before, during, and after dental work, childbirth, genitourinary and GI procedures.
3. Instruct client as to need to notify physician immediately if symptoms reappear.
V. Evaluation
A. Fever and signs of infection are absent.
B. Client remains free of complications.
C. Client maintains adequate cardiac output.
D. Client and family demonstrate an understanding of disease process, treatment, precautions, and home care.

Rheumatic Heart Disease

I. Description
A. Inflammatory process that may affect the myocardium, pericardium, and/or endocardium in the acute phase and in chronic valvular disease later
B. Severe pancarditis (involvement of myocardium, pericardium, and endocardium), which occasionally produces fatal congestive heart failure during acute phase

C. Usually resulting in distortion, scarring, and stenosis of valves; may lead to adhesions of adjacent tissue
D. Frequent cause of mitral stenosis
II. Data collection
A. Subjective symptoms
1. Prior history of rheumatic fever
2. General malaise, fatigue
3. Pain: may or may not be present
B. Objective symptoms
1. Temperature increase
2. Murmurs over affected valves
3. Dyspnea
4. Polyarthritis: red, swollen, painful large joints
5. Sydenham's chorea: abrupt, purposeless involuntary movements
III. Diagnostic tests and methods
A. Client history
B. Physical examination
C. WBC count and ESR
D. C-reactive protein
E. Cardiac enzymes
F. ECG
G. Chest x-ray
H. Echocardiography
I. Cardiac catheterization
IV. Implementation
A. Monitor vital signs.
B. Provide quiet, calm environment.
C. Provide adequate rest.
D. Administer prescribed medication (penicillin, digitalis, diuretics).
E. Provide prescribed nutrition.
F. Monitor I&O.
G. Explain disease process, treatment, and home care to client and family.
V. Evaluation
A. Client reports increased comfort.
B. Client remains free of complications.
C. Cardiovascular status remains within normal range.
D. Client and family demonstrate an understanding of disease process, treatment, and home care.

Valvular Heart Disease

I. Description
A. Valvular heart disease results in either stenosis or insufficiency of heart valves.
B. In valvular stenosis, the valve cusps become fibrotic and thicken, and may fuse together, hindering blood flow.
C. In valvular insufficiency, valve cusps become inflamed and scarred, and no longer close completely.
D. Alteration of blood flow through the heart results in a decrease in cardiac output, systemic and pulmonary congestion, and dilation of heart chambers.
E. Any of these conditions can lead to heart failure.
F. Types
1. Mitral stenosis: mitral valve becoming calcified and stiff; leading to left atrial hypertrophy with an increase in left atrial and pulmonary pressures; resultant right-sided heart failure

a. Causes
   1) Rheumatic fever
   b. Complications: atrial fibrillation, thrombus formation, and congestive heart failure
2. Mitral regurgitation: insufficient valves allowing blood to backflow from ventricle to atria during systole, with resultant atrial and left ventricular hypertrophy
   a. Causes
      1) Rheumatic fever
      2) MI
      3) Ventricular aneurysm
      4) Papillary muscle rupture
      5) Endocarditis
   b. Complications: atrial fibrillation, elevated left-sided heart pressures, CHF, systemic embolization
3. Aortic stenosis: aortic valve becoming stiffened and fibrotic, impeding blood flow during left ventricular emptying; resultant left ventricular hypertrophy, increased oxygen demands, and pulmonary congestion
   a. Causes
      1) Rheumatic fever
      2) Congenital valve defects
      3) Atherosclerosis
   b. Complications: right-sided heart failure, pulmonary edema, atrial fibrillation
4. Aortic regurgitation: aortic valve becoming insufficient owing to deformed or contracted valve cusps; inability of valves to close completely, resulting in backflow of blood into left ventricle; resultant left ventricular hypertrophy
   a. Causes
      1) Rheumatic fever
      2) Congenital defects
      3) Endocarditis
   b. Complications: left-sided heart failure, arrhythmias
5. Tricuspid stenosis: chordae tendinae becoming fused and shortened, resulting in a narrowing of the valvular opening; blood flow obstruction to the right atrium, causing right-sided heart failure and decreased cardiac output
   a. Causes
      1) Rheumatic fever
      2) Right atrial myxomata
6. Tricuspid regurgitation: valve becoming insufficient as a result of papillary muscle dysfunction or dilation of the valvular ring; blood flow returning to the right atrium, with resultant venous overload and decreased cardiac output
   a. Causes
      1) Rheumatic fever
      2) Congenital defect
      3) Dilation of right ventricle
      4) Endocarditis

II. Data collection
   A. Subjective symptoms
      1. Fatigue, weakness
      2. General malaise
      3. Dyspnea on exertion
      4. Dizziness
      5. Chest pain, discomfort
      6. Weight gain
      7. Prior history of rheumatic fever
   B. Objective symptoms
      1. Orthopnea
      2. Dyspnea, rales
      3. Pink-tinged sputum (mitral stenosis)
      4. Heart murmurs
      5. Palpitations
      6. Cyanosis, capillary refill
      7. Edema
      8. Arrhythmias
      9. Restlessness
      10. Left- or right-sided elevated pressures
III. Diagnostic tests and methods
   A. Client history
   B. Physical examination
   C. ECG
   D. Chest x-ray to determine size of heart
   E. Cardiac catheterization: identification of pressure changes
   F. Echocardiogram for information regarding structure and function of valves
IV. Implementation
   A. Assess, report, and record signs and symptoms and any reaction to treatment.
   B. Elevate head of bed.
   C. Give oxygen as prescribed.
   D. Provide emotional support to client and family.
   E. Administer prescribed medication (antibiotics, digitalis, diuretics, and anticoagulants); assess results and any side effects.
   F. Check digitalis toxicity reports.
   G. Provide quiet, calm environment to conserve client's energy.
   H. Monitor and record vital signs.
   I. Monitor I&O.
   J. Check for edema and capillary refill.
   K. Weigh daily.
   L. Provide sodium-restricted diet as prescribed.
   M. Provide progressive activity based on client's limitations.
   N. Explain disease process, treatment including medication and need for compliance, precautions, and home care including diet and activity to client and family.
V. Evaluation
   A. Client maintains adequate cardiac output.
   B. Client maintains effective breathing pattern.
   C. Client reports increased comfort.
   D. Anxiety and edema are reduced.
   E. Client demonstrates an understanding of disease process, treatment including medication and need for compliance, precautions, and home care.

Acute Pulmonary Edema

I. Description
   A. In cardiogenic pulmonary edema, fluid accumulation in alveoli, bronchioles, and bronchi is a result of elevations in pulmonary venous and capillary pressures. Gas exchange is decreased.

B. Pulmonary edema is a common complication of cardiac disorders; it can occur as a chronic condition or develop quickly with rapidly fatal consequences.

C. Causes
1. CHF
2. Valvular heart disease
3. Fluid overload
4. Inhalation of irritating chemicals
5. Nephrosis, extensive burns, liver disease, and nutritional deficiency owing to decreased serum colloid osmotic pressure
6. Hodgkin's disease: impaired lung lymphatic drainage

II. Data collection
A. Subjective symptoms
1. Difficulty in breathing
2. Anxiety, apprehension
3. Weakness
4. Cough
B. Objective symptoms
1. Dyspnea
2. Restlessness, confusion
3. Productive cough with frothy pink sputum
4. Weak, rapid pulse
5. Wheezing
6. Cyanosis
7. Increased CVP readings
8. Tachycardia
9. Orthopnea
10. Arrhythmias
11. Cold, clammy skin
12. Decreased BP

III. Diagnostic tests and methods
A. Client history
B. Physical examination
C. ABGs
D. Chest x-ray
E. Pulmonary artery catheterization

IV. Implementation
A. Provide complete bedrest.
B. Place client in high-Fowler's position.
C. Monitor vital signs.
D. Monitor breath sounds.
E. Check for peripheral edema.
F. Give oxygen as ordered.
G. Administer prescribed medications such as morphine, diuretics, digitalis, and vasodilators.
H. Observe effects of medications, including side effects.
I. Assess client's condition frequently.
J. Monitor ABG values.
K. Check cardiac monitor frequently; report any changes.
L. Assist with rotating tourniquets if prescribed; record sequence and timing.
M. Provide reassurance to client and family; explain procedures.
N. Explain disease process, treatments, prevention, and home care.

V. Evaluation
A. Venous return decreases.
B. Client maintains effective gas exchange.

C. Client maintains effective cardiovascular function.
D. Client reports increased comfort and decreased anxiety and apprehension.
E. Client demonstrates an understanding of disease process, treatment, prevention, and home care.

Cardiopulmonary Arrest

I. Description
A. Sudden cessation of the heart's pumping function, stopping ventilation and circulation; rapidly fatal if untreated; delay in treatment of 3–5 minutes possibly producing irreversible brain damage
B. Condition accounting for >350,000 deaths in the United States each year, with most occurrences outside of the hospital
C. Prompt, aggressive treatment and early hospitalization necessary to prevent death
D. Causes
1. Severe MI with necrosis
2. Ventricular fibrillation resulting from MI, heart failure, anesthetics, electrolyte disturbances (hyperkalemia and hypokalemia, acidosis), acute hemorrhage, electrical shock, ventricular irritation (from cardiac pacing wires, cardiac catheterization)

II. Data collection
A. Objective symptoms
1. Unconsciousness
2. Absence of pulse and respiration
3. Absence of heart sounds
4. Pupillary dilation
5. Cyanosis

III. Diagnostic tests and methods
A. Client history
B. Physical examination
C. ECG and enzyme studies, after emergency treatment

IV. Implementation
A. Perform basic life support measures (cardiopulmonary resuscitation [CPR]):
1. ABCs
2. Establish airway, begin breathing, assist with ventilation measures.
3. Assist with circulation measures:
a. Continue ventilation and circulation measures.
4. Interrupt ventilatory and circulatory measures (CPR) when:
a. Client begins to breathe spontaneously
b. Another person giving CPR replaces you
c. Client is transferred (resume CPR during transport to hospital)
5. Stop CPR when client is pronounced dead by physician or resuscitation is effective.
B. During recovery from cardiac arrest
1. Keep IV lines open as ordered to allow administration of IV drugs.
2. For clients with ventricular arrhythmias, keep IV lidocaine at bedside for bolus administration.
3. Monitor ABGs frequently.
4. Watch for arrhythmias, hypoxia, acidosis, and hypokalemia.

5. Assess renal status: monitor urine output and specific gravity hourly.
6. Monitor electrolyte, BUN, and creatinine levels daily.
7. Administer osmotic diuretics, if prescribed.
8. Assess cardiac status (level of consciousness, skin color, temperature, peripheral pulses; also monitor pulmonary artery catheter readings and cardiac output).
9. Assess neurological status (signs of cerebral edema, elevated temperature, wide pulse pressures, decreased responsiveness, or presence of seizures, changes in level of consciousness, pupil changes).
10. Observe for complications of CPR (rib or sternal fractures, cardiac tamponade, pneumothorax).
11. Give emotional support to family.

V. Evaluation
A. Spontaneous ventilation and circulation return successfully.
B. Client remains free of injury or complications.
C. Client and family are instructed in CPR; provide for return demonstration.

Peripheral Vascular System

Basic Information

Peripheral vascular disease refers to vascular disorders other than those specifically affecting the heart. Blood flow is decreased because of narrowed or obstructed blood vessels. The underlying factor is the arteriosclerotic process. The decreased blood flow causes changes in the tissues.

I. Basic data collection
A. Subjective symptoms
1. Aching calves
2. Numbness in legs
3. Leg cramps
4. Loss of sensation in legs
5. Pain in legs during exercise (intermittent claudication)
6. History of diabetes mellitus, thrombophlebitis, hypertension, alcoholism
B. Objective symptoms
1. Skin of lower extremities
a. Cold or blue feet
b. Redness of leg in dependent position
c. Sparse hair distribution
d. Edema
e. Stasis ulcers
f. Varicose veins
g. Diminished or absent pulses
h. Delay in capillary filling
i. Bruits heard in major arteries
j. Differences in circumference of legs

Major Peripheral Vascular Diagnoses

Raynaud's Disease (Thromboangiitis)

I. Description
A. Disease characterized by episodic vasospasm in

small peripheral arteries and arterioles, resulting in interruptions of blood flow to distal parts of affected extremities
B. Occurring bilaterally, usually affecting hands; feet less often affected
C. Most prevalent in women, especially between puberty and age 40 years
D. Precipitating factors
1. Cold, stress, smoking
2. Associated with collagen diseases in women
E. Contributing factors
1. Pressure to fingertips: typists, pianists, users of hand-held vibrating equipment

II. Data collection
A. Subjective symptoms
1. Numbness, coldness of hands or feet
2. Pain in hands or feet
B. Objective symptoms
1. Hands or feet feel cold to touch
2. Color changes: pallor, cyanosis, rubor
3. Numbness and tingling
4. Dryness and atrophy of nails
5. Ulcerations or gangrene, especially on fingertips

III. Diagnostic tests and methods
A. Client history
B. Physical examination
C. Arteriography
D. ECG
E. Doppler ultrasonography
F. Chest x-ray

IV. Implementation
A. Record location and characteristics of pain.
B. Administer prescribed vasodilators and analgesics; record results and any side effects.
C. Observe affected areas every shift for color, sensation, diminished pulse.
D. Keep extremities warm and protected.
E. Provide safe environment to prevent injury.
F. Instruct client to avoid exposure of hands and feet to cold and to use gloves and warm socks.
G. Instruct client to avoid constrictive clothing and to maintain adequate caloric intake.
H. Encourage rest after exercise.
I. Discourage smoking.
J. Provide emotional support.
K. Explain disease process, avoidance of cold, protection from trauma, cessation of smoking, and prevention of spasms to client and family.

V. Evaluation
A. Client verbalizes relief of pain.
B. Client maintains effective tissue perfusion and good skin hygiene.
C. Client and family demonstrate an understanding of disease process, treatment including medication, and prevention.

Thrombophlebitis

I. Description
A. Thrombophlebitis: characterized by inflammation and thrombus formation; may occur in deep or superficial veins

1. Superficial thrombophlebitis begins with localized inflammation alone (phlebitis); thrombus formation is frequently provoked by the inflammatory process.
2. Platelets, red blood cells (RBCs), and fibrin form a clot within the vein, which potentially can break loose and lead to emboli.
3. Deep vein thrombophlebitis frequently leads to pulmonary embolism.
4. Causes of deep vein thrombophlebitis:
   a. Damage to vessel lining
   b. Venous pooling and stasis
   c. Increased clotting ability of blood
5. Predisposing factors:
   a. Prolonged bedrest
   b. Trauma
   c. Surgery
   d. Prolonged periods of standing
   e. Increased abdominal pressure: pregnancy, obesity
   f. Use of oral contraceptives
6. Causes of superficial thrombophlebitis:
   a. Trauma
   b. Infection
   c. IV drug abuse
   d. Chemical irritation: extensive use of IV route for medications and diagnostic tests

II. Data collection
   A. Subjective symptoms
      1. Pain in affected extremity
      2. History of causes and contributing factors
   B. Objective symptoms
      1. Warmth and redness of extremity
      2. Elevation of body temperature
      3. Swelling
      4. Positive Homans' sign (pain on dorsiflexion of foot)
      5. Area sensitive to touch
      6. Quality of pulse in affected extremity

III. Diagnostic tests and methods
   A. Client history
   B. Physical examination
   C. Homans' sign
   D. Doppler ultrasonography
   E. Venography
   F. Phlebography
   G. Laboratory studies: CBC, ESR, coagulation studies
   H. Lung scan to rule out pulmonary embolism

IV. Implementation
   A. Assess, report, and record signs and symptoms and any reaction to treatment.
   B. Provide bedrest.
   C. Use moist heat as prescribed to reduce swelling and to provide comfort.
   D. Elevate affected limb to decrease swelling and to prevent blood stasis.
   E. Administer analgesics as ordered; monitor for side effects.
   F. Monitor thigh and calf measurements daily.
   G. Monitor vital signs every 4 hours.
   H. Avoid massaging affected leg.
   I. Use antiembolism stocking on unaffected leg.
   J. Administer anticoagulants, vasodilators, and anti-inflammatory medications as prescribed; monitor results.
   K. Assist with ROM exercises to unaffected extremity.
   L. Monitor for bleeding tendencies:
      1. Check gums.
      2. Check skin for bruises and petechiae.
      3. Watch for nosebleeds.
      4. Monitor Hgb and Hct levels.
   M. Monitor for signs and symptoms of complications such as embolism.
   N. Explain to client and family:
      1. Avoidance of long periods of sitting or standing
      2. Routine exercise plan
      3. Avoidance of tight, constrictive clothing
      4. Use of elastic or support hose for extended periods of sitting or standing

V. Evaluation
   A. Client reports increased comfort and decreased anxiety.
   B. Swelling is decreased or absent.
   C. Redness along affected superficial vein disappears.
   D. Pain is relieved.
   E. Client maintains effective tissue perfusion.
   F. Client and family demonstrate an understanding of disease process, treatment, prevention, and home care.

Varicose Veins

I. Description
   A. Dilated, tortuous leg veins owing to backflow of blood caused by incompetent venous valve closure, resultant venous congestion, and further vein enlargement
   B. Condition usually affecting subcutaneous leg veins (saphenous veins and branches)
   C. Causes
      1. Basic cause unknown
      2. Contributing factors
         a. Congenital weakness of venous valves or venous wall
         b. Diseases of venous system, such as thrombophlebitis
         c. Conditions that produce venostasis: pregnancy, prolonged standing
         d. Familial tendency

II. Data collection
   A. Subjective symptoms
      1. Aching
      2. Cramping and pain
      3. Heavy feeling in legs
   B. Objective symptoms
      1. Palpable nodules
      2. Ankle edema
      3. Dilated veins
      4. Pigmentation of calves and ankles

III. Diagnostic tests and methods
   A. Client history
   B. Physical examination

C. Venography
D. Trendelenburg's test
IV. Implementation
  A. Provide adequate rest with client's legs elevated.
  B. Apply support stockings.
  C. Discourage prolonged standing, sitting, and crossing legs.
  D. Encourage weight management.
  E. Instruct client to avoid constrictive clothing.
  F. Prepare client for surgical procedure (surgical vein stripping, ligation, vein sclerosing).
  G. After surgical procedure
    1. Administer analgesics as prescribed to alleviate pain.
    2. Elevate affected leg.
    3. Check circulation in toes frequently (color and temperature).
    4. Observe elastic bandages for bleeding.
    5. Rewrap bandage once per shift if ordered (wrap from toe to thigh with leg elevated).
    6. Watch for signs of complications:
      a. Sensory loss in leg (indicative of saphenous nerve damage)
      b. Calf pain (indicative of thrombophlebitis)
      c. Fever (indicative of infection)
V. Evaluation
  A. Pain is relieved.
  B. Client reports increased comfort.
  C. Client maintains adequate tissue perfusion.
  D. Client remains free of complications.
  E. Client demonstrates an understanding of the condition, prevention, and home care.

Aneurysms

I. Description
  A. The enlargement or ballooning of an artery.
  B. Some aneurysms progress to serious and eventually fatal complications, such as rupture.
  C. Types:
    1. Dissecting aneurysm: a hemorrhagic separation of the inner layer of the arterial wall
    2. Saccular aneurysm: an outpouching of one side of the arterial wall with a narrow neck
    3. Fusiform aneurysm: a spindle-shaped enlargement including the entire circumference of the artery
  D. Causes
    1. Arteriosclerosis primary cause: plaque formation causing degenerative changes, with resultant loss of vessel elasticity, weakness, and dilation
    2. Infections
    3. Congenital disorders
    4. Trauma
    5. Syphilis
    6. Hypertension
II. Data collection
  A. Thoracic aneurysm involves the transverse or descending portion of the aorta and is most common in men 50–70 years old. Dissecting aneurysms are most common in blacks.

1. Subjective symptoms
  a. Possibly asymptomatic
  b. Dyspnea
  c. Severe chest pain
  d. Dysphagia (difficulty in swallowing)
  e. Hoarseness or cough
  f. Dizziness
2. Objective symptoms
  a. Diaphoresis
  b. Increased pulse rate
  c. Cyanosis
  d. Neck vein distention
  e. Leg weakness or transient paralysis
  f. Diastolic murmur caused by aortic regurgitation
  g. Abrupt loss of femoral and radial pulses or wide variations in pulses of arms and legs
  h. Shock appearance, but systolic BP often normal or significantly increased
  i. Varying symptoms according to size and location of defect, the effects of compression, and erosion of surrounding structures
B. Abdominal aneurysm usually occurs between the renal arteries and iliac branches; is approximately four times more common in white men 50–80 years old than in the general population.
  1. Subjective symptoms
    a. Tenderness or pain in abdomen or back
    b. Chest pain in dissecting aneurysms
  2. Objective symptoms
    a. Pulsating mass in periumbilical area of abdomen
    b. Systolic bruit over aorta
    c. Elevated BP
    d. Pulse changes in lower extremities
    e. Possibly mimicking renal calculi, lumbar disk disease, or duodenal compression, if large
III. Diagnostic tests and methods
  A. Client history
  B. Physical examination
  C. Angiograph to determine location of aneurysm
  D. X-ray
  E. Ultrasonography
  F. Routine ECG
  G. Laboratory studies: Hgb, Hct
IV. Implementation
  A. Monitor vital signs and peripheral pulses every 15 minutes until stable.
  B. Monitor for signs of decreased tissue perfusion: low BP, bleeding, rapid weak pulse.
  C. Assess pain; respirations; and carotid, radial, and femoral pulses.
  D. Administer prescribed medications to decrease pain.
  E. Administer prescribed antibiotics.
  F. Listen to lung and bowel sounds at least every 4 hours.
  G. Monitor for arrhythmias.
  H. Apply antiembolism stockings; do not massage lower extremities.
  I. Compare extremities for warmth and color.
  J. Administer IV fluids as ordered.

K. Monitor oxygen therapy.

L. Assist with monitoring of CVP.

M. Monitor I&O for fluid balance.

N. Provide emotional support to client and family.

O. Provide information in regard to postoperative care, activity, and incisional management.

P. Encourage coughing and deep-breathing exercises.

Q. Maintain bedrest.

R. Encourage prescribed leg exercises to prevent venous stasis.

V. Evaluation

A. Client reports increased comfort and decreased anxiety.

B. Vital signs remain stable.

C. Fluid balance remains stable.

D. Pain is relieved.

E. Client remains free of complications.

F. Client demonstrates an understanding of disease process, surgical treatment, and home care.

Hematological System

Basic Information

- Blood is a major body fluid tissue that continuously circulates through the heart and blood vessels, carrying vital elements to all parts of the body.
- Erythrocytes (RBCs) carry oxygen to the tissues and remove carbon dioxide from them.
- Leukocytes (WBCs) assist in inflammatory and immune responses.
- Plasma carries antibodies and nutrients to tissues and wastes from tissues.
- Coagulation factors found in plasma along with thrombocytes (platelets) control blood clotting.
- The average individual has 5–6 L of circulating blood, which constitute 5–7% of body weight.
- The pH of blood ranges from 7.35–7.45 and is either dark red (venous blood) or bright red (arterial blood), depending on the level of Hgb and the degree of oxygen saturation.
- Malfunction of the hematological system has far-reaching effects on the body.

I. Basic data collection

A. Subjective symptoms

1. Weakness, fatigue
2. Nausea
3. Dyspnea
4. Irritability
5. Bleeding from nose and mouth
6. Headache
7. Numbness, burning of feet
8. Headache

B. Objective symptoms

1. Tachycardia
2. Pallor and jaundice
3. Pruritus
4. Incoordination
5. Mouth ulcerations
6. Smooth tongue
7. Hypotension

Major Hematological Diagnoses

Anemia Caused by Decreased Red Blood Cell Production

I. Description

A. Deficiency of RBCs (anemia) because of conditions affecting production of RBCs

B. Types

1. Pernicious anemia

   a. Condition caused by lack of intrinsic factor in GI system, which is required for the absorption of vitamin B_{12}.

   b. Deficiency of mucosal surface of GI tract, which secretes intrinsic factor.

   c. Those who have had gastrectomies and small bowel resections are at risk.

2. Folic acid deficiency

   a. Folic acid necessary for synthesis of DNA; DNA required for production of RBCs

   b. Condition caused by poor nutrition (lack of citrus fruits, liver, grains, leafy green vegetables), drugs, and malabsorption disorders, which interfere with absorption of folic acid

3. Iron-deficiency anemia

   a. Condition caused by insufficient intake of dietary iron, necessary for production of Hgb and RBCs

   b. Condition possibly caused by malabsorption, hemolysis of RBCs, and blood loss

II. Data collection

A. Subjective symptoms

1. Pallor
2. Fatigue
3. Dyspnea
4. Anginal pain
5. Blurred vision
6. Vertigo
7. Irritability
8. Depression
9. Nausea
10. Anorexia
11. Weight loss
12. Bone pain
13. Numbness, tingling of feet

B. Objective symptoms

1. CHF
2. Positive bone marrow findings
3. Incoordination
4. Confusion
5. Vomiting
6. Splenomegaly
7. Hepatomegaly
8. Signs of bleeding

III. Diagnostic tests and methods

A. Client history

B. Physical examination

C. Routine chest x-ray, ECG

D. CBC

E. Schilling test

F. Bone marrow biopsy

IV. Implementation
  A. Assess, report, and record signs and symptoms and any reaction to treatments.
  B. Monitor vital signs, I&O, and skin color.
  C. Provide planned activity; schedule rest periods.
  D. Administer prescribed supplemental oxygen.
  E. Administer prescribed medications such as iron supplements, vitamin B_{12}, and oral folic acid.
  F. Assist with comfort and hygienic needs.
  G. Monitor blood transfusions; check for reactions.
  H. Provide mouth care.
  I. Provide prescribed diet and fluid intake.
  J. Support client; allay anxiety.
  K. Provide emotional support.
  L. Explain condition, diagnostic procedures, treatment, prevention, home care including planned activities, and follow-up care to client and family.
V. Evaluation
  A. Client reports increased comfort and decreased anxiety.
  B. Client maintains adequate cardiac output and tissue perfusion.
  C. Laboratory values remain within normal range.
  D. Client and family demonstrate an understanding of disease process, diagnostic procedures, treatments, prevention, home care, and follow-up care.

Anemia Caused by Red Blood Cell Destruction

I. Description
  A. Condition caused by RBCs being destroyed faster than they are being produced
  B. Causes
    1. Infections
    2. Drugs, chemicals
    3. Snake venom
    4. Antigen-antibody reactions
    5. Disorders of the spleen
    6. Organic compounds
    7. Congenital disorders
II. Data collection
  A. Subjective symptoms
    1. Weakness, fatigue
    2. Pallor
    3. Weight loss
    4. Painful episodes; history of stress (sickle cell anemia)
  B. Objective symptoms
    1. Positive Coombs' test result: acquired anemia caused by drugs or autoimmune disorder
    2. Elevated serum bilirubin level
    3. Elevated reticulocyte count
    4. Enlarged spleen
    5. Low-grade fever
    6. Renal insufficiency
    7. Jaundice
III. Diagnostic tests and methods
  A. Client history
  B. Physical examination
  C. Laboratory studies: serum bilirubin, CBC, Coombs' test
  D. Renal studies to check renal status

  E. Routine chest x-ray
  F. Routine ECG
  G. Bone marrow biopsy
  H. Presence of abdominal sickle cells in blood or other abnormal cells (macrophytic, microcytic, hypochromic)
IV. Implementation
  A. Assess, report, and record signs and symptoms and any reaction to treatment.
  B. Schedule rest periods to avoid fatigue.
  C. Protect client from exposure to infection sources.
  D. Monitor for bleeding and bruising.
  E. Assist in administration of blood transfusions; check reaction to transfusion.
  F. Administer prescribed medications; check for side effects.
  G. Give oxygen as prescribed.
  H. Monitor fluid I&O.
  I. Monitor laboratory studies.
  J. Provide for genetic counseling.
  K. Caution client to avoid postural hypotension; advise him or her to get up slowly.
  L. Explain disease process, treatment, prevention, home care, and follow-up care to client and family.
V. Evaluation
  A. Client reports increased comfort and decreased anxiety.
  B. Client maintains adequate gas exchange.
  C. Client maintains adequate cardiac output and tissue perfusion.
  D. Client verbalizes feelings regarding disease.
  E. Client and family demonstrate an understanding of disease process, treatment, prevention, home care, and follow-up care.

Leukemia

I. Description
  A. Disorder of the hematological system characterized by an overproduction of immature WBCs
  B. Fewer normal WBCs produced as disease progresses
  C. Increase in abnormal WBCs, infiltrating and damaging bone marrow, lymph nodes, spleen, and other organs
  D. RBC production disrupted, leading to anemia, immature cells, thrombocytopenia, and decline in immunity
  E. Cause unknown; considered to be a neoplastic process.
  F. Predisposing factors
    1. Viral origin
    2. Exposure to radiation
    3. Exposure to chemicals
    4. Familial tendency
    5. Congenital disorders such as Down's syndrome, Fanconi's anemia, and congenital agammaglobulinemia
    6. All forms fatal if untreated
  G. Classification as acute or chronic, and according to cell type
    1. Acute lymphocytic leukemia (ALL)
      a. Lymphoblasts mostly present in bone marrow.

b. Incidence peaks at 2–4 years of age.
c. Remission induced in 40–65% of adults, through treatment.
d. Average survival 1–2 years.
2. Acute myelogenous leukemia (AML)
a. Myeloblasts are present mostly in bone marrow.
b. Incidence peaks at 12–20 and >55 years of age.
c. Average survival rate is 1 year after diagnosis, even with aggressive therapy.
3. Chronic myelogenous leukemia (CML)
a. Granulocytes mostly present in bone marrow.
b. Incidence peaks at 30–50 years of age.
4. Chronic lymphocytic leukemia (CLL)
a. Lymphocytes mostly present in bone marrow.
b. Incidence peaks at 50–70 years of age.
II. Data collection
A. Subjective symptoms: ALL and AML
1. Sudden onset of high fever
2. Abnormal bleeding such as nosebleeds, easy bruising, prolonged menses
3. Fatigue
4. Chills
5. Recurrent infections
6. Dyspnea
7. Abdominal or bone pain
8. Confusion, lethargy, headache when leukemic cells cross blood-brain barrier
B. Subjective symptoms: CLL and CML
1. Fatigue
2. Weakness
3. Anorexia
4. Weight loss
5. Lymph node enlargement
6. Recurrent infections
7. Bone tenderness
C. Objective symptoms: ALL and AML
1. Anemia
2. Elevated temperature
3. Abnormal bleeding
4. Lymphadenopathy
5. Ecchymoses
6. Tachycardia
7. Palpitations
8. Systolic ejection murmur
9. Positive bone marrow biopsy
10. Normal, elevated, or decreased WBC count
D. Objective symptoms: CLL and CML
1. Skin lesions
2. Elevated WBC count
3. Anorexia
4. Enlarged spleen and liver
5. Petechiae
6. Positive bone marrow biopsy
7. Anemia
8. Dyspnea
9. Tachycardia
10. Palpitations
11. Recurrent opportunistic fungal, viral, and bacterial infections

III. Diagnostic tests and methods
A. Client history
B. Physical examination
C. Laboratory studies: CBC, Hgb, Hct, platelet count
D. Differential leukocyte count for determination of cell type
E. Bone marrow biopsy
F. Routine chest x-ray
G. Routine ECG
H. Lumbar puncture for detection of meningeal involvement
IV. Implementation
A. Assess, report, and record signs and symptoms and any reaction to treatment.
B. Provide comfort measures.
C. Monitor laboratory data.
D. Check for signs of bleeding or infection.
E. Monitor vital signs.
F. Assist in administration of prescribed medications such as chemotherapeutic drugs, antiemetics, analgesics, IV fluids, and blood or blood-product transfusions.
G. Monitor for side effects of medications and transfusions.
H. Minimize side effects of chemotherapy.
I. Monitor fluid I&O.
J. Prevent exposure to infection.
K. Assist client with activities; schedule rest periods.
L. Provide emotional support.
M. Allay anxiety and fears.
N. Monitor supplemental oxygen, if ordered.
O. Provide and encourage prescribed diet.
P. Provide oral hygiene.
Q. Provide skin care; use protective devices.
R. Provide environment that allows client to verbalize feelings.
S. Request discharge planning regarding available community resources and support groups.
T. Explain disease process, treatment including medication, home care including diet, activity, avoidance of injury and infection, and checking for abnormal bleeding, and follow-up care.
V. Evaluation
A. Client reports increased comfort and decreased anxiety.
B. Client maintains adequate tissue perfusion and gas exchange.
C. Client remains free of injury or infection.
E. Client demonstrates an understanding of disease process, treatment including medication and side effects, home care, and follow-up care.

Multiple Myeloma

I. Description
A. A disseminated neoplasm of immature plasma cells that infiltrate bone to produce tumors throughout the skeleton (vertebrae, skull, pelvis, flat bones, ribs)
B. During the late stages, infiltrates body organs (lungs, liver, spleen, adrenals, lymph nodes, GI tract, kidneys, skin)

C. Men 50–70 years old mostly affected

D. Prognosis poor because diagnosis often made after widespread skeletal destruction

E. Vertebral collapse without treatment

F. In approximately 50% of clients, death within 3 months of diagnosis; in 90%, death within 2 years.

G. Life prolonged for 3–5 years with early treatment

H. Death usually after complications such as infection, fractures, hypercalcemia, hyperuricemia, or renal failure

I. Cause unknown

II. Data collection

A. Subjective symptoms
1. Bone pain
2. Fatigue
3. Achiness
4. Joint swelling
5. Tenderness
6. Fever
7. Weight loss
8. Decreased body height

B. Objective symptoms
1. Anemia
2. Deformities of thorax
3. Renal complications: pyelonephritis resulting from tubular damage
4. Elevated serum calcium and uric acid levels
5. Severe recurrent infections, such as pneumonia, as a result of damaged nerves associated with respiratory function
6. Pathological fractures
7. Symptoms of vertebral compression
8. Decreased platelet count
9. Elevated ESR
10. Hypercalciuria possibly present
11. Presence of Bence Jones protein in urine
12. Positive bone marrow aspiration for myeloma cells
13. Elevated globulin

III. Diagnostic tests and methods

A. Client history

B. Physical examination

C. CBC: determines presence of anemia

D. ESR

E. Urine studies

F. Bone marrow biopsy

G. Serum electrophoresis for abnormal globulin

H. X-rays of skeleton

I. IV pyelography (IVP)

IV. Implementation

A. Assess, report, and record signs and symptoms and any reaction to treatment.

B. Monitor vital signs, I&O, and laboratory studies.

C. Check for bleeding, infection, or presence of fractures.

D. Encourage fluid intake.

E. Monitor I&O (immediately report daily output of <1500 ml).

F. Encourage client to ambulate (decreases potential for bone demineralization and pneumonia).

G. Assist client in walking with use of walker or other supportive devices to prevent falls.

H. Protect client from others with infections.

I. Administer prescribed medications such as melphalan and prednisone, cyclophosphamide, antibiotics, and analgesics.

J. Assist with good hygienic measures to prevent infection.

K. Provide emotional support to client and family.

L. Prevent complications; watch for presence of fever or malaise.

M. If client is to receive complete bedrest, turn him or her every 2 hours.

N. Give passive ROM and deep-breathing exercises.

O. Ensure that blood is drawn as ordered for platelet count and WBC count before administration of melphalan (derivative of nitrogen mustard, which depresses bone marrow).

P. Prepare client and family for laminectomy if spinal cord compression occurs.

Q. Prepare client and family for dialysis if renal complications occur.

R. Provide comfort measures.

S. Provide information regarding appropriate community resources for additional support.

T. Explain disease, treatment including medication, prevention, and home care.

V. Evaluation

A. Client remains free of avoidable infections or injuries.

B. Client reports increased comfort and decreased anxiety.

C. Client maintains adequate I&O.

D. Client has access to community resources for support.

E. Client maintains adequate urine output.

F. Client demonstrates an understanding of disease process, treatment including medication, prevention, home care, and follow-up care.

Hodgkin's Disease

I. Description

A. Neoplastic disease with painless progressive enlargement of lymph nodes, spleen, and other lymphoid tissue.

B. Disease results from proliferation of Reed-Sternberg giant cells, lymphocytes, eosinophils, and histocytes.

C. Disease potentially curable because of recent advances in therapeutic measures.

D. Prognosis dependent on stage of the disease.

E. Four stages defined by the Ann Arbor clinical staging classification of Hodgkin's disease.

F. Five-year survival rate in approximately 54% of clients with treatment.

G. Disease occurs most often in young adults, with a higher incidence in men than in women.

H. Disease occurs in all races but is slightly more common in whites.

I. Incidence peaks in two age groups (15–38 and >50 years of age).

II. Data collection

A. Subjective symptoms
1. Fatigue

2. Loss of appetite
3. Weakness
4. History of recent upper respiratory infection
5. Persistent fever
6. Night sweats
7. Weight loss
8. Malaise
9. Pruritus
   B. Objective symptoms
   1. Enlarged lymph nodes, spleen, and liver
   2. Positive biopsy of lymph nodes: cervical nodes most often affected
   3. Anemia
   4. Positive CAT scan of liver and spleen
   5. Elevated temperature
   6. Thrombocytopenia
   7. Elevated serum alkaline phosphatase level: indicating liver or bone involvement
   8. Evaluation of stage by results of lymphangiography and laparotomy
   9. Positive bone marrow biopsy (if affected)
III. Diagnostic tests and methods
   A. Client history
   B. Physical examination
   C. Lymph node biopsy
   D. Bone marrow, liver, and spleen biopsies
   E. CAT scan of lung, bone, liver, spleen
   F. Lymphangiography for detection of involved lymph nodes or organ involvement
   G. Hematological tests: CBC, blood chemistries to check serum alkaline phosphatase levels
   H. Staging laparotomy for clients <55 years old· or with no obvious stage III or IV disease or other medical contraindications
   I. Measures to rule out other disorders that also cause enlarged lymph nodes
IV. Implementation
   A. Assess, report, and record signs and symptoms and any reaction to treatment.
   B. Assist with comfort measures for night sweats, itching, and fever.
   C. Prepare and explain to client and family treatments such as radiation, chemotherapy, and surgical procedures, if needed.
   D. Monitor vital signs and I&O.
   E. Protect client from contact with others who have infections.
   F. Provide safe environment.
   G. Provide emotional support to client and family.
   H. Monitor for signs of infection and changes in skin integrity.
   I. Minimize radiation side effects by good nutrition.
   J. Monitor for radiation and chemotherapeutic side effects (anorexia, nausea, vomiting, diarrhea, hair loss).
   K. Administer good oral hygiene using a soft toothbrush, cotton swab, or anesthetic mouthwash (if prescribed) to control pain and bleeding from stomatitis.
   L. Provide appropriate counseling and reassurance.
   M. Provide information regarding local chapter of American Cancer Society to assist in financial matters and supportive counseling, if needed.
   N. Explain disease, diagnostic procedures, treatment including medication, home care, and follow-up care to client and family.
V. Evaluation
   A. Client remains free of injury or infection.
   B. Client reports increased comfort and decreased anxiety.
   C. Client maintains good hygienic measures and skin integrity.
   D. Client uses effective coping strategies.
   E. Client and family demonstrate an understanding of disease process, treatment, home care, and follow-up care.

Thrombocytopenia

I. Description
   A. Most common cause of hemorrhagic disorders
   B. Condition characterized by a decreased number of circulating platelets
   C. Posing a serious threat to hemostasis
   D. Prognosis good if thrombocytopenia is drug induced by withdrawing drug
   E. Prognosis in other cases dependent on response to treatment of underlying cause
   F. Abnormally low platelet count (normal range 150,000–400,000/mm^3)
   G. Causes
   1. Congenital or acquired
   2. Condition usually results from:
      a. Decreased production of platelets in marrow (leukemia, aplastic anemia, or toxicity of certain drugs)
      b. Increased destruction of platelets outside the marrow (cirrhosis of liver, DIC, severe infections)
      c. Reduction in platelet survival time
      d. Collection of blood (sequestration) in spleen
      e. Acquired thrombocytopenia possibly caused by certain drugs, such as quinine, quinidine, chlorothiazide, sulfisoxazole, phenylbutazone, rifampin, heparin, and cyclophosphamide)
II. Data collection
   A. Subjective symptoms
   1. History of current medication intake
   2. Bleeding from oral cavity and nose
   3. Easy bruising
   4. Malaise
   5. Fatigue
   6. General weakness
   B. Objective symptoms
   1. Petechiae
   2. Ecchymoses
   3. Epistaxis or gingival bleeding
   4. Low platelet count
   5. Blood-filled bullae in oral cavity
   6. Presence of megakaryocytes (platelet precursors) in bone marrow aspirations
   7. Hematuria
   8. Tachycardia, dyspnea, loss of consciousness, and death from hemorrhage
III. Diagnostic tests and methods
   A. Client history

B. Physical examination

C. Laboratory (coagulation) tests, platelet count, Hgb, Hct

D. Bone marrow biopsy

IV. Implementation

  A. Assess, report, and record signs and symptoms and any reaction to treatment.

  B. Monitor for signs of bleeding.

  C. Protect from injury or trauma.

  D. Avoid invasive procedures such as venipuncture, intramuscular injections, urinary catheterization, and taking rectal temperature readings, if possible.

  E. If venipuncture is used, exert pressure on puncture site for at least 20 minutes, or until bleeding stops.

  F. Assist in administration of prescribed platelet transfusions.

  G. Monitor vital signs.

  H. Monitor platelet count, blood count, and bleeding times.

  I. Test stool for presence of blood; use a dipstick to test urine and emesis for blood.

  J. Instruct client to avoid aspirin and other drugs that decrease clotting.

  K. Instruct client to avoid straining at stool or when coughing (increases intracranial pressure [ICP] with potential for causing cerebral hemorrhage); provide stool softener, if necessary.

  L. Enforce bedrest if bleeding occurs.

  M. Provide safe environment.

  N. Provide emotional support.

  O. Explain disease process, diagnostic procedures, treatment including medication, prevention, home care, and follow-up care to client and family.

V. Evaluation

  A. Client reports increased comfort and decreased anxiety.

  B. Client remains free of injury.

  C. Client maintains adequate tissue perfusion.

  D. Client maintains good skin integrity.

  E. There is no bleeding.

  F. Client and family demonstrate an understanding of disease process, diagnostic procedures, treatment including medication, prevention, home care, and follow-up care.

Acquired Immunodeficiency Syndrome

I. Description

  A. Human immunodeficiency virus (HIV): disorder that disrupts T lymphocytes, eventually destroying them and causing an immune deficiency

  B. Disease resulting in inability of body to defend itself against infection

  C. Progressive and fatal, death occurring as result of opportunistic complications

  D. Causes

    1. HIV is spread by sexual contact, sharing of infected needles, and transfusions using blood or blood product containing HIV.

    2. The virus may also be transmitted by contaminated blood or body fluids in contact with broken skin surfaces.

    3. Infected mothers can pass the virus to their unborn infant.

II. Data collection

  A. Subjective symptoms

    1. Recurrent fever and night sweats

    2. Weight loss

    3. Anorexia

    4. Chronic diarrhea

    5. Fatigue, weakness

  B. Objective symptoms

    1. Swollen lymph glands

    2. White spots or lesions in oral cavity

    3. Dry cough

    4. Shortness of breath

    5. Presence of opportunistic infections such as Kaposi's sarcoma (purplish skin lesions) and *Pneumocystis carinii* pneumonia

III. Diagnostic tests and methods

  A. Client history

  B. Physical examination

  C. HIV or human T-cell lymphotropic virus type III (HTLV III) in serum

  D. Presence of opportunistic infections

  E. Lumbar puncture

  F. CAT scan

  G. Bronchial biopsy

IV. Implementation

  A. Assess, report, and record signs and symptoms and any reaction to treatment.

  B. Protect client from opportunistic infections.

  C. Administer azidothymidine (AZT) and other prescribed medications; check for side effects.

  D. Provide nutritional support.

  E. Monitor vital signs.

  F. Use blood and body fluid precautions:

    1. Protective clothing (gloves, masks, gowns, and so forth)

    2. Good handwashing technique

    3. Careful labeling of specimens

    4. Appropriate disposal of contaminated articles

  G. Encourage physical independence.

  H. Monitor oxygen therapy.

  I. Administer analgesics for pain.

  J. Schedule rest periods.

  K. Provide emotional support to client and family.

  L. Provide information for support network.

  M. Explain disease, mode of spread, protective measures, home care, and community resources.

V. Evaluation

  A. Client reports increased comfort.

  B. Client remains free of injury.

  C. Client maintains adequate tissue perfusion.

  D. Client demonstrates an understanding of disease process, mode of spread, protective measures, home care, and follow-up care.

Gastrointestinal System

Basic Information

• Breaks down food—carbohydrates, fats, and proteins—into molecules small enough to pass through cell membranes.

- Provides cells with necessary energy to function properly; prepares food for cellular absorption by altering its physical and chemical composition.
- Influenced by other systems: the endocrine, central nervous, and autonomic nervous systems, which serve as regulators.
- Malfunction of the GI tract has far-reaching metabolic effects on the body.
  I. Basic data collection
     A. Subjective symptoms
        1. Nausea and vomiting
        2. Difficulty in swallowing
        3. Difficulty in chewing
        4. Weight changes
        5. Indigestion
        6. Appetite change
        7. Gas
        8. Changes in bowel habits
        9. Intolerance to certain foods
        10. Personal and family history of GI-related problems
     B. Objective symptoms
        1. Stomatitis
        2. Hematemesis
        3. Abdominal distention
        4. Jaundice
        5. Constipation or diarrhea
        6. Edema
        7. Hemorrhoids
        8. Stool changes: clay-colored, black, frothy
        9. Dark urine

Major Gastrointestinal Diagnoses

Esophageal Varices

  I. Description
     A. Dilatation of blood vessels (varicose veins) at lower end of esophagus
     B. Causes
        1. Elevated pressure in portal vein (vessel bringing blood into liver) because of:
           a. Cirrhosis of the liver
           b. Mechanical obstruction of portal vein by blood clot or tumor or obstruction of the hepatic veins
     C. Possibility that varices may rupture, causing hemorrhage and shock
     D. Death from hemorrhage approximately 67%
  II. Data collection
     A. Subjective symptoms
        1. Anxiety
        2. History of cirrhosis, portal hypertension
        3. Weakness, vertigo
     B. Objective symptoms
        1. Blood in emesis
        2. Melena (black, tarry stools caused by bleeding)
        3. Low Hgb and Hct values
        4. Elevated SGOT, SGPT, amylase, bilirubin levels; low albumin level
        5. Hypotension
        6. Tachycardia

        7. Decreased level of consciousness
        8. Signs of shock
  III. Diagnostic tests and methods
     A. Client history
     B. Physical examination
     C. Endoscopy to identify bleeding site
     D. Laboratory studies: Hct, Hgb, liver function tests
     E. Angiography
  IV. Implementation
     A. Monitor for hemorrhage and hypotension.
     B. Monitor emesis and stool for presence of blood.
     C. Monitor laboratory test results, and report abnormal findings.
     D. Give oxygen, if prescribed.
     E. Monitor vital signs at least every 4 hours (every half-hour if bleeding occurs).
     F. Monitor I&O and CVP for volume determination.
     G. Evaluate level of consciousness.
     H. Provide emotional support and reassurance to client and family.
     I. Provide mouth care.
     J. Administer prescribed medications and monitor for side effects.
     K. Administer and monitor IV infusion and blood transfusions as prescribed.
     L. Keep client quiet and comfortable.

NOTE: Tolerance to sedatives and tranquilizers may be decreased because of liver disease.

     M. Control bleeding by:
        1. Giving ice water lavages
        2. Assisting with insertion of Sengstaken-Blakemore tube if ordered (keep scissors taped to head of bed in case of emergency)
        3. Administering vitamin K as prescribed
        4. Monitoring vasopressin (Pitressin) effects (used to constrict splanchnic vessels)
     N. Monitor client with Sengstaken-Blakemore tube for:
        1. Bleeding in gastric drainage
        2. Signs of asphyxiation
        3. Tube displacement
        4. Proper inflation of balloons
        5. Correct traction to keep tube in correct placement
     O. Assist with injection of sclerosing agent to control bleeding as ordered.
     P. Monitor for signs of hepatic encephalopathy.
     Q. Prepare client for surgery, if required to control bleeding.
     R. Provide postoperative care; explain care to client and family.
     S. Assist with preparation of client for discharge and self-care.
     T. Explain disease process, prevention, and home care.
  V. Evaluation
     A. Client reports increased comfort and decreased anxiety.
     B. Hemetemesis is decreased or absent.
     C. Melena is decreased or absent.
     D. Vital signs remain stable.

E. Client maintains adequate fluid I&O.
F. Client maintains adequate nutritional intake.
G. Laboratory values remain within normal range.
H. Client demonstrates an understanding of disease process, prevention, and home care.

Hiatal Hernia

I. Description
   A. Protrusion of part of stomach through weakened area of diaphragm into thoracic cavity
   B. Gastric reflux (regurgitation) when the lower esophageal sphincter (muscle) pressure is less than the pressure in the stomach
   C. Possibility of gastric reflux entering esophagus, resulting in inflammation and ulceration
   D. Causes
      1. Congenital weakness of diaphragm
      2. Trauma
   E. Related factors
      1. Increased abdominal pressure
      2. Relaxed esophageal sphincter
      3. Pregnancy
      4. Obesity
      5. Smoking and alcohol and caffeine ingestion
II. Data collection
   A. Subjective symptoms
      1. Heartburn
      2. Regurgitation
      3. Dysphagia (difficulty in swallowing)
      4. Feeling of fullness
      5. History of trauma, obesity, pregnancy
      6. Anxiety
   B. Objective symptoms
      1. Dyspnea (difficulty in breathing)
      2. Discovered via diagnostic methods
III. Diagnostic tests and methods
   A. Client history
   B. Physical examination
   C. Chest x-ray
   D. Upper GI series (barium swallow)
   E. Esophagoscopy
IV. Implementation
   A. Provide small, frequent meals (bland diet: high protein, low fat).
   B. Keep head of bed elevated when client is eating and up to 3 hours after meal.
   C. Administer medications such as bethanechol (Urecholine), cimetidine (Tagamet), and antacids as prescribed.
   D. Instruct client not to perform activities that increase abdominal pressure, such as lifting heavy objects, bending over, and wearing tight clothing around waist.
   E. Instruct obese clients regarding weight management.
   F. Keep head of bed slightly elevated during sleep periods.
   G. Instruct client to avoid alcohol and caffeine.
   H. Prepare client and family for surgical intervention, if conservative measures fail.
   I. Provide postoperative care:

      1. Assist with administration of and monitor IV therapy and blood transfusions.
      2. Assist in insertion of NG tube and monitor effects.
      3. Administer analgesics and antiemetics as prescribed.
      4. Monitor medications for side effects.
      5. Monitor fluid I&O.
      6. Monitor vital signs.
      7. Report incidence of gastric reflux immediately.
   J. Explain condition and medication compliance to client and family.
V. Evaluation
   A. Client reports increased comfort and decreased anxiety.
   B. Client maintains adequate nutritional intake.
   C. Symptoms disappear.
   D. Client and family demonstrate an understanding of condition and medication compliance.

Peptic Ulcer

I. Description
   A. Ulcerations in the gastric mucosal membrane.
   B. Ulcerations can develop in lower esophagus, stomach, pylorus, duodenum, or jejunum:
      1. Duodenal ulcer: approximately 80% occur in this area (proximal part of small intestine)
         a. Ulcer occurs most often in men 20–50 years old.
         b. Ulcer often becomes chronic, with remissions and exacerbations.
         c. Complications requiring surgical intervention possible.
      2. Gastric ulcer (stomach)
         a. Ulcer occurs most often in middle-aged and elderly men.
         b. Especially common among poor and undernourished.
         c. Tendency of benign gastric ulcers to recur.
   C. Both types of ulcers possibly asymptomatic.
   D. Complications:
      1. Penetration to pancreas, causing severe back pain
      2. Perforation of area involved
      3. Hemorrhage
      4. Pyloric obstruction
   E. Possible causes:
      1. Decreased mucus resistance
      2. Inadequate mucosal blood flow
      3. Defective mucus
      4. Acid hypersecretion, possibly from overactive vagus nerve, likely to contribute to duodenal ulcer formation
      5. Bacteria in stomach lining (*Helicobacter pylori*)
   F. Related factors:
      1. Chronic use of aspirin and alcohol
      2. Cigarette smoking
      3. Heredity
      4. Emotional stress
      5. Chronic use of drugs such as ibuprofen and corticosteroids

II. Data collection
  A. Subjective symptoms
    1. Gastric ulcer
      a. Heartburn
      b. Indigestion
      c. Feeling of fullness and distention after a large meal
    2. Duodenal ulcer
      a. Heartburn
      b. Pain (gnawing, burning) in middle-upper abdomen relieved by food ingestion
      c. Sensation of water bubbling in back of throat
      d. "Attacks" approximately 2 hours after meals or when stomach is empty
      e. Ingestion of citric juices, coffee, aspirin, or alcohol causing pain
  B. Objective symptoms
    1. Gastric ulcer
      a. Loss of appetite
      b. Possible repeated episodes of GI bleeding
      c. Weight loss
      d. Anemia
      e. Melena
      f. Vomiting: coffee-ground appearance with bleeding
    2. Duodenal ulcer
      a. Weight gain from eating to relieve discomfort
      b. Vomiting and other digestive symptoms rare
      c. Possibility of complications: watch for GI bleeding, melena
III. Diagnostic tests and methods
  A. Client history
  B. Physical examination
  C. Upper GI series
  D. Gastric analysis
  E. Gastroscopy
  F. Laboratory studies: Hct, Hgb, electrolytes, CBC
  G. Biopsy of tissue to rule out malignancy
IV. Implementation
  A. Assess, report, and record signs and symptoms and any reactions to treatment.
  B. Provide quiet environment, and assist with comfort measures.
  C. Administer prescribed medications such as analgesics, sedatives, antacids, anticholinergics, histamine receptor antagonists (ranitidine [Zantac], cimetidine) to neutralize or inhibit gastric secretions, sedatives, and bismuth preparations.
  D. Monitor and report medication side effects such as dizziness, rash, mild diarrhea, muscle pain, leukopenia, gynecomastia, dry mouth, blurred vision, headache, constipation, and urinary retention.
  E. Monitor vital signs.
  F. Monitor laboratory test results (Hct, Hgb, CBC, electrolytes).
  G. Watch for signs of bleeding:
    1. Changes in vital signs
    2. Vomiting (coffee-ground appearance)
    3. Anemia
    4. Black and tarry or bloody stools
  H. Provide prescribed diet: avoid irritating foods such as coffee and spices.

I. Discourage cigarette smoking.
J. Assist with preparation of client and family for surgical intervention, if required for recurrent ulcers, perforation, or hemorrhage.
K. Provide preoperative care:
  1. Assist in administration of blood replacement.
  2. Assist with insertion of nasogastric tube for gastric decompression.
  3. Provide reassurance to client and family.
L. Explain surgical intervention:
  1. Closure if perforation has occurred
  2. Total or partial resection of stomach or duodenum to remove ulcerated area(s)
  3. Pyloroplasty and vagotomy if gastric outlet is obstructed
M. Provide postoperative care:
  1. Monitor vital signs (report abnormalities immediately).
  2. Administer narcotics and analgesics as prescribed for pain.
  3. Monitor fluid I&O.
  4. Assess for signs of dehydration, sodium deficiency, and metabolic alkalosis (may occur secondary to gastric suction).
  5. Assist in administration of blood transfusions and IV infusions, and monitor for side effects.
  6. Monitor patency of nasogastric tube; check, record, and report characteristics of drainage.
  7. Monitor and report signs of bleeding.
  8. Encourage coughing and deep breathing.
  9. Monitor elimination. Check bowel sounds. Keep client nothing by mouth (NPO) until peristalsis resumes and NG tube is removed or clamped.
  10. Watch for complications:
    a. Hemorrhage, shock
    b. Iron folate, or vitamin B_{12} deficiency anemia (from continued blood loss or malabsorption)
    c. Dumping syndrome (weakness, nausea, diarrhea, gas pains, distention, and palpitations within 30 minutes after a meal)
  11. Begin nursing interventions if complications such as hemorrhage occur:
    a. Monitor vital signs every half-hour, and report abnormalities immediately.
    b. Monitor fluid I&O.
    c. Provide complete bedrest, and keep client NPO as ordered.
    d. Provide quiet environment; allay anxiety.
    e. Monitor NG drainage, presence of vomitus, bloody stools; report changes immediately.
    f. Assist in administration of blood, IV fluids, and medications as prescribed.
N. Instruct client in prevention of dumping syndrome:
  1. Eating four to six small, high-protein, low-carbohydrate meals during the day
  2. Sitting up or standing after meals
    a. Drink fluids between rather than with meals.
    b. Avoid eating large amounts of carbohydrates.
O. Instruct client that magnesium-containing antacids may cause diarrhea and that aluminum-containing antacids may cause constipation.

P. Instruct client to avoid drugs containing aspirin, as they irritate gastric mucosa.

Q. Advise client to avoid excessive use of coffee and alcohol and to avoid stressful situations.

R. Advise client to stop smoking, as it stimulates gastric secretions.

S. Explain condition, treatment including need for compliance, and home care.

V. Evaluation

A. Client reports increased comfort and decreased anxiety.

B. Client maintains adequate nutritional intake.

C. Symptoms disappear.

D. Laboratory values remain within normal range.

E. Client and family demonstrate an understanding of condition, treatment including need for compliance, and home care including lifestyle modification.

Crohn's Disease (Regional Enteritis)

I. Description

A. Inflammation of any part of the GI tract (usually the terminal ileum)

1. Lacteal blockage in intestinal wall, leading to edema.

2. Disease eventually leads to inflammation, ulceration, stenosis, abscess, and fistula formation.

B. Inflammation extending through all layers of the intestinal wall

C. "Cobblestone" ulcerations in intestinal lining, forming scar tissue

D. Bowel becoming thick and narrow

E. Possibly also involving regional lymph nodes and the mesentery

F. Possibility that ulcerations may perforate, resulting in fistulas leading to colon, bladder, vagina, and perianal area, as well as perirectal abscesses and perforations

G. Normal absorption of nutrients decreased owing to scar tissue formation

H. Possibility that strictures may develop, with potential for intestinal obstruction

I. Most prevalent in adults 20–40 years old

J. Two to three times more common in Jews and least common in blacks

K. In up to 5% of affected clients, pattern of one or more affected relatives (inheritance pattern is not clear)

L. Possible causes (exact cause unknown)

1. Allergies and other immune disorders

2. Lymphatic obstruction

3. Infection

4. Environmental or genetic factors

5. Emotional stress

6. Heredity (genetic cause)

II. Data collection

A. Subjective symptoms

1. Abdominal pain and cramping

2. Tenderness

3. Gas pains

4. Nausea

5. Loss of appetite

6. Malaise, weakness, fatigue

7. Anxiety

8. Inability to cope with everyday stress

B. Objective symptoms

1. Elevated temperature

2. Diarrhea (four to six stools a day) containing pus, mucus, or blood

3. Marked weight loss

4. Anemia

5. Laboratory test results

a. Elevated WBC count and ESR

b. Hypokalemia

c. Hypocalcemia

d. Hypomagnesemia

e. Depressed Hgb

6. Signs of dehydration (poor skin turgor, dry mucous membranes)

7. Results of stool specimen studies

8. Lower right quadrant tenderness

III. Diagnostic tests and methods

A. Client history

B. Physical examination

C. Stool specimen examination for occult blood

D. Laboratory studies: CBC, ESR, electrolytes, Hgb, Hct

E. Barium enema showing string sign (segments of stricture separated by normal bowel)

F. Endoscopy

G. Sigmoidoscopy or colonoscopy: patchy areas of inflammation possible (helps rule out ulcerative colitis)

H. Biopsy: for definitive diagnosis

I. Colonoscopy

IV. Implementation

A. Assess, report, and record signs and symptoms and any reaction to treatment.

B. Provide emotional support and adequate rest.

C. Record I&O (include amount of stool).

D. Weigh daily.

E. Watch for dehydration (decrease in urinary output, poor skin turgor).

F. Monitor fluid and electrolyte balance.

G. Monitor vital signs every 4 hours.

H. Watch for signs of intestinal bleeding (bloody stools):

1. Check stools daily for occult blood.

I. Provide prescribed diet:

1. Restricted fiber diet with no fruit or vegetables for intestinal stenosis

2. Low-fat diet to decrease fatty stools as ordered

3. Elimination of dairy products for lactose deficiency

J. Administer prescribed medications, and monitor for side effects:

1. Sulfasalazine for anti-inflammatory effects

2. Steroids to reduce inflammation (watch for GI bleeding, as steroids mask signs of infection)

3. Antibiotics to reduce risk of infection from peritoneal irritation, abscess, or fistulas

4. Sedatives

5. Analgesics

6. Anticholinergics

7. Bulk hydrophilic drugs to treat diarrhea

K. Check Hgb and Hct daily:
 1. Administer iron supplements and blood transfusions as prescribed.
L. Provide mouth care.
M. Provide good skin care after each bowel movement.
N. Keep clean, covered bedpan within client's reach.
O. Ventilate room to eliminate odors.
P. Monitor client for fever or pain on urination (may indicate a bladder fistula).
Q. Monitor client for abdominal pain, fever, and hard, distended abdomen (may indicate intestinal obstruction).
R. Provide information regarding surgical intervention and postoperative course, if required (colectomy with ileostomy often required in clients with extensive disease of large intestine and rectum).
 1. Before ileostomy, request that an enterostomal therapist visit client.
S. Care during postoperative period:
 1. Monitor IV infusion and NG tube for proper functioning.
 2. Monitor fluid I&O.
 3. Monitor vital signs.
 4. Watch for wound infection.
 5. Provide meticulous stoma care.
 6. Teach stoma care to client and family.
 7. Provide reassurance and emotional support (ileostomy changes client's body image).
T. Encourage reduction in stress (may need to refer client for counseling).
U. Explain disease process, diagnostic procedures, treatment including medication, home care including diet and bedrest, stoma care, sexuality, and follow-up care.
 V. Evaluation
A. Client reports increased comfort and decreased anxiety.
B. Client maintains adequate nutritional and fluid intake.
C. Client tolerates progressive activity.
D. Client verbalizes concerns and problems.
E. Client uses effective coping strategies.
F. Client demonstrates an understanding of disease process, treatment, prevention, home care, and follow-up care.

Ulcerative Colitis

 I. Description
A. Inflammatory, often chronic, disorder of the large bowel, with rectal and sigmoid colon mucosae and submucosae becoming edematous and developing small bleeding lesions that result in ulcerations
B. Inflammation often extending upward into entire colon; rarely affecting small intestine, except for the terminal ileum
C. Condition producing congestion, edema (resulting in mucosal friability)
D. Ulcerations developing into abscesses
E. Eventual loss of elasticity of colon, with a reduction in nutrient absorptive capability
F. Severity ranging from a mild, localized condition to

a severe disease that may result in a perforated colon, progressing to potentially fatal peritonitis and toxemia
G. At risk for development of colorectal cancer
H. Condition occurring primarily in young adults, especially women
I. More prevalent in Jews and upper socioeconomic groups
J. Overall, incidence rates increasing
K. Causes unknown
L. Possible predisposing factors
 1. Family history of disease
 2. Bacterial infection
 3. Allergic reaction to food, milk, or substances that release inflammatory histamine in the bowel
 4. Overproduction of enzymes that break down mucous membrane
 5. Autoimmune reactions such as arthritis and hemolytic anemia
 6. Environmental factors
 7. Emotional stress
 II. Data collection
A. Subjective symptoms
 1. Abdominal cramping pain
 2. Nausea
 3. Loss of appetite
 4. Irritability
 5. Anxiety
 6. Weakness
B. Objective symptoms
 1. Bloody diarrhea containing pus and mucus
 2. Spastic rectum and anus
 3. Weight loss
 4. Vomiting
 III. Diagnostic tests and methods
A. Client history
B. Physical examination
C. Stool examination
D. Sigmoidoscopy: shows increased mucosal friability; thick inflammatory exudate
E. Colonoscopy with biopsy to determine extent of disease and evaluate strictures and pseudopolyps
F. Barium enema to assess extent of disease and detect complications
G. Laboratory studies: electrolytes, CBC, Hgb, Hct, ESR
 IV. Implementation
A. Assess, report, and record signs and symptoms and any reaction to treatment.
B. Provide emotional support and adequate rest.
C. Provide good skin care to prevent anal excoriation.
D. Monitor the number, amount, time, and characteristics of stools.
E. Provide client with air mattress or sheepskin to prevent skin breakdown.
F. Monitor bowel sounds every 4 hours in all four quadrants.
G. Administer prescribed medications, and monitor for side effects:
 1. Corticosteroids (prolonged therapy causing "moonface," hirsutism, edema, gastric irritation)
H. Monitor vital signs.

I. Monitor I&O.
J. Watch for signs of dehydration (dry skin and mucous membranes, sunken eyes, fever).
K. Monitor Hgb, Hct, and electrolyte levels.
L. Assist with blood transfusions and IV therapy as prescribed.
M. Provide mouth care for those kept NPO.
N. Weigh daily.
O. Provide prescribed diet.
P. Assist with ADLs.
Q. Monitor for signs of complications such as perforated colon or peritonitis:
    1. Fever
    2. Severe abdominal pain
    3. Rigid and tender abdomen
    4. Cool, clammy skin
    5. Abdominal distention and decreased or absent bowel sounds
    6. Preparation of client for surgery if complications occur:
        a. Arrange for visit by an enterostomal therapist.
R. Provide postoperative care:
    1. Give meticulous care and teach correct stoma care to client and family.
    2. Monitor NG tube for patency.
    3. After NG tube removal, provide a clear-liquid diet; advance to low-residue diet.
S. Prepare client for discharge; encourage regular physical examinations.
T. Explain disease process, treatment including compliance, prevention, and home care to client and family.

V. Evaluation
A. Client reports increased comfort and decreased anxiety.
B. Client maintains adequate nutritional and fluid intake.
C. Client continues progressive activity.
D. Client verbalizes concerns.
E. Client explains or demonstrates self-care.
F. Client and family demonstrate an understanding of disease process, treatment including compliance, prevention, home care, and follow-up care.

Diverticulosis and Diverticulitis

I. Description
A. Bulging pouches (diverticula) found in the GI wall.
B. Mucosal lining pushed through surrounding muscle by diverticula.
C. Most common site is sigmoid colon, although it may develop from proximal end of pharynx to anus.
D. Diverticular disease of ileum (Meckel's diverticulum) most common congenital anomaly of GI tract.
E. Two clinical forms of diverticular disease:
    1. Diverticulosis
        a. Diverticula present but do not cause symptoms
        b. Possibly asymptomatic; usual occurrence before age 35 years

    2. Diverticulitis
        a. Diverticula are inflamed and may cause severe obstruction, infection, or hemorrhage.
            1) Retained, undigested food mixing with bacteria in diverticular sac, resulting in a hard mass.
            2) Blood supply cut off to thin walls of the diverticular sac, becoming susceptible to bacteria found in the colon.
            3) Inflammation results.
        b. Condition usually occurs between 50 and 70 years of age and may result in spasms, obstruction, perforation, or bleeding.
        c. Inflamed colon segment possibly results in a fistula leading to the bladder or other organs.

II. Data collection
A. Subjective symptoms
    1. Diverticulosis
        a. Usually asymptomatic
        b. In elderly persons, rare possibility of hemorrhage from diverticula in rectum (usually mild) as complication
    2. Diverticulitis
        a. Recurrent pain in lower left quadrant relieved by bowel movement or passage of gas
        b. Mild nausea
        c. Vomiting when obstruction is present
B. Objective symptoms
    1. Alternating constipation and diarrhea
    2. Irregular bowel movements
    3. Low-grade fever
    4. Increased WBC count
    5. Occult bleeding
    6. If rupture occurs, abdominal rigidity, severe lower left quadrant pain, signs of sepsis and shock (high fever, chills, hypotension)
    7. Rupture near blood vessel: mild to severe hemorrhage based on size of affected blood vessel
    8. Constipation, ribbonlike stools, intermittent diarrhea, abdominal distention (signs of incomplete bowel obstruction) usually a result of chronic condition
    9. Abdominal rigidity, decreased or absent bowel sounds, nausea, vomiting, abdominal pain (signs of increasing bowel obstruction)

III. Diagnostic tests and methods
A. Client history
B. Physical examination
C. Laboratory studies: CBC, ESR, Hgb, Hct, RBC count
D. Stool for occult blood
E. X-ray series: to reveal possible spasms of the colon
F. Upper GI series: for diverticulosis of esophagus and upper bowel
G. Barium enema: for diverticulosis of lower bowel
    1. In acute diverticulitis, enema may rupture bowel.
H. Sigmoidoscopy
I. Colonoscopy

IV. Implementation
A. Continuously assess, report, and record signs and symptoms and any reaction to treatment.
B. Provide emotional support.

C. For diverticulosis with pain, constipation, mild GI distress, or difficulty with bowel movements:
1. Provide prescribed diet (liquid or soft) during acute phase (helps to relieve symptoms, decrease irritation, and decrease progression to diverticulitis).
2. Administer stool softeners and medications as prescribed.
3. Monitor stools: check frequency, color, and consistency.
4. Monitor vital signs (changes may indicate progression of condition).
5. Encourage fluid intake.
6. Provide high-roughage diet and bulk-forming agents once pain subsides.
D. For mild diverticulosis without complications:
1. Provide quiet environment and bedrest.
2. Provide a liquid diet.
3. Administer prescribed medications such as stool softeners, broad-spectrum antibiotics, analgesics for pain, smooth muscle relaxants, antispasmodics.
4. Observe stools and record and report abnormalities.
5. Monitor vital signs for changes.
6. Monitor fluid I&O.
E. For hemorrhage:
1. Assist with administration of blood transfusions and IV therapy as prescribed.
2. Monitor fluid and electrolyte balance.
F. For surgical treatment for diverticulitis that does not respond to conservative therapy:
1. Prepare client for colon resection.
2. Prepare client for temporary colostomy in cases of perforation, peritonitis, obstruction, or fistula formation (to drain abscesses and rest colon before anastomosis).
3. For postoperative care:
a. Provide meticulous wound care.
b. Watch for signs of infection.
c. Check drain sites frequently (observe for pus, foul odor, or fecal drainage).
d. Change dressings as necessary.
e. Monitor fluid I&O.
f. Observe for postoperative bleeding (decreased Hgb and Hct).
g. Monitor other laboratory values (electrolytes; WBC, RBC counts).
h. Instruct client to cough and breathe deeply (to prevent atelectasis).
i. Monitor IV therapy.
j. Monitor patency and placement of NG tube.
G. Education
1. Assist with teaching of colostomy care, if needed; arrange for visit by enterostomal therapist.
2. Instruct client to avoid any activity that increases abdominal pressure, such as bending, wearing tight clothing around waist, and straining during bowel movement.
3. Explain disease process, treatment, prevention, home care including diet and stress management, and follow-up care.

V. Evaluation
A. Client reports increased comfort and decreased anxiety.
B. Client maintains adequate nutritional and fluid intake.
C. Signs and symptoms disappear.
D. Client demonstrates an ability to perform colostomy care if needed.
E. Client demonstrates an understanding of disease process, treatment, prevention, home care, and follow-up care.

Intestinal Obstruction

I. Description
A. Partial or complete blockage of the lumen in the small or large intestine
B. Decreased or absent peristaltic movement of intestinal contents because of mechanical or neurological disorders
C. Mechanical disorders including such conditions as scar tissue, strangulated hernias, and tumors
D. Neurological disorders including paralytic ileus, which interferes with innervation, preventing normal peristaltic activity
E. Pressure increasing as peristaltic activity attempts to move intestinal contents within intestine, resulting in:
1. Dilation, atonicity of smooth muscle
2. Prevention of flatus because of edema and decreased blood supply for elevated pressures
3. Collection of gas occurring in distended intestine
F. Complete obstruction if untreated, possibly causing death within hours from ischemia, necrosis, shock, and vascular collapse
G. Intestinal obstruction more likely to occur after abdominal surgery or in persons with congenital defects of the bowel
H. Causes
1. Adhesions and strangulated hernias usual causes of small bowel obstruction
2. Carcinomas and tumors usual causes of large bowel obstruction
3. Obstruction caused by mechanical disorders
a. Presence of foreign bodies such as fruit pits, gallstones, worms
b. Compression of intestinal wall caused by:
1) Stenosis
2) Intussusception (telescoping of bowel)
3) Volvulus (twisting) of sigmoid or cecum
4) Tumors
5) Atresia
4. Obstruction caused by physiological disturbances
a. Electrolyte imbalances
b. Toxicity (uremia, generalized infections)
c. Paralytic ileus
d. Spinal cord lesions
e. Thrombosis or embolism of mesenteric blood vessels

I. Three forms of intestinal obstruction
   1. Simple: intestinal contents blocked from passing; no other complications
   2. Strangulated: blockage of intestinal lumen, with lack of blood supply to part or all of obstructed section
   3. Close-looped: occlusion of both ends of the bowel section, isolated from rest of intestine
II. Data collection
   A. Subjective symptoms: small bowel obstruction
      1. Nausea
      2. Colicky pain
      3. Drowsiness
      4. Thirst
      5. Aching
      6. Dry mucous membranes
      7. Intestinal spasms
      8. Persistent epigastric pain
      9. Malaise, fatigue
   B. Subjective symptoms: large bowel obstruction
      1. Constipation
      2. Colicky abdominal pain with spasms
      3. Continuous hypogastric pain
      4. Nausea
   C. Objective symptoms: small bowel obstruction
      1. Vomiting
      2. Constipation
      3. Abdominal distention
      4. Presence of bowel sounds, borborygmi (rumbling in bowels)
   D. Objective symptoms: large bowel obstruction
      1. Constipation
      2. Leakage of liquid stool around obstruction: common in partial obstruction
      3. Intestinal spasms
      4. Fecal vomiting: usually absent at first
      5. Severe abdominal distention
III. Diagnostic tests and methods
   A. Client history
   B. Physical examination
   C. X-rays: flat plate of abdomen showing presence and location of intestinal gas or fluid
   D. Upper GI series
   E. Barium enema
   F. Laboratory studies: electrolytes, WBC count, amylase levels
IV. Implementation
   A. Continuously assess, report, and record signs and symptoms and any reaction to treatment.
   B. Provide emotional support.
   C. Keep client NPO.
   D. Monitor vital signs at least every 4 hours and report changes immediately.
   E. Assist with gastric or intestinal decompression to decrease nausea and vomiting.
   F. Monitor decompression tube; check and report amount and characteristics of drainage.
   G. Monitor patency of decompression tube; irrigate with normal saline, if ordered.
   H. Listen for presence or absence of bowel sounds; report presence of flatus or mucus through the rectum.
   I. Place client in Fowler's position to facilitate breathing and to decrease respiratory distress from abdominal distention.
   J. Monitor for signs of metabolic alkalosis (changes in consciousness; slow, shallow respirations; hypertonic muscles; tetany).
   K. Monitor for signs of metabolic acidosis (shortness of breath, disorientation; and later, deep, rapid breathing, malaise, and weakness).
   L. Monitor urinary output (assessment of circulating blood volume, renal function, possible urinary retention resulting from bladder compression by distended intestine).
   M. Assist with administration of and monitor IV therapy and electrolyte supplements.
   N. Provide mouth and nose care.
   O. Monitor for signs of dehydration.
   P. Administer medications as prescribed.
   Q. Prepare client and family for surgery and postoperative course, if required.
   R. Provide postoperative care:
      1. Encourage coughing, turning, and deep-breathing exercises to promote ventilation.
      2. Monitor bowel sounds (return of peristalsis) and elimination.
      3. Monitor fluid and electrolyte balance.
      4. Administer pain medication as prescribed.
      5. Assist with hygiene needs.
      6. Provide quiet, restful environment.
      7. Monitor nutritional status.
      8. Encourage early ambulation.
      9. Teach client and family colostomy care if required.
   S. Explain disease process, diagnostic procedures, treatment, home care, and follow-up care to client and family.
V. Evaluation
   A. Client reports increased comfort and decreased anxiety.
   B. Client maintains adequate hydration and electrolyte balance.
   C. Client maintains adequate nutritional intake.
   D. Abdominal distention is decreased or absent.
   E. Adequate bowel sounds are present.
   F. Signs and symptoms disappear.
   G. Client maintains normal bowel movement pattern.
   H. Client demonstrates an understanding of disease process, diagnostic procedures, treatment, home care, and follow-up.

Hernias

I. Description
   A. Protrusion of an organ or structure through an abnormal opening of the containing wall of its cavity
   B. Categories of hernias
      1. Reducible: relatively easily returned back to its normal position
      2. Irreducible: unable to be returned to its normal position
      3. Incarcerated: unable to be reduced because of formation of adhesions in hernial sac, causing an obstruction of intestinal flow

4. Strangulated: part of herniated intestine becomes twisted or edematous, cutting off blood supply and interfering with peristalsis (may lead to intestinal obstruction and necrosis)

C. Types
  1. Umbilical hernia
    a. Caused by abnormal muscular structures around umbilical cord
    b. Common in infants, often closing spontaneously
    c. Severe congenital hernia in which abdominal viscera protrude—requires immediate repair
    d. Possibly occurring in women who are obese or who have had several pregnancies
  2. Inguinal hernia
    a. Large or small intestine, omentum, or bladder protruding into inguinal canal
    b. Caused by increased abdominal pressure
    c. May be direct or indirect
    d. More common in men
  3. Femoral hernia
    a. Occurs where femoral artery passes into femoral canal
    b. Caused by increase in abdominal pressure from pregnancy or obesity
    c. Is more common in women
    d. Usually appears as a swelling or bulge at the pulse point of the femoral artery
    e. Usually is soft, reducible, nontender mass; may become incarcerated or strangulated
  4. Incisional hernia
    a. Protrusion of intestine or other structure through a previous incision
    b. Caused by increased abdominal pressure and weakened abdominal wall

D. Causes
  1. Congenital weakness in containing wall
  2. Weakness in containing wall because of previous incisional infections or the aging process
  3. Increased intra-abdominal pressure: heavy lifting, pregnancy, obesity, or straining
  4. Improper closure of opening in peritoneal sac in male clients

II. Data collection
  A. Subjective symptoms
    1. Presence of abdominal or inguinal mass after straining, coughing, or exertion
    2. Possible pain
    3. Swelling relieved by lying down
    4. Sharp, steady pain in groin (inguinal hernia)
    5. Severe pain and nausea (strangulated hernia)
    6. Signs of intestinal obstruction (strangulated hernia)
    7. Anorexia
  B. Objective symptoms
    1. Palpable mass in umbilical, inguinal, or femoral area
    2. Signs of intestinal obstruction
      a. Vomiting
      b. Irreducible mass
      c. Diminished or absent bowel sounds
      d. Shock

      e. Increased temperature
      f. Bloody stools
    3. Undescended testicle or hydrocele in infants

III. Diagnostic tests and methods
  A. Client history
  B. Physical examination

IV. Implementation
  A. Continuously assess, record, and report signs and symptoms and any reaction to treatment.
  B. Monitor vital signs.
  C. Restrict client's activities.
  D. Monitor I&O.
  E. Instruct client in use of truss, if prescribed, to keep hernia in place.
  F. Observe for signs of strangulation:
    1. Onset of pain
    2. Nausea and vomiting
    3. Abdominal distention
    4. Signs of shock
    5. Presence of blood in stools
  G. Prepare client for surgical intervention if required:
    1. Report symptoms of sneezing or upper respiratory tract infections before surgery (may cause tension and pressure on surgical repair site).
  H. Types of surgical intervention:
    1. Herniorrhaphy
      a. Surgical replacement of protruding part into its containing cavity
    2. Hernioplasty
      a. Surgical reinforcement of the containing wall to prevent recurrence
  I. Postoperative care:
    1. Monitor vital signs.
    2. Apply ice packs as ordered to control pain and swelling.
    3. Monitor urinary output after inguinal hernia repair.
    4. Monitor I&O.
    5. Encourage deep-breathing exercises. *Do not let client cough.*
    6. Administer pain medications as prescribed.
    7. Monitor incision site for signs of infection.
    8. Assist with ambulation.
    9. Explain condition, treatment, and home care to client and family:
      a. Take care of incision.
      b. Check for signs of infection.
      c. Restrict driving for at least 2 weeks.
      d. Restrict activities such as heavy lifting, pulling, or pushing for 6 weeks.
      e. Assure client that sexual activity is not affected.

V. Evaluation
  A. Client reports increased comfort and decreased anxiety.
  B. Client maintains adequate nutritional and fluid intake.
  C. Signs and symptoms disappear.
  D. Client remains free of postoperative complications.
  E. Client and family demonstrate an understanding of condition, treatment, and home care including activity restrictions.

Hemorrhoids

I. Description
   A. Presence of varicosities or dilated hemorrhoidal veins in the rectal and anal area that interfere with venous return
   B. Possibly occurring internally, externally, or both
   C. Incidence highest between ages of 20 and 50 years and involves both sexes
   D. Types
      1. First-degree hemorrhoids: may itch because of poor anal hygiene
      2. Second-degree hemorrhoids: may prolapse (usually painless) and return to anal canal after a bowel movement
      3. Third-degree hemorrhoids: cause constant discomfort and prolapse because of increased intra-abdominal pressure; must be manually returned to anal canal
   E. Sudden rectal pain caused by thrombosis of external hemorrhoids
   F. Severe or recurrent rectal bleeding, possibly leading to secondary anemia with signs of pallor, fatigue, and weakness
   G. Probable cause: increased intravenous pressure in hemorrhoidal vessels
   H. Predisposing factors
      1. Occupation: extended periods of sitting or standing
      2. Pregnancy
      3. Heredity
      4. Straining caused by constipation, diarrhea, coughing, sneezing, or vomiting
      5. Heart failure
      6. Hepatic disease such as cirrhosis, amebic abscesses, or hepatitis
      7. Alcoholism
      8. Anorectal infections
      9. Loss of muscle tone (aging patterns)
      10. Rectal surgery
      11. Episiotomy
      12. Anal intercourse
II. Data collection
   A. Subjective symptoms
      1. Rectal pain or itching or both
      2. History of prior episodes
      3. Painless intermittent rectal bleeding on defecation
III. Diagnostic tests and methods
   A. Client history
   B. Physical examination
   C. Digital examination
   D. Proctoscopy
IV. Implementation
   A. Assess, report, and record signs and symptoms and any reaction to treatment.
   B. Provide privacy and time for bowel elimination.
   C. Administer topical medications as prescribed to shrink mucous membranes (local anesthetic agents such as lotions, creams, or suppositories), astringents, or cold compresses.
   D. Administer stool softeners to keep stool soft and to avoid straining.

E. Assist with sitz bath to relieve pain.
F. Assist with comfort measures and supportive care.
G. Provide high-fiber diet to keep stools soft.
H. Assist with injection of sclerosing agent to produce scar tissue as ordered.
I. Assist with manual reduction of hemorrhoids as ordered.
J. Provide postoperative care:
   1. Check for signs of prolonged rectal bleeding.
   2. Administer analgesics as prescribed for pain.
   3. Assist with sitz baths as prescribed.
   4. Promote elimination (check stool).
   5. Monitor vital signs.
   6. Resume oral feedings as ordered (administer bulk medications after evening meal).
   7. Instruct client not to use stool softeners soon after hemorrhoidectomy (firm stool helps to dilate blood vessels and prevent anal strictures from forming scar tissue).
   8. Provide meticulous wound care.
K. Before discharge, assist with instruction of client and family about importance of high-fiber foods, regular bowel habits, and good anal hygiene.
L. Instruct client to use medicated astringent pads and white toilet paper (chemicals in colored toilet tissue may irritate skin).
M. Explain disease process, treatment, prevention of constipation, and home care including increased fluid intake and high-fiber diet.
V. Evaluation
   A. Client reports increased comfort and decreased anxiety.
   B. Client has no pain, bleeding, or constipation.
   C. Client maintains adequate hydration and nutritional status.
   D. Client and family demonstrate an understanding of disease process, treatment including medication, and home care including diet and hygiene.

Appendicitis

I. Description
   A. Inflammation of the appendix
   B. Possibly resulting in edema, abscess, necrosis, and rupture causing peritonitis, the most common emergent complication of appendicitis
   C. Occurring at any age and affecting both sexes
   D. Most prevalent in men between puberty and age 30 years
   E. Decreased incidence and death rate because of use of antibiotics
   F. Fatal if untreated
   G. Causes
      1. Obstruction to lumen of appendix because of kinking, fecal mass, barium ingestion, viral infections, or foreign bodies
      2. Decreased resistance to organisms within body (intestinal flora)
II. Data collection
   A. Subjective symptoms
      1. Abdominal pain in lower right abdomen (McBurney's point)

2. Anorexia
3. Nausea
4. Increased tenderness in area

NOTE: Sudden cessation of abdominal pain indicates rupture of appendix.

B. Objective symptoms
1. Vomiting
2. Abdominal rigidity
3. Retractive respirations
4. Severe abdominal spasms
5. Rebound tenderness

NOTE: Rebound tenderness on left side indicates rupture or infarction of appendix.

6. Constipation
7. Slight fever
8. Decreased bowel sounds
9. Tachycardia
10. Elevated WBC count: 12,000–15,000 mm^3

III. Diagnostic tests and methods
   A. Client history
   B. Physical examination
   C. WBC count
   D. Routine urinalysis
   E. Evaluation to rule out illnesses with similar symptoms: gastritis, colitis, diverticulitis, pancreatitis, renal colic, bladder infection, ovarian cyst, and uterine disease

IV. Implementation
   A. Assess, report, and record signs and symptoms and any reaction to treatment.
   B. Maintain bedrest.
   C. Place client in Fowler's position to decrease pain.
   D. Use ice packs to abdomen as prescribed.
   E. Keep client NPO.
   F. Assist with the administration of and monitor IV fluids to prevent dehydration.
   G. Monitor electrolytes.
   H. Administer sedatives and antibiotics as prescribed (remember that narcotics can mask symptoms).
   I. Monitor vital signs.
   J. Do not apply heat to abdomen, as it may cause appendix to rupture.
   K. Do not administer cathartics or enemas, as these may cause rupture.
   L. Prepare client and family for surgical intervention.
   M. Provide postoperative care:
      1. Monitor vital signs.
      2. Monitor I&O.
      3. Administer analgesics and antibiotics as prescribed.
      4. Monitor, report, and record bowel sounds (sign of return of peristalsis, indicating readiness to resume oral fluid intake).
      5. Encourage deep breathing, coughing, and changing position.
      6. Monitor dressing and operative site for drainage and for signs of infection.
      7. Encourage ambulation as soon as possible.
      8. Encourage progressive nutrition.

9. Observe for complications:
   a. Continuing pain may be caused by abscess formation.
   b. Complaint of "something gave away" may be indicative of wound dehiscence.
   c. Symptoms suggestive of peritonitis may occur.

V. Evaluation
   A. Client reports increased comfort.
   B. Client remains free of infection or avoidable complications.
   C. Client demonstrates an understanding of disease process, nature of surgery, and postoperative care.

Peritonitis

I. Description
   A. Acute or chronic inflammation of the peritoneum (membrane lining the abdominal cavity and covering the visceral organs)
   B. Inflammation that may extend throughout peritoneum or be localized
      1. Possibly affecting organs of abdominal cavity (adhesions, abscesses, and obstruction)
   C. Decreasing intestinal motility, resulting in intestinal distention with gas
   D. Approximately 10% mortality, most often caused by bowel obstruction
   E. Mortality rate much higher before advent of antibiotics
   F. Causes
      1. Bacterial invasion of peritoneum, usually from inflammation and perforation of GI tract:
         a. Appendicitis, diverticulitis, peptic ulcer, ulcerative colitis, volvulus, strangulated obstruction, abdominal neoplasm, or stab wound
         b. Common organisms including streptococci, staphylococci, *Escherichia coli,* pneumococci, and gonococci
      2. Chemical inflammation: rupture of ovarian tube or bladder, perforation of gastric ulcer, or release of pancreatic enzymes.
      3. In both bacterial and chemical inflammation, the body's normal immune response results in redness, edema, accumulation of fluids containing protein and electrolytes, adhesions, and abscess.

II. Data collection
   A. Subjective symptoms
      1. Sudden, severe, and diffuse abdominal pain
      2. Nausea
      3. Weakness
      4. Oliguria
      5. Thirst
      6. Shoulder pain: inflammation of diaphragmatic peritoneum
   B. Objective symptoms
      1. Excessive sweating
      2. Vomiting
      3. Cold skin caused by excess loss of fluid, electrolytes, and protein into abdominal cavity

4. Decreased or absent bowel sounds caused by effect of bacterial toxins on intestinal muscles
5. Hypotension
6. Signs of dehydration: dry swollen tongue, pinched skin
7. Abdominal rigidity
8. Rebound tenderness
9. Increased temperature: 103°F (39.4°C) or higher
10. Hiccups (inflammation of diaphragmatic peritoneum)
11. Abdominal distention with upward displacement of diaphragm
12. Decreased respiratory capacity: tendency to breathe shallowly
13. Symptoms of shock
14. Elevated WBC count: >20,000/mm^3

III. Diagnostic tests and methods
  A. Client history
  B. Physical examination
  C. Laboratory studies: WBC count, electrolytes, blood cultures
  D. Abdominal x-rays
  E. Chest x-rays: may show elevated diaphragm
  F. Paracentesis: reveals bacteria, exudate, blood, pus, or urine
  G. Laporatomy: may be required to identify underlying cause

IV. Implementation
  A. Assess, report, and record signs and symptoms and any reaction to treatment.
  B. Maintain bedrest.
  C. Place client in semi-Fowler's position.
  D. Assist with intestinal decompression: explain NG tube insertion.
  E. Assist with administration of and monitor IV infusion and electrolytes.
  F. Administer antibiotics as prescribed.
  G. Keep client NPO.
  H. Monitor fluid I&O.
  I. Monitor amount and characteristic of NG drainage or vomitus.
  J. Provide mouth care.
  K. If surgery is required, assist with explanation of surgical procedure to client and family.
  L. Administer preoperative analgesics as prescribed.
  M. Provide postoperative care:
    1. Administer postoperative analgesics, antibiotics, and sedatives as prescribed; monitor for side effects.
    2. Monitor IV infusion and electrolytes.
    3. Accurately record and report fluid I&O, including NG and incisional drainage.
    4. Provide emotional support and allay anxiety.
    5. Observe client for disorientation; keep siderails up.
    6. Encourage and assist with ambulation as ordered.
    7. Watch for signs of dehiscence and abscess.
    8. Assess bowel sounds frequently for peristaltic motility (abdomen soft, distended) to determine peristaltic status.

9. After return of peristalsis, normal temperature, and pulse rate, increase oral fluids as prescribed.
N. Explain disease process, treatment, postoperative care, and home care to client and family.

V. Evaluation
  A. Client reports increased comfort and decreased anxiety.
  B. Client remains free of infection.
  C. Client remains free of complications from surgery.
  D. Client and family demonstrate an understanding of disease process, treatment, and home care.

Colorectal Cancer and Polyps

I. Description
  A. Cancer of the colon and rectum that may be in the form of a well-defined tumor or cancerous polyp
  B. Incidence equally distributed between men and women   .
  C. Tending to progress slowly and remaining localized for a long time
  D. Potentially curable in 80–90% of clients if diagnosed early
  E. Early treatment allowing for resection before nodes become involved
  F. Causes
    1. Unknown
  G. Potential predisposing factors
    1. Relationship to diet high in animal fats and low in fiber
    2. Other diseases of GI tract
    3. Age >40 years
    4. History of ulcerative colitis
    5. History of familial polyps

II. Data collection
  A. Subjective symptoms
    1. Initially vague
    2. Abdominal aching
    3. Abdominal pressure or cramps
    4. Weakness
    5. Fatigue
    6. Dizziness
    7. Loss of appetite
    8. Nausea
    9. Change in bowel habits and shape of stool
    10. Signs of obstruction in left colon
      a. Intermittent abdominal fullness or cramping
      b. Rectal pressure
      c. Dull and constant ache in rectal or sacral region
      d. Relief of pain after passage of gas or stool
  B. Objective symptoms
    1. Black tarry stools
    2. Presence of anemia
    3. Exertional dyspnea
    4. Diarrhea, obstipation
    5. Vomiting
    6. Signs of intestinal obstruction
    7. Possible palpable tumor on right side
    8. Rectal bleeding
    9. Ribbon- or pencil-shaped stool

10. Dark-red blood and mucus in feces
11. Cachexia

III. Diagnostic tests and methods
  A. Client history
  B. Physical examination
  C. Digital examination for presence of abnormalities
  D. Hemoccult test (guaiac) to detect blood in stools
  E. Proctoscopy or sigmoidoscopy
  F. Colonoscopy to permit visual inspection and access for biopsy of tissue
  G. IVP to evaluate kidney function
  H. Barium x-ray to detect lesions
  I. Tumor biopsy to verify disease

IV. Implementation
  A. Assess, report, and record signs and symptoms and any reaction to treatment.
  B. Monitor vital signs at least every 4 hours.
  C. Monitor I&O.
  D. Provide emotional support.
  E. Administer medications as prescribed, and monitor for side effects.
  F. Prepare client and family for surgical intervention.
  G. Provide postoperative care:
    1. Explain to family the importance of positive reaction to client's adjustment.
    2. Monitor IV therapy and electrolytes.
    3. Monitor I&O.
    4. Monitor dressings and wound drainage.
    5. Administer medications to relieve pain as prescribed.
    6. Provide emotional support.
    7. Monitor perineal area if drain or packing was inserted.
    8. Assist with sitz baths, if ordered.
    9. Arrange for visit by enterostomal therapist if client has had a colostomy:
      a. Encourage client to examine stoma and to participate in its care as soon as possible.
      b. Teach good hygiene and skin care.
      c. Encourage client to shower or bathe as soon as incision heals.
      d. Arrange for visit by dietitian regarding diet.
      e. Instruct client regarding physical activities.
      f. Request that a visit be made by home health nurse to check on client's physical condition and ability to care for self.
      g. Encourage sexual counseling, if needed.
    10. Encourage yearly screening and follow-up testing.
    11. Explain disease process, treatment including medications, and home care to client and family.

V. Evaluation
  A. Client reports increased comfort and decreased anxiety.
  B. Client demonstrates ability to irrigate and care for stoma, if present.
  C. Client verbalizes concerns.
  D. Client and family demonstrate an understanding of disease process, treatment, home care including diet, and follow-up care.

Cholelithiasis, Choledocholithiasis, Cholangitis, and Cholecystitis

I. Description
  A. Cholelithiasis
    1. Presence of stones or calculi (gallstones) in the gallbladder
    2. Prognosis usually good with treatment unless infection occurs
    3. With infection, prognosis according to severity and response to antibiotics
    4. Causes
      a. Inflammation of biliary tract resulting in increased absorption of bile salts, which in turn decrease the solubility of cholesterol
      b. Metabolic alterations resulting from periods of sluggishness in gallbladder as a result of pregnancy, diabetes mellitus, oral contraception, celiac disease, cirrhosis of the liver, or pancreatitis
  B. Choledocholithiasis
    1. Gallstones in hepatic and bile duct
    2. Obstruction of bile flow into duodenum
    3. Condition leading to elevated bilirubin level, jaundice, and interference with fat and fat-soluble vitamin absorption
    4. Prognosis usually good unless infection occurs
  C. Cholangitis
    1. Infection of the bile duct
    2. Frequent association with choledocholithiasis
    3. Possible occurrence after percutaneous cholangiography
    4. Inflammatory process possibly causing fibrosis and stenosis of common bile duct
    5. Poor prognosis
    6. Predisposing factors
      a. Bacterial alteration of bile salts
      b. Metabolic alterations of bile salts
  D. Cholecystitis
    1. Acute or chronic inflammation of gallbladder
    2. Usual association with impacted gallstone in the cystic duct
    3. Painful distention of gallbladder
    4. Acute form common in middle-aged, overweight adults
    5. Chronic form common among older persons
    6. Prognosis good with treatment

II. Data collection
  A. Subjective symptoms
    1. Acute abdominal pain in right upper quadrant after high-fat meals
    2. Pain radiating to back, between shoulders, or front of chest
    3. Fat intolerance
    4. Indigestion
    5. Flatulence
    6. Nausea
    7. Chills
    8. Weakness
    9. Fatigue
    10. Pruritus

B. Objective symptoms
   1. Belching
   2. Profuse sweating
   3. Vomiting
   4. Jaundice
   5. Abdominal distention
   6. Absence of bowel sounds in severe cholangitis
   7. Elevated WBC count
   8. Elevated bilirubin level
   9. Clay-colored stool
   10. Dark urine
   11. Increase in temperature, heart rate, respiration, and BP
   12. Calculi observed on cholecystogram
   13. Prolonged PT resulting from interference with vitamin K absorption
   14. Easy bruising
III. Diagnostic tests and methods
   A. Client history
   B. Physical examination
   C. Laboratory studies: WBC count, total bilirubin, urine bilirubin, icteric index, alkaline phosphatase, PT
      1. Serum amylase levels to differentiate between gallbladder disease and pancreatitis
      2. Serial enzyme tests and ECG to rule out heart disease
   D. Oral cholecystography
   E. IV cholangiography
IV. Implementation
   A. Assess, report, and record signs and symptoms and any reaction to treatment.
   B. Administer analgesics for pain as prescribed.
   C. Administer antibiotics and antispasmodics as prescribed.
   D. Monitor for medication side effects.
   E. Keep client NPO.
   F. Provide mouth care.
   G. Assist with administration of and monitor IV therapy.
   H. Monitor I&O.
   I. Monitor laboratory studies.
   J. Monitor vital signs and any incidence of bleeding (e.g., urine, gums).
   K. Explain and assist with diagnostic procedures.
   L. Provide postoperative care:
      1. Monitor dressing.
      2. Monitor T-tube drainage (if T-tube present).
      3. Monitor NG tube for drainage.
      4. Assist with administration of and monitor IV therapy.
      5. Administer medications as prescribed.
      6. Assist in ambulation if ordered.
      7. Provide prescribed diet if ordered.
      8. Encourage deep breathing, coughing, and turning.
   M. Explain disease process, treatment including medication, prevention, and home care including dietary restrictions:
      1. Diet: low-fat, maintain calories
      2. Activity
      3. Caring for T-tube, if present

   4. Observing for signs of infection
   5. Follow-up care
V. Evaluation
   A. Client reports increased comfort and decreased anxiety.
   B. Client remains free of infection or complications.
   C. Client maintains adequate nutritional intake.
   D. Client resumes activity gradually.
   E. Client and family demonstrate an understanding of disease process, treatment including surgical intervention, prevention, and home care.

Hepatitis A, B, C, D, and E

I. Description
   A. Viral inflammation of the liver caused by hepatotoxins, viral agents, or drugs.
   B. Marked liver destruction, necrosis, and autolysis
   C. More than 70,000 cases reported annually
   D. Complications
      1. Chronic persistent hepatitis (may be benign)
      2. Chronic aggressive hepatitis
         a. Fatal in approximately 25% of cases (from hepatic failure)
      3. Fulminating hepatitis
         a. Life-threatening complication
         b. Development in about 1% of clients, causing hepatic failure with encephalopathy
         c. Progression to coma and death in approximately 2 weeks
   E. Preventive measures
      1. Enteric isolation
      2. Good handwashing technique
      3. Vaccination and immune globulin therapy
      4. Avoiding contact with blood or body fluids
   F. Five forms
      1. Hepatitis A
         a. Highly infectious (short-incubation hepatitis)
         b. Cause: hepatitis A virus (HAV)
         c. Usually transmitted by contact with feces or contaminated water or food
         d. Occasionally transmitted parenterally
         e. Outbreaks often following ingestion of contaminated seafood
         f. Incubation period 15–50 days
         g. Tending to be benign and self-limiting
         h. High-risk individuals: children, travelers to developing countries, health-care personnel
      2. Hepatitis B
         a. Serum (long-incubation hepatitis)
         b. Cause: hepatitis B virus (HBV)
         c. Rare occurrence in epidemics
         d. Higher mortality than hepatitis A
         e. Generally parenteral transmission: blood transfusion, direct contact
         f. Possible spread through contact with human secretions and feces
         g. Incidence rising among homosexuals: oral and sexual contact
         h. Incubation period 5–10 weeks
         i. High-risk individuals: parenteral drug users,

health-care workers in contact with contaminated blood or body fluids
3. Non-A, non-B hepatitis (hepatitis C)
   a. Mildest course of all types of hepatitis
   b. Cause: virus other than HAV or HBV
   c. Transmission by blood contact: usually from commercial blood donations
   d. Incubation period 14–150 days
   e. No specific diagnostic tests
   f. High-risk individuals: those receiving blood transfusions or those who come in contact with contaminated blood
4. Hepatitis D
   a. Cause: incomplete virus
   b. Complication of hepatitis B
5. Hepatitis E
   a. Cause: RNA virus
   b. Incubation period 2–9 weeks

II. Data collection
   A. Subjective symptoms: preicteric phase (lasts 1 week)
      1. Chills
      2. Anorexia
      3. Nausea
      4. Malaise, weakness
      5. Fatigue
      6. Headache
      7. Photophobia
      8. Pharyngitis
      9. Cough
      10. Respiratory difficulty, especially in hepatitis A
      11. Arthralgia, especially in hepatitis B
      12. Alterations in sense of taste and smell
      13. Loss of desire to smoke or to drink alcohol
   B. Subjective symptoms: icteric phase (lasts 2–6 weeks)
      1. Mild weight loss
      2. Continued anorexia
      3. Discomfort and pain in right upper abdominal quadrant
      4. Increased nausea
      5. Increased malaise and weakness
      6. Increased respiratory difficulty
      7. Pruritus
      8. Irritability
   C. Subjective symptoms: posticteric phase (lasts 2–6 weeks, with full recovery in 6 months)
      1. Decline in nausea, anorexia, and dyspnea
      2. Increased comfort
      3. Decreased weakness
   D. Objective symptoms: preicteric phase
      1. Dyspnea
      2. Vomiting
      3. Cough, coryza
      4. Elevated temperature
      5. Liver and lymph node enlargement
   E. Objective symptoms: icteric phase
      1. Dark urine
      2. Clay-colored stools
      3. Yellow sclera
      4. Liver that remains tender and enlarged
      5. Pain in right upper quadrant
      6. Splenomegaly
      7. Cervical adenopathy

8. Bile obstruction
9. Onset of jaundice
10. Elevated serum bilirubin levels
11. Elevated bilirubin and urobilinogen in urine
12. Prolonged PT and partial thromboplastin time (PTT)
13. Elevated aspartate aminotransferase (AST) (SGOT), alanine aminotransferase (ALT) (SGPT), alkaline phosphate levels
14. Decreased serum albumin level
   F. Objective symptoms: posticteric phase
      1. Decreased jaundice
      2. Decreased dyspnea and anorexia
      3. Resolution of abnormal laboratory test results
   G. Posticteric phase
      1. Lasts 2–6 weeks
      2. Relapse may occur
      3. Remains fatigued, liver decreases

III. Diagnostic tests and methods
   A. Client history
   B. Physical examination
   C. Presence of hepatitis B surface antigens (HBsAg) and hepatitis B antibodies (anti-HBs) to confirm hepatitis B
   D. Presence of anti-HAV antibody to confirm hepatitis A
   E. Absence of anti-HAV, HBsAg, and anti-HBs to confirm non-A, non-B hepatitis
   F. PT
   G. SGOT and SGPT levels, serum alkaline phosphatase level
   H. Serum albumin, globulin, and bilirubin levels
   I. Urine bilirubin level
   J. Liver biopsy
   K. CAT scan of liver

IV. Implementation
   A. Assess, report, and record signs and symptoms and any reaction to treatment.
   B. Provide restful environment.
   C. Assist with comfort measures.
   D. Provide emotional support.
   E. Monitor I&O.
   F. Monitor body weight.
   G. Provide and encourage adequate caloric intake (orally or IV).
   H. Limit visitors and impose Universal Precautions.
   I. Encourage fluid intake.
   J. Observe feces for color, consistency, frequency, and amount.
   K. Watch for signs of dehydration, pneumonia, vascular problems, decubitus ulcers, and hepatic coma.
   L. Administer prescribed medications such as antiemetics, antibiotics, vitamin K, antihistamines, corticosteroids, and fluid and electrolyte replacement.
   M. For clients with fulminant hepatitis:
      1. Maintain electrolyte balance.
      2. Maintain patent airway.
      3. Control bleeding.
      4. Administer prescribed medications to correct hypoglycemia.
   N. Schedule rest periods.
   O. Monitor laboratory results.

P. Monitor for signs of bleeding.
Q. Check skin integrity.
R. Explain disease process, diagnostic procedures, treatments, prevention, Universal Precautions, home care, and follow-up care to client and family.

V. Evaluation
A. Client reports increased comfort and decreased anxiety.
C. Client remains free of infection.
D. Client maintains adequate nutritional and fluid intake.
E. Client demonstrates an understanding of disease process, diagnostic procedures, treatment, prevention, enteric isolation procedure, and home care.

Cirrhosis of the Liver

I. Description
A. Chronic hepatic disease with diffuse destruction and fibrotic regeneration of liver cells
B. Liver structure and vasculature altered, resulting in impaired blood and lymph flow, leading to hepatic insufficiency
C. Prevalent among malnourished chronic alcoholics >50 years of age
D. Fifty percent more common in men than in women
E. High mortality rate
F. Six types of cirrhosis
1. Portal, nutritional, or alcoholic cirrhosis (Laënnec's type)
a. Most common: occurs in 30–50% of clients; 90% of clients have history of alcoholism
b. Liver damage primarily from malnutrition, especially lack of protein
2. Biliary cirrhosis
a. Affects 15–20% of clients
b. Results from bile duct diseases that disrupt bile flow
3. Postnecrotic (posthepatic) cirrhosis
a. Affects 10–30% of clients
b. Results from various types of hepatitis
4. Idiopathic cirrhosis
a. Affects about 10% of clients
b. Has no known cause

II. Data collection
A. Subjective symptoms
1. GI system: anorexia, indigestion, nausea, constipation, flatus, dull abdominal ache
2. Respiratory difficulties
3. CNS: lethargy, mental changes
4. Hematological: easy bruising
5. Endocrine: menstrual irregularities
6. Skin: itching
7. Miscellaneous: fatigue, pain in upper right abdomen
B. Objective symptoms
1. GI system: vomiting, constipation, and diarrhea or constipation
2. Respiratory system: decreased thoracic expansion as a result of abdominal ascites
3. Decreased gas exchange: hypoxia

4. CNS: slurred speech, asterixis, peripheral neuritis, hallucinations, unconsciousness, and coma
5. Hematological: nosebleeds, bruising, bleeding gums, anemia, increased bleeding time
6. Endocrine: testicular atrophy, menstrual irregularities, loss of hair on chest and axillary region
7. Skin: pruritus, poor tissue turgor, extreme dryness, spider angiomas, palmar erythema, jaundice
8. Hepatic: jaundice, ascites, edema of legs, enlarged liver, hepatorenal syndrome, hypoglycemia
9. Miscellaneous: enlarged superficial abdominal veins, muscle atrophy, palpable liver or spleen, elevated temperature, bleeding from esophageal varices resulting from portal hypertension, hypernatremia, hypoalbuminemia
10. Elevated SGOT, SGPT, LDH, bilirubin, ammonia levels

III. Diagnostic tests and methods
A. Client history
B. Physical examination
C. Laboratory studies: WBC count, Hgb, Hct, albumin, bilirubin, alkaline phosphatase, serum ammonia, serum electrolytes, globulin, thymol turbidity, SGOT SGPT, LDH, PT, and PTT
D. Bromsulphthalein (BSP) excretion test
E. Glucose tolerance test
F. Urine bilirubin level
G. Fecal urobilinogen level
H. Liver biopsy
I. Cholecystography
J. Cholangiography

IV. Implementation
A. Assess, report, and record signs and symptoms and any reaction to treatment.
B. Monitor skin, gums, stools, and emesis for bleeding tendencies.
C. Apply pressure to injection sites to prevent bleeding.
D. Advise client not to take aspirin, blow nose, strain during bowel movement, or sneeze.
E. Monitor weight daily.
F. Measure abdominal girth daily.
G. Monitor sacrum, legs, and ankles for presence of dependent edema.
H. Monitor vital signs.
I. Monitor electrolytes and other laboratory results.
J. Monitor I&O accurately.
K. Assist with comfort measures.
L. Provide emotional support.
M. Provide counseling on alcoholic consumption.
N. Provide mouth care.
O. Place in high-Fowler's position to assist in breathing when ascites is present.
P. Prepare client for paracentesis, if necessary.
Q. Administer prescribed medication such as diuretics; vitamins A, C, and K; folic acid; electrolyte supplements; IV fluids; antiemetics; antihistamines; and albumin.
R. Use lubricating lotion in place of soap when giving skin care to prevent skin breakdown in clients who have edema and pruritus.

S. Monitor skin integrity; avoid intramuscular injections.
T. Provide diet high in protein, high in carbohydrates, and containing vitamins. (High-protein diet is contraindicated in presence of portal system encephalopathy (PSE) because liver is not able to metabolize amino acids or ammonia; proteins are broken down to amino acids.)
U. Explain disease process, diagnostic procedures, treatment including medications, prevention, home care, and follow-up care to client and family.

V. Evaluation
   A. Client reports increased comfort and decreased anxiety.
   B. Client maintains adequate fluid and electrolyte balance.
   C. Client maintains effective breathing pattern.
   D. Ascites and edema are reduced.
   E. Client remains free of injury or infection.
   F. Client maintains good skin integrity.
   G. Client maintains adequate nutritional intake.
   H. Client and family demonstrate an understanding of disease process, diagnostic procedures, treatment, prevention, home care, and follow-up care.

Pancreatitis

I. Description
   A. Inflammation of the pancreas
   B. Acute and chronic forms
      1. Acute form: sudden occurrence, with one attack or recurrent attacks; followed by resolution
      2. Chronic form: continuous inflammation and destruction of pancreas, with proliferations of scar tissue in place of normal pancreatic tissue
   C. Common association with edema, necrosis, or hemorrhage
   D. Common association with alcoholism, trauma, or peptic ulcer in men
   E. Common association with biliary tract disease in women
   F. Prognosis poor when cause is alcoholism
   G. Prognosis good when cause is biliary tract disease
   H. Mortality up to 60% when condition associated with necrosis and hemorrhage
   I. Causes
      1. Most common causes are biliary tract disease and alcoholism.
      2. Other causes include pancreatic carcinoma, trauma, certain drugs, complication of peptic ulcer, mumps, or hypothermia.
   J. Increased permeability of the vascular bed, leading to further edema
   K. Damaged islets of Langerhans, possibly leading to complications including diabetes mellitus.
   L. Fulminant pancreatitis, causing massive hemorrhage and destruction of pancreatic tissue, ending in diabetic acidosis, shock, coma, and/or death

II. Data collection
   A. Subjective symptoms
      1. Abdominal discomfort or pain centered close to umbilicus and unrelieved by vomiting
      2. Severe attack: severe abdominal pain
      3. Relief of pain by drawing knees up
      4. Malaise
      5. Restlessness
      6. Nausea
      7. History of alcohol intake, previous trauma, surgery, gallbladder disease
      8. Chills
      9. Weight loss
   B. Objective symptoms
      1. Severe attack: persistent vomiting, abdominal rigidity, diminished bowel sounds, rales at bases of lungs, left pleural effusion
      2. Dehydration
      3. Elevated temperature
      4. Tachycardia
      5. Cold, sweaty extremities
      6. Elevated enzyme levels
      7. Elevated WBC count, bilirubin, blood glucose, serum amylase, serum lipase, Hct
      8. Decreased serum calcium level
      9. ECG changes: prolonged QT segment, normal T wave
      10. Abdominal x-ray: dilation of small or large intestine
      11. GI series: pressure on duodenum or stomach because of edema of pancreas head
      12. Paracentesis: exceedingly high amylase levels
      13. Positive stool test results for meat fibers, fat in chronic pancreatitis
      14. Chronic form showing calcification on CAT scan or ultrasound

III. Diagnostic tests and methods
   A. Client history
   B. Physical examination
   C. Laboratory tests: serum amylase, serum lipase, serum calcium, WBC count, serum glucose, Hct
   D. Routine ECG
   E. Abdominal x-rays
   F. GI series
   G. Chest x-rays
   H. Paracentesis

IV. Implementation
   A. Position client to relieve pain.
   B. Keep client NPO to allow pancreas to rest.
   C. Explain and assist in insertion of NG tube to allow pancreas to rest.
   D. Monitor I&O.
   E. Monitor vital signs continuously.
   F. Provide meticulous supportive care.
   G. Monitor pulmonary artery pressure closely, if present.
   H. Monitor CVP line closely, if present.
   I. Monitor fluid I&O.
   J. Monitor electrolyte, BUN, and creatinine levels.
   K. Assist in administration of IV fluids or blood as ordered.
   L. Assist in administration of plasma to maintain BP, if ordered.
   M. Assess for rales and decreased breath sounds.
   N. Maintain constant NG suctioning to decompress bowel, if required.

O. Provide good oral and nose hygiene.

P. Provide emotional support.

Q. Start client on clear liquids, progressing to bland low-fat diet in small feedings daily once oral intake is ordered.

R. Monitor for signs and symptoms of complications such as hyperglycemia or hypoglycemia and respiratory difficulties.

S. Explain condition, diagnostic procedures, treatment including medication, health maintenance procedures such as avoidance of alcohol and adequate nutrition, home care, and follow-up care to client and family.

V. Evaluation

A. Client reports increased comfort and decreased anxiety.

B. Client maintains adequate nutritional intake.

C. Client maintains fluid and electrolyte balance.

D. Client and family demonstrate an understanding of disease process, treatment including medications, health maintenance procedures, home care, and follow-up care.

Integumentary System (Skin)

Basic Information

The skin acts as the body's barrier and protector against the environment. The functions of the skin include temperature regulation, sensation, and excretion of small amounts of water and sodium chloride. It protects the body tissues and organs from external insults such as injury. Proper nutrition, hydration, exercise, rest, and electrolyte balance are required to maintain a healthy integumentary system.

I. Basic data collection

A. Subjective symptoms

1. History: onset of problem, changes, presence of pain, burning, itching sensations
2. Allergic reactions
3. Changes in lifestyle: diet, medications, environment, detergents, and so on
4. Change in body image
5. Changes in activities because of disease or condition

B. Objective symptoms

1. Skin
   a. Color: deviations from normal such as pallor, jaundice, cyanosis
   b. Temperature: differences in feeling of warmth, coolness
   c. Turgor: elasticity (hydration)
   d. Pressure sores: location, size, odor, color, edema, open wound
   e. Cleanliness of skin
2. Hair
   a. Texture: coarse, fine
   b. Lice
   c. Absence of body hair
3. Scalp
   a. Scars
   b. Parasites

4. Nails
   a. Shape
   b. Cleanliness
   c. Brittleness

Major Integumentary Diagnoses

Burns

I. Description

A. Injury to the skin from dry or moist heat, chemicals, electrical currents, or radiation that destroys the skin's normal protective function

B. Physiological changes
1. Depend on the severity of the burn
   a. Loss of protective barrier against infection
   b. Decreased sensory perception
   c. Loss of body fluids and electrolytes
   d. Loss of body temperature regulation
   e. Damage to sweat and sebaceous glands

C. Two stages of physiological changes
1. Hypovolemic stage
   a. Intravascular fluid shifting into interstitial space around burn, resulting in increased permeability of capillaries and cells; resultant vasodilation
   b. Leakage of protein and sodium into area, with edema and blister formation
   c. Occurring at onset of injury
   d. Lasting 48–72 hours
   e. Possibly leading to dehydration of healthy tissue, oliguria, hypoproteinemia, hypovolemic shock, hyperkalemia, hyponatremia, respiratory distress, and metabolic acidosis, depending on burn severity
2. Diuretic stage
   a. Beginning approximately 48–72 hours after initial injury
   b. Intravascular volume and capillary integrity restored
   c. Resulting in increased blood volume, increased renal function, and diuresis
   d. Possibly causing hypokalemia, fluid overload, sodium deficit, metabolic acidosis, anemia, and malnutrition

D. Classification of burns
1. First-degree
   a. Superficial partial-thickness burn limited to epidermis
   b. Presence of erythema (redness), edema, and pain
2. Second-degree
   a. Deep partial-thickness burn involving epidermis and part of dermis
   b. Presence of blisters and mottled, white, or red skin
   c. Mild or moderate edema and pain
   d. Heals with undamaged epithelial cells
3. Third-degree
   a. Full-thickness burn involving both epidermis and dermis
   b. Presence of white, leathery tissue (eschar) and thrombosed blood vessels

    c. Possibly extending through subcutaneous tissue to muscle and bone (fourth-degree)

    d. Presence of charred, white, dark, black, or red skin

    e. Absence of pain because of total nerve damage

    f. Requiring skin grafting to repair injury because of extent of damage

E. Use of "Rule of Nines" chart, taking into account client's age

    1. Measured by percent of body surface area (BSA) covered by burn

    2. Allows estimate of size of burn

    3. Correlation of size and depth of burn allows estimation of severity

F. Classification of severity of burn

    1. Minor

      a. Third-degree burn on <2% of BSA

      b. Second-degree burn on <15% of adult BSA (10% in children)

    2. Moderate

      a. Third-degree burn on 2–10% of BSA

      b. Second-degree burn on 15–25% of adult BSA (>10% in children)

    3. Major

      a. Third-degree burn on >10% of BSA

      b. Second-degree burn on >25% of adult BSA (>20% in children)

      c. Burns of eyes, ears, face, hands, feet, or genitalia

      d. Electrical burns

      e. Burns in presence of fractures or with respiratory damage

      f. All burns in poor-risk clients

        1) Children <4 years old; adults >60 years old

        2) Clients with history of complicating medical problems (e.g., disorders that impair peripheral circulation, such as diabetes and coronary artery disease)

II. Data collection

A. Subjective symptoms

    1. Pain (depending on degree of burn)

    2. Anxiety

    3. Confusion

B. Objective symptoms

    1. Skin appearance: indicative of type of burn

    2. Disfigurement

    3. Infection

    4. Loss of body tissue (protein)

    5. Hypoproteinemia (protein shifts into tissue space around injury)

    6. Electrolyte imbalance

    7. Decreased serum sodium levels

    8. Dehydration

    9. Edema

    10. Oliguria

    11. Hypovolemic shock caused by fluid loss or shift

    12. Hematuria caused by hemolysis of RBCs and decreased blood flow

    13. Signs of neurogenic shock

    14. Respiratory distress caused by hypovolemic shock, inhalation injury, or airway obstruction

III. Diagnostic tests and methods

A. Client history

B. Physical examination

IV. Implementation

A. Anticipate and prevent respiratory distress:

    1. Maintain airway (may be intubated if head or neck or both are involved, or for inhalation injury).

    2. Monitor breathing every hour; then every 4 hours when stable.

    3. Keep tracheostomy equipment available.

B. Keep client NPO for first 24 hours as ordered.

C. Monitor vital signs and CNS status frequently.

D. Insert catheter and urinary drainage as ordered.

E. Assist in insertion of CVP lines and other IV lines.

F. Assist in administration of rapid fluid replacement as prescribed.

G. Monitor I&O hourly.

H. Monitor for presence of hematuria.

I. Monitor serum and urine electrolytes and Hct.

J. Monitor weight daily.

NOTE: Weight gain of 15–20% is expected in first 72 hours.

K. Administer analgesics for pain as prescribed.

L. Avoid heavy sedation to prevent respiratory complications.

M. Administer prophylactic tetanus as prescribed.

N. Monitor burn site for appearance, fluid loss, infection, and damage extent.

O. Monitor pulses in all extremities if possible.

P. Monitor oxygen.

Q. Dress burned area and change dressings:

    1. Administer analgesic for pain before dressing changes.

    2. Clean and debride burn area with antiseptic agents and prescribed dressing.

    3. Apply appropriate wet dressings as prescribed.

R. Anticipate infection: maintain asepsis; reverse isolation; administer antibiotics; monitor vital signs frequently.

S. Anticipate shock: assess level of consciousness and mental state; monitor vital signs.

T. Prevent complications of immobilization: provide proper alignment to prevent deformities; prevent skin surfaces from touching by use of turning frames, cradles.

U. Assess for GI distress or bleeding.

V. Administer topical agents such as mefenide acetate (Sulfamylon cream), silver sulfadiazine (Silvadene cream), or silver nitrate to prevent infection and assist in the healing process as ordered.

W. Monitor for presence of paralytic ileus and impaction.

X. Assist with preparation of client for skin grafts if required.

Y. Provide adequate nutritional intake (after acute phase) (diet high in protein, vitamins, carbohydrates, fat, and calories).

Z. Provide frequent mouth and skin care.

AA. Encourage coughing and deep-breathing exercises.

BB. Assist in use of coping measures.

CC. Allow client to discuss feelings regarding condition.
DD. Explain home care and follow-up care:
    1. Caring for burn
    2. Skin care
    3. Medications
    4. Protective measures against irritants and infection
    5. Signs of complications
    6. Need for follow-up care
EE. Provide for counseling.
V. Evaluation
  A. Client remains free of infection or injury.
  B. Client reports increased comfort and decreased anxiety.
  C. Client maintains effective airway and breathing patterns.
  D. Client maintains fluid and electrolyte balance.
  E. Client maintains adequate cardiac output.
  F. Client maintains adequate I&O.
  G. Client maintains adequate nutritional intake.
  H. Client resumes social interaction.
  I. Client adapts to change in family process.
  J. Client demonstrates an understanding of condition, treatment including medication, home care, and follow-up care.

Neoplasms of the Skin

I. Description
  A. Malignant lesions of the skin
  B. May or may not metastasize to other tissues
  C. May cause destruction of cells
  D. May result in infection
  E. Types of neoplasms
    1. Basal cell epithelioma
      a. Slow-growing destructive skin tumor
      b. Usually occurs in individuals >40 years old
      c. Is more prevalent in blond, fair-skinned men
      d. Appears as an opaque light pink or tan nodule
      e. Seen mostly on hairy skin areas
      f. Usually does not metastasize but may become invasive
      g. Causes
        1) Prolonged sun exposure
        2) Radiation
        3) Burns
        4) Vaccinations
    2. Squamous cell carcinoma
      a. Invasive tumor of the epidermal surface with metastatic potential
      b. Usually located on arms or face
      c. May develop from pre-existing skin lesions such as keratosis or leukoplakia
      d. Occurs most often in white men >60 years old
      e. Risk increased in occupations necessitating outdoor employment in sunny, warm climate
    3. Malignant melanoma
      a. Most serious type of skin neoplasms
      b. Relatively rare: accounts for only 1–2% of all malignancies

      c. Slightly more common in women than in men; rare in children
      d. Peak incidence occurs between ages 50 and 70 years
      e. Occurrence mostly on skin areas exposed to sunlight
      f. Color of lesion varies (blue, black, or yellow) with irregular shapes and pigmentation
      g. Spreads through the lymphatic and vascular systems
      h. Metastasizes to regional lymph nodes, liver, lungs, and CNS (course unpredictable)
      i. Prognosis according to tumor thickness
      j. Superficial lesions generally curable; deeper lesions tending to metastasize
      k. Prognosis better for involvement on an extremity (drained by one lymphatic network) than for involvement of head, neck, or trunk (drained by several lymphatic networks)
II. Data collection
  A. Subjective symptoms
    1. History of prior skin tumors or lesions
    2. Soreness around site
    3. Itching
  B. Objective symptoms
    1. Presence of skin lesions
    2. Change in appearance, size, or shape of existing mole or nodule
    3. Drainage or bleeding from lesion
    4. Positive biopsy of lesion
III. Diagnostic tests and methods
  A. Client history
  B. Physical examination
  C. Skin biopsy with histological examination
  D. Baseline laboratory studies: CBC with differential, ESR, platelet count, urinalysis, liver function studies
  E. Chest x-rays
  F. CAT scan of body
IV. Implementation
  A. Assess, report, and record signs and symptoms and any reaction to treatment.
  B. Monitor skin lesions for appearance, size, shape, color, and drainage.
  C. Administer prescribed topical agents such as chemotherapeutic drugs and antibiotics.
  D. Provide skin care to lesion:
    1. Avoid use of metal-containing powders or creams.
    2. Use aseptic technique in cleaning area.
    3. Monitor for local reaction to topical medications.
  E. Explain condition, treatment such as irradiation, chemotherapy, and other medication, prevention, home care, and follow-up care.
V. Evaluation
  A. Client reports increased comfort and decreased anxiety.
  B. Client maintains good skin integrity.
  C. Client demonstrates an understanding of condition, diagnostic procedures, and treatment, prevention, home care, and follow-up care.

Renal and Urological Systems

Basic Information

The renal system maintains homeostasis through the production and elimination of urine. The kidneys regulate the volume, acid-base balance, and electrolyte balance of body fluids. This system is responsible also for detoxification of the blood, elimination of wastes, aiding in erythropoiesis, and regulating BP. Body wastes are eliminated by the kidneys via urine formation, tubular reabsorption, and tubular excretion. Disorders of these systems affect the body's normal function.

  I. Basic data collection
   A. Subjective symptoms
       1. Problems with elimination
       2. Changes in voiding habits
       3. Discharge from the urethra
       4. Pain in the suprapubic area
       5. Burning sensation on voiding
   B. Objective symptoms
       1. Bladder distention (rigid, tender abdomen)
       2. Urine color, odor, cloudiness, presence of mucus, sediment, blood
       3. Genital irritation
       4. Amount of urinary output
       5. Electrolyte studies
       6. Edema of extremities, scrotum
       7. Vital signs
       8. History of:
           a. Previously normal urinary habits
           b. Health problems with urinary system and other body systems
           c. Presence and location of edema
           d. Medications
           e. Food or medication allergies
           f. Spasms or pain (or both) in bladder region
           g. Presence of discharge

Major Renal and Urological Diagnoses

Renal Calculi (Kidney Stones)

  I. Description
   A. Most commonly develop in renal pelvis or calyces of the kidney but possible anywhere in the urinary tract
   B. Result from precipitation of substances such as calcium oxalate, calcium phosphate, urate, or cystine, which are normally dissolved in the urine
   C. Vary in size and may be solitary or multiple
   D. May stay in renal pelvis or descend into ureter
   E. Result in possible damage to renal and urinary tract tissue
   F. Possibly produce large calculi, causing pressure necrosis
   G. May cause obstruction along urinary tract, resulting in hydronephrosis
   H. Tend to recur
   I. Are more common in white men 30–50 years old; rare in blacks
   J. Are more prevalent in southeastern United States (the "stone belt"), possibly because of:

       1. Regional dietary habits
       2. Dehydration as a result of hot climate
   K. Unknown cause
   L. Predisposing factors
       1. Dehydration: decrease in urine production, allowing concentration of calculus-forming substances
       2. Prolonged immobilization: causing urinary stasis with accumulation of calculus-forming substances
       3. Infection: pH changes resulting in a medium favorable for calculus formation
       4. Obstruction: allowing calculus-forming substances to collect; promoting infection and further obstruction
       5. Metabolic factors: excessive intake of calcium or vitamin D; hyperparathyroidism; renal tubular acidosis; elevated uric acid; defective metabolism of oxalate
 II. Data collection
   A. Subjective symptoms
       1. Severe pain in flank area, suprapubic area, pelvis, or external genitalia (renal colic)
       2. Urgency, frequency of urination
       3. Nausea
       4. Chills
   B. Objective symptoms
       1. Increased temperature
       2. Pallor
       3. Hematuria
       4. Abdominal distention
       5. Pyuria
       6. Anuria (from bilateral obstruction)
       7. Evidence of urinary tract infection (UTI) via diagnostic procedures
       8. Evidence of presence of calculi via diagnostic procedures
III. Diagnostic tests and methods
   A. Urinalysis
   B. Urine culture
   C. 24-hour urine examination
   D. Kidney-ureter-bladder (KUB) x-ray
   E. Calculi analysis
   F. IVP
   G. Kidney ultrasonography
   H. Cystoscopy
   I. Serial blood calcium and phosphorus levels to detect hyperparathyroidism and increased calcium level compared with normal serum protein
 IV. Implementation
   A. Assess, report, and record signs and symptoms and any reaction to treatment.
   B. Maintain a 24- to 48-hour record of urine pH (test with nitrazine pH paper) as ordered.
   C. Strain all urine through gauze.
   D. Save all solid material in urine for analysis.
   E. Provide and encourage intake of fluids for a urinary output of 3–4 L/day.
   F. Offer fruit juices—especially cranberry juice—to acidify alkaline urine.
   G. Assist with administration of supplemental IV fluids as prescribed.

H. Record I&O accurately.

I. Weigh client and record weight daily.

J. Have dietitian instruct client regarding importance of proper diet.

K. Instruct client regarding need for compliance with drug therapy.

L. Prepare client for:
   1. Cystoscopy or passage of ureteral catheter surgery for crushing or dislodging calculi
   2. Transcutaneous shockwave lithotripsy: with client sitting in large warm bath, ultrasound waves delivered to area of calculus to disintegrate it

M. Prepare client for surgery to remove ureteral or kidney stone:
   1. Nephrolithotomy: incision through kidney and removal of calculus
   2. Pyelolithotomy: removal of calculi from renal pelvis
   3. Ureterolithotomy: removal of calculus in the ureter

N. Provide general preoperative and postoperative nursing care.

O. Provide analgesics as ordered.

P. Maintain patency of catheters: do not irrigate renal or ureteral catheters.

Q. Maintain gravity urinary drainage from catheter: do not clamp ureteral or nephrostomy catheters.

R. Record output from ureteral and nephrostomy catheters separately; report and record urine output from each.

S. Monitor for bleeding, vital signs, and signs of urinary obstruction.

T. Keep client NPO if nausea, vomiting, or abdominal distention occurs.

U. Assist with comfort measures.

V. Protect against infection.

W. Encourage activity.

X. Explain disease process, treatment, prevention, home care, and follow-up care.

V. Evaluation
   A. Client reports increased comfort and decreased anxiety.
   B. Client remains free of infection.
   C. Client maintains adequate urinary elimination pattern.
   D. Client demonstrates an understanding of condition, diagnostic procedures, treatment, prevention, home care, and follow-up care.

Acute Renal Failure

I. Description
   A. Sudden interruption of kidney function resulting from obstruction, reduced circulation, or disease of renal tissue
   B. Results in retention of toxins, fluids, and end products of metabolism
   C. Usually reversible with medical treatment
   D. May progress to end-stage disease, uremic syndrome, and death without treatment
   E. Causes

1. Prerenal failure associated with decreased blood flow to kidneys
   a. Hypovolemia
   b. Shock
   c. Blood loss
   d. Embolism
   e. Pooling of fluid because of ascites or burns
   f. Cardiovascular disorders: CHF, arrhythmias
   g. Sepsis

2. Intrinsic (parenchymal) renal failure owing to damage to kidneys
   a. Acute tubular necrosis
   b. Acute poststreptococcal glomerulonephritis
   c. Sickle cell disease
   d. Bilateral renal vein thrombosis
   e. Nephrotoxins
   f. Ischemia
   g. Renal myeloma
   h. Acute pyelonephritis

3. Postrenal failure caused by bilateral obstruction of urinary outflow
   a. Renal calculi
   b. Blood clots
   c. Benign prostatic hypertrophy
   d. Urethral edema from catheterization

II. Data collection
   A. Subjective symptoms
      1. Nausea
      2. Loss of appetite
      3. Headache
      4. Lethargy
      5. Tingling in extremities
   B. Objective symptoms
      1. Oliguric phase
         a. Vomiting
         b. Disorientation
         c. Edema
         d. Hyperkalemia
         e. Hyponatremia
         f. Elevated BUN and creatinine levels
         g. Acidosis
         h. Arrhythmias
         i. CHF, pulmonary edema
         j. Hypertension caused by hypervolemia
         k. Anorexia
         l. Sudden drop in urine output
         m. Convulsions, coma
         n. Pruritus
         o. Altered clotting mechanisms
         p. Diarrhea or constipation
         q. Stomatitis
         r. Hematemesis
         s. Uremic breath
      2. Diuretic phase
         a. Increased urine output: 4–5 L/day
         b. Gradual decline in BUN and creatinine levels
         c. Hyponatremia
         d. Hypokalemia
         e. Tachycardia
         f. Improved level of consciousness

III. Diagnostic tests and methods
   A. Client history

B. Physical examination
C. Laboratory blood studies: BUN, serum creatinine, sodium, potassium, pH, bicarbonate, Hgb, and Hct
D. Urine studies
E. Ultrasound of kidneys
F. Plain films of abdomen
G. KUB x-rays
H. IVP
I. Renal scan
J. Retrograde pyelography
K. Nephrotomography

IV. Implementation
A. Assess, report, and record signs and symptoms and any reaction to treatment.
B. Monitor fluid I&O:
   1. Oral fluids
   2. All body fluids, such as wound drainage, NG output, diarrhea
C. Monitor laboratory test results.
D. Assist in administering parenteral blood products as ordered.
E. Monitor vital signs.
F. Check for signs of pleuritic chest pain, tachycardia, and pericardial friction rub indicative of pericarditis.
G. Monitor electrolyte study results:
   1. Observe for symptoms of hyperkalemia, such as malaise, anorexia, paresthesia, or muscle weakness and changes in ECG readings (and report immediately).
   2. Watch for signs of hyperglycemia or hypoglycemia in clients receiving hypertonic glucose and insulin infusions.
H. Maintain nutritional status; provide high-calorie, low-protein, low-sodium, and low-potassium diet with vitamin supplements as ordered:
   1. Provide small, frequent meals to clients with anorexia.
I. Provide good mouth care (dry mucous membranes):
   1. Administer antibiotics for stomatitis as prescribed.
J. Check stools for blood.
K. Prevent complications from immobilization:
   1. Encourage frequent coughing and deep-breathing exercises.
   2. Assist the client to ambulate when ordered.
L. Use safety measures, such as siderails, for clients who are confused or dizzy.
M. Prepare client for peritoneal dialysis, if ordered:
   1. Elevate head of bed to reduce pressure on diaphragm and aid respiration.
   2. Monitor for signs of infection (elevated temperature, cloudy drainage).
   3. Monitor blood glucose periodically; administer insulin as ordered.
   4. Monitor for complications, such as peritonitis, hypokalemia, pneumonia, and shock.
N. Prepare client for hemodialysis, if ordered:
   1. Check site of arteriovenous shunt every 2 hours for patency and presence of clot.
   2. Use opposite arm for drawing blood or taking BP readings.

   3. Have clips available at bedside to clamp off shunt in case of disconnection.
   4. Monitor vital signs, clotting time, vascular access site, arterial and venous pressures, and blood flow during dialysis procedure.
   5. Monitor for complications such as embolism, hepatitis, septicemia, and electrolyte loss.
O. After hemodialysis
   1. Monitor vital signs.
   2. Monitor vascular access site.
   3. Observe for signs of fluid and electrolyte imbalance.
P. Provide reassurance and emotional support to client and family.
Q. Explain condition, diagnostic procedures, treatment, prevention, home care, and follow-up care to client and family.

V. Evaluation
A. Client reports increased comfort and decreased anxiety.
B. Client remains free of infection.
C. Client maintains adequate renal perfusion.
D. Client maintains adequate urinary elimination pattern.
E. Client maintains good skin integrity.
F. Client maintains adequate nutritional and fluid intake.
G. Client demonstrates an understanding of disease process, diagnostic procedures, treatment, prevention, home care, and follow-up care.

Chronic Renal Failure

I. Description
A. Resulting from a gradually progressive loss of renal function
B. Occasionally caused by rapidly progressive disease of sudden onset
C. Symptoms apparent once 75% of glomerular filtration is lost
D. Progressive destruction of the nephrons, resulting in cellular hypertrophy, retention of fluid and waste products with resultant loss of renal function
E. Accumulation of uremic toxins, producing physiological changes in major organ systems if not treated
F. Maintenance dialysis and transplantation to support life temporarily
G. Causes
   1. Recurrent infections, pyelonephritis
   2. Congenital anomalies such as polycystic kidneys
   3. Vascular disorders such as renal nephrosclerosis
   4. Toxic agents such as antibiotics overdose
   5. Endocrine disorders such as diabetic neuropathy
   6. Urinary obstruction such as calculi and strictures
   7. Chronic glomerular disease such as glomerulonephritis
   8. Acute renal failure that does not respond to treatment

II. Data collection
A. Subjective symptoms
   1. Anorexia

2. Nausea
3. Lethargy
4. Headache
B. Objective symptoms
1. Renal
   a. Hyponatremia
   b. Initially resulting in hypotension, dry mouth, loss of skin turgor
   c. Progression to confusion, salt overload, accumulation of potassium with muscle irritability and muscle weakness
   d. Fluid overload and metabolic acidosis
   e. Proteinuria
   f. Glycosuria
   g. Erythrocytes (RBCs), leukocytes (WBCs), and casts
2. Cardiovascular
   a. Hypertension
   b. Arrhythmias
   c. Pericardial effusion
   d. CHF
   e. Peripheral edema
3. Neurological
   a. Restless leg syndrome with burning, pain, and itching
   b. Paresthesia
   c. Motor nerve dysfunction
   d. Muscle cramping
   e. Shortened memory span
   f. Apathy
   g. Drowsiness
   h. Confusion
   i. Convulsions
   j. Coma
   k. Electroencephalographic (EEG) changes
4. GI
   a. Stomatitis, gum ulceration, and bleeding
   b. Parotitis
   c. Esophagitis, gastritis, duodenal ulcers
   d. Ulcerative lesions on small and large bowel
   e. Pancreatitis
   f. Ammonia smell to breath (uremic fetor)
   g. Vomiting
   h. Constipation
5. Respiratory
   a. Pulmonary changes with increased susceptibility to infection
   b. Pulmonary edema
   c. Pleural friction rub and effusion
   d. Pleural pain
   e. Uremic pneumonitis
   f. Dyspnea caused by CHF
   g. Kussmaul's respirations caused by acidosis
6. Endocrine
   a. Stunted growth patterns in children
   b. Amenorrhea and cessation of menses
   c. Male impotence
   d. Increased aldosterone secretion
   e. Impaired blood glucose levels because of impairment of carbohydrate metabolism
7. Hemopoietic
   a. Anemia

b. Decrease in RBC survival time
c. Blood loss from dialysis and GI bleeding
d. Platelet deficits
e. Bleeding and clotting disorders: purpura, hemorrhage from body orifices, ecchymoses
8. Skeletal
   a. Muscle and bone pain
   b. Bone demineralization
   c. Pathological fractures
   d. Calcifications in blood vessels, myocardium, joints, gums, eyes, and brain
9. Cutaneous
   a. Pallid, yellowish-bronze, scaly skin
   b. Pruritus
   c. Purpura
   d. Uremic frost
   e. Thin, brittle fingernails
   f. Dry, brittle hair: may change color and fall out
III. Diagnostic tests and methods
   A. Client history
   B. Physical examination
   C. Creatinine clearing test
   D. BUN, serum creatinine, potassium levels
   E. Arterial pH and bicarbonate
   F. Hgb and Hct
   G. Urine specific gravity
   H. Urinalysis
   I. KUB x-rays
   J. IVP
   K. Renal scan
   L. Renal arteriography
   M. Nephrotomography
   N. Kidney biopsy
IV. Implementation
   A. Assess, report, and record signs and symptoms and any reaction to treatment.
   B. Provide emotional support.
   C. Provide meticulous skin care.
   D. Provide good perineal care.
   E. Pad siderails to prevent ecchymoses.
   F. Turn client often; use egg-crate mattress.
   G. Provide mouth care.
   H. Offer small nutritious meals high in calories.
   I. Instruct client and family to avoid high-potassium and high-sodium foods.
   J. Monitor for signs of hyperkalemia (leg and abdominal cramps, diarrhea, muscle irritability, and weak pulse rate and ECG changes).
   K. Monitor for bone and joint complications, such as pathological fractures.
   L. Monitor hydration status:
      1. Check jugular vein distention.
      2. Auscultate lungs for rales.
      3. Measure I&O, including all drainage.
      4. Record daily weight.
      5. Assess for thirst.
      6. Monitor for signs of hypertension.
      7. Check for peripheral edema.
      8. Encourage deep breathing and coughing to prevent pulmonary congestion.

M. Monitor for signs of pulmonary edema (dyspnea, restlessness, rales).
N. Administer diuretics and other prescribed medications.
O. Maintain strict aseptic technique.
P. Watch for signs of infection (increased temperature, leukocytosis, malaise).
Q. Monitor for convulsions and coma:
   1. Assist with administration of IV sodium bicarbonate for acidosis.
   2. Administer sedatives or anticonvulsants as ordered.
   3. Keep padded tongue blade and suction at bedside.
   4. Assess neurological status frequently.
   5. Check for Trousseau's and Chvostek's signs (indicates low serum calcium).
R. Monitor for signs of bleeding (ecchymoses, petechiae):
   1. Check IV sites for prolonged bleeding.
   2. Monitor Hgb and Hct values.
   3. Monitor stool, urine, and emesis for blood.
S. Prepare client for hemodialysis, if required:
   1. Instruct client regarding care of arteriovenous shunt, if present.
   2. Check vascular access site every 2 hours for patency.
   3. Check upper extremity (temperature, pulse rate, capillary refill, and sensation to determine blood supply; nervous function).
   4. If shunt is present, check for bright-red blood pulsating in tube and listen for bruit on auscultation.
   5. Notify charge nurse if clotting is suspected.
   6. Avoid using arm with vascular access for drawing blood or taking BP.
   7. Keep clamps attached to shunt dressing in case of disconnection.
   8. Monitor Hgb and Hct values.
T. After dialysis
   1. Monitor for disequilibrium syndrome caused by sudden correction of blood chemistry abnormalities (headache, seizures).
   2. Check dialysis site for excessive bleeding.
   3. Apply pressure dressing as ordered.
   4. Monitor BP readings.
U. Prepare client for kidney transplantation, if indicated:
   1. Selection criteria
   2. Immediate postoperative period
   3. Reverse isolation and protection against infection
   4. Fluid balance maintenance
   5. Use of immunosuppressive drugs and their side effects
V. Refer client and family to appropriate counseling for assistance in coping with condition.
W. Explain disease process, treatment, health maintenance procedures, home care, and follow-up care:
   1. Preventive measures
   2. Dietary restrictions
   3. Skin care
   4. Treatment (dialysis, transplant, medication)

V. Evaluation
   A. Client reports increased comfort and decreased anxiety.
   B. Client remains free of infections.
   C. Client maintains adequate nutritional intake.
   D. Client maintains adequate fluid and electrolyte balance.
   E. Client maintains adequate urinary elimination pattern.
   F. Client maintains good skin hygiene.
   G. Client demonstrates an understanding of disease process, treatment, health maintenance procedures, home care, and follow-up care.

Lower Urinary Tract Infection (Cystitis and Urethritis)

I. Description
   A. Two forms of lower UTIs: cystitis and urethritis
   B. Usually responding well to treatment
   C. Possibly recurring because of presence of resistant bacteria
   D. More common in women than in men
   E. Prevalent in children—especially girls
   F. Frequent association with anatomic or physiological abnormalities in children and men
   G. Causes
      1. Gram-negative bacterial infection caused by organisms such as *Proteus, Enterobacter, Pseudomonas,* and *E. coli* ascending from the urethra
      2. Contamination of lower urinary tract during catheterization or instrumentation
      3. Breakdown in bladder's defense mechanisms, allowing bacteria to invade bladder mucosa
      4. Bacterial flare-up caused by resistance of organisms to antimicrobial therapy
      5. If recurrent, majority caused by reinfection by same or new pathogen
      6. Small number of recurrent cases caused by perseverant infection from conditions such as kidney stones or chronic prostatitis
      7. High incidence in women possibly caused by shortness of urethra
      8. Bacterial invasion from vagina, perineum, rectum, or sexual partner
II. Data collection
   A. Subjective symptoms
      1. Urgency
      2. Frequency of urination
      3. Cramps or bladder spasms
      4. Dysuria
      5. Itching
      6. Nocturia
      7. Burning on urination
      8. Low back pain
      9. Malaise
      10. Nausea
      11. Abdominal or flank pain
      12. Chills
   B. Objective symptoms
      1. Hematuria
      2. Increased temperature

3. Vomiting
4. Tenderness over bladder region
5. Purulent urine

III. Diagnostic tests and methods
   A. Client history
   B. Physical examination
   C. Routine urine examination
   D. Urine culture and sensitivity to identify pathogen and correct antimicrobial agent to use
   E. Culture of discharge from urethra (especially in men)
   F. IVP to detect congenital abnormalities that may be a cause for recurrent UTIs

IV. Implementation
   A. Assess, report, and record signs and symptoms and any reaction to treatment.
   B. Force fluids unless contraindicated.
   C. Provide diet that acidifies urine as ordered.
   D. Monitor temperature and administer antipyretics as prescribed.
   E. Administer antimicrobial agent as prescribed.
   F. Monitor results of urine examination and culture.
   G. Provide perineal care.
   H. Provide sitz baths.
   I. Prepare client for dilatation if stricture is present.

V. Evaluation
   A. Client reports increased comfort and decreased anxiety.
   B. Client remains free of infection.
   C. Client maintains adequate elimination pattern.
   D. Client demonstrates an understanding of condition, diagnostic procedures, and treatment including medication.

Cancer of the Bladder

I. Description
   A. Malignant lesions of the bladder
   B. Possibly developing on surface of bladder wall (papillomas, benign or malignant) or growing within bladder (usually more virulent)
   C. Invasion of underlying muscles
   D. More prevalent in individuals >50 years old; more common in men than women
   E. Incidence increased in densely populated industrial areas with high number of chemical plants
   F. High-risk individuals: rubber workers, weavers, aniline dye workers, hairdressers, petroleum workers, spray painters, and leather finishers
   G. Accounting for about 2–4% of all cancers
   H. Predisposing factors
      1. Specific environmental carcinogens such as benzidine, tobacco, and nitrates (latent period between exposure and development of symptoms about 18 years)

II. Data collection
   A. Subjective symptoms
      1. Urinary urgency
      2. Dysuria
   B. Objective symptoms
      1. Signs of cystitis
      2. Gross, painless, intermittent hematuria

3. Suprapubic pain after voiding (when invasive lesions occur)
4. Signs of renal failure
5. Positive bladder biopsy
6. Positive cystoscopic examination
7. Urinary frequency, nocturia, and dribbling

III. Diagnostic tests and methods
   A. Client history
   B. Physical examination
   C. Cystoscopy
   D. Bladder tissue biopsy
   E. IVP
   F. Urinalysis
   G. Excretory urography
   H. Pelvic arteriography
   I. CAT scan

IV. Implementation
   A. Assess, report, and record signs and symptoms and any reaction to treatment.
   B. Provide emotional support.
   C. Monitor urine output for evidence of bleeding.
   D. Obtain urine specimen for culture and sensitivity.
   E. Prepare client and family for surgical procedure:
      1. Transurethral fulguration or excision: removal of small tumors with little tissue-layer infiltration
      2. Cystectomy: various types of complete removal of bladder with permanent alteration of urinary elimination
         a. Uterostomy: excision of ureters from bladder and connection of ureters to abdominal wall to form stomas for urinary drainage
         b. Colonic conduit: excision of ureters from bladder to a resected portion of the colon, which is passed through abdominal wall to construct a stoma for urinary drainage
         c. Ileal conduit: similar to colonic conduit, except a portion of the ileum is used instead of the colon
         d. Ureterosigmoidostomy: anastomosis of ureters to sigmoid colon for urinary drainage through the rectum
         e. Nephrostomy: insertion of catheter into kidney for drainage
   F. Provide postoperative care, if required:
      1. Monitor urinary drainage and patency of conduits.
      2. Monitor for abdominal distention owing to hemorrhage.
      3. Monitor for signs of hemorrhage.
      4. Assist in promotion of adequate respiratory ventilation.
      5. Provide frequent meticulous skin care around stomas.
      6. Encourage fluid intake when ordered.
      7. Protect client from infection.
   G. Prepare client for radiation treatment and/or chemotherapy.
   H. Assist with and explain care of stoma and skin care.
   I. Explain drainage equipment and application.
   J. Provide visit with ostomy therapist.
   K. Provide information regarding local ostomy organization.

L. Explain disease process, diagnostic procedures, treatment, and home care to client and family.
V. Evaluation
  A. Client reports increased comfort and decreased anxiety.
  B. Client remains free of infection.
  C. Client maintains adequate urinary elimination pattern.
  D. Client uses effective coping strategies.
  E. Client and family demonstrate an understanding of condition, diagnostic procedures, treatment, home care, and follow-up care.

Male Genitourinary System

Benign Prostatic Hypertrophy

I. Description
  A. Slow enlargement of prostate gland (hypertrophy) with extension into bladder
  B. Obstruction of urinary outflow through the urethra
  C. Urinary stream decreasing, with dysuria
  D. Stasis of urine in bladder
  E. Gradual dilation of ureters and kidneys because of the obstruction
  F. Possible hydronephrosis, calculi formation, or cystitis
  G. Acute urinary retention if obstruction is complete
  H. Frequent occurrence in men >50 years old
  I. Cause unknown
  J. Theoretical causes
    1. Link between benign prostatic hypertrophy (BPH) and hormonal activity: androgenic hormone decreases with age, causing an imbalance between androgen and estrogen levels and high levels of dihydrotestosterone
    2. Neoplasms
    3. Arteriosclerosis
    4. Inflammation
    5. Metabolic or nutritional disturbances
II. Data collection
  A. Subjective symptoms
    1. Urgency, frequency, burning, and hesitancy on urination
    2. Decreased force on urination
    3. Nocturia
  B. Objective symptoms
    1. Voiding small amounts
    2. Hematuria possible
    3. Urinary retention
    4. Infection
    5. Enlarged prostate gland on palpation and proctoscopic examination
    6. Renal insufficiency secondary to obstruction
III. Diagnostic tests and methods
  A. Client history
  B. Physical examination
  C. IVP
  D. BUN and creatinine levels
  E. Urinalysis and urine culture
  F. Cystourethroscopy immediately before surgery
IV. Implementation
  A. Assess, report, and record signs and symptoms and any reaction to treatment.

B. Monitor urinary elimination pattern, intake, output, and characteristics of urine.
C. Prepare client for surgical intervention (transurethral prostatectomy [TURP] or suprapubic, retropubic, or perineal prostatectomy).
D. Assist with explanation of postoperative course, including bladder spasms, hemorrhage, pain, and catheter.
E. Provide postoperative care:
  1. Explain reason for sensation of bladder fullness from retention balloon on catheter.
  2. Instruct client to avoid attempting to urinate around catheter.
  3. Monitor three-way irrigation catheter patency; keep bladder free of clots.
  4. Keep catheter system sterile.
  5. Monitor urine output and characteristics (red to light pink for first 24 hours).
  6. Monitor and maintain accurate I&O; record all drainage tubes separately.
  7. Change dressing around suprapubic catheter frequently.
  8. Administer analgesics or antispasmodics as prescribed.
  9. Avoid use of rectal thermometer.
  10. Administer analgesics for pain as prescribed.
  11. After catheter removal, monitor urinary output, retention, and continence.
  12. Encourage oral fluid intake.
F. Explain disease process, diagnostic procedures, treatment, prevention, home care, and follow-up care.
V. Evaluation
  A. Client reports increased comfort and decreased anxiety.
  B. Client remains free of infection.
  C. Client maintains adequate urinary elimination pattern.
  D. Client demonstrates an understanding of diagnostic process, diagnostic procedures, treatment, prevention, home care, and follow-up care.

Cancer of the Prostate

I. Description
  A. Malignant tumor of the prostate gland
  B. After skin cancer, prostatic cancer most common neoplasm found in men >50 years old
  C. Seldom produces symptoms until well advanced
  D. Seldom results from BPH
  E. Accounts for 17% of all cancers
  F. Five-year survival rate 70% when treated in its localized form
  G. Five-year survival rate <35% if treatment occurs after metastases
  H. Fatal when widespread bone metastasis occurs
  I. Cause unknown
II. Data collection
  A. Subjective symptoms
    1. Early tumor: no symptoms
    2. Back pain
    3. Symptoms from metastases

B. Objective symptoms
1. Difficulty in starting urinary stream
2. Dribbling
3. Urinary retention
4. Unexplained cystitis
5. Hematuria (rare)
III. Diagnostic tests and methods
A. Client history
B. Physical (rectal) examination
C. Biopsy examination
D. Serum acid phosphatase levels
1. Elevated in prostatic cancer
2. Used as baseline to determine effectiveness of treatment
E. Serum alkaline phosphatase levels
1. Elevated levels point to bone metastasis
F. Bone scan
IV. Implementation
A. Assess, report, and record signs and symptoms and any reaction to treatment.
B. Provide emotional support to client and family.
C. Explain expected effects of surgery, such as possible incontinence, impotence, and treatment of radiation side effects.
D. Encourage client to express his fears.
E. Explain postoperative procedures such as dressing changes and placement of tubes.
F. Teach perineal exercises to decrease incontinence.
G. After prostatectomy:
1. Monitor dressing, incision, and drainage system for excessive bleeding.
2. Monitor for signs of bleeding (cold, clammy skin; pallor; restlessness; decreasing BP readings; and rising pulse rate).
3. Administer antispasmodics as ordered (control of postoperative bladder spasms).
4. Monitor for signs of infection (chills, increased temperature, inflamed incisional site).
5. Maintain adequate fluid intake (minimum of 2000 ml daily).
6. Provide good skin care (incontinence is a frequent problem).
H. After suprapubic prostatectomy:
1. Encourage family's psychological support.
2. Keep skin around drain clean and dry.
3. Encourage perineal exercises 24–48 hours after surgery.
4. Provide meticulous catheter care (check tubing for kinks, mucus plugs, clots).
5. Explain reason for avoiding pulling on tubes or catheter.
I. After perineal prostatectomy:
1. Avoid taking temperature rectally or inserting rectal tubes.
2. Provide frequent sitz baths to relieve pain and inflammation.
3. Use pads to absorb urinary drainage.
J. After transurethral resection:
1. Monitor for abdominal distention (caused by urethral stricture or blockage of catheter by blood clot).
2. Irrigate catheter as ordered.

3. Monitor for signs of urethral stricture (straining to urinate, dysuria).
K. Monitor for radiation effects, such as nausea and vomiting, dry skin, and alopecia.
L. Watch for side effects of diethylstilbestrol (DES) (estrogen therapy), such as gynecomastia, fluid retention, nausea, and vomiting.
M. Monitor for presence of thrombophlebitis in clients receiving DES.
N. Explain condition, diagnostic procedures, treatment, home care, and follow-up care.
V. Evaluation
A. Client reports increased comfort and decreased anxiety.
B. Client maintains adequate urinary elimination pattern.
C. Client remains free of infection.
D. Client demonstrates an understanding of condition, diagnostic tests, treatment, home care, and follow-up care.

Female Reproductive System

Basic Information

Nursing care of the gynecological client is a reflection of the interest in improving the quality of health for women. Multiple gynecological abnormalities may occur at the same time. For example, a client with vaginitis may also have dysmenorrhea, dysuria, and infertility. There may also be complications associated with the urological disorders because of the proximity of the reproductive system to the urinary system. Disorders of the reproductive system may interfere with sexuality, conception, and self-image.
I. Basic data collection
A. Subjective symptoms
1. Lower abdominal pain and cramping
2. Backache
3. Urinary frequency and urgency
4. Stress incontinence
5. Tenderness and burning of breasts
6. Tenderness and burning of nipples
7. Itching and burning of external genitalia
8. Burning, itching, tenderness, and pain during intercourse
9. Pain, headache, irritability, depression, and insomnia related to menstrual cycle
B. Objective symptoms
1. General appearance
2. Vital signs
3. Weight
4. Breasts
a. Shape
b. Skin dimpling
c. Presence of nodules
1) Size
2) Consistency
3) Fixed or mobile
d. Nipples
1) Asymmetry
2) Discharge

3) Retraction
4) Ulceration
5. External genitalia
    a. Irritation
    b. Redness
    c. Excoriation
6. External vaginal orifice
    a. Irritation
    b. Redness
    c. Nodules
    d. Excoriation
7. Vaginal discharge
    a. Color
    b. Consistency
    c. Odor

Major Female Reproductive System Diagnoses

Endometriosis

I. Description
  A. Presence of endometrial tissue outside the lining of the uterine cavity
  B. Endometrial cells bleeding into nearby spaces, to cause inflammation, adhesions, tumor, or cystic formation as a result of stimulation by ovarian hormones
  C. Condition usually confined to the pelvic area, most commonly around the ovaries, the cul-de-sac, uterosacral ligaments, and the uterovesical peritoneum but can appear anywhere in the body
  D. Usually occurring between the ages of 30 and 40 years, especially in women who postpone pregnancy; uncommon before age 20 years
  E. Severe endometriosis with abrupt onset or with slow development over a period of years
  F. Usually becoming progressively severe during the menstrual years
  G. Treatment variable depending on stage of the disease
    1. Conservative treatment in stages 1 and 2 possible in young women who wish to have children
    2. Surgical intervention conducted in stages 3 and 4 when ovarian masses are present, in order to rule out malignancy
    3. Possible conservative surgical intervention conducted to resect cysts and remove adhesions
    4. For women not wishing to bear children, or when the condition is in stages 3–5, total abdominal hysterectomy with bilateral salpingo-oophorectomy performed as treatment of choice
  H. Usually subsides after menopause
  I. Direct cause unknown
  J. Predisposing factors
    1. Familial susceptibility or recent surgery necessitating opening of the uterus, such as cesarean section
II. Data collection
  A. Subjective symptoms
    1. Abdominal fullness
    2. Dysmenorrhea: constant pain in lower abdomen, vagina, posterior pelvis, and back
      a. Begins approximately 5 days before menses; lasts 2–3 days

      3. Different from primary dysmenorrhea, which is more cramplike and located in the midline of the abdomen
    4. Affecting ovaries or cul-de-sac: dyspareunia
    5. Affecting ovaries and oviducts: profuse menses
    6. Affecting cervix, vagina, and perineum: bleeding from endometrial implants
    7. Affecting rectovaginal septum and colon: nausea
    8. Affecting small bowel: nausea, worsening before menses; abdominal cramps
    9. Irregular menses
    10. Menorrhagia
  B. Objective symptoms
    1. Infertility
    2. Nodular, tender uterosacral ligaments; enlarged uterus per pelvic examination
    3. Positive findings on laparoscopy
III. Diagnostic tests and methods
  A. Client history
  B. Physical examination
  C. Pelvic examination
  D. Palpitation
  E. Laparoscopy
  F. Cul-de-sac aspiration
  G. Barium enema to rule out bowel disorders
IV. Implementation
  A. Assess, report, and record signs and symptoms and any reaction to treatment.
  B. Allow client to verbalize feelings.
  C. Administer prescribed medication that suppresses ovulation, such as danazol or oral contraceptives.
  D. Advise adolescents to use sanitary napkins in place of tampons to assist in prevention of retrograde (backward) flow in girls who have a narrow vagina or small introitus (external vaginal orifice).
  E. Reassure client that condition is not normally life threatening.
  F. Prepare client and family for surgical intervention such as hysterectomy, salpingectomy, or oophorectomy, if needed.
  G. Provide appropriate postoperative care:
    1. Monitor vaginal packing.
    2. Monitor for signs of hemorrhage.
  H. Monitor urinary output for dysuria.
  I. Recommend an annual pelvic examination and Papanicolaou (Pap) smear to all female clients for early diagnosis and more effective treatment.
  J. Explain condition, diagnostic procedures, treatment, home care, and follow-up care to client and family:
    1. Medications
    2. Hygiene
    3. Activity
    4. Estrogen therapy, if premenopausal
V. Evaluation
  A. Client reports increased comfort and decreased anxiety.
  B. Client remains free of injury or infection.
  C. Client uses effective coping strategies.
  D. Client demonstrates an understanding of condition, diagnostic procedures, treatment, home care, and follow-up care.

Carcinoma of the Cervix

I. Description
  A. Malignant lesion of the cervix, classified as either preinvasive or invasive
  B. Preinvasive carcinoma ranging from minimal cervical dysplasia to carcinoma in situ
  C. Cervical dysplasia: cervical intraepithelial neoplasis (CIN) divided into three stages
    1. CIN I: mild to moderate dysplasia
    2. CIN II: moderate to severe dysplasia
    3. CIN III: severe to malignant
  D. Preinvasive carcinoma curable 75–90% of the time with early detection and proper treatment
  E. Preinvasive carcinoma if untreated possibly progressing to invasive cervical cancer
  F. In invasive carcinoma, spread of cancer cells directly to adjacent pelvic structures or to distant sites via lymphatic system
  G. Invasive carcinoma responsible for approximately 8000 deaths per year in the United States
  H. About 95% of all cases squamous cell carcinomas; only 5% adenocarcinomas
  I. Invasive carcinoma generally occurring between ages 30 and 50 years; rarely before age 20 years
  J. Mortality declining with early detection and Pap smear examinations
  K. Asymptomatic in early stages; treatment dependent on stage of disease, health status, age, and presence of complications
  L. Related risk factors
    1. Sexual intercourse at early age
    2. Lower socioeconomic status
    3. Contact with herpes virus type 2, and other bacterial or viral venereal infections
    4. Several sexual partners (no correlation with incidence of cancer)
II. Data collection
  A. Subjective symptoms
    1. Mild bleeding after intercourse or between menstrual cycles
    2. Back pain
    3. Pelvic pain
    4. Anorexia
    5. Weight loss
  B. Objective symptoms
    1. Watery discharge
    2. Foul vaginal discharge with disease progression
    3. Leakage of urine and feces from a fistula
    4. Evidence of malignancy via Pap smear: CIN III
    5. Evidence of dysplasia via Pap smear: CIN I or CIN II, indicating need for follow-up studies
III. Diagnostic tests and methods
  A. Client history
  B. Physical examination
  C. Pap smear
  D. Cervical biopsy examination
  E. Conization
  F. Schiller test
IV. Implementation
  A. Assess, report, and record signs and symptoms and any reaction to treatment.
  B. Allow client to verbalize feelings in regard to condition.
  C. Assist with preparation of client for appropriate treatment, such as hysterectomy, cryosurgery, radiotherapy, and chemotherapy.
  D. Provide appropriate postoperative care for simple or radical hysterectomy:
    1. Monitor I&O; patency of Foley catheter.
    2. Monitor for postoperative complications, such as thrombophlebitis and abdominal distention, vaginal hemorrhage, or vaginal discharge other than serosanguineous.
    3. Monitor for urinary retention if Foley catheter is not used.
    4. Change perineal pads every 3–4 hours and as needed.
    5. Monitor for return of bowel sounds.
  E. For clients who receive an internal radium implant
    1. Provide radiation precautions.
    2. Instruct client to maintain a sidelying or supine position to prevent displacement of implant.
    3. Provide perineal hygiene.
    4. Monitor for radiation sickness (nausea, vomiting, malaise, fever, diarrhea).
    5. Administer prescribed medications, including antiemetics.
    6. Provide a high-protein, low-residue diet to avoid straining during defecation as ordered.
    7. Encourage high fluid intake (2000–3000 ml daily).
    8. Explain to client, family, and visitors that time spent with client will be limited in order to avoid overexposure to radiation.
    9. Provide emotional support for feelings of alienation.
    10. Monitor patency of Foley catheter and I&O.
    11. Monitor vaginal packing used to protect bladder and rectum from radiation.
    12. Monitor for complications such as cystitis, hemorrhage, and vaginal fistula.
  F. Explain condition, diagnostic procedures, treatment, home care, and follow-up care:
    1. Avoidance of heavy lifting for approximately 2 months
    2. Avoidance of sexual intercourse for 4–6 weeks after surgery
    3. Checking for vaginal discharge or bleeding, which may appear after irradiation
    4. Engaging in activities that do not cause straining
    5. Keeping appointment for follow-up care
V. Evaluation
  A. Client reports increased comfort and decreased anxiety.
  B. Client remains free of complications.
  C. Client remains free of injury or infection.
  D. Client maintains good skin integrity.
  E. Client develops a positive self-image.
  F. Client demonstrates an understanding of condition, diagnostic procedures, treatment, home care, and follow-up care.

Ovarian Cancer

I. Description
   A. Primary ovarian cancer: fourth most common cause of cancer deaths among women in United States, after those of cancer of the breast, colon, and lung
   B. Metastatic ovarian cancer more common than cancers at other sites in women who have had previously treated breast cancer.
   C. Rapid spread by local extension, surface seeding, and occasionally via the lymph system and the bloodstream
   D. Prognosis generally poor because ovarian tumors tend to spread rapidly
   E. Five-year survival in about 25% of women
   F. Incidence higher in women who are:
      1. Between ages 40 and 65 years
      2. In the upper socioeconomic status
      3. Single
   G. Exact causes unknown
II. Data collection
   A. Symptoms variable according to size of tumor
   B. In early stages
      1. Vague abdominal discomfort
      2. Dyspepsia
      3. Other mild GI disturbances
   C. In later stages
      1. Urinary frequency
      2. Constipation
      3. Pelvic discomfort
      4. Abdominal distention
      5. Weight loss
      6. Palpable mass
   D. Advanced stage
      1. Ascites
      2. Symptoms relating to metastatic sites, such as symptoms of pleural effusion
      3. Rarely causes postmenopausal bleeding or pain
III. Diagnostic tests and methods
   A. Client history
   B. Physical examination
   C. X-rays of abdomen
   D. Chest x-rays for distant metastasis and pleural effusion
   E. CBC, blood chemistry, and ECG
   F. Culdoscopy
   G. Ultrasonography
   H. Lymphangiography to determine lymph node involvement
   I. Mammography to rule out primary breast cancer
   J. Liver function tests or liver scan for clients with ascites
   K. Ascites fluid aspiration for identification of cells by histology
   L. Biopsy examination
   M. Barium enema for clients with GI symptoms to determine presence of obstruction and size of tumor
   N. Exploratory laparotomy for accurate diagnosis: includes tumor resection and lymph node evaluation
   O. Histological studies

IV. Implementation
   A. Assess, report, and record signs and symptoms and any reaction to treatment.
   B. Prepare client for surgical intervention.
   C. Provide emotional support.
   D. Allow client to verbalize feelings regarding condition.
   E. Provide appropriate postoperative nursing care (oophorectomy, panhysterectomy):
      1. Monitor vital signs frequently.
      2. Monitor IV fluid therapy.
      3. Monitor I&O.
      4. Maintain patent Foley catheter.
      5. Check dressings for excessive bleeding or drainage.
      6. Observe for signs of infection.
      7. Provide abdominal support, and check for signs of abdominal distention.
      8. Administer prescribed analgesics for pain.
      9. Administer prescribed chemotherapeutic drugs; monitor for side effects.
      10. Reposition client at least every 2 hours.
      11. Encourage coughing and deep-breathing exercises.
      12. Encourage and assist with ambulation as necessary.
   F. Monitor and treat side effects of radiation and chemotherapy, if applicable:
      1. Provide emotional support for client and family.
      2. Request supportive care from chaplain, social worker, and other health-care team members as appropriate.
      3. Assist client in dealing with changes of body image.
      4. Assist client in developing coping strategies.
   G. Explain condition, diagnostic procedures, treatment including medication, home care management, and follow-up care.
V. Evaluation
   A. Client reports increased comfort and decreased anxiety.
   B. Client remains free of complications.
   C. Client remains free of injury or infection.
   D. Client maintains good skin integrity.
   E. Client develops a positive self-image.
   F. Client demonstrates an understanding of condition, diagnostic procedures, treatment, home care, and follow-up care.

Breast Mass

I. Description
   A. Nodule or mass in the breast, which may or may not be malignant
   B. Nonmalignant breast lesion
      1. Fibroadenomas
         a. Round, encapsulated, movable, firm, and nontender on palpation
      2. Dysplasia
         a. Thick, nodular lumps within the breast
         b. Association with pain during menses
         c. Nodule is soft, movable, and tender on palpation

      d. Possibly multiple nodules

      e. Occurring most often in women between 30 years of age and menopause

C. Malignant breast tumors

  1. Most common form of cancer in women

  2. Incidence increases with age

  3. Affecting whites more than blacks

  4. High-risk factors

      a. Women who have not nursed

      b. Presence of fibrocystic breast disease

      c. Family history

      d. Early menarche

      e. Prolonged menstrual history

      f. First pregnancy after age 25 years or women who have never had children

  5. Possibly firm, nonmovable, tender, and nontender on palpation

  6. Most frequently located in upper, outer portion of the breast.

  7. Metastasis occurring early, transported by lymph system, spreading to lung, bone, and/or brain

II. Data collection

A. Subjective symptoms

  1. Small mass felt during breast self-examination

B. Objective symptoms

  1. Palpable mass in breast tissue

  2. Presence of tumor on mammography

  3. Nipple retraction or elevation

  4. Skin dimpling

  5. Nipple discharge

  6. Abnormal findings on thermography

  7. Positive xeromammogram results

  8. Positive benign or malignant breast biopsy through needle aspiration or surgical removal of tumor and microscopic examination for malignant cells

III. Diagnostic tests and methods

A. Client history

B. Physical examination

C. Mammography: x-ray of breast tissue

D. Thermography: measures heat from breast tissue

E. Xenography: type of mammography using an electrically charged aluminum plate with a selenium layer; has ability to detect carcinoma 1–2 years before formation of a palpable 1-cm lesion

F. Hormonal reception assay tests: conducted on tumor tissue to determine if tumor is estrogen or progesterone dependent; useful in determining therapy strategies

IV. Implementation

A. Assess, report, and record signs and symptoms and any reaction to treatment.

B. Allow client to verbalize feelings regarding condition.

C. Provide emotional support.

D. Provide frequent contact and encourage illness adjustment.

E. Provide for visit of individuals from Reach to Recovery with approval of physician.

F. Prepare client for biopsy procedure.

G. Prepare client for surgical intervention, if required:

  1. Provide preoperative teaching.

  2. Explain type of surgical intervention:

      a. Lumpectomy: excision and removal of nodule

      b. Partial mastectomy: removal of tumor with small amount of adjacent tissue

      c. Simple mastectomy: removal of breast tissue, leaving anterior skin, underlying chest muscle, and axillary lymph nodes intact

      d. Subcutaneous mastectomy: removal of breast tissue, leaving skin, nipple, and areola intact

      e. Modified radical mastectomy: total removal of breast tissue and nipple with partial excision of skin, surrounding tissue, and lymph nodes

      f. Radical mastectomy: total removal of breast tissue and nipple with partial removal of overlying skin, chest muscles, axillary lymph tissue, and surrounding adipose tissue

      g. Oophorectomy, adrenalectomy, or hypophysectomy: to remove source of estrogen and hormones that stimulate the breast

H. Provide postoperative care:

  1. Administer prescribed analgesics.

  2. Monitor dressing and drainage and/or Hemovac drainage system; check client's back for pooling of blood.

  3. Empty Hemovac and measure every 8 hours.

  4. Elevate affected arm above level of right atrium of heart to prevent edema.

  5. Monitor circulatory status of affected arm.

  6. Measure upper arm and forearm of affected arm twice daily to detect presence of edema.

  7. Avoid drawing blood, administering parenteral fluids, or taking BP in affected arm.

  8. Encourage exercises of affected arm when ordered; avoid abduction:

      a. Squeezing ball

      b. Brushing hair

      c. Feeding self

      d. "Climbing" wall with fingertips

      e. Rope pull

      f. Elbow spread

      g. Arm swing

  9. Encourage adequate nutritional intake when appropriate.

  10. Administer prescribed corticosteroids, androgens, and antiestrogens to alter cancer that is dependent on specific hormones.

  11. Request representative from Reach to Recovery to revisit client with approval of physician.

  12. Provide information on breast prosthesis if requested.

  13. Provide emotional support; assist with adjustments to body image.

  14. Assist in development of coping strategies.

I. Provide appropriate nursing care for clients receiving radiation therapy:

  1. Apply prescribed lotion to skin.

  2. Monitor for skin problems such as radiation burns.

J. Administer adjuvant chemotherapeutic agents, if prescribed (vincristine, doxorubicin [Adriamycin], methotrexate, 5-fluorouracil, prednisone).

K. For clients receiving radiation and chemotherapeutic therapy:
  1. Explain and assist with potential side effects:
     a. Nausea and vomiting
     b. Anorexia
     c. Stomatitis
     d. Malaise
     e. Hair loss
     f. Itching
     g. Reduced energy
     h. Heartburn
     i. Cough
     j. Bone marrow depression
     k. Anemia
L. Prepare client for breast reconstruction, if indicated.
M. Explain condition, diagnostic procedures, treatment, prevention, home care, and follow-up care to client and family:
  1. Correct technique for breast examination
  2. Arm exercises and activity level
  3. Resumption of sexual activity
  4. Medication
  5. Information on community resources such as Reach to Recovery

V. Evaluation
A. Client reports increased comfort and decreased anxiety and fear.
B. Client remains free of injury or infection.
C. Client maintains adequate level of mobility.
D. Client develops a positive self-image.
E. Client and family demonstrate an understanding of condition, diagnostic procedures, treatment, home care, and follow-up care.

Endocrine System

Basic Information

Together with the nervous system, the endocrine system regulates and integrates the metabolic activities of the body. The hypothalamus controls endocrine organs by hormonal and neural pathways. Hormones are chemical transmitters that are released from certain types of cells in the bloodstream and then carried to its organ-receptor cells. These latter cells respond to the specific hormone.

The pathways of the nervous system connect the hypothalamus to the posterior pituitary gland. Neural stimulation causes the posterior pituitary gland to secrete two hormones: antidiuretic hormone (ADH) and oxytocin.

The hypothalamic hormones stimulate the anterior pituitary to emit the following tropic hormones: adrenocorticotropic hormone (ACTH), thyroid-stimulating hormone (TSH), follicle-stimulating hormone (FSH), and luteinizing hormone (LH). The hypothalamic hormones are also responsible for the release or inhibition of the human growth hormone (HGH) and prolactin. The atropic hormones in turn stimulate the adrenal cortex, thyroid, and gonads.

The endocrine system is regulated by a negative simple or complex feedback system. In a simple feedback system, the level of one substance regulates the secretion of a hormone.

For example, high serum calcium inhibits the secretion of the parathyroid hormone (PTH), while low serum calcium levels stimulate the secretion of PTH. An example of the complex feedback system is that of the stimulation of the release of ACTH as a result of the secretion of the hypothalamic corticotropin-releasing hormone (CRH). ACTH then stimulates the adrenal gland to secrete cortisol. Once serum cortisol rises, it inhibits the secretion of ACTH by decreasing CRH.

Careful evaluation of each level of the endocrine system is necessary in clients whose clinical condition suggests endocrine dysfunction owing to the involvement of the complex hormonal sequence. A disturbance in one of the secreting endocrine glands can affect the regulation of another gland. The client with an endocrine dysfunction may experience multiple problems.

I. Basic data collection
A. Subjective symptoms
  1. Pain: skeletal, back, abdominal, muscle spasms, headache
  2. Weakness
  3. Lethargy
  4. Numbness
  5. Mood swings
  6. Tingling
  7. Intolerance to cold or heat
  8. Polyuria, dysuria, nocturia
  9. Impotence, infertility, decreased libido
  10. Menstrual disturbances
  11. Anorexia or polyphagia
  12. Frequent infections
  13. Nausea
B. Objective symptoms
  1. General appearance
  2. Skin color
     a. Flushed
     b. Pale
     c. Bronze pigmentation
     d. Yellow pigmentation
  3. Skin temperature
     a. Excess perspiration
     b. Dry
     c. Moist
  4. Poor wound healing
  5. Nails
     a. Thin
     b. Thick
     c. Brittle
     d. Dry
  6. Hair
     a. Brittle
     b. Thin
     c. Dry
  7. CNS
     a. Alterations in consciousness
        1) Lethargy
        2) Decreased cognition
        3) Seizures
        4) Confusion
        5) Stupor
        6) Coma
     b. Personality changes

   c. Abnormal reflexes: Chvostek's or Trousseau's sign
   d. Slowed, sluggish speech
8. Eyes
   a. Protruding eyeball (exophthalmos)
   b. Drooping eyelids (ptosis)
   c. Edema around eyes (periorbital)
9. Respiratory system
   a. Kussmaul's respirations
   b. Acetone breath
   c. Tachypnea
10. Cardiovascular system
    a. Tachycardia
    b. Bradycardia
    c. Hypertension
    d. Hypotension
11. GI system
    a. Anorexia
    b. Polyphagia
    c. Polydipsia
    d. Diarrhea
    e. Constipation
12. Renal system
    a. Oliguria
    b. Anuria
    c. Polyuria
13. Musculoskeletal system
    a. Weight loss or gain
    b. Stature (excessive or delayed growth)
14. Vital signs

Major Endocrine Diagnoses

Hyperthyroidism (Graves' Disease; Thyrotoxicosis)

I. Description
   A. Metabolic imbalance caused by thyroid hormone overproduction
   B. Most common form, Graves' disease, in which thyroxine production is increased, with enlargement of the thyroid gland, resulting in multiple system changes
   C. Thyroid storm: an acute exacerbation of this condition, possibly leading to life-threatening cardiac, renal, or hepatic failure if not treated immediately
   D. Incidence highest in individuals between the ages of 30 and 40 years
   E. Incidence high in individuals with a family history of thyroid disorders
   F. Possible for most clients to lead normal life with treatment
   G. Causes and predisposing factors
      1. Presence of genetic and immunological factors
      2. Abnormal iodine metabolism
      3. Other endocrine disorders such as thyroiditis, hyperparathyroidism, and diabetes mellitus
      4. Excessive dietary iodine intake
      5. Stressful conditions: surgery, infection, toxemia of pregnancy, and diabetic ketoacidosis, especially in clients with untreated or inadequately treated hyperthyroidism, possibly precipitating thyroid storm

II. Data collection
   A. Subjective symptoms
      1. Fatigue
      2. Weakness
      3. Vision problems
      4. Intolerance to heat
      5. Increased appetite
      6. Diarrhea
      7. Palpitations
      8. Nervousness
      9. Menstrual abnormalities
      10. Difficulty in concentrating
      11. Clumsiness
      12. Nausea
      13. Loss of appetite
      14. Irritability
   B. Objective symptoms
      1. Enlarged thyroid gland (goiter)
      2. Weight loss
      3. Profuse diaphoresis
      4. Diarrhea
      5. Tremors
      6. Exophthalmos
      7. Shaky handwriting
      8. Smooth, warm, flushed skin
      9. Fine, soft hair
      10. Premature graying with increased hair loss
      11. Friable nails
      12. Thickened skin
      13. Tachycardia
      14. Bounding pulse
      15. Cardiomegaly
      16. Dyspnea on exertion and at rest
      17. Increased defecation
      18. Liver enlargement
      19. Muscle atrophy
      20. Oligomenorrhea or amenorrhea
      21. Gynecomastia in men caused by increased estrogen levels
      22. Increased serum T_4 and T_3 concentrations
      23. Thyroid storm: extreme irritability, hypertension, tachycardia, vomiting, temperature up to 106°F (41.1°C) delirium, and coma

III. Diagnostic tests and methods
   A. Client history
   B. Physical examination
   C. Radioimmunoassay
   D. Thyroid scan for evaluation of ^{131}I uptake
   E. Thyroid suppression test for evaluation of pituitary control of thyroid gland
   F. Thyroid-releasing hormone (TRH) stimulation test for evaluation of TSH levels
   G. Basal metabolism rate (BMR)
   H. Serum protein-bound iodine (PBI)
   I. Serum cholesterol and total lipids
   J. Ultrasonography to evaluate subclinical ophthalmopathy

IV. Implementation
   A. Assess, report, and record signs and symptoms and any reaction to treatment.
   B. Monitor vital signs and neurological status.
   C. Monitor weight daily.

D. Monitor serum electrolytes.
E. Monitor for signs of hyperglycemia and glycosuria.
F. Monitor cardiac function.
G. Monitor fluid I&O.
H. Monitor pregnant women for signs of spontaneous abortion (spotting, occasional mild cramps).
I. Mix prescribed iodine medication with milk to prevent GI distress.
J. Administer prescribed iodine medication through a straw to prevent tooth discoloration.
K. Administer other prescribed medications, such as digitalis, propranolol (Inderal), sedatives, and sleep aids.
L. Assist with comfort measures.
M. Assist with activities as needed.
N. Encourage adequate intake of high-calorie, high-carbohydrate, high-protein, and high-vitamin diet.
O. Explain and understand mood swings.
P. Monitor for signs of thyroid storm:
  1. Tachycardia
  2. Elevated temperature
  3. Tremors and restlessness
  4. Vomiting
  5. Hypertension
  6. Delirium
  7. Coma
Q. Treat thyroid storm as prescribed:
  1. Administer medications as prescribed:
    a. SSKI or ^{131}I to inhibit thyroid hormone (instruct client to expectorate or cough freely after ^{131}I therapy; saliva remains radioactive for 24 hours)
    b. Glucocorticoids to inhibit release of thyroid hormone
    c. Beta-adrenergic blockers for increased adrenergic stimulation
    d. Medications for CHF
  2. For clients taking methimazole:
    a. Monitor CBC periodically to detect leukopenia, thrombocytopenia, and agranulocytosis.
    b. Instruct client to take medication with meals to decrease GI distress.
    c. Instruct client to avoid over-the-counter cough preparations because they may contain iodine.
    d. Instruct client to report signs of blood dyscrasia, such as enlarged cervical lymph nodes, fever, mouth sores, sore throat, skin rash, or skin eruptions.
  3. Monitor BP and cardiac rate and rhythm.
  4. Monitor temperature.
  5. Administer hypothermic measures for high fever (sponging, hypothermia blankets, and acetaminophen; avoid aspirin as it raises thyroxine levels).
  6. Maintain IV line.
R. For clients with exophthalmos:
  1. Advise use of sunglasses, shields, or eye patches to protect eyes.
  2. Moisten conjunctivas with isotonic eyedrops.
  3. Advise client with severe lid retraction to avoid sudden movement (may cause lid to slip behind eyeball).
  4. Monitor for corneal damage.
S. Prepare client and family for surgical intervention, if required.
T. Provide postoperative care:
  1. Monitor for signs of respiratory distress frequently.
  2. Keep thoracotomy tray at bedside.
  3. Monitor for signs of hemorrhage into neck, such as tight dressing with absence of blood.
  4. Change dressing and perform wound care as ordered (check back of dressing for drainage).
  5. Place client in semi-Fowler's position (support head and neck with sandbags to ease tension on the incision).
  6. Monitor for signs of thyroid storm.
  7. Monitor for signs of hypoparathyroidism (tetany, numbness) caused by accidental removal of parathyroid gland during surgery.
  8. Emphasize importance of follow-up care after discharge (hypothyroidism may develop 2–4 weeks postoperatively).
  9. Emphasize importance of repeated measurement of serum thyroxine levels.
U. Explain condition, diagnostic procedures, treatment including medication, home care, and follow-up care to client and family.
V. Evaluation
A. Client reports increased comfort and decreased anxiety.
B. Client remains free of injury or infection.
C. Client maintains adequate nutritional intake.
D. Client maintains adequate rest and undisturbed sleep pattern.
E. Client participates in self-care activities.
F. Client uses effective coping strategies.
G. Client and family demonstrate an understanding of condition, diagnostic procedures, treatment including medication, home care, and follow-up care.

Hypothyroidism (Myxedema)

I. Description
A. Condition characterized by low serum thyroid hormone level resulting from hypothalamic, pituitary, or thyroid insufficiency
B. Leads to a decline in the metabolic rate and affects almost all systems
C. Clinical effects ranging from mild fatigue and loss of appetite to life-threatening myxedema coma
D. Most prevalent in women
E. Incidence rising in individuals between the ages of 40 and 50 years
F. Infection, use of sedatives, and exposure to cold may precipitate myxedema coma
G. Causes
  1. Dysfunction of thyroid gland caused by:
    a. Thyroidectomy
    b. Irradiation therapy (especially ^{131}I)
    c. Inflammation
    d. Chronic autoimmune thyroiditis
    e. Inflammatory conditions such as sarcoidosis and amyloidosis

2. Failure of pituitary gland to produce TSH
3. Failure of hypothalamus to produce TRH
4. Inborn errors of thyroid hormone synthesis
5. Iodine deficiency: usually dietary, resulting in inability to synthesize the hormone
6. Use of antithyroid medications such as propylthiouracil

II. Data collection
   A. Subjective symptoms
      1. Fatigue
      2. Forgetfulness
      3. Sensitivity to cold
      4. Loss of appetite
      5. Decreased libido, menstruation changes
      6. Muscle stiffness and pain
      7. Chest pain
      8. Headache
      9. Drowsiness or apathy
      10. Numbness or tingling
      11. Decreased mental status
   B. Objective symptoms
      1. Weight gain
      2. Decreased bowel sounds
      3. Constipation
      4. Dry, flaky, cool, coarse, inelastic skin
      5. Puffy face, hands, and feet
      6. Sparse body hair
      7. Immature body development
      8. Decreased BMR
      9. Bradycardia
      10. Hoarseness
      11. Periorbital edema
      12. Dry, sparse, brittle hair
      13. Upper eyelid droop
      14. Thick, brittle nails
      15. Abdominal distention
      16. Infertility
      17. Ataxia
      18. Intention tremor
      19. Nystagmus
      20. Reflexes: delayed reaction time
      21. Decreased urine output
      22. Low body temperature
      23. Decreased T_4, T_3, ^{131}I
      24. Pleural effusion on chest x-ray
      25. Elevated serum cholesterol, carotene, alkaline phosphatase, and triglyceride levels
      26. Signs of myxedema coma
         a. Progressive stupor
         b. Hypoventilation
         c. Hypoglycemia
         d. Hypotension
         e. Hyponatremia
         f. Hypothermia

III. Diagnostic tests and methods
   A. Client history
   B. Physical examination
   C. Radioimmunoassay: T_4, T_3, and ^{131}I uptake
   D. TSH levels
   E. Serum cholesterol, carotene, alkaline phosphatase, and triglyceride levels
   F. CBC with differential

   G. For myxedema coma
      1. Serum sodium levels (decreased)
      2. ABGs (decreased pH and elevated P_{CO_2})

IV. Implementation
   A. Assess, report, and record signs and symptoms and any reaction to treatment.
   B. Monitor vital signs, respirations, GI functions, and neurological status.
   C. Orient to environment as needed.
   D. Provide safe, warm environment.
   E. Provide a high-bulk, low-calorie diet.
   F. Encourage activity to promote weight loss and to combat constipation.
   G. Administer prescribed thyroxine replacement, analgesics for pain, laxatives or stool softeners for constipation, and IV fluids.
   H. Monitor for signs of hyperthyroidism caused by thyroxine replacement:
      1. Restlessness
      2. Nervousness
      3. Sweating
      4. Excessive weight loss
   I. Instruct client to report signs of cardiovascular diseases such as chest pain and tachycardia.
   J. Instruct client to report signs of infection immediately.
   K. Encourage fluid intake.
   L. Provide meticulous skin care; monitor for skin breakdown.
   M. Monitor for signs of myxedema coma:
      1. Decreased urinary output (sign of decreased cardiac output)
      2. Decreased temperature (hypothermia)
         a. Provide extra blankets and clothing.
         b. Provide a warm room.
         c. Avoid rapid rewarming as it may cause vasodilation and vascular collapse.
      3. Monitor daily I&O and weight.
      4. Turn client every 2 hours.
      5. Provide meticulous skin care.
      6. Avoid sedation or reduce dosage (hypothermia delays metabolism of many drugs).
      7. Maintain patent IV line:
         a. Monitor serum electrolytes while client is receiving IV therapy.
         b. Monitor vital signs—especially if client is receiving levothyroxine (too-rapid correction of hypothyroidism may cause adverse cardiac effect).
      8. Report chest pain or tachycardia immediately.
      9. Monitor elderly clients for hypertension and CHF.
      10. Monitor ABGs for signs of hypoxia and respiratory acidosis.
      11. Monitor for need of ventilatory assistance.
      12. Monitor urine and sputum for sources of infection.
      13. Check possible sources of infection (blood, urine, sputum), as coma may have been triggered by infection.
   N. Explain condition, diagnostic procedures, treatment, home care, and follow-up care to client and family:

1. Monitor vital signs, elimination, activity, skin care, reaction to medications.
2. Emphasize compliance to prescribed treatment.
3. Emphasize need for follow-up visits to physician.

V. Evaluation
   A. Client reports increased comfort and decreased anxiety.
   B. Client remains free of injury or infection.
   C. Client maintains good skin integrity.
   D. Client maintains adequate level of mobility.
   E. Client maintains adequate cardiac output.
   F. Client maintains adequate elimination pattern.
   G. Client demonstrates improvement in thought process.
   H. Client develops positive self-image.
   I. Client complies with thyroid medication routine.
   J. Client and family demonstrate an understanding of condition, diagnostic procedures, treatment including medication, home care, and follow-up.

Hyperparathyroidism

I. Description
   A. Condition characterized by overactivity of one or more of the four parathyroid glands, which results in an abnormal increase in the secretion of PTH
   B. Increased levels of PTH, which promotes resorption of bone and results in hypercalcemia (elevated serum calcium levels) and hypophosphatemia (diminished levels of phosphorus)
   C. Resultant increase in renal and GI absorption of calcium
   D. Classification as either primary or secondary hyperparathyroidism
   E. Primary type: increased PTH secretion caused by the enlargement of one or more of the parathyroid glands, which results in increased serum calcium levels
   F. Secondary type: increased PTH secretion caused by a hypocalcemia-producing abnormality excluding the parathyroid gland, which causes resistance to the metabolic action of PTH

II. Data collection
   A. Subjective symptoms
      1. Fatigue
      2. Weakness
      3. Anorexia
      4. Nausea
      5. Chronic low back pain
      6. Bone tenderness
      7. Constipation
      8. Abdominal pain
      9. Pruritus
      10. Marked muscle weakness
   B. Objective symptoms
      1. Elevated PTH levels
      2. Marked muscle atrophy
      3. Elevated serum calcium, chloride, and alkaline phosphatase levels
      4. Diminished serum phosphorus levels
      5. Elevated urine calcium levels
      6. Bone fractures or cysts on x-rays because of osteoporosis
      7. Polyuria
      8. Polydipsia
      9. Arrhythmias
      10. Hypertension
      11. Renal calculi
      12. Polynephritis
      13. Hematemesis
      14. Vomiting
      15. Signs of pancreatitis, peptic ulcer
      16. Stupor, coma
      17. Necrosis of skin
      18. Cataracts
      19. Calcium microthrombi in lungs and pancreas
      20. Positive Trousseau's or Chvostek's signs
      21. Subcutaneous calcification
      22. Memory loss
      23. Symptoms of secondary hyperparathyroidism
         a. Decreased serum calcium levels
         b. Variable serum phosphorus levels
         c. Skeletal deformities
         d. Symptoms of underlying disease

III. Diagnostic tests and methods
   A. Client history
   B. Physical examination
   C. Radioimmunoassay for PTH
   D. Total serum calcium
   E. Serum phosphorus
   F. Quantitative urinary calcium
   G. Uric acid and creatinine levels
   H. Tests for underlying disease for secondary hyperparathyroidism

IV. Implementation
   A. Assess, report, and record signs and symptoms and any reaction to treatment.
   B. Monitor vital signs, respiratory, and cardiovascular status frequently.
   C. Monitor skeletal, renal, and neurological status frequently.
   D. Administer prescribed diuretics and medications to inhibit bone resorption.
   E. Provide safe environment; assist with comfort measures.
   F. Administer prescribed analgesics for pain.
   G. Record I&O.
   H. Encourage fluid intake of 3000 ml daily; include cranberry juice to acidify urine.
   I. To help prevent spontaneous fractures:
      1. Assist with ambulation.
      2. Keep bed at lowest position with siderails up.
      3. Lift immobilized client carefully to decrease stress on bones.
      4. Check x-ray reports to determine which bones are the weakest.
   J. Explain rationale for low-calcium, low-phosphorus diet.
   K. Strain urine to monitor for presence of stones; check for signs of hematuria.
   L. Prepare client and family for surgical intervention (parathyroidectomy), if indicted.
   M. Explain condition, diagnostic procedures, and treatment.

V. Evaluation
   A. Client reports increased comfort and decreased anxiety.
   B. Client remains free of injury or infection.
   C. Client maintains adequate cardiac output.
   D. Client maintains adequate nutritional intake.
   E. Client maintains adequate elimination patterns.
   F. Client demonstrates an understanding of condition, diagnostic procedures, and treatment.

Hypoparathyroidism

I. Description
   A. Condition characterized by a deficiency of PTH
   B. Resultant decrease in bone resorption because low serum calcium levels (hypocalcemia) and increase in levels of phosphorus (hyperphosphatemia)
   C. Hypocalcemia producing neuromuscular symptoms ranging from paresthesia to severe tetany
   D. Clinical effects generally corrected with PTH replacement therapy
   E. Some complications, such as cataracts, possibly irreversible
   F. Either idiopathic or acquired
II. Data collection
   A. Subjective symptoms
      1. Numbness and tingling
      2. Dyspnea
      3. Depression or irritability
      4. Confusion
      5. Headache
      6. Visual problems, photophobia
      7. Muscle cramps and spasms
      8. Muscle pain
      9. Difficulty in walking
      10. Abdominal pain
   B. Objective symptoms
      1. Positive Trousseau's and Chvostek's signs (tetany)
      2. Convulsions
      3. Laryngeal stridor
      4. Arrhythmias
      5. CHF
      6. Calcification of skull on x-ray
      7. Dry, scaly skin
      8. Decreased calcium levels
      9. Elevated serum phosphorus levels
      10. Decreased urine calcium levels
      11. Increased bone density on x-ray
      12. Increased QT interval and ST segment on ECG as a result of hypocalcemia
      13. Cataracts
III. Diagnostic tests and methods
   A. Laboratory serum values: calcium, phosphorus
   B. Qualitative urinary calcium (Sulkowitch's) test
   C. X-rays of skeletal system
   D. ECG
   E. Trousseau's and Chvostek's tests
IV. Implementation
   A. Assess, report, and record signs and symptoms and any reaction to treatment.
   B. Monitor vital signs; maintain patent airway.
   C. Monitor serum calcium and phosphorus levels and urinary calcium levels.
   D. Maintain patent IV line; keep IV calcium available.
   E. Maintain seizure precautions.
   F. Keep tracheotomy tray and endotracheal tube at bedside (in case of laryngospasm).
   G. Assist in administration of prescribed IV diazepam; monitor vital signs frequently to ascertain BP and heart rate.
   H. Monitor for cardiac rhythm, if indicated.
   I. Monitor for signs of tetany; check Trousseau's or Chvostek's sign.
   J. Assist in administration of calcium gluconate or calcium chloride, and vitamin D as prescribed.
   K. Monitor I&O.
   L. Monitor for signs of heart block and signs of decreasing cardiac output.
   M. Provide adequate nutrition with high-calcium, low-phosphate diet.
   N. Apply prescribed cream to soften scaly skin.
   O. Explain condition, diagnostic procedures, treatment including medication compliance, home care, and follow-up care to client and family.
V. Evaluation
   A. Client reports increased comfort and decreased anxiety.
   B. Client remains free of injury or infection.
   C. Client maintains effective breathing pattern.
   D. Client maintains adequate cardiac output.
   E. Client maintains adequate nutritional and fluid intake.
   F. Client shows improvement in thought process.
   G. Client demonstrates an understanding of condition, diagnostic procedures, treatment including medication compliance, home care, and follow-up care.

Addison's Disease (Adrenal Hypofunction)

I. Description
   A. Condition characterized by hyposecretion of cortisol by the adrenal cortex
   B. Classification as primary or secondary
   C. Occurring at any age and in both sexes
   D. Incidence of secondary type increasing with use of steroid therapy
   E. Prognosis good with early diagnosis and appropriate treatment
   F. Adrenal crisis (addisonian crisis) a result of extreme deficiency of mineralocorticoids and glucocorticoids because of acute stress in individuals with chronic Addison's disease
   G. Adrenal crisis: requires immediate emergency treatment
   H. Causes
      1. Fungal infections such as histoplasmosis
      2. Bilateral adrenalectomy
      3. Hemorrhage into adrenal gland
      4. Tuberculosis
      5. Adrenal carcinoma
      6. Idiopathic atrophy
      7. Impaired circulation
      8. Autoimmune response (circulating antibodies react against adrenal tissue)

II. Data collection
   A. Subjective symptoms
      1. Weakness
      2. Fatigue
      3. Nausea
      4. Anorexia
      5. Inability to concentrate
      6. Muscle pain
      7. Menstrual changes, impotence
      8. Decreased tolerance for minimal stress
      9. Craving for salty food
   B. Objective symptoms
      1. Lethargy
      2. Bronze skin
      3. Weight loss
      4. Vomiting
      5. Chronic diarrhea
      6. Areas of absent skin pigmentation
      7. Decreased plasma ACTH
      8. Low serum sodium levels
      9. High serum potassium and BUN levels
      10. Elevated Hct, lymphocyte, and eosinophil counts
      11. Evidence of small heart and adrenal calcification on x-ray
      12. Hypoglycemia (fasting blood glucose)
      13. Poor skin turgor, sunken eyeballs, dry mucous membrane as a result of dehydration
      14. Hypotension
      15. Weak, irregular pulse
      16. Decreased concentration of corticosteroids in plasma or urine
      17. Decreased 17-hydroxysteroid and 17-ketosteroid and 17-hydroxycorticosteroid (17-OHCS) in 24-hour urine test
      18. Sparse body hair in women
III. Diagnostic tests and methods
   A. Client history
   B. Physical examination
   C. Plasma and urine corticosteroid levels
   D. Serum sodium, potassium, and BUN levels
   E. Fasting blood glucose test
   F. Metyrapone test
   G. X-rays
IV. Implementation
   A. Assess, report, and record signs and symptoms and any reaction to treatment.
   B. Monitor for electrolyte imbalance and hypoglycemia.
   C. For clients with diabetes, check blood glucose level periodically (steroid replacement therapy may require an adjustment of insulin dosage).
   D. Provide diet that maintains sodium and potassium balance.
   E. Administer prescribed glucocorticoid and mineralocorticoid replacement.
   F. Administer antacids to prevent ulcers.
   G. Provide safe, calm environment, limit visitors, avoid potential stressors.
   H. Provide emotional support.
   I. Monitor client receiving steroids for cushingoid symptoms, such as edema of face and around eyes.

   J. Observe client for signs of petechiae.
   K. Monitor for facial growth and other masculinization signs in female clients who are on testosterone injections for muscle weakness and decreased libido.
   L. Explain need for lifelong therapy and need to watch for symptoms of overdosage and underdosage.
   M. Advise client to avoid infections, injury, or heat, which may precipitate an adrenal crisis.
   N. Monitor for signs of addisonian crisis:
      1. Acute hypotension
      2. Profound weakness
      3. Nausea or vomiting
      4. Vascular collapse
      5. Shock
      6. Renal failure
      7. Coma
      8. Death
   O. Provide care for addisonian crisis:
      1. Assist in administration of prescribed IV hydrocortisone immediately.
      2. Administer prescribed intramuscular (IM) hydrocortisone IM after initial IV therapy or assist in administration of prescribed hydrocortisone diluted with IV saline or dextrose until condition stabilizes.
      3. Monitor vital signs every 15 minutes.
      4. Monitor urine output hourly.
      5. Monitor weight.
      6. Monitor serum sodium levels.
      7. Monitor fluid intake.
   P. Instruct client to carry a medical identification card.
   Q. Instruct client and family on how to inject hydrocortisone.
   R. Advise client and family to keep hydrocortisone in a prepared syringe for use in case of stress.
   S. Provide comfort measures, such as backrubs and relaxation techniques.
   T. Assist with gradual return to activities.
   U. Explain condition, diagnostic procedures, treatment, home care, and follow-up care to client and family.
V. Evaluation
   A. Client reports increased comfort and decreased anxiety.
   B. Client remains free of injury or infection.
   C. Client maintains adequate fluid balance.
   D. Client maintains adequate nutritional intake.
   E. Client uses effective coping strategies.
   F. Client and family demonstrate an understanding of condition, diagnostic procedures, treatment including medication compliance, home care, and follow-up care.

Cushing's Syndrome and Disease

I. Description
   A. Syndrome or disease characterized by a cluster of abnormalities caused by excessive levels of adrenocortical hormones (especially cortisol), androgens, and aldosterone
   B. Affecting women more than men

C. Affecting:
  1. Protein, carbohydrate, and fat metabolism
  2. Inflammatory and immune response
  3. Mineral and water metabolism
  4. Blood components
  5. Emotional status
D. Prognosis depends on underlying cause: poor in individuals who have not received treatment and in those with metastatic adrenal malignancy or untreatable ectopic ACTH-producing malignancy
E. Causes
  1. Overproduction of ACTH with resultant hyperplasia of adrenal cortex (Cushing's syndrome)
  2. Overproduction of ACTH from pituitary hypersecretion
  3. ACTH-producing tumor (ectopic ACTH secretion) in another organ external to the adrenal gland such as pancreatic or bronchogenic carcinoma
  4. Administration of synthetic glucocorticoids or ACTH
  5. Cortisol-secreting adrenal tumor: usually benign
II. Data collection
A. Subjective symptoms
  1. Fatigue
  2. Muscle weakness
  3. Irritability
  4. Insomnia
  5. Poor wound healing
  6. Changes in menstrual cycle and libido
  7. Bone pain
  8. Emotional disturbances
B. Objective symptoms
  1. Evidence of steroid diabetes: decreased glucose tolerance, glucosuria, and fasting hyperglycemia
  2. Moon face (from fat deposits)
  3. Buffalo hump: fat pads over upper back
  4. Fat pads over clavicle
  5. Truncal obesity with slender arms and legs
  6. Little or no scar formation
  7. Acne and hirsutism in women
  8. Muscle atrophy caused by increased catabolism
  9. Pathological fractures caused by decreased bone mineral
  10. Skeletal growth retardation in children
  11. Striae (stretch marks on skin)
  12. Evidence of peptic ulcer, resulting from increased gastric secretions and production of pepsin
  13. Hypertension caused by sodium and water retention
  14. Left ventricular hypertrophy
  15. Capillary weakness caused by protein loss: leads to petechiae and ecchymosis
  16. Infections caused by suppressed antibody formation and decreased lymphocyte production
  17. Sodium (and secondary fluid) retention
  18. Increase in potassium excretion
  19. Ureteral calculi caused by increased bone demineralization
  20. Elevated urine calcium levels
  21. Enlargement of breasts in men and clitoral hypertrophy, virilism, and amenorrhea in women
III. Diagnostic tests and methods
A. Client history
B. Physical examination
C. Plasma and urinary steroid levels
D. Low-dose dexamethasone suppression test for Cushing's syndrome
E. High-dose dexamethasone suppression test for Cushing's disease
F. Ultrasound, CAT scan, and angiography to localize adrenal tumors
G. CAT scan of head to identify presence of pituitary tumors
IV. Implementation
A. Assess, report, and record signs and symptoms and any reaction to treatment.
B. Monitor vital signs and neurological status every 4 hours.
C. Monitor serum electrolyte, blood glucose, and cortisol levels.
D. Monitor urinary glucose levels.
E. Monitor daily weight and check for edema.
F. Monitor I&O carefully.
G. Provide diet high in protein and potassium and low in calories, sodium, and carbohydrates.
H. Monitor for signs of infection:
  1. Check temperature every 4 hours.
  2. Check skin, oral cavity, and lungs for signs of infection.
  3. Encourage coughing and deep-breathing exercises.
  4. Turn client frequently.
  5. Provide proper hygienic measures.
  6. Avoid individuals with upper respiratory infections.
I. Assist in reducing stressors:
  1. Maintain continuity of nursing care.
  2. Avoid excessive noise or temperature changes.
  3. Limit visitors.
  4. Provide privacy.
  5. Allow adequate rest periods.
J. Monitor and record instances of emotional lability.
K. Provide a restful environment; allow client to verbalize feelings.
L. Administer prescribed medications, such as potassium replacements and inhibitors of cortisol production or release; monitor for side effects.
M. Prepare client and family for surgical intervention, if indicated:
  1. Bilateral adrenalectomy
  2. Total hypophysectomy
  3. Trans-sphenoidal adenectomy
N. Provide postoperative care:
  1. Monitor wound drainage or fever immediately.
  2. Use strict aseptic technique in changing dressings when ordered.
  3. Administer analgesics and replacement steroids as ordered.
  4. Monitor urinary output.
  5. Monitor vital signs; check for shock symptoms

(decreased BP, increased pulse rate, pallor, cold clammy skin):

    a. Administer prescribed vasopressors and increase IV flow rate as ordered.

    b. Monitor for decreased mental alertness and for signs of physical weakness.

    c. Assess neurological and behavioral status.

    d. Monitor for signs of nausea, vomiting, and diarrhea.

  6. Monitor laboratory reports for signs of hypoglycemia caused by removal of cortisol source (cortisol maintains normal blood glucose levels).

  7. Monitor for signs of adrenal hypofunction indicative of inadequate steroid replacement:

    a. Orthostatic hypotension

    b. Apathy, weakness, fatigue

  8. Monitor for signs of abdominal distention and recurrence of bowel sounds.

  9. For clients undergoing pituitary surgery, monitor and report signs of increased ICP (agitation, changes in level of consciousness, confusion, nausea, vomiting).

O. Advise client to take steroid replacements with antacids or meals to decrease gastric irritation.

P. Advise client to carry a medical identification card.

Q. Advise client to monitor for and immediately report signs of inadequate steroid dosage (weakness, vertigo, fatigue).

R. Instruct the client and family that discontinuation of the steroid replacement medications may produce a fatal adrenal crisis.

S. Encourage a positive self-image.

T. Explain condition, diagnostic procedures, treatment including medication, home care including activities and prevention of complications, and follow-up care to client and family.

V. Evaluation

A. Client reports increased comfort and decreased anxiety.

B. Client remains free of injury or infection.

C. Client maintains adequate activity.

D. Client maintains adequate fluid balance.

E. Client uses effective coping strategies.

F. Client develops a positive self-image.

G. Client maintains adequate nutritional intake.

H. Client maintains compliance with medication replacement therapy.

I. Client and family demonstrate an understanding of condition, diagnostic procedures, treatment including medications, prevention, home care, and follow-up.

Diabetes Mellitus

I. Description

A. Condition characterized by insulin deficiency or resistance, with disturbances in carbohydrate, protein, and fat metabolism followed by chronic neuropathies and microvascular change

B. Insulin responsible for transporting glucose into body cells for use as energy and for storing glycogen

C. Insulin causing stimulation of protein synthesis and free fatty acid storage

D. Deficiency in insulin that jeopardizes access of body cells to essential nutrients

E. Incidence approximately equal in men and women, rising with age

F. Predisposing client to renal failure, as well as to peripheral vascular, cerebrovascular, and coronary artery disease.

G. A leading cause of blindness

H. Two forms

  1. Insulin-dependent diabetes mellitus (IDDM, ketosis-prone, or juvenile diabetes)

    a. Usually occurring before age 30 years (although may occur at any age)

    b. Individual usually thin, requiring endogenous insulin and dietary management

  2. Non-insulin-dependent diabetes mellitus (NIDDM, ketosis-resistant, or maturity-onset diabetes)

    a. Most prevalent among obese adults (occurs occasionally in children)

    b. Responds to dietary treatment alone or in combination with hypoglycemic agents or insulin

I. Effects of insufficient endogenous insulin or action, including:

  1. Elevated serum blood glucose level as a result of impaired intake by liver; high blood levels of glucose pulling fluid from body tissues, causing osmotic diuresis

  2. Lipolysis resulting from changes in fat metabolism causing ketone formation, possibly leading to ketonuria

J. Glucose content in epidermis (skin) and urine, stimulating bacterial growth

K. Causes

  1. Heredity

  2. Environmental

  3. Autoimmune factors

  4. Precipitating factors

    a. Obesity: causes resistance to endogenous insulin

    b. Physiological or emotional stress: causes prolonged increased levels of cortisol, epinephrine, glucagon, and growth hormone, which in turn raise blood glucose levels, thereby increasing demands on the pancreas

    c. Pregnancy and use of oral contraceptives: increase levels of estrogen and placental hormones, which are antagonists of insulin

    d. Use of other insulin antagonists such as thiazide diuretics and renal corticosteroids

II. Data collection

A. Subjective symptoms

  1. Fatigue

  2. Polyphagia

  3. Polydipsia

  4. Nocturia, polyuria

  5. Visual disturbances as a result of edema and sugar deposits, which cause changes in lens

  6. Anxiety

  7. Weight loss

B. Objective symptoms
1. Lethargy
2. Weight loss (IDDM); obesity (NIDDM)
3. Elevated fasting serum glucose level
4. Glycosuria
5. Dehydration
6. Dry mucous membranes
7. Poor skin turgor
8. Long-term effects
  a. Retinopathy
  b. Nephropathy
  c. MI
  d. Stroke
  e. Peripheral neuropathy
  f. Nocturnal diarrhea
  g. Skin infections
  h. UTIs
  i. Vaginitis
  j. Anal pruritus

III. Diagnostic tests and methods
A. Client history
B. Physical examination
C. Fasting blood glucose test
D. Urinalysis
E. Urine tests for glucose and acetone
F. Postprandial blood glucose
G. Twenty-four-hour urine quantitative glucose specimen
H. Blood insulin level determination

IV. Implementation
A. Assess, report, and record signs and symptoms and any reaction to treatment.
B. Emphasize importance of compliance with prescribed program.
C. Provide safe and hazard-free environment.
D. Provide comfort measures.
E. Monitor I&O.
F. Monitor serum glucose, urine glucose levels, and electrolytes.
G. Monitor vital signs every 4 hours or as needed as condition warrants.
H. Monitor for signs of insulin shock (hypoglycemia: abnormally low blood glucose levels caused by an excess of insulin or oral hypoglycemic medication in relation to activity or dietary intake or the result of insufficient glucose to supply CNS needs):
1. Pallor
2. Weakness, numbness
3. Confusion or irritability
4. Fatigue
5. Vertigo
6. Blurred vision
7. Tachycardia
8. Diaphoresis
9. Hunger
10. Seizures
11. Coma
I. Instruct client and family on carbohydrate foods to treat hypoglycemia:
1. Fruit juice
2. Hard candy
3. Honey
4. Cola
J. If unconscious, assist in administration of IV glucogen or dextrose.
K. Continue to monitor vital signs and neurological status frequently.
L. Monitor blood glucose level frequently.
M. Provide safe, hazard-free environment.
N. Continue to monitor I&O and nutritional status.
O. Facilitate use of effective coping strategies.
P. Explain self-care and prevention.
Q. Monitor for signs of diabetic coma (ketoacidosis: acute or gradual insulin deficiency precipitated by emotional stress, infection, trauma, or other stressors; occurs in clients with insulin-dependent diabetes; leads to protein catabolism, release of potassium and urea nitrogen, and ketone formation from fat breakdown):
1. Increased thirst
2. Nausea, vomiting
3. Abdominal pain
4. Drowsiness
5. Headache
6. Acetone breath: fruity breath odor from respiratory compensation for elevated serum acetone level
7. Elevated serum glucose level
8. Elevated serum acetone level and osmolarity
9. Decreased arterial pH and bicarbonate level
10. Dehydration
11. Weak, rapid pulse
12. Kussmaul's respirations
13. Osmotic diuresis
14. Electrolyte imbalance
R. Monitor for signs of hyperglycemic nonketonic coma:
1. Polyuria
2. Thirst
3. Neurological abnormalities
4. Stupor
S. Both diabetic ketoacidosis and hyperosmolar coma are hyperglycemic crises:
1. Assist in administration of prescribed IV fluids.
2. Assist in administration of prescribed insulin and electrolyte replacement.
3. Assist in administration of potassium replacement, if required.
4. Monitor for signs of hypoglycemia as a result of insulin administration.
5. Monitor vital signs every 4 hours.
6. Monitor I&O hourly.
7. Monitor serum glucose levels, electrolytes, and ABGs.
8. Monitor for correction of dehydration.
9. Provide a safe, calm environment.
10. Monitor for diabetic effects on the cardiovascular system:
  a. Symptoms of cerebrovascular disease
  b. Symptoms of coronary artery and peripheral vascular disease
T. Monitor for and treat all injuries, cuts, and blisters (especially on lower extremities) as prescribed.

U. Monitor for signs of UTI and renal failure.
V. Assess client for diabetic neuropathy:
  1. Numbness
  2. Pain in arms and legs
  3. Footdrop
  4. Neurogenic bladder
  5. Instruct client to avoid trauma; client may injure himself or herself unknowingly because of decreased sensation in arms and legs.
W. Assist with instruction of client and family about insulin and explain that it is administered to control serum glucose metabolism and thereby control diabetes:
  1. Types of insulin
    a. Rapid-acting (Regular, Semilente): action begins within 1 hour, with peak action in 1–4 hours; solution appears clear.
    b. Intermediate-acting (neutral protamine Hagedorn [NPH], Lente): initial action begins in 2–4 hours, with peak action in 8–12 hours; solution appears cloudy.
    c. Long-acting (protamine zinc, Ultralente): initial action begins in 4–8 hours, peak action in 16–18 hours; solution appears cloudy.
  2. Strength or concentration
  3. Source: pork, beef, Humulin insulin
  4. Purity
  5. Regimen prescribed
  6. Rotation sites and subcutaneous injection
  7. Mixing of different types
X. Explain condition, diagnostic procedures, complications, treatment including medication, prevention, and home care including self-care and activity.
V. Evaluation
A. Client reports increased comfort and decreased anxiety.
B. Client remains free of injury or infection.
C. Client maintains adequate serum glucose level.
D. Client maintains adequate fluid and nutritional intake.
E. Client maintains adequate fluid balance and tissue perfusion.
F. Client maintains good skin integrity.
G. Client develops a positive self-image.
H. Client reports reduction in feeling of powerlessness.
I. Client verbalizes plan for compliance.
J. Client uses effective coping strategies.
K. Client demonstrates an understanding of condition, diagnostic procedures, complications, and treatment including medication, prevention, and home care including self-care and activity.

Musculoskeletal System

Basic Information

The musculoskeletal system is a complex system of bones, muscles, ligaments, tendons, and other connective tissue. This system gives the body shape and form. It also makes movement possible, protects vital organs, provides the site for hemopoiesis, and stores calcium and other minerals.

Muscle tissue has contractility that makes movement of bones and joints possible. Muscles also move food through the intestines, pump blood through the blood vessels of the body, and make breathing possible. The activity of muscles aids in temperature regulation by producing heat. Muscles also assist in maintaining body position such as standing and sitting. Muscles are classified as skeletal (attached to bones), visceral (provide function of internal organs), and cardiac (forming the wall of the heart). Muscles are also classified as voluntary and involuntary. Involuntary muscles are controlled by the autonomic nervous system, which includes the cardiac and visceral muscles. Voluntary muscles are controlled by deliberate intention and influenced by the somatic nervous system. These latter muscles are classified as skeletal muscles. Muscle mass accounts for about 40% of the weight of humans.

The human skeleton has 206 bones composed of organic salts, such as calcium and phosphate, which are imbedded in fibers of collagen. Bones are classified as long, short, flat, or irregular. Musculoskeletal disorders can be either acute or chronic. Acute problems are usually caused by simple injuries; chronic conditions often result in loss of mobility and changes in self-image.

I. Basic data collection
A. Subjective symptoms
  1. Weakness
  2. Pain
  3. Complaints of joint stiffness
  4. Weight loss
  5. Anorexia
  6. Limited movement
B. Objective symptoms
  1. General appearance
  2. Abnormal gait
  3. Impaired neurovascular status
  4. Differences between affected and unaffected sides
  5. Absence of extremity
  6. Decreased handgrip
  7. Abnormal spinal curvature
  8. Joint enlargement
  9. Presence of edema, redness, warmth over affected area
  10. Decreased ROM
  11. Changes in vital signs
  12. Nonalignment of extremities
  13. Inability to move a body part

Major Musculoskeletal Diagnoses

Systemic Lupus Erythematosus

I. Description
A. A chronic inflammatory disorder of connective tissues
B. Usually affecting multiple organ systems as well as the skin
C. Possibly fatal
D. Condition characterized by recurring remissions and exacerbations
E. Affecting women eight times as often as men; incidence increases during childbearing years
F. Exacerbations more common during the spring and summer

G. Prognosis improved with early detection and treatment
H. Prognosis poor for clients who develop complications: severe infections, renal and neurological problems
I. Causes unknown
J. Theoretical causes
  1. Autoimmune: antibodies entering tissue suppress normal immunity response of body
  2. Certain predisposing factors causing susceptibility
    a. Physical or mental stress
    b. Streptococcal or viral infections
    c. Immunization
    d. Exposure to sunlight or ultraviolet light
    e. Pregnancy
    f. Genetic predisposition
  3. Triggered or aggravated by certain drugs
    a. Anticoagulants
    b. Hydralazine
    c. Procainamide
    d. Sulfa drugs
    e. Penicillin
    f. Oral contraceptives

II. Data collection
A. Subjective symptoms
  1. Photosensitivity
  2. Fatigue
  3. Weakness
  4. Weight loss
  5. Joint pain and stiffness of hands, feet, or large joints
  6. Tenderness of affected joints
  7. Anorexia
  8. Abdominal pain
  9. Nausea
  10. Irregular menstrual periods
  11. Headaches, irritability
B. Objective symptoms
  1. Nondeforming arthritis
  2. Facial erythema (butterfly rash)
  3. Oral or nasopharyngeal ulcerations
  4. Pleuritis, pericarditis, neuritis, glomerulonephritis, peritonitis
  5. Convulsions
  6. Hemolytic anemia thrombocytopenia, leukopenia
  7. Positive antinuclear antibody (ANA) or systemic lupus erythematosus (SLE) cell test result
  8. Proteinuria
  9. UTIs
  10. Increased cellular casts in urine
  11. Alopecia
  12. Chronic false-positive serological test result for syphilis
  13. Increased temperature
  14. Vomiting
  15. Lymph node enlargement
  16. Diarrhea or constipation or both
  17. Dyspnea
III. Diagnostic tests and methods
A. Client history

B. Physical examination
C. CBC with differential
D. Platelet count
E. ESR
F. Serum electrophoresis
G. ANA and SLE cell tests
H. Urine studies
I. Chest x-ray
J. ECG
K. Kidney biopsy
IV. Implementation
A. Assess, report, and record signs and symptoms and any reaction to treatment.
B. Provide emotional support to client and family.
C. Monitor for dyspnea, chest pain, and edema of extremities.
D. Note size, type, and location of skin lesions.
E. Monitor urine for signs of hematuria.
F. Monitor scalp for hair loss (alopecia).
G. Monitor skin and oral mucous membrane for bleeding, ulceration, petechiae, and bruising.
H. Provide a well-balanced diet.
I. Provide a low-sodium, low-protein diet if renal disorder is present.
J. Administer prescribed medications such as:
  1. Ointments or creams for rash
  2. Corticosteroids for inflammatory response and renal or neurological complications
  3. Analgesics for arthritic pain
  4. Cytoxic drugs, if prescribed
K. Prepare client and family for dialysis or kidney transplant if renal failure occurs.
L. Advise use of protective clothing, screening agent, and sunglasses when out in sun.
M. Apply heat packs for relief of joint pain and stiffness.
N. Encourage full ROM exercises to prevent contractures.
O. Arrange for physical therapy and occupational counseling.
P. Provide frequent skin and mouth care.
Q. Monitor vital signs, I&O, laboratory reports, and weight.
R. Monitor GI secretions and stools for presence of blood.
S. Monitor for signs of renal involvement (hypertension, weight gain).
T. Assess for signs of neurological involvement (personality changes, ptosis, double vision, seizures).
U. Explain use of cosmetics to women (hypoallergenic cosmetics).
V. Refer client to Lupus Foundation of America and Arthritis Foundation.
W. Explain diagnostic condition, diagnostic procedures, treatment, home care, and follow-up care.
V. Evaluation
A. Client reports increased comfort and decreased anxiety.
B. Client remains free of injury or infection.
C. Client maintains good skin integrity.
D. Client uses effective coping strategies.
E. Client remains free of organ-specific complications.

F. Client demonstrates an understanding of condition, diagnostic procedures, treatment, home care, and follow-up care.

Rheumatoid Arthritis

I. Description
   A. Chronic, systemic, inflammatory disease that primarily involves peripheral joints and surrounding muscles, tendons, ligaments, and blood vessels
   B. Eventual depletion of joint cartilage results in joint dislocation
   C. Condition characterized by spontaneous remissions and unpredictable exacerbations
   D. Usually requiring lifelong treatment and occasionally surgery
   E. Possible for majority of clients to carry on with normal activity
   F. Occurring worldwide; affecting women three times more than men
   G. Occurring at any age but most prevalent in women aged 20 to 60 years, with peak onset between ages 35 and 45 years
   H. Inflammatory process within joints occurring in four stages if left untreated:
      1. First stage: synovitis developing from congestion and edema of synovial membrane and joint capsule
      2. Second stage: formation of thickened layers of granulation tissue, in which thickened layers cover and invade cartilage, destroying joint capsule and bone
      3. Third stage: formation of fibrous ankylosis; fibrous invasion of thickened layers of granulation tissue with scar formation, which occludes the joint space; visible deformities caused by bone atrophy and malalignment, resulting in muscle atrophy and imbalance
      4. Fourth stage: calcification of fibrous tissue, with bony ankylosis causing total immobility
   I. Cause unknown
   J. Theoretical causes
      1. Susceptibility caused by genetic defects impairing autoimmune system
      2. Bacterial or viral infection
      3. Environmental factors
      4. Endocrine, nutritional, and metabolic factors
      5. Occupational and psychosocial influences
II. Data collection
   A. Subjective symptoms
      1. Morning stiffness of joints
      2. Sore, stiff, swollen joint(s)
      3. Weakness
      4. Fatigue
      5. Malaise
      6. Numbness, tingling in feet, hands
      7. Loss of sensation in fingers and toes
      8. Inability to perform usual activities
      9. Pain with ROM
      10. Loss of appetite
   B. Objective symptoms
      1. Limited ROM of joint

2. Weakened grip
3. Low-grade fever
4. Anemia
5. Weight loss
6. Subcutaneous nodes
7. Enlarged lymph nodes
8. Muscle atrophy
9. Appearance of joints bilaterally
10. Elevated ESR
11. Positive rheumatoid factor (RF) or latex fixation test
12. X-ray evidence of joint deterioration
13. Spindle-shaped fingers
14. Flexion deformities of affected joints
15. Skin lesions and leg ulcers as a result of vasculitis
16. Peripheral neuropathy
17. Complications such as infection, osteoporosis, and temporomandibular disease (which impairs chewing and causes earaches)

III. Diagnostic tests and methods
   A. Client history
   B. Physical examination
   C. X-rays of joints
   D. Rheumatoid factor (RF) test
   E. ANA and SLE cell tests
   F. Synovial fluid analysis
   G. CBC with differential
   H. Serum protein electrophoresis
   I. ESR

IV. Implementation
   A. Assess, report, and record signs and symptoms and any reaction to treatment.
   B. Provide emotional support.
   C. Encourage adequate nutritional intake; assist with meals as needed.
   D. Schedule undisturbed rest periods.
   E. Administer heat applications such as paraffin dip, hot packs, and warm tub baths or showers for relief of pain and muscle relaxation as ordered.
   F. Administer analgesics and anti-inflammatory medications as ordered.
   G. Allow verbalization of feelings and support positive body image.
   H. Provide ROM exercises within limits of pain tolerance.
   I. Provide meticulous skin care; use lotion or cleaning oil in place of soap for dry skin.
   J. Apply splints correctly, if ordered; observe for pressure sores.
   K. Encourage mobility:
      1. Encourage client to perform ADLs with assistance as necessary.
      2. Assist with active ROM exercise.
      3. Instruct client to protect joints and conserve energy.
      4. Encourage client to ambulate with assistance as necessary.
      5. Coordinate care with physical therapy department.
   L. Explain disease process and chronic pain, as well as medical or surgical treatment (synovectomy, arthrotomy, arthroplasty, or arthrodesis).

V. Evaluation
  A. Client reports increased comfort and decreased anxiety.
  B. Client participates in ADLs.
  C. Client develops a positive self-image.
  D. Client maintains adequate nutritional intake.
  E. Client remains free of injury or infection.
  F. Client demonstrates an understanding of disease process, diagnostic procedures, treatment, home care, and follow-up care.

Osteoarthritis

I. Description
  A. Most common form of arthritis, a progressive disorder causing deterioration of the joint cartilage and formation of reactive new bone at margins of joints
  B. Most often affecting weight-bearing joints such as the hips and knees
  C. Incidence rising among older people
  D. Earliest symptoms generally beginning in middle age, becoming progressively severe with advancing age
  E. Affecting both sexes
  F. Prognosis that depends on site and severity of involvement; may range from minor limitations involving the fingers to severe disability involving knees and hips
  G. Varying rate of progression
  H. Causes
    1. Primary osteoarthritis: resulting from genetic predisposition, a normal part of aging
    2. Secondary osteoarthritis: an acquired form resulting from joint damage caused by trauma, stress, excessive "wear and tear," infection, underlying joint disease, and/or metabolic disorders

II. Data collection
  A. Subjective symptoms
    1. Pain after exercise or weight bearing
    2. Morning stiffness
    3. Aching during changes in weather
    4. "Grating" of joint during movement
  B. Objective symptoms
    1. Limited ROM
    2. Crepitant joint
    3. Prominent bony enlargement
    4. Heberden's nodes on distal joints of phalanges and Bouchard's nodes on proximal joints of phalanges: initially painless; then red, swollen, and tender

III. Diagnostic tests and methods
  A. Client history
  B. Physical examination
  C. X-rays of affected joints

IV. Implementation
  A. Assess, report, and record signs and symptoms and any reaction to treatment.
  B. Encourage client to verbalize feelings about condition.
  C. Provide adequate rest, especially after activity.
  D. Assist with physical therapy.
  E. Care for affected joint.
    1. Hand: Apply hot soaks and paraffin dips to relieve pain as ordered.
    2. Spine (lumbar and sacral): Provide firm mattress or bedboard to decrease morning pain.
    3. Spine (cervical): Provide cervical collar for constrictions; monitor for signs of redness.
    4. Hip
      a. Apply moist heat pads to relieve pain.
      b. Administer antispasmodic medications as ordered.
      c. Assist with ROM and strengthening exercises.
      d. Check assistive devices such as crutches, braces, and walker for proper fit.
      e. Advise use of elevated toilet seat and cushions when sitting.
    5. Knee
      a. Assist with prescribed ROM exercises.
      b. Encourage exercises to maintain muscle tone.
  F. Explain condition, diagnostic procedures, treatment, home care, and follow-up care:
    1. Avoid overexertion.
    2. Take medications as prescribed.
    3. Obtain adequate rest.
    4. Wear well-fitting supportive shoes.
    5. Use guardrails in bathroom:
      a. Minimize weight-bearing activities.

V. Evaluation
  A. Client reports increased comfort and decreased anxiety.
  B. Client remains free of injury or infection.
  C. Client participates in self-care activities.
  D. Client develops a positive self-image.
  E. Client demonstrates an understanding of condition, diagnostic procedures, treatment, home care, and follow-up care.

Gout

I. Description
  A. A metabolic disease resulting in an acute inflammation of synovial tissue characterized by deposits of urate crystals
  B. Increased concentration of uric acid resulting in urate deposits (tophi) in joints and tissues, causing local necrosis or fibrosis
  C. Primary gout occurring in men, with onset at approximately age 50 years, and in postmenopausal women
  D. Secondary gout occurring in elderly clients
  E. Following an intermittent course, with most clients free of symptoms for years between attacks
  F. Possibly leading to chronic disability
  G. In rare instances, possibly leading to severe hypertension and progressive renal disease
  H. Affecting any joint, but found mostly in joints of feet and legs
  I. Development in four stages: asymptomatic, acute, intercritical, and chronic
  J. Prognosis good with treatment
  K. Causes

1. Primary gout
   a. Exact cause unknown
   b. Condition linked to a genetic defect in purine metabolism, resulting in an overproduction of uric acid (hyperuricemia), retention of uric acid, or both
2. Secondary gout
   a. Follows course of other diseases such as polycythemia vera or multiple myeloma
   b. Caused by breakdown of nucleic acid
   c. May also follow drug therapy, such as hydrochlorothiazide, which interferes with urate excretion

II. Data collection
   A. Subjective symptoms
      1. Onset of pain in joint of the great toe, feet, ankles, or knees
      2. Pruritus
      3. Headache
      4. Malaise
      5. Severe back pain
   B. Objective symptoms
      1. Elevated serum uric acid level
      2. Normal or elevated 24-hour urinary uric acid level
      3. Positive for monosodium urate crystals in synovial fluid
      4. Inflamed joints
      5. Elevated WBC count and ESR
   C. Asymptomatic stage: serum urate levels increase with no apparent symptoms
      1. Acute stage
         a. Hypertension, kidney stones: attack sudden, peaking quickly
         b. Affected joints: hot, inflamed, dusky-red, cyanotic
         c. Joint of great toe usually affected first, followed by the instep, ankle, heel, knee, or wrist joints
      2. Intercritical stage: symptom-free between gout attacks
      3. Chronic stage
         a. Persistent painful polyarthritis
         b. Large, subcutaneous tophaceous deposits in cartilage, synovial membranes, tendons, and soft tissues (urate deposits above earlobe, fingers, hands, knees, feet, and ulnar sides of forearms)
         c. Ulcerations over tophi, with presence of chalky white exudate or pus
         d. Joint degeneration or deformity, and disability
         e. Kidney involvement, resulting in symptoms of chronic renal dysfunction
         f. Urolithiasis (urinary calculi)

III. Diagnostic tests and methods
   A. Client history
   B. Physical examination
   C. Serum uric acid levels
   D. Urinary uric acid levels
   E. WBC count
   F. ESR

G. Analysis of aspirated synovial fluid or of tophaceous material
H. X-rays of joints
I. RF test to rule out rheumatoid arthritis

IV. Implementation
   A. Assess, report, and record signs and symptoms and reaction to treatment.
   B. Provide bedrest during acute attacks.
   C. Provide adequate fluid to prevent calculi formation; monitor I&O.
   D. Monitor appearance of joints (ROM ability).
   E. Administer analgesics such as aspirin or acetaminophen as prescribed to relieve pain of mild attacks.
   F. Provide bedrest; use bed cradle to keep bedcovers off affected joints.
   G. Position affected joint in mild flexion position during acute attack; assist with mobility.
   H. Administer prescribed medications such as colchicine, anti-inflammatory drugs such as phenylbutazone (Butazolidin), probenicid (Benemid), indomethacin (Indocin), or sulfinpyrazone (Anturane) to facilitate uric acid secretion; allopurinol (Zyloprim) to decrease formation of uric acid; monitor for side effects.
   I. Administer corticosteroids for resistant inflammation as prescribed.
   J. Assist with joint aspiration and injection of intra-articular corticosteroid injection, if needed.
   K. Apply hot or cold packs to inflamed joints as ordered; monitor serum uric acid levels on a regular basis.
   L. Encourage weight loss in obese clients (obesity places additional stress on painful joints).
   M. Prepare client for excision and drainage of infected or ulcerated tophi.
   N. Monitor for acute gout attacks 24–96 hours after surgery.
   O. Explain disease process, diagnostic procedures, treatment, prevention, and home care:
      1. Checking serum uric acid levels periodically
      2. Avoiding use of high-purine foods such as anchovies, kidneys, sweetbreads, lentils, and alcoholic beverages
      3. Dieting to gradually decrease weight in obese clients
      4. Complying with prescribed medication regimen
      5. Reporting side effects of medications immediately

V. Evaluation
   A. Client reports increased comfort and decreased anxiety.
   B. Client remains free of injury or infection.
   C. Client maintains adequate nutritional and fluid intake.
   D. Client maintains adequate level of mobility.
   E. Client demonstrates an understanding of disease process, diagnostic procedures, treatment including medication, prevention, and home care.

Osteoporosis

I. Description
   A. Metabolic bone disorder with an acceleration of

bone resorption rate and a slowing down in the rate of bone formation, resulting in loss of bone mass
  B. Calcium and phosphate salts lost from affected bones
  C. Affected bones becoming brittle, vulnerable to fractures
  D. Either primary or secondary to an underlying disease
  E. Primary osteoporosis (senile or postmenopausal): most common in postmenopausal women
  F. Usually affected sites: vertebrae, pelvis, and femur
  G. Causes of primary osteoporosis
    1. Unknown
  H. Predisposing factors involving primary osteoporosis
    1. Prolonged negative calcium balance because of inadequate dietary intake of calcium
    2. Decline in gonadal adrenal function
    3. Faulty protein metabolism resulting from estrogen deficiency and sedentary lifestyle
  I. Causes of secondary osteoporosis
    1. Prolonged therapy with steroids or heparin
    2. Total immobilization or disuse of bone, as with hemiplegia
    3. Alcoholism: malnutrition
    4. Lactose intolerance
    5. Hyperthyroidism
    6. Scurvy
    7. Osteogenesis imperfecta
II. Data collection
  A. Subjective symptoms
    1. Backache
    2. Pain radiating around trunk
  B. Objective symptoms
    1. Vertebral compression
    2. Kyphosis
    3. Loss of height
    4. Pathological fractures: neck, femur, hip, Colles' fracture
    5. Changes in skull, ribs, and long bones owing to severe or advanced osteoporosis, as in hyperthyroidism or Cushing's syndrome
III. Diagnostic tests and methods
  A. Client history
  B. Physical examination
  C. Skeletal x-rays
  D. Serum calcium, phosphorus, and alkaline phosphatase levels within normal limits
  E. Elevated parathyroid hormone level
  F. Bone biopsy
IV. Implementation
  A. Assess, report, and record signs and symptoms and any reaction to treatment.
  B. Encourage exercise and other physical activity to prevent disuse atrophy.
  C. Administer estrogen replacement as ordered to improve calcium balance.
  D. Administer fluoride as ordered to stimulate bone formation.
  E. Provide diet high in protein and calcium.
  F. Administer vitamin D supplements and calcium as ordered to support normal bone metabolism.
  G. Encourage fluid intake of 2000–3000 ml daily to avoid formation of renal calculi (unless contraindicated).
  H. Provide support of spine with brace or corset as ordered.
  I. Monitor daily for redness, warmth, and new sites of pain.
  J. Perform passive ROM exercises as appropriate.
  K. Coordinate care with physical therapist.
  L. Provide safety precautions such as siderails, moving client gently and carefully.
  M. Administer analgesics as prescribed for pain.
  N. Encourage use of walker or cane to stabilize balance when client is ambulating.
  O. Encourage early mobilization after surgical procedure or trauma.
  P. Monitor for signs of malabsorption.
  Q. Encourage avoidance or decrease of alcohol consumption.
  R. Instruct client and family in importance of following prescribed daily activity.
  S. Advise client and family on importance of sleeping on a firm mattress and avoiding excessive bedrest.
  T. For women receiving estrogen, emphasize need for routine gynecological checkups, including Pap smears. Instruct client to report any abnormal bleeding and presence of breast lumps.
  U. Instruct client regarding good body mechanics, such as stooping before lifting and avoiding twisting motions and prolonged bending.
  V. Explain disease process, diagnostic procedures, treatment, prevention, home care, and follow-up care.
V. Evaluation
  A. Client reports increased comfort and decreased anxiety.
  B. Client remains free of injury or infection.
  C. Client maintains adequate level of mobility.
  D. Client maintains adequate nutritional and fluid intake.
  E. Client participates in self-care activities.
  F. Client demonstrates an understanding of disease process, diagnostic procedures, treatment, prevention, home care, and follow-up care.

Herniated Nucleus Pulposus (Slipped or Ruptured Disk)

I. Description
  A. Protrusion of the nucleus pulposus (soft, mucoid central portion of an intervertebral disk), resulting in compression of nerve roots of spinal cord or spinal cord itself
  B. Nucleus pulposus forced through the disk's weakened or torn outer ring
  C. Compressed nerve roots or spinal cord, resulting in back pain and other signs of nerve root irritation
  D. Usually occurring in adults (mostly men) under age 45 years
  E. Occurring anywhere along the spine; however, sites usually affected between L4 and L5, L5 and sacrum, C5 and C6, and C6 and C7

F. After trauma in lumbosacral area: pain possibly beginning suddenly, subsiding briefly, recurring at shorter intervals with progressive intensity; sciatic pain following; Valsalva maneuver, sneezing, coughing, or bending magnifying pain, accompanied by muscle spasms

G. Possibly causing sensory and motor loss in area innervated by compressed spinal nerve root followed by weakness and atrophy of affected muscles

H. Causes
1. Severe trauma or strain
2. Intervertebral joint degeneration
3. Congenitally small lumbar spinal canal

II. Data collection
A. Subjective symptoms
1. Cervical disk
a. Stiff neck
b. Shoulder pain descending down arm into hand
c. Numbness of arm and hand
2. Lumbosacral disk: severe low back pain radiating down buttocks, legs, and feet—usually unilaterally

B. Objective symptoms
1. Cervical disk: sensory disturbances of neck, arm, and hand
2. Lumbosacral disk
a. LeSegue's signs: pain in back and legs, loss of ankle or knee-jerk reflex with client lying flat, thighs and knees flexed 90 degrees while raising heel with knee straight
b. Straight-leg raising test: pain in posterior leg (sciatic pain) with client lying supine, examiner placing one hand on client's ilium and other hand under ankle, while slowly raising client's leg
c. Difficulty in ambulating
d. Numbness of leg and foot

III. Diagnostic tests and methods
A. Client history
B. Physical examination
C. Neurological examination
D. X-rays of spine
E. CAT scan of spine
F. Peripheral vascular status check: posterior tibial and dorsalis pedis pulses, and skin temperature of extremities to rule out ischemic vascular disease
G. Myelography
H. Electromyography

IV. Implementation
A. Assess, report, and record signs and symptoms and any reaction to treatment.
B. Encourage verbalization of fears and other feelings related to immobility.
C. Assess allergies to iodides (such as seafood) before myelography (may indicate sensitivity to radiopaque dye used in diagnostic test).
D. After myelography
1. Have client remain supine in bed.
2. Provide increased fluid intake to prevent renal stasis; monitor I&O.
3. Monitor for allergic reaction to dye.

E. Encourage deep breathing, coughing, and use of blow bottles to prevent pulmonary complications.
F. Provide meticulous skin care.
G. Assess bowel function and use fracture bedpan when client is receiving complete bedrest.
H. Monitor for abnormal neurological signs.
I. Apply antiembolism stockings as ordered.
J. Observe traction (cervical traction for cervical disk involvement; traction to lower extremities for lumbosacral disk involvement):
1. Check that weights are hanging free and have not fallen.
2. Observe for frayed ropes and loosened knots.
3. Maintain proper body alignment.
K. Provide diet high in fiber with adequate fluid intake to prevent constipation and straining.
L. Encourage client to move legs, if allowed.
M. Provide high-topped sneakers to prevent footdrop.
N. Coordinate prescribed exercises with physical therapist to ensure consistent regimen.
O. Prepare client for surgical intervention, if required (laminectomy or spinal fusion).
P. Provide postoperative care:
1. Enforce bedrest.
2. Monitor for leakage of cerebrospinal fluid (CSF) on surgical dressing; reinforce dressing until checked by physician.
3. Log-roll client to change position to prevent motion of spinal column.
4. Check tubing of Hemovac blood-draining system for kinks and patent vacuum.
5. Empty Hemovac at end of each shift; record amount and color of drainage.
6. Monitor neurovascular status of involved extremities; color, temperature, sensation, and mobility.
7. Monitor bowel sounds and abdomen for distention.
8. Administer prescribed analgesics.
9. Assist client during first ambulation attempt.
10. Instruct client with spinal fusion on how to wear a brace.
11. Assist with straight-leg raising and toe-pointing exercises as ordered.
Q. Prepare client for chemonucleolysis, if required:
1. Check for allergic reaction to radiopaque dyes or meat tenderizers, which are similar to chemical used (chymopapain) for procedure.
R. After chemonucleolysis procedure
1. Enforce bedrest.
2. Administer analgesics for pain as prescribed.
3. Apply heat to area, if ordered.
4. Assist with special exercises as prescribed.
S. Instruct client and family regarding proper body mechanics.
T. Advise client to use a firm mattress and to sleep on side rather than abdomen.
U. Encourage weight loss if client is obese to prevent lordosis.
V. Explain condition, diagnostic procedures, treatment, prevention, and home care.

V. Evaluation
  A. Client reports increased comfort and decreased anxiety.
  B. Client remains free of injury or infection.
  C. Client maintains adequate elimination patterns.
  D. Client maintains adequate level of mobility.
  E. Client verbalizes feelings and devlops a positive self-image.
  F. Client understands reason for weight reduction if obese.
  G. Client demonstrates an understanding of condition, diagnostic procedures, treatment, prevention, home care including activity, and follow-up care.

Fractures

I. Description
  A. Usually resulting from trauma and often causing substantial muscle, nerve, and other soft-tissue damage
  B. Prognosis varies with:
    1. Extent of disability or deformity
    2. Amount of tissue and vascular damage
    3. Adequacy of reduction and immobilization
    4. Client's health status, age, and nutritional status
  C. Possibility of bones of adults in poor health, along with impaired circulation, not to heal properly
  D. Severe open fractures, especially those involving the femoral shaft, possibly causing considerable bleeding and life-threatening hypovolemic shock
  E. Types of fractures
    1. Incomplete: break extending only partially through bone
    2. Complete: bone breaking into two or more pieces.
    3. Closed (simple): overlying skin remaining unbroken
    4. Open (compound): wound present over fractured area; fractured bone breaking through skin
    5. Nondisplaced: fractured bone remaining in proper alignment
    6. Transverse: break running transversally (straight across) the bone shaft
    7. Spiral: break encircling bone like a coil
    8. Oblique: bone broken at a diagonal angle
    9. Comminuted: bone shattered or compressed into bone fragments
    10. Impacted: bone ends driven into each other
    11. Compression: bone (vertebrae) collapsing under excessive pressure
    12. Linear: break running length of bone
    13. Greenstick: bone splintering fibers on one side of bone, leaving other side intact
    14. Avulsion: overexertion resulting in tearing of a muscle or ligament from a bone, pulling a small bone fragment with it
    15. Depression: bone fragments driven inward by trauma (usually referring to fracture of the skull)
  F. Complications of fractures of the extremities
    1. Permanent deformity and dysfunction caused by failure of bones to heal (nonunion) or bones healing improperly (malunion)
    2. Hypovolemic shock as a result of blood vessel damage
    3. Muscle contractures
    4. Aseptic necrosis of bone segments because of decreased circulation
    5. Renal calculi forming decalcification because of prolonged immobilization
    6. Fat embolism
  G. Causes
    1. Most fractures occur from major trauma.
    2. Pathological fractures occur because of underlying conditions of osteoporosis, bone tumors, or metabolic disease.
    3. Prolonged standing, walking, or running may cause stress fractures of foot and ankle (usually seen in postal workers, nurses, soldiers, and joggers).

II. Data collection
  A. Subjective symptoms
    1. Pain: usually intense and acute; worsening with pressure or movement
    2. Loss of movement of affected extremity
    3. Loss of sensory perception distal to fracture site
    4. Point tenderness
    5. Numbness and tingling
  B. Objective symptoms
    1. Pallor
    2. Limited motion or paralysis of affected limb distal to fracture site
    3. Deformity of affected limb
    4. Edema; discoloration
    5. Crepitus on movement of limb
    6. Warmth over site
    7. Possible arterial compromise or nerve damage
      a. Mottled cyanosis
      b. Cool skin at end of extremity
      c. Loss of pulses distal to injury
      d. Signs of shock
    8. Evidence of fracture on x-ray

III. Diagnostic tests and methods
  A. Client history
  B. Physical examination
  C. X-ray of suspected fracture sites and associated joints

IV. Implementation
  A. Assess, report, and record signs and symptoms and any reaction to treatment.
  B. Splint or immobilize injured area.
  C. Monitor vital signs; observe for shock symptoms (rapid pulse, decreased BP, cool clammy skin, and pallor).
  D. Assist in administration of IV fluids as ordered.
  E. Administer analgesics and/or muscle relaxants as prescribed.
  F. Apply ice compress to injured area as ordered.
  G. Discuss use of relaxation techniques.
  H. Prepare client for surgical intervention and provide postoperative care as indicated.
  I. Assist with passive and active ROM of unaffected limbs; maintain mobility.
  J. Assist with appropriate exercise to affected limb as ordered.

K. Encourage client to participate in self-care activities.
L. Provide a well-balanced nutritional diet: high in protein and vitamins, high in bulk.
M. Encourage adequate fluid intake to prevent bowel and urinary problems.
N. Monitor for signs of fat embolism (apprehension, sweating, fever, tachycardia, pallor, dyspnea, petechial rash on chest and shoulders, pulmonary effusion, tissue hypoxia, cyanosis, convulsions, coma).
O. Turn client, if not contraindicated, every 2 hours, maintaining proper alignment.
P. Encourage use of isometric exercises to prevent muscle atrophy.
Q. Types of traction
  1. Buck's traction: used to ease muscle spasm and immobilize limb by maintaining a straight pull on limb using weights
  2. Russell's traction: used to alleviate muscle spasm and immobilize limb by maintaining a pull at knee and foot with use of knee sling
  3. Skeletal traction: direct application of traction to bone with use of wires or pins (Steinmann pin, Kirschner wire) that are pulled by traction weights
  4. Crutchfield tongs: tongs inserted into shallow holes in the skull and joined to skeletal traction for fractures of the cervical vertebrae
R. Care for long-term immobilization with traction:
  1. Reposition client often to increase comfort and to prevent formation of decubitus ulcers.
  2. Assist with ROM exercises to prevent muscle atrophy.
  3. Encourage deep breathing and coughing to prevent pulmonary complications.
  4. Encourage adequate fluid intake to prevent urinary stasis and constipation.
  5. Monitor for signs of renal colic (flank pain, nausea, and vomiting).
  6. Maintain proper body alignment.
  7. Check ropes and weights for proper placement (weights should hang freely).
  8. Provide meticulous skin care.
  9. Avoid bumping into or manipulating traction device.
  10. Inspect site of pins and affected limb frequently.
  11. Monitor site of cervical tongs: provide meticulous skin care using aseptic technique.
  12. Use Posey footboard to prevent footdrop; use high-topped sneaker on unaffected leg.
  13. Monitor circulation; check for signs of thrombophlebitis.
S. Cast care:
  1. Support cast with pillows while still wet.
  2. Observe for skin irritation near cast edges.
  3. Check for foul odors or discharge.
  4. Instruct client to report signs of decreased circulation to the part (skin coldness, tingling, numbness, discoloration of toes or fingers).
  5. Instruct client to keep cast dry.
  6. Instruct client to avoid inserting foreign objects under the cast.

T. Encourage movement as soon as possible.
U. Assist with ambulation.
V. Demonstrate the correct method of walking with crutches (placing weight on hands and not on axillary region) to prevent damage to nerves.
W. After cast removal, refer to physical therapist for assistance in restoring limb mobility.
X. Explain condition, diagnostic procedures, treatment, prevention, home care including activity, and follow-up care.
V. Evaluation
  A. Client reports increased comfort and decreased anxiety.
  B. Client remains free of injury or infection.
  C. Client maintains safe environment.
  D. Client maintains adequate level of mobility.
  E. Client maintains good skin integrity.
  F. Client maintains adequate elimination pattern.
  G. Client maintains adequate tissue perfusion.
  H. Client maintains adequate nutritional intake.
  I. Client demonstrates an understanding of condition, diagnostic procedures, treatment, prevention, home care, and follow-up care.

Amputation

I. Description
  A. Two types: surgical and traumatic
  B. Surgical amputation: surgical removal of part or all of an extremity.
    1. Majority resulting from vascular disorders causing an inadequate oxygen supply to the tissue
    2. Other reasons for amputation: septic wounds, gas gangrene, malignant tumors, severe trauma, burns
  C. Traumatic amputation: the accidental loss of a body part, such as an arm, leg, finger, or toe
    1. In complete amputation, the part is completely severed.
    2. In partial amputation, some soft tissue remains.
    3. Prognosis has improved because of:
      a. Improved emergency and critical care management
      b. New surgical techniques
      c. New prosthetic designs
      d. Early rehabilitation
      e. Innovative limb reimplantation techniques used but their usefulness limited by incomplete nerve regeneration
    4. Causes: accidents involving farm, factory, motor vehicles, use of power tools, or war
II. Data collection
  A. Subjective symptoms (surgical amputation)
    1. Peripheral vascular diseases: pain, tingling
    2. Septic wounds and gas gangrene: pain
  B. Objective symptoms (surgical amputation)
    1. Peripheral vascular diseases
      a. Pallor
      b. Edema
      c. Diminished pulses
      d. Cyanosis

e. Ulcer formation
f. Hyperpigmentation
2. Septic wounds, gas gangrene
  a. Foul odor
  b. Blackened wound
  c. Edema
  d. Fever
  e. Necrosis
C. Subjective symptoms (traumatic amputation)
  1. Pain
D. Objective symptoms (traumatic amputation)
  1. Profuse bleeding
  2. Hypovolemic shock:
    a. Hypotension
    b. Narrowing pulse pressure
    c. Tachycardia
    d. Rapid, shallow respirations
    e. Oliguria
    f. Cold, clammy skin
    g. Metabolic acidosis

III. Diagnostic tests and methods
A. Both surgical and traumatic amputations
  1. Client history
  2. Physical examination
B. Surgical amputations
  1. Arteriography
  2. Oscillometry
  3. X-ray
  4. Skin temperature studies

IV. Implementation
A. Surgical amputation
  1. Assess, report, and record signs and symptoms and any reaction to treatment.
  2. Prepare client and family for surgical intervention.
  3. Encourage verbalization of feeling.
  4. Provide emotional support.
  5. Explain phantom pain (pain in amputated limb).
  6. Explain postoperative plan:
    a. Program of exercises
      1) Exercises for strengthening upper extremities
      2) Transferring from bed to chair and vice versa
      3) Ambulating with walker or crutches
  7. Provide postoperative care:
    a. Provide routine postoperative care.
    b. Provide reassurance to help client cope with altered body image.
    c. Apply Ace bandages in a figure-eight pattern only.
    d. Monitor for signs of bleeding; have a tourniquet at bedside for emergency use.
    e. Elevate stump 8–12 hours on a pillow.
    f. Remove pillow after 12 hours to prevent hip contracture.
    g. Place client in prone position every 4 hours to prevent hip contracture.
    h. Place trochanter roll along outer side of stump to prevent outward rotation.
    i. Instruct client to massage the stump to improve vascularity.
    j. Instruct client regarding conditioning of the stump to prepare for application of a prosthesis:
      1) Push stump against a pillow.
      2) Progress by pushing stump against a harder surface.
    k. Instruct client to avoid letting stump hang over edge of bed or chair to prevent stump contracture.
      1) Use transcutaneous electrical nerve stimulator (TENS) for relief of phantom pain, if ordered.
  8. Explain condition, diagnostic procedures, treatment, prevention, home care, and follow-up care.
B. Traumatic amputation
  1. Emergency treatment
    a. Monitor vital signs.
    b. Cleanse wound.
    c. Administer prescribed tetanus prophylaxis, antibiotics, and analgesics.
    d. After complete amputation
      1) Preserve extremity in cooled sterile normal saline solution within a sterile plastic bag.
      2) Notify reimplantation surgeon.
    e. After partial amputation
      1) Position limb in normal alignment.
      2) Drape with sterile towels soaked in sterile normal saline solution.
  2. Preoperative care: assist with thorough wound irrigation and debridement.
  3. Postoperative care
    a. Change dressing using sterile technique.
    b. Provide reassurance to help client cope with altered body image.
    c. Provide rehabilitation as in postoperative care of surgical amputation.

V. Evaluation
A. Client reports increased comfort and decreased anxiety.
B. Client remains free of injury or infection.
C. Client maintains adequate level of mobility.
D. Client maintains good skin integrity.
E. Client verbalizes feelings, develops positive self-image and self-concept.
F. Client uses effective coping strategies to cope with altered body image.
G. Client participates in self-care activities.
H. Client demonstrates an understanding of condition, treatment, home care, and follow-up care.

The Eyes

Basic Information

Visual acuity depends on general good health, CNS regulation of movement and conduction, and condition of eye structures. Vision disorders frequently indicate systemic disease. Disorders that affect the eye usually lead to impairment or loss of vision. Routine eye examination can provide information regarding diseases in other body systems. The incidence of visual impairment and blindness increases with age; however, individuals of all ages can be affected. Vision has recently been the focus of innovative medical and surgical treatment. Routine and early eye examinations, along with early treatment, are essential.

I. Basic data collection
   A. Subjective symptoms
      1. Double vision
      2. Blurred or clouded vision
      3. Decreased or absent vision
      4. Sensitivity to light
      5. Spots, halos around lights
      6. Flashes of light
      7. Problems seeing in dark
      8. Itching, pain, tearing, burning, headache
   B. Objective symptoms
      1. Tearing, discharge: clear or purulent
      2. Color of sclera: white, yellow, or pink
      3. Glasses or contact lenses
      4. Accuracy and range of vision
      5. Crusts, blinking, rubbing
      6. Edema of eyelids
      7. Squinting or drooping of lid
      8. Symmetry
      9. History of:
         a. Trauma to eyes
         b. Contact lenses
         c. Eye medications
         d. Changes in vision
         e. Systemic medications in use

Major Diagnoses Related to the Eyes

Cataract

I. Description
   A. Clouding or opacity of the lens, which prevents light rays from reaching the retina
   B. Commonly occurring bilaterally, with each progressing independently
   C. Most prevalent in persons over age 70 years, as part of aging process
   D. Surgical improvement of vision in 95% of affected individuals
   E. Causes
      1. Aging process (senile cataract)
      2. Injury to eye (traumatic cataract)
      3. Resulting from another eye disease (secondary cataract)
      4. Inherited trait (congenital cataract)
      5. Metabolic disease such as diabetes mellitus
      6. Infections
II. Data collection
   A. Subjective symptoms
      1. Progressive blurred vision
      2. Hazy vision
      3. Poor reading vision
      4. Seeing halos around lights
      5. Perceiving blinding glare from headlights
      6. Poor vision in sunlight
      7. Improvement of vision in dim light when pupils dilate (for clients with central opacities)
      8. Loss of vision

   B. Objective symptoms
      1. Opaque or cloudy-white pupil
      2. Less than 20/200 on visual testing
III. Diagnostic tests and methods
   A. Client history
   B. Physical examination
   C. Examination with ophthalmoscope
   D. Slit-lamp examination
IV. Implementation
   A. Assess, report, and record signs and symptoms and any reaction to treatment.
   B. Provide a safe environment; keep necessary items in specific areas within reach.
   C. Administer prescribed preoperative eye medication to dilate pupil for surgery.
   D. Provide postoperative care to prevent increased intraocular pressure:
      1. Position client on unoperative side.
      2. Administer prescribed analgesics and medication.
      3. Instruct client to avoid any actions that may increase intraocular pressure, such as straining, bending, or performing rapid head movements.
      4. Administer stool softener as ordered to prevent straining during bowel movement.
      5. Administer prescribed antiemetic to prevent vomiting.
      6. Monitor dressing: check for bleeding.
      7. Keep client supine or in low-Fowler's position as ordered.
      8. Prevent infection; administer antibiotic ointment or drops.
      9. Administer prescribed steroids to reduce inflammation.
      10. Monitor eye shield or dressing, if appropriate.
   E. Assist with self-care activities and ambulation.
   F. Instruct client and family in correct instillation of eyedrops.
   G. Monitor for complications such as prolapse of iris or sudden sharp pain in eye.
   H. Explain condition, diagnostic procedures, and treatment, home care, and follow-up care:
      1. Avoiding heavy lifting for several weeks
      2. Activity
      3. Use of eye shield
      4. Medications
V. Evaluation
   A. Client reports increased comfort and decreased anxiety.
   B. Client remains free of injury or infection.
   C. Client maintains adequate sensory perception.
   D. Client demonstrates an understanding of condition, diagnostic procedures, treatment, home care, and follow-up care.

Retinal Detachment

I. Description
   A. Sensory layer of the retina pulling away from pigmented layer
   B. Vitreous humor possibly leaking into space between the separated layers

C. Usually unilateral; most commonly affects men
D. New surgical techniques used to reattach retinal layers in about 90% of clients
E. Causes
  1. Degenerative changes of aging, resulting in a spontaneous retinal hole caused by shrinkage and pulling away of the vitreous framework
F. Predisposing factors
  1. Myopia
  2. Cataracts
  3. Surgery
  4. Trauma
  5. Result of systemic diseases
    a. Severe hypertension
    b. Chronic glomerulonephritis
    c. Diabetes mellitus
    d. Vascular changes in retina (retinal vein occlusion)
II. Data collection
  A. Subjective symptoms
    1. Floating spots from blood or retina cells as a result of tears
    2. Recurrent flashes of light
    3. Gradual, painless loss of vision
  B. Objective symptoms
    1. Loss of vision
    2. Retina separation on ophthalmoscopic exam
III. Diagnostic tests and methods
  A. Client history
  B. Physical examination
  C. Ophthalmoscopy after full pupil dilation
IV. Implementation
  A. Assess, report, and record signs and symptoms and any reaction to treatment.
  B. Provide bedrest; position head to relieve stress on tear.
  C. Restrict activity; use eye patch or eye shield to limit eye movement.
  D. Provide emotional support.
  E. Provide a calm, safe, restful environment, with siderails up and call signal within easy reach.
  F. Apply cool compresses as ordered to decrease swelling and discomfort.
  G. Instruct client to avoid activities that cause sudden movement of head, such as sneezing, coughing, or vomiting.
  H. Administer cough medications or antiemetics as ordered.
  I. Assist client with ADLs.
  J. Administer prescribed eye medications, such as mydriatics, antibiotics, or steroids.
  K. Administer prescribed analgesics.
  L. Prepare client and family for surgical intervention:
    1. Wash client's face with prescribed surgical soap preparation.
    2. Cut off eyelashes to decrease risk of infection.
    3. Administer antibiotics and mydriatic eyedrops as prescribed.
  M. Provide postoperative care:
    1. Position client as ordered (usually by elevating head of bed about 30 degrees).
    2. Instruct client to avoid bending over, straining, or rubbing eyes.
    3. Assist with ambulation when ordered.
    4. If restricted to prolonged bedrest, encourage leg exercises to prevent thrombophlebitis.
    5. Cleanse eye with warm compresses and instill prescribed ophthalmic medications.
    6. Monitor for possible complications, such as signs of bleeding or retinal detachment.
    7. Instruct client and family in instillation of eyedrops and ointments.
    8. Advise client to use dark glasses in bright light.
  N. Explain condition, diagnostic procedures, treatment, home care, and follow-up care.
V. Evaluation
  A. Client reports increased comfort and decreased anxiety.
  B. Client maintains adequate sensory perception.
  C. Client demonstrates an understanding of condition, diagnostic procedures, treatment, home care, and follow-up care.

Glaucoma

I. Description
  A. Abnormal increase in intraocular pressure, which may result in severe and permanent vision defects
  B. Increased intraocular pressure caused by disturbance in circulation of aqueous humor resulting from imbalance between production and drainage, as the angle of drainage closes
  C. Possibly secondary to injuries and infections
  D. Most preventable cause of blindness
  E. Affecting approximately 2% of individuals >40 years old in the United States
  F. Affecting women more often than men
  G. Accounting for 15% of all cases of blindness in the United States
  H. Normal intraocular pressure ranges from 10–21 mm Hg
  I. Requiring early diagnosis to prevent damage to the optic nerve and blindness
  J. Prognosis usually good with early diagnosis and treatment
  K. Several forms
    1. Chronic open-angle (most common)
      a. Caused by overproduction of aqueous humor or obstruction to its outflow
      b. Frequently familial in origin, affecting 90% of all individuals with glaucoma
      c. Usually bilateral, with insidious onset
      d. Symptoms usually appearing late in the disease
    2. Acute closed-angle (narrow-angle): obstruction to outflow of aqueous humor
      a. Resulting from:
        1) Anatomically narrow angle between anterior iris and posterior corneal surface
        2) Shallow anterior chamber
        3) Bulging iris that presses on the trabeculae (fibrous cords of connective tissue), closing the angle

              4) Thickened iris causing closure of the angle on pupil dilation
           b. Rapid onset; produces blindness in 3–5 days if not treated promptly
           c. Symptoms possibly misinterpreted as GI distress
        3. Chronic closed-angle
           a. Resulting from:
              1) Untreated acute closed-angle glaucoma
              2) Mild, recurring acute attacks resulting in adhesions in the trabeculae
           b. Gradual onset
           c. Progressing to absolute glaucoma with pain and blindness
           d. Enucleation possibly necessary to relieve extreme pain
 II. Data collection
     A. Subjective symptoms (chronic open-angle glaucoma)
        1. Asymptomatic early in disease
        2. Mild aching in eyes
        3. Loss of peripheral vision
        4. Seeing halos around lights
        5. Reduced visual acuity, especially at night (not corrected with glasses)
     B. Subjective symptoms (acute closed-angle glaucoma)
        1. Unilateral pain
        2. Pressure over eye
        3. Blurred vision
        4. Decreased visual acuity
        5. Seeing halos around lights
        6. Nausea
     C. Subjective symptoms (chronic closed-angle glaucoma)
        1. Usually producing no symptoms
        2. Blurred vision possible
        3. Seeing halos around lights possible
        4. Severe pain if not treated
     D. Objective symptoms
        1. Elevated intraocular pressure with tonometry
        2. Inflammation
        3. Decreased peripheral vision with testing
        4. Photophobia
        5. Optic-disk cupping on ophthalmoscopic examination
        6. Vomiting
        7. Loss of vision
III. Diagnostic tests and methods
     A. Client history
     B. Physical examination
     C. Tonometry
     D. Gonioscopy: to differentiate between chronic open-angle and acute or chronic closed-angle glaucoma
     E. Ophthalmoscopy
     F. Slit-lamp examination
     G. Fingertip tension: to check whether one eye feels harder than other (as occurs in acute closed-angle glaucoma) on gentle palpation of closed eyelids
     H. Perimetry or visual field tests: to evaluate extent of chronic open-angle or closed-angle deterioration
 IV. Implementation

     A. Assess, report, and record signs and symptoms and any reaction to treatment.
     B. Explain and administer prescribed eyedrops to decrease aqueous humor production or facilitate drainage (miotic agent pilocarpine; beta-blocker timolol maleate).
     C. Explain the need for lifetime compliance in the use of eye medications to prevent disk changes, loss of vision, and need for surgery.
     D. Prepare client and family for surgical intervention, if required.
     E. Provide postoperative care:
        1. Administer cycloplegic eyedrops to affected eye:
           a. Decrease inflammation and relax ciliary muscle.
           b. Prevent adhesions.
        2. Administer prescribed analgesics for eye pain.
        3. Administer prescribed eye medications to dilate pupil.
        4. Administer prescribed steroids to rest the pupil.
        5. Protect eye with eye patch or eye shield.
        6. Assist with positioning on unoperative side.
        7. Provide safe environment, with siderails up and call signal within easy reach.
     F. Educate client and family in the importance of glaucoma screening for early detection and prevention.
     G. Explain condition, diagnostic procedures, treatment, home care, and follow-up care:
        1. Explain lifetime medication regimen.
        2. Explain type of medication, including any side effects.
        3. Instruct client to report to physician any eye pain, changes in vision, or seeing halos around lights immediately.
  V. Evaluation
     A. Client reports increased comfort and decreased anxiety.
     B. Client remains free of injury or infection.
     C. Client maintains adequate sensory perception.
     D. Client demonstrates an understanding of condition, diagnostic procedures, treatment, home care, and follow-up care.

Conjunctivitis

  I. Description
     A. Infection or inflammation of the conjunctiva because of infection, allergy, or chemical reactions
     B. Usually benign and self-limiting
     C. Possibly chronic, indicative of degenerative changes or damage from repeated attacks
     D. Most common eye disorder in the Western Hemisphere
     E. Very contagious (especially in young children)
     F. Usually beginning in one eye and spreading to other eye via contaminated towels, washcloths, or client's own hands
     G. Causes
        1. Bacterial infections
        2. Chlamydial infections

3. Viral infections
4. Allergic reactions to pollen, grass, air pollutants (e.g., smoke), topical medication, unknown seasonal allergens, occupational irritants, and rickettsial and parasitic diseases

II. Data collection
  A. Subjective symptoms
    1. Itching
    2. Burning
    3. Sensation of foreign body in eye
    4. Pain
  B. Objective symptoms
    1. Photophobia
    2. Tearing
    3. Sticky, mucopurulent discharge
    4. Profuse, purulent discharge if caused by *Neisseria gonorrhoeae*
    5. Enlarged preauricular lymph node if caused by viral infection

III. Diagnostic tests and methods
  A. Client history
  B. Physical examination
  C. Conjunctival scrapings
  D. Culture and sensitivity tests for bacterial infections

IV. Implementation
  A. Assess, report, and record signs and symptoms and any reaction to treatment.
  B. Apply warm compresses to affected eye.
  C. Cleanse affected eyelid, using warm compresses and removing crusts, before administering eye medications.
  D. Administer prescribed ointment or drops.
  E. Instruct client in correct instillation of eyedrops and ointments.
  F. Advise client to wear safety glasses when working near chemical irritants.
  G. Educate client and family regarding spread of infection:
    1. Teach proper handwashing technique.
    2. Avoid sharing washcloths, towels, and pillows.
    3. Isolate personal items (washcloths, towels, pillows).
    4. Instruct client to avoid rubbing affected eye.
    5. Instruct client not to irrigate eye.
    6. Use clean washcloths and towels frequently to avoid infecting other eye.
  H. Explain condition, diagnostic procedures, treatment, and home care including medication.

V. Evaluation
  A. Client reports increased comfort and decreased anxiety.
  B. Client remains free of injury or infection.
  C. Client demonstrates an understanding of condition, treatment, infection control, and home care.

The Ears

Basic Information

Hearing is initiated by sound waves reaching the tympanic membrane, causing a vibration of the ossicles in the middle ear. The stapes transmit the vibrations to the perilymphatic fluid in the inner ear by vibrating against the oval window. These vibrations then pass across the cochlea's fluid receptor cells, stimulating movement of the hair cells of the organ of Corti and initiating auditory nerve impulses to the brain.

The inner ear structure also maintains the equilibrium and balance of the body. The fluid in the semicircular canals is set into motion by body movement and stimulates nerve cells lining the canal. These cells transmit impulses to the brain via the vestibular branch of the acoustic nerve.

The sense of hearing contributes to well-being and safety. Initially, hearing problems are usually not as obvious as other disorders. Many individuals refuse to wear hearing aids because they associate hearing loss with dependency or disfigurement. Hearing should be assessed for each client.

Conductive hearing loss is a result of injury, obstruction, or disease that interferes with sound wave conduction to the inner ear (e.g., wax in the ear canal). Sensory hearing loss is a result of a malfunction of the inner ear, the auditory nerve, or the auditory center in the brain.

I. Data collection
  A. Subjective symptoms
    1. Difficulty in hearing
    2. Vertigo
    3. Pain
    4. Blurred vision
    5. Headache
    6. Itching, pressure (or "full" feeling)
    7. Ringing, popping, buzzing
  B. Objective symptoms
    1. Drainage
    2. Hearing loss
    3. Nonresponse to loud noises
    4. Vomiting
    5. Tenderness
    6. Dried secretions
    7. Deformities of ear
    8. Presence of hearing aid
    9. Notation of history of:
      a. Ear infections
      b. Ear surgery
      c. Head injury
      d. Medications

Major Diagnoses Related to the Ears

Ménière's Disease

I. Description
  A. Chronic disease of the inner ear characterized by sudden attacks of vertigo, tinnitus (ringing in the ears), and hearing loss, which results in alterations in body equilibrium and balance
  B. Attacks lasting a few minutes to several weeks
  C. Usually affecting men more often than women, between the ages of 30 and 60 years
  D. Possibly leading to residual tinnitus and hearing loss if attacks continue over time
  E. Symptoms possibly not apparent between attacks (except for tinnitus, which worsens during an attack)
  F. Attacks several times per year or remissions possible, which can last several years

G. Attacks eventually becoming less frequent with increasing hearing loss
H. Attacks possibly ceasing entirely with total hearing loss
I. Surgical destruction of the affected labyrinth possibly required to relieve symptoms permanently if disorder persists for >2 years of treatment or produces constant vertigo (resulting in permanent, irreversible hearing loss)
J. Unknown causes
K. Precipitating factors
    1. Autonomic nervous system dysfunction resulting in a temporary constriction of blood vessels that supply inner ear
    2. Premenstrual edema
    3. Viral infection
II. Data collection
  A. Subjective symptoms
    1. Vertigo
    2. Nausea
    3. Tinnitus, hearing loss
    4. Headache
    5. History of ear infection
    6. Fullness or blocked feeling in ear
    7. Loss of balance
  B. Objective symptoms
    1. Nystagmus
    2. Vomiting
    3. Diaphoresis
    4. Sensorineural hearing loss demonstrated with audiometry and vestibular testing
III. Diagnostic tests and methods
  A. Client history
  B. Physical examination
  C. Neurological assessment
  D. Caloric testing
  E. X-ray
IV. Implementation
  A. Assess, report, and record signs and symptoms and any reaction to treatment.
  B. Provide bedrest during attacks.
  C. Advise client to avoid reading and exposure to bright lights to minimize vertigo.
  D. Provide a safe environment; keep siderails up.
  E. Assist with ADLs and ambulation.
  F. Instruct client to move slowly to prevent vertigo.
  G. Instruct client to avoid sudden position changes.
  H. Administer prescribed medications, such as diuretics, vasodilators, antibiotics, antiemetics, and steroids.
  I. Provide a low-sodium diet.
  J. Provide care same as that for client with limited hearing (see under Basic Information).
  K. Prepare client and family for surgical intervention, if necessary.
  L. Provide postoperative care:
    1. Give general postoperative care.
    2. Record fluid I&O.
    3. Advise client to expect vertigo and nausea for 1–2 days.
    4. Administer prophylactic antibiotics and antiemetics as ordered.
    5. Instruct client to move slowly.

    6. Assist with ambulation while equilibrium is impaired.
  M. Assist with coping and comfort measures.
  N. Explain condition, diagnostic procedures, treatment, and home care including activities.
V. Evaluation
  A. Client reports increased comfort and decreased anxiety.
  B. Client remains free of injury or infection.
  C. Client maintains adequate auditory sensory perception.
  D. Client use effective coping strategies.
  E. Client demonstrates an understanding of condition, diagnostic procedures, treatment, and home care.

Otosclerosis

I. Description
  A. Disorder of the middle ear characterized by a slow formation of spongy bone around the stapes
  B. Prevents normal movement of the stapes, resulting in disruption of the conduction of vibrations from the tympanic membrane to the cochlea, which causes progressive hearing loss of the affected ear, possibly progressing to the unaffected ear
  C. Affects approximately 10% of whites between the ages of 15 and 30 years
  D. Prevalence 50% higher in women than in men
  E. Prognosis good with surgery
II. Data collection
  A. Subjective symptoms
    1. Hearing loss
    2. Tinnitus
    3. Ability to hear conversation better in a noisy environment than a quiet one (paracusis of Willis)
  B. Objective symptoms
    1. Positive findings on audiometric testing
    2. Conductive loss, as demonstrated by Weber's and Rinne's tests
III. Diagnostic tests and methods
  A. Client history
  B. Physical examination
  C. Rinne's test
  D. Weber's test
  E. Audiometric testing
IV. Implementation
  A. Assess, report, and record signs and symptoms and any reaction to treatment.
  B. Monitor for degree of hearing loss.
  C. Provide a safe environment, and assist with ADLs as necessary.
  D. Prepare client and family for stapedectomy (removal of stapes) and insertion of plastic or stainless steel prosthesis for the purpose of restoring hearing in the middle ear.
  E. Provide postoperative care:
    1. Keep client flat with head turned so that affected ear is turned upward (which assists in maintaining position of the prosthesis).
    2. Instruct client to avoid sneezing, coughing, blowing nose (if sneezing unavoidable, instruct

client to keep mouth open to equalize ear pressure).
3. Administer prescribed antibiotics, analgesics, and antiemetics.
4. Instruct client to move slowly to decrease vertigo episodes.
5. Monitor for presence of nausea, vomiting, vertigo, headache, or abnormal ear sensations.
6. Assist with activities as necessary.
7. Reassure client that hearing will improve when packing is removed and edema disappears.
F. Prepare client for use of a hearing aid (air conduction aid with molded ear insert receiver) as a substitute procedure if stapedectomy is not possible; it enables one to hear conversations in normal surroundings, although it is not as effective as a stapedectomy.
G. Provide discharge instructions:
1. Instruct client to avoid loud noises and sudden pressure changes (flying or diving) until healing is complete (usually 6 months).
2. Instruct client to avoid blowing nose for at least 1 week to prevent contaminated air and bacteria from entering the eustachian tube.
3. Advise client to protect ears against cold.
4. Advise client to avoid contact with individuals who have upper respiratory infections.
5. Instruct client to avoid any activities that produce vertigo, such as bending, heavy lifting, straining.
6. Teach client and family to change the external ear dressing and care for the surgical incision.
7. Advise the client and family of the necessity to complete the prescribed antibiotic regimen.
H. Explain condition, diagnostic procedures, treatment, home care, and follow-up care.
V. Evaluation
A. Client reports increased comfort.
B. Client remains free of injury or infection.
C. Client maintains adequate auditory perception.
D. Client demonstrates an understanding of condition, diagnostic procedures, treatment, home care, and follow-up care.

Neurological System

Basic Information

The neurological system consists of the communication network responsible for coordinating and organizing the functions of all body systems. There are three main divisions: the CNS, which is the control center of the body (brain and spinal cord); the peripheral nervous system, which includes nerves communicating with distant body parts, relaying and receiving messages from them; and the autonomic nervous system, regulating involuntary functions of the internal organs.

The pathology involving the CNS arises from injuries, vascular insufficiency, tumors, infections, and disorders from other diseases. Neurological medical problems are caused by interference with normal functioning of the affected cells.

I. Basic data collection
A. Subjective symptoms
1. History of head injury, vertigo, weakness, headache, loss of consciousness, paralysis, seizures, double vision
2. Pain, numbness, difficulty concentrating, memory loss, drowsiness, difficulty with elimination
B. Objective symptoms
1. Orientation to person, time, and place
2. Mental status (drowsiness, lethargy)
3. Level of consciousness (arousal status to verbal and physical stimuli)
a. Use of Glasgow coma scale to describe level of consciousness
1) Eye opening
2) Verbal response
3) Motor response
4. Emotional response
5. Speech: presence of aphasia, appropriate speech patterns
6. Behavior: appropriate for situation
7. Ability to follow simple instructions
8. Vital signs (temperature, pulse, respirations, and BP)
9. Motor function: gait, balance, coordination, strength, posture, and function
10. Eyes
a. Movement of lids and pupils
b. Size, configuration, and reaction of pupils to light
c. Comparison from baseline assessment
11. Ears: drainage
12. Facial symmetry
13. Sensation for pain, smell, and light
14. Bladder and bowel control

Major Neurological Diagnoses

Cerebrovascular Accident (Stroke)

I. Description
A. Sudden impairment of the circulation in one or more of the blood vessels supplying the brain; blood vessels occluded, stenosed, or ruptured
B. Oxygen supply to the affected brain tissue interrupted or diminished, often causing severe damage or necrosis of the involved tissue
C. Sudden or gradual onset
D. Symptoms related to location and size of brain area affected
E. Approximately 50% of survivors permanently disabled
F. High proportion experiencing recurrence within weeks to years
G. Chances for complete recovery depending on the circulation returning to normal soon after the initial episode
H. Third most common cause of death in the United States and most common cause of neurological disability
I. Predisposing factors
1. History of transient ischemic attacks (TIAs)

2. Hypertension
3. Arrhythmias
4. Atherosclerosis
5. Rheumatic heart disease
6. Myocardial enlargement
7. Diabetes mellitus
8. High serum triglyceride levels
9. Lack of exercise
10. Cigarette smoking
11. Family history

J. Causes
  1. Thrombosis
     a. Obstruction of blood vessel by blood clot formed within vessel
     b. Most common cause of CVA in middle-aged and elderly individuals
     c. Tendency to develop while individual is awake or shortly after awakening
     d. Individuals at risk including clients with a history of atherosclerosis, diabetes, and hypertension
     e. Risk increasing with smoking or obesity or both
  2. Embolus
     a. Occlusion of blood vessel in brain by a fragmented clot, tumor, fat, air, or bacteria
     b. Can occur at any age and is the second most common cause of CVA
     c. Individuals at risk include clients with a history of rheumatic heart disease, myocardial fibrillation, other arrhythmias, or endocarditis, or clients who have just undergone open-heart surgery
     d. Usually developing rapidly (10–20 seconds) and without warning
     e. Most often affecting middle cerebral artery
     f. If embolus septic, infection may extend beyond blood vessel wall, with development of abscess or encephalitis
        1) Infection within blood vessel wall may develop into an aneurysm, with potential cerebral hemorrhage.
  3. Hemorrhage
     a. Sudden rupture of a cerebral blood vessel
     b. Occurring at any age and is the third most common cause of CVA
     c. Individuals at risk including clients with chronic hypertension or aneurysms, which rupture cerebral artery
     d. Blood supply to the affected brain tissue decreasing with accumulation of blood deep within brain substance, with subsequent compression of nerve tissue and further damage

K. Classification of CVA (least severe to complete stroke)
  1. TIA
     a. "Little stroke" caused by temporary interruption of blood flow
     b. Occurring most often in carotid and vertebrobasilar arteries

2. Progressive stroke
   a. Thrombus in evolution begins with slight neurological deficit.
   b. Condition exacerbates within 1–2 days.
3. Complete stroke: maximum neurological deficits occur immediately at onset

II. Data collection
  A. Depending on artery affected, area of brain involved, severity of damage, and extent of collateral circulation, which develops to compensate the brain for diminished blood supply
  B. Left hemisphere involvement resulting in symptoms on right side of body; right hemisphere in symptoms on left side of body
  C. CVA causing cranial nerve damage, which produces neural dysfunction on same side of the body
  D. Subjective symptoms
     1. Changes in sensation and strength
     2. Headache
     3. Dizziness
     4. Difficulty in speaking
     5. Visual disturbances
  E. Objective symptoms
     1. Middle cerebral artery
        a. Aphasia, hemiparesis, visual field cuts
        b. Hemiparesis more severe in face and arm than in leg
     2. Anterior cerebral artery
        a. Numbness, confusion, weakness (especially lower limb)
        b. Incontinence
        c. Personality changes
        d. Loss of coordination
        e. Impaired motor and sensory functions
     3. Posterior cerebral artery
        a. Visual field cuts
        b. Dyslexia
        c. Cortical blindness
        d. Sensory impairment
        e. Usually paralysis absent
     4. Carotid artery
        a. Weakness, paralysis
        b. Sensory changes
        c. Altered level of consciousness
        d. Headache
        e. Aphasia
        f. Ptosis
        g. Visual disturbances on affected side
     5. Vertebrobasilar artery
        a. Numbness around lips
        b. Weakness on affected side
        c. Double vision
        d. Slurred speech
        e. Dysphagia
        f. Poor coordination
        g. Vertigo
        h. Amnesia
        i. Ataxia

III. Diagnostic tests and methods
  A. Client history
  B. Physical examination
  C. Neurological assessment

D. Brain scan
E. CAT scan
F. Lumbar puncture
G. EEG
H. Cerebral angiography
I. Ophthalmoscopy
J. Baseline laboratory studies
  1. Coagulation studies
  2. Urinalysis
  3. Serum osmolality
  4. CBC
  5. Triglycerides
  6. Serum electrolytes
  7. Creatinine and BUN levels

IV. Implementation
A. Assess, report, and record signs and symptoms and any reaction to treatment.
B. Provide bedrest; provide complete care.
C. Maintain patent airway and oxygen therapy.
D. Check for ballooning of cheek with respiration (side affected by stroke).
E. Keep unconscious client in a lateral (sidelying) position to allow secretions to drain by gravity or use suction as necessary (prevents aspiration of saliva).
F. Monitor vital signs and neurological status.
G. Monitor BP, voluntary and involuntary movements, changes in pupils, level of consciousness, speech, skin color, sensory function, and neck rigidity or flaccidity.
H. Monitor for signs of pulmonary emboli, such as chest pain, shortness of breath, increased temperature, and tachycardia; and check ABGs for signs of increased PCO_2 or decreased PO_2.
I. Monitor for signs of increased ICP.
J. Keep precautionary respiratory equipment at bedside.
K. Provide a safe environment and elevate siderails.
L. Administer prescribed medications such as antihypertensives, diuretics, and anticoagulants; monitor for side effects.
M. Maintain fluid and electrolyte balance:
  1. Encourage fluid intake orally as ordered.
  2. Assist in IV administration as ordered.
N. Monitor ability to swallow (check gag reflex).
O. Place bedside stand in client's visual field so that client can see what is on stand.
P. Provide meticulous mouth care; clean and care for dentures.
Q. Provide meticulous eye care; patch affected eye if client cannot close lid.
R. Maintain adequate nutritional intake (make sure gag reflex has returned):
  1. Place food in client's visual field so that client can see what is on tray.
  2. Assist in insertion of NG feeding tube if unable to intake food by mouth.
S. Position client, align extremities correctly; use turning sheet to turn client every 2 hours.
T. Use padded (Posey) footboard to prevent footdrop and contracture.
U. Assist client with ROM exercises for both affected and unaffected sides.
V. Instruct client in how to use unaffected side to exercise affected side.
W. Provide egg-crate, pulsating, or flotation mattress to prevent skin breakdown (decubiti).
X. Facilitate communication with client:
  1. Allow client sufficient time to communicate.
  2. Anticipate needs; speak slowly and clearly.
  3. If client is aphasic, set up other means of communication such as drawing, writing, use of pictures, gestures.
  4. Assure client that intellect has not been impaired; include family members in communicating methods.
  5. Encourage speech therapy.
Y. Involve family members in client's care when possible.
Z. Monitor elimination pattern:
  1. Offer bedpan frequently for urinary or fecal incontinence.
  2. Assist client as necessary; provide privacy by not exposing client.
  3. Be alert for signs of straining at stool (which increases ICP).
  4. Check with dietitian to modify diet and to administer stool softener and/or prescribed laxatives.
  5. Encourage adequate fluid intake.
  6. Provide roughage in diet.
AA. Begin rehabilitation of client on admission:
  1. Amount of teaching varies depending on neurological deficit present.
  2. If necessary, teach client to bathe, comb hair, and dress.
  3. Encourage client to begin speech therapy as soon as possible (if needed).
  4. Involve family in all aspects of rehabilitation.
  5. Coordinate care with physical therapist; use walking frames, handbars on toilet, and ramps.
BB. Instruct client and family regarding signs of CVA.
CC. Instruct client and family to watch for possible GI bleeding if aspirin is prescribed to decrease the risk of emboli stroke.
DD. Explain disease process, treatment, home care, and follow-up to client and family.
EE. Explain prevention of CVAs:
  1. Stress:
    a. Need to control diseases such as hypertension or diabetes mellitus
    b. Emphasis on importance of eating a low-salt, low-cholesterol diet
    c. Need to control weight
    d. Need to increase activity
    e. Avoidance of smoking and prolonged bedrest

V. Evaluation
A. Client reports increased comfort and decreased anxiety.
B. Client remains free of injury or infection.
C. Effective communication is established.
D. Client maintains effective airway clearance and breathing pattern.
E. Client maintains effective elimination (urinary and bowel) patterns.

F. Client maintains good skin integrity.

G. Client maintains adequate cerebral tissue perfusion.

H. Client and family demonstrate an understanding of disease process, diagnostic procedures, treatment, home care, and follow-up care.

Increased Intracranial Pressure

I. Description
  A. Fluid accumulation or lesion taking up space in the cranial cavity, producing ICP
  B. Resulting in gradual compression of the brain, with potential cessation of life-sustaining functions
  C. Progressing slowly or occurring suddenly
  D. Causes
    1. Edema from trauma and abscesses
    2. Tumors
    3. Hematoma
II. Data collection
  A. Subjective symptoms
    1. Related to primary disorder
    2. Headache, anxiety
    3. Blurred or double vision
    4. Lethargy
    5. Weakness
  B. Objective symptoms
    1. Vomiting: projectile, recurrent, unrelated to nausea
    2. Irregular, Cheyne-Stokes, or Kussmaul's respirations
    3. Seizures
    4. Altered level of consciousness: confusion, slurred speech, decreased level of response
    5. Change in pupil response to light
    6. Elevation of BP; wide pulse pressure
    7. Initial increase in pulse followed by decrease to 40–60 bpm
    8. Progressive signs of paralysis
    9. Loss of consciousness, coma, and death
III. Diagnostic tests and methods
  A. Client history
  B. Physical examination
  C. Neurological assessment
  D. ICP monitoring
IV. Implementation
  A. Assess, report, and record signs and symptoms and any reaction to treatment.
  B. Elevate head to semi-Fowler's position (do *not* place client in Trendelenburg position).
  C. Maintain patent airway; provide oxygen therapy.
  D. Prevent aspiration; position client on side.
  E. Monitor vital signs every 15 minutes.
  F. Monitor neurological responses frequently.
  G. Monitor laboratory values.
  H. Monitor I&O.
  I. Turn client every 2 hours.
  J. Provide hygienic care frequently, including mouth care, skin care, and hair care.
  K. Provide passive ROM exercises.
  L. Use footboard or hightop sneakers for prevention of footdrop and contractures.
  M. Use splints to prevent wrist deformities.
  N. Monitor pupillary response (usually unequal and may not react to light).
  O. Provide safe environment (elevate siderails).
  P. Report any change in level of consciousness immediately.
  Q. Assist in administration of prescribed medications or devices.
  R. Provide usual care and observation for unconscious client or one with seizures.
  S. Explain condition, diagnostic procedures, treatment, home care, and follow-up care to client and family.
V. Evaluation
  A. Client reports increased comfort and decreased anxiety.
  B. Client remains free of injury or infection.
  C. Client maintains adequate cerebral tissue perfusion.
  D. Client maintains adequate airway clearance, breathing patterns, and gas exchange.
  E. Client maintains adequate cardiac output.
  F. Client maintains adequate fluid and electrolyte balance.
  G. Client maintains adequate nutritional intake.
  H. Client maintains adequate elimination pattern.
  I. There are no deformities or contractures.
  J. Client and family demonstrate an understanding of condition, treatment, home care, and follow-up care.

Intracranial Tumors

I. Description
  A. Malignant or benign lesion within the brain that may displace or destroy adjacent structures or increase ICP
  B. Either lesion originating within brain tissue (primary lesion) or one originating elsewhere in the body and metastasizing to the brain (secondary lesion)
  C. ICP possible because of displacement of space by tumor, cerebral edema, and vasodilation resulting from impairment of the cerebral blood flow
  D. More common in men than in women
  E. Occurring at any age; in adults, incidence usually highest between the ages of 40 and 60 years
  F. Classification according to tissue origin
    1. Gliomas: arise in cerebral connective tissue; unencapsulated
      a. Characterized by rapid growth with infiltration of the brain tissue
      b. Are not well defined for surgical removal
      c. Occur most often in cerebral hemispheres, especially frontal and temporal lobes
      d. Prognosis: mean survival rate 6 months; maximum 1–2 years
    2. Meningiomas: originate within meningeal layers
      a. Constituting 15% of primary brain tumors
      b. Peak incidence among 50-year-olds; rare in children, more common in women than in men

c. Occurring most often in sphenoidal ridge, anterior part of the base of the skull, and spinal canal

d. Tumors benign, well circumscribed, and highly vascular

e. Compression of adjacent underlying brain tissue by invading overlying skull

f. Prognosis: median survival rate 1–2 years or less; if treated, neurological deficits potentially completely reversible

3. Neuromas: originate on cranial nerves

a. Benign but often classified as malignant because of growth pattern: slow-growing, present for years before symptoms appear

b. Accounting for approximately 10% of all intracranial tumors

c. Incidence higher in women

d. Onset of symptoms approximately 30–60 years of age

e. Affecting craniospinal nerve sheath: usually eighth cranial nerve; also affecting fifth and seventh cranial nerves, although to a lesser extent

f. Prognosis: if adequately treated, potential for permanent cure

4. Pituitary tumors: originate most often in anterior pituitary gland

a. Accounting for 10% of intracranial tumors

b. Occurring in adults of both sexes ages 30–50 years

c. Three types: chromophobe adenoma, basophilic adenoma, and eosinophilic adenoma

d. Amenable to surgical treatment

e. Prognosis: fair to good, depending on extent of tumor spread beyond sella turcica

5. Metastatic tumors: originate elsewhere in body, often from lung

a. Prognosis: poor

G. Gliomas and meningiomas most common type among adults

H. Brain tumors one of the most common causes of death from cancer in children

1. Incidence usually highest <1 year old and then 2–12 years of age

2. Astrocytoma (type of glioma), medulloblastomas (rare type of glioma), and brainstem gliomas most common types

I. Cause unknown

II. Data collection

A. Subjective symptoms

1. Alterations in judgment or personality
2. Visual disturbances
3. Headache
4. Numbness, tingling sensations
5. Difficulty and loss of hearing
6. Family or personal history

B. Objective symptoms

1. Vomiting
2. Orientation to person, place, and time
3. Movement and strength of extremities
4. Reaction of pupils to light
5. Changes in vital signs
6. Changes in level of consciousness

7. Presence of papilledema
8. Presence of seizures
9. Abnormal cranial nerve reflexes
10. Signs of increased ICP
11. Presence of protein and decreased glucose and occasional tumor cells in spinal fluid
12. Signs associated with tumor location

a. Frontal lobe: personality changes, hemiparesis, visual problems

b. Temporal lobe: visual hallucinations, seizures, changes in sense of taste, odor

c. Parietal lobe: visual disturbances, jacksonian seizures related to tumor involving precentral gyrus, inability to differentiate between left and right

d. Occipital lobe: visual problems, convulsions

III. Diagnostic tests and methods

A. Client history
B. Physical examination
C. Neurological assessment
D. CAT scan
E. Skull x-ray
F. Brain scan
G. EEG
H. Biopsy of lesion
I. Cerebral angiography
J. Lumbar puncture

IV. Implementation

A. Assess, report, and record signs and symptoms and any reaction to treatment.

B. Monitor and record baseline information regarding neurological status.

C. Check continuously for changes in neurological status:

1. Watch for and immediately report sudden unilateral dilation of pupil with loss of light reflex (indicates transtentorial herniation).

D. Monitor for signs of increased ICP:

1. Rising systolic pressure
2. Widening pulse pressure
3. Decrease in pulse rate
4. Changes in level of consciousness
5. Abnormal respiratory patterns
6. Elevation of temperature

E. Assist with mobility and exercise.

F. Monitor respiratory changes (anoxia, abnormal respiratory rate and depth), which may indicate rising ICP or herniation of cerebellar tissue from expanding mass.

G. Monitor temperature (increased temperature often follows hypothalamic anoxia and might also indicate meningitis).

1. Use hypothermia blankets, if prescribed, to decrease temperature and decrease metabolic demands of brain tissue.

H. Discuss effects of treatment with client and family.

I. Document seizure activity.

J. Maintain patent airway.

K. Provide safe and hazard-free environment (elevate siderails).

L. Administer anticonvulsants, diuretics, and steroids as prescribed.

M. Assist with administration and monitoring of IV therapy.
N. Monitor fluid I&O and electrolyte balance; restrict fluids as ordered (rapid diuresis may lead to heart failure).
O. Prepare client and family for surgical intervention.
P. Monitor for side effects of radiation therapy, if ordered (check for wound breakdown, infection, signs of rising ICP).
Q. Monitor for side effects of prescribed medication adjuncts to radiotherapy and surgery:
   1. Cause delayed bone marrow depression (watch for signs of infection or bleeding)
R. Assist with instruction of client and family in early signs of recurrence; encourage compliance with therapy.
S. Begin rehabilitation early; encourage independence in ADLs.
T. Provide aids for self-care, if necessary.
U. Arrange for consultation with speech therapist if client is aphasic.
V. Explain diagnosis, treatment, potential disabilities, lifestyle alterations, home care, and follow-up care to client and family.

V. Evaluation
A. Client reports increased comfort and decreased anxiety.
B. Client remains free of injury or infection.
C. Client maintains adequate cerebral tissue perfusion.
D. Client maintains adequate airway clearance and breathing pattern.
E. Client participates in rehabilitation therapy (exercise, ambulation, ADLs).
F. Client demonstrates an understanding of disease process, diagnostic tests, treatment including medication, prevention, and home care.

Parkinson's Disease

I. Description
A. Condition characterized by progressive muscle rigidity, akinesia, and involuntary tremor
B. Caused by damage to neurons in the substantia nigra, located within the basal ganglia
C. Unknown cause
D. Predisposing factors
   1. Deficiency in dopamine, which interferes with inhibition of excitatory impulses
   2. May be related to certain viruses, drugs, arteriosclerosis
E. Progression of deterioration for an average of 10 years
F. Death usually caused by aspiration pneumonia or other infection
G. More common in men than in women

II. Data collection
A. Subjective symptoms
   1. Drooling
   2. Fatigue
   3. Intolerance to heat
   4. Muscular pain
   5. Problems with coordination
   6. Changes in emotion and judgment
B. Objective symptoms
   1. Muscle rigidity: resistance to passive muscle stretching ("lead pipe" or jerky)
   2. Akinesia (loss of movement) causing shuffling gait, loss of posture control, altered reflexes, masklike facial expression, high-pitched monotone voice, and dysphagia
   3. Difficulty performing ADLs
   4. Tremors of fingers (unilateral "pill-roll" tremor) increasing with stress

III. Diagnostic tests and methods
A. Client history
B. Physical examination
C. Neurological assessment
D. Urinalysis (dopamine levels)

IV. Implementation
A. Assess, report, and record signs and symptoms and any reaction to treatment.
B. Encourage client to maintain independence in ADLs as much as possible.
C. Assist client while eating; have him or her use utensils with large handles for easy grip.
D. Encourage client to continue with previous work, social, and diversionary activities as much as possible.
E. Maintain effective airway clearance.
F. Provide safe, hazard-free environment.
G. Administer levodopa (dopamine replacement) as prescribed; monitor for side effects.
H. Administer alternate drug therapy such as anticholinergics and antihistamines as prescribed.
I. Assist in establishment of a regular bowel routine (encourage fluid intake, high-bulk foods).
J. Provide emotional support to client and family.
K. Prepare client and family for stereotactic neurosurgical procedure (electrical coagulation, freezing, radioactivity, or ultrasound to destroy the ventrolateral nucleus of thalamus to prevent involuntary movement), if necessary.
L. After surgery, monitor for signs of hemorrhage and increased ICP.
M. Coordinate care with physical therapist (used to assist in maintenance of normal muscle tone and function).
N. Instruct family members how to prevent contracture formation (use of firm mattress without a pillow; lying in prone position to facilitate proper posture during rest).
O. Maintain good skin integrity, and instruct client and family in prevention of skin breakdown.
P. Instruct family to establish long- and short-term goals, awareness of need for intellectual stimulation and diversion for client.
Q. Explain disease process, treatment, home care, and follow-up care.

V. Evaluation
A. Client reports increased comfort and decreased anxiety.
B. Muscular tremors and rigidity are reduced.
C. Client maintains good skin integrity.

D. Client maintains effective airway clearance.
E. Client maintains adequate nutritional and fluid intake.
F. Client performs some ADLs and participates in physical therapy.
G. Client demonstrates an understanding of disease process, treatment, home care, and follow-up care.

Paraplegia

I. Description
  A. Spinal cord trauma or disease resulting in motor or sensory loss in the lower extremities with or without involvement of abdominal and back muscles
  B. Possibly complete or incomplete paralysis, which may be flaccid or spastic, permanent or temporary, and symmetrical or asymmetrical
  C. Complete severing of spinal cord resulting in permanent paralysis of body parts below site of injury
  D. Approximately 50% of spinal cord injuries resulting in paraplegia
  E. More prevalent in men than in women; incidence highest between ages 16 and 35 years
  F. Causes
    1. Trauma: automobile, diving, motorcycle, gunshot wounds, falls, other sporting accidents
    2. Nontraumatic lesions such as spina bifida, spinal tumors, scoliosis, and chordoma
II. Data collection
  A. Subjective symptoms
    1. Loss of sensation
    2. Loss of voluntary movement
  B. Objective symptoms
    1. Immediate phase
      a. Areflexia as a result of spinal shock
      b. Complete loss of sensation
      c. Complete loss of voluntary (motor) function
      d. Flaccid paralysis below site of injury
      e. Hypotonia
    2. Later phase
      a. Spasticity of muscles below site of injury
      b. Hyperreflexia: hyperactive responses
    3. Level of injury
      a. Lower thoracic level
        1) Loss of movement of bowel, bladder, and lower extremities, depending on level of injury
        2) Paralysis of legs
      b. Lumbar and sacral level
        1) Loss of movement and sensation of lower extremities
        2) S2–4 center of micturation: injury or lesion above this level permitting bladder to empty involuntarily; lesions below this level resulting in bladder contraction without emptying (autonomous neurogenic bladder)
    4. Injury above S2 (in men): allowing erection to occur without ejaculation because of sympathetic nerve damage
    5. Injury between S2 and S4: prevention of erection or ejaculation because of damaged sympathetic and parasympathetic nerves
    6. Associated injuries such as fractures, hemorrhage, shock
III. Diagnostic tests and methods
  A. Client history
  B. Physical examination
  C. Neurological assessment
  D. Lumbar puncture
  E. Laboratory studies: CBC, PT, electrolytes, urinalysis
  F. After stabilization: hip, knee, chest x-rays, IVP to provide baseline information for detection of pathological changes
  G. Weekly urine culture and sensitivity tests
IV. Implementation
  A. Emergency care
    1. Assess for:
      a. Pain, tenderness
      b. Numbness, tingling
      c. Weakness
      d. Alterations of sensation and motor function below level of injury
    2. Monitor for signs of shock.
    3. Provide supportive treatment to control systemic shock and hemorrhage.
    4. Immobilize client (movement may further damage spinal cord).
    5. Stabilize head and spine by strapping client on board.
    6. Place client on stretcher in emergency department without removing him or her from board.
    7. Insert Foley catheter to ensure uninterrupted urine drainage.
  B. Phase after emergency intervention
    1. Assess, report, and record signs and symptoms and any reaction to treatment.
    2. Provide meticulous catheter care; use intermittent catheterization to re-establish bladder capacity and to prevent infection once spinal shock period is over.
    3. Maintain proper body alignment and position to prevent contractures in immobilized client.
    4. Provide meticulous skin care, inspect pressure areas daily, and have client shift position at least every 15 minutes while sitting in wheelchair.
    5. Administer prescribed medications, such as corticosteroids, to reduce spinal cord edema, and analgesics for pain.
    6. Monitor fluid I&O; restrict fluids to 2000–2500 ml/day if client is on an intermittent catheterization program. Increase fluids for clients with indwelling Foley catheters to 4000 ml/day.
    7. Assist with active and passive ROM exercises; coordinate care with physical therapist.
    8. Monitor for symptoms of orthostatic hypotension as client progresses from bedrest to wheelchair; use antiembolism hose to assist in compensation for a sitting position after being restricted to a lying position for a long time.

9. Provide a high-bulk diet to prevent constipation; give protein supplements to build up body tissues.
10. Establish a bowel elimination routine:
    a. Provide stool softeners, suppositories, and laxatives as ordered.
    b. Administer stool softeners and suppositories on a regular timed schedule.
    c. Use digital stimulation, if necessary.
    d. Teach muscle strengthening.
    e. Monitor for abdominal distention, flatus, and fullness in rectum, which indicates need to defecate.
    f. Teach client to use intra-abdominal compression by leaning forward and use of Valsalva's maneuver, except if cardiac problems are present.
11. Monitor for UTIs.
12. For autonomic or spastic bladder reflex, instruct client regarding possible stimuli to initiate urination; use external catheters for men. Teach client to report signs of UTI.
13. For atonic or areflexic bladder, instruct client to observe for distention. Use intermittent catheterization. Teach use of Credé's maneuver or abdominal straining to initiate urination.
14. Provide postoperative wound care if a laminectomy is performed.
15. Encourage family involvement in rehabilitation.
16. Monitor for psychological problems (altered body image, loss of self-esteem, denial, anger).
17. Provide emotional support to client and family.
18. Provide counseling on sexual dysfunction or alterations.
19. Provide client and family with information regarding community resources.
20. Explain condition, treatment including medication, home care, and follow-up care.

V. Evaluation
A. Client reports increased comfort and decreased anxiety.
B. Client remains free of injury or infection.
C. Client maintains good skin integrity.
D. Client maintains adequate (bowel and bladder) elimination patterns.
E. Client copes effectively with alterations in sensory and motor function.
F. Client verbalizes feelings regarding self-image, self-concept, and sexual concerns.
G. Client participates in self-care activities.
H. Client demonstrates an understanding of condition, diagnostic procedures, treatment including medications, home care, and follow-up care.

Quadriplegia

I. Description
A. A permanent injury that affects all body systems
B. Condition characterized by paralysis of the arms, legs, and body below the level of injury to the spinal cord

C. Affecting 150,000 individuals in the United States
D. Incidence highest in men ages 20–40 years
E. Causes flaccidity of the arms and legs and loss of movement and sensation below the level of injury
F. Injury above the fifth cervical vertebra also causes blockage of the sympathetic nervous system, which allows the parasympathetic system to dominate; complications that may result from this phenomenon include:
   1. Hypotension with BP <90/60 caused by vasodilation allowing blood to pool in veins of extremities, resulting in slowing of the venous blood return to the heart
   2. Bradycardia (decreased heartbeat) as a result of stimulation of the heart by the vagus nerve and the absence of the inhibiting effects of the sympathetic system
   3. Decrease in body temperature because of inability of blood vessels to constrict effectively; allows blood vessel to contact with body surface; results in heat loss
   4. Respiratory complications: caused by damage to upper cervical cord
   5. Decreased peristalsis
   6. Autonomic dysreflexia (injuries above the fourth thoracic vertebra): connections between the brain and spinal cord are severed; produces an exaggerated autonomic response to specific stimuli such as distended bladder or bowel, presence of infection, decubitus ulcers, and/or surgical manipulation; key symptom is severe hypertension
G. Causes
   1. Spinal cord injury; especially involving the fifth to seventh cervical vertebrae
   2. Vertebral pressure from tumors, degenerative spinal cord lesions
II. Data collection
A. Subjective symptoms
   1. Loss of sensation
   2. Difficulty in breathing
   3. Pain
   4. Nature of injury
   5. Orientation
B. Objective symptoms
   1. Symptoms of spinal shock
   2. Complete loss of sensation below level of injury
   3. Complete loss of movement below level of injury
   4. Unconsciousness
   5. Flaccid paralysis
   6. Hypotonia
   7. Respiratory difficulty
   8. Level of injury
      a. Cervical lesion with paralysis of trunk and all extremities
      b. Possible shoulder movement if at C5 or below
      c. Decreased perspiration
      d. Decrease in touch sensation
      e. Respiratory failure at level of C4 or above

III. Diagnostic tests and methods
   A. Client history
   B. Detailed history of trauma
   C. Physical examination
   D. Neurological assessment
   E. Spinal x-rays
   F. Myelography to identify fractures, dislocations, subluxation, and blockage in spinal cord
   G. X-rays of head, chest, and abdomen to rule out underlying injuries
   H. Laboratory studies to assess respiratory, hepatic, and pancreatic function
IV. Implementation
   A. Assess, report, and record signs and symptoms and any reaction to treatment.
   B. Monitor respirations, chest movement, and vital signs frequently (injury at C4 or above requires permanent ventilatory support).
   C. Monitor PCO_2 and pH for signs of respiratory insufficiency.
   D. Assist with administration of IV therapy (do not overhydrate if vasodilation and venous pooling are present below level of injury).
   E. Assist with insertion of NG tube, if needed.
   F. Observe for signs of GI complications, such as paralytic ileus, bleeding, and pancreatic dysfunction:
      1. Listen for bowel sounds every 8 hours.
      2. Record amount and type of NG drainage; check for coffee-ground secretions.
   G. Assist with intubation and ventilatory support as ordered.
   H. Connect client to cardiac monitor if bradycardia occurs.
   I. Place client in slight Trendelenburg position if signs of hypotension occur (constantly assess respiratory function).
   J. Use abdominal binder and antiembolism stockings when placing client in upright position (aid venous return and prevent orthostatic hypotension).
   K. Warm client with blankets if hypothermia occurs (temperature <90°F [32.2°C]). Do not use hot-water bottles or mechanical heat devices, as these may result in burning caused by sensory deficit.
   L. Maintain proper body alignment and immobilization of spine.
   M. Monitor neurological status, level of consciousness, sensations, movement, and pupil response frequently.
   N. Monitor for severe hypertension, which may lead to heart failure, intracranial bleeding, and retinal hemorrhage (sign of autonomic dysreflexia in client with injury above C4):
      1. In presence of hypertension
         a. Elevate head of bed to decrease BP.
         b. Check for bladder distention; obstructed catheter.
         c. Check for fecal impaction; do not manipulate rectum, as it worsens symptoms.
            1) Before removal of impaction, apply topical anesthetic ointment, which decreases risk of further increasing the BP.

            2) Administer a smooth muscle relaxant or antihypertensive, if prescribed.
            3) Administer a ß-adrenergic blocking agent for persistent hypertension as prescribed.
   O. Maintain skeletal traction, tongs, or CircOlectric bed or Stryker frame.
   P. Prepare client for surgical intervention such as spinal decompression; provide postoperative care.
   Q. Administer medications as prescribed.
   R. Provide frequent skin care to prevent formation of decubitus ulcers and infection.
   S. Turn client every 2 hours.
   T. Maintain firm mattress support.
   U. Assist with passive ROM exercises; coordinate care with physical therapist.
   V. Assist with urinary elimination.
   W. Explain condition, diagnostic procedures, treatment, home care, follow-up care, and community resources.
V. Evaluation
   A. Client reports increased comfort and decreased anxiety.
   B. Client remains free of injury or infection.
   C. Client maintains effective breathing pattern and gas exchange.
   D. Client maintains adequate level of mobility in wheelchair.
   E. Client maintains good skin integrity.
   F. Client participates in self-care activities.
   G. Client copes effectively with alterations in sensory perception and motor function.
   H. Client maintains adequate elimination pattern.
   I. Client demonstrates an understanding of condition, treatment, home care, follow-up care, and community resources.

Nursing Care of the Older Adult
Kathleen R. Culliton, RN, CS, MS, GNP

I. Facts about older people
   A. The population of older adults is the fastest growing segment of the U.S. population.
   B. More than 13% of the population is >65 years old.
   C. Older adults consume >70% of health-care services.
   D. Older adults commonly suffer from one or more chronic diseases requiring long-term treatment and life changes.
   E. Most of the older population live in the community.
   F. Only 5% of the people >65 years old live in long-term care facilities (nursing facilities).
   G. Forty percent of the residents in nursing facilities are >85 years old.
II. Beliefs about aging
   A. Society often discriminates against older people because of the value it places on youth, appearance, work performance, and functional independence.
   B. Television, greeting cards, and advertisements often portray a negative image of older people and aging.
   C. Many false beliefs about aging exist that can have an

Table 5–1. False Beliefs about Aging

All old people are sick.
All old people are alike.
All old people are senile.
Most old people are in nursing homes.
All old people are depressed.
Nurses who are not good enough to work in hospitals work in nursing homes.

impact on the health care that an older person receives (Table 5–1).

III. Loss related to aging
  A. Physical changes of aging (Table 5–2)
    1. All body systems are affected by the aging process.
    2. It is often difficult to differentiate the normal process of physical aging from disease processes.
    3. Healthy lifestyle choices regarding diet, exercise, chemical exposure, stress management, and genetic exploration may change or slow the normal aging process.
  B. Social changes of aging
    1. Role changes
      a. Retirement can be a stressful life change if not thought out and planned.
      b. Widowhood can lead to loneliness and isolation.
      c. Acting as caregiver to a spouse may be a stressful burden.
      d. Moving out of one's home and into an apartment or health-care facility often means leaving social contacts, family, and valued responsibilities, which can be stressful.
      e. Loss of income or having a low income may place older adults in situations in which they have to choose among eating, buying medications, and maintaining their living situation.
  C. Factors associated with loss
    1. Older adults may have problems with loneliness in response to multiple losses.
      a. Encourage socialization through community groups, senior centers, senior volunteer opportunities, shared living situations, and pets.
      b. Identify social support network of family, friends, and neighbors.
    2. Depression is common in older adults who have experienced multiple losses, such as loss of spouse, disability, social isolation, loneliness, and inability to function in previous roles.
      a. Be alert for signs of potential suicide: expressing hopelessness, giving things away, saying goodbye to friends and family, and having a plan for taking one's life.
      b. Refer client to professional counseling or crisis management.
    3. Older people often fear dependence more than they fear death.
      a. Encourage them to talk about their views and beliefs about death.
      b. Encourage future planning using living wills, estate planning, and funeral planning so client's wishes are made known.

IV. Ethics and aging
  A. Social policy issues
    1. Informed consent
      a. Client or resident has the basic right to information that will allow him or her to make appropriate choices for care.
      b. When informed, the older adult has the right to refuse care.
      c. Informed consent implies that the older adult has received complete information regarding the type of procedure being done, potential complications, expected outcomes, and alternatives to the procedure.
      d. LPNs often sign as witnesses to the older person's signature, implying that the person was competent (mentally able to understand and give consent), that the person was not coerced into signing, and that his or her signature was valid.
      e. Family members and others can sign consent forms if they have legal guardianship or power of attorney related to health care.
    2. Living will (advanced directives)
      a. Older people may choose to make their wishes known regarding the type and amount of treatments and care they want to receive if they are found to be terminally ill.
      b. Some states recognize a living will as a legal expression of the person's wishes.
      c. Because living wills serve only as a general guideline for care, dilemmas regarding what the older person would really want done in a specific care situation may develop.
  B. Family and family caregiver issues
    1. Caregiver burden
      a. Family caregiving can be a stressful and negative experience, as well as a rewarding and positive experience.
      b. Stress is related to the amount of care required, past relationship with the frail relative, financial burden, and change in the caregiver's and family's lifestyle.
      c. Support for family caregivers is provided through caregiver support groups, in-home respite care volunteers, and community-based respite and adult daycare centers.
    2. Elder abuse
      a. Elder abuse is an increasing problem, with victims most often being dependent, isolated, and frail older adults.
      b. Clues that nurses need to be aware of as indicating possible abuse include malnutrition, dehydration, bruises, fractures, pressure ulcers, burns, overmedication, cuts, scratches, and bite marks.
      c. Adult protective services should be notified of any suspected abuse situations.

Table 5–2. **Physical Changes: Implications of Normal Physiological Aging**		
Age-Related Changes by Body System	Impact on Functional Ability	Nursing Interventions to Promote Function and Decrease Disability
Vision Dry eyes ↓Macular acuity ↑Lens size Lens yellowed ↓Upper gaze	Increased risk of falling Increased risk of making errors in taking medications	Provide artificial tears as needed. Increase lighting. Color-code medications using reds and yellows. Use medication dosage boxes. Organize furniture, avoid clutter. Encourage eye exams and glasses.
Hearing ↓Function of cochlear ↓Movement of ossicles	Decreased ability to hear spoken words Increased risk of confusion	Speak clearly but do not shout. Maintain eye contact when giving instructions. Check batteries on hearing aid. Repeat instructions. Perform audiology exam.
Smell ↓Acuity	Inability to smell smoke	Smoke detector: instruct what to do in a fire emergency.
Taste ↓Number of taste buds	Potential weight loss	Visually stimulate appetite. Use spices to enhance food flavor.
Neurological ↓Reaction time Mild short-term memory loss	Frustration with forgetfulness Increased errors when rushed	Reassure and allow time to remember and perform tasks. Use memory aids (calendars, pill-reminder boxes).
Respiratory Kyphosis ↓Alveoli ↑Inelastic tissue ↑Dead air space	Decreased tolerance of activity	Evaluate tolerance of activity without shortness of breath. Encourage rest periods. Teach deep-breathing exercises.
Cardiovascular ↓Vessel elasticity ↑Peripheral resistance ↓Stroke volume Thickening of heart valves	Increased risk of falls related to orthostatic hypertension Decreased response to exercise and stress	Assess blood pressure in lying, sitting, and standing positions. Encourage to stop between position changes and report if feeling dizzy. Encourage regular exercise and stress-reduction techniques.
Digestive ↓Saliva Gum atrophy ↓Metabolism Slowed stomach emptying ↓Intestinal motility Slowed absorption	Potential decreased food intake, weight loss Potential adverse drug effects with ↓metabolism Potential constipation	Encourage regular dental exams. Make sure that dentures are in good repair. Food should be appropriate for dentition. Fluid intake is at least 1500 ml. Monitor drug effects. Prevent constipation through: Fluid intake Dietary fiber, bulk Exercise
Urinary ↓Renal blood flow ↓Filtration rate ↓Urge feeling	Potential adverse drug reactions with ↓ excretion Potential inconsistence	Monitor effects of drugs. Maintain good fluid intake. Monitor urine output. Encourage regular toileting (toilet before leaving room, going to activities, and going to bed). Provide bladder training.
Muscular ↓Muscle strength ↓Muscle mass	Potential for decreased mobility	Provide full ROM exercises. Maintain physical exercise and activity (use least restrictive assistance).

Table 5–2. Physical Changes: Implications of Normal Physiological Aging continued		
Age-Related Changes by Body System	Impact on Functional Ability	Nursing Interventions to Promote Function and Decrease Disability
Skeletal Bone loss Cartilage thinning Kyphosis	Potential for falls and fractures	Encourage weight bearing. Assist in ambulating with assistive devices (cane, walker). Monitor gait, balance, and transfer ability.
Skin Thinning of skin and hair Loss of subcutaneous fat ↓Sweat Fragile blood vessels	Increased risk of bruises and skin tears Slowed wound healing	Use soap on skin minimally. Use nonscented creams and lotions. Monitor for skin breakdown and wound healing. Use a gait belt. Do not grab skin areas during transfers.

Common Nursing Care Issues of Older Adults (Table 5–3)

LPNs are nursing care providers for older adults in the community, hospitals, and nursing facilities. Their primary role is assisting older adults to achieve their highest functional ability through chronic disease management, rehabilitation, and promoting function through nursing interventions. Knowledge of medical-surgical nursing practice and of the common problems associated with aging enables the nurse to fulfill this role.

Confusion

I. Not a disease per se but often a symptom of an underlying problem or disease process; two types being delirium and dementia.
   A. Delirium: confusion related to a specific cause, such as medications, infection, distended bladder, fecal impaction, pain, or change in environment
      1. Related medical diagnoses
         a. Infection
         b. Fever
         c. Dehydration
         d. Circulatory, respiratory, or metabolic diseases
      2. Data collection
         a. Sudden onset, commonly at night
         b. Memory, alertness, and thinking ability changes through the day
         c. Misinterpretation of environment and care
         d. Sleepiness during the day, wakefulness at night
         e. Mood swings and agitated pacing or fidgeting
         f. Hallucinations and delusions
      3. Implementation
         a. Identify cause and initiate treatment for full recovery.
         b. Often all medications are stopped, as they are a common cause of delirium.
         c. Ensure safety by close nursing supervision, possibly even one-on-one supervision.
         d. Decrease environmental stimuli such as noise, too-bright or too-dim lighting, and number of people in care area.
         e. Develop a toilet-training program.
         f. Assess for fecal impaction.
         g. Orient client to environment.
            1) Open blinds so client can look out of the window.
            2) Encourage sitting up in chair and ambulating during the day.
            3) Dress client in his or her own clothes.
            4) Place calendars and clocks in the room.
            5) Encourage family members to visit.
         h. Treat symptoms of pain.
         i. Talk in soft, reassuring tones, using simple commands and questions.
         j. Use physical and chemical restraint only if other care approaches have not worked.
   B. Dementia: irreversible progressive loss of mental functioning; can be worsened by medications, pain, bowel or bladder distention, infections, physical restraints, changes in environment or environmental stimuli; most often accompanied by problem behaviors
      1. Related medical diagnoses
         a. Delirium
         b. Alzheimer's disease
         c. Multi-infarct dementia
      2. Data collection
         a. Onset usually over months or years
         b. Usually gradual steady loss of memory over time
         c. Often denial of memory problems and made-up responses to mask memory problems
         d. Identification of problems and seeking of medical care by family members rather than by client
         e. Deterioration of skills related to work, finances, and social behavior before functional ability

f. Client generally healthy and lacking underlying disease processes

3. Implementation
   a. Rule out any reversible cause for the change in mental functioning, such as causes of delirium.
   b. Approaches to problem behaviors are found in Table 5–4.
   c. Reassure client and orient to environment.
   d. Support family members and caregivers.
      1) Provide information about Alzheimer's disease.
      2) Refer to caregiver support groups and the Alzheimer's association.
      3) Discuss respite care and adult daycare.
      4) Discuss nursing home placement.

C. Physical and chemical restraints (see Chapter 6)
   1. Physical and chemical restraints have often been used to manage problem behaviors—especially with confused or mentally ill older adults.
   2. Recent federal and state mandates have identified the use of restraints as only a last resort when other nursing or medical interventions have failed and the client is at risk of endangering himself or herself or others.
   3. Physical restraints have been related to loss of mobility, increased risk of pressure ulcers, incontinence, social isolation, falls, and deaths.
   4. The use of restraints requires a physician's order.
   5. All other nursing measures used to manage the problem behavior must be documented.
   6. The type of restraint, when it was applied, when it was released, and the client's response to the restraint must be documented.
   7. The nurse must assess skin condition and proper application of restraints.
   8. Client should be toileted, given skin care, walked, and repositioned before restraint is reapplied.
   9. When chemical restraints such as psychoactive drugs are used, the client must have a documented medical diagnosis that fits the drug being used.
      a. Sedatives: documented insomnia
      b. Psychotropics: psychotic behavior, hallucinations
   10. Most agencies require that a consent form related to restraint use be signed by the client or guardian.
   11. Alternatives to restraints
      a. Increased involvement in appropriate activities
      b. Involvement of family and volunteers
      c. Initiation of behavioral approaches (Table 5–4)
      d. Secure environment
      e. Wedge cushions and postural supports
      f. Use of reclining chairs
      g. Decreasing clutter and confusion in the environment

II. Communication problems
   A. Altered visual function

Table 5–3. Common Problems of Older Adults and Related Nursing Diagnoses

Problem	Related Nursing Diagnoses
Confusion (delirium and dementia)	Potential for injury
	Impaired verbal communication
	Impaired social interaction
	Social isolation
	Altered role performance
	Altered family processes
	Altered sexuality patterns
	Sleep pattern disturbance
	Self-care deficit
	Altered thought process
	Potential for violence
	Anxiety
Altered communication	Impaired verbal communication
	Impaired social interaction
	Sensory and perceptual alterations
Functional ability	Potential for injury
	Altered sexual patterns
	Impaired physical mobility
	Activity intolerance
	Diversion activity deficit
	Impaired home maintenance management
	Self-care deficit
	Body image disturbance
	Self-esteem disturbance
	Unilateral neglect
Bowel problems	Constipation
	Perceived constipation
	Diarrhea
	Bowel incontinence
Urinary dysfunction	Altered patterns of urinary elimination
	Urinary retention
	Incontinence (stress, reflex, urge, functional, or total)
Skin breakdown	Potential for infection
	Impaired skin integrity
Nutritional problems	Altered nutrition: more or less than body requirements
	Fluid volume deficit or excess
	Altered oral mucous membrane
	Feeding self-care deficit
	Impaired swallowing
Altered mood and behavior	Impaired social interaction
	Spiritual distress
	Ineffective individual coping
	Impaired adjustment
	Altered thought process
	Potential for violence
	Anxiety
	Fear
Chemical and physical restraints	Altered nutrition: less than body requirements
	Altered patterns of urinary elimination
	Diarrhea
	Potential fluid volume deficit
	Potential for injury
	Potential for poisoning
	Impaired social interaction
	Impaired physical mobility
	Sleep disturbance
	Self-care deficit

Table 5–4. Approaches to Problem Behaviors

Problem Behavior	Intervention

Striking out or hitting
Yelling and swearing
Sexual aggression
	Prevention the best intervention
	Positive and receptive attitude
	Environment
	    Decrease noise level and room temperature; adjust lighting to decrease glare and maximize vision; decrease clutter and crowding; do not change room arrangements.
	Consistent daily routine
	Cues for orientation (clock, calendar)
	Diversional activities
	    Walking, soft music, snack or drink, moving to another area or room, one-on-one talking

Constant requests or cries for help	Encouraging involvement in activities One-on-one visits with staff and volunteers Offering real choices in care Pet therapy Scheduling times for nursing interventions
Refusal to eat	Offering food and fluid choices Allowing choices of where to eat meals, time to eat, and amount of food desired Finger foods or "carry-along" foods for clients who do not sit down long enough to finish meal Small meals, with between-meal snacks Record of intake and weight daily

Refusal to perform personal hygiene	Minimizing confusion by breaking down tasks into specific instructions (task segmentation)
	Example: "Brush your teeth" changes to:
	  1. Wet your toothbrush.
	  2. Put toothpaste on your toothbrush.
	  3. Put the toothbrush in your mouth.
	  4. Brush up and down.
	  5. Take a drink of water.
	  6. Swish and spit.
	  7. Rinse your toothbrush.
	Allowing choices such as when to bathe and type of bath desired, what to wear, whether to dress in bathroom or at bedside
	Leaving and requesting again later, if patient refuses
	Evaluating plan of care if activity is necessary at specific time or day
	Consistent care provider
	Share care
	    Example: "You put your shirt on while I help you with your socks and shoes."

Wandering	Providing secure and safe areas to wander Closing doors to discourage going into other clients' rooms Hanging "Stop" signs or placing Velcro strips across open doorways Disguising doorways with wallpaper Placing doorknobs and latches high on the door, out of the line of vision Using door buzzers or bells that sound when door is opened Electronic beeper for client Medical alert bracelet with address and phone number and pertinent disease information Physical activities to use up energy to wander Removing clutter and other potential factors that contribute to falls Providing diversional activities: sorting tasks, laundry, music, reminiscing support groups Monitoring for toileting, hunger, pain, signs of infection

1. Related medical diagnoses
   a. Diabetes
   b. Cataracts
   c. Glaucoma
   d. Macular degeneration
   e. Dry eyes
   f. Eye surgery
2. Data collection
   a. Complaints of inability to see
   b. Unsteady ambulation; holding onto furniture, walls, and doorframes when walking
   c. Isolation, refusing to leave room
   d. Wearing of mismatched or soiled clothing
   e. Making mistakes in taking medications
   f. Lack of eye contact
3. Implementation
   a. Promote function and minimize disability.
   b. Encourage regular eye examinations and updating of glasses.
   c. Encourage use of visual aids: magnifying glass, page magnifier.
   d. Refer to agencies that support the blind.

e. Recommend use of tape recorders, dictation machines, and tape players for letter dictating; "talking books"; and music activities.
f. Organize room and belongings so client can find things easily and risk of falling will be minimized.
g. Assist in clothing selection.
h. Provide large color cues rather than written instructions to identify medications.
i. Place medications in different-sized bottles or use medication box to assist in medication identification.

B. Communication
1. Related medical diagnoses
   a. Alzheimer's disease
   b. CVA
   c. Parkinson's disease
   d. Deafness or hearing impairment
2. Assessment
   a. Slurred or difficult-to-understand speech
   b. No verbalization or making repetitive sounds
   c. "Word salad," use of words that do not make sense
   d. Inability to respond to commands or sounds
   e. Use of hearing aid
3. Implementation
   a. Use hearing aid in working condition with battery.
   b. Encourage client to wear hearing aid.
   c. Use word or picture board so client can point out requests.
   d. Ask client to restate communication to ensure that message was received.
   e. Break complex tasks and commands into smaller parts.
   f. Reassure clients when they become frustrated with inability to speak or communicate.

III. Functional ability and rehabilitation potential
A. Functional ability
1. Related medical diagnoses
   a. Hip, wrist, and vertebral fractures
   b. Paralysis
   c. CVA
   d. Arthritis
   e. Alzheimer's disease and other dementias
2. Assessment
   a. Inability to ambulate, transfer, bathe, toilet, eat, or perform personal care independently
   b. Unkempt appearance
   c. Isolation
   d. Skin breakdown
   e. Malnourishment and dehydration
3. Implementation
   a. Set rehabilitative goals:
      1) To restore function to maximum self-sufficiency
      2) To replace assistance with task segmentation and verbal cuing
      3) To restore ability to support client function with fewer supports
      4) To shorten time required to provide assistance

      5) To expand the space in which self-sufficiency can be practiced
      6) To avoid or delay additional loss of independence
      7) To support the client who is certain to decline in order to lessen the likelihood of complications
   b. Select clothing that is easier to dress in (jogging suits, slip-on shoes, two-piece underwear).
   c. Help resident to use assistive devices that reduce energy expenditure and promote independence in dressing (garter ropes to pull on socks, rigid sock sleeve).
   d. Ask client to identify things that may support independence in dressing, grooming, bathing, toileting, transfers, ambulation, and eating.
   e. Encourage strengthening exercises for weakened muscle groups that client can do independently or with assistance.
   f. Instruct in use of ambulation and mobility aids (walker, cane, wheelchair).
   g. Encourage client to ambulate to and from activities and meals.
   h. Monitor respiratory rate, pulse rate, and BP with increase in client's activity and any complaints of exhaustion.
   i. Make home visits to assess appropriateness of discharge to the home environment and to instruct or recommend changes to family members (number of steps; main-floor bathroom; doorways and rooms that will accommodate walker or wheelchair).
   j. Allow client and family to verbalize concerns about discharge and ability to meet functional needs.
   k. Discuss slower recovery time from major illness associated with aging.

B. Falls
1. Related medical diagnoses
   a. Hip fracture and vertebral fractures
   b. Paralysis
   c. CVA
   d. Arthritis
   e. Alzheimer's disease and other dementias
   f. Orthostatic hypotension
   g. Peripheral neuropathy
2. Assessment
   a. Reduced hearing or vision or both
   b. Dizziness or syncope
   c. Impaired balance
   d. Confusion
   e. Impaired physical mobility
   f. Orthostatic hypotension
   g. Use of psychoactive (sedating) drugs
   h. Use of diuretics, antihypertensives, anticonvulsants, cardiac antiarrhythmics, and alcohol
   i. History of falls
3. Implementation
   a. Assess medications for appropriate dosages and dosage times.

b. Consult with physician for medication-reduction strategy.
c. Living area is free of clutter.
d. Railings and grab bars are available in halls, stairwells, and bathrooms.
e. Bed is in low position.
f. Call signal is within easy reach at all times.
g. Personal items are within safe reach (water, television controls, radio, phone, comb, toothbrush, reading material).
h. Well-lighted rooms and night lights are available.
i. Nonskid floor surfaces are available.
j. Instruct client to move from lying to sitting to standing positions, slowly pausing at each position change.
k. Electronic bed or chair alarms are available.
l. Self-releasing seatbelts are available when client sits up in chair (if client can release them independently, they are not restraints).
m. Siderails and chest or belt restraints are available in chair and bed with a physician's order; be careful of their use, as it may lead to agitation, decreased mobility, incontinence, and skin breakdown.
n. Keep wheelchairs locked during transfers.
o. A bedside commode is present.
p. Elevated toilet seats and high-seated chairs are available.

IV. Urinary incontinence; indwelling catheter
A. Related medical diagnoses
1. Fecal impaction
2. Atrophic vaginitis
3. Prostatic hypertrophy
4. UTI
5. Dehydration
6. Use of diuretics or psychoactive drugs
7. Alzheimer's disease or other dementias
B. Data collection
1. Inability to recognize and/or respond to the urge to void
2. Loss of urine
3. Inability to get to the toilet in time to void
4. Foul-smelling urine
5. Small amounts of concentrated urine
C. Implementation
1. Document an incontinence record to identify times or patterns of incontinence.
2. Perform urine culture to rule out UTI.
3. Perform a rectal check to assess for fecal impaction.
4. Monitor fluid intake, and encourage 1500–3000 ml of fluid per 24 hours.
5. Identify most appropriate method for toileting.
6. Toilet every 2 hours, or as appropriate for client's pattern of incontinence.
7. Monitor urine characteristics.
8. Urinary indwelling catheters are indicated only when a client is documented to be terminally ill, has stage 3 or 4 buttocks or coccyx skin breakdown, or has no spontaneous voiding.

V. Nutritional status
A. Factors related to nutritional problems
1. Physiological factors
a. Aging process
b. Chronic diseases
1) Diabetes mellitus
2) CVA, COPD, alcoholism
3) Alzheimer's disease and other dementias
4) Nutrient deficiencies (iron, vitamin B_{12}, protein, caloric)
c. Side effects of medical treatment
d. Functional status
2. Psychosocial factors
a. Social interaction
b. Long-established food habits
c. Mental status and behavior
d. Financial need
3. Environmental factors
a. Dining room atmosphere
b. Staffing during meal times
c. Food preparation and serving
d. Alternatives to meals being served
B. Data collection
1. Loss of teeth or gum disease
2. Poorly fitting dentures
3. Refusal to eat
4. Eating <75% of meals
5. Refusal to eat in public dining area
6. Weight loss
C. Implementation
1. Provide meals with texture and appearance that are pleasing to the client yet are appropriate to the client's chewing and swallowing ability.
2. Promote a pleasant dining room environment.
3. Offer alternatives to clients who do not finish at least 75% of their meals.
4. Provide between-meal nutritional supplements.
5. Use universal cuffs and utensils with built-up handles to promote independence in feeding.
6. Allow client the opportunity to feed himself or herself before you feed him or her.
7. Encourage finger foods that may allow independence in feeding.
8. Allow client to choose foods.
9. Provide feeding tubes for clients with severely compromised nutritional status. Monitor for:
a. Aspiration and respiratory distress
b. Placement of tube and potential dysfunction
c. Nasal irritation
d. Distended abdomen
e. Gastric ulcers or hemorrhage
f. Pain
g. Client pulling tube out

VI. Dehydration, fluid maintenance
A. Related medical diagnoses
1. Alzheimer's disease and other dementias
2. Diabetes mellitus, COPD
3. Terminal disease (cancer)
4. Urinary incontinence
B. Data collection
1. Confusion
2. Weakness

3. Poor skin turgor
4. Dry mouth, tongue, and skin
5. Concentrated urine, low urine output
6. Poor fluid intake to control incontinence

C. Implementation
1. Explain necessity of 2000–3000 ml of fluid intake a day.
2. Increase amount of fluid served with meals.
3. Give 8 oz of fluid with medications.
4. Provide water pitcher and glass at bedside.
5. Assist functionally disabled clients to drink recommended amount of fluid daily.
6. Monitor fluid intake and urinary output.

VII. Pressure ulcers
A. Related medical diagnoses and risk factors
1. Hip, wrist, and vertebral fractures
2. Paralysis, arthritis, CVA, Parkinson's disease
3. Alzheimer's disease and other dementias
4. Diabetes mellitus
5. Spasms and contracture
6. Incontinence
7. Pressure, shear, moisture, and friction
8. Terminal disease

B. Data collection
1. Areas of redness or open wounds over areas of pressure
2. Coccyx, hip, heel, and buttocks the most common areas for pressure ulcers
3. Low serum albumen level, Hgb or Hct

C. Implementation
1. Prevention is the key to treatment because pressure ulcers are very difficult to heal.
2. Turn and reposition client every 2 hours or more when in bed and even when sitting up in chair.
3. Instruct client to do small weight shifts that can change pressure over bony areas.
4. Keep skin dry and immediately remove any urine and feces from skin.
5. Do not massage reddened area of skin, as it may further traumatize or even break down the fragile capillary system under the skin.
6. Monitor and document size of wound, signs of healing, any drainage or odor, and type of treatment used.
7. Follow Agency for Health Care Policy and Research protocol.

1. A 49-year-old woman was admitted to a physical rehabilitation unit 2 weeks after surgery for a below-the-knee amputation on her right leg. She asks, "Why do I have to keep wrapping my stump?" The nurse's best response is:

   A. "You will have to shrink and shape the residual limb to fit the prosthesis."
   B. "You want to increase the size of the residual limb to fit the prosthesis."
   C. "You need to because it is what your physical therapist wants."
   D. "You need to speak to your doctor."

2. To prevent flexion contraction of the hip after a below-the-knee amputation, the nurse should encourage the client to be:

   A. In supine position with a pillow between the legs
   B. In a semi-Fowler's position most of the day
   C. In supine position with a pillow under the knees
   D. In prone position

3. After a below-the-knee amputation, a client states, "Please tell me I am not crazy because it still feels like my right foot is still there." The nurse's best response is:

   A. "Since your leg is not there, you should not feel anything."
   B. "You are experiencing phantom limb sensation, which is normal."
   C. "It might be best for you to see a psychiatrist to help you deal with your loss."
   D. "Next you will be telling me you can see your toes."

4. In caring for a residual limb after a below-the-knee amputation, the nurse knows that which of the following statements by the client indicates a need for further teaching? "I should

   A. Inspect the stump for redness and abrasions."
   B. Apply lotion or alcohol to the stump."
   C. Use a stump sock or Ace bandage."
   D. Clean the stump with mild soap."

5. A 65-year-old man with hypertension has suffered a stroke and has right hemiplegia. When assessing the client, the nurse expects to find:

   A. Weakness on one side of the body
   B. Paralysis of the lower extremities
   C. Total body paralysis
   D. Paralysis of one side of the body

6. A client has dysphagia. The nurse would include in the plan of care which of the following?

   A. Promote exercises to decrease facial rigidity.
   B. Allow extra time for speaking.
   C. Institute special feeding precautions.
   D. Increase light in the environment.

7. When assessing a client after a stroke, the nurse notes that there is an impairment of the ability to read, write, speak, listen, and comprehend. The nurse identifies this as:

   A. Ataxia
   B. Aphasia
   C. Dysphagia
   D. Agnosia

8. A client's entire posterior chest and buttocks have full-thickness burns. Using the Rule of Nines, the nurse would calculate the BSA burned as:

   A. 9
   B. 18
   C. 27
   D. 36

9. Which of the following is the most characteristic symptom of the disequilibrium syndrome associated with hemodialysis?

   A. Seizures
   B. Hypertension
   C. Chest pain
   D. Shortness of breath

10. A wife whose husband has suffered an MI states, "My husband's favorite foods are fried chicken and french-fried potatoes. Would it be okay for me to bring him some?" The nurse's best response is:

    A. "That's a good idea; he has a hearty appetite."
    B. "If you bring him only a small amount, it will be okay."
    C. "First let's speak to the dietitian about his diet."
    D. "No, you can't bring food into the hospital."

11. The nurse is preparing a 42-year-old man for hospital discharge after an MI. Which of the following statements indicates the need for further teaching?

    A. "I will take my medications as prescribed."
    B. "I will follow a low-cholesterol, low-fat diet."
    C. "I can exercise as much as I want."
    D. "I can have a small glass of wine with the evening meal."

12. A wife whose husband has suffered a stroke notices that he cries and laughs inappropriately. She asks, "Why does he do that?" The nurse's best response is:

    A. "He is experiencing emotional lability, which is common after a stroke."
    B. "Ignore him; he likes to play games."
    C. "Don't you also cry when something is funny and laugh when it is not?"
    D. "I don't know; maybe he needs a psychiatrist."

13. A 17-year-old girl was injured in a car accident. She now has paraplegia secondary to a T11 spinal cord injury. The nurse identifies the four divisions of the spinal column as:

    A. Coccygeal, cranial, thoracic, lumbar
    B. Cervical, thoracic, lumbar, sacral

C. Cervical, trochanter, ischial, sacral
D. Thoracic, coccygeal, femur, ulnar

14. The nurse assesses for which of the following symptoms in a T11 spinal cord injury?
    A. Loss of movement in both the upper and lower extremities
    B. Loss of bladder control
    C. Loss of movement in the upper extremities
    D. Loss of respiratory control

15. Humulin NPH insulin is administered at 7 AM. At what time would the nurse anticipate the peak action to take place?
    A. 9 AM
    B. 12 noon
    C. 5 PM
    D. 11 PM

16. While the client is in the prone position, which site is most likely to develop a pressure area?
    A. Occiput
    B. Buttocks
    C. Heels
    D. Toes

17. When performing endotracheal suctioning, suctioning should be limited to how many seconds?
    A. 5
    B. 10
    C. 20
    D. 30

18. A 56-year-old man is walking down the hall and complains of chest pain. Before administering nitroglycerin sublingually, what action should be performed first?
    A. Call for a stat 12 lead ECG.
    B. Lower the head of the bed.
    C. Start oxygen with a nasal cannula.
    D. Tell client to stop and rest.

19. Which position facilitates the greatest expansion of the lungs for the client restricted to bedrest?
    A. High-Fowler's
    B. Low-Fowler's
    C. Sims'
    D. Trendelenburg

20. For adults, the diastolic BP is recorded when:
    A. The first sound is heard during cuff deflation
    B. The muffled sound is heard during cuff deflation
    C. The muffled sound is heard during cuff inflation
    D. The last sound is heard during cuff deflation

21. When teaching a female client the proper technique for cleaning the perineum before intermittent self-catheterization, the nurse would teach her to separate the labia and:
    A. Wipe from back to front
    B. Wipe in a circular motion
    C. Wipe from side to side

D. Wipe from front to back

22. When administering which medication does the nurse frequently obtain peak-and-trough levels?
    A. Digoxin
    B. Heparin
    C. Aminophylline
    D. Vancomycin

23. What is the minimum time established for a health-care worker to properly wash the hands?
    A. 10 seconds
    B. 30 seconds
    C. 45 seconds
    D. 60 seconds

24. Which of the following is a common symptom of constipation?
    A. Increase in appetite
    B. Suprapubic distention
    C. Vomiting
    D. Firm abdomen

25. What directions should the nurse give a client who has just been given a suppository for complaints of constipation?
    A. Get up and go to the toilet immediately.
    B. Wait 5–10 minutes before going to the toilet.
    C. Wait 20–30 minutes before going to the toilet.
    D. Remain in the prone position before getting up and going to the toilet.

26. The physician has ordered povidone-iodine (Betadine) for wound care. When pouring povidone-iodine onto the 4 × 4 bandages, the nurse should:
    A. Hold the bottle with the label facing the sterile field
    B. Pour while holding the bottle high over the sterile field
    C. Pour 1–2 ml into another container before pouring onto the sterile bandages
    D. Pour some into a cap and then over the sterile bandages

27. The major cause of nosocomial infection in the hospital setting is:
    A. Excessive use of disposable equipment
    B. Proximity of beds in a semiprivate room
    C. Infrequent handwashing
    D. Excessive use of oral antibiotics

28. A surgical incision has become infected and now requires wound care every 8 hours. When packing the incision with saline-soaked 4 × 4 bandages, the nurse accidentally drops the dressing on the client's chest. The nurse should:
    A. Use the bandage if the client has just bathed
    B. Resoak the bandage in sterile saline and place it in the incision
    C. Discard that bandage and prepare a fresh one
    D. Use the bandage on top of other sterile bandages

29. The nurse knows the best place to assess for pallor in a very dark-skinned person is:

A. The sclera
B. The nailbed
C. The mucous membranes
D. The lips

30. While charting, the nurse makes an error while writing in the nurse's notes. The nurse should:

A. Write with erasable ink to easily correct the entry
B. Draw lines through the entry until the entry is no longer readable
C. Draw one straight line through the erroneous entry, initial it, and write "error"
D. Draw one straight line through the erroneous entry and initial it

31. Your client has left-leg weakness and needs to use a cane. You observe proper ambulation with the cane when the client:

A. Keeps one point of support on the floor at all times
B. Keeps two points of support on the floor at all times
C. Leans slightly to the left with the cane in the left hand
D. Uses the proper-length cane—the top of the cane should be at waist level

32. To measure BP accurately, the nurse should:

A. Position the client's arm above the level of the heart
B. Position the cuff at least 2 inches above the site of the radial artery pulsation
C. Position the client's arm extended, with the palm down
D. Center the arrow marker on the cuff over the brachial artery pulsation

33. The most accurate technique used to assess the apical pulse is:

A. Inspection
B. Palpation
C. Auscultation
D. Percussion

34. The nurse is giving discharge instructions to a client who will be receiving oxygen at home, including placing a "No Smoking" sign at all entrances to the home. The rationale for using the sign is:

A. Oxygen can cause a fire to ignite.
B. Oxygen can cause an explosion.
C. The sign alerts visitors to enter the home at their own risk.
D. Smoking causes lung cancer.

35. The nurse plans to give a complete bed bath to a 70-year-old woman. When cleansing the face area, the nurse should use:

A. Warm water only
B. Tissues instead of a washcloth
C. Liquid soap on all areas except the eyes and lips
D. The client's preference of facial soap and warm water

36. While receiving a soapsuds enema, the client complains of abdominal cramps. The nurse should:

A. Temporarily stop the flow of the enema
B. Tell the client to breathe slowly through the mouth

C. Raise the height of the enema container
D. Clamp the tubing and withdraw the rectal tube

37. The nurse auscultates a BP of 180/99 in the right arm and decides to double-check the reading. Before reinflating the cuff, the nurse should wait:

A. 10 seconds
B. 30 seconds
C. 1 minute
D. 2 minutes

38. The nurse obtains a report from the laboratory stating her client's serum potassium is 4.3 mEq/L. Which action should she perform next?

A. Notify the doctor immediately, because the value is dangerously low.
B. Note the value in her notes, and notify the doctor when he makes rounds.
C. This is a panic value. The level is dangerously high, and the doctor must be notified immediately.
D. Offer the client potassium-rich foods such as orange juice and bananas.

39. Postoperatively, a client has not voided in more than 8 hours. The nurse feels the lower abdomen and finds it to be distended. The method of physical examination used by the nurse is termed:

A. Auscultation
B. Percussion
C. Palpation
D. Inspection

40. A sterile specimen would be obtained from an indwelling Foley catheter by:

A. Taking urine from the urinometer
B. Taking urine from the drainage bag
C. Disconnecting the catheter from the drainage tubing
D. Withdrawing urine from the latex port

41. The nurse knows that an enteric-coated oral medication:

A. Dissolves rapidly when placed under the tongue
B. Needs to be shaken before being administered
C. Does not dissolve until it reaches the small intestine
D. Needs to be chewed and taken with a full glass of water

42. A client is ordered to receive an IM injection by the Z-track method. The rationale for the use of this method is that it:

A. Prevents the drug from irritating the skin
B. Allows faster absorption of the drug
C. Eliminates discomfort caused by the needle
D. Allows slower absorption of the drug

43. Medications are absorbed most rapidly through which of the following routes?

A. Topical
B. IV
C. IM
D. Oral

44. After abdominal surgery, your client has a Salem sump tube that is draining excessive amounts of fluid. Which acid-base disturbance is most likely to occur?

    A. Metabolic acidosis
    B. Metabolic alkalosis
    C. Respiratory acidosis
    D. Respiratory alkalosis

45. Your client is being discharged and has been instructed how to lift objects to avoid lower back strain. Which of the following statements made by the client is correct? "I must

    A. Narrow my base of support."
    B. Move away from the object to be lifted."
    C. Position my center of gravity high above the object to be lifted."
    D. Maintain alignment of the head, neck, and back while lifting."

46. The nurse knows that evaluation is:

    A. The final phase of the nursing process
    B. Not related to client goals of care
    C. The first phase of the nursing process
    D. A continuous and ongoing process

47. To administer oral care to an unconscious client, the nurse should:

    A. Use a toothbrush and floss after every meal
    B. Squirt 30 ml of mouthwash into the mouth and then suction the oral cavity
    C. Scrape secretions from inside the mouth with a tongue blade
    D. Use a padded tongue blade to keep the mouth open

48. According to the AHA, which of the following is the most prevalent form of cardiovascular disease?

    A. Stroke
    B. CAD
    C. Hypertension
    D. Rheumatic heart disease

49. A 65-year-old man is admitted to the hospital with the diagnosis of congestive heart failure (CHF). Which of the following is an expected symptom of CHF?

    A. Shortness of breath
    B. Decrease in tissue turgor
    C. Flat neck veins
    D. Left upper quadrant abdominal tenderness

50. Which of the following would be an appropriate nursing intervention for a client in CHF?

    A. Assess daily weight.
    B. Encourage fluids.
    C. Position the head of the bed <30 degrees upright.
    D. Teach the importance of a diet enriched with sodium.

51. Which of the following is the usual adult daily dose of digoxin?

    A. 0.025 mg
    B. 0.25 mg

C. 2.5 mg
D. 25 mg

52. Which symptom represents a toxic side effect of digoxin?

    A. Ringing in the ears
    B. Fluid retention
    C. Anorexia, nausea, vomiting
    D. Hair loss

53. Which of the following is a symptom of thrombophlebitis of the leg?

    A. Negative Homans' sign
    B. Weak or absent pedal pulses
    C. Cool temperature and mottled appearance of the foot
    D. Calf pain with dorsiflexion of the foot

54. Which intervention would be indicated for a client with thrombophlebitis of the leg?

    A. Encourage fluids by mouth.
    B. Gently massage the affected leg.
    C. Keep the leg positioned below the level of the heart.
    D. Start antibiotic therapy.

55. The rationale for starting a heparin infusion for a client with thrombophlebitis is:

    A. Heparin dissolves blood clots.
    B. Heparin dilates the vessels to increase blood flow in the leg.
    C. Heparin prevents additional clots from forming.
    D. Heparin constricts the vessels to increase blood flow in the leg.

56. A heparin drip consists of 25,000 units of heparin in 250 ml D_5W. The infusion is being delivered via an infusion pump at a rate of 10 ml/hr. How many units per hour are infusing?

    A. 10
    B. 100
    C. 1000
    D. 2500

57. Your client will be discharged from the hospital on warfarin (Coumadin). Which of the following statements do you want to include in teaching about this drug?

    A. Decrease your dietary intake of green leafy vegetables.
    B. When you have a headache, aspirin may be taken to relieve the discomfort.
    C. You will need to have periodic PTT drawn.
    D. Shave with a straight-edge razor.

58. Which of the following is the best site for assessing skin turgor in an 80-year-old client?

    A. Dorsal hand
    B. Forearm
    C. Sternum
    D. Ankles

59. When would you advise someone with unknown heart disease who is experiencing chest pain to seek emergency care?

A. If the chest pain persists more than 2 minutes
B. If three nitroglycerin tablets taken 3–5 minutes apart do not relieve the pain
C. If more than six nitroglycerin tablets are taken in a 24-hour period
D. When the chest pain goes away

60. A 55-year-old female client has been diagnosed with CAD. Which therapeutic intervention would offer a cure for this disease?

A. Coronary artery bypass graft (CABG) surgery
B. Placement of a coronary artery stent
C. Balloon angioplasty of the coronary artery blockage
D. No cure currently available

61. Which of the following would be a major modifiable risk factor for the development of CAD?

A. Obesity
B. Family history of CAD
C. Cigarette smoking
D. Diabetes

62. Which of the following is the best site to assess for edema in a client confined to bed?

A. Ankles
B. Pretibial
C. Hands
D. Sacrum

63. The nurse is teaching a client nutritional aspects of a low-cholesterol diet. Which statement made by the client indicates understanding of the diet?

A. "Broiled chicken, with the skin removed, contains no cholesterol."
B. "Eat fish rather than red meat because it contains no cholesterol."
C. "It is permissible to use polyunsaturated oils to fry food."
D. "Egg whites do not contain cholesterol."

64. The discomfort of angina pectoris most commonly radiates to what area of the body?

A. Left arm
B. Both arms
C. Neck bilaterally
D. Jaw unilaterally

65. The nurse is caring for a client 2 days after percutaneous coronary angioplasty (PTCA). During the morning assessment, a pulse deficit is detected. A pulse deficit is best described as:

A. The absence of a particular pulse
B. The difference between the systolic and diastolic BP
C. The difference between the apical and radial heart rates
D. The radial pulse minus the apical pulse rate

66. Which nursing intervention is appropriate when caring for a client immediately after cardiac catheterization?

A. Allow to ambulate to bathroom with assistance only.
B. Monitor pedal pulses frequently.

C. Maintain the head of bed in a high-Fowler's position.
D. Restrict fluids.

67. Which pulse is located behind the medial malleolus?

A. Radial
B. Popliteal
C. Dorsalis pedis
D. Posterior tibial

68. A 38-year-old man has hypertension. He is interested in starting an exercise program. What form of exercise would be best for him?

A. Bicycling
B. Water skiing
C. Weight lifting
D. Calisthenics

69. Which condiment would the nurse recommend to a client who is on a low-sodium diet?

A. Catsup
B. Lemon juice
C. Garlic salt
D. Soy sauce

70. A 39-year-old man was admitted to the hospital 4 days ago with an acute MI. He is expected to be discharged tomorrow. Suddenly he calls you to his room and complains of chest pain. Which action should you perform first?

A. Assess the vital signs.
B. Administer nitroglycerin sublingually stat.
C. Raise the head of the bed to a 30–45-degree angle.
D. Call the physician stat.

71. A 56-year-old woman was placed on strict I&O. Her diagnosis is renal insufficiency. The I&O for the last 24 hours was 3000 cc in and 1000 cc out. Based on this information, the nurse anticipates her weight to:

A. Increase by 2 kg
B. Increase by approximately 2 lb
C. Decrease by approximately 2 lb
D. Remain the same

72. A client with chronic CHF is being discharged on furosemide (Lasix). The dietitian advises a diet high in potassium. Which food choice listed below has the most potassium content?

A. Peanuts
B. Peaches
C. Broccoli
D. Milk

73. A 60-year-old man has an ileostomy. He is admitted to the hospital with nausea, vomiting, diarrhea, and severe dehydration. What IV fluids would this nurse expect the physician to order?

A. 0.9 normal saline (NS) with added potassium
B. 0.9 NS
C. 0.45 (½ NS) with added potassium
D. 3% NS with added potassium

74. Which of the following would be included in the routine care of an ileostomy?
    A. Bowel training, thus eliminating need to wear appliance
    B. Irrigating the stoma daily to promote continence
    C. Providing a skin barrier around the stoma
    D. Administering a stool softener daily

75. A 75-year-old man has a diagnosis of oat cell cancer of the lung. After several courses of chemotherapy, the tumor has not responded. There are no other treatment options available, and he is dying. Which of the following is the most appropriate action for the nurse to take while caring for this dying client?
    A. Limit visitors to no more than two at a time.
    B. Request frequent reassignments to prevent becoming too attached to client and family.
    C. Advise the client and family to settle unfinished business.
    D. Request reassignments when client displays angry behavior.

76. A client with a diagnosis of terminal cancer states, "If I can just beat this thing, I'll go back to church every Sunday." Which stage of the dying process does this statement represent?
    A. Denial
    B. Anger
    C. Depression
    D. Bargaining

77. For which of the following infusions must the nurse use an electronic controlling device delivery system?
    A. Dopamine
    B. Packed RBCs
    C. Vancomycin
    D. One liter D$_5$W with 40 mEq KCl

78. A breathing pattern in which respirations gradually wax and wane in a regular pattern (increase and decrease in rate and depth) with periods of apnea is known as:
    A. Kussmaul's
    B. Biot's
    C. Cheyne-Stokes
    D. Eupnea

79. While a nurse is bathing a terminally ill client, he stops breathing. He has told the nurse many times that he does not want to live on machines. The physician has not written a "do not resuscitate" order. The nurse's best response is to:
    A. Continue bathing him for 5 minutes and then call a full code.
    B. Start CPR immediately and then call a full code.
    C. Start artificial respiration, but if asystole occurs, stop trying to revive him.
    D. Stop the bath, and consult with the charge nurse for further instructions.

80. While providing postmortem care, the nurse will:
    A. Place an incontinence pad under the buttocks
    B. Place the body in a flat position

C. Remove the dentures
D. Remove the hospital armband

81. The most characteristic assessment finding for the client in pulmonary edema is:
    A. Nondistended neck veins
    B. Anxiety
    C. Generalized edema
    D. Pink, frothy sputum

82. Vancomycin 500 mg in 250 cc of IV solution is to be administered over 90 minutes IV piggyback. Calculate the rate in drops per minute using a drop factor of 20 gtts/ml.
    A. 20 gtts/min
    B. 56 gtts/min
    C. 83 gtts/min
    D. 90 gtts/min

83. A 76-year-old female client informs you that she has been having vaginal bleeding for the last several days. Which of the following is the most appropriate response?
    A. Reassure her that vaginal bleeding is normal for her age.
    B. Explain that the bleeding will stop in a few days.
    C. Encourage her to notify her doctor.
    D. Encourage her to notify her daughter.

84. A 60-year-old man is scheduled for suprapubic resection of the prostate in the morning. He discusses with you that he is worried about his sexual functioning after surgery. Your most appropriate response would be:
    A. Assume he is joking and chuckle at his statement.
    B. "Don't worry, the surgery will not affect your sexual functioning."
    C. "I understand your concern, but most men do not experience a problem after surgery."
    D. "I understand your concern. Most men do experience sexual functioning problems after this type of surgery."

85. Which of the following interventions would be appropriate when caring for a client with hypercalcemia?
    A. Encourage fluids.
    B. Promote bedrest.
    C. Administer calcium supplement tablets.
    D. Administer antibiotics.

86. Which of the following would be an appropriate food choice for a neutropenic client?
    A. Bananas
    B. Carrot sticks
    C. Garden salad
    D. Canned pears

87. Which of the following does the nurse recognize as being the only diagnostic parameter for cancer?
    A. Elevated carcinoembryonic antigen (CEA) level
    B. Positive tissue biopsy
    C. Sore that does not heal
    D. Nagging cough or hoarseness

88. A 40-year-old man has developed stomatitis after chemotherapy treatment. He should be encouraged to:

   A. Eat hot, spicy foods
   B. Brush his teeth after each meal and at bedtime
   C. Rinse his mouth with commercial mouthwash after each meal
   D. Drink plenty of orange juice

89. When irrigating a descending colostomy with 1000 ml of warm tap water, the nurse would expect:

   A. Complete return of the solution plus soft or formed feces
   B. Complete return of the solution mixed with liquid stool
   C. Evacuation of soft and formed feces only
   D. Evacuation of tap water only

90. Which acid-base disturbance would be most characteristic of a narcotic overdose?

   A. Metabolic acidosis
   B. Respiratory acidosis
   C. Metabolic alkalosis
   D. Respiratory alkalosis

91. The nurse recognizes which of the following as early signs of hypoxemia?

   A. Restlessness, yawning, tachycardia
   B. Dyspnea, restlessness, hypotension
   C. Yawning, confusion, bradycardia
   D. Bradycardia, hypotension, dyspnea

92. In compliance with standard (Universal) blood and body fluid precautions, the nurse would wear which of the following when giving an IM injection?

   A. Mask, gown, gloves, goggles
   B. Gloves and gown only
   C. Gloves
   D. Gloves and goggles

93. Before beginning intermittent feeding via NG tube, the nurse will first:

   A. Auscultate for bowel sounds and instill 100 cc of air
   B. Auscultate for bowel sounds and instill 10 ml of tap water
   C. Confirm tube placement with an abdominal x-ray
   D. Aspirate and reinstill the stomach contents

94. What side effects would you expect a client to experience receiving external beam irradiation for esophageal cancer?

   A. Nausea, dysphagia, bone marrow suppression
   B. Diarrhea, dysphagia, bone marrow suppression
   C. Alopecia, nausea, dysphagia
   D. Dysphagia, alopecia, constipation

95. A female client is receiving external beam irradiation for squamous cell cancer of the lung. After 2 weeks of treatment, her skin in the treatment field is red and warm to touch. Your best response would be to apply which of the following?

   A. Solarcaine, and notify the doctor
   B. A&D ointment, and notify the doctor
   C. Desitin, and notify the doctor
   D. Nothing, but notify the doctor

96. A 49-year-old Jehovah's Witness was recently given a diagnosis of multiple myeloma. The Hgb level is 6.3 and the doctor writes an order to infuse 4 units of RBCs. The client refuses the transfusion on religious grounds. The nurse's most appropriate response would be to:

   A. Do nothing
   B. Notify the doctor of the client's refusal
   C. Convince the client to take the transfusion
   D. Administer the transfusion as ordered

97. A 50-year-old female client is thrombocytopenic (decreased platelets) secondary to chemotherapy. She complains of nausea and vomiting. All of the following medications are ordered on an as-needed basis. Which medication would be the most appropriate for the client to receive?

   A. Promethazine (Phenergan) 25 mg PO
   B. Thiethylperazine maleate (Torcan) 10 mg IM
   C. Promethazine 25 mg suppository
   D. Prochlorperazine maleate (Compazine) 10 mg IV push

98. Your client is receiving continuous enteral nutrition via an NG tube. Which of the following interventions is the most important to prevention aspiration?

   A. Adding blue food coloring to the formula
   B. Keeping the head of the bed elevated
   C. Administering at rates less than 50 ml/hr
   D. Hanging no more formula than the client will receive in a 4-hour period

99. While assisting a client with right-sided hemiparesis to ambulate, the nurse should stand on the client's:

   A. Left side and hold the left hand
   B. Right side and hold the right hand
   C. Left side and hold one arm around the client's waist
   D. Right side and hold one arm around the client's waist

100. After an eye operation, the client may experience partial loss of sight. The nurse should assist at mealtime by:

   A. Feeding the client everything on the tray
   B. Encouraging the family to feed the client
   C. Orienting the client to the location of all foods on the tray
   D. Encouraging the client to use a spoon only

101. A 33-year-old client has pneumonia. When the nurse assesses this client, the following data will receive highest priority:

   A. Size of pupil, presence of sneezing, location of pain
   B. Presence of hiccups, amount of sweating, BP
   C. Capillary refill, amount of sputum, trembling
   D. Restlessness, chest wall movement, color of nails

102. A 42-year-old client has pneumonia and is receiving oxygen by nasal cannula. The quickest way to obtain an accurate reading of his temperature is to take it by:

A. Mouth
B. Axilla
C. Rectum
D. Feeling the forehead

103. The nurse is teaching a first-aid class for parents. The topic is treatment for a nosebleed. One of the parents indicates a need for further teaching with the following statement:

 A. "Pinch the soft part of the nose firmly."
 B. "Administer some warm milk or cocoa."
 C. "Apply ice to the back of the neck or to the nose."
 D. "Consult a physician as needed."

104. A 56-year-old client is scheduled for a partial laryngectomy. The nurse recognizes that he needs more preparation for surgery when the following statement is heard:

 A. "I will be able to talk by covering the tracheostomy tube."
 B. "I will be fed through a tube for a few days after surgery."
 C. "My bed should be in Fowler's position."
 D. "I should hold my head still after surgery."

105. A 26-year-old client is experiencing an attack of asthma. The following outcome will receive the highest priority in the care of this client:

 A. The client's anxiety level will be reduced.
 B. The client should maintain an open airway with adequate gas exchange.
 C. The client should talk about how he feels about his disease.
 D. The client should maintain adequate fluid balance.

106. A 46-year-old client is on a ventilator and is receiving positive-end-expiratory pressure. He starts sweating profusely, the pulse increases to 122 bpm, the trachea is deviated to the right, and breath sounds on the left are diminished. The nurse would prepare for a possible:

 A. Cor pulmonale
 B. Cardiac tamponade
 C. Pneumothorax
 D. Pleural effusion

107. The following laboratory test result indicates that a client is infectious for pulmonary tuberculosis:

 A. A positive Mantoux
 B. A negative Gram stain
 C. Lesion seen on x-ray
 D. Positive sputum for acid-fast bacillus

108. The nurse is teaching a 56-year-old client about hypertension. This nurse recognizes a need for more instruction when the client makes the following statement:

 A. "I need to learn to manage stress better."
 B. "As long as my pressure gets no higher than 140/90, I'm OK."
 C. "High blood pressure can lead to heart attack and/or stroke."

 D. " I can stop taking my blood pressure medicine when I feel all right."

109. A friend calls and states that he has taken three nitroglycerin tablets for his chest pain, but the pain is still there. The nurse advises him to:

 A. Call his doctor
 B. Drive to the nearest emergency room
 C. Lie down and rest to see if the pain goes away
 D. Call 911

110. A 47-year-old client is in acute CHF after an MI. The goal of highest priority for this client at this time is to:

 A. Decrease the workload of the heart
 B. Breathe easily
 C. Decrease edema
 D. Know his medications

111. This is the second postoperative day for a 54-year-old client who had a CABG. At 8 AM her BP is normal; the pulse rate is 123 bpm (normally 82 bpm) and weak. The client is cold, clammy, and confused. Her respiratory rate is 44/min; bowel sounds are absent, and the urinary output is 22 cc/hr. The nurse prepares for the treatment of:

 A. CHF
 B. MI
 C. Shock
 D. Cardiac tamponade

112. The nurse is about to administer a dose of digoxin to a client. The client states that she has not eaten her breakfast and complains of being nauseated and having visual changes. After checking her apical and radial pulses and the serum digoxin level, the nurse would:

 A. Call the physician
 B. Check tissue perfusion
 C. Review the latest electrolyte report
 D. Administer an ordered antiemetic

113. A 33-year-old client is admitted to a nursing unit complaining of pain and swelling in her left leg. She has a positive Homans' sign and is diagnosed with deep vein thrombosis (DVT). An appropriate nursing intervention would be:

 A. Apply antiembolism stockings to both legs.
 B. Administer aspirin for pain.
 C. Massage both legs to promote comfort.
 D. Provide bedrest.

114. A 46-year-old client recently had a radical mastectomy. She will not look at the surgical site and refuses to see her visitors. An appropriate action for the nurse to suggest is:

 A. See a minister.
 B. Talk about her feelings.
 C. Join a support group.
 D. Face reality.

115. A 48-year-old client with leukemia is receiving chemotherapy. Depression of bone marrow is a possible

side effect. The nurse would assess for any signs of infection and/or anemia. The nurse would also observe for:

A. Decrease in cardiac output
B. Drop in urinary output
C. Broken bones
D. Bleeding

116. A client with AIDS indicates that more teaching about the condition is needed when the nurse hears the following statement:

A. "This disease is spread by sexual contact."
B. "I'm afraid to touch anyone; I might give them my disease."
C. "The virus may also be spread through body fluids."
D. "Infected mothers can pass the virus to their unborn infants."

117. A nurse explains to a family that the Sengstaken-Blakemore tube is used for the treatment of:

A. Esophageal varices
B. Cirrhosis of the liver
C. Renal stones
D. Hiatal hernia

118. The nurse recognizes that a client needs more teaching about prevention of peptic ulcer disease (PUD) after he states:

A. "I shouldn't use aspirin-like drugs too often."
B. "I will miss my morning coffee so much."
C. "I have to stop smoking."
D. "I need to manage stress better."

119. A 36-year-old client recently returned from the operating room after having a partial gastrectomy for peptic ulcer disease. He has an NG tube that has been connected to low, intermittent suction for 2 days. A nurse would observe for:

A. High serum potassium level
B. Respiratory alkalosis
C. Metabolic alkalosis
D. Metabolic acidosis

120. A 46-year-old client has his first meal after a Billroth II surgical procedure. About 30 minutes after the meal, he becomes nauseated, feels very weak, and complains of severe gas pains and distention. The nurse prepares for treatment of:

A. Shock after perforation of the GI tract
B. Paralytic ileus
C. GI obstruction
D. Dumping syndrome

121. A 34-year-old client is hospitalized for Crohn's disease; the nurse should assess this client frequently for:

A. Vital signs, bleeding, and diarrhea
B. Skin turgor, urinary output, and electrolyte report results
C. Breath sounds, pupil size, and change in mental status
D. Peripheral perfusion, skin color, and muscle twitching

122. A 39-year-old client has an ileal conduit after recent surgery for cancer of the bladder. The nurse assesses the amount and characteristics of the drainage, the fluid and electrolyte balance of the client, and the condition of the stoma and surrounding skin and for:

A. Adventitious lung sounds
B. Pulse deficits
C. Renal stones
D. Bowel sounds

123. A 27-year-old client has chest tubes connected to a Pleuravac after a stab wound to the left chest. When the client goes to radiology via wheelchair, the nurse would manage the Pleuravac in the following way:

A. Disconnect the Pleuravac from the drainage tubing.
B. Clamp the drainage tubing before disconnecting the Pleuravac.
C. Replace wall suction with a portable suction machine.
D. Attach the Pleuravac to the side of the wheelchair.

124. While assessing a client who has a possible bowel obstruction, the nurse hears very loud, rumbling bowel sounds (a stethoscope is not needed). The nurse would chart these sounds as:

A. Excess flatus
B. Acini
C. Hypoactive
D. Borborygmi

125. A 33-year-old client recently had an inguinal hernia repair. The nurse modifies postoperative care from that given most general surgery clients as follows:

A. Antiembolism stockings are not used for this client.
B. Hemorrhage is not as likely in this client.
C. This client should not cough.
D. Infection is less likely in this client.

126. A 27-year-old client returns to the hospital room after a barium enema. An important part of his nursing care at this point in time is to:

A. Obtain an order for a cleansing enema
B. Observe for signs of renal damage
C. Maintain bedrest until a physician orders otherwise
D. Observe for an allergic reaction to the barium

127. A 16-year-old client complains of abdominal pain. The nurse:

A. Recommends a laxative
B. Checks for rebound tenderness
C. Applies a heating pad
D. Calls the physician

128. A 44-year-old client is diagnosed with peritonitis after a small bowel obstruction. The nurse would:

A. Encourage ambulation
B. Place the client in a supine position
C. Check the mouth for ulcerations
D. Keep the client NPO

129. A client admitted for a diagnostic workup passes a stool that is of normal size in some areas but stringlike in others. The nurse would:

A. Document the finding on the chart
B. Ignore the appearance of the stool
C. Obtain an order for a laxative
D. Check for fecal impaction

130. A nurse is teaching a client about choledocholithiasis. The nurse explains that the term means:

A. Infection of the bile duct
B. Stones in the hepatic and bile duct
C. Inflammation of the gallbladder
D. Stones in the gallbladder

131. When the nurse is giving emotional support to a comatose client, this nurse would:

A. Disturb the client as little as possible
B. Explain all nursing actions to the family
C. Encourage the client to express feelings
D. Explain all nursing actions to the client

132. A nurse is doing preoperative teaching for a client who will have a cholecystectomy. The nurse teaches that special care must be taken to prevent the following postoperative complication:

A. Hypostatic pneumonia
B. Thrombosis
C. Hemorrhage
D. Paralytic ileus

133. A nurse is teaching a client with newly diagnosed hepatitis A. The client asks, "How did I catch this disease?" The best response by the nurse is which of the following?

A. Blood or contaminated needles
B. Body fluids
C. Sexual intercourse
D. Feces or contaminated food or water

134. A client has been given a diagnosis of hepatitis A. The nurse would use which of the following precautions for preventing transmission of the disease to self and others?

A. Reverse isolation
B. A mask and gown
C. Universal Precautions
D. Isolation precautions for trash

135. A 44-year-old client has cirrhosis of the liver with severe ascites. The nurse plans for the following intervention:

A. Apply prolonged pressure to injection sites.
B. Administer aspirin for headache as needed.
C. Measure abdominal girth weekly.
D. Provide a low-protein, high-carbohydrate diet.

136. A client has been given a diagnosis of acute pancreatitis. The nurse will assess this client for:

A. Hyperkalemia
B. Metabolic acidosis
C. Hypocalcemia
D. Hyperglycemia

137. A nurse assesses the surgical wound of a client who recently had an appendectomy. The wound is red and

swollen with pus oozing from the lower edge. The nurse would:

A. Clean the wound with an antibiotic solution
B. Report the findings to a physician
C. Clean the wound with hydrogen peroxide
D. Irrigate the wound with NS

138. A 34-year-old client has third-degree burns on 10% of the BSA. A dressing change is scheduled for 10 AM. The nurse would:

A. Force fluids by mouth
B. Use clean technique for changing the dressing
C. Administer the analgesic as needed at about 9 AM
D. Monitor I&O each shift

139. A 23-year-old client received multiple superficial injuries in a motorcycle accident. The nurse in the emergency room will:

A. Ask when the client had the last tetanus shot
B. Administer a tetanus injection as prescribed
C. Treat the injuries and send the client home
D. Administer morphine as prescribed for pain

140. A 47-year-old man enters the emergency room complaining of severe pain in the left flank, which radiates to the suprapubic area. He is nauseated and gives a history of renal stones. The nurse would:

A. Save all of the client's urine
B. Keep the client NPO
C. Record I&O
D. Strain all urine through gauze

141. A 41-year-old client has a ureteral catheter because of a stone in the left lower ureter. The nurse would:

A. Clamp the catheter and change the drainage tubing as needed
B. Record output from the ureteral catheter separately
C. Irrigate the ureteral catheter every 4 hours
D. Maintain bedrest until the catheter is removed

142. A client with chronic renal failure in the early stage of uremia is instructed on diet. The nurse recognizes a need for more instruction when the following statement is heard:

A. "I will need meat three times a day and all the milk I can drink."
B. "I need a lot of calories to provide energy for healing."
C. "I need to avoid foods high in potassium, like bananas and raisins."
D. "I can't add salt to my food or eat foods high in salt."

143. A 33-year-old client is undergoing peritoneal dialysis for acute renal failure. To prevent one of the most common complications of peritoneal dialysis, the nurse

A. Makes certain that the drain time is adequate
B. Checks the dwelling time to see that it is precise
C. Uses strict aseptic technique
D. Adds calcium gluconate to the solution

144. A 44-year-old client with chronic renal failure has an arteriovenous shunt in the right arm for access to hemodialysis. The nurse would:

A. Check BP in the left arm
B. Start an IV in the right arm
C. Irrigate the shunt every 4 hours
D. Draw blood from the shunt

145. A 46-year-old client is scheduled to go for hemodialysis at 9:30 AM. The physician has ordered cimetidine, digoxin, and docusate for 9 AM. The nurse would:

A. Give all medications as ordered
B. Hold all medications until dialysis has been completed
C. Check to see which medications are removed by dialysis
D. Check with the physician

146. A nurse is writing a care plan for a 45-year-old client with chronic renal failure. An important goal would be to:

A. Detect fluid or electrolyte imbalances
B. Protect the perianal area from excoriation
C. Detect respiratory changes caused by alkalosis
D. Observe for signs and symptoms of hypokalemia

147. A 56-year-old client just returned from the operating room after having a TURP for cancer. The nurse will give highest priority to assessing for:

A. Urinary output
B. Bowel sounds
C. Abnormal lung sounds
D. Clot formation in an extremity

148. A 62-year-old client is receiving radiation treatments for lung cancer. The field for radiation therapy is clearly outlined with purple ink. The nurse would treat this field as follows:

A. Bathe it the same as any other part of the body.
B. Apply moisturizing lotion to prevent dryness.
C. Wipe it with clear water and pat dry as needed only.
D. Treat as a stage I decubitus ulcer.

149. A 49-year-old client just returned from the operating room after having a total abdominal hysterectomy. The nurse will:

A. Encourage the client to void
B. Apply antiembolism stockings PRN
C. Change perineal pads every 8 hours
D. Change the abdominal dressing to check for bleeding

150. Ken Shaw, a 44-year-old male client, recently had a lumbosacral laminectomy to repair a herniated nucleus pulposus. The nurse would:

A. Get the client out of bed the first day of surgery
B. Apply a brace before getting the client out of bed
C. Teach the client not to raise his legs or point his toes
D. Log-roll the client when changing his position in bed

151. A client has a diagnosis of epiglottitis. It would be most important for the nurse to keep which of the following at the bedside?

A. Oxygen
B. An oral airway

C. Suction equipment
D. Tracheostomy set

152. After a liver biopsy, the nurse should place the client in which of the following positions?

A. Right side
B. Left side
C. High-Fowler's
D. Trendelenburg

153. A 50-year-old man complains of chills, low back pain, and nausea 10 minutes after a blood transfusion has begun. An hour later, his temperature increases to 102°F (38.8°C), he is hypotensive, and he voids urine red in color. Which type of blood transfusion reaction is occurring?

A. Febrile
B. Allergic
C. Septic
D. Hemolytic

154. An 18-year-old client is experiencing a sickle cell crisis. Which of the following interventions is indicated for this client?

A. ROM exercises every 2 hours
B. Fluid restriction of <1 L/day
C. Administration of antidiarrheal medications
D. Pain assessments every 4 hours

155. An 80-year-old client who had a left cerebrovascular accident (CVA) is experiencing continuous oozing of small amounts of liquid stool and has not had a bowel movement in 4 days. He eats only 20% of meals served to him. The oozing of stool is most likely a result of:

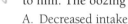

A. Decreased intake
B. Spinal cord trauma
C. Fecal impaction
D. Dehydration

156. A client has been diagnosed with epilepsy. Which of the following is an appropriate action for the nurse to take when a client is having a seizure?

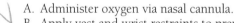

A. Administer oxygen via nasal cannula.
B. Apply vest and wrist restraints to prevent injury.
C. Pry the jaw open to maintain an airway.
D. Place the client on the side with the head flexed forward.

157. A client who has received continuous enteral tube feedings for a week has pulled her NG tube out. Within an hour, she develops tachycardia, diaphoresis, and tremors of her hands. The nurse correctly identifies her symptoms as:

A. Hypoglycemia
B. Hyperglycemia
C. Hypokalemia
D. Hyperkalemia

158. A client in a nursing home is at high risk to develop pressure ulcers because of immobility, incontinence, and low serum albumin. Which of the following would the nurse assess for as a first sign of a pressure ulcer?

A. Breakdown of the skin
B. Erythema of the skin
C. Clear-colored drainage
D. Exposure of underlying muscle

159. A client has been placed on oral anticoagulants after an MI. Which of the following instructions should the nurse give to the client?

   A. The client will need to have a PTT monitored periodically.
   B. The client should carry identification indicating that he or she is taking an anticoagulant.
   C. The client should take aspirin instead of acetaminophen for headaches and minor pain.
   D. One or two alcoholic beverages per week will not interfere with the effectiveness of the anticoagulant.

160. A client is scheduled to receive morphine sulfate. Which of the following is an appropriate nursing action?

   A. Monitor the pulse rate and withhold administration if <60 bpm.
   B. Monitor the respiratory rate and withhold administration if <12/min.
   C. Monitor the temperature and administer if >101°F (38.3°C).
   D. Monitor the BP and administer if <90/60 mm Hg.

161. A 74-year-old woman is admitted with symptoms of vaginal bleeding. The nurse identifies this bleeding as most likely a result of:

   A. An irregular menstrual cycle
   B. An increase in estrogen production
   C. A sexually transmitted disease
   D. Uterine cancer

162. The nurse is assessing a client who has recently been found to be hyperthyroid. The nurse would expect to find which of the following symptoms?

   A. Progressively gains weight
   B. Cannot tolerate cold temperatures
   C. Has a rapid pulse on rest and exertion
   D. Often develops myxedema

163. The nurse is teaching a class on wound healing. Which of the following is an accurate statement concerning wound healing?

   A. Accumulation of blood in a wound becomes a growth medium for infection.
   B. A tight dressing increases the blood supply carrying nutrients to the area.
   C. Clients taking steroids have a heightened inflammatory response.
   D. Activity promotes wound healing.

164. The nurse is assessing the client for hypovolemic shock. Which of the following symptoms would the nurse expect to find?

   A. A slow, thready pulse
   B. Deep, slow respirations
   C. Cold, moist skin
   D. Urinary output of 100 cc/hr or more

165. A client with a DVT suddenly cries out with sharp, stabbing pains in the chest and becomes dyspneic, anxious, and cyanotic. The nurse correctly identifies this as which of the following?

   A. MI
   B. Anaphylaxis
   C. Pulmonary embolism
   D. Bronchopneumonia

166. A client has been given a diagnosis of esophageal stricture. It is important for the nurse to teach him to:

   A. Eat hot, spicy foods to relax the stricture.
   B. Lie supine after eating.
   C. Eat just before bedtime.
   D. Eat small amounts frequently.

167. When planning for care of the client with a percutaneous endoscopic gastrostomy (PEG) tube, it would be important for the nurse to include which of the following:

   A. Nasal assessment for skin irritation from the tube
   B. Securing the tube to the client's cheek
   C. Assessing for tube displacement after coughing or suctioning
   D. Assessing bowel elimination patterns

168. A client has a bowel movement that consists of dark, tarry stools. The nurse would expect that the client is experiencing bleeding from:

   A. Hemorrhoids
   B. The stomach
   C. The rectum
   D. The sigmoid colon

169. A client is admitted with a diagnosis of peptic ulcer disease (PUD). Which of the following symptoms would alert the nurse that the ulcer has perforated?

   A. The client complains of chronic continuous pain persisting for a week.
   B. Bowel movements are painful and the stool is white.
   C. Pain is noted in the right shoulder.
   D. Gastric pain is noted after eating.

170. A client has light-colored stools and dark urine. The nurse correctly identifies these symptoms as being associated with:

   A. Hepatitis B
   B. PUD
   C. Renal failure
   D. Small bowel obstruction

171. Four units of regular insulin are given subcutaneously to a client at 4 PM for an elevated glucose level. The client is at greatest risk for rebound hypoglycemia at:

   A. 4:01 PM
   B. 8 PM
   C. Midnight
   D. 6 AM the following morning

172. Which of the following statements made by a client indicates a need for additional diabetic teaching?

A. "If I ever get shaky, hungry, and sweaty, I should drink some juice or eat some sugar."
B. "I could go blind from the diabetes."
C. "My blood sugar level will remain the same throughout the day now that I am on insulin."
D. "I draw up the regular insulin first, then the intermediate-acting NPH insulin when I put them both in one syringe."

173. After a thyroidectomy, a client develops spasms of the hands and feet accompanied by muscle twitching. The nurse identifies these symptoms as signs of:

A. Hypocalcemia
B. Hypercalcemia
C. Hypokalemia
D. Hyperkalemia

174. A client has received steroid therapy for 1 year. Which of the following is caused by long-term steroid therapy?

A. Weight loss
B. Masking of signs of infection
C. Addison's disease
D. Improvement in facial acne

175. The nurse is developing a plan of care for a client who has a diagnosis of acute pancreatitis. The rationale for maintaining the client on bedrest is to:

A. Reduce pancreatic and gastric secretions
B. Minimize the effects of hypoglycemia
C. Reduce the risk of DVT
D. Decrease the likelihood of orthostatic hypotension

176. The physician has ordered a urinalysis for a client. The nurse gives which of the following instructions?

A. Women should cleanse the perineum from back to front.
B. Hands should be washed before collecting the specimen.
C. The container should be pressed gently against the genitalia.
D. The first portion of the voiding should not be collected.

177. The nurse is doing discharge planning with a quadriplegic client. Which of the following instructions should be given to the client with an indwelling urinary catheter connected to gravity drainage?

A. The drainage bag should be placed above the level of the heart when the client is in bed.
B. The drainage bag should rest on the floor while the client is sitting in a chair.
C. The drainage bag should be emptied when completely full.
D. The tubing of the drainage bag should be inspected for kinks or twists frequently.

178. Which of the following statements made by a client indicates that a complication of peritoneal dialysis is occurring?

A. "The dressing around the peritoneal catheter is completely dry."

B. "A little bit of blood comes out of the peritoneal catheter on the days I menstruate."
C. "The drainage from my catheter is cloudy and white in color."
D. "I haven't gained any weight over the past week."

179. A client with a history of recurrent UTIs is being evaluated in the clinic. Which of the following actions indicates that the client is adhering to instructions?

A. Limits fluids to 32 oz/day
B. Voids every 2–3 hours while awake
C. Discontinues antibiotics when symptom-free
D. Takes daily tub baths

180. A client is placed on hemodialysis. The nurse would best assess the client's progress by:

A. Monitoring the client's weight
B. Performing a calorie count
C. Measuring the client's exercise tolerance
D. Inspecting the client's skin for bruising

181. A client is evaluated in the clinic 2 years after having a kidney transplant. The nurse expects this client to be most concerned about:

A. Fear of kidney rejection
B. Developing an infection
C. Uncertainty about the future
D. Effects of immunosuppressive therapy

182. Which of the following is an applicable nursing diagnosis for a client admitted with renal stones?

A. Impaired gas exchange
B. Fluid volume deficit
C. Risk for infection
D. Disturbance in self-concept

183. A 34-year-old recently married man is admitted for an ileal conduit urinary diversion. The nurse should:

A. Teach the client how to perform intermittent urinary catheterization
B. Explore the client's self-concept and self-esteem before surgery
C. Explain the rationale for peritoneal dialysis
D. Inform the client that urine and stool will be redirected to a stoma on the abdominal wall

184. A male client has a diagnosis of herpes genitalis infection. The nurse should instruct him to:

A. Avoid condom use to reduce irritation
B. Take all prescribed antibiotic doses
C. Avoid touching the blisterlike lesions
D. Apply antifungal cream sparingly

185. An 80-year-old man states that he experiences dribbling of clear yellow urine, hesitancy in starting urination, and a sensation of incomplete emptying of the bladder. The nurse identifies which of the following as the most likely cause of the symptoms?

A. The aging process
B. An enlarged prostate gland

C. A UTI
D. Chronic constipation

186. A client with AIDS is unable to cough because of weakness and fatigue. The client is at risk for:

A. Impaired gas exchange
B. Pain
C. Altered thought processes
D. Ineffective airway clearance

187. The nurse is changing the dressing covering an infected abscess that has been drained. The gauze is saturated with a foul-smelling yellow exudate. The nurse removes the dressing:

A. With bare hands
B. After donning nonsterile gloves
C. After donning sterile gloves
D. After double-gloving

188. A client states that his eyes and skin itch 10 minutes after a penicillin derivative is administered. Hives are noted on the client's arms, trunk, and legs. The nurse can anticipate that which of the following may occur?

A. Hypertensive crisis
B. Laryngeal edema
C. Paralytic ileus
D. Liver failure

189. During the physical assessment of a woman with an exacerbation of systemic lupus erythematosus (SLE), the nurse is likely to note which of the following?

A. Bulging eyes
B. Butterfly-shaped rash across the bridge of the nose
C. Jaundice
D. Kaposi's lesions

190. A nurse is conducting a physical assessment on a client. Which of the following characteristics of a mole on the skin warrants further evaluation by a physician?

A. Brown color
B. Irregular shape
C. Located on the neck
D. Skin around area sunburned

191. A child sustains a burn injury when a boiling pot of water is knocked off a stove. The skin on the child's chest appears sunburned and is dry. The nurse describes the burn injury as a:

A. Smoke inhalation injury
B. Superficial (first-degree) injury
C. Partial-thickness (second-degree) injury
D. Full-thickness (third-degree) injury

192. The nurse identifies which of the following as care of the client during the rehabilitation phase of burn care:

A. Monitoring urine output hourly
B. Maintaining NG suction
C. Applying topical antibacterials
D. Applying pressure garments

193. A medication is ordered to be administered "1 gtt to OD." The nurse administers 1 drop to:

A. The right eye
B. The left eye
C. Both eyes
D. Each ear

194. To reduce intraocular pressure in the client who has undergone retinal surgery, the nurse would:

A. Apply a hot compress to the eye
B. Provide bright lighting and teaching tools in large print
C. Instruct the client to gently press on the eye if discomfort occurs
D. Elevate the head of the bed 30 degrees or higher

195. A client has undergone ear surgery. The nurse should instruct the client to:

A. Blow nose frequently
B. Shampoo on the day after surgery
C. Report altered taste and mouth dryness
D. Keep the ear packing moist

196. A client has sustained a head injury from a motor vehicle accident. The nurse would assess for which of the following early signs of increasing ICP?

A. Reaction only to loud auditory or painful stimuli
B. Absence of reflexes and flaccidity of extremities
C. Fixed and dilated pupils
D. Lethargy and changing levels of consciousness

197. A client is unconscious after a severe head injury. The nurse's most important action is to:

A. Provide meticulous skin care
B. Maintain an airway and adequate ventilation
C. Turn the client every 2 hours to reduce infection risk
D. Elevate the head of the bed to prevent aspiration of secretions

198. After a CVA, a client experiences memory loss, inability to concentrate, altered judgment, and impaired decision making. The nurse identifies these as which type of deficit?

A. Sensory
B. Verbal
C. Cognitive
D. Emotional

199. The nurse is planning a bowel program for a client with multiple sclerosis. This would include:

A. Fluid restriction
B. A high-fiber diet
C. Daily irrigation of the colostomy
D. Intermittent self-catheterization

200. After a total hip replacement, the nurse should assess the neurovascular status of the leg by:

A. Monitoring vital signs
B. Noting the amount of wound drainage
C. Assessing capillary refill of the toes
D. Performing ROM exercises

ANSWERS

1. **(A)** Nursing process phase: implementation; client need: basic care and comfort; content area: medical-surgical.
   RATIONALE
   (A) Shrinking the residual limb and shaping it into a conical form help to ensure the comfort and fit of the prosthetic device; wrapping helps to shrink the size. **(B)** The residual limb needs to be decreased, not increased in size. **(C)** Telling a client that it is what the therapist wants is not a sufficient answer. **(D)** It is inappropriate to tell her to call her doctor when the nurse can answer the question.

2. **(D)** Nursing process phase: implementation; client need: reduction of risk potential; content area: medical-surgical.
   RATIONALE
   (A) Lying supine with a pillow between the legs does not prevent flexion contraction of the hip. **(B)** A semi-Fowler's position promotes development of flexion contraction. **(C)** Although the limb should be elevated the first 24 hours to reduce swelling and edema around the incision site, placing a pillow under the knees not only promotes venous stasis but also contributes to flexion contraction. **(D)** Lying prone stretches the flexor muscles and prevents flexion contraction of the hip.

3. **(B)** Nursing process phase: implementation; client need: coping and adaptation; content area: medical-surgical.
   RATIONALE
   (A) Although the leg has been severed, the nerve tracts sending messages to the brain are still functioning. **(B)** This response explains phantom limb sensation, which is pain in the amputated limb. It is a real sensation caused by nerve tracts that register pain still sending their messages to the brain. **(C)** Most people are able to get over the loss of a body part without severe emotional problems necessitating the help of a psychiatrist. **(D)** This response demonstrates the nurse's unfamiliarity with the phantom limb phenomenon.

4. **(B)** Nursing process phase: implementation; client need: prevention and early detection of disease; content area: medical-surgical.
   RATIONALE
   (A) Redness can be a sign of infection, and abrasions are susceptible to the development of infection. **(B)** Alcohol dries and cracks the skin, and lotion softens the skin too much; therefore, both create a risk for safe prosthesis use. No ointments, antiseptics, or lotions should be used unless ordered by the physician. **(C)** The stump sock helps to prevent skin breakdown; ACE bandages are used the first 24–48 hours to prevent swelling and edema. **(D)** The stump should be cleaned with a mild soap and a soft cloth.

5. **(D)** Nursing process phase: data collection; client need: physiological adaptation; content area: medical-surgical.
   RATIONALE
   (A) This response is the definition of hemiparesis, not hemiplegia. **(B)** Paraplegia is the paralysis of the lower extremities. **(C)** Quadriplegia is total body paralysis. **(D)** Hemiplegia is the paralysis of one side of the body.

6. **(C)** Nursing process phase: data collection; client need: physiological adaptation; content area: medical-surgical.
   RATIONALE
   (A) Exercises to decrease facial rigidity would not help the dysphagia problem. **(B)** Dysarthria, not dysphagia, is the lack of coordination in speech. **(C)** Dysphagia is inability to swallow or difficulty in swallowing; therefore, instituting special feeding precautions would need to be included in the plan of care. **(D)** Increasing the light in the environment would have absolutely no influence on the dysphagia problem.

7. **(B)** Nursing process phase: data collection; client need: physiological adaptation; content area: medical-surgical.
   RATIONALE
   (A) Ataxia is unsteady gait. **(B)** Aphasia is the inability to express oneself through speech and language. **(C)** Dysphagia is difficulty swallowing. **(D)** Agnosia is difficulty smelling.

8. **(B)** Nursing process phase: data collection; client need: reduction of risk potential; content area: medical-surgical.
   RATIONALE
   (A) This response represents a miscalculation of the percent burned. **(B)** The Rule of Nines is a quick method to calculate the percentage of BSA burned. The entire posterior chest and buttocks represent 18%. The total body is divided into nine sections of multiples of nine. The head and neck equals 9%, each arm 9%, each leg 18%, anterior chest 18%, posterior chest including buttocks 18%, perineum 1%. **(C)** This response represents a miscalculation of the percent burned. **(D)** This represents a miscalculation of the percent burned.

9. **(A)** Nursing process phase: data collection; client need: reduction of risk potential; content area: medical-surgical.
   RATIONALE
   (A) The disequilibrium syndrome is caused by rapid fluid shifts occurring as the result of hemodialysis, especially during one of the first treatments. When solutes such as urea and sodium are removed from the blood faster than from the CSF, seizures are most likely to occur. Other associated symptoms are nausea and vomiting, headache, restlessness, and confusion. **(B)** Hypertension is not commonly associated with the syndrome. **(C)** Chest pain is not associated with the syndrome; but it can occur with cardiac clients if the speed of blood flow is high. **(D)** Shortness of breath is not associated with the syndrome. If present, it usually represents a symptom of fluid overload.

10. **(C)** Nursing process phase: planning; client need: prevention and early detection of disease; content area: medical-surgical.
    RATIONALE
    (A) A hearty appetite is no reason to eat high-fat foods. **(B)** The diet to prevent coronary artery disease (CAD) is lifelong. Clients and spouses should be encouraged to eat foods low in fat, cholesterol, and sodium. **(C)** The client and his wife need diet instruction. A diet high in fat and cholesterol will further contribute to the CAD process. **(D)** Some hospitals allow foods to be brought in, but often times a doctor's order is needed.

11. **(C)** Nursing process phase: evaluation, client need: prevention and early detection of disease; content area: medical-surgical.
    RATIONALE
    (A) Taking medications as prescribed is a desired response. **(B)** This is the recommended post-MI diet. **(C)** Although exercise is recommended after MI, it is usually done in a cardiac rehabilitation program where the client is monitored. Exercise is gradually increased over several weeks. **(D)** Consuming a small glass of wine with the evening meal complies with the current literature.

12. **(A)** Nursing process phase: implementation; client need: coping and adaptation; content area: medical-surgical.

RATIONALE

(A) Emotional lability (inappropriate laughing and crying) is an emotional change that is common after a stroke and may or may not be appropriate to the situation. (B) Ignoring a client would not be a correct action; nor should the nurse assume he is playing games. (C) This is a nonsense answer. People do not typically cry when something is funny or laugh when it is not. (D) The emotional lability after a stroke does not typically warrant a psychiatric consultation.

13. **(B)** Nursing process phase: data collection; client need: physiological adaptation; content area: medical-surgical.

    RATIONALE

    (A) Cranial is not a division of the spinal canal. (B) The four divisions of the spinal column are cervical (neck), thoracic (upper back), lumbar (lower back), and sacrum and coccyx (tailbone). (C) Trochanter and ischial are not divisions of the spinal canal; they refer to parts of a bone. (D) Femur and ulnar are not divisions of the spinal canal; they refer to bones.

14. **(B)** Nursing process phase: data collection; client need: physiological adaptation; content area: medical-surgical.

    RATIONALE

    (A) The client would have movement of the upper extremities. An injury above C5 would indicate loss of control of the arms. (B) The client with a T11 injury is paraplegic and loses all function below this level. (C) Movement in the upper extremities would remain intact. (D) Respiratory control would remain intact.

15. **(C)** Nursing process phase: data collection; client need: pharmacological and parenteral therapies; content area: medical-surgical.

    RATIONALE

    (A) Peak action of NPH insulin would not occur within 2 hours (9 AM). (B) Peak action of NPH insulin would not occur within 5 hours (12 noon). (C) NPH is an intermediate-acting insulin. The peak action takes place 8–12 hours after administration. If NPH were given at 7 AM, the peak action would occur between 3 PM and 7 PM. (D) Peak action of NPH insulin would not take this long to occur (11 PM).

16. **(D)** Nursing process phase: data collection; client need: reduction of risk potential; content area: medical-surgical.

    RATIONALE

    (A) The occiput is a posterior structure. (B) The buttocks are located on the posterior surface. (C) The heels are located on the posterior surface. (D) When the client is prone, the anterior structures of the body receive pressure. The toes are the only anterior features among the choices.

17. **(B)** Nursing process phase: implementation; client need: reduction of risk potential; content area: medical-surgical.

    RATIONALE

    (A) Five seconds is too little time spent suctioning. The result would not be effective. (B) To prevent hypoxemia, time spent suctioning should be no longer than 10–15 seconds, and no more than 80–120 mm Hg suction should be used. (C) Twenty seconds exceeds the recommended time and is more likely to result in hypoxemia. (D) Thirty seconds greatly exceeds the acceptable limits of time spent suctioning.

18. **(D)** Nursing process phase: implementation; client need: physiological adaptation; content area: medical-surgical.

    RATIONALE

    (A) Although a 12-lead ECG is important to obtain when a client is having chest pain, the question focuses on what should be done before administering nitroglycerin. (B) Based on the information that has been given, there is no reason to lower the head of the bed. (C) Although a client experiencing chest pain should receive supplemental oxygen, the question focuses on what should be done before administering nitroglycerin. (D) Rest reduces the need for oxygen.

19. **(A)** Nursing process phase: implementation; client need: physiological adaptation; content area: medical-surgical.

    RATIONALE

    (A) High-Fowler's position allows gravity to assist in dropping the diaphragm. If the client is allowed to dangle the legs at the bedside, chest expansion would be facilitated even further because posterior chest movement is not inhibited by the bed. (B) The gravitational pull on the diaphragm is not as great in the low-Fowler's position because the head of the bed is elevated to only 30 degrees. (C) Sims is a sidelying position and therefore restricts chest movement on the dependent side. (D) Trendelenburg is a head-down, feet-up position. As a result, abdominal contents tend to be pushed up on the diaphragm, thus resulting in less chest expansion.

20. **(D)** Nursing process phase: implementation; client need: basic care and comfort; content area: medical-surgical.

    RATIONALE

    (A) The first sound heard when the cuff is deflating is the systolic pressure. (B) In children, the diastolic pressure is the muffled sound heard when deflating the cuff. (C) One does not listen to the sounds as the cuff inflates. (D) For adults, the diastolic pressure is recorded when the last sound is heard during cuff deflation.

21. **(D)** Nursing process phase: implementation; client need: basic care and comfort; content area: medical-surgical.

    RATIONALE

    (A) Wiping from back to front greatly increases the chance of fecal contamination and consequent development of a urinary tract–vaginal infection. (B) Circular motion increases risk of fecal contamination when movement, especially with the swing from back to front, occurs. (C) Side to side does not indicate whether the swab is progressing from front to back or back to front. (D) Wiping from front to back decreases fecal contamination of the vagina and urinary meatus. Fecal contamination greatly increases the chance of developing an infection.

22. **(D)** Nursing process phase: implementation; client need: pharmacological and parenteral therapies; content area: medical-surgical.

    RATIONALE

    (A) Digoxin has a narrow therapeutic margin; therefore, periodic serum levels are drawn. (B) The therapeutic effect of heparin is monitored by drawing periodic partial thromboplastin time (PTT). (C) Serum theophylline levels are often drawn when a client is receiving aminophylline, especially the IV form. (D) For the choices given, only vancomycin requires the periodic drawing of peak-and-trough levels. When a peak-and-trough level is ordered, the trough is drawn immediately before the administration of the scheduled dose. Peak levels are usually drawn 30 minutes after the medication has completely infused.

23. **(A)** Nursing process phase: evaluation; client need: safety and infection control; content area: medical-surgical.

    RATIONALE

    (A) Proper handwashing by health-care workers reduces the risk of nosocomial infections. Ten seconds of vigorous handwashing will remove most transient flora and is the minimum amount of time one should spend washing. (B) Although washing for 30 seconds will remove more flora, it does not represent the minimum time one should spend washing. (C) Forty-five seconds is longer than the minimum acceptable time. (D) Sixty seconds is longer than the minimum acceptable time.

24. **(D)** Nursing process phase: data collection; client need: basic care and comfort; content area: medical-surgical.

RATIONALE

(A) Constipation tends to cause a decrease rather than an increase in appetite. **(B)** Suprapubic distention is a symptom associated with bladder fullness. **(C)** Nausea may infrequently be associated with constipation, but vomiting is a rare occurrence. **(D)** Symptoms of constipation include abdominal firmness, distention, hard-formed stools, fewer stools than normal, headache, and a decrease in appetite.

25. **(C)** Nursing process phase: implementation; client need: pharmacological and parenteral therapies; content area: medical-surgical.

RATIONALE

(A) Getting up and going to the toilet immediately causes premature, ineffective evacuation of the bowel. **(B)** Waiting 5–10 minutes results in less effective evacuation of the bowel, when compared to waiting 20–30 minutes. **(C)** Waiting 20–30 minutes gives the suppository time to dissolve and irritate the colon, and the irritation stimulates the bowel evacuation. **(D)** Being in the prone position may or may not help retention of the suppository.

26. **(C)** Nursing process phase: implementation; client need: safety and infection control; content area: medical-surgical.

RATIONALE

(A) The label is obliterated when the fluid is poured facing the sterile field. The bottle is held with the label in the palm of the hand. **(B)** To avoid splashing the fluid when poured, the bottle is held rather low over the sterile field. **(C)** Before pouring sterile solution onto a sterile field, 1–2 ml of the fluid is discarded to remove organisms from the lip of the bottle. **(D)** The cap is in contact with the lip and may harbor organisms.

27. **(C)** Nursing process phase: implementation; client need: safety and infection control; content area: medical-surgical.

RATIONALE

(A) Disposable equipment does not cause nosocomial infections. **(B)** Semiprivate rooms do not cause nosocomial infections. **(C)** The most common cause of nosocomial infections is infrequent handwashing by health-care workers. **(D)** Oral antibiotics do not cause nosocomial infections.

28. **(C)** Nursing process phase: implementation; client need: safety and infection control; content area: medical-surgical.

RATIONALE

(A) The bandage became contaminated once it touched the skin. **(B)** Placing the bandage in the sterile saline would contaminate the sterile saline. **(C)** To maintain surgical asepsis, remember: sterile touching clean becomes contaminated; sterile touching contaminated becomes contaminated. **(D)** Once a sterile item is contaminated, the only option is to discard it and prepare a fresh one. Using the contaminated bandage would contaminate the other sterile bandages.

29. **(C)** Nursing process phase: data collection; client need: basic care and comfort; content area: medical-surgical.

RATIONALE

(A) Pallor can be assessed in the conjunctiva, not the sclera. **(B)** Assessing pallor in the nailbeds is not as reliable as assessing the mucous membranes. **(C)** It is more difficult to assess changes such as pallor (paleness indicating decreased amounts of oxygen-carrying Hgb) in clients with dark skin tones. Pallor is most easily perceived in the buccal mucous membranes of the mouth. **(D)** Assessing pallor of the lips is not as reliable as assessing the mucous membranes.

30. **(D)** Nursing process phase: implementation; client need: management of care; content area: medical-surgical.

RATIONALE

(A) Black, permanent ink is used, not erasable ink or pencil. **(B)** Inking over an entry may appear to be an attempt to hide information. **(C)** Writing "error" is no longer advised because it can be interpreted to mean an error or mistake was made in the client's care. **(D)** The acceptable method of correcting an erroneous entry is to draw one straight line through the erroneous entry and initial it. A nurse can be charged with fraud for otherwise altering a client's record.

31. **(B)** Nursing process phase: evaluation; client need: safety and infection control; content area: medical-surgical.

RATIONALE

(A) Keeping one point of support does not provide enough stability to prevent the client from falling. **(B)** Two points of support are on the floor at all times. The cane is kept on the stronger (right side). First the cane is moved forward, keeping body weight on both legs. Second, the weaker left leg is moved forward to the cane (body weight evenly divided between the stronger leg and the cane). Third, the stronger right leg is advanced past the cane (weaker leg and body weight are supported by the cane and weaker leg). **(C)** The client should stand upright, not leaning to the side. The cane should be in the right hand if the left leg is weak. **(D)** The top of the cane should be at the level of the greater trochanter of the client's femur.

32. **(D)** Nursing process phase: data collection; client need: prevention and early detection of disease; content area: medical-surgical.

RATIONALE

(A) The client's arm should be positioned at the level of the heart. If the arm is above the heart level, the measurement results in a falsely low reading. If the arm is positioned below the heart level, the measurement results in a falsely high reading. **(B)** The cuff is traditionally positioned 1 inch above the brachial, not the radial, artery. If the BP is obtained at the radial site, the cuff is placed 1 inch above the artery. **(C)** The client's arm should be extended with the palm up. **(D)** To ensure an accurate BP measurement, proper pressure is applied to the brachial artery by inflating the bladder of the cuff directly over the artery.

33. **(C)** Nursing process phase: data collection; client need: prevention and early detection of disease; content area: medical-surgical.

RATIONALE

(A) Although in some individuals the pulsatile force of the heart can be seen, it is not easily visible. **(B)** Although the apical pulse can be palpated (felt), especially in thin people, it is not as accurate as the amplified sound heard with the stethoscope. **(C)** The stethoscope amplifies the sound of the heart (apical pulse) when placed over the precordium. **(D)** Percussion is performed by tapping to produce sounds in underlying organs and tissues. The apical pulse cannot be obtained with this method.

34. **(A)** Nursing process phase: implementation; client need: safety and infection control; content area: medical-surgical.

RATIONALE

(A) Oxygen is a highly combustible gas. Oxygen can easily cause a fire to ignite if it contacts a spark. **(B)** Oxygen does not spontaneously burn or cause an explosion. **(C)** Oxygen use in the home does not represent a health risk to others who may visit. **(D)** The statement that smoking causes lung cancer is true, but it is not the correct rationale in this specific example.

35. **(D)** Nursing process phase: planning; client need: basic care and comfort; content area: medical-surgical.

RATIONALE
(A) The nurse should use warm water only if it is the client's preference. (B) Using tissues may be a preference for some people. (C) The nurse should use soap if it is the client's preference. (D) Whenever possible, the client should be asked about personal preferences of skin care and hygiene products. The client's preference determines the regimen to be followed when washing the face.

36. **(A)** Nursing process phase: implementation; client need: basic care and comfort; content area: medical-surgical.

RATIONALE
(A) Cramping is temporarily relieved by lowering the container and/or clamping the tubing to temporarily stop the flow of enema solution. Once cramping passes, the enema is continued until the entire amount of fluid is administered. (B) Mouth breathing may help to relax the client, but it does not relieve cramping. (C) Raising the height of the enema container would increase the rate of flow and increase the degree of cramping. (D) It is not appropriate to clamp and withdraw the tube; cramping is very commonly experienced. The nurse simply stops the flow until the cramping subsides and then resumes the enema.

37. **(D)** Nursing process phase: implementation; client need: prevention and early detection of disease; content area: medical-surgical.

RATIONALE
(A) Waiting only 10 seconds increases venous congestion and may make the reading erroneous. (B) Waiting only 30 seconds tends to increase venous congestion in the arm and may make the reading erroneous. (C) The American Heart Association (AHA) recommends waiting 2 minutes, not 1 minute, before repeating the pressure. (D) The AHA recommends waiting 2 minutes before repeating a BP reading in the same arm. This decreases venous congestion.

38. **(B)** Nursing process phase: implementation; client need: reduction of risk potential; content area: medical-surgical.

RATIONALE
(A) The value is not low; it is within normal limits. (B) A normal serum potassium level is 3.8–5.0 mEq/L; therefore, a potassium level of 4.3 is within the normal limits. Unless ordered to notify the physician of a laboratory value, the nurse would note the potassium result in her notes and inform the physician when he makes rounds. (C) The value is not high; it is within normal limits. (D) It is not necessary to offer potassium-rich foods because the potassium value is well within the normal limits.

39. **(C)** Nursing process phase: data collection; client need: prevention and early detection of disease; content area: medical-surgical.

RATIONALE
(A) Auscultation uses the sense of hearing to assess clients. The stethoscope is used with this technique. (B) Percussion uses a striking motion to elicit sounds and thus assess underlying structures. (C) Palpation uses the sense of touch to perform physical assessments. The nurse when feeling the lower abdomen is using the palpation technique. (D) Inspection uses the sense of sight to assess clients.

40. **(D)** Nursing process phase: implementation; client need: prevention and early detection of disease; content area: medical-surgical.

RATIONALE
(A) The urinometer is considered contaminated. The urinometer rapidly grows bacteria as urine collects and therefore should not be used as a site for collecting a urine specimen for culture. (B) The drainage bag, like the urinometer, is considered contaminated. Bacteria grow rapidly as urine collects in the bag. (C) Disconnecting the catheter disrupts the closed sterile system and allows introduction of additional bacteria into the system. (D) The correct procedure for collecting a sterile urine specimen is to use a sterile needle and syringe and use the latex sampling port on the tubing.

41. **(C)** Nursing process phase: implementation; client need: pharmacological and parenteral therapies; content area: medical-surgical.

RATIONALE
(A) The enteric coating does not dissolve in the mouth. (B) This is a nonsense answer. Enteric coatings are placed on pills and do not apply to liquids. (C) The enteric coating on an oral medication consists of materials that do not dissolve in the mouth or the stomach. The coating dissolves in the intestine, where the medication is absorbed. (D) The enteric coating is destroyed when it is chewed. The medication is then absorbed from the stomach and not from the intestine as designed.

42. **(A)** Nursing process phase: planning; client need: pharmacological and parenteral therapies; content area: medical-surgical.

RATIONALE
(A) By displacing the tissue laterally using the Z-track method, the needle track is sealed as the needle is removed. The medication cannot escape from the deep muscle, and irritation to sensitive tissues is avoided. (B) The Z-track method does not affect the speed of absorption of the medication into the body. (C) The Z-track method does not eliminate discomfort caused by the needle. (D) The Z-track method does not affect absorption rate from the muscle.

43. **(B)** Nursing process phase: implementation; client need: pharmacological and parenteral therapies; content area: medical-surgical.

RATIONALE
(A) Topical absorption is usually the slowest. (B) A medication administered IV begins to act immediately as it directly enters the bloodstream. (C) IM absorption is slower than IV, but usually faster than oral. (D) Oral absorption is slower than IM, but usually faster than topical.

44. **(B)** Nursing process phase: data collection; client need: physiological adaptation; content area: medical-surgical.

RATIONALE
(A) Metabolic acidosis is caused by an excessive amount of acid or not enough base in the body. The GI tract is predominately "base." When excessive base is lost (diarrhea), metabolic acidosis usually results. (B) The Salem sump tube drains stomach contents that are acidic because of the hydrochloric acid. The loss of stomach acid sets up a situation in which the body then has too much base for the amount of acid present. This situation can also occur when excessive vomiting occurs. This is a metabolic problem; thus, metabolic alkalosis occurs. (C) The primary cause of respiratory acidosis is a respiratory problem. When too much acid (carbon dioxide) accumulates, as with hypoventilation, respiratory acidosis occurs. (D) The primary cause of respiratory alkalosis is also a respiratory problem. The problem now is not enough acid (carbon dioxide). This occurs in hyperventilation states.

45. **(D)** Nursing process phase: evaluation; client need: prevention and early detection of disease; content area: medical-surgical.

RATIONALE
(A) An enlarged base of support maintains better body balance. (B) By moving close to the object to be lifted, one increases body balance. (C) The center of gravity should be low, not high.

(D) The head, neck, and back should be maintained in proper alignment, along with a low center of gravity and a wide base of support. The muscle groups can then work in a synchronized manner, and risk of injury to the lumbar spine and muscles is reduced.

46. **(D)** Nursing process phase: evaluation; client need: management of care; content area: medical-surgical.

    RATIONALE

    (A) Evaluation is not final; it is ongoing and continuous. (B) Evaluation is always related to client goals of care. (C) Data collection is considered the first phase. (D) Evaluation is a continuous and ongoing process that interacts with other phases of the nursing process. Evaluation indicates effectiveness of the care plan through assessment of the client's response.

47. **(D)** Nursing process phase: implementation; client need: basic care and comfort; content area: medical-surgical.

    RATIONALE

    (A) Unconscious clients are not able to chew food; therefore, food particles would not get trapped between teeth, necessitating the need to floss. Putting food in the mouth of an unconscious person would greatly increase the risk of aspiration. (B) 30 ml of fluid squirted into the mouth is a large volume and could easily cause aspiration. (C) Scraping secretions with a tongue blade is not recommended. Not only is it ineffective, but it could cause mucosal trauma. (D) A padded tongue blade keeps the mouth open and teeth separated during oral care without traumatizing the oral cavity. The teeth are cleaned with a sponge, toothbrush, or gauze-wrapped tongue blade to gently stimulate the gums and mucosa. To prevent aspiration, the sponge or gauze is moistened (not soaked).

48. **(C)** Nursing process phase: data collection; client need: reduction of risk potential; content area: medical-surgical.

    RATIONALE

    (A) Stroke is not the most prevalent form of cardiovascular disease. (B) CAD is not the most prevalent form of cardiovascular disease. (C) The AHA states the most prevalent form of cardiovascular disease is hypertension, followed in descending order by CAD, rheumatic heart disease, and stroke. (D) Rheumatic heart disease is not the most prevalent form of cardiovascular disease.

49. **(A)** Nursing process phase: data collection; client need: prevention and early detection of disease; content area: medical-surgical.

    RATIONALE

    (A) Shortness of breath is an expected symptom with CHF. The heart is an ineffective pump and less blood is ejected with each beat. The extra volume of blood left in the heart exerts a pressure. As the pressure increases, it is exerted backwards from the left ventricle to the left atrium and finally to the lungs. The alveoli start to fill with fluid as the capillary pressure increases, leading to shortness of breath. (B) There is a decrease in tissue turgor with hypovolemic, not hypervolemic, states. (C) Neck veins become distended as the pressure on the left side of the heart is exerted backwards to the right heart. More blood (volume) stays in the peripheral circulation, eventually leading to systemic edema. (D) Right, not left, upper quadrant abdominal tenderness develops as the liver becomes engorged with extra circulation volume from the right side of the heart.

50. **(A)** Nursing process phase: implementation; client need: basic care and comfort; content area: medical-surgical.

    RATIONALE

    (A) Fluid lost or gained would be reflected as a loss or gain in weight. One liter equals 1 kg (2.2 lb). A rapid rise in weight would indicate that the CHF is getting worse. (B) Fluids are usu-

ally limited or restricted (not encouraged) because of the hypervolemia. (C) To help alleviate the shortness of breath, most clients are more comfortable in an upright position (head of bed elevated >30–45 degrees). (D) Sodium in the diet should be limited, not enriched. Sodium fosters the retention of fluid, thus making the volume overload problem worse.

51. **(B)** Nursing process phase: implementation; client need: pharmacological and parenteral therapies; content area: medical-surgical.

    RATIONALE

    (A) This dose is well below the usual adult daily dose. (B) The usual dose of digoxin for adults is 0.25 mg every day. (C) This dose well exceeds the usual dose. (D) This dose well exceeds the usual dose and would probably result in death.

52. **(C)** Nursing process phase: implementation; client need: pharmacological and parenteral therapies; content area: medical-surgical.

    RATIONALE

    (A) Ringing in the ears is not a typical symptom of digoxin toxicity. (B) Fluid retention is not a typical sign of digoxin toxicity. (C) Digoxin has a very narrow therapeutic margin, and toxic effects are frequently seen. Anorexia, nausea, and vomiting are often the first signs of developing toxicity. (D) Hair loss is not a typical symptom of digoxin toxicity.

53. **(D)** Nursing process phase: data collection; client need: prevention and early detection of disease; content area: medical-surgical.

    RATIONALE

    (A) A positive, not negative, Homans' sign is a symptom of thrombophlebitis. (B) Thrombophlebitis involves the venous system. Because the arterial flow is not impaired, the pedal pulses would not be affected. (C) Cool temperature of the extremity and a mottled appearance indicate impaired arterial flow. Arterial circulation is not the problem. (D) Calf pain on dorsiflexion of the foot (positive Homans' sign) is a symptom of thrombophlebitis. Other common symptoms include stiffness and redness over the inflamed site.

54. **(A)** Nursing process phase: implementation; client need: reduction of risk potential; content area: medical-surgical.

    RATIONALE

    (A) Efforts should be made to ensure that clients are adequately hydrated. Dehydration and/or fluid volume deficit increase the viscosity of the blood. The increased viscosity is a causative factor in the development of thrombophlebitis. (B) Massaging the affected leg is never done because this action can dislodge a thrombus and cause an embolus. The nurse should be alert for the signs and symptoms of a pulmonary embolus. (C) The leg should be positioned above, not below, the level of the heart to aid venous return. (D) Antibiotics are not usually indicated in thrombophlebitis.

55. **(C)** Nursing process phase: data collection; client need: pharmacological and parenteral therapies; content area: medical-surgical.

    RATIONALE

    (A) Heparin cannot dissolve existing clots. (B) Heparin has no vasoactive properties; therefore, it cannot dilate vessels. (C) Heparin prevents additional clots from forming. (D) Heparin has no vasoactive properties; therefore, it cannot constrict vessels.

56. **(C)** Nursing process phase: data collection; client need: pharmacological and parenteral therapies; content area: medical-surgical.

    RATIONALE

    (A) This answer indicates a miscalculation. (B) This answer indicates a miscalculation. **(C)** 25,000 : 250 : : x : 10; 250x = 25,000; x = 1000 units/10 ml. **(D)** This answer indicates a miscalculation.

57. **(A)** Nursing process phase: implementation; client need: pharmacological and parenteral therapies; content area: medical-surgical.

RATIONALE

(A) Green leafy vegetables and other foods high in vitamin K (asparagus, broccoli, cabbage, brussels sprouts) should be limited. Vitamin K counteracts the therapeutic effects of warfarin. **(B)** Aspirin inhibits platelet aggregation by decreasing the synthesis of substances that mediate platelet aggregation. Aspirin can thus cause bleeding and is contraindicated in connection with other anticoagulant medications. **(C)** PTT values monitor the therapeutic effects of heparin. PT monitors the effects of warfarin. **(D)** Cuts are more likely to occur when shaving with a straight-edge razor and should be discouraged.

58. **(C)** Nursing process phase: data collection; client need: prevention and early detection of disease; content area: medical-surgical.

RATIONALE

(A) The skin elasticity over the dorsal hand is lost early in the aging process and therefore is not a reliable indicator of turgor in the elderly client. **(B)** The skin elasticity of the forearm is lost during the aging process and is not a reliable indicator of turgor in the elderly client. **(C)** The elasticity of the skin decreases as one ages. The skin over the sternum retains elasticity longer than the skin on other areas of the body. **(D)** The skin is normally very taut over the ankle, making it difficult to pinch and painful for the client of any age.

59. **(A)** Nursing process phase: implementation; client need: pharmacological and parenteral therapies; content area: medical-surgical.

RATIONALE

(A) A person with no history of heart disease should seek emergency care if chest pain persists longer than 2 minutes. **(B)** This is the recommended procedure for people with a history of CAD who have been prescribed nitroglycerin. **(C)** A person with undiagnosed heart disease should not be taking nitroglycerin that has been prescribed for someone else. **(D)** It would be absolutely wrong to wait until the chest pain goes away before seeking care.

60. **(D)** Nursing process phase: data collection; client need: reduction of risk potential; content area: medical-surgical.

RATIONALE

(A) CABG surgery is not a cure. This disease in the native vessels continues to progress. The disease can also occur in the bypass graft vessels. **(B)** Coronary artery stent is not a cure. It is a mechanical device to keep the coronary artery patent at the blockage site. **(C)** Angioplasty is not a cure. The balloon dilation at the blockage site reduces the severity of the lesion. **(D)** CAD is a lifelong process that currently has no cure. Risk factor modification will help to slow the disease process.

61. **(C)** Nursing process phase: data collection; client need: prevention and early detection of disease; content area: medical-surgical.

RATIONALE

(A) Obesity is a modifiable risk factor, but not considered a major risk factor. **(B)** Family history, gender, sex, and age are the nonmodifiable risk factors. **(C)** The three major modifiable risk factors in the development of CAD are hypertension, hypercholesteremia, and cigarette smoking. **(D)** Diabetes is a contributing factor in the development of CAD. Diabetes can be controlled, but it is not considered one of the major modifiable risk factors.

62. **(D)** Nursing process phase: data collection; client need: prevention and early detection of disease; content area: medical-surgical.

RATIONALE

(A) The ankles are one of the first places for edema to accumulate when a client is predominantly in the upright position. **(B)** In the upright position, edema first accumulates in the ankles. As the condition advances, edema starts accumulating in the legs (distal to proximal). **(C)** The hands become edematous as the edema accumulates, but the edema first appears in the sacrum of the bedridden client. **(D)** The sacrum is the most dependent area of the body for the client confined to bedrest. Edema accumulates in dependent area first.

63. **(D)** Nursing process phase: implementation; client need: prevention and early detection of disease; content area: medical-surgical.

RATIONALE

(A) Broiled chicken does contain cholesterol, but less than red meat. **(B)** Fish also contains cholesterol, but in much smaller amounts than red meat. **(C)** Polyunsaturated oils are recommended for use, but heating them changes their polyunsaturated states. Fried foods are not recommended. **(D)** Egg yolks contain cholesterol; egg whites do not.

64. **(A)** Nursing process phase: data collection; client need: prevention and early detection of disease; content area: medical-surgical.

RATIONALE

(A) The discomfort of angina most commonly radiates to the left arm, along with feelings of arm numbness and heaviness. Radiation to both arms, the jaw, and the neck does occur but less frequently than to the left arm. **(B)** Although radiated pain may be in both arms, it is most often in the left arm. **(C)** Although radiated pain may be in the neck, it is usually unilateral. **(D)** Although radiated pain may be in the jaw, it is most often in the left arm.

65. **(C)** Nursing process phase: data collection; client need: prevention and early detection of disease; content area: medical-surgical.

RATIONALE

(A) Although certain beats in the peripheral pulse cannot be palpated (felt) when a pulse deficit is present, it is not the absence of a pulse. **(B)** The difference in systolic and diastolic pressures is known as the pulse pressure. **(C)** The difference in the apical and radial heart rates is known as a pulse deficit. The heartbeat can be auscultated apically but cannot be felt in the radial (peripheral) pulse. **(D)** Because it is the peripheral pulse that has a deficit, the peripheral pulse rate is subtracted from the apical rate.

66. **(B)** Nursing process phase: implementation; client need: reduction of risk potential; content area: medical-surgical.

RATIONALE

(A) Bedrest is maintained for 4–6 hours after this procedure because the clot that has sealed the insertion site may burst with activity. **(B)** Immediately after the procedure vital signs are assessed every 15 minutes. Assessing distal circulation (pedal pulses), especially in the cannulated leg, is performed as frequently as assessment of vital signs. **(C)** The head of the bed is usually ordered to be no higher than 30 degrees (low-Fowler's position). **(D)** Fluids are encouraged to aid in eliminating the dye used in the procedure.

67. **(D)** Nursing process phase: data collection; client need: prevention and early detection of disease; content area: medical-surgical.

RATIONALE

(A) The radial pulse lies just medial to the radius at the wrist. (B) The popliteal pulse lies in the posterior fossa behind the knee. (C) The dorsalis pedis runs along the anterior surface of the foot. (D) The posterior tibial pulse is located behind the medial malleolus (ankle bone).

68. **(A)** Nursing process phase: evaluation; client need: prevention and early detection of disease; content area: medical-surgical.

RATIONALE

(A) Of the choices given, bicycling represents the only isotonic (dynamic) exercise, which is the form recommended for hypertensive clients. There are two types of exercise: isotonic and isometric. Isotonic exercise involves change in the muscle length, shortening of muscle fibers, and moving joints and bones. Isometric exercise involves development of tension within the muscle length, which increases BP during the process. (B) Water skiing represents a form of isometric exercise. (C) Weight lifting represents a form of isometric exercise. (D) Calisthenics represents a form of isometric exercise.

69. **(B)** Nursing process phase: implementation; client need: prevention and early detection of disease; content area: medical-surgical.

RATIONALE

(A) Catsup is high in sodium content. (B) Lemon juice represents the only choice that has no sodium; all of the other choices are high in sodium content. (C) Garlic salt is very high in sodium content. (D) Soy sauce is very high in sodium content.

70. **(A)** Nursing process phase: implementation; client need: prevention and early detection of disease; content area: medical-surgical.

RATIONALE

(A) Although nitroglycerin is indicated for clients with chest pain, before it is administered the BP should be assessed. If the pressure is low, nitroglycerin is contraindicated. (B) Nitroglycerin has vasodilating properties and will lower the BP. Before administering nitroglycerin, the BP should be taken. If the client is hypotensive, nitroglycerin should not be given because it lowers the pressure even further. (C) Raising the head of the bed may ease the effort of breathing if shortness of breath and dyspnea are present, but the question does not give this information. (D) Before calling the physician, additional assessment data must be obtained, such as vital signs.

71. **(A)** Nursing process phase: data collection; client need: physiological adaptation; content area: medical-surgical.

RATIONALE

(A) Intake greater than output would reflect an increase in weight. One liter of fluid is equal to 1 kg (2.2 lb) in weight. Intake exceeds output by 2000 cc (2 kg). The nurse would anticipate the weight to increase by 2 kg or 4.4 lb. (B) The weight would be increased by approximately 4.5 lb, not 2. (C) The weight would increase, not decrease, because more fluid was taken in. (D) The weight would not remain the same because there is a difference in the 24-hour I&O.

72. **(B)** Nursing process phase: implementation; client need: basic care and comfort; content area: medical-surgical.

RATIONALE

(A) Peanuts are high in magnesium content. Depending on the preparation, peanuts may also be high in sodium. (B) The following foods are rich in potassium: bananas, cantaloupe, apricots, peaches, dates, raisins, orange juice, tomato juice, avocados, navy beans, potatoes, squash, carrots, and cauliflower. (C) Broccoli is high in calcium content. (D) Milk is not a potassium-rich food.

73. **(C)** Nursing process phase: planning; client need: pharmacological and parenteral therapies; content area: medical-surgical.

RATIONALE

(A) Although potassium is needed, NS is not the needed solution. NS exerts equal pressure on the cell and does not aid in rehydration. (B) NS is not the needed solution, as stated in rationale A. (C) Because of fluid loss from vomiting and diarrhea, the client needs a hypotonic solution (.45 NS). Hypotonic fluids allow fluid to re-enter the cell. Potassium should be added because of the loss of potassium-rich fluid through vomiting and diarrhea. (D) Hypertonic solutions (3%) pull additional fluid out of the cell, thus making the dehydration worse.

74. **(C)** Nursing process phase: implementation; client need: basic care and comfort; content area: medical-surgical.

RATIONALE

(A) Bowel training is not done with ileostomies because the contents are liquid and contain digestive enzymes. The client must wear an appliance to collect the fluid. (B) Ileostomies are not routinely irrigated; doing so always makes the client incontinent. (C) To maintain skin integrity, the nurse would ensure that the skin is clean and dry and then apply a skin barrier and a properly fitting appliance. (D) Because the contents of the ileum are liquid, stool softeners are not necessary.

75. **(C)** Nursing process phase: implementation; client need: coping and adaptation; content area: medical-surgical.

RATIONALE

(A) Instituting steadfast rules limiting visitors should not be done routinely. Restricting visitors can be done at intervals if the client seems to be adversely affected. (B) Although caring for dying clients can be extremely difficult, consistent nursing assignments are imperative for the development of therapeutic relationships with the terminally ill. (C) Once the nurse, terminally ill client, and family establish a therapeutic relationship, the nurse is often the one to advise completion of unfinished business. (D) Anger is one of the stages in the dying process. Although difficult for some clients to identify, their outward behavior is often indicative of internal emotions. The nurse assists the client and family to understand these emotions.

76. **(D)** Nursing process phase: data collection; client need: coping and adaptation; content area: medical-surgical.

RATIONALE

(A) There is no evidence of denial in the statement. (B) There is no evidence of anger in the statement. (C) There is no evidence of depression in the statement. (D) Kubler-Ross has identified five stages in the dying process: denial, anger, bargaining, depression, acceptance. By promising to return to church every Sunday, the client is bargaining with God to prolong life.

77. **(A)** Nursing process phase: implementation; client need: pharmacological and parenteral therapies; content area: medical-surgical.

RATIONALE

(A) Dopamine is a very potent vasopressor and must always be delivered via an electronic device. (B) Electronic pumps should not be used to infuse RBCs; damage to the cells can occur, causing hemolysis. (C) Vancomycin, although a very potent antibiotic, does not have to be infused via an electronic pump. (D) Only very strong concentrations of KCl should be administered via a pump. Forty mEq in 1 L is not a strong concentration; therefore, a pump is not mandatory.

78. **(C)** Nursing process phase: data collection; client need: prevention and early detection of disease; content area: medical-surgical.

RATIONALE

(A) Kussmaul's respiration is a hyperventilation pattern. There is an increase in both rate and depth. (B) Biot's breathing is similar to Cheyne-Stokes, except the pattern is irregular. (C) The observed breathing pattern is known as Cheyne-Stokes. (D) Eupnea is normal breathing: regular, quiet, effortless.

79. (B) Nursing process phase: implementation; client need: management of care; content area: medical-surgical.

    RATIONALE

    (A) The nurse could be charged with murder or manslaughter because there is no written "no-code" order. (B) Although it is always preferable to obtain a no-code order before an emergency situation occurs, in its absence, unless a living will has been signed, the nurse's only legal recourse is to begin CPR and call a code. (C) In the absence of a written no-code order, if the client stops breathing but has a pulse, artificial respiration alone is in order. Once the client becomes pulseless or asystole occurs, both breathing and compressions must be performed. (D) Consulting with the charge nurse is wasting time. In the absence of a written no-code order, the nurse must begin CPR and call a code.

80. (A) Nursing process phase: implementation; client need: basic care and comfort; content area: medical-surgical.

    RATIONALE

    (A) Incontinence pads should be placed under the deceased individual's buttocks because bowel and bladder evacuation may continue even after death has occurred because of relaxation of the bowel and bladder muscles. (B) The deceased client's head should remain slightly elevated to prevent pooling of blood and interstitial fluid in the head or face or both. (C) Dentures should not be removed. If the client dies not wearing dentures, they should be placed in the mouth during postmortem care. It is very difficult to open the mouth after rigor mortis occurs. (D) The identification armband should not be removed because positive identification is required before the body can be released to the morgue.

81. (D) Nursing process phase: data collection; client need: prevention and early detection of disease; content area: medical-surgical.

    RATIONALE

    (A) The neck veins would be distended in pulmonary edema. (B) Clients do display anxiety when in pulmonary edema. There are many causes of anxiety; therefore it is not the most characteristic symptom. (C) Clients in pulmonary edema often do have peripheral edema, but this is not always the case. (D) Pink, frothy sputum is the characteristic finding with pulmonary edema.

82. (B) Nursing process phase: implementation; client need: pharmacological and parenteral therapies; content area: medical-surgical.

    RATIONALE

    (A) This answer indicates a miscalculation. (B) x gtts/min = 250 cc/90 min × 20 gtts/cc. (C) This answer indicates a miscalculation. (D) This answer indicates a miscalculation.

83. (C) Nursing process phase: implementation; client need: prevention and early detection of disease; content area: medical-surgical.

    RATIONALE

    (A) Vaginal bleeding is not normal after menopause. (B) The bleeding is abnormal at her age; she needs to see her physician. (C) Vaginal bleeding after menopausal onset is highly abnormal and usually indicates the presence of gynecological malignancy. Although the bleeding may become intermittent, continue, or get worse, the most appropriate response would be to recommend that she consult her physician for medical follow-up. (D) Notifying her daughter could be done if the client wishes, but doing so does not solve the vaginal bleeding problem. Physician notification is the most appropriate answer.

84. (C) Nursing process phase: implementation; client need: coping and adaptation; content area: medical-surgical.

    RATIONALE

    (A) It is inappropriate to joke and chuckle. Doing so may inhibit expression of his feelings. (B) It is inappropriate to tell him not to worry; there is a chance that sexual functioning will be influenced by surgery. (C) When the suprapubic or retropubic approach is used in the removal of the prostate gland, erectile function is preserved. However, if a perineal prostatectomy is performed, innervation of the penile shaft can possibly be affected and impotence ensue. (D) It is inappropriate to tell him that most men do have sexual functioning problems after surgery; this is not true.

85. (A) Nursing process phase: implementation; client need: reduction of risk potential; content area: medical-surgical.

    RATIONALE

    (A) Hypercalcemia is a condition in which serum calcium is elevated. By providing increased amounts of fluid, calcium excretion is promoted and the amount of circulating calcium decreased. (B) When caring for client with hypercalcemia, ambulation, not bedrest, should be encouraged. During periods of bedrest and immobility, the bone releases calcium into the peripheral circulation. (C) Administering calcium supplements would only make the condition worse. (D) Antibiotics have no effect on hypercalcemia.

86. (D) Nursing process phase: implementation; client need: basic care and comfort; content area: medical-surgical.

    RATIONALE

    (A) A banana is a raw fruit and not allowed on this diet. (B) Raw vegetables such as carrot sticks are not allowed on the diet. (C) Garden salads are made of raw vegetables and are not allowed on the diet. (D) Neutropenic clients have a decreased number of circulating WBCs and therefore have an increased potential for developing an infection. Raw fruits and vegetables are not allowed on a neutropenic diet because they may contain microbial contamination. All fruits and vegetables must be thoroughly cooked before the client eats them. Canned fruits and vegetables are permitted. The safety of dairy products remains controversial.

87. (B) Nursing process phase: data collection; client need: prevention and early detection of disease; content area: medical-surgical.

    RATIONALE

    (A) Although some clients with malignant disease processes have an elevated CEA level, it is not diagnostic. (B) A positive tissue biopsy is the only reliable diagnostic measure. (C) A sore that does not heal is an early warning sign of cancer, but not diagnostic. (D) A nagging cough or hoarseness is an early warning sign of cancer, but not diagnostic.

88. (B) Nursing process phase: implementation; client need: basic care and comfort; content area: medical-surgical.

    RATIONALE

    (A) Eating spicy food causes further oral discomfort for clients with stomatitis. (B) Stomatitis is inflammation of the mucous membranes of the mouth. Although the oral mucosa might be tender, clients with stomatitis should be encouraged to brush their teeth after each meal and before bedtime with a soft toothbrush or toothettes to prevent secondary infections. (C) Although commercial mouthwashes may kill the germs commonly found in the oral cavity, they are not recommended because of their alcohol content and irritating nature. (D) Orange juice is acidic and will cause further oral discomfort.

89. **(A)** Nursing process phase: evaluation; client need: reduction of risk potential; content area: medical-surgical.

    RATIONALE

    (A) Complete return of the solution should occur with the evacuation of soft or formed feces. Soft or formed stool is found in the descending colon. **(B)** Liquid or semisoft stool is found in the ascending and transverse colon. **(C)** Lack of irrigation return could signal irrigant absorption, potentiating hypervolemia. **(D)** Evacuation of irrigant could signal only possible fecal impaction.

90. **(B)** Nursing process phase: evaluation; client need: pharmacological and parenteral therapies; content area: medical-surgical.

    RATIONALE

    (A) This acidosis is caused by hypoventilation (respiratory) and not by metabolic causes. **(B)** A narcotic overdose slows the rate and depth of breathing. This leads to the retention of carbon dioxide (acid). Hypoventilation problems produce respiratory acidosis. **(C)** Hypoventilation produces acidosis, not alkalosis. **(D)** Respiratory alkalosis is produced when too much carbon dioxide is blown off. The problem is retention of carbon dioxide.

91. **(A)** Nursing process phase: data collection; client need: prevention and early detection of disease; content area: medical-surgical.

    RATIONALE

    (A) Restlessness, yawning, tachycardia, and hypertension are all early signs of hypoxemia. As the oxygen deprivation continues, dyspnea, confusion, and impaired judgment occur. With the development of severe hypoxemia, tachycardia, hypotension, and bradycardia are seen. **(B)** Hypotension is a sign of severe hypoxemia. **(C)** Bradycardia is a sign of severe hypoxemia. **(D)** Bradycardia and hypotension are signs of severe hypoxemia.

92. **(C)** Nursing process phase: implementation; client need: safety and infection control; content area: medical-surgical.

    RATIONALE

    (A) Mask, gown, and goggles are not necessary because excessive contamination is not possible in this situation. **(B)** Gowns are necessary when soiling of clothes is likely from splashes of blood and body fluids. This is not likely when giving an IM injection. **(C)** A small amount of blood may ooze from the needle puncture site after an IM injection. Therefore, the nurse should wear gloves for self-protection when massaging, holding pressure, and wiping the site. **(D)** Goggles are necessary in procedures likely to generate droplets of blood and body fluids.

93. **(D)** Nursing process phase: data collection; client need: reduction of risk potential; content area: medical-surgical.

    RATIONALE

    (A) Although instillation of air assists in assessment of tube placement, it does not provide the nurse with a residual volume. Very high residual volumes mean the client is not absorbing and is more likely to aspirate the tube's contents. It is advisable to auscultate for bowel sounds, but no more than 20 cc of air should be used; otherwise, gastric distention is likely to occur. **(B)** One does not instill fluid first without checking placement with air and the residual volume. If the tube is not in the stomach, aspiration may occur. **(C)** Although an abdominal x-ray will confirm tube placement, it is costly and placement can be checked by other means. **(D)** It is best for the nurse to aspirate stomach contents to ascertain tube placement as well as absorption of the tube feeding. The gastric contents are reinstilled to prevent electrolyte imbalance.

94. **(A)** Nursing process phase: data collection; client need: reducti0n of risk potential; content area: medical-surgical.

RATIONALE

(A) Because radiation therapy affects fast-growing cells, the hemopoietic and GI systems would be affected. Because the treatment field incorporates the throat, esophagus, and stomach, the GI symptoms most commonly seen would include nausea and dysphagia. Bone marrow suppression would occur because the treatment field includes the sternum. **(B)** Diarrhea would not be seen because the small bowel is not included in the treatment field. **(C)** Alopecia is observed only in brain irradiation. **(D)** Radiation does not cause constipation.

95. **(D)** Nursing process phase: implementation; client need: reduction of risk potential; content area: medical-surgical.

    RATIONALE

    (A) Notify the physician; this is an over-the-counter agent. **(B)** Notify the physician; this is an over-the-counter agent. **(C)** Notify the physician; this is an over-the-counter agent. **(D)** You should never apply an over-the-counter medication to a radiation treatment field. Most of these products contain petroleum derivatives or metallic fragments, which may actually intensify the burning process. Therefore, you should notify the physician and obtain orders for a water-based emollient such as Aquaphor.

96. **(B)** Nursing process phase: implementation; client need: management of care; content area: medical-surgical.

    RATIONALE

    (A) It would be inappropriate for the nurse to do nothing. An Hgb level of 6.3 is critical; some course of action needs to be taken. The physician needs to be notified promptly. **(B)** Jehovah's Witnesses are opposed to blood transfusions and organ donations. The physician should be informed because the client's refusal may be life-threatening. **(C)** It is inappropriate for the nurse to try to convince the client to take blood and go against religious practices. **(D)** It is very inappropriate for the nurse to administer the blood without the client's consent.

97. **(D)** Nursing process phase: planning; client need: pharmacological and parenteral therapies; content area: medical-surgical.

    RATIONALE

    (A) Because the client is already vomiting, the oral route in this situation would not facilitate maximum absorption of the drug. **(B)** IM medications are not administered because of the potential for bleeding and hematoma formation. **(C)** Rectal suppositories are not administered to thrombocytopenic clients because of the vascularity of the rectal mucosa and the potential for bleeding if the area were injured during the suppository insertion. **(D)** Antiemetics should be administered only IV or by mouth when the client is thrombocytopenic. The nurse would administer the IV push medication.

98. **(B)** Nursing process phase: implementation; client need: pharmacological and parenteral therapies; content area: medical-surgical.

    RATIONALE

    (A) Blue food coloring only helps to detect aspiration once it has occurred. **(B)** The head of the bed should always be elevated at least 30 degrees when continuous enteral feedings are infusing. The flat or low positions facilitate gastric reflux, which increases the risk of aspiration. **(C)** Enteral feedings are often prescribed at rates greater than 50 ml/hr. As long as the gastric residuals are not high, higher infusion rates are acceptable. **(D)** This intervention helps to decrease microbial proliferation in the formula; it does not influence aspiration risk.

99. **(D)** Nursing process phase: implementation; client need: basic care and comfort; content area: medical-surgical.

    RATIONALE

    (A) The nurse stands on the weaker (right) side, not on the stronger (left) side. **(B)** Holding the client's hand does not give stability to the gait. **(C)** The nurse stands on the client's right (weaker) side, not on the stronger (left) side. **(D)** Hemiparesis is slight paralysis affecting one side of the body. The nurse always stands on the client's affected side and supports the client by holding one arm around the client's waist and the other arm around the client's upper arm, so that the nurse's hand supports the client's axilla. A client with right-sided weakness requires the nurse to stand on the right side.

100. **(C)** Nursing process phase: implementation; client need: basic care and comfort; content area: medical-surgical.

    RATIONALE
    (A) There is no need for the nurse to feed the client. **(B)** There is no need for the family to feed the client. The client is capable and should be encouraged to feed himself or herself. **(C)** A client with recent visual impairment is encouraged and assisted to participate in regular ADLs. The nurse assists the client by preparing the food tray (open containers, cut meat, and so on) and orienting the client to the location of all items on the food tray. **(D)** There is no reason to encourage use of the spoon exclusively.

101. **(D)** Nursing process phase: data collection; client need: prevention and early detection of disease; content area: medical-surgical.

    RATIONALE
    (A) None of the areas is the most important respiratory assessment to make, with the possible exception of pain. **(B)** BP and sweating are important, but not the most important assessments to make. **(C)** Capillary refill is more directly related to perfusion. Trembling is irrelevant. Amount of sputum is important, but not the most important assessment. **(D)** All three of these assessments are the most essential areas to cover during a respiratory assessment; restlessness could indicate a lack of oxygen to the brain.

102. **(C)** Nursing process phase: data collection; client need: prevention and early detection of disease; content area: medical-surgical.

    RATIONALE
    (A) The oxygen would affect a temperature reading taken orally. **(B)** An axillary temperature is not very accurate. **(C)** A rectal temperature would give the most accurate reading of body temperature. **(D)** Feeling the forehead would not give an accurate measure of body temperature.

103. **(B)** Nursing process phase: implementation; client need: physiological adaptation; content area: medical-surgical.

    RATIONALE
    (A) Pinching the soft tissue applies pressure to stop the bleeding. **(B)** Warm liquids should be avoided; dilatation of blood vessels could exacerbate the bleeding. **(C)** Cold constricts blood vessels and helps to stop the bleeding. **(D)** A physician should be consulted as part of follow-up care unless the cause of the bleeding is obvious.

104. **(A)** Nursing process phase: planning; client need: prevention and early detection of disease; content area: medical-surgical.

    RATIONALE
    (A) The client should save his voice until his physician tells him to use it. **(B)** The client will receive tube feedings for a few days after surgery. **(C)** The bed should be in a Fowler's position to promote an open airway. **(D)** The client should be taught that he will have to hold his head still following surgery.

105. **(B)** Nursing process phase: planning; client need: physiological adaptation; content area: medical-surgical.

RATIONALE
(A) Reducing anxiety is a desired outcome but should not receive highest priority. **(B)** An open airway with adequate gas exchange takes the highest priority because it is essential to the life of the client. **(C)** Talking about feelings is an important outcome but does not take highest priority. **(D)** Maintaining fluid balance is important but not the most essential outcome to maintain life.

106. **(C)** Nursing process phase: planning; client need: prevention and early detection of disease; content area: medical-surgical.

    RATIONALE
    (A) The presence of cor pulmonale would be indicated by signs and symptoms of right-sided heart failure. **(B)** Pulsus paradoxus or distant heart sounds would indicate cardiac tamponade. **(C)** The data support pneumothorax. **(D)** The trachea would more likely be deviated with a pneumothorax.

107. **(D)** Nursing process phase: data collection; client need: prevention and early detection of disease; content area: medical-surgical.

    RATIONALE
    (A) A positive Mantoux test result means only that the client has had the tubercle bacillus in the body at one time; it does not mean that the client is infectious. **(B)** The tubercle bacillus is Gram-positive. **(C)** The lesion could be walled off; unless the organism is in the sputum, the client will not be infectious. **(D)** Pulmonary tuberculosis is spread by way of airborne droplets of sputum; the organism must be in the sputum before the infection can be spread.

108. **(D)** Nursing process phase: evaluation; client need: prevention and early detection of disease; content area: medical-surgical.

    RATIONALE
    (A) A client with hypertension should learn how to manage stress. **(B)** A BP of 140/90 is the upper limit of normal. **(C)** Stroke and heart attack can result from untreated hypertension. **(D)** Antihypertensives should not be discontinued because the client feels OK.

109. **(D)** Nursing process phase: implementation; client need: reduction of risk potential; content area: medical-surgical.

    RATIONALE
    (A) The client may be having an MI; calling the physician will delay treatment. **(B)** Driving could cause injury to himself and others. **(C)** Emergency care is needed. **(D)** A rescue squad is best equipped to give emergency treatment.

110. **(A)** Nursing process phase: planning; client need: physiological adaptation; content area: medical-surgical nursing.

    RATIONALE
    (A) Decreasing any strain on the heart is the highest priority in restoring the health of the client at this time. **(B)** Breathing easily is only one component of reducing the workload on the heart. **(C)** Decreasing edema is only one component of reducing the workload on the heart. **(D)** Learning about the medications is not the highest priority at this time.

111. **(C)** Nursing process phase: data collection; client need: reduction of risk potential; content area: medical-surgical.

    RATIONALE
    (A) No mention is made of data indicating either left or right heart failure. **(B)** The data do not indicate presence of an MI. **(C)** The signs are classic for shock; the BP can be normal. **(D)** Signs of cardiac tamponade are absent.

112. **(C)** Nursing process phase: data collection; client need: pre-

vention and early detection of disease; content area: medical-surgical.

RATIONALE

(**A**) It would be helpful to know the electrolyte report results when talking with the physician. (**B**) Signs of digoxin toxicity are present; treatment could be delayed. (**C**) Digoxin toxicity can occur while serum levels of the drug are normal when electrolyte imbalances occur. (**D**) Administering an antiemetic could mask the symptoms and delay treatment.

113. (**D**) Nursing process phase: implementation; client need: physiological adaptation; content area: medical-surgical.

    RATIONALE

    (**A**) Antiembolism stockings should be applied only to the unaffected leg. (**B**) Aspirin inhibits platelet aggregation and might interfere with heparin therapy. (**C**) The clot could be dislodged and cause a pulmonary embolus. (**D**) Bedrest helps to prevent a pulmonary embolus.

114. (**B**) Nursing process phase: implementation; client need: coping and adaptation; content area: medical-surgical.

    RATIONALE

    (**A**) The question does not state the client's spiritual foundation. (**B**) She needs most of all to talk about her feelings. (**C**) She may not be quite ready for a support group. (**D**) She needs to face the problem when she is ready to face it.

115. (**D**) Nursing process phase: data collection; client need: pharmacological and parenteral therapies; content area: medical-surgical.

    RATIONALE

    (**A**) No indication is given that one of the drugs might affect the heart. (**B**) Chemotherapy can be nephrotoxic, but nephrotoxicity is not part of bone marrow depression. (**C**) No data are given to indicate a need to assess for the integrity of bones. (**D**) Platelets could be depressed when bone marrow is depressed; therefore, assessment needs to be made for signs of bleeding.

116. (**B**) Nursing process phase: evaluation; client need: prevention and early detection of disease; content area: medical-surgical.

    RATIONALE

    (**A**) HIV can be spread by sexual contact. (**B**) The virus is not spread by touching, and the client needs to touch others. (**C**) The virus can be spread by way of body fluids. (**D**) A mother can pass the virus to her unborn infant.

117. (**A**) Nursing process phase: implementation; client need: physiological adaptation; content area: medical-surgical.

    RATIONALE

    (**A**) The Sengstaken-Blakemore tube is used to control bleeding for a client with esophageal varices. (**B**) A client with cirrhosis of the liver would not need a Sengstaken-Blakemore tube unless esophageal varices were present. (**C**) The Sengstaken-Blakemore tube is not used to treat renal stones. (**D**) This tube is not used to treat hiatal hernia.

118. (**B**) Nursing process phase: evaluation; client need: prevention and early detection of disease; content area: medical-surgical.

    RATIONALE

    (**A**) Nonsteroidal anti-inflammatory drugs (NSAIDs) have been associated with the occurrence of peptic ulcer disease in several research studies. (**B**) Coffee in moderation has not been shown to be associated with PUD. (**C**) Smoking has been associated with causing PUD. (**D**) Stress has also been associated with the development of PUD.

119. (**C**) Nursing process phase: data collection; client need: reduction of risk potential; content area: medical-surgical.

    RATIONALE

    (**A**) No data exist to suggest that hyperkalemia could be a problem. (**B**) No data exist to suggest that an acid-base disorder of respiratory origin might be a problem. (**C**) Loss of gastric acid by suction for several days could lead to metabolic alkalosis. (**D**) No data exist to suggest that acidosis might occur.

120. (**D**) Nursing process phase: planning; client need: reduction of risk potential; content area: medical-surgical.

    RATIONALE

    (**A**) A rigid abdomen would be present if perforation of the GI tract occurred. (**B**) Absence of bowel sounds would be needed to support a diagnosis of paralytic ileus. (**C**) Data do not give strong support for an obstruction. (**D**) The signs and symptoms are classic for dumping syndrome.

121. (**B**) Nursing process phase: data collection; client need: prevention and early detection of disease; content area: medical-surgical.

    RATIONALE

    (**A**) Vital signs may be taken routinely, bleeding should not be a problem, and diarrhea would be monitored as it occurs. (**B**) Fluid volume deficit and electrolyte imbalances could occur; they need to be detected early. (**C**) The data do not indicate that these assessments should be made frequently. (**D**) Perfusion could be a reflection of fluid balance, and muscle twitching could indicate electrolyte imbalance, but the variables listed in rationale B would be more likely to detect fluid and electrolyte imbalances earlier.

122. (**D**) Nursing process phase: data collection; client need: prevention and early detection of disease; content area: medical-surgical.

    RATIONALE

    (**A**) The data do not call for more than routine assessment of lung sounds. (**B**) The data do not suggest a need to assess for a pulse deficit. (**C**) The data do not suggest a need to assess for renal stones. (**D**) Assessment for bowel sounds needs to be made frequently because a section of the GI tract was removed.

123. (**D**) Nursing process phase: implementation; client need: reduction of risk potential; content area: medical-surgical.

    RATIONALE

    (**A**) The lung would collapse because the pleural cavity would be exposed to atmospheric pressure. (**B**) The tubing should not be clamped because pressure could build up in the pleural cavity or a spontaneous, closed pneumothorax could occur. (**C**) Excess suction could cause a closed pneumothorax. (**D**) The Pleuravac should be attached to the side of the wheelchair to avoid damage to the closed chest drainage system.

124. (**D**) Nursing process phase: implementation; client need: prevention and early detection of disease; content area: medical-surgical.

    RATIONALE

    (**A**) The sounds are probably caused by peristalsis and the obstruction; excess flatus would be misleading. (**B**) Acini are small saclike structures usually found at the end of a gland. (**C**) Hypoactive would be misleading. (**D**) The loud, rumbling sounds are called borborygmi.

125. (**C**) Nursing process phase: planning; client need: reduction of risk potential; content area: medical-surgical.

    RATIONALE

    (**A**) The client does need antiembolism stockings after hernia repair. (**B**) Signs of hemorrhage should be assessed the same as for other types of general surgery. (**C**) The client should not cough because the increase in pressure in the abdominal cavity could injure the repair. (**D**) Precautions against infection are just as important for the client with a hernia repair.

126. (**A**) Nursing process phase: implementation; client need: reduction of risk potential; content area: medical-surgical.

    RATIONALE

    (**A**) A cleansing enema is needed to clean all of the barium out of the GI tract; it can obstruct the appendix. (**B**) Barium does not usually cause renal damage. (**C**) Activity helps to eliminate the barium. (**D**) Barium does not usually cause an allergic reaction.

127. (**B**) Nursing process phase: data collection; client need: prevention and early detection of disease: content area: medical-surgical.

    RATIONALE

    (**A**) If the client has appendicitis, a laxative could cause the appendix to rupture. (**B**) Checking McBurney's point for rebound tenderness would be appropriate; it would provide more data about possible appendicitis. (**C**) A heating pad could cause an inflamed appendix to rupture. (**D**) More data are needed before calling a physician.

128. (**D**) Nursing process phase: implementation; client need: reduction of risk potential; content area: medical-surgical.

    RATIONALE

    (**A**) Bedrest should be maintained. (**B**) A semi-Fowler's position is needed to facilitate respiratory movement. (**C**) The data do not support a need to check the mouth for ulcerations. (**D**) Food in the GI tract would make the obstruction worse, and the client should be prepared for surgery.

129. (**A**) Nursing process phase: data collection; client need: prevention and early detection of disease; content area: medical-surgical.

    RATIONALE

    (**A**) The stool is indicative of regional enteritis, or Crohn's disease; documentation of the stool would aid diagnosis. (**B**) The stool should not be ignored for the reason given under rationale A. (**C**) A laxative is not indicated. (**D**) The stool is more indicative of a regional enteritis than a fecal impaction.

130. (**B**) Nursing process phase: implementation; client need: prevention and early detection of disease; content area: medical-surgical.

    RATIONALE

    (**A**) *Cholangitis* is the appropriate term for infection of the bile duct. (**B**) *Choledocholithiasis* means that stones are present in the hepatic and bile duct. (**C**) *Cholecystitis* means inflammation of the gallbladder. (**D**) *Cholelithiasis* means stones in the gallbladder.

131. (**D**) Nursing process phase: implementation; client need: coping and adaptation; content area: medical-surgical.

    RATIONALE

    (**A**) All nursing actions should be explained to the client. (**B**) The client's anxiety is lessened if all actions are explained. (**C**) Encouraging someone to do something he or she is not ready to do could increase anxiety. (**D**) The client's anxiety is lessened if all actions are explained.

132. (**A**) Nursing process phase: implementation; client need: prevention and early detection of disease; content area: medical-surgical.

    RATIONALE

    (**A**) The incision is located below the rib cage; therefore, the

coughing and deep breathing necessary to prevent hypostatic pneumonia are especially difficult postoperatively. (**B**) The data do not indicate special precautions to prevent thrombosis. (**C**) The ordinary precautions to prevent hemorrhage are sufficient. (**D**) No special precautions are needed to prevent paralytic ileus.

133. (**D**) Nursing process phase: implementation; client need: physiological adaptation; content area: medical-surgical.

    RATIONALE

    (**A**) Hepatitis A is only occasionally transmitted parenterally. (**B**) Hepatitis A is not usually transmitted through body fluids. (**C**) Hepatitis A is not usually transmitted through sexual intercourse. (**D**) Hepatitis A is usually transmitted through feces or contaminated food or water.

134. (**C**) Nursing process phase: implementation; client need: safety and infection control; content area: medical-surgical.

    RATIONALE

    (**A**) Reverse isolation is used to prevent infection in the client. (**B**) A mask and gown are not required because the disease is not spread by way of the respiratory tract. (**C**) Universal Precautions provide protection except in unusual circumstances. (**D**) Trash should be isolated, but Universal Precautions are more important.

135. (**A**) Nursing process phase: implementation; client need: reduction of risk potential; content area: medical-surgical.

    RATIONALE

    (**A**) The client may have a tendency to bleed easily because clotting factors are formed in the liver. (**B**) Aspirin should not be given because it inhibits aggregation of platelets, and clotting factors may be inadequate because of a diseased liver. (**C**) The abdominal girth should be measured daily. (**D**) Unless portal system encephalopathy is present, the client needs a high-protein and high-carbohydrate diet.

136. (**D**) Nursing process phase: data collection; client need: physiological adaptation; content area: medical-surgical.

    RATIONALE

    (**A**) The data do not indicate a need to assess for hyperkalemia. (**B**) No data suggest metabolic acidosis. (**C**) Hypocalcemia is not likely. (**D**) Hyperglycemia or hypoglycemia could occur if damage is done to the islets of Langerhans.

137. (**B**) Nursing process phase: implementation; client need: reduction of risk potential; content area: medical-surgical.

    RATIONALE

    (**A**) Signs of infection indicate a need for medical treatment. (**B**) A physician needs to prescribe treatment. (**C**) A physician needs to prescribe treatment. (**D**) A physician needs to prescribe treatment.

138. (**C**) Nursing process phase: planning; client need: pharmacological and parenteral therapies; content area: medical-surgical.

    RATIONALE

    (**A**) Fluids are given parenterally. (**B**) Aseptic technique is needed to prevent infection. (**C**) An analgesic should be timed so that the client experiences minimal pain during the dressing change. (**D**) I&O should be monitored hourly.

139. (**B**) Nursing process phase: implementation; client need: reduction of risk potential; content area: medical-surgical.

    RATIONALE

    (**A**) Even if the client had a tetanus injection within the last 10 years, it will be more important to give a tetanus booster. (**B**) A booster is necessary after injuries to ensure inactivation of any tetanus toxin produced by entry of the tetanus bacillus. **(C)** Someone should be with the client to observe for signs of head injury. **(D)** Heavy sedation should be avoided in the event of a head injury.

140. **(D)** Nursing process phase: implementation; client need: basic care and comfort; content area: medical-surgical.
    RATIONALE
    (A) Saving all urine would not be necessary. **(B)** Forcing fluids would be more appropriate. **(C)** Recording I&O would be important but not as important as straining urine. **(D)** The data indicate that the client may have a renal stone; it would be most important to strain the urine to obtain the stone for analysis.

141. **(B)** Nursing process phase: implementation; client need: basic care and comfort; content area: medical-surgical.
    RATIONALE
    (A) A ureteral catheter should never be clamped. **(B)** The output from the ureteral catheter should be recorded separately in order to assess drainage from the left kidney. **(C)** The catheter is irrigated only with a physician's order and then with strict aseptic technique and with no more than 5 ml of solution. **(D)** Activity should be encouraged.

142. **(A)** Nursing process phase: evaluation; client need: prevention and early detection of disease; content area: medical-surgical.
    RATIONALE
    (A) A low-protein diet is needed to reduce metabolic products causing the uremia. **(B)** A high-calorie diet is indicated in chronic renal failure. **(C)** A low-potassium diet is needed. **(D)** A low-sodium diet is needed.

143. **(C)** Nursing process phase: implementation; client need: reduction of risk potential; content area: medical-surgical.
    RATIONALE
    (A) Major complications of peritoneal dialysis are not related to drainage time. **(B)** Dwelling time needs to be accurate, not precise. **(C)** Infection is perhaps the most common complication of peritoneal dialysis; it can be prevented by using strict aseptic technique. **(D)** Calcium is not usually added to the dialysis solution unless hypocalcemia is problem.

144. **(A)** Nursing process phase: data collection; client need: basic care and comfort; content area: medical-surgical.
    RATIONALE
    (A) BP should be checked in the left arm to preserve the shunt. **(B)** An IV should not be started in the right arm. **(C)** The shunt should not be irrigated. **(D)** Blood should not be drawn through the shunt.

145. **(C)** Nursing process phase: implementation; client need: pharmacological and parenteral therapies; content area: medical-surgical.
    RATIONALE
    (A) Some medication might be removed by dialysis. **(B)** If these drugs are not removed by dialysis, they should be given. **(C)** Medications not removed by dialysis should be given. **(D)** It is not necessary to bother the physician.

146. **(A)** Nursing process phase: planning; client need: reduction of risk potential; content area: medical-surgical.
    RATIONALE
    (A) Detecting fluid or electrolyte imbalances would be a high priority in the care of a client with chronic renal failure. **(B)** Constipation is more likely than diarrhea in chronic renal failure. **(C)** Acidosis is more likely in chronic renal failure. **(D)** Hyperkalemia is more likely in chronic renal failure.

147. **(A)** Nursing process phase: data collection; client need: reduction of risk potential; content area: medical-surgical.
    RATIONALE
    (A) Urinary output should get highest priority because a urethral stricture or clot in the catheter could be detected early. **(B)** Urinary output would take a higher priority for reasons explained in rationale A. **(C)** Urinary output would take a higher priority for reasons explained in rationale A. **(D)** Urinary output would take a higher priority for reasons explained in rationale A.

148. **(C)** Nursing process phase: implementation; client need: physiological adaptation; content area: medical-surgical.
    RATIONALE
    (A) Nothing should be done to irritate the skin in the field of radiation therapy. **(B)** No lotions or creams are to be applied without a physician's order. **(C)** Most authorities allow cleaning the skin in the field of radiation therapy with water and patting dry as needed. **(D)** A physician's order is needed before any lotion or cream is applied.

149. **(B)** Nursing process phase: implementation; client need: physiological adaptation; content area: medical-surgical.
    RATIONALE
    (A) The client should have a Foley catheter in place. **(B)** If antiembolism stockings are not in place, they should be applied immediately; thrombus formation is one of the biggest complications of a hysterectomy. **(C)** Perineal pads should be changed every 3–4 hours, and bleeding should be assessed. **(D)** The physician usually likes to make the first dressing change; until then, nurses reinforce the dressing.

150. **(D)** Nursing process phase: implementation; client need: reduction of risk potential; content area: medical-surgical.
    RATIONALE
    (A) The client should remain on bedrest until the physician writes an order for him to be up. **(B)** A brace is used only when a spinal fusion is done. **(C)** Raising the legs and pointing the toes may be ordered as exercises after surgery. **(D)** The client should be log-rolled to prevent manipulation of the spinal column and possible injury to the cord.

151. **(D)** Nursing process phase: planning; client need: reduction of risk potential; content area: medical-surgical.
    RATIONALE
    (A) Epiglottitis, or inflammation of the flap of cartilage that covers the larynx, causes airway obstruction. Oxygen is indicated if hypoxia occurs and is effective only if a patent airway is present. **(B)** An oral airway assists in preventing the tongue from obstructing the airway, but it does nothing to alleviate the obstruction caused by epiglottitis. **(C)** Respiratory distress from the epiglottitis is caused by airway obstruction and not accumulation of secretions. **(D)** A tracheostomy set contains instruments that a physician can use to create an opening in the trachea below the epiglottis, thus restoring airway patency.

152. **(A)** Nursing process phase: implementation; client need: reduction of risk potential; content area: medical-surgical.
    RATIONALE
    (A) When the client is placed on the right side, the biopsy site of the liver capsule is compressed against the chest wall, and the escape of blood or bile is impeded. **(B)** When the client is placed on the left side, the biopsy site of the liver capsule is not compressed against the chest wall, and bleeding may occur. **(C)** After a liver biopsy, the client should remain recumbent and immobile. **(D)** When feet are raised as in the Trendelenburg position, venous return is increased. The increased blood flow may cause bleeding from the biopsy site.

153. **(D)** Nursing process phase: data collection; client need: pharmacological and parenteral therapies; content area: medical-surgical.

RATIONALE

(A) Febrile reactions are characterized by fevers and shaking chills that occur within 30 minutes of the start of the blood transfusion. **(B)** Hives, generalized itching, and occasionally wheezing or anaphylaxis occur during allergic reactions. **(C)** Septic reactions result from transfusion of blood contaminated with bacteria and cause rapid onset of chills and high fever, vomiting, diarrhea, and hypotension. **(D)** Hemolytic reactions, which occur when the donor blood is incompatible with that of the client, cause chills, low back pain, headache, and nausea within the first 10 minutes of a transfusion. Hypotension and vascular collapse follow, and hemoglobinuria (red urine) occurs.

154. **(D)** Nursing process phase: implementation; client need: basic care and comfort; content area: medical-surgical.

RATIONALE

(A) Severe joint pain occurs during a sickle cell crisis; careful movement, positioning, and support of painful areas are indicated. **(B)** Fluids should be encouraged because they promote hemodilution and reverse the clumping of sickled cells in small vessels, which causes pain. **(C)** Diarrhea is not associated with sickle cell crisis; constipation often occurs as a result of immobility and narcotic analgesic use. **(D)** Pain from sickle cell crisis, caused by clumping of sickled cells in small blood vessels, is often severe and requires narcotic analgesics. Frequent assessments of pain assist in monitoring the client's response to hydration and pain control, the mainstays of treatment for sickle cell crisis.

155. **(C)** Nursing process phase: data collection; client need: basic care and comfort; content area: medical-surgical.

RATIONALE

(A) A decrease in intake causes smaller stools but does not cause seepage of liquid stool. **(B)** Spinal cord trauma is not associated with CVAs; constipation often occurs in the CVA client as a result of immobility. **(C)** Fecal impactions cause continuous oozing of liquid stool because the liquid portion of feces located high in the colon seeps around the edges of the impacted mass. **(D)** Dehydration causes hard stools and constipation.

156. **(D)** Nursing process phase: implementation; client need: reduction of risk potential; content area: medical-surgical.

RATIONALE

(A) Clients having seizures are at risk for airway obstruction when the tongue occludes the airway. If they become hypoxic during a seizure, opening the airway will relieve the hypoxia; oxygen is not indicated. **(B)** Clients with seizures should not be restrained. Because muscular contractions are strong during a seizure, restraint can produce injury. **(C)** The jaw of a client having a seizure should not be pried open because broken teeth and injury to the lips and tongue may result. **(D)** When the client is placed on one side with head flexed forward, the tongue falls forward, which assists in maintaining a patent airway, and drainage of saliva and mucus is facilitated.

157. **(A)** Nursing process phase: data collection; client need: physiological adaptation; content area: medical-surgical.

RATIONALE

(A) Enteral feedings contain glucose; abrupt discontinuation of glucose feedings will cause the blood glucose to drop rapidly, resulting in symptoms of hypoglycemia such as an increased heart rate, sweating, and tremors. The symptoms can progress to slurred speech, incoordination, double vision, and drowsiness. **(B)** Hyperglycemia, or high blood glucose, may occur while a client receives enteral feedings. Withdrawal of glucose causes the

opposite condition, hypoglycemia. **(C)** Enteral feedings are not associated with alterations in potassium levels. Administration of parenteral fluids (IV fluids) may cause alterations in potassium levels. **(D)** Enteral feedings are not associated with alterations in potassium levels. Administration of parenteral fluids (IV fluids) may cause alterations in potassium levels.

158. **(B)** Nursing process phase: data collection; client need: prevention and early detection of disease; content area: medical-surgical.

RATIONALE

(A) A breakdown of the skin occurs in the second stage of pressure ulcer development. **(B)** The first stage of pressure ulcer development consists of redness of the skin that blanches with pressure, complaints of discomfort, and swelling. **(C)** Drainage of pressure ulcers occurs in stages II, III, and IV. **(D)** A stage IV pressure ulcer is characterized by extension to underlying muscle and bone, infection, necrosis, and drainage.

159. **(B)** Nursing process phase: implementation; client need: prevention and early detection of disease; content area: medical-surgical.

RATIONALE

(A) A PTT is used to monitor response to heparin therapy. A PTT or PT is used to monitor response to oral anticoagulants. **(B)** Carrying information about oral anticoagulant therapy is helpful in an emergency situation and provides information for other health-care providers, such as dentists. **(C)** Aspirin has anticoagulation action and should not be used concurrently with other anticoagulants because it increases the risk of bleeding. **(D)** Alcohol interferes with platelet function, which increases the risk of bleeding, and therefore should be avoided.

160. **(B)** Nursing process phase: data collection; client need: pharmacological and parenteral therapies; content area: medical-surgical.

RATIONALE

(A) Morphine sulfate is a respiratory depressant. Digoxin is a medication that is withheld if the pulse rate is <60 bpm. **(B)** When administering morphine sulfate, a respiratory depressant, the nurse should assess the respiratory rate; if it is less than 12 bpm, the nurse should withhold the drug and call the physician. **(C)** Antipyretics, or temperature-lowering drugs, are usually administered for elevated temperatures. Morphine sulfate is a respiratory depressant. **(D)** Morphine sulfate does not increase BP; it has a hypotensive effect, and respiratory depression is its most common effect.

161. **(D)** Nursing process phase: data collection; client need: physiological adaptation; content area: medical-surgical.

RATIONALE

(A) The median age of menopause is 51 years; it may occur in some women as young as 42 years or as late as 55 years. A 74-year-old woman is considered to be postmenopausal and therefore would not be menstruating. **(B)** Estrogen production decreases with advancing age and is not a cause of vaginal bleeding. **(C)** Sexually transmitted diseases cause a variety of vaginal discharges but do not cause vaginal bleeding. **(D)** Any vaginal bleeding that occurs 1 year after cessation of menses should be evaluated; the most likely cause of vaginal bleeding in a postmenopausal woman is uterine cancer.

162. **(C)** Nursing process phase: data collection; client need: prevention and early detection of disease; content area: medical-surgical.

RATIONALE

(A) Progressive loss of weight occurs with hyperthyroidism. **(B)** Hyperthyroid clients tolerate heat poorly and perspire freely;

cool to cold temperatures are preferred. **(C)** The primary function of the thyroid hormones are to control cellular metabolic activity. The pulse rate, at rest and on exercise, is rapid and clients with hyperthyroidism may experience palpitations. **(D)** Myxedema occurs with hypothyroidism.

163. **(A)** Nursing process phase: data collection; client need: physiological adaptation; content area: medical-surgical.
    RATIONALE
    (A) Accumulation of blood creates dead spaces and dead cells that become media for infection. **(B)** Tight dressings reduce the blood supply carrying nutrients and oxygen to the wound. **(C)** Steroids may mask the presence of infection by impairing normal inflammatory response. **(D)** Activity prevents approximation of wound edges; rest favors healing.

164. **(C)** Nursing process phase: data collection; client need: prevention and early detection of disease; content area: medical-surgical.
    RATIONALE
    (A) Hypovolemic shock is caused by decreased fluid volume from blood or fluid loss. The pulse rate is rapid and may be irregular. **(B)** Respirations are shallow and rapid in hypovolemic shock. **(C)** In hypovolemic shock, the skin is cool, pale, and moist. The lips and nails may be cyanotic. **(D)** Urine output decreases in hypovolemic shock and may progress from 50 cc/hr to <10 ml/hr (anuria).

165. **(C)** Nursing process phase: data collection; client need: physiological adaptation; content area: medical-surgical.
    RATIONALE
    (A) An MI may cause chest pain, but dyspnea as a primary symptom indicates a cause other than an MI. **(B)** Anaphylaxis occurs as a response to an allergic agent. **(C)** A serious complication of a DVT is pulmonary embolism. When the embolus travels to the right side of the heart and occludes the pulmonary artery, the symptoms are sudden. The client experiences chest pain and becomes breathless and cyanotic. Sudden death may occur. **(D)** Bronchopneumonia does not have a sudden onset and is characterized by an elevated temperature.

166. **(D)** Nursing process phase: implementation; client need: prevention and early detection of disease; content area: medical-surgical.
    RATIONALE
    (A) Hot, spicy foods should be avoided in clients with an esophageal stricture because they stimulate esophageal spasm. **(B)** The client should remain upright for 1–4 hours after each meal to prevent reflux by using gravity to decrease an elevated gastroesophageal pressure gradient. **(C)** Eating should be avoided just before bedtime to prevent reflux. **(D)** Small, frequent feedings are recommended because large quantities of food overload the stomach and promote gastric reflux.

167. **(D)** Nursing process phase: data collection; client need: basic care and comfort; content area: medical-surgical.
    RATIONALE
    (A) A PEG tube exits from the GI tract via an abdominal incision. An NG tube, not a PEG tube, could potentially cause skin irritation of the nares. **(B)** Securing feeding tubes to the client's cheek is only applicable for nasogastrically inserted tubes. **(C)** Assessment for NG tube displacement is necessary after coughing, tracheal or NG suctioning, and airway intubation. Because a PEG tube is surgically inserted, checking for displacement after coughing, suctioning, and intubation is not indicated. **(D)** Assessment of bowel elimination patterns is indicated for the client fed via a PEG tube since feedings are often hyperosmolar and may cause diarrhea.

168. **(B)** Nursing process phase: data collection; client need: prevention and early detection of disease; content area: medical-surgical.
    RATIONALE
    (A) Hemorrhoids are located near or external to the anus; they usually bleed on defecation and the blood is red to bright red. **(B)** The passage of dark, tarry stools (melena) indicates bleeding from the upper GI tract. Stools appear dark and tarry because they contain digested Hgb. **(C)** The rectum and sigmoid colon are parts of the lower GI tract; dark, tarry stools are characteristic of bleeding from the upper GI tract. **(D)** The rectum and sigmoid colon are parts of the lower GI tract; dark, tarry stools are characteristic of bleeding from the upper GI tract.

169. **(C)** Nursing process phase: data collection; client need: prevention and early detection of disease; content area: medical-surgical.
    RATIONALE
    (A) Pain associated with a perforated peptic ulcer is sudden and severe in the upper abdominal area. **(B)** Stools are dark and tarry in PUD. **(C)** Pain, which is referred to the shoulders, especially the right shoulder, occurs when a peptic ulcer perforates because of irritation of the phrenic nerve. **(D)** Pain is relieved by eating when a peptic ulcer is located in the duodenum.

170. **(A)** Nursing process phase: data collection; client need: prevention and early detection of disease; content area: medical-surgical.
    RATIONALE
    (A) Jaundice, light-colored stools, and dark urine are associated with hepatitis B and caused by the inability of the diseased liver cells to clear bilirubin from the blood. **(B)** Dark, tarry stools are associated with PUD. **(C)** Although the urine may appear dark with renal failure, stools are not light-colored. **(D)** With small bowel obstructions, there may be no stool, and the urine would not be dark-colored.

171. **(B)** Nursing process phase: data collection; client need: pharmacological and parenteral therapies; content area: medical-surgical.
    RATIONALE
    (A) Short-acting regular insulin has an onset of action of ½–1 hour. At 4:01 PM, the insulin has not yet begun to act. **(B)** The peak action of regular insulin is 2–4 hours; during this time, clients are at greatest risk for developing rebound hypoglycemia. **(C)** Regular insulin has a duration of 6–8 hours; rebound hypoglycemia would not occur at midnight. **(D)** Regular insulin has a duration of 6–8 hours; rebound hypoglycemia would not occur at 6 AM the following day.

172. **(C)** Nursing process phase: evaluation; client need: prevention and early detection of disease; content area: medical-surgical.
    RATIONALE
    (A) Immediate treatment of hypoglycemia, characterized by sweating, tremor, tachycardia, nervousness, and hunger, is administration of a fast-acting sugar such as glucose tablets, fruit juice, hard candies, sugar, or honey. **(B)** Diabetic retinopathy is the leading cause of blindness in adults in the United States; annual eye examinations for adults with diabetes are recommended. **(C)** Variations in blood glucose levels are expected throughout the day, with the lowest levels before meals and the highest levels 1–2 hours after eating. The goal of diabetes treatment is to minimize wide swings in glucose levels, not to eliminate normal variations. **(D)** Regular (short-acting) insulin should be drawn up before the NPH insulin when combined in one syringe to keep the regular insulin vial "pure"; this practice eliminates the chance that the longer-acting NPH insulin would be introduced into the regular insulin vial.

173. **(A)** Nursing process phase: data collection; client need: reduction of risk potential; content area: medical-surgical.

RATIONALE

(A) During thyroid surgery, the parathyroid glands may be injured or removed, producing a decrease in calcium production. Hyperirritability of the nerves, spasms of the hands and feet, and muscular twitching are a group of symptoms called *tetany,* and are caused by hypocalcemia. **(B)** Hypocalcemia causes the symptoms of tetany. **(C)** Although hypokalemia can cause muscular weakness, it does not cause spasms and twitching. **(D)** Symptoms of hyperkalemia include dysrhythmia, paresthesia, and nausea.

174. **(B)** Nursing process phase: data collection; client need: pharmacological and parenteral therapies; content area: medical-surgical.

RATIONALE

(A) Changes in metabolism occur as a result of long-term steroid therapy, and weight gain results. **(B)** Because of suppression of the immune system and inflammatory response from long-term steroid therapy, infections may occur with minimal or no symptoms. **(C)** Addison's disease is caused by chronic adrenocortical insufficiency; clients on long-term steroid therapy are at risk for developing Cushing's syndrome from excessive adrenocortical activity. **(D)** As a result of long-term steroid use, facial skin becomes oily and acne flares.

175. **(A)** Nursing process phase: data collection; client need: reduction of risk potential; content area: medical-surgical.

RATIONALE

(A) Bedrest decreases body metabolism and thus reduces pancreatic and gastric secretions in the client with acute pancreatitis. **(B)** Impairment of endocrine function of the pancreas from pancreatitis results in increased serum glucose levels. **(C)** Bedrest increases the risk of a DVT. **(D)** The rationale for bedrest for the client with pancreatitis is to reduce pancreatic and gastric secretions; clients are still at risk for orthostatic hypotension.

176. **(D)** Nursing process phase: implementation; client need: reduction of risk potential; content area: medical-surgical.

RATIONALE

(A) Cleansing from the anus toward the urethra results in the introduction of rectal bacteria in the urethral area. **(B)** It is not necessary to wash hands before collecting the specimen. **(C)** The collection container should not come in contact with the genitalia; contamination may result. **(D)** Midstream urine collections are the most accurate. Because the distal portion of the urethral orifice is colonized by bacteria, voiding washes away the urethral contaminants.

177. **(D)** Nursing process phase: implementation; client need: basic care and comfort; content area: medical-surgical.

RATIONALE

(A) A urinary drainage bag connected to an indwelling urinary catheter should never be raised above the level of the bladder; contaminated urine from the drainage bag would flow into the client's bladder. **(B)** The drainage bag should not lie on the floor; contamination may result. The bag should be hung from the bed frame or chair frame. **(C)** The drainage bag should be emptied at least every 8 hours to lessen the risk of bacterial growth. **(D)** A free flow of urine reduces the risk of infection. When the drainage tubing is kinked or twisted, pools of urine are allowed to collect in the loops of the tubing.

178. **(C)** Nursing process phase: evaluation; client need: reduction of risk potential; content area: medical-surgical.

RATIONALE

(A) Dry peritoneal catheter dressings are desired; a wet dressing may indicate the complication of leakage. **(B)** A bloody effluent (drainage) may be observed occasionally, especially in young, menstruating female clients. **(C)** Peritonitis is the most common complication of peritoneal dialysis; indications of peritonitis include cloudy drainage and abdominal pain. **(D)** Rapid weight gain in clients on peritoneal dialysis occurs from fluid volume overload. A stable weight indicates that the peritoneal dialysis is effectively eliminating waste products.

179. **(B)** Nursing process phase: evaluation; client need: prevention and early detection of disease; content area: medical-surgical.

RATIONALE

(A) Drinking 8–10 glasses or more of fluids daily is recommended to flush out bacteria that cause UTI. **(B)** Voiding every 2–3 hours during the day prevents overdistention of the bladder and compromised blood supply to the bladder wall, which predispose clients to UTI. **(C)** Antibiotics should be taken for as long as they are prescribed; premature discontinuation (even if symptom-free) may result in repeated infection as a result of inadequate antibiotic therapy. **(D)** Showers are preferable to tub baths because bacteria in the bath water can enter the urethra.

180. **(A)** Nursing process phase: evaluation; client need: reduction of risk potential; content area: medical-surgical.

RATIONALE

(A) Hemodialysis is indicated for clients with chronic renal failure who experience fluid volume excess and electrolyte imbalances. Removal of the excess fluid during the dialysis process results in weight loss. Monitoring a client's weight is a simple indirect way to assess a client's fluid balance. **(B)** A calorie count provides information about the client's nutritional intake but is not of value for assessing response to hemodialysis. **(C)** Measuring exercise tolerance does not assist in assessing a client's response to hemodialysis as much as measuring the client's weight; most clients with chronic renal failure experience anemia and, as a result, are chronically fatigued. **(D)** Assessing for skin bruising is not a means of assessing response to hemodialysis. A skin alteration commonly associated with chronic renal failure is uremic frost, a white powdery substance that appears on the skin because of elevated urates.

181. **(D)** Nursing process phase: data collection; client need: pharmacological and parenteral therapies; content area: medical-surgical.

RATIONALE

(A) Kidney rejection is most likely to occur early (within 24–72 hours) or may occur within a few day or a few months. **(B)** Infection by bacterial or fungal pathogens is most likely to occur during the first few weeks following transplant. Immunosuppressive agents are gradually tapered over a period of several weeks, depending on the client's immunologic response to the transplant. **(C)** Although clients can experience uncertainty about the future at any time, the feeling of uncertainty in the kidney transplant recipient is greatest before receipt of the transplanted kidney. **(D)** Two years after a kidney transplant, a client is most likely to express concerns about the long-term effects of immunosuppressive therapy, such as developing diabetes, glaucoma, cataracts, and osteoporosis.

182. **(C)** Nursing process phase: data collection; client need: physiological adaptation; content area: medical-surgical.

RATIONALE

(A) Symptoms associated with renal stones include pain, nausea, hematuria, and symptoms of infection. Impairment of gas exchange is not associated with renal stones. **(B)** A renal stone obstructs flow of urine; it does not impair renal function. **(C)** Because of blockage of the urinary tract, clients are at risk for infection. **(D)** Self-concept disturbances are associated with alterations in how clients perceive themselves. Presence of an internally located renal stone would not be likely to alter a client's self-concept.

183. **(B)** Nursing process phase: implementation; client need: reduction of risk potential; content area: medical-surgical.

    RATIONALE

    (A) In an ileal conduit, the urine is diverted by implanting the ureter into a loop of ileum that is led out through the abdominal wall. An ileostomy bag is used to collect the urine. Intermittent urinary catheterization is not indicated. **(B)** Changes in physical structure and function occur with an ileal conduit procedure; the ability to cope with these changes depends to a great degree on the client's self-concept and self-esteem. **(C)** Peritoneal dialysis is used when renal failure occurs; an ileal conduit is used when urinary diversion is needed. **(D)** Only urine is diverted via an ileal conduit; the ends of the remaining intestine are connected to provide an intact bowel.

184. **(C)** Nursing process phase: implementation; client need: physiological adaptation; content area: medical-surgical.

    RATIONALE

    (A) Because herpes genitalis is a sexually transmitted disease, condoms should be used to reduce the likelihood of disease transmission to the female partner. **(B)** The herpes virus causes herpes genitalis; antibiotics are indicated for bacterial infections. **(C)** Herpes genitalis causes vesicular (blisterlike) lesions in the perineum. Complications such as extragenital spread can result from touching lesions and then touching the buttocks, thighs, eyes, or other areas. **(D)** Because herpes genitalis is caused by a virus, antifungal preparations are not indicated.

185. **(B)** Nursing process phase: data collection; client need: physiological adaptation; content area: medical-surgical.

    RATIONALE

    (A) Symptoms of dribbling, difficulty in starting urination, and sensations of incomplete emptying indicate that an obstruction is occurring between the bladder and meatus, and these symptoms are not characteristic of the normal aging process. **(B)** The prostate gland is a walnut-sized gland that is located at the base of the bladder. Enlargement causes symptoms of obstruction, such as dribbling, difficulty in starting urination, and sensations of incomplete emptying. **(C)** Enlarged prostate glands often cause stasis of urine in the bladder, which subsequently becomes infected. However, when a UTI occurs, the urine is concentrated and cloudy, and may be bloody. **(D)** Chronic constipation does not cause urinary symptoms.

186. **(D)** Nursing process phase: data collection; client need: prevention and early detection of disease; content area: medical-surgical.

    RATIONALE

    (A) Inability to cough results in pooling of secretions and ineffective airway clearance. Gas exchange is not impaired (the airway is impaired). **(B)** Pain may result from coughing, but inability to cough results in inability to clear the airway. **(C)** Altered thought processes may occur with hypoxia (decreased oxygen supply). However, inability to cough results in airway impairment. **(D)** Inability to cough causes secretions to pool and obstruct the airway. Coughing is a mechanism for clearing an airway; when coughing is impaired, ineffective airway clearance results.

187. **(B)** Nursing process phase: implementation; client need: safety and infection control; content area: medical-surgical.

    RATIONALE

    (A) Because the exudate is a body fluid, Universal Precautions, which mandate gloving before contact with body fluids, should be instituted. **(B)** Nonsterile gloves should be used to remove dirty dressings that contain exudate, considered a body fluid. Wearing gloves reduces the risk that the nurse could acquire the infection from the client. **(C)** Sterile gloves are not indicated for removing "dirty" dressings; nonsterile gloves are sufficient, readily available, and much more cost effective. **(D)** Double gloving is not a recommended principle of Universal Precautions. Donning a single pair of nonsterile gloves is considered sufficient protection when changing soiled dressings.

188. **(B)** Nursing process phase: planning; client need: pharmacological and parenteral therapies; content area: medical-surgical.

    RATIONALE

    (A) Hypotension and shock occur with anaphylactic (immediate hypersensitivity) reactions as a result of the release of mast cell mediators. Penicillin and its derivatives have known anaphylactic potential. **(B)** Laryngeal edema, bronchospasm, cyanosis, and even cardiac arrest can occur with an anaphylactic reaction. Because less severe symptoms such as hives can progress to a life-threatening event, anticipation of this possibility enables the nurse to be prepared. **(C)** Paralytic ileus does not occur during an anaphylactic reaction. **(D)** Liver failure is typically a chronic process. Anaphylactic events occur suddenly and are usually of short duration. Liver failure is therefore unlikely.

189. **(B)** Nursing process phase: data collection; client need: prevention and early detection of disease; content area: medical-surgical.

    RATIONALE

    (A) Bulging eyes (exophthalmos) are commonly associated with Graves' disease (hyperthyroidism) and do not occur in systemic lupus erythematosus. **(B)** A butterfly-shaped erythematous rash across the nasal bridge is a classic sign of SLE. **(C)** Jaundice, or yellowing of the skin, may occur when liver function is impaired and does not occur with SLE. **(D)** Kaposi's lesions are cutaneous lesions that are brown to purple and occur in Kaposi's sarcoma, an AIDS-related malignancy.

190. **(B)** Nursing process phase: data collection; client need: prevention and early detection of disease; content area: medical-surgical.

    RATIONALE

    (A) Nevi (moles) are typically brown. Colors of concern include blue-black, gray, and purple. **(B)** An irregularly shaped mole warrants further evaluation, particularly if the mole was once circular and has changed. **(C)** Moles can be located all over the body. Location is of concern only when a mole is located in an area of mechanical trauma or friction, such as under a bra strap. **(D)** Sun rays, which are ultraviolet rays, cause sunburns, which increase the risk of skin cancer. However, the characteristics of the mole need to be examined, not the surrounding skin. Clients should be taught to avoid sun exposure.

191. **(B)** Nursing process phase: data collection; client need: prevention and early detection of disease; content area: medical-surgical.

    RATIONALE

    (A) Smoke inhalation injury results from the inhalation of the products of incomplete combustion. The injury is a result of chemical irritation of the pulmonary tissues at the alveolar level. Burns involving boiling water are topical and do not result in smoke inhalation. **(B)** In first-degree burns, the epidermis is destroyed or injured and a portion of the dermis may be injured. The area may be painful, appear red and dry, or it may be blistered. **(C)** In second-degree burns, the epidermis and the dermis are injured. The area is painful, appears red, and exudes fluid. **(D)** In third-degree burns, there is total destruction of epidermis and dermis; the color of the wound may be white to red to black. The burn is painless because of destruction of nerve fibers and has a leathery appearance.

192. **(D)** Nursing process phase: implementation; client need: physiological adaptation; content area: medical-surgical.

    RATIONALE

    (A) Monitoring hourly urine output is performed during the immediate phase of burn care. **(B)** NG suction is maintained during the immediate phase of burn care because burn injury often produces paralytic ileus. **(C)** Topical antibiotic agents are applied during the intermediate phase of burn care to reduce the risk of bacterial colonization. **(D)** Elastic bandages or pressure garments are applied over healed areas prone to scarring to prevent hypertrophic scarring and to achieve an optimal cosmetic effect during the rehabilitation or long-term phase of burn care.

193. **(A)** Nursing process phase: implementation; client need: pharmacological and parenteral therapies; content area: medical-surgical.

    RATIONALE

    (A) The abbreviation *OD* refers to "oculus dexter," or "right eye." **(B)** The abbreviation *OS* refers to "oculus sinister," or "left eye." **(C)** The abbreviation *OU* refers to "oculus unitas," or "both eyes." **(D)** The abbreviation *AU* refers to "both ears."

194. **(D)** Nursing process phase: implementation; client need: reduction of risk potential; content area: medical-surgical.

    RATIONALE

    (A) Cold compresses, not hot, should be applied to reduce pain and intraocular pressure. **(B)** To decrease intraocular pressure, light levels should be reduced (lights dimmed, drapes drawn), and clients should be instructed to wear dark glasses in strong light. **(C)** Pressing or rubbing the eye should be avoided to facilitate healing and reduced intraocular pressure. **(D)** Head elevation and avoiding lying on the operative side decrease eye edema and intraocular pressure.

195. **(C)** Nursing process phase: implementation; client need: reduction of risk potential; content area: medical-surgical.

    RATIONALE

    (A) The client should be reminded not to blow nose or sneeze because such actions my force organisms through the auditory canal to the middle ear. **(B)** Shampoos are discouraged for about 2 weeks; moisture helps transmit organisms. **(C)** The client should be instructed to report facial paralysis, drooping of the mouth on the affected side, altered taste, drooling when drinking, and mouth dryness, which may indicate surgical trauma to the seventh cranial nerve. **(D)** Ear packing should be kept clean and dry; moist environments promote microbial growth.

196. **(D)** Nursing process phase: data collection; client need: prevention and early detection of disease; content area: medical-surgical.

    RATIONALE

    (A) Reaction only to loud noises and pain indicates serious impairment of brain circulation and is a late sign of increasing ICP. **(B)** Absence of reflexes and flaccid extremities are late signs of ICP. **(C)** Fixed and dilated pupils are very late signs of ICP; a fatal outcome is usually inevitable. **(D)** Lethargy, changing levels of consciousness, slowing of the speech, and delay in response to verbal stimuli are early indicators of increasing ICP.

197. **(B)** Nursing process phase: implementation; client need: reduction of risk potential; content area: medical-surgical.

    RATIONALE

    (A) An unconscious client is at risk for developing pressure ulcers and therefore requires skin care; however, the most important nursing action is to maintain an airway. **(B)** Maintaining an airway is the most important nursing action when caring for an unconscious client because the epiglottis and tongue may relax and occlude the oropharynx. If the airway becomes occluded, the brain is deprived of oxygen. **(C)** Turning a client who is unable to turn is necessary to prevent pressure ulcers and reduce infection risk, but maintaining an airway takes higher priority. **(D)** The head of the bed of an unconscious client should be elevated 30 degrees to reduce aspiration risk; however, maintaining a patent airway is the most important nursing action.

198. **(C)** Nursing process phase: data collection; client need: physiological adaptation; content area: medical-surgical.

    RATIONALE

    (A) Sensory deficits caused by a CVA include paresthesia (numbness and tingling) and difficulty with proprioception. **(B)** Verbal deficits caused by a CVA include various types of aphasia, such as expressive, receptive, and global (both expressive and receptive). **(C)** Short- and long-term memory loss, decreased attention span, inability to concentrate, poor abstract reasoning, and altered judgment are examples of cognitive deficits caused by a CVA. **(D)** Emotional deficits after a CVA include loss of self-control, decreased tolerance to stress, depression, withdrawal, fear, hostility, and anger.

199. **(B)** Nursing process phase: implementation; client need: basic care and comfort; content area: medical-surgical.

    RATIONALE

    (A) Clients with multiple sclerosis experience altered bowel elimination because of spinal cord dysfunction. Neurogenic impairment typically causes constipation. Adequate fluid intake, not fluid restriction, is needed to prevent constipation. **(B)** A high-fiber diet increases bulk and reduces the likelihood of constipation and is a component of bowel programs designed for clients with multiple sclerosis. **(C)** Clients with multiple sclerosis have an intact bowel; they experience neurogenic impairment and do not require colostomies. **(D)** Intermittent self-catheterization is recommended as part of a bladder program for some clients with multiple sclerosis.

200. **(C)** Nursing process phase: implementation; client need: reduction of risk potential; content area: medical-surgical.

    RATIONALE

    (A) Vital signs are monitored after a total hip replacement to assess for hemorrhage. **(B)** The wound of a client who has undergone total hip replacement is monitored for blood loss and infection. **(C)** After a total hip replacement, neurovascular status is assessed by observing the capillary refill of the toes. Rapid return of pink color indicates good capillary perfusion. **(D)** Performing ROM of the hip after a total replacement is not indicated; the hip should be kept in an abducted position and in neutral rotation to prevent dislocation.

CHAPTER 6

Psychiatric–Mental Health Nursing: Content Review and Test

Diane Hamilton, RN, PhD
Eileen W. Keefe, RN, CMS

Nursing Care of Psychiatric–Mental Health Clients

The psychiatric nurse promotes health through caring for and about the client. The health promotion is accomplished through understanding, observing, teaching, and physical care skills.

1. **Care of physiological needs:** Psychiatric clients are often unable to complete activities of daily living (ADLs) independently. The nurse monitors and supervises their performance.

   Feeding: Quantity and quality of food intake are observed and recorded. Calorie counts are recorded. Intake and output (I&O) of fluids are monitored. Confused, severely depressed, and severely retarded clients are fed by the nurse. Appetite is observed and documented.

   Sleep: Amount and quality of sleep are observed and recorded. Clients are checked every 30 minutes throughout the night. Sleep charts are recorded. Often clients are not allowed to sleep in the daytime, to stabilize sleep patterns.

   Vital signs: Psychiatric medications may cause wide fluctuations in blood pressure and temperature. Vital signs are checked and recorded as the physician orders, usually four times daily. Orthostatic blood pressure measurements (checking the blood pressure with the client lying down and 1 minute later with the client standing) give physicians information about how medication is being metabolized in the client. A high temperature is a side effect of neuroleptic (antipsychotic) medication.

   Hygiene: Psychiatric clients, particularly those who are very confused, depressed, or withdrawn, need assistance with bathing, bed making, and dental care. Encourage the client to complete as many of the hygiene tasks as possible. The nurse assists the client in completing daily hygiene.

   Elimination: Psychiatric medications may alter elimination habits. Information about bowel and urinary function is gathered and documented by the nurse daily.

   Activity: The client's energy level is observed. Clients are encouraged to attend therapeutic activities (e.g., art therapy, music therapy). Mobility, gait, and coordination are observed. The nurse assists clients who cannot ambulate independently.

2. **Safety:** Psychiatric clients' safety is the responsibility of the nurse. Specific psychiatric nursing procedures include the following:

   Admission: The nurse ensures the client's safety by removing guns, knives, sharp instruments, glass objects, and medications on admission. Often, very confused or disturbed clients are dressed in pajamas on admission. Most clients are allowed to wear street clothes, but belts and sharp jewelry are removed from the client to ensure safety.

   Restraints: When clients are assessed to be harmful to themselves or others, the physician may order restraints. All other measures must be exhausted before restraints are used. An order for restraints is *written* for a specified period not to exceed 12 hours (differs from state to state). The health-care team organizes the procedure before approaching the client. A *minimum* of five people is needed to restrain a client. Each team member is assigned a limb (arm or leg) to restrain. The team leader explains the procedure to the client and directs the team. With very violent clients, a waist restraint may be added. A client in restraints is monitored constantly by a nurse to provide a calm and safe environment, to attend to physiological needs, and to observe reactions. Restraints are removed each hour to ensure circulation.

Seclusion: Clients who are assessed to be harmful to themselves or others are sometimes placed in seclusion (a bare room with a mattress) to decrease environmental stimuli. Seclusion allows the client to retain or regain control of behavior. The team escorts the client to seclusion (a minimum of three personnel) *after* a physician's order is obtained. Sharp objects, belts, and jewelry are removed from the client to ensure safety. Clients may be placed in various forms of seclusion:

- **Locked-door seclusion:** The door is locked and the client and the mattress remain in the room. The client is constantly observed.
- **Open-door seclusion:** The client remains in the room with the door unlocked and open. The client is observed constantly or every 5 minutes.
- **Room program:** The client remains in the room 30 minutes but is allowed out of the room 30 minutes each hour. The client's reaction and behavior are observed. If the client resumes control of his or her behavior, the in-and-out time is altered accordingly (e.g., 45 minutes out, 15 minutes in).

Mobility: Psychiatric medication may cause dizziness (vertigo). All psychiatric clients are checked frequently (e.g., at 15, 30, or 60 minutes) to assess their safety.

Environmental: No cords over pathways, sharp corners on furniture, loose rugs, or items that are hard and can be thrown to cause harm are permitted.

Management: The nurse is responsible for the safety of the clients and staff. The psychiatric nurse observes client-client, client-family, and client-staff interactions to prevent outbursts.

3. The psychiatric nurse encourages and assists clients to interact and communicate with others. The nurse observes:

Emotional reactions: Does the client laugh or cry inappropriately? Does the client talk with clients and staff? Can he or she carry on a social conversation? Does the client react appropriately? Does he or she smile? Can the client demonstrate caring for others? Does he or she participate in activities? Can the client enjoy himself or herself?

Communication: What are the client's nonverbal and verbal communication skills? Is the client's behavior similar to the communication skills? Does he or she sound and look pleasant, or sound happy *and* look angry?

Family: What are the interactions of the client with the family, spouse, and/or children? What pattern have they developed (are they sullen, silent, happy, fighting)?

4. **Self-esteem:** The psychiatric nurse promotes the maintenance and development of a client's self-esteem.

Self relationship: Assess for client self-worth, strengths, goals, problem-solving ability, motivation, state of independence, ability to participate in daily care, and discharge planning.

The Health-Care Team

1. A psychiatrist is a physician who specializes in the care of clients having mental disorders.
2. A psychiatric nurse is a nurse who specializes by experience and/or education in the care of psychiatric clients. A psychiatric clinical specialist has a master's degree in nursing or doctoral degree in nursing.
3. A psychologist specializes in psychological testing, counseling, and therapy.
4. An occupational therapist specializes in teaching leisure, occupational, or daily skills to clients (e.g., cooking, art, typing).
5. A recreational therapist teaches clients recreational and leisure skills (e.g., painting, needlework, model cars).
6. A social worker specializes in working with the family, in community resources, and in counseling and therapy.
7. A molecular psychiatrist specializes in biochemical aspects of the brain, a neurophysiologist specializes in the physiology of the body's nervous systems, and a neuropsychiatrist specializes in the neurological system and behavior.
8. A psychopharmacologist specializes in psychotropic medications and drugs that affect behavior.

Psychiatric Terminology

Affect: Refers to mood or emotion; seen on one's face and described as blunted, flat, inappropriate, or bland

Ambivalence: Two feelings together (love-hate, pleasure-pain, like-dislike) toward a person, object, or idea

Behavior: Any observable, recordable act, movement, or response of an individual

Blocking: Interruption of flow of speech owing to distracting thoughts

Body language: Transmission of a message by body movements

Catatonia: State of immobilized stupor that can quickly swing to extreme agitation

Catharsis: Release that occurs when clients talk openly

Cathexis: Freud's term for attachment to an object or idea; when one connects to a person or idea, there is a strong bond

Circumstantial: Digression of thought into unnecessary details (e.g., explaining pain, but talking about one's mother's surgery)

Claustrophobia: Fear of closed places

Compulsion: Irresistible urge to perform some act (e.g., handwashing)

Congruent: Verbal communication that matches nonverbal communication

Delirium: Medical diagnostic term that describes rapidly occurring onset of confusion

Delusion: Fixed false belief (e.g., one believes that he is Christ)

Depression: Can be a sign, symptom, disease, or reaction of sadness or grief

Dissociation: Separation of mental processes from a person's consciousness

Diurnal mood: Changes in mood because of time of day

Echolalia: Imitation of another's words

Echopraxia: Imitation of another's body position

Ego boundaries: Person's perception of the boundaries between self and environment

Endogenous: Occurring within; refers to a type of depression

Environment: Circumstances, people, objects, and conditions that surround and have an impact on one's life

Ethnocentrism: Imposing of one's beliefs and values on other cultural groups

Fantasy: Daydreaming

Flight of ideas: Rapid shift of ideas while speaking (e.g., speaking of weather, to mother, to pain with no connection between subjects)

Grandiose: Ideas of fame, wealth, or importance that are unfounded or untrue (e.g., a woman thinking that she is Elizabeth Taylor)

Hallucination: Seeing, hearing, smelling, or feeling something that is not a result of external stimuli (e.g., seeing or feeling bugs crawl on the skin)

Hostility: An attitude of negativity or anger

Hypochondriasis: Belief that one is ill with no organic cause, such as pain with no cause

Hypomania: An older clinical term that refers to "less than severe manic" behavior (generally, behavior that is unfocused or hyperactive is called "manic"; if the client is excited and exhausted it is called "full-blown mania")

Illusion: Misinterpretation of sensory—usually visual—input (e.g., seeing water in the desert that is really sand)

Insight: Awareness and understanding of behavior

Institutionalized syndrome: Characterized by apathy, withdrawal, and submission to authority

Labile: Frequent and rapid change of emotions

Limit setting: Communicating the rights, responsibilities, and expectations to a person so that expected normal limits and rules can be identified

Manic-depressive illness (MDI): A psychotic state characterized by excited or severely depressed behavior; bipolar disorder

Neologism: Invention of a new word (e.g., "alzopra" instead of "chair")

Neurotic: Behavior or dysfunction that is characterized by anxiety but no distortion of reality

Nihilism: False belief that part of one's self is dead

Obsession: Recurring unstoppable thought

Orientation: Knowing correctly the time, place, and person

Panic: Extreme anxiety that involves dread and loss of rational thought

Phobia: Extreme persistent fear that is out of proportion to reality

Psychosis: Severely dysfunctional behavior characterized by anxiety, reduced functioning, limited awareness, and personality distintegration; out of touch with reality

Reminiscence: Systematic review of life experiences

Repression: Involuntary exclusion of painful memories

Self-disclosure: Revealing information about one's ideals, feelings, and values in the context of a therapeutic or specific goal

Somnambulism: Sleepwalking

Transference: Response of a client to a nurse that was originally associated with an important figure in early life (e.g., a client treating a nurse like his or her mother)

Word salad: Jumbled disconnected words (e.g., down far black strip grass)

Types of Treatment Distinctive to Psychiatric Settings

The psychiatric nurse promotes a therapeutic environment for the client by assisting in the different types of treatment.

Somatic Therapy

1. Antipsychotic drugs
   Action: Stopping or diminishing disabling symptoms such as aggression, hallucinations, irritability, delusions
   Use: Psychotic disorders such as organic disorders, affective disorders, and schizophrenia
   Agents: Chlorpromazine (Thorazine), haloperidol (Haldol), loxapine (Loxitane), fluphenazine (Prolixin), molindone (Moban)
   Major side effects: Extrapyramidal side effects such as restlessness, shuffling gait, muscle rigidity, urinary retention, low blood pressure, sedation, and high temperature
   Nursing care: Reporting of observations of high temperature or movements; checking frequency of elimination patterns; monitoring vital signs lying down and standing
2. Antidepressants
   Action: Stimulating the limbic system (tricyclics and heterocyclics) or inhibiting the oxidase enzyme (monamine oxidase inhibitors, or MAOIs); mood elevated
   Use: Clinical depression; depressive cycle of MDI
   Agents: Isocarboxazid (Marplan [MAOI]), tranylcypromine (Parnate [MAOI]), amitriptyline (Elavil), desipramine (Norpramin), imipramine (Tofranil)
   Nursing care: Intramuscular (IM) administration not recommended as absorption is slow and erratic; quickly absorbed sublingually. Observe for inhibition and excitement after multiple doses. Observe for withdrawal symptoms after long-term use. Monitor vital signs. Teach client not to consume alcohol while taking anxiolytics.

Electroconvulsive Therapy

Electroconvulsive therapy (ECT) is a series of controlled electrical currents applied to the brain to produce grand mal seizures; it is given under anesthesia. Nursing care of the client undergoing ECT includes:

1. Provide preoperative care (keep client on nothing by mouth [NPO], remove dentures, empty bladder).
2. Give preoperative muscle relaxer IM.
3. Complete preoperative checklist.
4. Accompany client to ECT room.
5. Monitor vital signs.
6. Prevent aspiration as needed.
7. Observe for complications of fractures.
8. Assist in recovery, anticipate confusion; help to reorient.
9. Document recovery.
10. ECT is now used only as a last resort when all other treatments of certain depressions do not help the client.
11. Provide safety measures and reorientation if client is confused.

Milieu Therapy

The environment can promote recovery and health.
1. Manage physical and psychological aspects of the client's environment to promote behavioral changes.
2. Increase or decrease environmental stimuli to promote client's interactions, monitor activity, protect the client, enhance the client's personality.
3. Assist with adjunct therapies:
   Occupational therapy
   Recreational therapy
   Group therapy
   Client education groups
   Discharge groups
   Family therapy groups
   Music therapy
   Dance therapy
   Pet therapy
   Movement therapy
   Psychodrama
   Reminiscence therapy

The Nurse-Client Relationship

The psychiatric nurse uses self as a tool to assist the client in healing. Nursing care includes:
1. Understanding of self, needs, and feelings
2. Awareness of personal strengths and limitations
3. Respect for the client
4. Ability to listen
5. Being genuine
6. Offering support, reassurance
7. Maintaining a calm attitude
8. Using empathy (understanding), which is more effective than sympathy (pity)
9. Understanding of the client's cultural beliefs
10. Understanding that the nurse-client relationship is goal oriented, time limited, and composed of three phases (introduction, working, ending)

Mental health nursing occurs in the following environments:
1. Inpatient hospital
2. Outpatient clinic
3. Day (or night) care
4. Assisted living
5. Homeless shelter
6. Nursing home

Communication

Communication is a process of sending and receiving verbal (spoken) and nonverbal (body language) messages. The nurse uses communication to gather information, establish a relationship with the client, and provide nursing care.
1. Effective communication between the nurse and client is encouraged by:
   - Finding a private place to talk
   - Making sure the client is comfortable
   - Reducing distractions (television, radio, noise)
   - Stating sentences clearly
   - Listening to the client's words
   - Listening to what the client means
   - Maintaining eye contact with the client
   - Sitting no farther than 3 feet away from the client
   - Treating the client like a person
   - Smiling; looking concerned
   - Behaving in a caring manner
   - Using language the client will understand
2. Nurses communicate in many ways:
   Verbal (spoken or written) communication, including voice tone, vocabulary, speed of speech
   Nonverbal communication, including the body and facial expression (kinesis), how close or far the nurse sits to the client (proxemics)
   Effective communication is:
   - Efficient and clear
   - Consistent (say and mean the same thing)
   - Open, friendly
   - Purposeful
   Communication may be blocked by:
   - Giving advice ("Mr. Jones, I think you *should.* . . .")
   - Changing topics quickly
   - Blaming the client ("You know it's bad to smoke.")
   - False reassurance ("Don't worry, it'll be OK.")
   - Saying something that is not true (lying)
   - Judging the client ("You're stupid to eat sweets.")
   - Asking "why" too often
   - Asking too many questions
   - Being angry with the client
   - Arguing with the client
   Therapeutic communication techniques include:
   - Open-ended statements: Saying "Tell me more about that."
   - Reflection: When the client feels depressed, the nurse reflects, "You feel depressed."
   - Finding the meaning: When the client says, "I feel depressed," the nurse says, "And 'depressed' means what to you?"
   - Silence.
   - Listening.
   - Identifying themes: Helping the client see a pattern of thought and feeling ("You're talking about death a lot.").
   - Accepting: Allowing the client to speak freely.
   - Attentiveness: Calling client by name; responding nonverbally.
   - Clarifying: "You mean. . . ."
   - Restating: Rearranging words in a different order to clarify meaning.
   - Focusing: Assisting client to stick to the topic.
   - Giving information: Giving the client facts about diagnostic test, and so on.
   - Providing feedback: "You have been speaking of anger against your Mom."
   - Making observations: "You look happy."
3. Therapeutic communication methods include:
   Become aware of and monitor own verbal and nonverbal communication patterns.
   - Recognize that your own cultural and subcultural values and customs influence perception and interpretation of another's behavior.
   Check on your interpretations of client behavior with client or with other professionals.

Operate on facts, not assumptions:
- State your observations ("You are talking about funerals. Are you thinking of death?").

Demonstrate acceptance of client:
- Remain objective in assessing client's behavior.
- Demonstrate concern, understanding, and respect.
- Remain genuine and nonjudgmental.

Allow sufficient time and avoid a hurried approach.

Focus on strengths of client.

Use therapeutic communication techniques.

Communicate openness and willingness to trust client and to share a nurse-client relationship.

Select an environment that provides privacy, comfort, and minimal distraction.

Express empathy by accurately understanding client's feelings. Your answers should reflect an awareness of and sensitivity to the client's culture, values, and life experiences.

Use resources of information (chart, family, physician).

Assist the client to become more aware of an aspect of his or her behavior or problem.

Development of Self

The self may include:
1. **Self-concept:** How one *thinks* of oneself
2. **Self-ideal:** One's ideal notion of who one should be
3. **Self-esteem:** How one feels about oneself
4. **Spiritual self:** Allows one the opportunity to connect

with a higher being and to find meaning and purpose in one's experiences
5. **Identity:** A general sense of who one is
6. **Character:** A person's pattern of discipline, moral constitution, and reputation
7. **Personality:** Behaviors specific to each individual (e.g., a general pattern of self-centeredness, kindness, suspiciousness, and so on)
8. **Role:** One's perception of how one fits into social settings (e.g., role of aunt, employee, sister)

The self is the sum total of thoughts, feelings, physical characteristics, socioeconomic status, ethnicity, and family-cultural factors. Self is affected by:
1. **Heredity:** Genetic impact on neurological system that influences behavior
2. **Environment:** External factors that influence behavior (family, culture, and so on)
3. **Developmental norms:** Level of development of self described by several theorists

Table 6–1 is an overview of three theories of development at each stage of life.

Nursing Care of Problem Behaviors

Anxiety

Anxiety is a generalized vague feeling of psychic pain that is associated with feelings of uncertainty and helplessness. It occurs as a result of a threat to a person's ideals, being, or self-esteem.

Table 6–1 Overview of three developmental theories

Approximate Age	Freud	Erikson	Piaget
Infant (0–1 yr)	Oral stage: Characterized by dependence and narcissism; exploration using mouth especially when area stimulated	Trust versus mistrust: Characterized by establishing a trusting relationship with another	Sensorimotor: Learning to recognize object permanence
Toddler (1–3 yr)	Anal: Defiant behavior, socialization control established	Autonomy versus shame: Characterized by negativism and exertion of self-will	Preoperational: Learning to think in terms of past, present, and future
Preschooler (3–5 yr)	Phallic: Beginning socialization, faculty, sexual identity, sexual deviations	Initiative versus guilt: Imitation of adults, development of a conscience	
School Age (6–11 yr)	Latency: Group identification, intellectual growth	Industry versus inferiority: Intellectual curiosity, learning rules and regulations	Concrete operations: Ability to classify, order, and sort facts
Adolescent (12–18 yr)	Genital: Sexual maturity, heterosexual relations	Identity versus role confusion: Establishment of identity, development of heterosexual relationships	Formal operations: Ability to think abstractly and logically
Young Adult (19–34 yr)		Intimacy versus isolation: Close personal relationships with adults and with both sexes	
Middle Adult (35–60 yr)		Generativity versus stagnation: Creativity and productivity, development of lasting, fulfilling relationships	
Older Adult (>60 yr)		Ego integrity versus despair: Accepting of death, adjustment to changes in body image	

Data Collection

1. Mild anxiety is associated with day-to-day living. Person is alert, motivated, creative, productive, and aware.
2. Moderate anxiety narrows the awareness of environment. Symptoms include tension in neck and shoulders, urinary frequency, headaches, perspiration, sleep disturbances, restlessness, being overly critical of self and others, and an inability to concentrate.
3. Severe anxiety is very uncomfortable. The person is unable to focus on anything but obtaining relief. Observe for clinical symptoms of chest pain, angry outbursts, mood swings, helplessness, physical complaints, and inability to complete ADLs.
4. Panic is a feeling of terror, pain, or helplessness. Individuals experience a loss of control of increased motor activity, loss of rational thought, and an inability to function as an organized human being. Darting eyes, dilated pupils, fixed stare, hypertension, and flushed face are common symptoms.

Planning and Implementation

1. Keep client safe.
2. Establish a trusting relationship.
3. Administer medications (lorazepam [Ativan], alprazolam [Xanax]).
4. Provide calm environment.
5. Use short, simple sentences.
6. Assist client to verbalize anxiety.
7. Encourage client to identify acceptable methods of coping.

Evaluation

1. Client remains free of anxiety symptoms.
2. Client is able to verbalize source of anxiety.

Loss (Grief)

Loss is a life event experienced by everyone, regardless of age, sex, race, or economic status. Loss is defined as any change in an individual's situation. One can experience loss of others (through death, divorce, or separation); loss of objects; loss of abstractions of self (pride, self-esteem); or loss of self (amputation, suicide, death).

Data Collection

1. Stages of dying (Kubler-Ross) include:
   A. **Shock and denial:** Person cannot believe that he or she will die; seeks second opinions, ignores facts, and is unable to accept own demise.
   B. **Anger:** Person realizes the truth and is enraged at this impending death; becomes demanding, dependent, or aggressive.
   C. **Bargaining:** Person bargains with God or authority for more time.
   D. **Depression:** Person feels sad, alone, and helpless to change fate; withdraws, cries, and ponders.
   E. **Acceptance:** Person is tranquil and ready for death; has made peace with the inevitable.

2. States of grief (Engel): Loss of self (dying) is only one manifestation of loss. Loss of others, objects, or abstractions can produce a grief response. These states of grief are also seen in surviving significant others.
   • **Shock and disbelief:** Person refuses to acknowledge or believe the loss.
   • **Developing awareness:** Person experiences physical symptoms such as nausea, diarrhea, crying, and anger.
   • **Restitution:** Person accepts that the loss has occurred; total resolution may take 1–2 years to adapt to new situation.

Planning and Implementation

1. Be empathetic and kind.
2. Offer support, listening, presence.
3. Use the techniques of life review and reminiscence.
4. Attend to physical needs.
5. Include family in process.
6. Use resources that client may need (priest, spiritual counselor, lawyer, social worker, and so on).

Evaluation

1. Client resolves loss and verbalizes meaning of experience.

Anger and Aggression

Anger is a *feeling* of resentment that occurs when a person feels a threat. Hostility is an *attitude* associated with anger. Aggression is a *behavior* aimed at hurting another psychologically or physically. Anger may be positive in that anger energizes people, encourages expression, increases self-esteem, protects the self, gives one a sense of control, and alerts one to the need for coping mechanisms. Aggression and rage are most often viewed as negative.

Data Collection

1. Observe what stimulates anger in the client; determine what threatens the client (husband or wife, job loss, boss, bankruptcy, pain).
2. Aggressive acts range from attacks on objects to homicide; assess the client's level of self-control, own safety, and the safety of others.
3. Diminished capacity to think and speak may be evident.
4. Physiological responses (tight jaw, clenched fist, hypertension) should be documented.

Planning and Implementation

1. Observe and document physical and verbal symptoms.
2. Keep client and staff safe.
3. Stay calm.
4. Set limits ("I understand your anger, but you may not throw the chair at me.").
5. State expectations in a positive way.
6. Help client to explore meaning of anger.
7. Help client to explore spiritual needs.
8. Teach client to express anger in appropriate way.
9. Medicate, if necessary.

10. *Never* see potentially violent client alone.
11. *Never* block your escape route.

Evaluation

1. Feelings are expressed without violence.
2. Client discovers source of anger and identifies coping mechanisms for future.

Self-Destruction and Suicidal Behavior

Suicide is self-inflicted death. A **suicidal gesture** is a suicide attempt that is planned to be discovered. A **suicidal threat** is a nonverbal or verbal warning of an individual's plan to attempt suicide (e.g., "Will you remember me when I'm gone?"). **Suicidal thoughts** are thoughts about killing oneself. Confused, alcoholic, chronic pain, insomniac, and severely depressed persons have a suicide potential. *All* types of suicidal behaviors (both threats and gestures) should be considered serious by the nurse.

Data Collection

1. Symptoms of severe depression with suicide potential include:
   A. Sleep disorders, appetite change, weight loss
   B. Despondency (severe sadness)
   C. Helplessness, hopeless feelings
   D. Poor impulse control
   E. Feelings of rage
   F. History of suicide threats
   G. Guilt, agitation
2. Behaviors that suggest suicide potential include:
   A. Giving away personal articles
   B. Early morning awakening (3 AM to 5 AM)
   C. Sudden changes in energy (depression to gaiety)
   D. Self-preoccupation
   E. Withdrawal from communication
   F. Putting things "in order" (will, personal files)

Planning and Implementation

1. Safety is the nurse's highest priority:
   A. Remove all sharp objects, matches, and belts.
   B. Ensure that medications are swallowed (*never* leave the medications in the room, and *do* check the client's mouth after giving medications).
   C. Keep eyes *on* the client, but remain sensitive to privacy.
   D. Temperature, level of bath water, and the client's bathing should be monitored by nurse.
   E. Temperature is taken rectally or by axillary means (not orally).
   F. Client's poor impulse control (e.g., head-banging) may require seclusion or restraint.
   G. Supervise smoking.
   H. Stairwells and windows must be kept locked.
2. Communication with suicidal clients includes:
   A. Face your own feelings about suicide.
   B. Display understanding ("I understand that you feel like hurting yourself.").
   C. Tell the client that you intend to protect him or her

by making statements such as "I am here to make sure that you are safe."
   D. Encourage the client to talk, but do not probe.
   E. Ask directly if the client has a plan ("Do you have a plan to hurt yourself?").
   F. Report and document the client's suicidal statements.
   G. Report and document client's mood change (e.g., depression to gaiety).
   H. Inform charge nurse when you are going to be with a suicidal client (charge nurse is responsible for safety of staff and client).
   I. Call for help if client becomes impulsive (e.g., if client begins to head-bang, get help).

Evaluation

1. Client expresses feelings of safety and remains safe.

Withdrawal

Clients who demonstrate withdrawn behavior may be psychotic, depressed, confused, or angry. Withdrawal may be seen as seclusive or isolative. Extreme withdrawal is a break from reality (psychosis). Withdrawal may be physical, psychological, and/or social.

Data Collection

Symptoms of withdrawal include:
1. Lack of attention to personal hygiene
2. Inability to experience pleasure (anhedonia)
3. Talking to self (or imaginary persons)
4. Suspicion of others; lack of trust
5. Poor eye contact
6. Lack of interest in surroundings
7. Lack of appetite
8. Preoccupation
9. Blank expression on face (flat affect)
10. Inability to make decisions
11. Fear of others
12. Thinking about one topic constantly (rumination)
13. Unwillingness or inability to communicate
14. Indifference, aloofness
15. Lack of interest in other's feelings

Planning and Implementation

1. Demonstrate a quiet, warm, accepting presence with the client.
2. Establish rapport through shared time and supportive companionship.
3. Offer assistance with activities.
4. Intervene when necessary to ensure client's physical health and safety.
5. Be cognizant of maintaining appropriate physical distance and using touch cautiously.
6. In an acute situation, reassure client and remain with him or her in a quiet setting.

Evaluation

1. Client responds appropriately and is able to interact with people and within the environment.

Psychosis

Psychosis occurs when the client loses contact with reality. Often the thought content and form, as well as the client's affect and relationships, are severely disturbed. Psychotic clients require accurate and constant observation.

Data Collection

1. Delusions
2. Hallucinations
3. Fear of staff
4. Loose thinking
5. Suspiciousness
6. Aggressive behavior
7. Blank stare on face
8. Rigid movement
9. Regressed, childlike behavior

Planning and Implementation

1. Provide safe environment (remove sharp objects).
2. Stay with client.
3. Provide reassurance.
4. Monitor hygiene and food intake.
5. Stay calm.
6. Do not support delusions ("I know you believe that, but I do not.").
7. Do not support hallucinations ("I know you're frightened, but I see nothing.").
8. Do not argue with the client.
9. Document sleep pattern.
10. Involve client in structured activity.
11. Provide reassurance.
12. Protect other clients from intrusion.
13. Administer medications (lithium or antidepressants such as Elavil, or both).
14. Be firm but kind.
15. Assist with diagnostic studies.
16. Obtain family history of mood disorder.
17. Document client's behavior.
18. Encourage family support.

Evaluation

1. Psychotic episodes have a cyclic pattern; improvement rather than cure is the goal.
2. Client remains safe, in a stable mood.
3. Client is able to return to work.

Personality Disorders

Manipulation is a hallmark of personality disorders. Personality disorders are diagnosed when personal traits are maladaptive and cause significant functional impairments or subjective distress. Types of personality disorders include:

1. **Paranoid:** Essential feature of suspicion
2. **Schizoid:** Pervasive pattern of strange thoughts, dress, and relationship deficits
3. **Antisocial:** Impulsive, self-centered pattern of behavior that concludes in frequent conflicts with society
4. **Passive-aggressive:** Characterized by passive resistance to demands in occupational and social settings

5. **Borderline:** Marked by instability of interpersonal behavior, mood, and self-esteem. (Instability "borders" between psychosis and neurosis.)

Data Collection

Chronic, maladaptive social responses according to DSM-IV category:

1. Cluster A (paranoid, schizoid): aloofness, anger, anxiety in social situations
2. Cluster B (social, borderline, histrionic, narcissistic): suicidal tendency, irritability, poor frustration tolerance, impulsiveness, controlling behavior, dramatization, erratic behavior
3. Cluster C (disorders of anxiety or of a fearful nature): isolation, compulsive work habits, extreme criticism of others

Planning and Implementation

1. Provide consistency of care, set limits, and teach self-responsibility for control.
2. Provide physical and psychosocial accessibility.
3. Include significant others in care.
4. Teach relaxation and alternative responses to anxiety-producing situations.
5. Protect client from, and prevent, serious physical harm.
6. Focus on client's strengths.
7. Develop behavioral contracts.

Evaluation

1. Client returns to adequate social functioning, although personality disorders frequently show only marginal improvement.

Psychiatric Illness

Thought Disorders

Thought disorders are a cluster of disorders that compose a syndrome in which thought content, thought form, affect, and relationships are severely impaired. Schizophrenia is one thought disorder. Types of schizophrenia include:

1. **Disorganized type:** Regressed childlike behavior, inappropriate affect
2. **Catatonic type:** Disturbed psychomotor behavior alternating between withdrawal and excitement and accompanied by hallucinations, delusions, rigidity, and posturing
3. **Paranoid type:** Delusions, grandiosity, suspiciousness, and hallucinations

Data Collection

Includes observations of:

1. Delusions
2. Hallucinations
3. Tangential thought
4. Negativism
5. Aggressive behavior
6. Diminished thinking ability
7. Diminished self-care activities

8. Inappropriate emotional response
9. Spiritual distress

Nursing diagnosis: alteration in thought, self-care deficit

Planning and Implementation

1. Provide safe environment.
2. Administer neuroleptic (haloperidol, chlorpromazine).
3. Assist client to decrease anxiety.
4. Provide reassurance.
5. Assist client to decrease hallucinations.
6. Monitor self-care patterns.
7. Monitor spiritual concerns.
8. Encourage family support.
9. Document behavior.

Evaluation

Psychotic episodes have a pattern; improvement rather than cure is the goal.

Affective Disorders

Affective disorders are disorders of mood, thought, and affect (feelings). Affective disorders have a distinctive pattern. Types include:

1. **Bipolar disorders (manic, depressive, or mixed):** mood swings from euphoria to profound depression
2. **Major depression (dysthmic disorder):** persistent despondency and withdrawal

Data Collection

Includes observations of:
1. Inappropriate dress
2. Inexhaustible energy or lack of energy
3. Grandiosity; spending money freely
4. Arrogance
5. Lack of self-care activities
6. Self-doubt
7. Sleep disturbances
8. Weight loss
9. Spending sprees or delusions of poverty
10. Suicidal ideation

Nursing diagnosis: potential for injury, self-care deficit, alteration in thought, sleep pattern disturbance

Planning and Implementation

1. Provide safe environment.
2. Monitor self-care activities.
3. Structure time.
4. Document sleep pattern.
5. Provide reassurance.
6. Administer medications (lithium or antidepressants such as Elavil, or both).
7. Assist with diagnostic studies (magnetic resonance imaging, stress test).
8. Obtain family history of mood disorder.
9. Document client's behavior.
10. Encourage family support.
11. Provide for spiritual well-being.

Evaluation

1. Absence of mood alteration
2. Structuring time
3. Encouragement of activities
4. Short, frequent visits
5. Frequent documentation

Abuse Disorders

In our society, use of certain substances without a prescription to modify mood or behavior is generally regarded as abuse. Commonly abused substances include coffee, tea, and nicotine. A pathological dependence on or aversion to food is called an eating disorder. Dependence on psychoactive substances (alcohol, marijuana, phencyclidine piperidine [PCP], lysergic acid diethylamide [LSD], cocaine) is considered a mental disorder called psychoactive substance abuse.

Characteristics of Psychoactive Substance Abuser

1. Client recognizes that substance use is excessive.
2. A great deal of time is spent to produce substance.
3. Client suffers withdrawal symptoms when substance is not used.
4. Despite psychological, social, and physical problems, client continues to abuse substance.
5. Significant tolerance occurs.

Data Collection

1. Dilated or contracted pupils depending on drug involved
2. Slurred speech
3. Convulsions
4. Restlessness, tremors
5. Occupational difficulties
6. Odor of alcohol
7. Inappropriate behavior
8. Little tolerance for frustration
9. Marital problems
10. Tendency to develop infections
11. History of blackouts
12. Poor attention span

Planning and Implementation

1. Provide emergency management for acute substance abuse.
2. Assess vital signs, output, and mental alertness.
3. Administer emergency drugs.
4. Assist in diagnostic studies.
5. Place in quiet environment.
6. Provide safe environment.
7. Assess pattern of substance abuse.
8. Teach new coping behavior.
9. Provide for spiritual well-being.

Evaluation

1. Client experiences withdrawal without physical complications.
2. Client seeks rehabilitation.

Eating Disorders

Eating disorders, characterized by a gross disturbance in eating behaviors, include anorexia nervosa and bulimia. Eating disorders can be thought of as a fear of obesity or an addiction to or drive toward thinness.

Data Collection

In anorexia, clients are 15% below normal weight in absence of organic disease.
1. Bradycardia
2. Electrolyte imbalance
3. Malnourished appearance

In bulimia, clients are usually of normal weight but purge (vomit) after overeating; however, both anorexics and bulimics:
1. Restrict food
2. Exercise vigorously
3. May have gastric ruptures or esophageal tears
4. May have black teeth (from stomach acid)
5. May use laxatives excessively

Planning and Implementation

1. Assess during meals.
2. Lock bathroom to prevent purging (for bulimia).
3. Remove wastebaskets.
4. Assess closely to prevent overvigorous exercising.
5. Teach about nutrition.
6. Administer antianxiety medication before meals as prescribed.
7. Weigh three times weekly.
8. Assess for suicidal gestures.
9. Assess for spiritual well-being.
10. Refer client to formal eating disorder program.
11. Assess hoarding of food and use of laxatives.
12. Assess elimination practices.
13. Involve family in therapy.

Evaluation

1. Client maintains goal of a certain weight.
2. Purging (frequent self-induced vomiting) and bingeing (eating huge quantities of food in small amount of time) are absent.

Confusion

Organic mental syndrome refers to a group of psychological or behavioral signs and symptoms without reference to etiology, such as organic anxiety syndrome and dementia organic brain syndrome. **Organic mental disorder** designates a particular mental syndrome in which the cause is known (e.g., Parkinson's disease, Huntington's chorea, multi-infarct dementia). Causes of organic mental disorders include:
1. Central nervous system infection
2. Head trauma
3. Intracranial lesions
4. Hepatic disease
5. Subarachnoid hemorrhage
6. Cerebral hypoxia
7. Thyroid, parathyroid, or adrenal dysfunction
8. Genetic (e.g., Down's syndrome predisposes client to Alzheimer's disease)

Data Collection

1. Weakness of limbs
2. Unstable shuffling gait
3. Tremors, slow speech
4. Seizures
5. Personality changes
6. Anxiety
7. Persistent hallucinations
8. Impaired memory; making up stories to fill in memory gaps
9. Rage reactions
10. Impaired social judgment, apathy
11. Tangential, circumstantial speech
12. Inability for self-care
13. Frequent falls, mobility impairment
14. Mental confusion
15. Repetitive movements

Planning and Implementation

1. Remove dangerous objects.
2. Pad siderails.
3. Administer neuroleptics as prescribed for agitation.
4. Reorient client frequently; provide external signs of orientation (calendars, clocks).
5. Attend to ADLs.
6. Prevent complications.
7. Provide calm, well-lighted, simple environment.
8. Limit number of people caring for client.

Evaluation

1. Client remains safe (impairment may be reversible or chronic).

Disorders of Youth (Children and Adolescents)

Although children and adolescents may suffer from thought disorders (schizophrenia), affective disorders (depression), and other psychiatric disorders commonly diagnosed in adults, some illnesses are specifically characteristic of these groups. These include mental retardation, learning and motor skill disorders, disruptive behavior and attention deficit disorders, feeding and eating disorders, and separation-anxiety disorders.

Mental Retardation

Characteristics

1. Measured IQ level 70 or below
2. Failure of developmental functioning
3. Types: mild (IQ 55–70), moderate (IQ 40–55), severe (IQ 20–40), and profound (IQ <20)
4. Social, sensimotor, or communication skills limited

Data Collection

1. Motor development
2. Self-care abilities

3. Communication abilities
4. Family resources
5. Family genogram
6. Physiological function
7. Spiritual development

Planning and Implementation

1. Maintain a consistent, caring approach.
2. Strive to develop potential of client.
3. Use community resources.
4. Meet client at own level.
5. Assess self-care needs.
6. Provide for spiritual well-being.
7. Develop and enhance strengths.

Evaluation

1. Client performs self-care activities.
2. Client engages in a living pattern reflective of his or her potential.
3. Community resources are used.

Coping Mechanisms and Defense Mechanisms

To deal with anxiety, loss, and anger, each individual uses a set of behaviors learned at an early stage of development to relieve tension. Coping mechanisms are action-oriented activities to increase one's ability to cope; defense mechanisms are unconscious reactions to protect oneself from feeling inadequate.

Coping Mechanisms

1. Seek out another person to gain comfort.
2. Use food to relax.
3. Express feelings (cry, scream, and so on).
4. Withdraw (become "couch potato").
5. "Talk it out."
6. "Think it out."
7. "Work it off" (walk, run, scrub floors).
8. Use symbolic comfort (religion).
9. Compromise (negotiate verbally).

Defense Mechanisms

1. Suppression
   - Suppression is voluntary and involuntary exclusion from conscious level of ideas and feelings.
   - For example, a student who receives a poor report card forgets to show it to his or her parents.
2. Sublimation
   - Sublimation is replacement of an unacceptable need, attitude, or emotion with one that is more acceptable.
   - For example, a woman who feels unattractive puts her energy into competitive sport.
3. Rationalization
   - Rationalization is an attempt to make unacceptable feelings and behaviors acceptable.

   - For example, a student fails an exam and complains that the lectures were disorganized.
4. Identification
   - An attempt to change oneself to resemble an admired person is called identification.
   - For example, a 6-year-old dresses like her mother.
5. Introjection
   - Intense identification in which one incorporates values of another into self is known as introjection.
   - For example, a child scolds her doll for spilling milk.
6. Displacement
   - Rejection of an emotional feeling from one idea, person, or objective to another is displacement.
   - For example, a frustrated nurse goes home and screams at the cat.
7. Projection
   - Projection is attributing one's own thoughts or impulses to another.
   - For example, a female physician denies her sexual feelings about a male nurse and accuses him of flirting with her.
8. Regression
   - Regression is retreating to an earlier stage of development.
   - For example, a 6-year-old girl begins wetting her pants when her new baby brother comes into the family.
9. Repression
   - Repression is the involuntary exclusion of a painful thought, impulse, or memory.
   - For example, after the loss of his spouse, a man cannot remember his marriage date.
10. Reaction formation
    - Development of conscious attitudes and behaviors opposite to those one really feels is called reaction formation.
    - For example, a male professor attracted to a female student treats her harshly.
11. Intellectualization
    - Intellectualization is excessive reasoning to avoid feeling.
    - For example, a battered wife talks about how her husband beats her and says that she should leave for her safety, but remains with her husband.
12. Conversion
    - Conversion is the expression of intrapsychic conflict through physical symptoms.
    - For example, an unprepared student develops abdominal pain before a test.
13. Compensation
    - The process by which a person makes up for his or her perceived deficiency is compensation.
    - For example, a 5-foot-tall male neurosurgeon becomes aggressive, forceful, and controlling at work.
14. Denial
    - Denial is disowning consciously intolerable thoughts and impulses.
    - For example, a terminal cancer client tells her husband that the results of the biopsy were negative.

1. A 21-year-old secretary with a history of anxiety reactions is admitted to the emergency room. The nurse should know that the most common symptoms of an anxiety reaction are:

   A. Hypotension, pain
   B. Lethargy, flat affect
   C. Confusion, hunger
   D. Increased pulse, tightness in the chest

2. An initial care plan for a client with a diagnosis of anxiety would include which of the following interventions?

   A. Monitoring vital signs, offering reassurance
   B. Monitoring I&O, obtaining weight
   C. Observation of nailbed color
   D. History of drug use, offering high-carbohydrate food

3. To help a client modify an anxiety reaction, the nurse should speak slowly and softly, asking the client if there is anything in his or her life that is upsetting. The client responds, "Nothing is wrong; everything is perfect." This may be an example of:

   A. Introjection
   B. Sublimation
   C. Denial
   D. Displacement

4. Which of the following pharmacological agents is prescribed to reduce anxiety?

   A. Imipramine (Tofranil)
   B. Lorazepam (Ativan)
   C. Lithium (Lithane)
   D. Amitriptyline (Elavil)

5. After administering an anxiolytic to an emergency room client, the nurse checks to see if the siderails are secure. The nurse realizes that one of the common side effects of anxiolytics is:

   A. Drowsiness
   B. Convulsions
   C. Blurred vision
   D. Fear of falling

6. A client is given a prescription for lorazepam. It is the nurse's responsibility to inform the client that anyone taking lorazepam should not:

   A. Work
   B. Consume herring
   C. Consume alcohol
   D. Spend prolonged time in the sun

7. After a client suffering from an anxiety reaction was safely discharged from the emergency room, the nurse documented that the client experienced a rapid pulse, tightness of the chest, discomfort, and an inability to focus on anything but obtaining relief. The nursing diagnosis may conclude:

   A. Panic-level anxiety
   B. Mild anxiety
   C. Moderate anxiety
   D. Severe anxiety

8. A 59-year-old man is admitted to a medical unit with symptoms of lethargy and withdrawal. He was forced into early retirement because of his company's merger with a larger sister company. On admission, the nurse observes that the client will not make eye contact with any member of the staff. Poor eye contact is an example of:

   A. Verbal communication
   B. Therapeutic communication
   C. Nonverbal communication
   D. Mass communication

9. A nurse observes that a client has poor eye contact, complains of nausea and diarrhea, and is crying about the death of his wife. The nurse realizes that this cluster of symptoms is common in:

   A. Anxiety disorders
   B. Grief reactions
   C. Panic attacks
   D. Eating disorders

10. In planning initial care for a newly admitted client, the nurse realizes that one establishes a therapeutic relationship by:

    A. Assessing the client, remaining subjective
    B. Judging the client, offering advice
    C. Respecting the client, offering presence
    D. Confronting the client, displaying sympathy

11. A client informs the nurse that his wife died 2 days ago. The nurse replies, "Tell me more about that." This is an example of the therapeutic communication technique of:

    A. Restating
    B. Providing feedback
    C. Identifying themes
    D. Open-ended statement

12. During a conversation between a client and the nurse, the physician enters the room accompanied by seven medical students. The nurse and the client end their discussion because:

    A. Physicians are important in status
    B. The physician's entry changed the context and psychosocial setting
    C. The content of the communication between the nurse and the client should remain private
    D. The type, quality, and purpose of nurses' and physicians' communication are totally different

13. A student nurse says to a client who has been grieving over the death of a spouse, "I think you should get on with life and stop mourning over the death." This is an example of communication called:

A. Omission of content
B. Offering personal opinion
C. Rejection
D. Faulty reassurance

14. In assessing a 61-year-old client, the nurse should know that the developmental stage is:

A. Industry versus inferiority
B. Intimacy versus isolation
C. Ego integrity versus despair
D. Generativity versus stagnation

15. A 60-year-old client becomes very upset after his sister visits. He throws a tray at the wall. The nurse's most effective response would be:

A. Maintain a calm and supportive manner.
B. Administer neuroleptic drugs.
C. Encourage the client to call his sister.
D. Report the incident to the hospital administrator.

16. A 75-year-old client tells the nurse that he wishes to see a priest because "it will help." The nurse realizes that this would be an example of:

A. A coping mechanism
B. A defense mechanism
C. Reaction formation
D. Intellectualization

17. A 39-year-old client has a diagnosis of depression. The physician prescribes ECT. The nurse must know that ECT:

A. Requires preoperative nursing care
B. Causes excessive weight gain
C. Is administered in conjunction with neuroleptics
D. Will result in mood suppression

18. A 14-year-old girl who displays symptoms of anorexia nervosa was brought to the clinic for an evaluation. She has a 15-year-old sister and lives with her parents, who are physicians. The client achieves well in school and is very active in sports activities. During the initial interview with the nurse, the client states that she is "just normal." Which of the following would suggest to the nurse that the client displays symptoms of anorexia nervosa?

A. She expresses a desire to gain weight.
B. She has episodes of overeating.
C. She has had severe weight loss due to dieting.
D. She uses large amounts of food to relax.

19. The nurse would know that the development stage of a 14-year-old adolescent is:

A. Trust versus mistrust
B. Autonomy versus shame and doubt
C. Initiative versus guilt
D. Identity versus role diffusion

20. The nurse should know that it is important to assess for which one of the following characteristics of anorexia nervosa?

A. Vigorous exercise
B. Increased libido

C. Average intelligence
D. Tachycardia

21. A 21-year-old client denies that she ever feels anxious, but the nurse observes her biting her fingernails. One component of nursing care for the client would be for the nurse to:

A. Administer neuroleptic medication
B. Assess the client's coping mechanisms
C. Encourage vigorous exercise
D. Make arrangements for sculptured nails

22. A client tells the nurse that when she gets upset, she kicks the cat. This is an example of which one of the following defense mechanisms?

A. Rationalization
B. Projection
C. Displacement
D. Regression

23. While interacting with a client with a diagnosis of anorexia nervosa, the client changes the conversation from talking about self to talking about the weather. The nurse must use which of the following communication techniques?

A. Refocusing
B. Restating
C. Silence
D. Summarizing

24. A 15-year-old female client with a diagnosis of anorexia is scheduled for an electrocardiogram (ECG). The nurse will:

A. Teach the client about the procedure
B. Tell the client that she has a heart problem
C. Explain that persons with anorexia nervosa suffer from tachycardia
D. Ask a male aide to accompany the client

25. An 18-year-old male client has serious problems with substance abuse. He has had difficulty with his school work and with school authority figures. He has come to the clinic for help. The nurse observes that the client is restless and pacing. Other physical characteristics of substance abusers that the nurse should pay special attention to include:

A. Dilated pupils
B. Increased concentration
C. Euphoria
D. Pale nailbeds

26. A 22-year-old admitted to the emergency room stated that 1 month previously he had been brought to the emergency room for an overdose of cocaine. What nursing actions in the emergency room would be most important in treating a client who has overdosed?

A. Monitoring vital signs and output
B. Obtaining weight and temperature
C. Inducing client to vomit
D. Obtaining a psychiatric evaluation

27. A client is admitted to an inpatient detoxification unit. During the acute phase of detoxification from drug abuse, which of the following would be the most important nursing action?

    A. Monitoring manipulative behavior
    B. Monitoring family dynamics
    C. Evaluating vocational abilities
    D. Monitoring vital signs frequently

28. A client in a substance abuse program tells the nurse during the first week of treatment that he has no drug problem. The nurse identifies this behavior as an example of the defense mechanism:

    A. Denial
    B. Projection
    C. Displacement
    D. Sublimation

29. When a client explains to the nurse that he does not have a drug abuse problem, the nurse replies, "What do you mean when you say you have no drug problem?" This communication technique is an example of:

    A. Focusing
    B. Clarifying
    C. Providing feedback
    D. Making an observation

30. Which of the following behaviors would the nurse expect to observe from a client who has successfully completed a substance abuse treatment program?

    A. Identifying positive ways to cope with anxiety
    B. Identifying ways to decrease but not discontinue drug use
    C. Identifying the family members responsible for the drug abuse
    D. Identifying methods of social isolation

31. A 48-year-old man is admitted to a surgical unit with the diagnosis of chronic cholecystitis. The client's chart reveals that he is scheduled for surgery the following morning and that he has lived in a sheltered residence home for 10 years and suffers from schizophrenia. As a nurse reads the chart, he or she should know that schizophrenia is:

    A. A thought disorder
    B. An affective disorder
    C. A personality disorder
    D. An adjustment disorder

32. With the diagnosis of schizophrenia, the nurse may anticipate which of the following cluster of symptoms?

    A. Stuttering, cluttering, passive behavior
    B. Delusions, tangential thought, hallucinations
    C. Hyperactivity, crying, violence
    D. Inexhaustible energy, absence of mood, altered sleep pattern

33. Clients who suffer from schizophrenia are most likely to be given a prescription for which of the following?

    A. Anxiolytic medications
    B. Antidepressant medications
    C. Antipsychotic medications
    D. Antiseizure medications

34. The nurse who cares for clients taking antipsychotic medication knows that:

    A. The nurse must monitor temperature closely
    B. The nurse must monitor vital signs
    C. The nurse must monitor diet closely
    D. The nurse must monitor blood levels

35. A hospitalized client recovering from surgery tells the nurse that "men from Mars are fixing get-well food to be put in my veins." The nurse knows that this is an example of:

    A. A delusion
    B. A hallucination
    C. Anxiety
    D. Tangential thought

36. As a 25-year-old male client suffering from schizophrenia recovers from surgery, he becomes more disorganized in his thinking and his behavior becomes more inappropriate. The nurse's best nursing action is to:

    A. Tell the client he is psychotic
    B. Alter medications as needed
    C. Tolerate the client's behavior
    D. Document the client's behavior

37. A 40-year-old woman is admitted to the emergency room. Her husband states that she has not slept in 48 hours, is irritable and uncooperative, and has made comments about ending her life. When the nurse attempts to take the client's vital signs, she strikes the nurse's hand. The thermometer breaks and the client bursts into tears. The nurse's first response is to:

    A. Comfort the client and hold her hand
    B. Tell the client to act appropriately
    C. Call for assistance
    D. Obtain vital signs

38. A client is given a diagnosis of bipolar disorder. Bipolar disorder is:

    A. A disorder of mood, affect, and thought
    B. A disorder of personality and self-care
    C. A disorder of interpersonal deficits
    D. A disorder of intelligence and ideation

39. Clients with the medical diagnosis of bipolar disorder are often placed on lithium. Before administering this medication, the nurse is aware of:

    A. The diet of the client
    B. The sleep pattern of the client
    C. The lithium blood level of the client
    D. The activity level of the client

40. A client who has been taking lithium for a number of months and has a lithium blood level mEq/l >1.2 may experience lithium toxicity. Lithium toxicity is characterized by:

    A. Painful eyes, nausea, vomiting
    B. Diarrhea, nausea, vomiting, tremors

C. Hypertension, swollen joints, fever

D. Hypotension, thirst, nausea, vomiting

41. A 90-year-old man who resides in a nursing home has been given a diagnosis of Alzheimer's disease. The nurse caring for this client would anticipate which of the following behaviors?

A. Overeating, overspending

B. Mood stability

C. Self-care deficits, impaired memory

D. Limb pain

42. In caring for clients with Alzheimer's disease, the nurse should:

A. Provide external signs of orientation

B. Provide increased environmental stimulation

C. Encourage frequent change

D. Encourage group therapy

43. A 75-year-old male client diagnosed with Alzheimer's disease becomes very agitated at night and begins tearing off the bed sheets. He tells the nurse that his suitcase is in the bed and he must catch a train to the office. The nurse's most appropriate response is to:

A. Restrain the client

B. Reorient and reassure the client

C. Provide a well-lighted environment

D. Observe the client

44. The nurse knows that a person in his 90th year is in the developmental stage of:

A. Trust versus mistrust

B. Ego integrity versus despair

C. Identity versus identity diffusion

D. Generativity versus stagnation

45. In caring for clients with Alzheimer's disease, the nurse's priority is:

A. Physiological care

B. Psychological care

C. Safety

D. Spiritual care

46. A 7-year-old girl is admitted to the pediatric unit. She is severely mentally retarded and is admitted for cellulitis. When admitting a retarded child, the nurse first assesses for:

A. Communication ability

B. Reading ability

C. Hobbies

D. Moral development

47. In caring for mentally retarded children, the nurse must:

A. Be aware of his or her own feelings

B. Minimize family contact

C. Interview the child extensively

D. Teach the child to cope with anxiety

48. The mother of a 10-year-old girl reports to the clinic nurse that her daughter has been acting "jumpy" lately. If the client is experiencing anxiety, the most important symptom that the nurse would likely observe is:

A. Withdrawal

B. Lethargy

C. Hunger

D. An increased heart rate

49. A 32-year-old client is receiving treatment for obsessive-compulsive disorder (OCD). Obsessive-compulsive behaviors manifest themselves as:

A. Reality orientation

B. Rigid perfectionism

C. A wide range of emotions

D. Ritualistic thoughts

50. A hospitalized client misses breakfast in the cafeteria three times in one week because of his ritualistic handwashing. His handwashing ritual may go on for 30 minutes. Which of the following nursing actions would be most appropriate for the client with an OCD?

A. Document the behavior, and work with the treatment team to design a treatment program to extinguish the behavior.

B. Tell the client to stop washing his hands and design a care plan to decrease anxiety.

C. Ask the client why he feels he must wash his hands and ask the physician for an order for an antianxiety agent.

D. Plan to bring a breakfast to the client's room and schedule three periods a day for handwashing activity.

51. A 14-year-old girl has been hospitalized by the court for psychiatric evaluation after running away from home repeatedly. The nurse finds the client in her room during school hours and asks why she is not in class. The client responds by stating that another nurse said she could miss class if she did not feel like going. The nurse knows the client's response is an example of:

A. Avoidance behavior

B. Manipulation

C. Rebellion

D. Projection

52. A 16-year-old girl who is hospitalized for running away from home refuses to attend class, stating that yesterday the other nurse told her she did not have to go to class if she did not want to. The nurse's best response would be:

A. "I know that you are lying."

B. "Missing class is against the rules."

C. "Why do you fight the system?"

D. "Fine, but you're confined to your room."

53. Acting-out behavior is exemplified by which one of the following?

A. Discussing sexual feelings

B. Attempting suicide

C. Attending treatment activities

D. Contracting for safety

54. Two 15-year-old boys are being treated on the psychiatric unit. During a card game in the recreation room, they begin fist-fighting. Nursing interventions for this incident would include:

A. Remove the boys to separate areas and set limits.

B. Obtain an order for seclusion.

C. Share observations with the boys.
D. Restrain each boy as punishment for fighting.

55. A 17-year-old male client is readmitted to the hospital for leukemia. He is angry and refuses to talk with staff. The nurse should know that:

A. Adolescents may find it difficult to talk about death
B. Adolescents see death as temporary
C. Adolescents feel that death is a punishment
D. Adolescents are looking forward to the future

56. A client is being discharged from the hospital after a below-the-knee amputation. Which statement by the client would indicate that the client is getting in touch with the loss?

A. "What is the use of going home with one leg?"
B. "Why me, God? If only I had changed my ways!"
C. "Are there support groups that help people like me?"
D. "Please leave me alone until my friend comes to take me home."

57. A 13-year-old client's history reveals that his cultural orientation discourages him from verbalizing his spiritual issues. Which one of the following is the best nursing intervention?

A. Reassure the client that it is all right to verbalize spiritual issues.
B. Question the client about his religious orientation needs.
C. Refer the client to a nondenominational group.
D. Discuss immortality with the client.

58. Which of the following concepts should the nurse be aware of when interacting with survivors of victims of sudden death?

A. Survivors have time to engage in anticipatory grief.
B. Survivors may feel guilty for not engaging in special activities with the deceased.
C. Survivors feel immediate detachment.
D. Survivors may experience an uncomplicated grief response.

59. During an interview, an 83-year-old male client confides in the nurse that his spiritual needs are not being met. Which one of the following is most important for the nurse to explore?

A. Source of strength and hope
B. Purpose and meaning in living
C. Spiritual orientation
D. Religious affiliation

60. A 55-year-old male client who has been a heavy drinker for 20 years presents at the emergency room in a state of agitation, delirium, and diaphoresis. It is reported that the client has not consumed any alcohol during the past 72 hours. The nurse should know that the client is suffering from:

A. Delirium tremens
B. Korsakoff's syndrome
C. Alcoholic hepatitis
D. Alcoholic hallucinosis

61. A 16-year-old boy was brought to the emergency room by his parents because he was abusing cocaine and out of control. The nurse should know that one of the signs of cocaine intoxication is:

A. Dry, cool skin
B. Hypotension
C. Bradycardia
D. Psychomotor agitation

62. Which one of the following drugs is used to inhibit impulsive abuse of alcohol?

A. Chlordiazepoxide (Librium)
B. Disulfiram (Antabuse)
C. Diazepam (Valium)
D. Lithium

63. Which one of the following is a contributing factor in the development of codependency?

A. Effective family dynamics
B. Difficulty in negotiating boundaries
C. Balanced internal ego states
D. Positive aspects of self

64. What is the nurse's greatest responsibility when intervening with an alcoholic family?

A. Instill hope in the family's future.
B. Maintain homeostatic balance.
C. Encourage cross-generational clinging.
D. Promote the use of defense mechanisms.

65. A woman is admitted to a psychiatric unit for evaluation after displaying recurring bizarre behavior. The nurse explains to the client's family that:

A. The mentally ill person has often learned inappropriate behaviors that must be unlearned or replaced with acceptable behaviors
B. Treatment is aimed at complete recovery, which can occur at any time during the therapy
C. Part of the mental illness is insensitivity of the person to how others react to him or her
D. Evaluation is based on known criteria from which the mentally ill rarely deviate

66. The family of a newly admitted client is concerned about the client's rights should commitment be necessary. It is important to remember that:

A. Initially commitment implies custodial care and therefore a client's rights are not compromised
B. A client has the right to therapeutic treatment, informed consent, and to refuse treatment
C. Although a client retains all right to participate in his treatment, the facility cannot be held liable if treatment is not provided
D. Treatment will not be initiated until the client and the legal guardian consent

67. A mother received a call from her daughter's teacher. The 7-year-old child seems withdrawn, does not interact with other children, and does not participate in class. The concern of the mother and the teacher is based on the fact that:

A. Children progress through the stages of development at a similar rate and react to school with predictable behaviors
B. This developmental period is psychologically stormy and changes in behaviors are considered significant
C. Seven-year-old children rely on peer approval rather than positive reinforcement from parents
D. This is usually a period during which the child makes great social and intellectual strides

68. An individual's personality and perception of self are key factors in determining behavior. The nurse recognizes that:
A. Events occurring throughout life affect emotional adjustment
B. It is not necessary to complete one developmental stage before the individual can progress to the next stage
C. Withdrawn behavior illustrates a person's inability to move from one developmental stage to the next
D. The most psychologically significant stage of development is birth to 12 months

69. A 70-year-old severely dehydrated woman was admitted to a medical unit. Her husband died a month ago and she lives alone. Her only child lives 200 miles away with his wife and son. The nurse notes that the client always gazes downward and does not respond to questions. This behavior is an example of:
A. Conversion reaction
B. Suppression
C. Depression
D. Reaction formation

70. The developmental stage for a 70-year-old client is:
A. Industry versus inferiority
B. Intimacy versus isolation
C. Integrity versus despair
D. Generativity versus stagnation

71. In trying to reassure a recently widowed client, the nurse says, "Don't worry, everything is going to be fine." According to the principles of therapeutic communication, this statement communicates:
A. Empathy and understanding
B. Clarification of a client's feelings
C. Devaluation of a client's own perception
D. Caring and concern

72. During his monthly therapy session, a 48-year-old father of an adolescent son tells you that his son is "impossible" and cannot make decisions. On the basis of your knowledge of adolescent behavior, you know that:
A. All adolescents are difficult to control and cannot make sound decisions
B. A hallmark of adolescence is ambivalence related to dependence and independence
C. Adolescents want to be dependent and rely on others to make decisions
D. At this developmental stage, the adolescent is primarily seeking parental approval

73. Sex education during adolescence is important because:
A. Adolescents are unaware of the physical and emotional changes that are occurring
B. The love object of an adolescent is primarily the parent of the same sex
C. Adolescents are more concerned about self than others, and this is the focus of their attention
D. As bodily changes occur, the adolescent has to feel comfortable discussing these changes

74. In response to failing courses in school, an adolescent boy says, "Well, if I were all brains and nothing else, I would make As in all of my courses." This is an example of which defense mechanism?
A. Repression
B. Compensation
C. Denial of reality
D. Rationalization

75. At the conclusion of a therapy session, a client says to the therapist, "I'm really grateful for your time; you're a great listener. You know, you remind me of my wife." An appropriate response by the therapist would be:
A. "She must be a great listener too."
B. "That's because she and I are both concerned about you and your son."
C. "What about me reminds you of your wife?"
D. "Do you want to talk about this some time?"

76. The major clinical use of antipsychotics (or neuroleptics) is in the treatment of psychoses. When used in the treatment of schizophrenia, neuroleptics:
A. Eliminate the need for psychotherapy by effectively curing social withdrawal and apathy
B. Provide symptomatic control by blocking the activity of dopamine
C. Heighten the sex drive and require weekly titers to assess peak and trough
D. Alter the client's response to reality and decrease paranoia

77. The nurse's plan of care for the client taking neuroleptics must include observing for side effects, which include:
A. Nausea, vomiting, diarrhea, weight loss
B. Heartburn, hypoglycemia, edema
C. Nasal congestion, seizures, urinary retention
D. Insomnia, drooling, agranulocytopenia

78. A 3- to 4-month-old infant who is allowed to cry for hours or who is neglected:
A. Will instinctively continue to cry until his or her needs are met and he or she no longer feels neglected
B. Begins to mistrust people and surroundings even though the infant is too young to distinguish himself or herself from others
C. Will withdraw from the world of reality to the world of fantasy, which feels less threatening
D. Will develop alternate ways to feel good about himself or herself and about the world

79. A nurse is teaching parenting classes. When teaching growth and development the nurse states, "The gradual realization in a child that neither the child nor his or her parent is omnipotent leads to . . .

    A. sadness and withdrawal."
    B. anger and displacement."
    C. mastery of more skills."
    D. developmental regression."

80. When the nurse is teaching the growth and development of a 2-year-old child, the nurse identifies that the child:

    A. Begins to develop a sense of autonomy
    B. Becomes dependent and less self-reliant
    C. Generally cannot master new challenges
    D. Cannot socialize and demonstrates fear of the environment

81. When teaching the growth and development of 3- to 5-year-old children, the nurse identifies:

    A. Little or no need for discipline
    B. Lack of concern for parental approval
    C. Increasing motor and intellectual skills
    D. Lack of social skills

82. A client who was raped 10 years ago is now unable to have a satisfying sexual relationship with her husband. The nurse identifies that the client may be exhibiting which defense mechanism?

    A. Reaction formation
    B. Displacement
    C. Repression
    D. Suppression

83. A man who was paralyzed from his waist down after an accident is asked what effect his paralysis will have on his previously active life. His response is, "no effect." The nurse identifies this as an example of:

    A. Denial of reality
    B. Compensation
    C. Fantasy
    D. Introjection

84. A 3- or 4-year-old child who has been toilet trained begins to have incontinent episodes and "talk baby talk" when her newborn sister is brought home from the hospital. This behavior demonstrates which defense mechanism?

    A. Displacement
    B. Regression
    C. Sublimation
    D. Reaction formation

85. A client experiences free-floating anxiety that has worsened since his recent divorce. He is taking a nonbarbiturate benzodiazepine agent. The nurse recognizes that this classification of drug:

    A. Is recommended because of its low potential for abuse, toxicity, and lethal overdose
    B. Works selectively on the limbic system of the brain, which is responsible for emotions such as rage and anxiety

    C. Has a tranquilizing effect without numbing emotions and produces reversible amnesia in the treatment of post-traumatic stress disorder (PTSD)
    D. Acts primarily by enhancing normal coping mechanisms, is well tolerated, and is nonaddictive

86. Antidepressants are used in the treatment of depressive disorders caused by emotional, physical, chemical, and/or environmental stressors. Regarding the classifications of antidepressants, the nurse knows that:

    A. Tricyclic antidepressants decrease the level of neurotransmitters in cases in which an increase in neurotransmitters causes depression
    B. MAOIs are effective when administered over a short period; they are less toxic than other classifications
    C. Tricyclic antidepressants are contraindicated in the treatment of depression associated with physiological symptoms such as insomnia, fatigue, and irritability
    D. Hypertensive crisis may result if MAOIs are taken with tyramine-rich foods, such as aged cheese, avocados, and chicken livers

87. Personality disorders are maladaptive patterns of seeing, relating to, and thinking about one's environment. Nursing care for clients with personality disorders should include:

    A. Reinforcing limits to counteract manipulative behavior
    B. Allowing hostile exchanges that foster open expression
    C. Assisting the client to focus by limiting diversional activities
    D. Helping the client to build self-esteem by ignoring inappropriate behaviors

88. During a therapeutic session, the client tells the nurse, "You're just like my mother, and you're never going to change. First you tell me to talk about how I feel, then when I talk, you cut me off and don't let me finish a sentence." This is an example of:

    A. Conversion reaction
    B. Blatant hostility
    C. Displacement
    D. Transference

89. A 40-year-old client with chronic schizophrenia and a history of multiple hospitalizations is readmitted for noncompliance with medication therapy. The most common reason for noncompliance with antipsychotic medications is:

    A. Neuroleptics tend to produce unpleasant side effects and adverse reactions.
    B. The medications are too expensive to purchase.
    C. The client improves and believes that he no longer requires medication.
    D. Neuroleptics are designed for short-term use only.

90. The nurse on the unit presents the client's medication in a pill cup already opened. The client refuses to take the medication, stating, "I don't know what that is." A nursing intervention to educate the client and promote compliance would be to:

    A. Tell the client what the medication is and encourage him or her to take it.

B. Obtain an unopened labeled dose and show the client the medication.

C. Reassure the client that it is the right medication and that it is important that it be taken.

D. Tell the client if he or she refuses to take the medication orally, it will be administered intramuscularly.

91. During dinner a client refuses to eat, stating, "You are serving me dog flesh." The best response for the nurse would be:

A. "Don't be silly, we don't eat dog meat here."
B. "What makes you think this is dog flesh?"
C. "Don't worry, I'll get you something else."
D. "If you don't want to eat, it's up to you."

92. For the client with a history of noncompliance with medication therapy, the physician has decided to prescribe decanoate neuroleptics. Client and family teaching for this medication should include the following:

A. These neuroleptic medications have few side effects.
B. A special diet is required while on this medication.
C. Blood levels to assess effectiveness must be drawn monthly.
D. The medication is given IM every 2–4 weeks.

93. A 23-year-old female client has been admitted to the inpatient psychiatric unit with a diagnosis of catatonic schizophrenia. She appears weak and pale. The nurse would expect to observe which behaviors in this client?

A. Scratching and catlike motions of the extremities
B. Exaggerated suspiciousness and excessive food intake
C. Stuporous withdrawal, hallucinations, and delusions
D. Sexual preoccupation and word salad

94. A 28-year-old male client with a history of antisocial personality disorder is admitted to the psychiatric unit because of a suicide attempt while in jail awaiting trial for assault. The client acts very disinterested in treatment and has developed a rapport with several clients whom he is influencing in negative ways. In evaluating his progress, the nurse recognizes that he:

A. Could make behavioral changes within a short time if motivated
B. May not be motivated to change his behavior or lifestyle
C. Manipulates others but does not manipulate family members
D. Usually requires intensive psychotropic drug therapy, which he refuses

95. A 15-year-old girl is admitted with a diagnosis of anorexia. She is an honor student and participates in school activities. She is 40% below expected weight, states that she is fat, and demonstrates uncooperative behavior during the admission process. In anorexia, the client has a distorted view of:

A. Self-esteem and self-worth
B. Ability to control

C. Self-image and intellect
D. Need to mature

96. A 7-year-old boy is admitted for evaluation. His history reveals multiple reports by teachers that he is unable to sit still in class, is aggressive with the other children, and cannot concentrate on a task more than 5 minutes. An appropriate nursing intervention for the first few days includes:

A. Set clear, concise behavior expectations with consistent limits.
B. Put him in time-out if he does not follow the rules.
C. Observe his behavior and assess for patterns.
D. Ask him why he is acting as he is.

97. A physician prescribes lithium for a client who was recently admitted to a unit. The nurse knows the following to be true of this medication:

A. Onset of therapeutic effect is 7–14 days; side effects include fine tremors and blurred vision.
B. Nausea and vomiting are common side effects that are treated symptomatically with daily low doses of antiemetics.
C. Therapeutic effect is minimal, and noncompliance is difficult to detect; blood levels are therefore drawn weekly.
D. IM administration results in immediate relief of symptoms, and effects usually last 27–48 hours.

98. Three weeks after beginning lithium therapy, a client appears lethargic and ataxic and has a decreased level of consciousness. These symptoms indicate:

A. A decrease in therapeutic levels
B. Toxic ranges of lithium
C. Maximum therapeutic effectiveness of lithium
D. Expected side effects of lithium

99. In the case of suspected lithium toxicity, the best intervention for the nurse is to:

A. Assess the most current laboratory values and force fluids
B. Hold the next dose and draw a serum level
C. Notify the physican and wait for instructions
D. Give the medication and assess for further side effects

100. In the United States, older adults are more frequently the recipients of health care than are other age groups because:

A. They are prone to chronic illness and depression and require long-term therapy
B. Single-adult households are more common among older people and this often means that family resources are less available
C. They are lonely, and health-care providers traditionally provide understanding and comfort
D. Physiological changes in older adults are irreversible and require planned health-care interventions

ANSWERS

1. **(D)** Nursing process phase: data collection; client need: coping and adaptation; content area: psychiatric nursing.
   RATIONALE
   (A) Hypotension and pain may be possible symptoms of anxiety but are not typical of a generalized anxiety reaction. **(B)** Lethargy and flat affect are not typical symptoms of anxiety. **(C)** Confusion and hunger are possible symptoms but not common features of an anxiety reaction. **(D)** Increased heart rate and tightness in the chest are common characteristics of anxiety.

2. **(A)** Nursing process phase: implementation; client need: basic care and comfort; content area: psychiatric nursing.
   RATIONALE
   (A) The initial care plan would include monitoring vital signs and providing support and reassurance. The initial priority is to deal with the current anxiety reaction. **(B)** There is no reason to measure I&O or obtain weight for an anxiety reaction. **(C)** Nailbed color would not change during an anxiety reaction. **(D)** The nurse might later explore a history of drug use and offer high-carbohydrate foods, but not as an initial plan.

3. **(C)** Nursing process phase: data collection; client need: coping and adaptation; content area: psychiatric nursing.
   RATIONALE
   (A) Introjection is identifying with another. **(B)** Sublimation is replacing an unacceptable need with one more acceptable. **(C)** The client is using denial. **(D)** Displacement is transferring feelings about one person onto another.

4. **(B)** Nursing process phase: implementation; client need: pharmacological and parenteral therapies; content area: psychiatric nursing.
   RATIONALE
   (A) Imipramine is an antidepressant. **(B)** Lorazepam is an anxiolytic. **(C)** Lithium is a mood stabilizer. **(D)** Amitriptyline is an antidepressant.

5. **(A)** Nursing process phase: implementation; client need: pharmacological and parenteral therapies; content area: psychiatric nursing.
   RATIONALE
   (A) Anxiolytics often have the side effect of drowsiness. **(B)** Some clients could experience convulsions; however, it is a more common side effect of an antipsychotic drug. **(C)** Although blurred vision may be experienced by some clients, it is not a common side effect of anxiolytics. **(D)** Fear of falling is not a common side effect of medications.

6. **(C)** Nursing process phase: implementation; client need: pharmacological and parenteral therapies; content area: psychiatric nursing.
   RATIONALE
   (A) Many persons work while taking psychiatric medications. **(B)** Persons taking antidepressants such as MAOIs should not consume herring. **(C)** A person taking lorazepam, an anxiolytic, should not consume alcohol. **(D)** Persons taking some antipsychotics such as phenothiazine should be cautious in the sun because of the possibility of sunburn.

7. **(D)** Nursing process phase: data collection; client need: coping and adaptation; content area: psychiatric nursing.
   RATIONALE
   (A) In panic-level anxiety, the person has dilated pupils, a feel-ing of terror, and loss of rational thought. **(B)** Mild anxiety is associated with day-to-day living. **(C)** Moderate anxiety manifests as tension in neck, headaches, hypercriticism, and inability to concentrate. **(D)** Severe anxiety is associated with the stated symptoms.

8. **(C)** Nursing process phase: data collection; client need: prevention and early detection of disease; content area: psychiatric nursing.
   RATIONALE
   (A) The medium of verbal communication is speech. **(B)** Therapeutic communication is a process of using specific techniques. **(C)** Poor eye contact is an example of nonverbal communication. **(D)** Mass communication is a component of journalism or marketing.

9. **(B)** Nursing process phase: data collection; client need: coping and adaptation; content area: psychiatric nursing.
   RATIONALE
   (A) Anxiety disorders manifest themselves with a different cluster of symptoms. **(B)** The cluster of symptoms is common in grief reactions, specifically the stage of developing awareness. **(C)** Panic attacks typically are characterized by a sudden onset of intense discomfort and often resemble symptoms of a heart attack. **(D)** The stated symptoms are not typical of eating disorders.

10. **(C)** Nursing process phase: implementation; client need: coping and adaptation; content area: psychiatric nursing.
    RATIONALE
    (A) The nurse does not want to remain subjective, but rather objective. **(B)** The nurse does not want to judge the client, nor offer advice. **(C)** Therapeutic communication requires that the nurse respect the client and offer presence. **(D)** Empathy, rather than sympathy, is a therapeutic technique.

11. **(D)** Nursing process phase: implementation; client need: management of care; content area: psychiatric nursing.
    RATIONALE
    (A) Restating is repeating the client's message using different words. **(B)** Providing feedback is making observations about the client's behavior. **(C)** Identifying a theme is helping the client see a pattern of thought. **(D)** The nurse is giving the client an opportunity to verbalize by using an open-ended statement.

12. **(B)** Nursing process phase: data collection; client need: coping and adaptation; content area: psychiatric nursing.
    RATIONALE
    (A) Obviously, the nurse does not stop communicating simply because physicians have status. **(B)** A one-to-one communication is altered when physical (e.g., noise) or psychosocial (e.g., visitors, physicians) factors change. **(C)** There is no overriding reason that the communication between nurse and client should be private. Usually, the content of the communication is charted and shared with the team. **(D)** The purpose of other health team members' communication with the client is generally similar. All health-care disciplines are concerned with caring and communicating with the client.

13. **(B)** Nursing process phase: implementation; client need: coping and adaptation; content area: psychiatric nursing.
    RATIONALE
    (A) Omission of content means failing to consider the entire conversation between the student and client. **(B)** The student offered

289

personal advice, which stops open, effective communication. **(C)** The student is not rejecting the client; she is offering personal advice. **(D)** There is no indication that the student is offering faulty reassurances by offering a personal opinion.

14. **(C)** Nursing process phase: data collection; client need: growth and development through the life span; content area: psychiatric nursing.

RATIONALE

(A) According to Erikson's theory, industry versus inferiority occurs between 6 and 11 years. **(B)** Intimacy versus isolation occurs between 19 and 34 years. **(C)** The developmental stage of a 61-year-old is ego integrity versus despair. **(D)** The generativity versus stagnation developmental stage occurs between 35 and 60 years.

15. **(A)** Nursing process phase: implementation; client need: coping and adaptation; content area: psychiatric nursing.

RATIONALE

(A) The nurse must offer calm support to maintain a relationship with the client and assess the situation. **(B)** Neuroleptic drugs are used to treat acute and chronic psychosis. **(C)** It is more important to help the client develop self-direction than to give advice. **(D)** Notifying the hospital administrator is inappropriate until more data are collected.

16. **(A)** Nursing process phase: data collection; client need: coping and adaptation; content area: psychiatric nursing.

RATIONALE

(A) Coping mechanisms are task-oriented behaviors to increase one's ability to cope. **(B)** Defense mechanisms are unconscious ego-oriented reactions for self-protection. **(C)** Reaction formation is a defense mechanism. **(D)** Intellectualization is also a defense mechanism.

17. **(A)** Nursing process phase: implementation; client need: reduction of risk potential; content area: psychiatric nursing.

RATIONALE

(A) ECT is administered to depressed clients and requires all the nursing care that an operative procedure requires (e.g., NPO, preoperative permit, denture removal). **(B)** ECT does not cause weight gain. **(C)** ECT is not usually given in conjunction with neuroleptics. **(D)** ECT usually increases rather than decreases mood.

18. **(C)** Nursing process phase: data collection; client need: prevention and early detection of disease; content area: psychiatric nursing.

RATIONALE

(A) Clients with a diagnosis of anorexia are frightened of being fat. **(B)** Clients with a diagnosis of anorexia do not eat large amounts of food. **(C)** Clients with anorexia are very thin because of starvation. **(D)** Clients with a diagnosis of anorexia do not perceive food as comforting or relaxing.

19. **(D)** Nursing process phase: data collection; client need: growth and development through the life span; content area: psychiatric nursing.

RATIONALE

(A) The trust versus mistrust stage of development occurs in infancy, according to Erikson. **(B)** The autonomy versus shame and doubt stage of development occurs in a 2-year-old child, according to Erikson. **(C)** The initiative versus guilt stage of development occurs during the preschool years, according to Erikson. **(D)** A 14-year-old struggles with identity versus role diffusion, according to Erikson.

20. **(A)** Nursing process phase: data collection; client need: prevention and early detection of disease; content area: psychiatric nursing.

RATIONALE

(A) Individuals with anorexia nervosa often exercise 3–4 hours daily. **(B)** Individuals with anorexia nervosa have decreased libido. **(C)** Individuals with anorexia nervosa usually are of above-average intelligence. **(D)** Individuals with anorexia nervosa suffer from bradycardia.

21. **(B)** Nursing process phase: data collection; client need: prevention and early detection of disease; content area: psychiatric nursing.

RATIONALE

(A) Neuroleptic drugs are used to treat thought disorders. **(B)** Coping mechanisms should be assessed to determine the client's pattern of coping with anxiety. **(C)** Vigorous exercise should be discouraged. **(D)** Nurses do not "prescribe" fingernail treatment.

22. **(C)** Nursing process phase: data collection; client need: coping and adaptation; content area: psychiatric nursing.

RATIONALE

(A) Rationalization is an attempt to make unacceptable feelings acceptable. **(B)** Projection is attributing one's own thoughts to another. **(C)** This is a classic case of displacement. **(D)** Regression is retreating to an earlier stage of life.

23. **(A)** Nursing process phase: implementation; client need: psychosocial adaptation; content area: psychiatric nursing.

RATIONALE

(A) The nurse must help the client stick to a theme of therapeutic value. **(B)** Restating talk about self when the topic is weather is less than useful. **(C)** Silence would be inappropriate in this case. **(D)** Summarizing may be used to link themes and feelings and to review important points in the interaction. Summarizing would be an inappropriate communication technique in this case.

24. **(A)** Nursing process phase: implementation; client need: prevention and early detection of disease; content area: psychiatric nursing.

RATIONALE

(A) Clients should receive information regarding procedures. **(B)** The implications of the procedure should not be exaggerated or overexplained. **(C)** This response does not meet the client at her level of understanding. **(D)** A male aide should not accompany a teenage girl suffering from anorexia nervosa for an ECG because of the client's development stage.

25. **(A)** Nursing process phase: data collection; client need: physiological adaptation; content area: psychiatric nursing.

RATIONALE

(A) Clients suffering from substance abuse often have dilated pupils. **(B)** Substance abusers have poor concentration and low tolerance for frustration. **(C)** Euphoria is a psychological characteristic. **(D)** The color of nailbeds is not generally affected by substance abuse.

26. **(A)** Nursing process phase: implementation; client need: physiological adaptation; content area: psychiatric nursing.

RATIONALE

(A) Drug overdose can lead to unstable vital signs and diminished urine output. **(B)** Obtaining weight and temperature is not an immediate concern. **(C)** Some drug overdoses would preclude inducing vomiting. **(D)** A psychiatric consultation may be obtained after the threatening situation is resolved.

27. **(D)** Nursing process phase: implementation; client need: physiological adaptation; content area: psychiatric nursing.

RATIONALE

(A) The nurse may consider monitoring manipulative behavior but not during the acute phase of detoxification. (B) Intervening in family dynamics is not an important issue during the acute phase of detoxification. (C) Evaluating vocational skills during the acute phase of detoxification is not an appropriate nursing action. (D) Monitoring a client's vital signs is an important nursing task during the acute phase of withdrawal.

28. **(A)** Nursing process phase: data collection; client need: coping and adaptation; content area: psychiatric nursing.
   RATIONALE
   (A) Denial is consciously disowning intolerable compulsions and thoughts. Denial is extremely common in substance abuse clients. (B) Projection is attributing one's own thoughts to another. (C) Displacement is shifting your emotions to another person or object. (D) Sublimation is substituting a socially acceptable goal for an unwanted drive.

29. **(B)** Nursing process phase: implementation; client need: coping and adaptation; content area: psychiatric nursing.
   RATIONALE
   (A) Focusing provides statements that help the client expand on the topic. (B) Clarifying is a communication technique that is effective in seeking consensual validation of the client's perception of reality and its significance and meaning to his or her life. (C) Providing feedback promotes exchange with the sender and the receiver. (D) Making an observation is the receiver telling the sender what he or she sees and thinks.

30. **(A)** Nursing process phase: evaluation; client need: coping and adaptation; content area: psychiatric nursing.
   RATIONALE
   (A) At the termination of therapy, the client will identify new modes of coping. (B) Clients must discontinue all drug use. (C) Clients must accept responsibility for their lives and actions. (D) Clients must find new ways of social interaction.

31. **(A)** Nursing process phase: data collection; client need: coping and adaptation; content area: psychiatric nursing.
   RATIONALE
   (A) Schizophrenia is a thought disorder characterized by disturbances of thought content, form, affect, and relationship. (B) Affective disorders are disorders of feeling or mood. (C) Personality disorders are disorders of personality traits that are inflexible and maladaptive. (D) An adjustment disorder is one in which psychological factors affect physical conditions; it is usually short lived and related to stress.

32. **(B)** Nursing process phase: data collection; client need: coping and adaptation; content area: psychiatric nursing.
   RATIONALE
   (A) Stuttering, cluttering, and passive behavior are not symptoms characteristic of schizophrenia. (B) Schizophrenia is characterized by delusions, hallucinations, grandiosity, suspiciousness, disorganized behavior, tangential thought, negativism, diminished self-care, and inappropriate emotional responses. (C) Hyperactivity, crying, and violence are symptoms of mood disorders. (D) These symptoms are characteristic of other mood disorders or thought disorders but not of schizophrenia.

33. **(C)** Nursing process phase: implementation; client need: pharmacological and parenteral therapies; content area: psychiatric nursing.
   RATIONALE
   (A) Anxiolytic medications are used for anxiety disorders. (B) Antidepressant medications are used for mood disorders. (C) Schizophrenia is a thought disorder that generally responds to antipsychotic medications such as haloperidol, trifluoperazine (Stelazine), or fluphenazine. (D) Antiseizure medications are used for various types of seizures (e.g., epilepsy).

34. **(B)** Nursing process phase: implementation; client need: pharmacological and parenteral therapies; content area: psychiatric nursing.
   RATIONALE
   (A) Less frequently, antipsychotic medications may cause neuroleptic malignant syndrome (NMS) in which the client experiences high temperatures (105°F [40.5°C]). (B) Antipsychotic medications frequently result in orthostatic hypotension, and therefore blood pressure measurements are taken lying and standing before the medication is administered. Although NMS is less common than orthostatic hypotension, it is important to monitor vital signs such as blood pressure and temperature. (C) There is no indication that antipsychotic medications have complex interactions with various foods in a client's diet. (D) Blood samples should be ordered by the physician at frequent intervals to determine the therapeutic level of the medication. The nurse should notify the physician of abnormal laboratory results.

35. **(A)** Nursing process phase: data collection; client need: prevention and early detection of disease; content area: psychiatric nursing.
   RATIONALE
   (A) This is an example of a delusion or a faulty thought process or belief. (B) A hallucination is a sensory response to something or someone not present. (C) Anxiety is a feeling of vague uneasiness that may cause physiological arousal. (D) Tangential thought is skipping from one topic to another.

36. **(D)** Nursing process phase: implementation; client need: psychosocial adaptation; content area: psychiatric nursing.
   RATIONALE
   (A) Telling the client that he is psychotic is not an acceptable nursing action. (B) Medications are altered by physician's orders, not by the nurse. (C) Tolerating the behavioral change is not an accountable action. (D) When a client's behavior changes, the nurse must document the assessment.

37. **(C)** Nursing process phase: implementation; client need: psychosocial adaptation; content area: psychiatric nursing.
   RATIONALE
   (A) The nurse must demonstrate respect for the client's personal space. An invasion of the client's space will likely escalate the agitated behavior. (B) Telling the client to act appropriately may lead to a communication barrier between nurse and client. Avoid giving advice. (C) When a client strikes a nurse, the client is displaying poor impulse control. Safety of self, the client, and the staff is a priority. Impulsive clients should not be managed alone. The nurse should call for assistance before any other nursing actions are planned. (D) Obtaining vital signs is important information but inappropriate at this time.

38. **(A)** Nursing process phase: data collection; client need: psychosocial adaptation; content area: psychiatric nursing.
   RATIONALE
   (A) In bipolar disorder, client behavior ranges from excitability to depression. Bipolar disorder is an alteration of mood, affect, and thought. (B) Many clients have personality problems and self-care deficits, but the central issue of the disorder is altered mood. (C) Interpersonal functioning may contribute to altered mood episodes. (D) Intelligence and ideation are not relevant.

39. **(C)** Nursing process phase: implementation; client need: pharmacological and parenteral therapies; content area: psychiatric nursing.
   RATIONALE
   (A) The nurse might monitor the diet but not specifically for administration of lithium. (B) The sleep pattern may also be monitored but not specifically for administration of lithium. (C)

Lithium is a salt; its blood level must be monitored. The range of normal blood levels is 1.0–1.2 mEq/l. If the lithium blood level is >1.2, the nurse will hold the medication and notify the physician. **(D)** The nurse might monitor the activity level as part of overall care but not specifically for administration of lithium.

40. **(B)** Nursing process phase: data collection; client need: prevention and early detection of disease; content area: psychiatric nursing.

    RATIONALE

    (A) Lithium toxicity usually does not cause painful eyes, nausea, or vomiting. **(B)** Lithium toxicity is a serious disorder characterized by diarrhea, tremors, nausea, and vomiting. Generally, toxicity is reversed by intravenous infusion. **(C)** These symptoms are not typical of lithium toxicity. **(D)** Hypotension, thirst, nausea, and vomiting usually are not common symptoms of lithium toxicity.

41. **(C)** Nursing process phase: data collection; client need: physiological adaptation; content area: psychiatric nursing.

    RATIONALE

    (A) Overeating and overspending are not characteristics of Alzheimer's disease. **(B)** Labile mood rather than mood stability is characteristic of Alzheimer's disease. **(C)** Alzheimer's disease is characterized by impaired memory, self-care deficits, anxiety, impaired judgment, rage reactions, and weakness of limbs. **(D)** Limb pain is not a characteristic of Alzheimer's disease.

42. **(A)** Nursing process phase: implementation; client need: psychosocial adaptation; content area: psychiatric nursing.

    RATIONALE

    (A) Clients with Alzheimer's disease are frequently confused and disoriented. Clocks, calendars, and open drapes help the client to know time, place, and person. **(B)** These clients need a stable environment and decreased environmental stimuli when they no longer can tolerate the sensory level. **(C)** Clients with Alzheimer's disease need a consistent care routine. **(D)** Because of the narrowed communication ability, these clients usually are unable to work in group situations.

43. **(B)** Nursing process phase: implementation; client need: psychosocial adaptation; content area: psychiatric nursing.

    RATIONALE

    (A) Restraints and medication may be necessary, but these are not the first line of intervention. **(B)** Clients with Alzheimer's disease often become confused at night. This is called "sundowning." The nurse should first reorient the client and offer reassurance. **(C)** Controlling the light is an important environmental factor and may enhance the client's ability to maintain orientation, but reassurance is most important. **(D)** Safety issues are the responsibility of the caregiver, and observation of all clients serves to eliminate unsafe conditions.

44. **(B)** Nursing process phase: data collection; client need: growth and development through the life span; content area: psychiatric nursing.

    RATIONALE

    (A) The development stage of trust versus mistrust occurs between 0 and 12 months of age. **(B)** The aged client's developmental stage is ego integrity versus despair. The wisdom, experience, and purpose of one's life should synthesize in old age to create an integration of the self or ego. **(C)** Identity versus identity confusion occurs in the teen years. **(D)** Generativity versus stagnation occurs in the middle years.

45. **(C)** Nursing process phase: implementation; client need: prevention and early detection of disease; content area: psychiatric nursing.

    RATIONALE

    (A) Nursing care must be planned to meet the physiological needs of the person, if the client is unable to meet these needs. Impaired cognition usually involves sensory and perceptual disorders that may endanger the client's safety. Meeting the client's safety need is the number one priority. **(B)** Alzheimer's disease is a progressive deterioration that robs the person of intellectual functioning with possible emotional changes. Falls become a safety concern in clients with Alzheimer's disease. **(C)** A safe environment allows for both simple activities and security. Attention span and the ability to concentrate may be impaired as a result of neurological brain disease. To promote and maintain optimal health, the nurse must attend to the client's safety. If priorities must be set, safety is of extreme importance to the care of the client with Alzheimer's disease. **(D)** Spiritual care must be appropriate for the client and should be included as part of holistic nursing interventions, but safety is the number one priority.

46. **(A)** Nursing process phase: data collection; client need: prevention and early detection of disease; content area: psychiatric nursing.

    RATIONALE

    (A) Although severely retarded children usually have an IQ between 20 and 40, it is important to assess for communication abilities so that their needs can be understood. **(B)** Severely retarded children usually do not read. **(C)** Children who are severely retarded do not usually participate in hobbies. **(D)** These children may not know right from wrong.

47. **(A)** Nursing process phase: implementation; client need: psychosocial adaptation; content area: psychiatric nursing.

    RATIONALE

    (A) Mentally retarded children are exceptional and need a great deal of care. Their handicaps often elicit feelings within nurses that should be recognized and processed. **(B)** It is important to have family contact. **(C)** The child's mental development precludes extensive interviewing. **(D)** Teaching coping skills may be attempted but may prove to be futile.

48. **(D)** Nursing process phase: data collection; client need: physiological adaptation; content area: psychiatric nursing.

    RATIONALE

    (A) Withdrawal is not typical of anxiety reactions. **(B)** Lethargy may exist without anxiety. **(C)** Hunger is not related to an anxiety reaction. **(D)** The nurse may see an increased heart rate, hypervigilance, a startled response, or irritability in children with anxiety.

49. **(B)** Nursing process phase: data collection; client need: coping and adaptation; content area: psychiatric nursing.

    RATIONALE

    (A) Reality orientation is not associated with OCD. **(B)** Persons with a diagnosis of obsessive-compulsive behavior disorder exhibit a preoccupation with rules, lack spontaneity, and are perfectionistic. **(C)** A wide range of emotions is not associated with OCD. **(D)** Ritualistic thought is the obsessive part of the disorder. Compulsion describes the action.

50. **(A)** Nursing process phase: implementation; client need: psychosocial adaptation; content area: psychiatric nursing.

    RATIONALE

    (A) The most appropriate nursing intervention would be to document the behavior and work with the treatment team to design a consistent treatment program. The treatment of OCD requires an interdisciplinary approach that addresses the anxiety, dread, and guilt of the client; extinguishes the behavior; allows a safe environment; and assists the client to understand his or her feelings and actions. Rituals are extinguished in a systematic time-step fashion over a period of weeks. **(B)** Asking the client to stop the ritualistic behavior may produce anxiety that the client is unable to manage. **(C)** Asking a "why" question is unrealistic and may cause the client to become defensive. **(D)** Reinforcing the behavior is ineffective.

51. **(B)** Nursing process phase: data collection; client need: psychosocial adaptation; content area: psychiatric nursing.

    RATIONALE

    (A) Avoidance is a conscious or unconscious defense mechanism used to manage anxiety-laden experiences through evasive behaviors. There is no indication that the client is exhibiting avoidance behavior. **(B)** The client is trying to manipulate the nurse by playing one staff member against the other (commonly called "splitting"). Manipulation is characterized by (1) having a conflict of goals, (2) consciously and intentionally trying to influence others, (3) practicing deception, and (4) feeling good about the act of manipulation. **(C)** The client is not opposing or resisting authority. She is playing one staff member against the other. **(D)** The client is not using the unconscious defense mechanism of projection. Projection is attributing one's own thoughts to another.

52. **(B)** Nursing process phase: implementation; client need: psychosocial adaptation; content area: psychiatric nursing.

    RATIONALE

    (A) Accusatory statements do not facilitate constructive communication. **(B)** Missing class is against the rules. Reinforcing the rule avoids a power struggle with the client. The client needs to understand rules and limitations, and that these rules and limitations will be reinforced consistently. **(C)** The question is inappropriate at this stage of the illness. **(D)** Closed-ended comments inhibit communication between the nurse and the client.

53. **(B)** Nursing process phase: data collection; client need: coping and adaptation; content area: psychiatric nursing.

    RATIONALE

    (A) A discussion of sexual feelings can increase knowledge and may decrease anxiety and facilitate problem solving. **(B)** Attempted suicide is an extreme form of acting out. Acting-out behavior is limit testing. Limits are challenged in an attempt to communicate feelings of fear or anger, which the client is unable to communicate directly. **(C)** Attending activities is not a form of acting-out behavior. **(D)** Contracting for safety suggests that the client is seeking security in the environment.

54. **(A, C)** Nursing process phase: implementation; client need: psychosocial adaptation; content area: psychiatric nursing.

    RATIONALE

    (A) To defuse the situation, the nurse should provide a safe, nonthreatening environment and remove the stimulus reinforcement. Limits are clearly reinforced in conversation. **(B)** Seclusion is viewed as control over personal freedom. **(C)** Sharing observations assists the client to problem-solve (e.g., "Fighting is against the rules. It doesn't solve the conflict. What happened to start the fight? How could it be handled differently?"). **(D)** Restraints should not be used as punishment. Clients are restrained if they are possibly harmful to themselves or others.

55. **(A)** Nursing process phase: data collection; client need: growth and development through the life span; content area: psychiatric nursing.

    RATIONALE

    (A) Adolescents find it difficult to engage in a discussion related to death. **(B)** It is the child who sees death as temporary. **(C)** School-age children feel that death is a punishment. **(D)** Adolescents are thinking about the future and realize that they might not participate.

56. **(C)** Nursing process phase: data collection; client need: coping and adaptation; content area: psychiatric nursing.

    RATIONALE

    (A) The client is angry and feels helpless and hopeless. **(B)** The client is in the bargaining stage of the grief process. **(C)** The client indicates that she is willing to move on with her life. **(D)** The client sounds depressed and continues to mourn over the loss.

57. **(A)** Nursing process phase: data collection; client need: psychosocial adaptation; content area: psychiatric nursing.

    RATIONALE

    (A) Spiritual development is an important aspect of the personality. A holistic approach to nursing care is provided within the framework of the nurse-client relationship and includes spiritual health. **(B)** Questioning may sort out the religious preoccupation, but the client may use it as a barrier for any further communication. **(C)** Because it is impossible to be informed about all religious traditions, it is important to discuss the client's spiritual issues with informed members of the health-care team before referring him to any group. **(D)** A discussion about immortality would be inappropriate.

58. **(B)** Nursing process phase: data collection; client need: coping and adaptation; content area: psychiatric nursing.

    RATIONALE

    (A) Survivors do not have time to engage in anticipatory grief, the progression through the phases of grief before the death. **(B)** Many survivors feel guilty for not having given something special or extra to the deceased. **(C)** Survivors' immediate responses to a sudden death are feelings of shock, disbelief, guilt, despair, desertion, or betrayal. Detachment takes place over time and is the process of "letting go." **(D)** An uncomplicated grief reaction is an essential emotional process that is a normal response to a loss. Survivors of victims of sudden death do not have time to prepare for the loss.

59. **(B)** Nursing process phase: data collection; client need: coping and adaptation; content area: psychiatric nursing.

    RATIONALE

    (A) Significant others and religious beliefs may serve as a source of help and strength, but often do not. Clients need to experience hope and support for the beliefs that give them strength. **(B)** Spirituality concerns, especially among elderly persons, cause them to question the meaning and purpose in living. Persons experiencing spiritual distress question their own existence and the reasons for suffering. **(C)** Information about the client's spiritual component is hard to obtain because it does not always lend itself to direct observation. **(D)** Religious affiliation may be most meaningful for the client, and it is an outlet for the expression of spirituality, but it is not the issue here.

60. **(A)** Nursing process phase: data collection; client need: physiological adaptation; content area: psychiatric nursing.

    RATIONALE

    (A) The symptoms indicated are associated with delirium tremens and usually develop 72 hours after the last drink. **(B)** Korsakoff's syndrome is a disturbance of short-term memory possibly related to thiamine deficiency. **(C)** Alcoholic hepatitis is a physical effect of chronic alcoholism. There is no observable evidence of hepatitis at this time. **(D)** Alcoholic hallucinosis refers to auditory hallucinations. The client did not present with hallucinations.

61. **(D)** Nursing process phase: data collection; client need: physiological adaptation; content area: psychiatric nursing.

    RATIONALE

    (A) A sign of cocaine intoxication is diaphoresis, not dry, cool skin. **(B)** Clients suffering from cocaine intoxication experience elevated blood pressure. (**C**) A common effect of cocaine detoxification on the body is a demand for oxygen and an increase in the heart rate. (**D**) A common sign of cocaine intoxication is psychomotor agitation.

62. (**B**) Nursing process phase: data collection; client need: pharmacological and parenteral therapies; content area: psychiatric nursing.

    RATIONALE

    (**A**) Librium is commonly used in the treatment of alcohol withdrawal. (**B**) Disulfiram is used as a deterrent to drinking, if the client wishes to stop drinking alcohol. Ingestion of alcohol while Antabuse is in the body results in an unpleasant physical reaction. (**C**) Valium is used to reduce the symptoms of alcohol withdrawal. (**D**) Lithium is the drug of choice for clients suffering from mood disorders.

63. (**B**) Nursing process phase: data collection; client need: psychosocial adaptation; content area: psychiatric nursing.

    RATIONALE

    (**A**) The harboring of family secrets and the inability to express true feelings are dysfunctional behaviors that may contribute to ineffective family dynamics rather than effective family dynamics. (**B**) A person who is codependent has difficulty with establishing a separate identity. Ego boundaries are weak and the diffuseness of boundaries inhibits the development of autonomy. (**C**) Codependency involves an imbalance in internal ego states. (**D**) Codependency involves negative messages about self that came from childhood experiences.

64. (**A**) Nursing process phase: implementation; client need: psychosocial adaptation; content area: psychiatric nursing.

    RATIONALE

    (**A**) Instilling hope in the family's future is one of the nurse's greatest responsibilities. (**B**) Alcoholic families are dysfunctional and lack homeostatic balance. (**C**) Cross-generational clinging is dysfunctional and should be discouraged. (**D**) Promoting defense mechanisms such as rationalization or blaming others for behaviors associated with alcohol abuse serves only to prolong the denial.

65. (**A**) Nursing process phase: data collection; client need: psychosocial adaptation; content area: psychiatric nursing.

    RATIONALE

    (**A**) Behavior modification therapy can be effective in facilitating coping skills and adaptive behaviors in certain mental illnesses. (**B**) Although complete recovery may be possible, the aim of treatment is to facilitate the client's ability to function more effectively. (**C**) Mentally ill persons are sensitive about how others will react to them. (**D**) Evaluation is based on observation of the individual's behavior. Diagnostic criteria are delineated in the *Diagnostic and Statistical Manual of Mental Disorders,* fourth edition (*DSM-IV*). This may not be significant to the family.

66. (**B**) Nursing process phase: planning; client need: management of care; content area: psychiatric nursing.

    RATIONALE

    (**A**) Clients have a right to therapeutic, not custodial, care. (**B**) A client's Bill of Rights ensures that a client has the right to therapeutic treatment, informed consent, and to refuse treatment. (**C**) Court cases have found in behalf of clients who did not receive therapeutic treatment and/or who were not treated humanely. The facility was held liable, and the client was released. (**D**) The courts can look at competency versus incompetency of the person. Competency is defined as the capability of making a decision. At times, the courts have appointed a guardian, by not always. Therefore, a client may not even have a guardian.

67. (**D**) Nursing process phase: data collection; client need: growth and development through the life span; content area: psychiatric nursing.

    RATIONALE

    (**A**) Individuals develop at their own rate although, in any stage, most individuals accomplish certain tasks within that stage. (**B**) This school-age period (6–16 years) is psychologically the quiet years. (**C**) During this developmental period, children usually get a sense of approval from positive reinforcement from the parent. (**D**) Sexual curiosity is replaced by intellectual curiosity; great social and intellectual strides are accomplished; group activities become more important.

68. (**A**) Nursing process phase: data collection; client need: growth and development through the life span; content area: psychiatric nursing.

    RATIONALE

    (**A**) Events occurring throughout life may affect emotional adjustment; most experts believe that events which occur in the first 20 years have the greatest impact; some believe the first 6 years are the most significant. (**B**) Every developmental stage is the foundation for the next. If a stage is completed successfully, the foundation is firm; if not, the personality structure may be weakened. (**C**) Inability to progress through a developmental stage does not always result in withdrawn behavior, and it is not the primary cause of withdrawn behavior. (**D**) Events occurring during the first 12 months of life primarily affect the development of trust versus mistrust, but this period is not the most psychologically significant.

69. (**C**) Nursing process phase: data collection; client need: coping and adaptation; content area: psychiatric nursing.

    RATIONALE

    (**A**) Conversion reaction occurs when unacceptable feelings disguised by repression manifest as physical symptoms. (**B**) Suppression is consciously keeping unacceptable feelings and thoughts out of awareness. (**C**) Symptoms of depression can include withdrawal, poor eye contact, and failure to perform ADLs such as eating and hygiene. (**D**) Reaction formation occurs when unacceptable feelings are disguised by repression of the true feelings and reinforcement of the opposite feelings.

70. (**C**) Nursing process phase: data collection; client need: growth and development through the life span; content area: psychiatric nursing.

    RATIONALE

    (**A**) This is the developmental stage for ages 6–12 years. (**B**) This is the developmental stage for ages 18–25 years. (**C**) This is the developmental stage for ages 65 years to death. (**D**) This is the developmental stage for ages 30–45 years.

71. (**C**) Nursing process phase: implementation; client need: coping and adaptation; content area: psychiatric nursing.

    RATIONALE

    (**A**) Empathy is the ability to feel the feelings of others so that one can relate to the situation in their terms. (**B**) The client is aware that everything will not be fine; she is alone and her spouse is deceased. (**C**) This communication block does not acknowledge the client's own perception of her situation. (**D**) Superficial reassurance denies the client's feelings and her grief.

72. (**B**) Nursing process phase: data collection; client need: growth and development through the life span; content area: psychiatric nursing.

    RATIONALE

    (**A**) This statement is all-inclusive; therefore, "all-or-none" cannot be correct. (**B**) Adolescents want independence without responsibility, and this accounts for ambivalent feelings. (**C**) The dependence versus independence conflict accounts for much of adolescents' irritable and erratic behavior; they long to be independent and self-sufficient. **(D)** Peer approval is very important to adolescents; they are deeply involved in their own feelings of self-worth and self-identity.

73. **(D)** Nursing process phase: planning; client need: growth and development through the life span; content area: psychiatric nursing.
    RATIONALE
    (A) Adolescents are aware of physical and emotional changes as well as of the sexual changes equated with maturity and the need to belong. **(B)** "Love" relationships are likely to be based on what the "loved" person does to strengthen the adolescent's own self-esteem; these love objects are found among peers and others outside the home setting. **(C)** Adolescents have a need to be accepted by others, as is evident by the development of language or cues unique to the group and the creation of inclusive situations that readily make the members identifiable. **(D)** The adolescent is keenly aware of body changes and maturation and shows a readiness to learn about them. Sex education during this period is important to prevent pregnancy and sexually transmitted diseases.

74. **(D)** Nursing process phase: data collection; client need: coping and adaptation; content area: psychiatric nursing.
    RATIONALE
    (A) Repression is unconsciously keeping unacceptable feelings out of awareness. **(B)** Compensation is overachievement in one area because of feeling of inadequacy in another. **(C)** Denial of reality involves the repression of a reality as though it does not exist (e.g., an alcoholic who says he does not have a drinking problem). **(D)** Rationalization is the falsification of experience through the creation of a logical or socially acceptable explanation of the behavior.

75. **(C)** Nursing process phase: implementation; client need: coping and adaptation; content area: psychiatric nursing.
    RATIONALE
    (A) This response makes assumptions about characteristics that may or may not be true or contribute to the client's perceptions. **(B)** This response makes inappropriate generalizations of emotions about family and/or significant others. **(C)** This response is an open-ended question that does not cue the client as to an expected response. **(D)** This response does not maintain the focus of the session or the direction of the interaction. In addition, the therapist is setting himself or herself up for a boundary violation.

76. **(B)** Nursing process phase: evaluation; client need: pharmacological and parenteral therapies; content area: psychiatric nursing.
    RATIONALE
    (A) Neuroleptics do not cure social withdrawal and apathy; they treat brain chemistry to aid in the reintegration and reorganization of thoughts. **(B)** Increased levels of dopamine increase the neurotransmitter activity in the brain and result in erratic behavior associated with schizophrenia. **(C)** Neuroleptics do not increase sex drive; in men, they cause ejaculation dysfunction. **(D)** Alteration of reality is unclear in terms of how the client's perception of reality changes. Paranoia does not occur in all schizophrenia; it is a component or symptom of some mental illnesses.

77. **(C)** Nursing process phase: evaluation; client need: pharmacological and parenteral therapies; content area: psychiatric nursing.
    RATIONALE
    (A) Neuroleptics cause weight gain secondary to decreased metabolism and gastric motility. **(B)** Neuroleptics may precipitate a *hyperglycemic* response in individuals who are predisposed but are not associated with precipitating diabetes. **(C)** Nasal congestion, seizures, and urinary retention are serious side effects that are believed to occur because of the additive anticholinergic properties of phenothiazine. **(D)** A common side effect of neuroleptics is hypersomnia.

78. **(B)** Nursing process phase: planning; client need: growth and development through the life span; content area: psychiatric nursing.
    RATIONALE
    (A) Infants will withdraw and no longer cue their needs through crying. **(B)** The developmental stage for this age group is trust versus mistrust. The unrelenting frustration of not having needs met can result in the negative outcome of mistrust. **(C)** Infants do not possess the cognitive ability to create an alternate or fantasy world. **(D)** Infants lack the cognitive ability to accomplish this.

79. **(C)** Nursing process phase: data collection; client need: growth and development through the life span; content area: psychiatric nursing.
    RATIONALE
    (A) This realization is a turning point in the infant's development of self and self-sufficiency. **(B)** The infant does not have the emotional ability to displace anger or frustration on others. **(C)** Gradually the child begins to master more skills that allow him or her to feel more in control of the environment and more secure. **(D)** As skills are developed and mastered, the infant progresses developmentally.

80. **(A)** Nursing process phase: data collection; client need: growth and development through the life span; content area: psychiatric nursing.
    RATIONALE
    (A) A 2-year-old's exploration of the environment leads to conquests and feelings of autonomy. **(B)** The 2-year-old child is independent and self-reliant. **(C)** New challenges, for example, toilet training, are mastered. **(D)** Social skills are increased, usually secondary to a curiosity about the environment.

81. **(C)** Nursing process phase: data collection; client need: growth and development through the life span; content area: psychiatric nursing.
    RATIONALE
    (A) Discipline is needed to provide the 3- to 5-year-old with structure and a sense of security. **(B)** Parental approval is important in the development of good self-esteem. **(C)** Motor and intellectual skills are increasing, and in 3- to 5-year-olds accomplishments such as the ability to ride a tricycle, run with only a few falls, and dress themselves boost their self-esteem. **(D)** This age group is becoming more aware of peers and group activities; socialization skills improve.

82. **(C)** Nursing process phase: data collection; client need: coping and adaptation; content area: psychiatric nursing.
    RATIONALE
    (A) Reaction formation is denial of unacceptable feelings and the adoption of the opposite behavior. If this were the case, the client would be promiscuous. **(B)** Displacement occurs when the client transfers hostile or unacceptable behavior from one object to another. **(C)** Repression is unconsciously keeping unacceptable feelings out of awareness. This client has repressed her feelings about the catastrophic sexual experience earlier in life. **(D)** Suppression is the conscious keeping of unacceptable feelings out of awareness.

83. **(A)** Nursing process phase: data collection; client need: coping and adaptation; content area: psychiatric nursing.

    RATIONALE

    (A) The reality in this situation is the paralysis. To deny that paralysis will change his previously active life is to deny its reality. **(B)** Compensation allows the individual to cover up a perceived area of inadequacy or weakness by overexcelling in another area. **(C)** Fantasy allows the temporary escape from a painful environment; it can also help the individual arrive at solutions to problems that he otherwise may not be able to solve. **(D)** Introjection occurs when the person incorporates into his own personality attributes of others, thus protecting him from threatening circumstances.

84. **(B)** Nursing process phase: data collection; client need: coping and adaptation; content area: psychiatric nursing.

    RATIONALE

    (A) Displacement occurs when a person transfers hostile and aggressive feelings from one object to another object or person. For example, a man who gets "chewed out" at work comes home and kicks the dog or yells at his wife and children. **(B)** Regression, displayed by this child, is a reaction against anxiety that allows the person to go back in development to a time when he or she felt more at ease and better able to cope with his environment. **(C)** Sublimation allows the person to divert unacceptable impulses and motives into socially acceptable ones. For example, persons with strong aggressive impulses participate in physically violent sports or other socially accepted activities. **(D)** Reaction formation occurs when one denies unacceptable feelings and impulses by adopting conscious behavior that appears (at least on the surface) to be contradictory to the feelings being denied.

85. **(B)** Nursing process phase: evaluation; client need: pharmacological and parenteral therapies; content area: psychiatric nursing.

    RATIONALE

    (A) This classification of drugs, which includes Librium, Valium, Tranxene, Ativan, and Serax, has a high potential for abuse, toxicity, and lethal overdose, and it is recommended that these drugs be used for a short time only (1–2 weeks). **(B)** By binding with γ-aminobutyric acid, the benzodiazepine agent decreases anxiety and produces a sedative effect by blocking the release of γ-aminobutyric acid. **(C)** Although drugs in this classification have a tranquilizing effect without sedation, they may also numb emotions and decrease one's enthusiasm for life. **(D)** Benzodiazepines interfere with normal coping mechanisms and may cause an increase in irritability, aggression, hostility, and depression.

86. **(D)** Nursing process phase: evaluation; client need: pharmacological and parenteral therapies; content area: psychiatric nursing.

    RATIONALE

    (A) Tricyclic antidepressants increase the level of the neurotransmitter serotonin or norepinephrine; a deficiency in neurotransmitters is thought to cause depression. **(B)** MAOIs prevent the metabolism of neurotransmitters; they must be given for long periods (2–6 weeks) and are more toxic. Those commonly used include Marplan, Nardil, and Parnate. **(C)** Tricyclic antidepressants are used to treat the symptoms of depression. In about 85% of the cases, individuals demonstrate an increase in mental alertness and physical activity within a few days of beginning treatment. **(D)** Hypertensive crisis may result if MAOIs are taken with tyramine-rich foods, such as aged cheese, avocados, bananas, and chicken livers. Clients should avoid drinking beer, red wine, and caffeine-containing beverages.

87. **(A)** Nursing process phase: implementation; client need: psychosocial adaptation; content area: psychiatric nursing.

    RATIONALE

    (A) Many personality disorder clients are manipulative and do not have appropriate personal and social boundaries. Limits must therefore be reinforced. **(B)** Interventions should encourage relaxed rather than hostile exchanges. **(C)** Planned diversional activities are recommended in the care of clients with personality disorders. **(D)** Commonly occurring inappropriate behaviors include blaming, accusing, and intimidating. The nurse should directly and clearly identify inappropriate behaviors that alienate others.

88. **(D)** Nursing process phase: evaluation; client need: coping and adaptation; content area: psychiatric nursing.

    RATIONALE

    (A) In conversion reaction, unacceptable thoughts and feelings are repressed and manifest as physical symptoms. **(B)** The client is not demonstrating hostility toward the nurse. The object of any hostility in this exchange would have to be the client's mother. **(C)** In displacement, a client transfers hostile or unacceptable behavior from one object to another. **(D)** Transference is the result of unresolved childhood experiences with significant others; the client transfers unresolved feelings to present relationships in an attempt to resolve them.

89. **(A)** Nursing process phase: data collection; client need: pharmacological and parenteral therapies; content area: psychiatric nursing.

    RATIONALE

    (A) The side effects include anticholinergic effects such as dry mouth, urinary retention, weight gain, and sexual dysfunction. **(B)** Neuroleptics are not considered cost prohibitive, and many clients are subsidized through mental health clinics. **(C)** In chronic mental illness, clients are usually aware of their need for medication therapy. **(D)** Neuroleptics are designed for long-term use in mental illness.

90. **(B)** Nursing process phase: implementation; client need: psychosocial adaptation; content area: psychiatric nursing.

    RATIONALE

    (A) The paranoid client is mistrustful; your explanations will not be accepted. **(B)** This action removes the stimulus on which this mistrust is based. **(C)** The paranoid client's feelings of mistrust are not helped by reassurance. **(D)** This is and will be perceived by the client as a threat and will further exacerbate the trust issues.

91. **(B)** Nursing process phase: implementation; client need: coping and adaptation; content area: psychiatric nursing.

    RATIONALE

    (A) This is a demeaning and superficial response that attacks the client's self-esteem. **(B)** This open-ended question allows the client to express his or her perception and provides an opportunity for intervention. **(C)** This response indicates that the nurse is contributing to the client's delusional structure. **(D)** This noninterventional response makes no attempt to assess the client's perception or to provide the client with the opportunity for reality orientation.

92. **(D)** Nursing process phase: planning; client need: pharmacological and parenteral therapies; content area: psychiatric nursing.

    RATIONALE

    (A) There are only two decanoate drugs: Haldol and Prolixin. Their delivery is different; both have side effects. **(B)** The client is not required to adhere to a special diet while taking neuroleptics. **(C)** Behavioral changes and improvement in thought reorganization are used to measure the effectiveness of neuroleptics. **(D)** The decanoate salt is slowly absorbed and has a sustained duration of action that decreases the need for frequent dosing. The dose amount and frequency are highly individualized and determined by the resolution of specific symptoms.

93. **(C)** Nursing process phase: data collection; client need: coping and adaptation; content area: psychiatric nursing.
RATIONALE
(A) This is not a characteristic of catatonic schizophrenia. **(B)** This is a characteristic of paranoid schizophrenia that is not generally seen in catatonic schizophrenia. The symptoms can result in an unwillingness or inability to eat. **(C)** Stuporous withdrawal, hallucinations, and delusions are characteristics of catatonic schizophrenia. **(D)** Sexual preoccupation is more a characteristic of sexual disorders and the manic phase of bipolar disorder. Word salad is a speech pattern in which words do not make sense and is not characteristic of catatonic schizophrenia.

94. **(B)** Nursing process phase: planning; client need: psychosocial adaptation; content area: psychiatric nursing.
RATIONALE
(A) Clients with antisocial personality disorder reject social norms as limits and exhibit poor impulse control. This client cannot be expected to monitor his own behavior effectively. **(B)** Establishing clear, consistent limits on behavior will contribute to this client's ability to interact appropriately on the unit. **(C)** Peer interaction offers the opportunity for the client to receive feedback about his interactions with others. Encouraging peer interaction also helps model social norms. **(D)** Clients with antisocial personality disorder come from dysfunctional families and have poor, often volatile, interpersonal relationships. The nurse cannot expect these families and significant others to participate effectively with the client in treatment.

95. **(C)** Nursing process phase: data collection; client need: psychosocial adaptation; content area: psychiatric nursing.
RATIONALE
(A) Although therapy serves to reinforce self-esteem and self-worth, this is not at the basis of the deficit. **(B)** Exerting control over eating habits and weight provides positive reinforcement; the client feels in control and able to live in an otherwise out-of-control environment. **(C)** Although the client may "see" herself as "fat," this is a figurative distortion and does not include intellect. **(D)** The need to mature is not a part of this struggle and does not enter into the consideration of how to deal with her environment.

96. **(C)** Nursing process phase: planning; client need: psychosocial adaptation; content area: psychiatric nursing.
RATIONALE
(A) Behaviors that he is currently exhibiting are usually accompanied by low frustration level and easy distractibility. Initially he will not be able to meet concise behavioral expectations and will react with increased agitation. **(B)** Isolation will not provide him with the feedback he needs. He may see this only as another step in ritualistic behavior without recognizing its relationship to inappropriate behavior. **(C)** This intervention is most important at this time. Even though he has a short attention span and appears unable to concentrate, the sequence of behaviors may provide insight. **(D)** Initially he will not know how to respond; at this point he lacks the insight to provide this information.

97. **(A)** Nursing process phase: planning; client need: pharmacological and parenteral therapies; content area: psychiatric nursing.
RATIONALE
(A) To minimize side effects, therapeutic levels of lithium are reached over 7–14 days. **(B)** These are not "common" side effects of lithium therapy, and prophylactic treatment is not required. **(C)** Noncompliance results in the reappearance of symptoms and is therefore observable. **(D)** Lithium is not a short-onset, fast-acting drug. It is intended for use in long-term care.

98. **(B)** Nursing process phase: planning; client need: pharmacological and parenteral therapies; content area: psychiatric nursing.
RATIONALE
(A) Decrease in therapeutic levels results in agitated behavior. **(B)** Toxic ranges are possibly a result of self-administration error or noncompliance. **(C)** Lithium therapy is intended to control symptoms while allowing maximum level of functioning. **(D)** Lethargy and other emotional blunting symptoms are not expected side effects of lithium therapy.

99. **(C)** Nursing process phase: implementation; client need: pharmacological and parenteral therapies; content area: psychiatric nursing.
RATIONALE
(A) Lithium levels would be the most significant laboratory value at this time. Forcing fluids would not be the priority intervention. **(B)** The concern is toxicity, which would require direct intervention to reverse, rather than passive intervention, such as withholding a dose of lithium. **(C)** This is the most appropriate and priority nursing intervention in this situation in which a toxic level appears to have accumulated. **(D)** This intervention would result in further elevation of lithium levels and more critical symptoms as toxicity worsens.

100. **(B)** Nursing process phase: data collection; client need: coping and adaptation; content area: psychiatric nursing.
RATIONALE
(A) This response is a prejudiced opinion that stereotypes older adults. Not all older adults are "prone" to depression, and not all require long-term care. **(B)** It is estimated that 20 to 25% of all US households are occupied by single adults. For the older adult, this means that there are fewer times when family members or significant others are in close enough proximity to respond to health-care needs. **(C)** This response is a stereotypical statement that is untrue. **(D)** Not all physiological changes in older adults are irreversible.

UNIT **III**

Related Sciences
Reviews and Tests

CHAPTER **7**

Procedures for the Licensed Practical Nurse*

Patricia Gauntlett Beare, RN, PhD

A very important part of nursing is the ability to perform certain skills and procedures. No matter what type of procedure is done, certain standards must be met to obtain the highest level of health possible for the client. The purpose of this chapter is to assist the practical nurse (PN) in carrying out common procedures. A brief description and purpose of each procedure is given. The steps in each procedure, along with the reasons for each step, are provided. Each procedure also includes a section on the nursing implications. The entire procedure should be read carefully before actually carrying it out. When the PN knows what the procedure should include, there is less chance of forgetting important steps.

New information may require some changes in the way a procedure is carried out. Each hospital or other health-care facility should have a procedures manual on hand and revise it as necessary when new information is obtained. Certain procedures may differ from one health-care institution to another; for example, the number of times the temperature, pulse, respirations, and blood pressure are taken after a blood transfusion. The procedures presented in this chapter are based on current knowledge.

Procedure: Placing a Nasal Cannula

Description: A nasal cannula is used to give oxygen to the client. The nasal tips (prongs) come out from the center of a plastic tube and are placed into the nose openings. This allows the client to breathe through the nose or mouth.

Purpose: To deliver low to moderate amounts of oxygen to clients with certain types of pulmonary disease, heart surgical procedures, and other illnesses.

STEP	RATIONALE
1. Collect necessary equipment: • Wall or tank oxygen source • Plastic nasal cannula with a connecting tube • Humidifier filled with sterile water • Flowmeter	Having the required equipment on hand makes it safer and quicker to start. A humidifier is a special container that, when filled with sterile water, provides moisture to the lining of the nose and upper respiratory system.
2. Connect flowmeter to oxygen. Attach humidifier with nasal cannula tubing.	Humidification helps to prevent drying of mucous membranes, which makes the client more comfortable.

*Content reviewed by Jeanne C. Scherer, RN, MS.

STEP	RATIONALE
3. Check physician's order for the rate of flow and check to make sure that the flow rate is correct. The usual dose is 1–6 L/min. There should be bubbling in the humidifier container.	Giving oxygen to a client requires a physician's order. Rates of flow >6 L/min do not increase the amount of oxygen the client is receiving and may cause extreme dryness of the lining of the nose and throat, as well as increase gastric bloating.
4. Gently place the nasal prongs into the nasal openings.	Oxygen enters the upper respiratory system directly through the nasal cannula.
5. Adjust the tubing around the back of the ears so that the nasal prongs fit comfortably. Slide the plastic adjuster up under the chin until the fit is correct.	The client is likely to be more comfortable and cooperative in keeping the nasal cannula in place.
6. Observe and record how the client responds to the treatment by checking his or her breathing and mental orientation to time and place. Check arterial blood gases (ABGs).	Indicates how well client is responding to the treatment. ABG testing is the best way of determining that adequate amounts of oxygen are being delivered and of allowing the physician to determine if changes need to be made in the medical plan.

Nursing Implications: Make sure that the level of sterile distilled water in the humidifier container is correct. Check the physician's orders in regard to the oxygen administration as well as the setup at least once every 8 hours. Observe the client's nasal openings and the back of the ears for irritation and skin breakdown. If the client complains of pressure behind the ears, apply clean 2 × 2 or 4 × 4 dressings over the pressure area.

Record the amount of oxygen being administered and observations at the beginning and end of each shift. Note any changes in client's response resulting from oxygen administration, as well as any changes in the physician's orders. Any changes or abnormal reactions should be reported to the head nurse and physician immediately. Place "No Smoking" signs over client's bed and on the door.

Procedure: Inserting a Nasal Catheter

Description: In this procedure, a plastic nasal catheter is placed into the nose (one nostril) and into the nasopharynx. The nasal catheter is usually used for a short time.

Purpose: To give oxygen at flow rates of 1–6 L/min to decrease oxygen needs of the client.

STEP	RATIONALE
1. Collect necessary equipment: • Wall or tank oxygen source • Flowmeter • Oxygen tubing • Nasal catheter (check for correct size) • Humidifier filled with sterile water • Water-soluble lubricant	Organizing necessary equipment allows quick and safe implementation. The oxygen catheter is a smooth, flexible tube with openings in the tip that allow the oxygen to pass through the nose into the lungs. The size of the catheter differs for children and adults.
2. Connect flowmeter with the wall or tank source of oxygen and attach the humidifier with the nasal catheter and tubing.	Humidification helps to prevent drying of the lining of the nose and throat.
3. Measure the length of the nasal catheter from the client's nose to earlobe. Mark this area with a small piece of tape.	The distance from nose to earlobe approximately equals the distance that the catheter needs to be placed through the nose to the area called the oropharynx.
4. Use the lubricant on the tip of the catheter.	Lubricating the tip allows easier placement and decreases the possibility of injuring the lining of the nose and back of mouth.
5. Set flow rate at 2–3 L/min and gently place catheter into one nostril. The catheter should enter and proceed easily. Stop placement when taped area is reached. If the nostril is obstructed, *do not* force catheter.	Allows oxygen flow to decrease risk of obstructing catheter by secretions in the nose.
6. Inspect placement of catheter by observing oral cavity. The tip of the catheter should be visible. Gently pull the catheter back about ¼ inch until the tip of the catheter can no longer be seen. Use a flashlight and a tongue depressor to help you see the nasal catheter tip.	Ensures that the catheter has been placed correctly and decreases chance of swallowing too much air.

STEP	RATIONALE
7. Set flow rate according to the physician's orders. The usual rate is 1–6 L/min.	Giving oxygen to a client requires a physician's orders. Flow rates >6 L/min may cause extreme dryness of the lining of the nose and throat as well as gastric bloating.
8. Attach catheter to nose with tape.	Tape prevents catheter from being moved out of place.
9. Observe and record how client responds to treatment by checking his or her breathing and mental orientation to time and place. Check ABG test results.	The client's breathing and orientation to time and place indicate the client's response to the treatment. ABG testing is the best way of determining whether adequate amounts of oxygen are delivered in needed amounts and of allowing the physician to determine if changes need to be made in the medical plan.

Nursing Implications: Change the nasal catheter at least once a day and transfer to opposite nostril. The catheter tip may become clogged with secretions, decreasing the amount of oxygen the client is receiving. Record the oxygen treatment, including rate of flow, at the beginning and end of each shift. Note changes in the client's response to oxygen treatment or the physician's orders. Any abnormal reaction or changes in response should be reported to the head nurse and physician immediately. Keep sterile distilled water in the humidifier container at the correct level. Check the physician's orders and oxygen setup at least once every 8 hours. Place a "No Smoking" sign on the client's door and above the bed.

Procedure: Applying a Venturi Mask

Description: A Venturi mask is an oxygen mask that fits comfortably over the client's mouth and nose to make sure that the oxygen the client is receiving is in the correct amount and concentration. The openings can be adjusted to allow oxygen to be given at 24–40% of concentration. Venturi masks are used for clients who keep more carbon dioxide in their system than normal (e.g., clients with chronic obstructive lung disease).

Purpose: To deliver a known depth of oxygen while delivering a high amount of moisture to the upper airway.

STEP	RATIONALE
1. Collect necessary equipment: • Wall or tank oxygen source • Venturi mask for correct mix of oxygen and air (24%, 28%, 31%, 35%, 40%) • Compressed air source (for high humidity) • Nebulizer with sterile water	Organizing necessary equipment allows quick and safe implementation.
2. Connect Venturi mask with tubing to flow gauge and wall or tank oxygen source.	
3. Turn on oxygen flow gauge (meter) and adjust dial on mask opening (port) to the rate ordered by the physician. The proper setting and depth (concentration) of oxygen is usually noted on the side of the mask.	The correct mix of air to oxygen must be provided so that the correct amount of oxygen is delivered. The Venturi mask mixes a fixed flow of oxygen with different amounts of air. Oxygen enters through an opening at a high speed. The larger the opening, the lower the amount of room air drawn into the mask.
4. Place Venturi mask gently over client's nose and mouth. Adjust the placement of the elastic strap. Make sure that openings for the entry of room air are not blocked by client's bedding.	Any obstruction in air openings will interfere with the air-oxygen mixture.
5. Observe and record client's response to the procedure by checking his or her breathing and mental status.	Observation can assist in deciding the success of the oxygen delivery procedure. Checking the ABGs is the best means of judging if adequate oxygen is being delivered and provides a reason for changes in the medical plan by the physician.

Nursing Implications: Change mask, tubing, and nebulizer every day. Check water level in the nebulizer often for proper amount. Drain tubing often to remove extra amount of water that has formed. This extra water will interfere with the correct amount of oxygen being delivered to the client. Document procedure, including amount of oxygen delivered, at the beginning and end of each shift. Place "No Smoking" signs on client's door and above the bed. Wash hands before and after the procedure.

Procedure: Applying a Simple Face Mask, with or without Aerosol

Description: A simple face mask is used to give oxygen in a low-flow system. The amount of oxygen the client gets depends on his or her breathing rate.

Purpose: To administer levels of oxygen at 35–40% concentration; aerosol given to assist in removal of secretions.

STEP	RATIONALE

1. Collect necessary equipment:
  • Wall or tank oxygen source
  • Nebulizer with distilled water
  • Plastic aerosol mask with tubing
  • Flowmeter (gauge)
	Organizing necessary equipment allows for quick and safe implementation.

2. Connect the flowmeter (gauge) with the wall or tank oxygen source and attach the nebulizer with aerosol mask and tubing.	The nebulizer helps to prevent extreme drying of the lining of the nose and upper airway of the client.
3. Set the correct amount of oxygen depth on the nebulizer bottle (check the physician's orders for the correct setting).	The percentage of oxygen to be inhaled by the client is 35–40% and is determined by the setting on the nebulizer.
4. Set the flow rate until the right amount of mist is seen (usual rate is 10–12 L/min).	The flow rate must meet or exceed the highest amount of breath that the client can take in. The client must get a good enough flow of oxygen so that he or she gets the correct amount and depth of oxygen.
5. Place mask gently over the client's nose and mouth. Make sure elastic strap fits comfortably and mask is in right position.	Correct placement of mask is required so that the correct amount and depth of oxygen is delivered to the client.
6. Observe and record the client's response to the oxygen procedure. Observe and report the client's breathing and mental status. Check and report ABG values to the head nurse and physician.	Good observation can help the physician's decision in making changes in the medical plan. The best means of deciding whether oxygen delivery is correct for the client is to pay attention to the ABG reports.

Nursing Implications: Change mask, tubing, and nebulizer every day. Check the water level in the nebulizer often for the correct amount of water. Drain tubing often to remove extra water that has formed in the tubing. This extra water will interfere with the correct amount of oxygen being delivered to the client.

Record the procedure and amount of oxygen being delivered at the beginning and end of each shift. Place "No Smoking" signs on the client's door and above the bed. If heating equipment is used, check the temperature often to prevent the client's airway from being burned.

Procedure: Performing Postural Drainage

Description: Places the client in certain positions to assist in removal of secretions from the lung. Different positions help to drain certain areas of the lung (bronchial tree). Suctioning the trachea (windpipe) or having the client cough will help to remove secretions.

Purpose: To clear secretions from the tracheobronchi (windpipe and main divisions leading to the lung) in the client having difficulty (abnormality) clearing his or her airway.

STEP	RATIONALE
1. Examine the client to determine areas of congestion (excess fullness) in the lungs. Check information recorded on the chart, including radiographic reports. Check the lungs with a stethoscope to determine areas of congestion.	Each client must be examined to determine the best position for drainage.
2. Place client in position so that the congested lung is highest. Maintain comfort and proper position with pillows.	Placing the client in the correct position allows secretions to drain from the affected area of the lung.
3. Keep client in same position for 10–15 minutes for an adult and 3–5 minutes for a child. Observe breathing.	Some clients having difficulty breathing are not able to stay in the same position for long.
4. After 10–15 minutes (adult) have client sit up and cough. If the client is unable to cough, suction trachea (windpipe).	Any secretions that collect because of the positioning should be expectorated (removed by coughing or suction) before placing the client in another position.

STEP	RATIONALE
5. After client has rested for a short time, change the client's position as needed to drain other congested areas of the lung.	A short period of rest can help to prevent fatigue (exhaustion).

Nursing Implications: Do the positioning before meals. In some cases, secretions may not be present after positioning. Some clients with fractures or severe softening of the bones may not be able to stay in all the positions required. The time for the entire procedure should not exceed 30–60 minutes.

Observe client for signs of difficulty in breathing or changes in pulse, respiratory rate, and blood pressure readings; evidence of chest pain; or complaints of discomfort, as well as any signs of not being able to stay in the position in which he or she has been placed. If any of these signs is present, stop the treatment. Have client cough secretions into a plastic container. Chart and record client's response to the procedure, including a description of the secretions.

Postural drainage is often accompanied by chest percussion (clapping the chest with cupped hands).

Procedure: Performing Percussion and Vibration (Chest Physiotherapy)

Description: Percussion involves clapping the chest with cupped hands while the client is in a postural drainage position (position that assists the congested lung area in removing secretions). Vibration involves using the flat part of the hand on the chest during exhalation (breathing out) during postural drainage.

Purpose: To help in the removal of secretions in the tracheobronchi (windpipe and major divisions leading to the lung).

STEP	RATIONALE
1. Check client for areas of lung congestion (fullness). Use information from the recorded radiographic reports and listen to the breath sounds using a stethoscope to determine which areas of the lung are congested. Do not perform procedure if the client has fractures of the ribs or any bleeding problems.	Each client must be checked to determine his or her best position for drainage.
2. Place client so that the congested lung is in the highest position.	Helps the secretions to drain from the lung.
3. Ask the client to take long, deep breaths and not to hold his or her breath.	Helps the client relax.
4. Percuss (clap chest with cupped hands) or vibrate (apply pressure on the affected lung area while the client is breathing out) for 5–7 minutes.	Helps to remove secretions from the affected areas of the lung.
5. After completion of each percussion or vibration, have client sit up and cough. If he or she is not able to cough, suctioning of the trachea (windpipe) may be required.	Helps to get rid of secretions that are a result of the treatment and helps to keep the client's airway open.

Nursing Implications: Always follow the way the ribs are moving when using vibration. Percussion (clapping) should not be painful; check with client if there is any feeling of discomfort. Observe client for any signs of breathing difficulty, changes in pulse and breathing rate, and changes in blood pressure readings. If any of these occurs, stop the treatment. Let client sit up and cough as needed.

Procedure: Bed Bath

Description: A total bath given to clients in bed who are unable to bathe themselves.

Purpose: To ensure personal cleanliness and make client comfortable; to remove secretions or excretions that have collected on the skin.

STEP	RATIONALE
1. Wash hands.	Prevents transfer of microorganisms to client's skin.
2. Collect necessary equipment: • Washcloth	Organizing necessary equipment allows quick and safe implementation.

STEP	RATIONALE

- Face towel
- Bath towel
- Cotton balls
- Clean gown
- Bath blanket
- Soap and soap dish
- Wash basin
- Bath thermometer

3. Arrange bath articles on overbed table or on top of bedside stand.
4. Draw the client's screen or curtain around bed.
5. Offer bedpan or urinal or assist client to commode or bathroom. Empty bedpan or help client back to bed.
6. Wash hands.
7. Remove spread and blanket. Discard in hamper or fold and place on chair.
8. Remove top sheet while placing bath blanket over the client. A top sheet or spread may be used if bath blanket is not available.
9. Check water with bath thermometer. Water temperature should be 115–120°F (46.1–48°C).
10. Fill wash basin two-thirds full of water.
11. Place basin on overbed table.
12. Remove the client's gown while placing bath towel over chest. Put on disposable gloves.
13. Dip cotton ball into water and squeeze out excess water. Wipe the client's eye from the inner to outer edge where the upper and lower eyelids meet. Repeat procedure for other eye, using a new cotton ball.
14. Wrap washcloth around your hand, folding extra cloth into the palm of your hand.
15. Place washcloth and your hand in wash basin. Wring out washcloth to remove excess water. Gently wash the client's face, ears, and neck, using soap if requested. Pat skin dry using towel on the client's chest.
16. Place bath towel under arm opposite from where you are. Keep bath blanket over the client's body.
17. Wash arm from shoulder to fingertips.
18. Rinse and dry each body part after washing. Cover with bath blanket.
19. Rinse washcloth and replenish soap periodically.
20. Wash, rinse, and dry axilla.
21. Place towel under arm nearest work area and repeat steps 17–20.
22. If the client wishes to wash own hands, position overbed table over the client's legs and place his or her hands in wash basin.
23. Gently wash and dry hands, especially between fingers. Check nails.
24. Place towel over chest and abdomen. Fold bath blanket to just above pubic area.
25. Wash chest and abdomen under towel. Dry, especially under the breasts of female client. Bring bath blanket back over chest and abdomen. Remove towel.
26. Remove bath blanket from leg and tuck blanket around pubic area.

Ensures privacy.
Assists in making client comfortable during the bath procedure.

Removes secretions, excretions, germ particles.
Prepares bed for changing of linen after bath is given.

Bath blanket keeps client warm and ensures privacy.

Water tends to cool rapidly. Washcloth absorbs considerable amount of heat from water.
Prevents spilling.
This keeps basin in a comfortable position for bathing client.
Prepares client for bath.

Bathes the eyes with clean water (may use clean washcloth).

Makes a wash mitt that prevents ends of cloth from hanging out.

Soap may dry facial skin. Patting skin reduces chances of harming skin than if rubbed dry.

Puts towel in place for drying area and decreases chance of contamination of arm nearest work area by nurse leaning over to reach opposite side.
Stimulates blood flow.
Removing soap decreases drying of skin. Use of bath blanket keeps client warm.
Cleans washcloth and provides more soap for bathing.

Cleanses remaining arm.

Lets client place hands in water for a refreshing handwash.

Stops moisture from collecting between fingers.
Determines whether special nail care is needed.
Ensures warmth and privacy.

Ensures warmth and privacy. Prevents moisture from collecting between skin surfaces, causing skin breakdown.

Cleanses body part farthest from work area and decreases chance of contaminating leg nearest work area by leaning over to reach opposite side. Tucking blanket around pubic area provides privacy.

STEP	RATIONALE
27. Wash leg from hip to ankle using long, firm strokes. Dry and cover with bath blanket.	Stimulates blood flow.
28. Repeat steps 26 and 27 for leg nearest work area.	
29. Place bath towel on bed. Place basin on bath towel. Uncover foot farthest from work area, place in basin, hold basin firmly.	Provides foot bath. Soaking helps soften skin and nails of foot. Helps to remove skin secretions.
30. Gently wash and dry foot, especially between toes. Check feet and toenails.	Determines whether special attention is needed.
31. Repeat steps 29 and 30 for opposite foot.	
32. Empty wash basin; rinse and fill with clean, warm water.	Removes dirty water and provides fresh, warm water.
33. Help client into a side-lying position. Keep covered with bath blanket.	Gets client ready for back wash and back rub.
34. Place towel lengthwise on bed next to the client's back. Fold bath blanket to just below buttocks.	Exposes back only; ensures privacy.
35. Wash back from shoulders to buttocks; include buttocks. Dry thoroughly; cover back, leaving buttocks uncovered.	Stimulates blood flow.
36. Rinse and apply soap on washcloth. Wash, rinse, and dry area between buttocks.	Cleanses area between buttocks. Decreases moisture collecting between skin surfaces; lessens chance of skin breakdown.
37. Help client to lie on back (supine position).	Positions client for care of genital area.
38. Empty, rinse, and refill basin with clean warm water.	Provides clean warm water after bathing between buttocks.
39. If client is able to wash genital area, position head of bed to a comfortable position. Place wash basin within reach of client. Let client complete washing, rinsing, and drying of genital area.	Allows client to wash own genital area; lessens embarrassment to the client.
40. If client cannot or does not wish to complete bath, place towel over chest and abdomen, folding back bath blanket from pubic area. Gently wash the pubic area. Wash between folds. Dry gently but thoroughly.	Reduces possible embarrassment and produces as little exposure as possible. Decreases moisture from collecting between skin surfaces, thus decreasing possible skin breakdown.
41. Reposition bath blanket over client's body. Remove towel and discard into laundry hamper.	Ensures warmth and privacy. Removes soiled towel.
42. Assist client in putting on gown.	
43. Make occupied bed.	
44. Proceed with hair, nail, and shaving needs.	See procedures for hair and nail care.
45. Raise siderails as necessary.	Ensures safety.
46. Remove soiled linens and place into laundry hamper. Remove basin; empty, rinse, replace.	Removes soiled articles from bedside. Cleans bath equipment.
47. Make sure call signal is within easy reach of client.	Enables client to call for assistance if necessary.
48. Open bedside curtains.	
49. Ensure comfort.	
50. Wash hands.	Prevents transfer of microorganisms.

Nursing Implications: Clients who need help to bathe or must be bathed by the nurse feel exposed and vulnerable. The nurse needs to be aware of the client's feelings and approach the client with a caring attitude. The bath gives the nurse the opportunity to observe the skin and body parts for any potential problems. Examination of the color of the skin may help in assessing the vascular system. By moving the extremities, the nurse may gain information about the musculoskeletal system. This procedure also provides an opportunity to establish communication with the client, as well as the opportunity to teach the client the principles of good hygiene if necessary.

Procedure: Mouth Care

Description: Mouth care is given to clients who are unable to give themselves mouth care.

Purpose: To ensure personal cleanliness for clients who have ineffective mouth care; are malnourished or dehydrated; have not had fluids by mouth for >24 hours; are continuously breathing through their mouths; have had contact with irritating chemicals; have injured the tissues in or around the mouth; or have an infection of the mouth.

STEP	RATIONALE
1. Wash hands.	Prevents transfer of microorganisms to client's skin.
2. Collect necessary equipment; place on bedside stand. (If client is up and about, place equipment near client's sink or on bedside within easy reach.)	Organizing necessary equipment allows quick and safe implementation.
• Fresh water or mouthwash	
• Cup	
• Emesis basin	
• Toothbrush	
• Toothpaste	
• Dental floss	
• Asepto bulb syringe	
• Gauze pad	
• Denture cup	
• Denture cream or powder	
• Water-soluble lubricant	
• Towel	
• Clean gloves	

Mouth Care for Conscious Client:

STEP	RATIONALE
1. Explain procedure.	Informs client of procedure.
2. Wash hands; put on clean gloves.	Prevents transfer of microorganisms.
3. Raise head of bed to sitting position.	Decreases chances of getting water into lungs.
4. Raise bed to a comfortable working position.	Decreases chances of straining nurse's back.
5. Place towel under client's chest and tuck under chin.	Protects client and linens from spillage of water.
6. Put fresh water into cup.	
7. Place toothpaste on toothbrush.	
8. Place emesis basin under chin.	Allows collection of rinse water and prevents spilling on bed linens.
9. Wrap moistened gauze pad around index finger and middle finger of hand not used in giving mouth care.	Allows gentle handling of tissues of the mouth cavity without slipping.
10. Instruct client to open mouth.	Prepares client for mouth care.

Mouth Care for Unconscious Client:

STEP	RATIONALE
1. Explain procedure to the client.	If hearing is intact, client may understand procedure.
2. Collect necessary equipment.	Organizing the equipment allows for safe and quick implementation.
3. Wash hands; put on gloves.	Decreases chances of contamination by germs.
4. Pour fresh water into cup. Fill Asepto bulb syringe with 30–50 ml of water. Place toothpaste on toothbrush. Attach suction catheter to suction source. Wrap gauze pads around tongue blade. Secure it with adhesive.	Allows for efficiency in giving care.
5. Place client on side, if not contraindicated, with head lowered.	Allows rinse water to drain from mouth to prevent swallowing or having water enter lungs.
6. Place towel under head and neck.	Protects bed linens.
7. Place suction tip under tongue or between cheek and lower jaw; if suction is unavailable, place emesis basin against cheek and neck under mouth.	Removes rinse water from mouth to prevent it from being swallowed or taken into lungs.
8. Wrap gauze pad moistened with water around index and middle fingers of hand to be used in giving mouth care.	Allows nurse to handle moist mouth tissues without slipping.
9. Insert tongue blade between upper and lower teeth; gently open jaws.	Opens jaws to let nurse examine inner surfaces of mouth and to allow insertion of toothbrush.
10. Squirt about 10 ml of water from Asepto bulb syringe into each side of the mouth. Allow rinse water to reach suction tip or drain into emesis basin.	Assists in removal of particles. Prevents water from being taken into the lungs.
11. Replace tongue blade; use moistened gauze pad around fingers and clean mouth tissues and tongue. (Special solutions may be ordered to clean the mouth. Check with team leader or head nurse.)	Removes remaining material from mouth when client is unable to eat or drink.

STEP	RATIONALE
12. Use Asepto bulb syringe to rinse mouth as necessary.	Ensures removal of remaining particles and other materials from mouth.
13. Remove emesis basin; dry mouth and chin with towel.	Prevents potential skin breakdown.
14. Place water-soluble lubricant to the lips.	Adds moisture to tissues.
15. Remove towel from under head and neck.	
16. Place client in correct alignment with head and mouth facing toward the bed for at least 15 minutes.	Prevents any remaining water from being taken into the lungs.
17. Remove, clean, rinse, and replace equipment.	Makes equipment ready for future use.
18. Remove gloves and wash hands.	Prevents transfer of microorganisms.

Mouth Care Using Floss in Conscious Client:

After Completion of Mouth Care:

STEP	RATIONALE
1. Wrap end of floss around the middle fingers of both hands. Tighten floss by stretching it with your thumbs.	Places the floss in the correct position.
2. Place the floss between upper teeth beginning at back of mouth. Slide floss back and forth between teeth from the tips of the teeth to the gum line. Continue around the mouth until all spaces between the teeth have been flossed.	Assists in removing plaque and food particles that have not been removed by brushing.
3. Use a new piece of floss and repeat steps 1 and 2 for the bottom teeth.	
4. Have client rinse mouth until returns are clear.	Completes removal of any particles.
5. Wipe face with washcloth.	Removes toothpaste and water.
6. Remove and discard rinse water. Clean and rinse emesis basin; store in proper place. Replace other equipment used.	Prepares equipment for future use. Tidies the area around client.
7. Secure call signal within reach. Place client in comfortable position.	Ensures ability to call nurse when needed.
8. Remove gloves and wash hands.	Prevents transfer of microorganisms.

Denture Care:

STEP	RATIONALE
1. Explain procedure.	Informs client of procedure.
2. Collect necessary equipment and place on overbed table within reach of client.	Organizing necessary equipment allows for quick and safe implementation.
If client is up and about, place equipment at client's sink if he or she has access to one.	Makes it convenient for the client to use.
3. Wash hands; put on gloves.	Prevents transfer of microorganisms.
4. Raise head of bed to a comfortable sitting position.	Makes it less likely for water to enter lungs.
5. Raise bed to a comfortable working position.	Decreases possibility of back strain for the nurse.
6. Place towel on chest and tuck under chin.	Protects client and bed linens from possible spillage of rinse water.
7. Position denture cup on overbed table within client's reach. Have him or her remove dentures.	Allows client to cleanse dentures.
8. If client needs assistance in removing dentures, hold upper denture with a gauze pad and gently move denture up and down until dentures are loose.	Gauze pad allows for a good grip on denture. Wiggling dentures helps break the suction between denture and gums.
9. Place denture in denture cup. Repeat step 8 for removal of lower denture.	Allows safety and security of denture.
10. Have client brush and rinse mouth in usual way.	Assists in removal of particles from mouth.
11. If client is unable to clean dentures, wrap gauze pad around fingers. Moisten with water or mouthwash.	Assists in cleaning inside the mouth.
12. Place emesis basin under client's chin.	Collects rinse water.
13. Wipe inside the mouth on all surfaces.	Removes particles.
or	
Gently brush gums, mouth, and tongue.	
14. If client cannot rinse mouth, place a suction tip under tongue and turn suction source on low.	Sucks out excess water and stops the client from swallowing water or inhaling it into the lungs.
15. Using an Asepto bulb syringe, squirt 30–50 ml of water to rinse out both sides of the mouth.	Used to help rinse out mouth.
16. Wipe dry face and chin. Remove suction tip.	Removes any spillage and helps to prevent possible skin breakdown.

STEP	RATIONALE
17. Take dentures in cup to a sink. Fill sink about one-third full of lukewarm water.	Helps to ensure safety of dentures; water acts as cushion in case dentures are dropped. Hot water may soften plastic denture material.
18. Place denture cleaning paste on toothbrush.	Denture cleaning paste is made especially for denture cleaning.
19. Remove denture from cup over water in sink. Rinse with lukewarm water.	Water in sink acts as cushion for denture if accidentally dropped.
20. Brush denture on all surfaces with toothbrush. Rinse and replace denture in cup.	Removes particles and used denture paste that may have collected on dentures.
21. Repeat steps 18–20 for remaining denture.	
22. Return dentures to client. Have client place dentures in his or her mouth.	Encourages wearing of dentures.
23. If client cannot replace dentures, place denture cream evenly over inner surface of denture.	Used to create a bond between inner surface of dentures and gums.
24. Have client open mouth, place denture on gum, and press gently to create bond between inner surface of denture and gums.	
25. Wipe and dry the client's face.	Removes any excess water and paste.
26. Place client in a comfortable position; place call signal within reach.	Leaves client comfortable and secure in knowledge that call signal can be used to call nurse if needed.
27. Clean and replace denture cup in proper place.	Denture cup is ready for next use.

Nursing Implications: Examination of the mouth helps in determining the type of mouth care to be done. If client is able to perform his or her own mouth care, then the procedure to be followed is that for a conscious client with the addition of flossing or denture care if required. Any complaints of pain, irritation, or other problems related to the oral cavity should be noted, reported, and documented. Further evaluation may be necessary. If the client does not drink or eat for more than 12–24 hours, the germs and other materials that build up could further damage the tissues in the mouth. Oil-soluble lubricants should never be used because these substances may be aspirated into the lungs, causing a specific type of pneumonia called lipid pneumonia. If the client is unconscious, a mouthwash such as hydrogen peroxide or potassium permanganate (weak antiseptics) may be used. These solutions are often part of commercially prepared mouthwashes. Check with the team leader or head nurse for specific mouth care lubricants and antiseptics.

Procedure: Nail Care

Description: Nail care includes cleaning and trimming.

Purpose: To ensure that nails are clean and trimmed and cuticles are smooth, without hangnails; to ensure that skin of hands and feet is smooth; and to examine condition of nails and surrounding skin of hands and feet.

STEP	RATIONALE
1. Wash hands.	Prevents transfer of microorganisms.
2. Collect necessary equipment: • Nail clippers or scissors • Emery board or nail file • Orange stick • Tissues • Water and soap • Small basin • Towel • Nailpolish remover	Organizing necessary equipment allows quick and safe implementation.
3. Explain procedure.	Informs client of procedure.
4. Arrange necessary equipment on bedside table or overbed table.	Organizes work area.
5. Fill basin with water about 105°F (40.5°C). For care of fingernails, place basin on overbed table; for toenails, place basin on floor covered with protective material or near client's feet on bed (cover sheet with protective material).	Temperature should be comfortable for client's hands and feet. Places basin in correct location for soaking hands and feet. Protects floor and linens from water spillage.

STEP	RATIONALE
6. Have client soak hands or feet in basin for about 15–20 minutes. Exchange water if it becomes cool.	Softens and prepares nails for trimming and cleaning.
7. Remove hand or foot, dry thoroughly, especially between fingers and toes. Remove other hand or foot from basin and repeat drying.	Prevents moisture from collecting between fingers and toes.
8. Push cuticles back gently with towel. Use nonpointed end of orange stick until cuticles are pushed back.	Prevents drying of cuticles, which prevents potential hangnails and inflammation.
9. Using orange stick or nail file, remove material that has collected under nails, wipe stick or file on tissue. Repeat until all nails are cleaned.	Removes collection of materials from under nails.
10. Remove basin.	
11. Clip or trim nails straight across. Do not cut surrounding skin.	Prevents splitting of nail margins, which can cause injury to surrounding skin.
12. File or shape fingernails with emery board. Smooth cut edges of nails.	Smooths and evens the cut edges of nails; prevents injury to surrounding skin.
13. Apply lotion to dry areas of hands and feet.	Softens and moisturizes dry skin.
14. Place the client in a comfortable position. Place call signal in client's reach.	Ensures comfort and safety.
15. Empty and clean basin. Store in appropriate place.	Prepares equipment for next use.
16. Wash hands.	Prevents transfer of microorganisms.

Nursing Implications: Record nail care. Report any unexpected problems to team leader or head nurse.

Procedure: Care of the Hair

Description: Combing or brushing the hair is considered part of the client's bath. The nurse is responsible for care of the client's hair if he or she is unable to care for it. Shampooing the hair is done by the nurse as needed.

Purpose: To keep the client's hair clean, fresh smelling, and arranged in a neat, attractive manner that is satisfying to the client.

STEP	RATIONALE
1. Collect necessary equipment for combing and brushing or shampooing hair: • Comb, brush, or pick • Shampoo, conditioner, moisturizer • Towels, washcloth • Mirror • Shampoo tray • Bath thermometer • Plastic sheet • Basin for discarding rinse water • Hairdryer, if available	Organizing necessary equipment allows for quick and safe implementation.

Combing and Brushing Hair:

1. Explain procedure.	Informs client of procedure; gains cooperation.
2. Wash hands.	Prevents transfer of microorganisms.
3. Place client's bed in an upright position or place client upright in chair. Place a mirror in front of client.	Position is convenient for the nurse and prevents back strain.
4. Put a clean towel around client's shoulders.	Keeps stray hairs from falling on client's clothes.
5. If hair is straight or slightly curly, comb hair from scalp to the ends of hair. Gently use the comb's teeth or brush bristles against the scalp.	Separates and smooths hair strands. Stimulates scalp.
6. For tangled hair, hold ends near scalp with hand and gently comb through tangled hair one section at a time.	Prevents pulling of hair follicles.
7. Arrange hair the way the client likes it. Use combs or rubber bands for long hair.	Makes the client comfortable with her or his appearance. Keeps long hair in place.

STEP	RATIONALE
8. If approved by client, braid hair, especially if client is bed-bound.	Prevents tangling.
9. If hair is tight and curly, remove tangles using fingers to free strands. Place fingers in hair and spread fingers apart.	Loosens tangles.
10. Divide hair into sections. Use a wide-toothed comb or pick for freeing tangles, beginning at ends and working toward scalp.	Makes it easier to free tangles close to scalp.
11. Brush hair from scalp to ends.	Makes client comfortable with his or her appearance.
12. Apply hair products as client desires if not contraindicated by client's condition.	
13. Remove towel; place in laundry hamper. Remove collected hair and hair products.	
14. Clean comb, brush, or pick. Place in client's bedside stand.	Prepares equipment for future use. Tidies client's immediate area.
15. Position client in a comfortable position. Secure call signal bell within easy reach.	Makes client feel comfortable and secure in ability to call nurse if needed.
16. Wash hands.	Decreases possibility of transfer of germs.

Shampooing the Hair:

STEP	RATIONALE
1. Explain procedure.	Informs client of procedure.
2. Collect necessary equipment; wash hands.	Organizing necessary equipment allows for quick and safe implementation. Handwashing prevents transfer of microorganisms.

For Client in Bed:

STEP	RATIONALE
3. Place bed in a flat position. Raise bed to comfortable working position. Place client on back near working position.	Places client with head down and keeps water from the client's face while the hair is washed and rinsed. Raising the bed and positioning client on side of bed nearest working area help to prevent back strain.
4. Place a plastic sheet covered with towel or sheet under client's head, neck, and shoulders.	Protects bed, linens, and client.
5. Position client's head on shampoo tray. Use folded washcloth or small towel between client's neck and rim of tray. Cover client's eyes with small towel.	Prepares client for shampoo. Protects neck muscles and underlying blood vessels and nerves from pressure against rim of tray. Protects eyes from water spillage and shampoo.
6. Place basin under tray drain.	Basin used for draining rinse water.
7. Fill pitcher with water at a temperature of about 105°F (40.5°C).	Water temperature of 105°F (40.5°C) prevents potential injury to scalp.
8. Wet hair with water. Distribute water through hair with fingers.	Allows for even distribution of water through hair.
9. Put small amount of shampoo in palm of hand. Make a lather by rubbing hands together.	Lather allows for even distribution of suds through hair.
10. Lather client's hair. Massage scalp lightly using tips of fingers in a circular motion.	Allows thorough distribution of suds through hair. Massage assists in circulation of blood to scalp and stimulates natural hair oils, which moisturize and aid hair growth.
11. Remove excess shampoo. Rinse with clean water, using pitcher. **NOTE:** Use hand-held spray, if available.	Removes excess shampoo, dirt, and other particles. Any shampoo remaining on hair is potentially irritating and may cause dryness of the scalp.
12. Repeat steps 9–11.	Ensures cleanliness of hair.
13. Wrap large bath towel around client's head. For clients in bed, remove shampoo tray. Dry hair by massaging with towel.	Removes excess moisture from hair. Prevents accidental spills.
14. Position another towel around client's shoulders. Remove towel from head. Place towel in laundry hamper.	Prepares client for completion of hair grooming.
15. Comb hair; be careful in removing tangles. If available, use hairdryer.	Hairdryer allows for speedier drying and prevents chilling.
16. Comb and arrange hair in manner requested by client.	Ensures comfort.
17. Remove towel, plastic sheet, and cover. Discard in an appropriate manner.	Keeps client's environment neat.
18. Wash hands.	Prevents transfer of microorganisms.

STEP	RATIONALE
For Client in Tub or Shower:	
19. Repeat previous steps 1 and 2.	
20. Place washcloth or small towel over client's eyes.	Prevents water and shampoo from getting into eyes.
21. Test water temperature.	Ensures that water is not too hot or too cold.
22. Rinse hair with clean water after bath is completed. Use clean warm water at about 105°F (40.5°C) temperature. (If available, use hand-held spray instead of pitcher.)	Prepares hair for even distribution of shampoo. Prevents burning scalp.
23. Repeat previous steps 9–18.	
For Client Sitting in Chair:	
24. Place chair so that it faces away from bathroom sink.	Places chair in best position for shampooing client's hair.
25. Assist client to sit in chair.	
Place towel around shoulders.	Protects client's bedclothes from accidental spillage of water.
26. Help client to hyperextend head and neck by putting head back as far as possible.	Places the client in a position for water draining from hair to drain into sink.
Place folded washcloth or small towel between neck and rim of sink. Place washcloth or small towel over eyes.	Prevents pressure on neck muscles, blood vessels, and nerves, thereby decreasing potential for injury. Prevents water and shampoo from entering eyes.
27. Make sure that water temperature is about 105°F (40.5°C).	Decreases potential to burn scalp.
28. Wet hair thoroughly.	Wetting hair strands helps to distribute shampoo.
29. Repeat previous steps 9–18.	Completes procedure.

Nursing Implications: Examine condition of hair and scalp. Determine whether there is any irritation, injury, or dryness of scalp. Report and document any problems. If hair and scalp are dry, request physician's order for special hair preparation if necessary. Use dry hair formula shampoo and rinse with conditioner. Request that hair shampooing be done less frequently.

Use cream rinse or an oil preparation, if available, to loosen tangles and snarls. Do not cut hair unless permission is received to do so. If a regular shampooing is not possible, see if a dry shampoo is available for use.

Procedure: Eye Care

Description: Cleansing of the eyes of clients is part of the bath when eye pathology is present, and includes cleansing of eyeglasses or care of contact lenses.

Purpose: To remove foreign particles, including microorganisms, from the eye; to give proper care to eyeglasses and contact lenses.

STEP	RATIONALE
1. Collect necessary equipment:	Organizing necessary equipment allows for quick and safe implementation.
• Fresh tap water or sterile water or saline	
• Sterile cotton balls or gauze pad	
• Small clean or sterile basin	
• Tissue wipes	
• Clean towel	
• Sterile lubricant and preparation prescribed by physician	
• Eyedropper (optional)	
• Cleansing solution and papers for lens	
• Contact lens suction cup	
Eye Cleansing:	
1. As part of bath, encourage client to wash eyes. If client is not able, explain procedure.	Gives client a sense of independence for own care. Prepares client for procedure.
2. Place required equipment on bedside table. Place bedside table next to bed for easy access to equipment by nurse.	Prepares for procedure.
3. Wash hands. Put on disposable gloves.	Prevents transfer of microorganisms.
4. Raise the bed to a comfortable working position.	Prevents back strain.
5. Place client in sitting position. Place pillow behind shoulders to allow client's head to fall backward and eyes and face to lift upward (hyperextension of neck).	Ensures comfort.

STEP	RATIONALE
6. Place towel over client's chest and under chin.	Prevents solution from dripping on bedclothes; towel is in position when needed.
7. Pour a small amount of water into basin.	Prepares client for cleansing.
8. Dip cotton ball or gauze into water and remove excess water.	Wets the cotton ball or gauze. Prevents excess water from dripping on client's clothes or bed linens.
9. Gently wipe eye from inner portion (inner canthus) of eye to outer portion (outer canthus) with cotton ball or sponge.	Prevents particles or secretions from entering lacrimal sac (tear duct), which is located in the inner canthus.
10. Repeat step 10 with other eye using clean cotton ball or sponge.	Prevents contamination from first eye.
11. If crusts or secretions are present, moisten gauze pad and place over closed eyes.	Softens and loosens crusts.
12. Leave gauze pads in place until crusts are softened. Remove and discard sponges.	Assists in removal of crusts.
13. If client is unconscious:	
• Lower siderails.	
• Raise eyelids; instill "artificial tears," if ordered. Gently pull lower eyelid downward to instill eyedrops in order not to injure the eyeball (cornea).	
• Moistens eyes. Unconscious clients lack the "blink reflex" and are unable to moisten eyeball.	
14. Close eyelids. Place eyepad over eyes and tape in position.	Protects eye from foreign particles that may injure the eye. Taping pad in position prevents eyes from opening further, thus protecting the eyes from injury as the blink reflex is absent.
15. Lower bed. Place client in a comfortable position. Raise siderails as necessary.	Ensures safety and comfort.
16. Wash hands.	Decreases chances of transfer of microorganisms.

Care of Eyeglasses:

STEP	RATIONALE
1. Collect necessary equipment.	Organizing necessary equipment allows for quick and safe implementation.
2. Wash hands.	Prevents transfer of microorganisms.
3. Ask client to remove glasses. If client is unable to remove glasses, explain procedure. Take hold of both earpieces above ears. Lift eyeglass frame up and out from ears. Move glasses down and away from face.	Allows for feeling of independence. Avoids pulling at client's ears; prevents twisting or bending eyeglass frames.
4. Examine the eyeglass lenses for any scratches or damage.	Determines condition of lenses and the amount of cleansing needed.
5. Wash and rinse lenses with slightly warm (tepid) water or cleansing solution. (Never use warm or hot water.)	Removes smudges, body oils. Use of very warm or hot water may soften and distort plastic frames.
6. Hold glasses by earpieces without twisting frame. Be careful not to drop glasses.	Prevents damage to frames or lenses.
7. Dry lenses with clean tissue or lens tissue. (Do not use rough material in wiping glasses or touch lenses with fingers.)	Prevents scratching of lens.
8. Fold frame and place in eyeglass case. Place in drawer of bedside table. If case not available, place eyeglasses between tissues; do not place glasses on any surface with lenses facing down.	Prevents accidental damage. Protects eyeglasses from smudging.
9. Cleanse eyes, if necessary, after eye-cleansing procedure (steps 1–16 under Eye Cleansing).	
10. Remove glasses from case or tissues; unfold frames.	
11. Hold eyeglass frames by both earpieces.	Prepares eyeglasses for placement over client's eyes.
12. Place earpieces just above each ear in correct position and nosepiece of frame over bridge of nose.	Prevents bending or twisting of frames. Prevents hitting client's face with earpieces.
13. Check to see whether glasses are in the correct position. Check with client as to whether glasses are in a comfortable position.	Places frames correctly.
14. Repeat steps 15 and 16 under Eye Cleansing.	

STEP	RATIONALE
Care of Contact Lenses (may differ with type of contact lenses):	
1. Collect necessary equipment.	Organizing necessary equipment allows for quick and safe implementation.
2. Ask client to remove lenses.	Prevents possible injury to eye.
3. If client is unable to remove lenses, then wash hands and separate upper and lower eyelids with thumbs.	Makes contact lens visible.
4. Gently push upper eyelid to the top edge of the lens. Hold upper lid in place by pressing against upper bony portion under eyebrow. Press lower lid against contact lens. *or* Use special lens suction cup. Attach cup on lens and remove lens.	Loosens lens from eye (cornea) by breaking the suction.
5. Catch lens in clean washcloth and store in correct lens container.	Prevents lens from falling out of view.
6. Repeat steps 3–5 for removal of remaining contact lens.	
7. Take lens container to sink. Close drain and fill with about 2 or 3 inches of water.	Provides cushion of water to catch lens if it accidentally falls.
8. Hold one lens between thumb and index finger over water. Squeeze a small amount of lens cleanser on each side of lens. Spread cleanser evenly over lens with finger.	Cleans and lubricates lens.
9. Rinse lens with tap or distilled water. Place in correct lens container.	Rinses cleanser from lens. Protects lens.
10. Repeat steps 8 and 9 for remaining lens.	
11. Cleanse client's eyes, if necessary.	See steps 1–16 under Eye Cleansing.
Reinsertion of Lenses:	
1. Remove one lens from container; hold between thumb and index finger.	Prepares lens for reinsertion.
2. Apply a drop of lens-wetting solution to inside of lens.	Moistens lens and creates correct amount of suction when lens is placed over eyeball (cornea).
3. Hold outside of lens in tip of index finger and place it gently over iris (colored portion of eye) and pupil.	Positions lens correctly.
4. Repeat steps 1–3 for replacement of remaining contact lens.	
5. Repeat steps 15 and 16 under Eye Cleansing.	

Nursing Implications: Record procedure. Report any unusual observations such as inflammation, redness, tearing, and swelling. Check whether pupils respond normally to light. Check to see if eyes move together. Watch for excessive secretions and for crusts, and note color of secretions. Report any client complaints such as irritation, burning, pain, or dryness, as well as any problems with eyeglasses or contact lenses.

Procedure: Applying Restraints

Description: Special devices are used to immobilize client or extremities (arms or legs). A physician's order is necessary.

Purpose: To prevent unwanted movement when giving certain treatments, when client is restless or confused; to control client from harming himself or herself or others; and to assist the client to support posture.

Use of Jacket or Vest: Prevents client from falling out of bed or chair; secures client but allows some freedom of movement

Use of Mitt: Prevents client from scratching skin and allows greater freedom than use of wrist restraint

Use of Wrist or Ankle Restraint: Prevents client from moving arm or leg when intravenous (IV) line or other devices are in place

Use of Belt Restraint: Prevents client from falling out of bed or stretcher

Use of Infant Restraint: Immobilizes infant while a treatment procedure is being done

STEP	RATIONALE

1. Collect necessary equipment.
  • Restraints: vest or jacket; safety wrist or ankle mitt; belt; blanket or sheet
  • Safety pins
  • Foam or cotton padding
  • Rolled bandage
	Organizing necessary equipment allows for quick and safe implementation.

Application of Vest or Jacket:

STEP	RATIONALE
1. Explain procedure.	Informs client of procedure and reason for restraint.
2. Using the vest, place client's arms through armholes. Check that overlapping vest pieces are to the front of client's body.	Places vest to allow for some movement but limits freedom.
3. Overlap front body pieces. Place ties through slots and loops on side of vest.	Secures vest restraint.

Applying Restraints:

STEP	RATIONALE
1. Criss-cross ties over front of vest.	Secures vest restraint.

For Client in Bed:

STEP	RATIONALE
2. Take ties and secure to the bed frame (movable part). Make a half-bow knot.	Secures vest restraint. Prevents tightness when bed is raised or lowered or when client moves. Half-bow knot makes it easier to untie vest from bed in an emergency.
3. Examine client and restraint.	Prevents injury and ensures client's safety.

For Client in Chair:

STEP	RATIONALE
4. Follow steps above up to and including step 1 under Applying Restraints.	
5. Cross vest straps behind chair seat and lower legs. Make sure that left strap is tied to right leg of chair, and right strap is tied to left leg of chair.	Secures client to chair
6. Follow step 3.	

Applying a Mitt Restraint:

STEP	RATIONALE
1. Explain procedure.	Informs client of procedure and reason for restraint.
2. Using a rolled bandage, place client's fingers around bandage.	Places client's fingers in a natural position to prevent strain on muscles and joints.
3. Place the client's hand into the mitt. Tie wrist ties.	Secures mitt to hand and wrist.
4. Tie ends of ties to movable part of bed frame and complete by using a half-bow tie.	Prevents tightness when bed is raised or lowered. Half-bow tie makes it easier to release restraint in case of an emergency.
5. Check client and restraint.	Prevents possible injury and ensures client's safety.

Application of Wrist or Ankle Restraint:

STEP	RATIONALE
1. Explain procedure.	Informs client of procedure and reason for restraint.
2. Place cotton or foam padding around wrist or ankle.	Protects skin by decreasing pressure against skin and by decreasing potential for skin breakdown.
3. Place wrist or ankle restraint around padding.	

Application of Restraint:

STEP	RATIONALE
4. Pull tie through opening on side of restraint.	Secures restraint on body part.
5. Attach end of tie to movable part of bed frame and tie with half-bow.	Prevents tightness when bed is raised or lowered. Prevents possible injury. Half-bow tie allows for easy release of restraint when necessary.
6. Examine client and restraint carefully.	Ensures safety.

Belt Restraint:

STEP	RATIONALE
1. Explain procedure.	Informs client of procedure and reason for restraint.
2. Place client in supine position (lying on back).	Prepares client for application of restraint.
3. Position the long part of belt under the client. Tie ends of belt to movable part of bed.	Attachment of belt to frame before securing belt to client helps to prevent problems when attaching belt to client.

STEP	RATIONALE
4. Take shorter part of belt and place it around client's waist. Secure ends of belt.	Secures restraint.
5. Examine client and restraint.	Ensures safety.

Infant Restraint:

STEP	RATIONALE
1. Explain procedure to family or significant others.	Informs family or significant others of procedure and reason for restraint.
2. Lay blanket or sheet on bed or other flat surface.	Prepares infant for restraint.
3. Fold down top corner of blanket, making sure tip is on the center of blanket.	Prepares restraint for infant's head.
4. Place infant on back (supine position) on blanket with head lying midway on the folded corner.	Prepares infant for restraint.
5. Fold one side corner of blanket over infant and tuck it under body just below axilla (armpit).	Restrains infant.
6. Repeat step 5 using remaining side corner of blanket.	
7. Raise the infant and fold bottom corner under body.	Completes restraint procedure.
8. Check infant and restraint.	Ensures safety.

Nursing Implications: Check client's behavior before, during, and after application of restraints. Record procedure and reasons for same. Indicate type of restraint, status of client, and any problems or complications that may have occurred. Report to team leader or head nurse.

Check the pulse, temperature, and skin color of extremities of restrained client. Check for ability of movement. If abnormal, may be sign of pressure on the nervous and vascular systems. Restraints must be loosened, and range of motion (ROM) performed, every 2 hours. Client must be checked every 30 minutes or per hospital policy.

Know the policies of the institution in regard to use of restraints. **The use of restraints requires a physician's order.** If client is confused or disoriented, use of restraints may be justified. However, use of inappropriate restraints or improper attachment of restraints may be considered imprisonment.

Procedure: Perineal Care

Description: In perineal care, the perineal area is cleansed in clients who are unable to bathe themselves.

Purpose: To ensure personal cleanliness, remove secretions from the urethra, vagina, and anus for clients who are unconscious or helpless or need special hygienic measures.

STEP	RATIONALE
1. Collect necessary equipment: • Bath blanket • Wash basin and water • Washcloth and towels • Soap • Bath thermometer • Plastic sheet • Toilet tissue • Clean gloves • Pitcher	Organizing necessary equipment allows for quick and safe implementation.
2. Explain procedure. State steps in a manner that does not embarrass client.	Informs client of procedure. Reassures client.
3. Obtain water; check temperature. Arrange equipment on overbed table. Have pitcher and wash basin with warm water.	Ensures warmth of water. Organizes work area.
4. Close curtains around client's bed. Close door to room.	Ensures privacy.
5. If client is conscious, check whether bedpan is needed. Give bedpan, if necessary; remove and discard urine appropriately; then clean and replace bedpan in proper place.	Ensures emptying of bladder before procedure.
6. Wash hands; put on clean gloves.	Prevents transfer of microorganisms.

STEP	RATIONALE
7. Raise bed to proper working position using proper body mechanics.	Prevents back strain.
8. If siderail is up, lower it on working side of bed and help client to a supine (back-lying) position.	Places client in position for the procedure.
9. Remove top covers while placing bath blanket over client. Pull top covers to bottom of bed, leaving bath blanket over client. Fold bed covers and place on chair.	Covers client for privacy.
10. Place plastic sheet covered with bed linen under client.	Protects bottom sheet and mattress.
11. Fold bath towel and place under hips. Place bedpan under buttocks.	Raises hips slightly so that perineal area is in correct position.
12. Flex client's knees and hips. Have client move, or move client's legs, so that toes point outward and heels inward (rotate legs toward the outside).	Positions perineal area correctly for perineal care.
13. Move the bath blanket so that the corners form a diamond. (Top corner points toward head of bed; two side corners point down each side of bed; lower corner drapes over client's legs.)	Covers client's body and legs, provides warmth, and protects privacy.
14. Wrap two side corners around client's legs and place corner under hips.	Prepares client for perineal care.
15. Place washcloth into basin of warm water, apply soap, and wring out excess water.	Prepares client for bathing.
16. Raise corner of blanket from between client's legs and place corner toward client's head.	Exposes perineal area only.
17. Wash and rinse upper thighs. Dry thoroughly.	Removes secretions from area near perineal area.

For the Female Client:

STEP	RATIONALE
1. Follow steps 1–17.	
2. Rinse washcloth and reapply soap. Wash labia majora (top outer part of the perineal area), moving the washcloth from front to back (anus). Do not wash over area that has already been washed. Redo procedure, if necessary, using clean washcloth, soap and water.	Bathes from the area of the least germs and secretions (the urethra, or opening from the bladder) to that of the most (the anus). Prevents contamination of urethra by germs from the anus. Decreases possibility of infection.
3. Rinse washcloth. Do not reapply soap. Spread labia majora (outer perineal area) with hand not being used to bathe perineal area.	Prevents irritation of sensitive tissues.
4. Wash the labia minora (inner perineal area) with a corner of washcloth, moving washcloth down toward the anus. Rinse. Use a fresh corner for each area. If client is menstruating or has a catheter in place, use cotton balls to clean the inner labia.	Prevents contamination of the labia with germs and secretions from other parts of perineal area.
5. Pour pitcher of warm water over perineal area. Remove bedpan when rinse is completed.	Rinses soap, water, germs, and secretions from perineum.
6. Dry perineal area gently but thoroughly. Apply dusting powder lightly.	Prevents moisture collection and growth of germs. Decreases possibility of infection. Use of powder (lightly) helps in absorbing moisture and prevents irritation caused by contact of two skin surfaces.
7. Remove towel pad from under hips. Position client on side with his or her back toward working area.	Prepares for bathing the anal area.
8. Inspect space between buttocks; remove any excretions with toilet tissue, if present.	Prevents possible contamination of wash water and surrounding skin.
9. Wash between buttocks, especially around the anus. Dry thoroughly. Apply powder lightly.	Decreases possibility of infection by removing secretions and germs.
10. Remove plastic sheet and cover. Place client in a comfortable position and replace top covers. Remove bath blanket. Place call signal in easy reach.	Disposes of used linens. Ensures comfort. Allows client to call nurse if necessary.
11. Place used linens in laundry hamper. Wash, rinse, dry, and replace equipment in proper place.	Disposes of contaminated linen. Prepares equipment for future use.
12. Discard gloves and wash hands.	Limits transfer of germs.

STEP	RATIONALE
For the Male Client:	
1. Follow steps 1–17.	
2. Raise and place towel under penis. Hold penis and move foreskin from tip of penis, if present, downward. Wash the area exposed, beginning with the tip of the penis and moving to the area to which the foreskin has been moved. Replace foreskin.	Protects scrotum and bed linens. Removes secretions and germs that may have collected under foreskin. Prevents contamination of the urethra with germs on the remainder of the penis.
3. Rinse and resoap washcloth; wash remainder of penis, using downward strokes.	Bathes remainder of penis.
4. Rinse, resoap, and wash the scrotum, especially between the folds of skin. Dry thoroughly.	Removes germs and moisture that may cause infection. Completes procedure.
5. Follow steps 5–11 under For the Female Client.	

Nursing Implications: Record procedure. Report and record any unusual findings or problems. Report and document any complaints of itching, pain, or discomfort. For female clients, check, report, and record any vaginal, urethral, or anal discharge or odor. Discharge, odor, or both may be signs of infection.

Report and record any signs of incontinence of urine or stool. If client has had perineal surgery, check for, report, and record amount, color, and odor of drainage, if present. Such drainage requires frequent assessment and perineal care to prevent irritation and infection.

Procedure: Handwashing

Description: Hands are washed correctly before and after performing any procedure.

Purpose: To limit transfer of microorganisms.

STEP	RATIONALE
1. Collect necessary equipment: • Soap • Running water • Clean towel or sterile towel	Organizing necessary equipment allows for quick and safe implementation.
2. Check hands for any skin breaks. If present, use clean sterile gloves to prevent contamination.	Prevents contamination.
3. Remove all hand jewelry except smooth-surfaced rings.	Prevents microorganisms from collecting in and under jewelry.
4. Slide watchband up arm.	Wrist needs to be washed to remove any germs that may have collected under watchband.
5. Stand in front of sink without touching sink surfaces.	Prevents back strain. Prevents contamination of uniform with organisms on sink surface.
6. Use a paper towel to turn on water faucet. Adjust flow and temperature. Use elbow, knee, or foot pedal, if available.	Prevents contamination of hands. Prevents hot water from injuring skin.
7. Wet lower arms, wrists, and hands, holding them under running water with fingers pointing downward.	Water flows from the area of least contamination (lower arms) to area of greatest contamination (fingertips).
8. Apply soap and produce a lather. If bar soap is used, rinse bar under running water before placing soap in soap dish.	Removes any microorganisms before use by another person.
9. Rub hands together using a back-and-forth and circular motion; cover all parts of hands, including fingers, area between fingers, palm, back of hand, and wrists. Continue procedure for about 3 minutes unless there is a potential for a greater risk of contamination; then continue washing hands for up to 3 minutes more.	Exposes hands and wrists to soap and water, including areas between fingers.
10. Rinse hands under running water with fingers pointing downward.	Soapy water flows downward from area of least contamination to area of greatest contamination.
11. Dry hands from fingers to wrist to lower arms with a paper towel. Use a clean, dry towel for each hand.	Dries skin from the cleanest area to the dirtiest. Removes moisture and prevents chapping.
12. Discard towel. Turn off water. Use a clean paper towel to close water flow if hand controls are used.	Prevents contamination of hands.

Nursing Implications: Routine handwashing is not usually recorded or reported. Check whether hands are dry or chapped; may need to use hand creams or other softening agents. Check for any cuts or abrasions or infection. Report same. Check whether client has any signs of infection. Report signs and symptoms to team leader or head nurse. Record same. Handwashing should be performed before and after caring for each client.

Procedure: Surgical Asepsis

Description: These methods establish and maintain sterility.

Purpose: To produce a relatively sterile field in order to remove harmful organisms from skin surfaces by washing, scrubbing, and disinfection; to create a sterile field using sterile protective clothing and sterile equipment, depending on type of sterile field required.

STEP	RATIONALE
1. Collect necessary supplies and equipment: • Antiseptic detergent • Scrub brushes • Orange stick • Sterile cap, gown, and mask • Sterile gloves • Sterile packages • Sterile solution	Organizing necessary supplies and equipment allows quick and safe implementation.

Surgical Hand Scrub:

STEP	RATIONALE
1. Remove all jewelry.	Prevents microorganisms from collecting on and under jewelry.
2. Examine hands for any skin breaks.	Check to see if other procedures may be necessary to protect nurse from possible exposure to harmful organisms.
3. Put on scrub clothes or make sure mid-upper arms are not covered.	Prepares for procedure.
4. Put on face mask.	Prevents organisms from mouth and nose from contaminating sterile field.
5. Turn on and adjust water flow and temperature using foot or knee controls.	Prepares for hand scrub.
6. Wet one arm thoroughly from upper arm to fingertips. Repeat with other arm. Keep arms bent with hands above elbows. Point fingers downward.	Allows water to drip from dirtiest part (fingers).
7. Lather hands with antiseptic detergent to above elbows.	Covers hands and arms with lather.
8. Use orange stick to clean under fingernails; rinse stick and fingers under running water.	Removes collected material and organisms from under nails.
9. Rinse each arm from fingertips to above elbows.	Allows lather and organisms to drain.
10. Reapply detergent and repeat step 9.	
11. Scrub each hand with brush, using a back-and-forth motion for about 45 seconds.	Friction along with action of detergent loosens and removes material and microorganisms from skin.
12. Scrub upper arms above elbows for 15–20 seconds.	Moves from the dirtiest area (hands) to the cleanest (upper arm).
13. Scrub lower arm thoroughly for 45 seconds.	
14. Dispose of brush. Rinse arms and hands from upper arms to fingertips. Keep arms bent so fingertips are above elbows.	Allows for water to drain from cleanest area (hands) toward arm.
15. Use second brush and scrub each hand for 1 minute.	Extra scrubbing allows removal of remaining organisms.
16. Discard brush and repeat step 14.	
17. Using knee or foot control, turn off water. Keep fingertips above elbows.	Holding hands and fingers up decreases chances of touching any surfaces.
18. Keep arms elevated; dry one hand and arm with a sterile towel by patting it dry. Discard towel. Repeat step for other hand and arm.	Patting prevents unnecessary injury to skin surfaces that may be irritated by detergent and scrubbing action.

Putting on Sterile Cap:

STEP	RATIONALE
1. Using the correct-size cap, separate elastic band with hands. Pull cap over back of head so that elastic band is below earlobes.	Allows good fit and complete coverage of hair.
2. Make sure that cap completely covers all hair.	Prevents contamination of sterile field by hairs.

STEP	RATIONALE

Putting on a Face Mask:
1. Choose a face mask. Locate top. Hold mask by the top two strings and place over face with nose strip over nose.

   Keeps clean the part of the mask that covers nose and mouth.
2. Place top strings or loops over the top of ears. Tie strings behind head or slip loops over ears.

   Prevents contamination of the mask; secures mask in place.
3. If mask has strings (not loops), tie bottom strings behind neck so that lower edge of mask is under chin.

   Makes edges of mask fit against face. Helps prevent escape of organisms from mouth and nose.
4. Make sure plastic or metal bridge (if present) is placed over bridge of nose and that mouth and nose are completely covered.

   Prevents escape of organisms from mouth and nose.

Putting on Sterile Gown:
1. Pick up gown, hold inside of neck surface. Hold gown away from body.

   Prevents contamination of outside of gown, keeping it sterile.
2. Lift gown so that it does not touch floor. Let gown unfold by holding inside neck surface with both hands. Do not touch outside of gown.
3. Open gown so that inside shoulder seams are visible.
4. Place one hand through armhole while holding inside neck surface with other hand. Place other hand through armhole.
5. Raise arm upward; place arms into sleeves.

   Allows placement of sleeves on arms without contaminating outside of gown.
6. Have another worker pull inside back of gown toward back so that back edges of gown overlap. Have worker tie neck ties.

   Keeps outside of gown sterile, and secures gown in position. Prevents touching of outside of gown.
7. Have worker tie waistband securely.

Putting on Sterile Gloves:
1. Open glove package by pulling apart the sides of package.
2. Remove inner package and place on clean surface.
3. Open package by touching only the corners.

   Prevents contamination of gloves and inside of package.
4. Check for right and left gloves; pick up inside cuff with the nondominant hand (the one you use less than the other).

   Prevents touching of outside of sterile glove. Inside of glove now contaminated.
5. Slip the other hand inside glove, making sure that thumb and fingers are lined up with the glove thumb and fingers. Do not touch outside of glove.
6. Push hand into glove, pulling the inside cuff with thumb and index finger of the nondominant hand. Make sure that only the inside of glove is touched.
7. Using the gloved hand, slip fingers under cuff of remaining glove and slip nondominant hand inside glove.

   Contamination of glove is prevented by using sterile gloved hand to put on second glove.
8. Push nondominant hand inside glove. With the gloved hand under the cuff, pull glove over nondominant hand.

   Prevents contamination of outside of gloved hand.
9. Interlock fingers of hands (place fingers of one hand between fingers of other hand).

   Allows free movement of fingers and thumb.

Opening a Sterile Package:
1. Collect necessary equipment.

   Organizing necessary equipment allows for quick and safe implementation.
2. Check label for contents, expiration date, and any instructions.

   Checks sterility of package.
3. Place package on clean surface at waist level.

   Places package in good working position.
4. Break seal, touching only edge of package. Open one flap away from you. Do not bend over package.

   Prevents contamination of inside of package. Prevents airborne dust particles from contaminating inside of package.
5. Open side flap, let fall flat on surface. Repeat same with other side flap.
6. Lift flap nearest you; open flap toward you and let it fall flat on surface.

STEP	RATIONALE
Pouring Sterile Liquid:	
1. Open sterile set. Locate empty sterile container.	
2. Open sterile solution bottle or package. Set cap or lid with the inside up on a clean surface.	Prevents inside bottle or cap from contamination.
3. Pick up bottle, holding it with label inside palm of hand.	Protects label from drainage while pouring solution.
4. Pour a small amount of solution into a disposable receptacle. (Do not touch disposable receptacle with bottle lip.) Discard solution in disposable receptacle.	Washes bottle lip with solution that is to be discarded.
5. Pour appropriate amount of solution into sterile container. Do not touch lip of bottle to sterile container. Avoid splashing and dripping solution on sterile field.	Prevents contamination of sterile field.
6. Place solution bottle on clean surface and replace cap.	Prevents microorganisms in air from entering solution bottle.

Nursing Implications: Check to see whether client has signs or symptoms or diagnosis of an infection. Report and record any signs of redness, pain, swelling, drainage, increased temperature, or elevated white blood count. Such signs may indicate that both nurse and client require protection from contamination.

Any break in surgical asepsis is considered dangerous. Change protective clothing and equipment if they become contaminated.

Procedure: Protective Asepsis

Description: This method controls infection for the protection of the client, health-care personnel, and any other people who may be exposed to the infection.

Purpose: Depending on the way the infection enters the body, to provide protection for the person(s) who get the disease and for those who come in contact with one who has the disease.

Category-Specific Precautions

Strict Isolation: Provides methods to prevent transmission of highly contagious infectious diseases that are spread through air or by direct contact. Examples include smallpox, chickenpox, and measles.

Respiratory Isolation: Provides methods to prevent transmission of diseases that are spread over short distances, such as particles or droplets containing the disease agent that are transferred through the air. Examples include many of the childhood diseases.

Contact Isolation: Provides methods to prevent transmission of highly contagious diseases that are spread by close or direct contact but that do not require strict isolation. Examples include impetigo, burn infections, and acute respiratory infections in infants and children.

Tuberculosis (TB) Isolation: Provides methods to prevent transmission of the tubercle bacillus, which is the infectious agent of TB. Method of isolation is specific for clients who have pulmonary (lung) TB as diagnosed by sputum smear or chest radiograph.

Drainage or Secretion Precautions: Provide methods of preventing direct or indirect contact with infected material or fluid draining from an infected site in the body. Examples include abscesses, infected burns, wounds, and pressure sores.

Blood or Body Fluid Precautions: Provide methods to prevent direct or indirect transfer of infectious agents through contact with blood or other body fluids. Examples include acquired immunodeficiency syndrome (AIDS), hepatitis B, syphilis, and gonorrhea.

Enteric Isolation Precautions: Provide methods to prevent transfer of infectious agents that are spread through direct or indirect contact with feces. Examples include cholera, viral hepatitis A, and gastroenteritis.

Standard Precautions: All nurses should use standard precautions at all times when caring for clients.

STEP	RATIONALE

1. Collect necessary equipment:
  • Protective face mask
  • Protective gown and gloves
  • Disposable dishes and eating utensils
  • Isolation cart
  • Plastic or special disposable laundry or trash bags
	Organizing necessary equipment allows for quick and safe implementation.

Isolation Room Preparation:	
1. Explain procedure. Include significant others in discussion.	Informs client of procedure and reason for use. Gains cooperation.
2. Use private room for isolation, if available. Equipment in room should include:	Provides a unit with necessary equipment for isolation.

STEP	RATIONALE

- Sink in room
- Adjoining private bathroom
- Rack to hang reusable gowns, if needed
3. Collect supplies to be kept in room:
   - Single-use antiseptic soap
   - Laundry hamper (considered dirty)
   - Waste container lined with plastic bags
   - Fresh linen
   - Tissues, soap, wash basin, other toiletries, water container, disposable cup or glass

Prevents transfer of disease agent by decreasing the number of times room is entered for bringing in supplies. Allows for disposal of trash and equipment.

4. Collect and place supplies outside the room door, including:
   - Supply cart
   - Clean gowns, gloves, masks
   - Large isolation laundry bags
   - Large plastic disposable trash bags
   - Specific disinfectants as required

Keeps protective clothing and equipment outside of infected or contaminated area.

5. Place precaution sign on door.

Informs staff that protective measures are needed.

6. Move client into room.
7. Place sign on room door requiring visitors to go to nurse's station for information.

Informs visitors of need for protective measures.

8. Show client the protective measures that need to be taken. Include family, if present. Answer questions.

Decreases anxiety and gains cooperation.

Putting on Protective Gown, Mask, and Gloves:

1. Remove jewelry.
2. If watch is needed, place in a clear plastic bag.
3. Wash hands.
4. Place mask on face.
5. Take clean gown from supply cart.
6. Hold gown up by inside neck surface and let gown unfold with open part of back facing nurse.
7. Slip one arm into sleeve, touching only neck of gown. Slip other arm into sleeve.
8. Working inside the sleeve with hand covered by gown, pull sleeve up on one arm and shoulder. Repeat with other arm.
9. Place fingers inside neck of gown at the back and fix gown so that it fits well over shoulders.
10. Tie neck ties. Do not touch hair.
11. Draw gown edges together at back so that edges overlap and entire back is covered.
12. Tie waist ties securely.
13. Put on clean or sterile gloves. See surgical asepsis procedure.
14. Collect necessary supplies and enter room.
15. Place watch (in plastic bag) near work area.

Prevents transfer of microorganisms in and out of room.
Protects watch from contaminated items if touched.
Prevents transfer of microorganisms.
See surgical asepsis procedure.

Protects uniform when in contact with client and contaminated materials.
Prevents hands from contacting outside gown.

Prevents contamination of hands with hair.
Provides total coverage of nurse's uniform.

Secures gown in place.
Protects hands from contact by infectious agent.

Prepares client for procedure.
Prevents contamination of watch.

Removal of Gown, Mask, and Gloves:

1. Remove gloves by bringing gloves down from wrist so that gloves are inside out when removed.
2. Remove mask by untying ties. Do not touch face part of mask.
3. Untie waist ties.
4. Wash hands.

Prevents outside gloves (contaminated side) from touching clean areas.
Face part of mask may contain organisms spread through air.

Prevents transfer of microorganisms that may have come in contact with hands during removal of mask and gloves and in untying waist ties.

5. Untie neck ties. Do not touch outside of gown.
6. Place index finger under cuff of one sleeve. Pull sleeve over hand without touching outside gown.
7. Using the hand covered by gown sleeve, pull other sleeve off the arm.

Prevents transfer of microorganisms that may be on gown.
Begins removal of contaminated gown.

STEP	RATIONALE
8. Remove gown without touching the outside gown or having gown touch uniform.	
9. Fold gown inside out. Do not shake gown.	Prevents transfer of microorganisms on gown into air.
10. Roll up gown and discard it into dirty laundry bag.	
11. Wash hands.	Removes any organisms that hands may have come in contact with during removal of gown.
12. Slip hand into plastic bag and get watch. Do not touch outside of bag. Keep hand in plastic bag and discard plastic bag.	
13. Open door with paper towel when leaving room.	Prevents transfer of disease agent that might be present on inside of door.

Taking Supplies and Equipment into Room:

STEP	RATIONALE
1. Collect necessary disposable equipment.	Prevents transfer of disease agent.
2. Place equipment and supplies on cart outside room.	
3. Put on protective clothing.	See procedure for Putting on Protective Gown, Mask, and Gloves.
4. Hold supplies or equipment in gloved hands. Push room door open with arms or back.	
5. When care of client is completed, discard contaminated disposable equipment and supplies into trash container. Empty liquids into toilet and flush.	Prevents transfer of disease agent.
6. Remove protective clothing and leave room.	See procedure for Removal of Gown, Mask, and Gloves.

Double Bagging for Removal of Discarded Supplies and Trash:

STEP	RATIONALE
1. Put on protective clothing and enter room.	See procedure for Putting on Protective Gown, Mask, and Gloves.
2. Empty waste materials into special bag in room. Seal bag. Place new bag in position.	Prevents transfer of microorganisms by closing bag tightly. Organizes supply for next time that it is needed.
3. Have a second person outside room hold a clean bag open with the top of the bag cuffed over her or his hands.	Protects second worker's hands from contamination.
4. Place sealed bag inside clean bag. Do not touch the outside clean bag.	
5. Have the second worker close, seal, and label outside bag for special disposal.	Prevents transfer of germs by placing contaminated items in two bags. Label identifies material as being contaminated.
6. Leave isolation room.	
7. Remove double-bagged container to appropriate place for disposal.	Prevents microorganism growth in contaminated items.
8. Wash hands.	

Removing a Specimen from the Room:

STEP	RATIONALE
1. Bring labeled specimen container and plastic bag into room when entering.	Prepares for efficient performance of procedure.
2. Collect specimen, close container, and place in plastic bag.	Allows specimen container to be seen by laboratory personnel.
3. Have another person outside room hold a large, clear plastic bag cuffed over hands.	Prevents transfer of disease agent.
4. Place bag containing specimen into bag held by second person. Do not touch outside bag held by second person.	
5. Have second person close, secure, and label bag with client's name, room number, and type of isolation precautions.	Protects worker who receives specimen.
6. Remove protective clothing; leave room.	See procedure for leaving (step 13 under Removal of Gown, Mask, and Gloves).
7. Take double-bagged specimen to laboratory.	

Transporting Client Who Is Isolated:

STEP	RATIONALE
1. Explain procedure and reason for leaving room to client.	Informs client of procedure.
2. Cover wheelchair or stretcher with a clean sheet before taking it into room.	Protects vehicle from contamination.
3. Help client to put on isolation gown, mask, and cap, if required (strict or respiratory isolation).	Protects other persons outside isolation room.
4. Help client into wheelchair or onto stretcher.	
5. Place a clean sheet or bath blanket over client's body, including shoulders and feet.	

STEP	RATIONALE
6. Leave room with client.	
7. Make sure that personnel receiving client know what isolation precautions are necessary.	Prepares personnel in other departments.

Nursing Implications: The type of protective isolation depends on how the microorganisms are transmitted. Check with institutional policy and team leader or head nurse. Each procedure is done to prevent the transfer of the microorganism responsible for the onset of the disease to others.

For Strict Isolation Procedures: The room should be private and the door kept closed. All persons entering the room must wear a protective gown, gloves, and mask. All contaminated articles need to be bagged and labeled before being discarded.

For Respiratory Isolation Procedures: A private room is usually designated for this type of isolation; however, room may be shared if both clients have the same respiratory condition. Check with team leader or head nurse and institutional policies. Gowns and gloves are not indicated. A mask should be worn.

For Contact Isolation Procedures: Usually the client is placed in a private room, although some institutions allow the room to be shared if both clients have the same infectious disease. If there is a possibility of soiling uniform, then a protective gown should be worn. Gloves should be worn if the nurse is in contact with infective material. Masks should be worn if there is close contact with the client. Contaminated articles that are to be discarded should be bagged and labeled.

TB Isolation Procedures: A private room is usually designated but may be shared if both clients have TB. The room should be specially ventilated and the door kept closed. Gowns are worn to prevent contamination of clothing. Gloves are not indicated but a mask should be used, particularly if the client is coughing.

Drainage or Secretions Precautions: Room may be shared. A gown and gloves are required if infective material is to be touched. A mask is usually not indicated.

Blood or Body Fluid Precautions: A private room may be used if necessary, especially if the client does not have good hygienic habits. A gown and gloves are indicated if infective material is to be touched. A mask is usually not indicated.

Enteric Isolation Precautions: The same precautions are taken as for blood and body fluid precautions.

Report and record any unusual findings, as well as type, amount, color, and odor of any secretions or excretions. Follow specific procedures carefully to prevent transfer of organisms to others.

Procedure: Chart Recording

Description: Care given to the client from admission to discharge is recorded.

Purpose: To describe accurately and completely objective and subjective information as it relates to client care, including mental and physical assessment of the client's condition, all treatments prescribed and given, and any treatments refused by the client or any care not given with the reason for same; to communicate information that is correct and important for health-care personnel to use in continuing effective client care.

STEP	RATIONALE
On Admission:	
1. Interview client.	Helps to determine client's understanding of his or her condition and complaints.
2. Ask client for information about pain, type, location, and changes in severity; other physical symptoms such as weakness, fever, chills, dizziness, fear, and mood changes; and onset of such symptoms.	Obtains subjective complaints.
3. Ask client for information on any changes in eating, swallowing, bowel habits, voiding, sleeping, walking, standing, hearing, vision, taste, and smell.	Helps to identify any changes that may show worsening of or improvement in the client's condition.
On Examination:	
1. Check level of consciousness.	Changes in level of consciousness may indicate changes in brain function.
2. Check on whether client displays any evidence of pain, anxiety, weakness, and the like.	Checks on client's statements made during interview.
3. Check for any signs of sweating, changes in skin color, temperature of skin, spasms.	Obtains physical evidence of problems.
4. Check vital signs (temperature, pulse, respiration, blood pressure).	Obtains information that may indicate changes occurring in body.

STEP	RATIONALE
5. Check for the following signs: • Bleeding • Tenderness and location • Stiffness in joints and deformities • Drainage location, type, amount, odor (describe in detail) • Difficulty in moving about • Problems in communication	Obtains information of changes that may be occurring in body functions. Type of drainage or excretions that are usual (urine or feces may show presence of bleeding, changes in color, and so on). Other drainage may be abnormal, for example, drainage from wounds.
6. Assess each body system for signs and symptoms indicating a problem.	Obtains systematic information from physical assessment.

Entering Information on Chart:

To Ensure Legality of Notes:

1. Write date and time of entry of information in ink (check with policy in regard to color of ink).	Legal requirement. Prevents changing of information in chart.
2. Do not leave blank spaces.	Prevents new information from being added at a later time.
3. Do not erase any information.	Prevents questions about information being changed or deleted. If error occurs, draw line through error and write in "error" with your initials.
4. Do not add more information after notations have been signed.	New information should be noted with time and labeled as a "late notation" and signed. For information that has been written earlier and is incorrect, begin new notation with corrected statement.
5. End notation with signature and abbreviated title (LVN or LPN).	Identifies notation by name and title of person doing the recording.

To Ensure Accuracy and Completeness of Charted Information:

1. Record all important information.	Ensures completeness.
2. Record any critical information immediately.	Ensures promptness.
3. Use institution's policy in regard to medical terms and abbreviations.	Prevents misunderstanding by reader.
4. Use proper grammar, spelling, and punctuation.	Demonstrates professionalism.
5. Record data obtained from assessment of client. Include: • Any changes in condition • Changes in behavior • New symptoms and signs • Information on drainage (type, amount, location, character, and so on) • Response to treatments • Decreases in or absence of earlier signs or symptoms	Ensures completeness of information, including any observations in regard to changes in client's physical and/or mental status.
6. Write information from your assessment in a logical, organized fashion.	Makes it easier to follow and ensures completeness.
7. Do not use terms such as "little" or "small." If exact size is unknown, use phrases such as "reddened area the size of a half-dollar noted on sacrum."	Such terms have different meanings to different people.
8. Make sure that body locations are correctly recorded.	Ensures accurate information.
9. Write notations in chart at regular intervals.	Provides accurate information on a continuous basis.
10. Record the following information with correct date and time: • Initial assessment • Changes in condition • Nursing care given such as treatments, helping with activities of daily living (ADLs), teaching	Provides accurate written information of client's progress. Keeps a record of treatment regimen and client's responses.
11. Record visits of physician and other health professionals.	Reports on visits that are necessary to obtain reimbursement funds from special outside agencies such as Medicare.
12. Record specific information, including laboratory data, vital signs, changes in client's condition, and physician's response.	
13. Record medications given after they have been given.	Ensures accuracy and completeness.

STEP	RATIONALE
Flow Sheet Recording:	
1. Obtain necessary information requested on flow sheet.	Ensures information requested is obtained.
2. Enter date and time of information.	Ensures time sequence.
3. Write information in correct location.	Ensures accuracy of information.
4. Sign signature or initials in correct spot (check institutional policy).	Identifies person recording information.

Nursing Implications: Written records are used to communicate accurate and complete data regarding care received by the client and must follow the policy in terms of the institutional and legal requirements. The Joint Commission on Accreditation of Healthcare Organizations (JCAHO) requires evidence of the nursing process. Information on charts is used in lawsuits and in reimbursement of funds from outside agencies and therefore must be accurate and complete. Charts are used by other health-care personnel to determine client's condition, treatment effects, and so on.

Procedure: Taking Vital Signs

Description: This is the procedure for taking the body temperature, pulse, respirations, and blood pressure measurements.

Purpose: To assess the vital signs in an accurate manner to determine the amount of heat stored in the body.

The temperature is taken on admission and as ordered by the physician, as well as when the client shows signs of a fever such as feeling cold, hot, or thirsty, or is shivering or perspiring.

The pulse is taken to obtain information about the function of the heart, the circulatory system, and the client's general physical state.

The respirations are taken to determine the rate per minute and its depth, quality, and pattern of respiration, and to assess if any changes occur over time.

The blood pressure is measured as systolic (upper figure) and diastolic (lower figure). It is taken to determine the relationship between the cardiac output (the amount of blood pumped out of the heart) and the resistance to the blood flow by the blood vessels outside the heart. The assessment of blood pressure assists health-care personnel in determining if the client is within the normotensive (normal), hypertensive (high blood pressure), or hypotensive (low blood pressure) state.

STEP	RATIONALE
1. Collect necessary equipment for taking the temperature: • Thermometer (glass or electronic) • Probe cover, tissues, lubricant • Paper towel and disposable gloves	Organizing necessary equipment allows quick and safe implementation.
Oral Temperature:	
1. Explain procedure.	Informs client of procedure.
2. Wash hands.	Prevents transfer of microorganisms.
When Using a Glass Thermometer:	
3. Hold at end opposite bulb part and rinse in cold water.	Avoids touching the bulb part that will be placed in client's mouth. Rinsing removes disinfectant and other material on thermometer. Hot water expands mercury and may break thermometer.
4. Wipe thermometer from fingers to bulb part with a clean tissue.	Removes water from area of greatest contamination (part not stored in disinfectant solution and touched by nurse's fingers) to area of least contamination (bulb part of disinfectant solution).
5. Hold thermometer lengthwise at eye level, turn until measuring scale can be seen, and read the number at the end of the mercury level.	Allows ease in viewing scale to make sure that mercury level is below body temperature.
6. Hold end opposite bulb and shake thermometer downward with a flick of the wrist until mercury reads 95°F (35°C).	Lowers mercury level so that it is below expected body temperature.
7. Before inserting an electronic thermometer, remove the portable unit from base. Check to make sure that the unit is charged.	Prepares thermometer for use.

STEP	RATIONALE
8. When using either thermometer: Instruct client to open mouth and hold tongue against upper teeth.	
9. Insert thermometer tip or probe gently under tongue.	Positions the mercury tip or probe in heat area of mouth.
10. Ask client to close mouth and hold tip or probe in place between his or her lips. Ask client not to bite down on glass thermometer.	Keeps thermometer in place until temperature is recorded. Prevents possible injury of mouth if thermometer breaks.
11. When using a glass thermometer, leave thermometer in place for 3–11 minutes, depending on your institution's guidelines. (At this time check other vital signs.)	Ensures adequate time for accurate temperature reading.
12. Once time interval is completed, hold the end of the thermometer and ask client to open his or her mouth.	Reduces possibility of dropping thermometer.
13. Remove thermometer; wipe with a tissue moving from end held in your fingers to bulb part.	Removes germs and other materials from area of least contamination to area of most contamination.
14. Read the thermometer and record.	Ensures accurate notation.
15. Wash thermometer with cool soapy water; rinse with cool water. Dry with tissue or clean paper towel. Replace in container.	Removes microorganisms and other material.
16. When using an electronic thermometer, check digital panel until a signal is heard indicating that the maximum temperature has been reached.	Provides evidence that indicates the thermometer is recording the temperature.
17. Hold end of probe and ask client to open his or her mouth. Remove probe.	Prevents probe from falling out of client's mouth.
18. Read the temperature on digital panel and record immediately.	Ensures accurate notation.
19. Eject probe cover into waste receptacle.	Discarding of probe cover prevents contamination of other clients.
20. After use of either thermometer, inform client of his or her temperature, if allowed.	Decreases anxiety.
21. Wash hands.	Prevents transfer of microorganisms.

Rectal Temperature:

STEP	RATIONALE
1. Explain procedure.	Decreases anxiety; gains cooperation.
2. Follow steps 1–7 for taking an oral temperature.	
3. When using a rectal glass thermometer or electronic thermometer, put on clean disposable gloves.	Protects hands from becoming contaminated with client's body excreta.
4. Place lubricant on bulb end of glass thermometer or on probe of electronic thermometer.	Allows for easier insertion of thermometer into the rectum.
5. Pull curtains around client's bed or close room door.	Ensures privacy.
6. Ask or assist client to lie on his or her side with upper leg bent.	Places client in position so that rectal area is visible.
7. Lower pajama bottom, if worn, and place bed linens so that only buttocks are visible.	Ensures privacy.
8. Separate buttocks gently with one hand.	Exposes the anus to view.
9. Touch tip of probe or bulb end of glass thermometer to anus, explaining what is being done. Ask client to take a deep breath.	Client feels the position of thermometer. Placing thermometer tip against the anal area relaxes the anal muscles. Deep breathing helps to relax the client.
10. Place probe or tip gently into anus point tip toward umbilicus (belly button) and guide it along rectal wall. Insert tip up to about 3 inches in the adult and about ½ inch in infants.	Placement of bulb against wall of rectum places tip close to blood vessels. Placing thermometer carefully in the proper area of the rectum helps to prevent injury to the rectal tissues.

When Using a Glass Thermometer:

STEP	RATIONALE
11. Hold thermometer in place for 2–4 minutes. Check institutional policies.	Gives enough time for correct reading.
12. Remove thermometer gently. Wipe the thermometer from fingers to bulb with clean tissue, turning the tissue around the thermometer.	Decreases discomfort. Removes germs and other material from thermometer from the area of least contamination to the area of most contamination. Turning the tissue allows for removal of fecal material.
13. Read thermometer; place it aside. Inform client of temperature if not contraindicated by institutional policy.	Decreases anxiety.

STEP	RATIONALE
14. Record temperature.	Allows prompt and accurate recording.
15. Remove any remaining lubricant from anal area with tissue. Client may wish to clean area himself or herself. Give client tissue.	Ensures personal hygiene.
16. Replace pajama bottoms, if worn, and replace bed linens. Place client in comfortable position. Raise siderails, if required.	Ensures comfort.
17. Wash thermometer with cool soapy water and rinse with cool water; dry with paper towel or tissue. Replace in storage container.	Removes remaining material and other organisms from thermometer before replacing in container.
18. Discard gloves; wash hands.	Prevents transfer of micoorganisms.
19. Open curtains or doors to room.	

When Using an Electronic Thermometer:

STEP	RATIONALE
20. Watch digital panel until unit signals that the maximum temperature has been reached.	Indicates that thermometer is recording the temperature.
21. Remove thermometer gently. Check the temperature readout on the digital panel of the thermometer.	Decreases discomfort. Obtains accurate reading.
22. Eject the probe cover into waste receptacle.	Prevents contamination of other clients.
23. Follow steps 14–19 for taking a rectal temperature with a glass thermometer.	

Axillary Temperature:

STEP	RATIONALE
1. Explain procedure.	Informs client of procedure. Decreases anxiety; gains cooperation.
2. Wash hands.	Decreases transfer of microorganisms.

When Using a Glass Thermometer or Electronic Probe:

STEP	RATIONALE
3. Follow steps 1–7 for taking an oral temperature.	
4. Draw curtain around bed or close room door.	Ensures privacy.
5. Place client on back or in sitting position.	Places client in best position for placement of thermometer.
6. Assist client to remove gown or other top clothing.	Prepares for exposing area under arm (axilla).
7. Raise client's arm or ask him or her to raise the arm; gently dry axilla.	Dries any moisture under arm that may lower the temperature readout because of evaporation.
8. Place bulb or probe tip into the center of the axilla. Hold in place.	Places thermometer near blood vessel supply.
9. Lower client's arm over thermometer and position his or her arm across chest.	Keeps thermometer in place.
10. Hold glass thermometer in place for 10 minutes; hold electronic thermometer in place until signal is heard.	Ensures accurate reading.
11. Raise client's arm, remove probe or glass thermometer. Replace gown or clothing.	
12. Wipe thermometer with a tissue, using a twisting motion toward bulb end.	Removes contaminants from thermometer from area of least contamination to area of greatest contamination.
13. Read and record temperature.	Ensures accurate information.
14. Wash thermometer with cool soapy water and rinse with cool water. Dry with clean paper towel or tissue; replace in storage container.	Removes any remaining materials from thermometer.
15. Inform client of temperature unless contraindicated.	Decreases anxiety.
16. Place client in a comfortable position. Open curtains or door.	Ensures comfort.
17. Wash hands.	Decreases transfer of microorganisms.

When Using an Electronic Thermometer:

STEP	RATIONALE
18. Remove portable unit from base. Check to ensure that unit is charged.	Prepares thermometer for use. A maximally charged unit produces an accurate temperature recording.
19. Place a probe cover over probe.	Prepares the thermometer.
20. Follow steps 4–17.	

Nursing Implications: Report any changes in temperature to team leader or head nurse. Document temperature on chart and flow sheet. Report elevated or subnormal temperature immediately. Such readings may signify an imbalance between heat produced and heat lost. Extremely low or high temperatures may cause damage to body cells and even death if these temperatures remain over a prolonged period of time. The body temperature may be measured in different sites, depending on the client's condition. The decision of the site depends on the client's condition, the order of the physician, and the decision of the team leader or head nurse. Such decisions are made based on the following:

- Nearness of major arteries, because arterial blood temperature is the closest measure of total body temperature
- Amount of accuracy required based on client's condition
- Age of client (e.g., infants and very young children cannot hold a thermometer in their mouths for the required time)
- Presence of inflammation (e.g., inflamed tissue having higher temperature than normal tissue)
- Client's overall condition (e.g., unconscious, paralyzed clients may not be able to have temperatures taken by mouth; in burned clients, location of temperature reading requires special decisions)

Temperature may be taken rectally instead of orally if client has recently eaten, drunk, or smoked. These conditions may raise or lower the temperature under the tongue, resulting in an incorrect temperature reading.

Procedure: Taking the Pulse

Description: Methods of measuring the pulse rate include radial, apical, and apical-radial measurements.

Purpose: To obtain information about the functioning of the heart, the circulatory system, and client's general physical state; to measure client's emotional state and body responses to stress, exercise, blood loss, fatigue, and injury to tissues; and to evaluate response to trauma, surgery, medications, and other treatments (including rate, rhythm, and depth).

STEP	RATIONALE
1. Collect necessary equipment: • Stethoscope • Antiseptic swabs • Watch with second hand or digital panel	Organizing necessary equipment allows quick and safe implementation.
Radial Pulse:	
1. Explain procedure.	Informs client of procedure. Decreases anxiety; gains cooperation.
2. Wash hands.	Prevents transfer of microorganisms.
3. For clients lying on their backs, place client's arm across chest, palm down. For those who are sitting, place arm on his or her lap, palm down.	Places wrist in a resting position.
4. Place first three fingers of your hand on client's radial artery, located just below client's thumb on his or her wrist.	Positions fingers over artery. *Never* use thumb to take a pulse. The pulse in your thumb may be felt instead of the client's pulse.
5. Feel for pulse sensations. Note rhythm and strength of pulse.	Check quality and rhythm of pulse.
6. Look at watch. Note location of second hand and wait until 15, 30, or 60 seconds have passed.	If taking routine pulse rate, a 15-second count is usually sufficient unless institutional policy differs. If any abnormalities are present, count for a full 60 seconds.
7. Multiply the count by 4 if pulse was taken for 15 seconds, by 2 if taken for 30 seconds.	Determines pulse rate for a full minute.
8. Inform client of pulse unless contraindicated.	Relieves anxiety.
9. Record pulse rate, rhythm, and quality.	Ensures accurate documentation.
10. Wash hands.	Prevents transfer of microorganisms.
Apical Pulse:	
1. Follow previous steps 1 and 2.	
2. Clean earpieces and diaphragm of stethoscope with an antiseptic swab.	Prevents transfer of possibly dangerous organisms from previous use.
3. Help client to a back-lying position or a low-Fowler's (sitting) position.	Places client in comfortable position. Prevents possible changes in heart rate by decreasing strain on the client.
4. Close room door or draw curtains around bed.	Ensures privacy.
5. Expose left chest by placing bed linens away from left chest and removing gown from left chest area.	Removes clothing and linens that may interfere with hearing heart sounds.
6. Rub bell or diaphragm of stethoscope with palm of hand.	Warms diaphragm before placement on chest wall.

STEP	RATIONALE
7. Place earpieces in your ears. Place stethoscope bell or diaphragm on the fourth or fifth rib space (intercostal space) on left chest.	Prepares to take apical pulse. Positions stethoscope near apex of heart.
8. Listen for a "lub-dup" sound. Move bell or diaphragm until sound is heard.	This sound identifies two normal heart sounds: S_1 (closure of semilunar valves of heart) and S_2 (closure of atrioventricular valves).
9. Check the rhythm of heart sound.	Evaluates rhythm.
10. Time the heart rate, rhythm, and quality using the second hand of watch or digital readout.	A full-minute count should be taken so that any abnormalities may be noted.
11. Remove stethoscope; replace gown and bed linens. Place client in a comfortable position.	Ensures comfort.
12. Record apical pulse.	Ensures accurate and prompt documentation.
13. Wash hands. Clean stethoscope earpieces, diaphragm, or bell with antiseptic swabs.	Prevents transfer of microorganisms.

Apical-Radial Pulse:

STEP	RATIONALE
1. Explain procedure: "One nurse will be counting heartbeats; a second nurse will count radial pulse to compare the rates." Answer any questions.	Informs client of procedure; decreases anxiety.
2. Prepare for measuring apical pulse; follow steps 1–9 for taking apical pulse.	
3. Have second nurse take the radial pulse after procedure for taking apical pulse.	
4. Watching the second hand or digital dial, let second nurse know when to begin counting radial pulse. Begin counting the radial and apical pulses at the same time.	Coordinates the count. This verifies if any differences exist between the apical and radial pulse counts.
5. Both nurses count the heart rate for one full minute.	Ensures accuracy.
6. Tell second nurse to stop when 1 minute has passed.	Ensures accuracy.
7. Place client in comfortable position.	Ensures comfort.
Record apical and radial pulse. Note and report any differences between apical and radial pulse rates.	Ensures prompt and accurate recording.
8. Wash hands; clean stethoscope earpieces, diaphragm, or bell with antiseptic swabs.	Prevents transfer of microorganisms.

Nursing Implications: Document pulse, report any changes in pulse rate, depth, rhythm, and quality to team leader or head nurse. Checking the pulse rate provides how many times the heart beats every minute, as well as the rhythm and the quality of heartbeats. Remember that many different factors can affect pulse rate. Age of the client affects pulse rate. For example, a newborn infant's pulse rate is normally between 120 and 140 bpm. A child of 6 or 7 years has a pulse rate of about 100, whereas the adult female pulse rate ranges from 55 to 90. The male pulse rate may range from 50 to 85. Other factors affecting pulse rate include exercise, emotions, body chemicals, body temperature, and diseases involving the heart and other body organs.

The quality of the pulse is affected by the function of the heart and the circulatory system. Conditions such as dehydration causes blood volume to decrease, thereby producing a weak, thready pulse.

Sites where the pulse rate may be measured, other than the apical and radial sites, include the temporal pulse, located between the outside of the eye and the hairline. This site is often used in infants and children and when other sites are not accessible, as in the presence of severe body burns, body casts, and so on.

The pulse may also be measured at the carotid artery (carotid pulse), located just below the angle of the jaw. This location is often used in times of emergencies. Because the carotid artery is located near the heart, the pulse may often be detected even when blood volume is low and other pulses cannot be felt.

The brachial pulse is taken over the brachial artery, which runs down the arm and is measured just below the inner side of the antecubital fossa. This pulse site is used to listen to sounds reflective of the arterial blood pressure.

Another site for monitoring the pulse is close to the pubis bone near the upper inner thigh. This site is often used to check the circulation of the lower extremities or to perform special circulatory tests.

The popliteal pulse is found under the knee. The knee needs to be flexed (bent) to locate the pulse. This site is used to check the circulation of the lower extremity and may be used to check the arterial blood pressure in the leg.

Another site that is used to check the circulation in the feet is the dorsalis pedis pulse. It is located on the top of the foot, a little toward the tendon of the big toe. It should be noted that this artery does not exist in a small percentage of individuals.

One final site is located on the inside of the ankle. It is at this site that the posterior tibial pulse may be monitored. This site is used to check the circulation of the lower extremities. It should be noted that this pulse is often difficult to find, especially if the individual is edematous or obese, and even may not be found in some instances.

Procedure: Taking the Respirations

Description: This measures the respiratory rate of clients.

Purpose: To measure the respiratory rate in order to obtain information reflecting the process of oxygen delivery to the cells and the return of oxygen to the outside air; to determine the client's usual pattern, rate, quality of respirations, and any changes that have occurred; to assist in the evaluation of pathological conditions that are reflected by abnormal rates.

STEP	RATIONALE
1. Collect necessary equipment: wristwatch with second hand or digital readout. **NOTE:** This procedure is done immediately after taking the radial pulse.	Organizing necessary equipment allows for quick and safe implementation.
2. Keep client's wrist over chest after taking radial pulse.	This position allows nurse to watch rise and fall of wrist and count respirations without having client control his or her respirations and in turn change rate.
3. Note rhythm, depth, quality, and pattern of respirations.	Checks for any abnormality.
4. Using watch, count respirations for one full minute.	Ensures accuracy of rate.
5. Record respiratory rate.	Ensures accurate and prompt recording.
6. Wash hands.	Prevents transfer of microorganisms.

Nursing Implications: Record findings. Report any unusual findings immediately to team leader or head nurse.

When Client's Respirations Are Slower Than Usual: If client is conscious, have him or her take deep breaths at about 10–12/min. Check other vital signs and report findings immediately to team leader or head nurse. Check if client has received depressant medication. Be prepared to assist in giving artificial respiration if required.

When Client's Respirations Are Faster Than Usual: Report to team leader or head nurse. If pain or fever is present, check with team leader about prescribed medications. If client is under emotional stress and consequently is hyperventilating, talk quietly to client for reassurance. If hyperventilation is caused by anxiety, try placing a paper bag over client's mouth and nose and ask him or her to breathe into it. The client rebreathes the exhaled carbon dioxide, thus decreasing the depth of the respiration and slowing its rate. If hyperventilation is a result of respiratory or nervous system disorders, report to team leader or head nurse immediately if it is a change from previous measurements of the respirations.

If client has stopped breathing, begin respiratory resuscitation immediately: 12 respirations per minute for adults and 20 respirations per minute for children. Call or have someone call for a respiratory arrest team.

The respiratory rate varies depending on age, exercise, disease or disorders, certain metabolic changes, medications, and emotions.

Age: Newborn infant's respirations are about 35/min; adult's are 14–20/min.

Exercise: When exercising, the body cells require more oxygen. To supply the need, respirations increase. Resting lowers the respiratory rate. It should be noted that respiratory rates in individuals who have been immobilized for a long time may be increased because of factors affecting the respiratory and circulatory systems.

Disease or Disorders: Certain diseases or disorders may cause a mild decrease of oxygen in the arterial blood circulation (hypoxic state) that will increase respiratory rates. If the hypoxic state is severe, the usual body mechanisms that control respirations may be affected and so increase the respiratory rates.

Certain Metabolic Changes: An example of metabolic changes is increases or decreases in thyroid hormones that regulate metabolism in the body. If these hormones decrease or increase, respiratory rates also decrease or increase.

Medications: Medicines that depress the central nervous system (brain) may decrease respiratory rates.

Emotions: Anger, anxiety, and fear induce a response from the autonomic nervous system causing an increase in respiratory rates.

Procedure: Measuring Blood Pressure

Description: This measures the compression against the brachial artery by an inflated cuff (part of sphygmomanometer) and the auscultation (listening to the first and last sounds of the blood flow through the artery when the cuff is slowly deflated, causing a decompression against the brachial artery).

Purpose: To assess the blood pressure reading of a client as a part of vital sign measurement; to determine any changes from the normal range or usual range for the client, which may indicate need for further treatment.

STEP	RATIONALE
1. Collect necessary equipment: • Sphygmomanometer: mercury or aneroid with inflation cuff • Stethoscope • Antiseptic swabs	Organizing necessary equipment allows for quick and safe implementation.
2. Explain procedure.	Informs client of procedure; decreases anxiety.
3. Wash hands.	Prevents transfer of microorganisms.
4. Place bedridden client in back-lying or side-lying position with arm resting at side, with upper arm at heart level with palm up. *or* Place sitting client's arm on his or her lap or armrest of chair, with upper arm at heart level with palm up.	Arm elevated above heart may cause ineffective compression of artery.
5. Make sure that mercury level or dial needle is at 0.	Ensures proper reading.
6. Measure cuff width against client's arms to check for accurate fit.	False reading may occur if cuff is too small because of ineffective compression over artery.
7. Make sure that the mercury meniscus is at eye level or aneroid dial is directly in front of eyes.	Prevents false readings by having accurate visualization of scale.
8. Palpate (feel) the brachial artery pulse.	Locates artery for correct placement of arm cuff.
9. Release valve lock to remove any air in inflation bladder located in the cuff.	Uneven inflation may give inaccurate readings.
10. Center the arrow on cuff over artery with lower edge of cuff about 1 inch above the antecubital fossa.	Ensures inflation bladder is over artery. Makes sure that lower edge of cuff does not cover brachial site where stethoscope will be placed.
11. Wrap cuff evenly around client's upper arm, making sure of a snug fit.	
12. Fasten Velcro or tuck end under cuff.	Secures cuff in correct position for inflation.
13. Wipe stethoscope earpieces and diaphragm or bell with antiseptic swabs.	Prevents transfer of microorganisms.
14. Place earpieces of stethoscope in ears and feel for the brachial artery pulse.	Prepares for taking blood pressure reading.
15. Hold hand pump in one hand and tighten valve lock with thumb.	Prevents air from leaking out. Ensures effective compression of artery.
16. Inflate cuff with a brisk pumping motion. Palpate artery and watch mercury level or needle of dial.	Ensures adequate amount of blood in artery during compression.
17. When brachial pulse disappears, remove fingers from artery area and place diaphragm or bell over brachial artery.	Indicates sufficient compression to stop blood flow through artery and time to begin listening (auscultating) for return of blood flow.
18. Stop inflating cuff when mercury level increases to 30 mm above the point where pulse disappeared.	Indicates that sufficient compression has occurred and prevents false readings if compression stops during auscultatory gap.
19. Loosen valve lock slowly and deflate cuff at a rate of 2–3 mm Hg per heartbeat.	Begins to decompress artery, allowing blood flow to restart. Decompressing the artery too fast makes it difficult to read the scale accurately. Decompressing too slowly may cause falsely high measurements and increase discomfort for client.
20. Listen carefully for the first "tap-tap" sounds (Korotkoff's sounds). Note the mercury level and read the measurement scale.	Indicates systolic reading.
21. Listen for changes in the sounds.	
22. When sounds disappear, note the measurement reading.	Indicates diastolic reading.
23. Open valve cock completely. Note diastolic sound; rapidly deflate and remove cuff.	Removes compression and discomfort.
24. Inform client of reading unless contraindicated.	Decreases anxiety.
25. Place client in comfortable position. Record reading immediately.	Ensures comfort. Ensures prompt and accurate recording.
26. Wash hands; cleanse stethoscope earpieces and diaphragm or bell with antiseptic swabs.	Decreases potential for transfer of microorganisms.

Nursing Implications: The most common method of taking the blood pressure is by auscultation (listening for sounds of blood flow with a stethoscope). Note usual blood pressure. Check and report any changes. Factors that control blood pressure include the amount of circulating blood. More blood flow increases blood pressure, whereas less blood volume circulation decreases blood pressure. If the heart muscle becomes damaged, the output from the heart chambers decreases and blood pressure decreases. The greater the resistance by the vessels outside of the heart, the higher the blood pressure. The greater the width of the blood vessel, the lower the pressure. Dilation (widening) of blood vessels decreases blood pressure. Narrowing of blood vessels, such as that caused by atherosclerosis, lessens the elasticity of the blood vessel walls and so increases resistance to blood flow, thereby increasing blood pressure. The viscosity (thickness or thinness) of blood affects blood pressure in that when the blood is thicker, blood flow slows down. If the tone of the smooth muscles of the blood vessels becomes impaired, the blood vessels lose their elasticity and become overdistended. This process affects the diastolic pressure.

Certain receptors found at several points in the arterial system send impulses to the vasomotor section of the brain in response to changes in blood volume and chemical composition. The brain, in turn, responds by causing either dilation or constriction of blood vessels.

Certain body chemicals, such as epinephrine, antidiuretic hormone, and histamine, cause vasodilation (widening) of blood vessels.

Output from the heart is affected by exertion, exercise, stress, and other emotions that raise blood pressure. Other factors that affect blood pressure include age (gradual increase in blood pressure with aging); gender (women have lower blood pressures than men between the beginning and end of menstruation and higher pressures after menopause); weight (obesity tends to raise blood pressure); and race (blacks have higher blood pressure than whites).

Generally, blood pressure is lowest in the morning and highest in the late afternoon or early evening in individuals who normally sleep at night. The average normal adult blood pressure reading is 120/80. A systolic blood pressure of 140 and a diastolic pressure of 90 are considered the upper limits of the range, according to the American Heart Association, although normal range may be up to 160/90. To determine that blood pressure is higher or lower than the normal range for individuals, one must have prior blood pressure readings for comparison.

If blood pressure reading is 20–30 mm Hg or more lower than previous readings, retake the blood pressure to make sure that the reading was accurate. If pressure is still low, recheck blood pressure in opposite arm.

Check client for other signs and symptoms such as changes in pulse rate, respiration, and temperature. Check for changes in skin color, skin temperature, chest pain, confusion, lethargy, or unconsciousness. If there is no evidence of other signs and symptoms, place client in a back-lying position, report findings immediately, and continue taking the blood pressure at regular intervals.

In cases when the blood pressure measurement is 20–30 mm Hg higher than the client's usual range, retake blood pressure and check findings using the correct techniques including an accurate cuff size for the client's arm. Retake blood pressure in opposite arm if findings still indicate a higher pressure than usual.

Check the client for other signs and symptoms suggestive of high blood pressure, such as changes in other vital signs, chest pain, difficulty breathing, and skin color and temperature changes.

If any of these signs and symptoms are present, report finding immediately. If no other signs and symptoms are present, retake the blood pressure in 15–20 minutes and recheck at regular intervals. Document and report all findings.

In cases when the sounds heard through the stethoscope are faint or absent, check all vital signs. Check equipment for proper working order. Have client raise arm above shoulder and rapidly inflate cuff. Lower arm and take reading. If difficulty still persists, inform team leader or head nurse immediately.

If other noises interfere with ability to hear Korotkoff's sounds, check to see that the stethoscope or blood pressure monitor tubings are not hitting against each other or against other objects. If sounds are caused by others making noise, such as loud talking or television or radio interference, request that such noise interference be muted until the procedure is completed.

Procedure: Intake and Output

Description: This is the process of measuring, recording, and reporting the intake of oral fluids, IV fluids, blood or blood products, total parenteral nutrition, and enteral nutrition. Measurement of output including urinary output (with or without indwelling catheter), vomitus, liquid stools, and drainage from nasogastric tube and other tubes such as chest tubes and T-tubes.

Purpose: To assess for signs of imbalance of both fluids and electrolytes (normally fluid intake is approximately equal to fluid output of the body; an imbalance suggests unusual or abnormal processes).

STEP	RATIONALE
1. Put intake and output (I&O) record in place, as indicated in institutional policies.	Alerts staff to necessity for measuring I&O.
2. Place I&O sign near client's bedside.	Alerts staff and client that I&O is to be measured.
3. Check, measure, and record intake from: • IV fluids • Blood and blood products • Total parenteral nutrition	Records all applicable fluid intake.

STEP	RATIONALE
• Oral fluid intake, including liquid supplements and semiliquid food such as sherbet, ice cream, gelatin.	
4. Check, measure, and record output from: • Urinary output (including indwelling catheter) • Vomitus • Liquid stools • Nasogastric tube drainage • Drainage from wounds (including bedsores) or other tubes	Records all applicable fluid output.
5. Explain that urine is measured as output.	Informs client of procedure.
6. Show client where urinary collection receptacle is and demonstrate method of collection.	Prepares client for measuring output.
7. Show client how to measure and record urinary output.	Demonstrates how to measure and record output.
8. Ask client to demonstrate how to measure and record urinary output.	Checks on client's ability to measure and record output accurately.
9. Explain to family and visitors reasons for monitoring I&O. Ask them to assist client, if needed.	Ensures understanding and possible assistance in measuring and recording fluid I&O.
10. Check on client's I&O recording periodically.	Ensures accuracy of recording.
11. Place completed I&O sheet in client's record according to policy.	Ensures completeness of record.
12. Report any unusual findings, such as blood in urine, very small (<30 cc/hr) or excessive amount of urine output.	Ensures immediate response.

Nursing Implications: Record I&O, reporting any unusual finding such as decreased or increased urine output, concentrated urine, weight loss, increased pulse, increased body temperature, decreased fluid intake, dry skin or mucous membranes, complaints of thirst or weakness, and confusion. These symptoms indicate an imbalance in fluid and electrolytes and suggest a fluid volume deficit.

Report any signs of edema, tightness of skin, weight gain, and increased blood pressure. These signs may indicate an imbalance in fluid and electrolytes suggestive of fluid volume excess.

Procedure: Assisting with IV Fluid Administration (LPN role varies according to state law.)

Description: The practical nurse assists in the procedure of starting an IV solution.

Purpose: Allows for the replacement of fluids and electrolytes resulting from decreased fluid volume, concentration, and makeup of electrolytes in the body; allows for potential replacement of lost fluids and electrolytes during surgical or other treatments.

STEP	RATIONALE
1. Obtain necessary supplies and equipment: • IV solution ordered by physician • IV administration set and tubing • Infusion tray • Clean gloves • Correct needle and catheter • Tourniquet • IV pole • Adhesive tape • Antiseptic swabs or other preparation equipment • Sterile 2 × 2 gauze pads • Armboard • Disposable razor • Label	Organizing necessary equipment allows quick and safe implementation.
2. Wash hands.	Prevents transfer of microorganisms.
3. Double-check IV solution for correct solution and expiration date with registered nurse (RN).	Ensures that client is receiving correct solution.
4. May shave excessive body hair from chosen site, if requested.	Prepares site for IV needle and catheter insertion.

STEP	RATIONALE
5. Hand tourniquet to RN, if requested.	Tourniquet will be used to compress vein and distend venipuncture site.
6. Hand antiseptic swab or other prep material to RN when ready to disinfect skin surface.	Prepares site for IV needle and catheter insertion.
7. If requested, may attach sterile needle to tip of tubing; run fluid through needle, and reclamp tubing. Replace sterile cap over needle.	Primes needle.
8. Hand tubing with needle (remove needle cap using aseptic technique) to RN.	Keeps needle tip sterile.
9. Open clamp on tubing on request, after correct insertion of needle into vein and removal of tourniquet.	Allows IV fluid to enter vein.
10. Hand adhesive strips to RN.	Ensures placement of needle.

When a Venous Catheter Is to Be Used:
11. Follow previous steps 1–6.
12. Hand needle and catheter to RN, who will remove cover.
13. Follow previous steps 9 and 10.

For Both Needle and Catheter Insertion:

14. Provide RN with iodine preparation or other authorized preparation.	Placement of prep at puncture site limits possible contamination of needle or catheter and the blood.
15. After completion of procedure, check site for swelling or return of blood in the tubing.	Checks for infiltration.
16. Discard used equipment; return unused supplies to proper place.	
17. Wash hands.	

Managing a Continuous Intravenous Infusion:

1. Check that correct amount and rate of flow of IV solution is being used. (Refer to physician's orders and nursing care plan.)	Ensures that correct solution is being administered within prescribed time.
2. Examine IV equipment and flow sheet at regular times (hourly checks are recommended) to check the following: • Presence of correct drip rate • Correct IV solution • Amount of IV fluid infused (compare with prescribed amount) • Intact IV system	Checks for accuracy.
3. Check site of IV needle or catheter for evidence of infiltration: • Swelling at site • Redness, warmth at site • Redness along vein path • Complaint of burning pain along venous pathway	Ensures immediate response in removal and/or replacement.
4. If solution is not dripping: • Check to see if clamp on tubing is too tight. • Check whether tubing is kinked or lying under client.	Catching problem early can make it easier to continue IV infusion at prescribed rate.
• Inspect IV site for infiltration. • Check height of IV solution container. • Check to see if drip chamber is half full. • Check tape over puncture site. • Check that tubing stays above puncture site.	Raising height increases gravity flow. Allows for ability to see the dripping solution. A tape that is too tight interferes with IV fluid entering vein. Gravity assists in IV flow.
5. Check for signs of dyspnea; edema; weak, rapid pulse; rapid and shallow respirations occurring on a regular basis.	Assessment of complications caused by overload of IV fluid.
6. Report any unusual problems to RN immediately.	Ensures continuation of IV infusion.

Changing Intravenous Solution Container (Based on Institutional Policy):

1. Check amount of IV fluid infused until less than 50 ml remains in container.	Keeps some IV solution in tubing. Traps any microorganisms that may be present on the surface of the solution (which may occur when using glass bottle containers).

STEP	RATIONALE
2. Check physician's orders and nursing care plan for correct IV solution rate of flow and amount to be infused.	Ensures correctness of order.
3. Obtain new correct IV container and take to client's bedside. Explain procedure.	Decreases anxiety.
4. Wash hands.	Prevents transfer of microorganisms.
5. Remove protective cover from new solution. Make sure that sterility is maintained.	Prevents contamination of solution.
6. Take used IV container from IV standard; clamp tubing; invert container (turn container so that top of container is opposite to what it was when infusing). Remove spike of tubing from container (maintain sterility of spike).	Removes used container.
7. Insert spike into stopper or top of the container without twisting tubing.	Attaches new IV container to IV tubing.
8. Hang the new container on the IV standard immediately.	Ensures gravity force to start flow rate.
9. Open clamp and check rate of solution flow.	
10. Check system on a regular basis.	Ensures proper functioning.

Discontinuing an Intravenous Infusion:

STEP	RATIONALE
1. Explain procedure.	Informs client of procedure.
2. Wash hands; put on gloves.	Prevents transfer of microorganisms.
3. Clamp IV tubing.	Stops IV flow.
4. Hold needle and catheter steady and loosen tape from IV site.	Decreases possibility of injury to vein.
5. Place antiseptic swab above IV site.	Prevents contamination.
6. Remove needle and catheter by gently pulling needle out.	Decreases possibility of injury to vein.
7. Press swab and gauze against site for 2–3 minutes or until bleeding stops.	Presses down on the vein so bleeding stops. *Do not rub IV site!* Rubbing may cause bleeding into tissues.
8. Apply bandage or dressing to site.	Prevents contamination.
9. Record the amount of solution infused on IV record.	Documents accurate amount infused.
10. Discard used solution container and tubing set.	
11. Leave client in comfortable position. Make sure call signal is within easy reach.	Ensures comfort.
12. Remove gloves; wash hands.	Prevents transfer of microorganisms.

Procedure: Applying an External Catheter

Description: Application of an external catheter (Texas or condom catheter) is for the incontinent or paralyzed or unconscious male client (physician's order required).

Purpose: Allows urine to empty into a bag attached to client's leg or a collecting bag attached to the bed frame.

STEP	RATIONALE
1. Collect necessary equipment: • Condom catheter with drainage tube • Adhesive strip • Leg or collecting bag • Alcohol wipes • Soap, water • Washcloth, towel • Disposable gloves	Organizing necessary equipment allows for quick and safe implementation.
2. Explain procedure.	Informs client of procedure.
3. Close curtains around bed or close room door.	Ensures privacy.
4. Place equipment on bedside table or overbed table.	Prepares for procedure.
5. Wash hands; put on clean gloves.	Prevents transfer of microorganisms.
6. Raise bed to a comfortable working position.	Prevents back strain.
7. Lower covers to expose genital area.	Prepares for procedure.
8. Using the soap and water, clean around penis with a circular movement. Rinse and dry. Wipe area with alcohol wipe. Allow to dry.	Removes material around penis. Helps in keeping condom catheter adhered in place.

STEP	RATIONALE
9. Attach collection bag to bed frame or client's leg as appropriate.	Prepares bag for use.
10. Hold penis along shaft with one hand.	Places the sheath of penis in a secure manner.
11. Place rolled condom catheter at tip of penis with other hand. Gently unroll condom sheath onto shaft of penis.	
12. Allow about 1 inch between tip of penis and end of condom catheter that empties into collecting bag.	Provides a space (reservoir) for urine to pass into before draining into tubing.
13. Position end of sheath of catheter and anchor it by placing the adhesive strip around the penis so that the adhesive does not touch skin or make the catheter too tight around the penis.	Provides a tight fit of the catheter to the penis and prevents the leakage of urine around the opening.
14. Attach catheter end to the drainage tubing.	Provides for drainage into the collecting bag.
15. Make a coil of excess tubing and attach to bottom bed sheet.	Allows straight drainage of urine.
16. Replace bed covers; place client in a comfortable position. Make sure call signal is within reach. Open curtains or room door.	Ensures comfort.
17. Discard washcloth and towel. Remove gloves; wash hands.	Prevents transfer of microorganisms.

Nursing Implications: Record procedure. Document reason for external catheter application. Record and report response of client to procedure. Report and record any skin irritation from urine. Check for presence of edema. Check and report any unusual urinary problems, including color and odor of urine collected. Watch for any signs of skin impairment. Be aware of potential embarrassment involving the procedure. Act professionally.

If catheter sheath is too tight, remove and replace sheath. Reapply adhesive strip and ensure that it is not too tight.

If urine leaks from upper part of catheter, remove catheter, wash penis. Dry with alcohol and replace catheter. Wrap adhesive firmly but not too tightly around base of penis, without allowing adhesive to touch skin. If the catheter sheath falls off, wash penis as previously indicated, and reapply catheter.

Procedure: Giving Enema Using Disposable Enema Equipment

Description: Enemas introduce a solution into the rectum.

Purpose: To stimulate peristalsis (intestinal mobility), to remove flatus (gas) or feces, or to instill prescribed medications.

STEP	RATIONALE
1. Collect necessary equipment: • Enema administration package or equipment • Clean pitcher • Protective covered plastic sheet or protective padding • Enema solution and prescribed solution • Bath thermometer • Lubricant • IV pole (standard) • Clean gloves • Toilet tissue • Bedpan • Disposable gloves	Organizing necessary equipment allows quick and safe implementation.
2. Wash hands.	Prevents transfer of microorganisms.
3. Open enema package; remove items.	Prepares for procedure.
4. Pour appropriate amount of warmed solution (water or saline) into enema administration container.	Prepares solution before placement into enema administration container.
5. Check solution with bath thermometer: 105–110°F (40.5–43.3°C). If saline is used, warm by placing saline container in basin of hot water.	Prevents cramping that may occur if solution is too cool. Decreases chances of tissue injury if temperature is too hot.
6. Add soap (for soapsuds enema) and mix into water.	Allows soap to dissolve evenly in solution. Addition of soap after water is prepared decreases bubbles in solution. The absence of bubbles decreases flatus in the bowel.

STEP	RATIONALE
7. Clamp enema administration tubing.	Prevents solution from passing through tubing when solution is placed in enema container.
8. Pour enema solution into enema bag.	Prepares for enema administration.
9. Close top of container.	
10. Explain procedure. Determine the amount of solution he or she can tolerate.	Informs client of procedure.
11. Bring prepared enema to bedside. Hang bag or container on IV pole next to client.	Places enema administration near client.
12. Draw curtain around bed and/or close room door.	Ensures privacy.
13. Raise bed to comfortable working position.	Prevents back strain.
14. Assist client into a left Sims' (side-lying) position to expose buttocks.	Permits solution to flow into the rectum by gravity.
15. Place protective pad or covered plastic sheet under buttocks and thighs.	Prevents soiling bed linens.
16. Position bedpan next to client.	Bedpan will be within easy reach if client cannot retain enema.
17. Put on disposable gloves.	Protects nurse's hands from possible soiling by feces.
18. Remove protective cap from enema tip or nozzle. Open clamp on tubing; let solution flow through tubing into bedpan.	Fills tubing with solution. Air is removed from tubing. Prevents air from entering rectum.
19. Lubricate 3–4 inches of rectal tube or nozzle.	Allows easier insertion.
20. Remove enema container from IV pole and hold at the same height as the client's rectum.	Decreases the pressure of the solution entering rectum and allows the solution to enter rectum slowly, thereby increasing retention of solution.
21. Separate buttocks and visualize anus.	Prepares for procedure.
22. Ask client to take a deep breath and at the same time insert nozzle or rectal tube into anus; point tip of tube or nozzle toward umbilicus for about 3–4 inches.	Relaxes the anus. Placing the nozzle or rectal tube into rectum and pointing same toward umbilicus allows the nozzle or rectal tube to stay inside the rectum without injuring the rectal mucosa (tissue).
23. Unclamp tubing; raise container until solution flows into rectum.	Gradual increase of pressure in enema tubing prevents injury to rectal tissue. If the container is too high, there will be increased pressure and rapid instillation, which can cause painful distention of rectum and early evacuation.
24. Tell client that the solution is being instilled. Ask him or her to let you know if there is any pain or cramping. If so, clamp tubing briefly until pain or cramping stops.	Informs client of procedure. Allows the client to let the nurse know if pain or cramping occurs.
25. Clamp tubing, remove rectal tube and nozzle when all solution is used or client is no longer able to hold solution.	Prevents accidental spilling of any remaining solution in container.
26. Wipe anal area with toilet tissue; remove gloves inside out and discard.	Removes any feces and solution from buttocks and surrounding area; decreases chances of irritating skin.
27. Set aside enema equipment. Place client on bedpan or assist to commode or bathroom when ready (if client uses bathroom, ask him or her not to flush toilet).	Readies client for evacuation of solution, flatus, and feces. Allows nurse to check results of enema procedure.
28. Place call signal within easy reach; ask client to use call signal when finished.	Ensures privacy and comfort.
29. Assist client to clean perianal area with soap and water; dry.	Decreases potential irritation of skin around anal area.
30. Assist client to a comfortable position in bed. Leave protective pad in place unless soiled. If soiled, replace with a clean protective pad.	Ensures comfort. Decreases chances of further soiling of bed linens.
31. Check the enema return before emptying bedpan or commode or flushing toilet.	Evaluates results of enema.
32. Wash hands.	Prevents transfer of microorganisms.
33. Wash, rinse, and hang enema equipment to dry.	Readies the equipment for later use by the same client. If equipment is reusable and is to be used for other clients, it must be sterilized.
34. Record results of enema in terms of amount, color, and odor of feces and of solution.	Ensures accurate recording of results.

Prepackaged Enema Administration:

STEP	RATIONALE
1. Follow previous steps 10–18.	
2. Inspect nozzle for lubricant (add lubricant, if needed).	Allows easier insertion of nozzle into rectum.

STEP	RATIONALE
3. Squeeze container gently.	Expels air before insertion.
4. Separate buttocks and locate anus.	Prepares for insertion of nozzle.
5. Follow previous steps 24–27.	
6. Record results of enema.	Ensures accurate recording of procedure and results.

Nursing Implications: Record and report any unusual problems, such as fresh blood in the returned enema solution and feces, inability to insert nozzle or rectal tube because of fecal impaction, client complaints of severe cramping, and distention with rigidity of the abdomen as noted during or following an enema. This last symptom may indicate perforation of the bowel. If this occurs, remove the tube immediately and check vital signs. If vital signs are within normal range and symptoms disappear, check with RN regarding reinsertion of rectal tube. If discomfort continues and vital signs indicate a problem, notify the RN in charge immediately.

If the client begins to expel the enema solution before the procedure is completed, place the client on a bedpan, reinsert rectal tube or nozzle, and *slowly* instill the remaining solution. This tends to stimulate peristalsis and assist in removal of feces and flatus (gas).

If the client does not expel the enema solution or feces after a small enema has been given, the enema may have been given to soften fecal material, as is the case with an oil retention enema. If so, the client is expected to expel feces within 12–24 hours. If the purpose of the enema was to stimulate peristalsis and the enema has not been expelled, the solution may have been absorbed in the stool without stimulating the walls of the rectum (peristalsis).

Report these findings to the RN or team leader to determine if another enema should be given. Document all findings.

Procedure: Inserting Rectal Tube

Description: A rectal tube is inserted into the rectum.

Purpose: Assists in the removal of feces or flatus (gas); must be ordered by the physician.

STEP	RATIONALE
1. Collect necessary equipment: • Disposable rectal tube • Plastic bag or plastic specimen container • Protective pad • Rubber band • Lubricant • Adhesive tape • Clean gloves	Organizing necessary equipment allows for quick and safe implementation.
2. Explain procedure.	Informs client of procedure.
3. Place rectal tube, end opposite the tip, into plastic bag or plastic specimen container.	Provides a container for liquid feces expelled.
4. Place within reach two pieces of tape, each about 6 inches long.	Prepares for later use.
5. Wash hands.	Prevents transfer of microorganisms.
6. Close curtains around bed or close room door.	Ensures privacy.
7. Assist client into a left-lying position.	Allows inserted tube to follow anatomic curve without injury to rectal tissue.
8. Put protective pad under buttocks and thighs.	Prevents soiling of bed linens.
9. Put on clean gloves.	Helps to keep hands from becoming contaminated with feces.
10. Lubricate the tip of rectal tube.	Allows easier insertion into rectum and decreases potential for injury to rectal tissue.
11. Ask client to take a deep breath and at the same time insert rectal tube about 4–6 inches into rectum. Point tube toward umbilicus while inserting.	Relaxes the anal musculature; decreases chances of injuring rectal tissues.
12. Place tapes in position to secure tube in rectal area.	Fixes the tube so that it stays in place.
13. If plastic bag is used, tape the plastic bag tightly around bag and rectal tube.	Decreases chances of accidental soiling of bed linen.
14. If specimen container is used, place tape around rectal tube near slit and anchor tape to container.	
15. Remove and discard gloves.	

STEP	RATIONALE
16. Replace client's bed linens. Make sure call signal is within easy reach.	Leaves client comfortable.
17. Leave rectal tube in place for 20–30 minutes.	Allows sufficient time to expel flatus.
18. Ask client if he or she has expelled flatus. Put on gloves; remove rectal tube and set aside.	Determines results of procedure.
19. Remove protective pad. Wash, rinse, and dry anal and surrounding skin area.	Removes fecal material from perianal area.
20. Take rectal tube and container to bathroom; examine contents.	Evaluates results of procedure.
21. Discard rectal tube and container.	
22. Remove gloves; wash hands.	Prevents transfer of microorganisms.

Nursing Implications: Document procedure and results. If the rectal tube cannot be inserted because of fecal impaction, notify the RN or team leader for instructions. Any complaints of severe cramping with obvious signs of distention and rigidity of the abdomen upon insertion of the rectal tube demand immediate attention; report to RN or team leader immediately. This situation may indicate a perforation of the bowel. If the symptoms disappear and vital signs are within normal range, check with RN or team leader about reinsertion of rectal tube. If vital signs are abnormal and symptoms remain, notify RN or team leader.

Document procedure and all findings.

Procedure: Managing Wounds

Description: Wound management includes the assessment, cleaning, and protection of wounds.

Purpose: To prevent infection so that healing can take place.

STEP	RATIONALE
Application of a Dry Dressing:	
1. Obtain necessary supplies and equipment: • Sterile gloves • Sterile dressing set • Sterile drape • Gauze pads • Abdominal pads • Cotton balls and swabs • Scissors • Forceps and hemostat • Small basin • Dressing materials (nonadherent or transparent dressings) • Ointment or powder if prescribed • Waterproof pad • Tape, ties, elastic bandages, Montgomery straps, butterflies • Bath blanket • Waterproof disposal bag	Organizing necessary supplies and equipment allows for quick and safe implementation.
2. Explain procedure.	Informs client of procedure.
3. Check whether client has pain; check with RN regarding administration of pain medication.	Decreases anxiety.
4. Bring supplies and equipment to bedside. Ask client not to touch any of the supplies during the procedure.	Prepares for procedure.
5. Pull curtains around bed or close room door.	Ensures privacy.
6. Position client so that wound can be accessed. Make client as comfortable as possible.	Allows care of wound.
7. Lower bedclothes; drape around wound area with sheet or bath blanket.	Ensures privacy.
8. Wash hands.	Prevents transfer of microorganisms.
9. Fold top of waterproof bag over back of straight chair or in easy reach.	Provides a container for disposal of used materials.

STEP	RATIONALE
10. Remove dressing binder or untie Montgomery straps, if used.	Prepares for procedure.
11. Loosen tape (if used). Hold skin and peel the edges of the tape.	Prevents injury to upper thin layers of skin.
12. Remove tape by pulling in a line with wound.	Prevents injury (peeling of upper layers of skin).
13. Put on clean gloves. Hold a corner of dressing at edge away from client's face; roll it off wound and remove old dressing.	Protects hands from contamination with microorganisms. Keeps contamination of airborne microorganisms from client's mouth and nose.
14. Check the amount, odor, color, and thickness of any drainage on dressing.	May indicate possible infection or excess drainage.
15. Fold the edges of the dressing inward and dispose of in waterproof container.	Prevents contamination.
16. Remove gloves and discard in bag.	Prevents transfer of microorganisms.
17. Wash hands.	Prevents transfer of microorganisms.
18. Place sterile dressing tray on overbed table; open tray using aseptic technique and add necessary supplies.	Prepares for wound management.
19. Fill sterile basin with sterile solution.	Prepares for wound cleansing.
20. Use sterile forceps to remove any remaining contact dressing over wound.	Prevents contamination of hands that may be present on dressing.
21. If dressing is stuck to wound, pour a small amount of solution from basin directly over dressing.	Prevents injury to skin and helps to loosen dressing from wound.
22. Check the odor, consistency, color, and amount of drainage. Check wound for signs of healing or complications.	Evaluates the condition of the wound.
23. Discard forceps.	
24. Put on sterile gloves.	Maintains sterility.
25. Using new forceps, pick up gauze or cotton balls; keep tips of forceps pointed downward.	Prevents potential contaminants from traveling up forceps.
26. Clean wound. Clean first over incisional area and then next to incision, using a circular motion.	Moves from area of least contamination to area of greatest contamination.
27. Discard cotton ball or gauze after one use.	Use of clean gauze or cotton balls prevents spread of microorganisms.
28. Dry wound in the same way, using dry cotton balls or gauze.	
29. Discard forceps.	
30. Apply prescribed ointment or solution using aseptic technique.	
31. Place enough sterile gauze directly over wound to absorb drainage.	Decreases the amount of drainage on surrounding skin areas or bandages.
32. Remove and discard disposable sterile gloves in bag.	Prevents transfer of microorganisms.
33. Touching only outside pad, place abdominal pad over dressing.	Absorbs drainage and prevents airborne microorganisms from contaminating wound.
34. Place tape, Montgomery straps, or binder over dressing.	Secures dressing.
35. Discard remaining materials and supplies.	
36. Remove drape and place the client in a comfortable position. Place call signal within easy reach.	Ensures comfort.
37. Wash hands.	Prevents transfer of microorganisms.

Nursing Implications: Document procedure and amount, color, odor, and viscosity of drainage. Report any unusual findings immediately to RN or team leader. Indicate location of wound and record drainage or moisture on outside of the dressing that was removed. Such findings may indicate excessive wound secretions, which will need more absorbent dressing materials. Check for any fresh blood on dressing, including amount in documentation. This may indicate hemorrhage, which will need immediate attention. A pressure dressing may be required. Determine if client is in pain and check with RN or team leader regarding pain medication before dressing application is started.

Procedure: Performing Passive Range-of-Motion Exercises

Description: Exercises of the joints are performed by the health-care worker three to four times a day to maintain joint function.

Purpose: To maintain joint function and prevent contractures of muscular groups of those joints that a client is unable to move or has restricted movement of.

STEP	RATIONALE
1. Explain procedure.	Informs client of procedure; gains cooperation.
2. Wash hands.	Prevents transfer of microorganisms.
3. Pull curtains around client's bed or close room door.	Ensures privacy.
4. Raise bed to a comfortable working position. Place bed in a flat position.	Prevents back strain. Places client in correct position for the procedure.
5. Remove top bed linens and any clothing that may restrict movement. Cover with bath blanket.	Makes it easier to do the exercises. Ensures privacy.
6. Lower siderails on one side of bed and move client's body toward that side of the bed.	Assists nurse in using good body mechanics and permits closer proximity to client.
7. Place hands under client's neck and back of head. Raise head, move chin toward chest, flexing (bending) the neck. Lower head so neck is in a resting position.	ROM exercise for neck. Repeat each step two times.
8. Lower client's head and turn head to one side. Repeat in other direction. Move head to normal resting position.	
9. Rotate head slowly three times. Put client's head in a normal resting position when neck exercises are completed.	
10. Explain steps and reason for exercise to client or significant other.	Teaches client and/or significant other.
11. Hold client's arm farthest away from you by the elbow and hand. Flex (bend) shoulder by raising his or her arm in an arc (circular motion) from bed to above his or her head. Extend (straighten) shoulder and lower arm to client's side of bed.	ROM exercise for shoulder. Repeat each shoulder exercise slowly two times.
12. Abduct (move away from midline of body) shoulder; hold wrist and elbow and move client's arm away from his or her side.	
13. Adduct (move toward midline of body) shoulder; return arm over client's body toward opposite side.	
14. Hold upper arm away and out from body at the level of the shoulder; hold elbow and grasp client's palm. Raise his or her hand above head level. Internally rotate shoulder by turning client's palm above his or her head toward the body.	
15. Externally rotate shoulder by moving client's palm (hand) away from the body. Keep hand over client's head during this step.	
16. Flex (bend) elbow by grasping client's palm; place other hand under client's elbow. Move client's forearm toward his or her upper arm.	Exercises elbow through its normal ROM. Repeat each step two times.
17. Extend elbow (straighten arm).	
18. Supinate forearm by holding palm and elbow upward.	Exercises wrist through its normal ROM. Repeat each step slowly two times.
19. Pronate forearm by moving forearm so that palm faces downward.	
20. Flex (bend) wrist by turning hand toward inner part of forearm.	
21. Extend (straighten) wrist.	
22. Hyperextend wrist by moving hand toward the back of arm.	
23. Rotate (turn) thumb toward the thumb (radial) side of hand. Then turn the opposite side of palm toward the little finger.	Exercises finger joints through their normal ROM. Repeat each step slowly two times.
24. Close your hand and fingers around the back of the client's hand while holding his or her wrist; flex (bend) client's finger joints.	
25. Extend (straighten) joints by opening client's hand.	
26. Move client's thumb toward his or her little finger and back again.	

STEP	RATIONALE
27. Repeat steps 11–26 for arm closest to you.	
28. Place one of your hands under knee and one hand under heel of leg farthest from you.	Exercises knee and hip through their normal ROM. Repeat steps slowly two times.
29. Raise lower leg, making sure that both hip and knee are flexed (bent). Lower leg and straighten (extend) hip and knee.	
30. Keeping one hand under knee and other hand under heel, abduct client's hip by moving leg away from midline of body. Adduct hip by moving leg toward the midline of body and over opposite leg.	
31. Holding the client's heel, rotate (turn) the entire leg internally (inward) and externally (outward).	
32. Put your hand under client's heel, and forearm against bottom of his or her foot. Bend (dorsiflex) the ankle so that toes point upward toward client's knee.	Exercises ankle through its normal ROM. Repeat steps 30–32 two times.
33. Plantar-flex (straighten) ankle so that toes point downward, away from knee.	
34. Hold client's heel with one hand and turn (invert) foot inward.	
35. Turn (evert) foot outward with other hand.	
36. Hold bottom of foot over arch with hand, flex (bend) toes forward. Extend (straighten) toes.	Exercises toe joints through their normal ROM. Repeat steps three times.
37. Move each toe separately by separating and placing them together.	
38. Repeat steps 28–37 for opposite leg.	
39. Remove drapes; replace client's clothing and bed linens. Place client in a comfortable position. Replace siderails, if required. Lower bed. Place call signal within easy reach.	Ensures comfort.
40. Open curtains and room door.	
41. Wash hands.	

Nursing Implications: Document procedure and level of ROM. Record and report any unusual signs and symptoms such as complaints of pain. If client complains of severe pain, check with RN or team leader about the possibility of administering pain medication and postpone exercises until client is more comfortable. Note limits of ROM for each joint.

In the presence of risk factors for potential contractures, as in clients who have had a stroke, ROM exercises are essential to prevent development of such contractures.

Check to see if any joints appear swollen or inflamed. On exercising specific joints, report and record any unusual sound or movement. Check muscles of extremities to determine if there is less or more muscle mass in one extremity than in the other. Report all findings to RN or team leader.

Teach joint exercises so that client, if able, may do his or her own active ROM exercises or may participate actively in the exercise as it is given by the nurse.

Procedure: Care of Decubitus Ulcer

Description: Management of stage I–IV decubitus ulcers.

Purpose: To decrease the potential for further breakdown of decubitus ulcers once they have occurred.

Stage I: Reddening of skin. Skin is pinkish-red and mottled. These signs disappear in about 5 minutes once pressure is relieved over the part. Black clients have purplish or darker discoloration. Skin is not broken. There is usually no remaining tissue damage if ulcer is taken care of properly.

Stage II: Superficial (outside) skin damage including superficial blood vessels. Reddening of skin does not disappear with release of pressure. The area is edematous, showing blistered, cracked, or broken skin. Damage to skin may be shallow or include destruction to skin layers (dermis and epidermis).

Stage III: Deep tissue involvement. Skin is broken, drainage is present. Area may be necrotic (black), draining (yellow), or granulating (red). Infection is more likely to occur in ulcers at this stage.

Stage IV: Advanced destruction of capillaries under skin layers and muscle. Large ulcerated areas penetrate to muscle and bone. Dead (necrotic) tissue is visible in the ulcerated area and extensive drainage is present. Infection at this stage is common.

STEP	RATIONALE

Management of Stage I Decubitus Ulcer:

1. Obtain necessary supplies and equipment:
   - Extra pillows
   - Air mattress, egg-crate or foam mattress, sheepskin, alternating-pressure mattress, or water bed
   - Turning sheet
   - Sterile culture tubes
   - Heating lamp (if ordered under supervision of RN)
   - Sterile culture tubes
   - Wound care supplies
   - Irrigating solution
   - Dressings
   - Asepto bulb syringe
   - Basin
   - Disposable gloves

   Organizing necessary supplies and equipment allows for quick and safe implementation.

2. Place client on protective mattress used in your institution. — Distributes body weight evenly to decrease amount of pressure over bony parts of the body.
3. Apply sheepskin heel or elbow protectors. — Protects bony areas against too much pressure over capillaries. These areas have very little fat or muscle.
4. Turn client every 2 hours or less. Use lift or turning sheet; ambulate; exercise as able. Get client up in chair, if ordered, but for not more than 1 hour. — Changes pressure areas.
5. Do not place client on affected area until signs of stage I bedsores disappear. — Decreases pressure on developing decubitus.
6. Check bony parts of body every 2–4 hours. — Checks for early signs.
7. Keep skin dry and free of excretions and secretions. — Excretions and secretions may help in developing bedsores.
8. Do not use soaps, perfumed lotions, or other products with an alcohol base. — Use of such products increases excess drying of skin surfaces.
9. Encourage fluid intake (240 ml every 2 hours, unless restricted). Monitor I&O. — Ensures sufficient fluids to maintain body fluid balance.
10. Encourage a well-balanced diet, especially with high-protein foods. — Ensures protein intake required for tissue rebuilding.
11. Do not massage the decubitus area. — Massage of decubitus area interferes with protective mechanism of hyperemia.
12. Place pillows to cushion bony areas when sitting in chair or wheelchair. — Protects skin from pressure over time.

Management of Stage II Decubitus Ulcer:

1. Use same measures as in stage I. Apply gloves. — Ensures continuation of care.
2. Cleanse the affected area using sterile technique. Use either half-strength hydrogen peroxide or other agent prescribed by physician. — Helps to remove harmful microorganisms or other materials.
3. Rinse area with normal saline. — Removes cleansing agents and other materials.
4. Be careful not to further injure the area of decubitus or surrounding skin area. — Broken skin encourages further breakdown of skin.
5. Apply prescribed medication to decubitus as prescribed by physician or institutional policy.
6. For dry treatment of decubitus ulcer (under RN supervision), dry ulcer after cleansing and expose area to a heat lamp for 20 minutes at 18–20 inches distance (see institutional policy). — Dries skin surface. Heat dilates (widens) blood vessels under skin, which increases blood supply to area and stimulates healing process.
7. Check skin every 5 minutes if heat lamp is used. Remove heat lamp if signs of beginning burn occur, or after 20 minutes. — Ensures that burns have not occurred.
8. Apply a sterile dressing (4 × 4 gauze pads) over broken skin area and about 2 inches around area. Secure with paper tape. — Protects open area from microorganisms; paper tape is less likely to injure skin than other types of tape.

or

Leave wound undressed (check institutional policy).

STEP	RATIONALE
For Wet Treatment:	
9. Clean wound as in step 3, and dry the area thoroughly.	Removes harmful microorganisms.
10. Place a transparent dressing over the area and about 2 inches around area. Leave in place until it falls off.	Covers entire surface of affected area. This dressing allows exchange of gases while keeping secretions under dressing.
Management of Stage III Decubitus Ulcers:	
1. Use the same processes as in stages I and II.	
2. Send a culture specimen of the wound secretions to laboratory.	Identifies organisms responsible for infection.
3. Use medications and treatment as ordered by the physician.	Provides comprehensive care.
4. Encourage diet with increased amount of proteins and vitamin C.	Adds extra protein and vitamin C to assist in tissue rebuilding.
5. Assess client's age and weight, and check about increasing fluid intake.	Lubricates body cells and tissues.
6. Cleanse wound as described in stage II management.	Removes wound secretions microorganisms and other waste material.
7. Irrigate ulcer with half-strength hydrogen peroxide or other solution prescribed by physician. Use sterile technique.	Loosens dead (necrotic) tissue and scabs. Stimulates new tissue growth.
8. Have RN debride necrotic tissue and scabs (eschar) using irrigation and cleansing with saturated gauze pads (sterile technique).	Removes necrotic tissue and other materials.
9. Apply sterile wet to dry dressing for continued debridement.	Helps to continue removal of dead tissue.
10. Apply medication to area as prescribed by physician.	
Management of Stage IV Decubitus Ulcers:	
1. Use same measures as in stages I–III.	
2. RN will consult with physician with regard to medical and/or surgical treatment.	Provides comprehensive treatment. If ulcerated areas are very deep and penetrate to muscle and bone, surgical closure may be necessary. The wound must first be free of infection before surgical treatment is attempted.

Nursing Implications: Assess client for risk of developing decubitus ulcers (e.g., low serum albumin, immobility, incontinence, anemia). Document findings and record measures taken to treat the decubitus ulcer. Report to RN any findings that may indicate the formation of new decubiti. Check to see if the decubitus has progressed from one stage to another; report such findings. Check to see if healing is taking place by determining whether wound secretions and size are decreasing and whether granulation is taking place at the edges of the wound.

Check with RN regarding pain medications if client complains of pain. Check vital signs. A temperature increase may suggest an increase in the decubitus size and development to a further stage.

Be careful when sitting the client up in bed. A shearing force occurs when the client's skin sticks to the bed linen as he or she slides down to the foot of the bed. The tissues underlying the outer skin surface slide simultaneously in the opposite direction, injuring the tissue.

Clients who are poorly nourished may lose muscle mass and subcutaneous tissue. This results in less padding between skin and bone. Fluid and electrolyte imbalances and loss of protein inhibit wound healing. Clients with impaired circulation or anemia and elderly clients are at high risk for development of decubitus ulcers.

Incontinence leads to continuous moisture on the skin and allows growth of bacteria that thrive in a moist, warm, dark environment. This environment is conducive to infection. Infection also increases body temperature, which in turn increases moisture on the skin.

Clients who are immobilized in bed, chair, or wheelchair are susceptible to pressure and the development of decubiti. Clients in traction or immobilized in a cast may develop decubitus ulcers from pressure from the equipment or cast. Note that pressure sores can also develop from pressure exerted by an improperly secured nasogastric tube or other catheters if present for prolonged periods.

Procedure: Performing Cardiopulmonary Resuscitation

Description: Cardiopulmonary resuscitation (CPR) is the basic emergency procedure for cardiopulmonary arrest and consists of artificial ventilation and manual external cardiac massage.

Purpose: To restore cardiac and respiratory function.

STEP	RATIONALE
1. Assess to determine responsiveness by gently tapping or shaking client's shoulder.	Confirms unconsciousness.
2. If client is unresponsive, call for help and access emergency medical system (EMS).	Assistance may be needed to notify the emergency system.
3. Position the victim by turning on back as a unit, supporting head and neck.	For CPR to be effective, the person must be supine and on a firm, flat surface.
4. Determine breathlessness by opening or maintaining the airway. Use head-tilt/chin-lift maneuver. Place ear over the person's mouth and observe the chest—look, listen, and feel for breathing. In infants (younger than 1 year), do not hyperextend the neck.	The most important action in successful resuscitation is immediate opening of the airway. Hyperextending the neck in infants blocks off the airway.
5. If no respirations are noted, deliver two ventilations at 1–1.5 seconds per inspiration. Observe chest rise and fall before delivering the second ventilation. Maintain head-tilt/chin-lift position during ventilations; pinch nose with one hand and seal mouth completely. Deliver only as much volume as needed to expand the chest.	An excess of air volume and fast inspiratory flow rates are likely to cause gastric distention.
6. Assess to determine pulselessness. **Adult:** Feel for carotid pulse for 5–10 seconds while maintaining head-tilt with the other hand. **Child (1–8 years):** Check carotid pulse 5–10 seconds. **Infant:** Check brachial pulse 5–10 seconds.	Chest compressions should not be performed on a person with a pulse. Time should be allowed for correct assessment of pulselessness.
7. If pulseless, begin chest compressions and repeat call for help: a. Kneel by victim's shoulders. b. Locate proper hand position and begin compressions. **Adults:** Compress 1½–2 inches with a rate of 80–100 per minute. **Child:** Compress 1–1½ inch with a rate of 80–100 per minute. **Infant:** Compress ½–1 inch with a rate of 100 per minute.	Proper hand position reduces risk of injury. Proper hand position and compression depth ensure adequate circulation of blood volume.
8. Compression-to-ventilation rate: **Adult—one-person CPR:** 15 compressions to two ventilations at 1.5–2 seconds per inspiration. **Adult—two-person CPR:** five compressions to one ventilation. **Child:** Five compressions to one ventilation. **Infant:** Five compressions to one ventilation.	
9. Assessment for pulse after: **Adult—one-person CPR:** Four cycles of 15 compressions to two ventilations (or 1 minute). **Adult—two-person CPR:** After 1 minute and at intervals thereafter. **Child:** 10 cycles of five compressions to one ventilation. **Infant:** 10 cycles of five compressions to one ventilation.	
10. Determine pulselessness by assessing for 5 seconds. If pulse and ventilations are absent, continue CPR. If pulse but no respiration is present, perform rescue breathing: **Adult:** 12 times per minute **Child:** 15 times per minute **Infant:** 20 times per minute	
11. If pulse and respirations are present, monitor the person and contact emergency medical personnel. Place in recovery position. Client lies on right side, with upper leg slightly drawn up and left arm crooked. Hand is under head.	All persons who undergo CPR need to be seen by a physician.

Nursing Implications: All nursing personnel need to be certified annually for basic life support (BLS). Support CPR efforts for as long as possible or until emergency personnel are on the scene. Do not interrupt CPR for more than 7 seconds except in special circumstances.

Procedure: Care of Client with Skeletal Traction

Description: Metal pins or nails are inserted into the tissue structure and attached to traction devices.

Purpose: To immobilize, position, or align a fractured bone and facilitate healing; to provide supportive care and safety measures.

STEP	RATIONALE
1. Examine traction for proper body alignment and weight. Check knots, ropes, and pulleys.	Ensures proper traction. Make sure that weights are free-swinging.
2. Assess client's response: note presence of pain, spasm, or sense of comfort.	Relief of pain or muscle spasms may not be immediate.
3. Administer narcotics or relaxants as ordered and needed.	Decreases anxiety and ensures comfort.
4. Check affected extremity for temperature, pulses, color, movement (of fingers or toes) and sensation every 1–2 degrees × 24 hours, then as ordered.	Provides information on neurovascular status.
5. Cleanse area around pin insertion sites with solution of normal saline and hydorgen peroxide every 8–24 hours. Apply small sterile dressing. (An ointment of Betadine or Neosporin may be applied before dressing.)	Reduces microorganisms at insertion sites. Check with physician before performing site care.
6. Observe insertion sites for signs of redness, swelling, or drainage.	Indicates presence of inflammation or infection.

Nursing Implications: Be alert for signs and symptoms of fat embolism: restlessness, mental status alterations, tachycardia, tachypnea, hypotension, dyspnea, and petchial rash over upper chest and neck. Clients at risk are those with long bone fractures. Fat embolism usually occurs within the first 72 hours.

Report any signs of swelling (edema), increased pain, or inability to move joints, which could indicate compartment syndrome. This leads to decreased perfusion and tissue anoxia.

Procedure: Applying an Abdominal Binder

Description: A snugly fitting wrap is secured across an abdominal incision.

Purpose: To provide support of the operative incision site and underlying musculature; to provide comfort and security with movement.

STEP	RATIONALE
1. Obtain abdominal binder of appropriate size. The binder should be large enough to wrap around abdomen and overlap for safe securing of Velcro closure. Measure abdomen with tape measure, if necessary.	Abdominal binder must be of appropriate size for fit and comfort.
2. Position client lying on side. Fold one end of binder and place against back toward midline.	This position is more comfortable for placement of binder.
3. Roll client in the other direction over the folded end of the binder. Pull out folded section and smooth.	Lessens the pull on abdominal incision and muscles.
4. Roll client on back over center of binder and position so that lower edge of binder is at level of symphysis pubis.	Centering ensures proper placement and support of underlying structures.
5. Pull distal end over abdomen and maintain tension while pulling proximal portion over. Secure with Velcro closure.	
6. Ask client whether binder feels secure and comfortable.	

Nursing Implications: A binder that is too tight may hinder breathing and limit circulation. A binder that is positioned incorrectly may pull on incision line and cause separation and bleeding. Assess respirations with binder on and readjust if necessary.

Procedure: Applying a Sling

Description: A triangular cloth is applied to securely hold the affected arm in a bent position across chest. Manufactured slings with Velcro closures are also used.

Purpose: To immobilize the affected arm, providing support and decreasing muscle strain.

STEP	RATIONALE
1. Obtain triangular bandage. Position open sling with binder center under arm, pointed end at wrist, and base of triangle at elbow.	Provides support at elbow.
2. Pull ends up, encasing arm in sling, bent at elbow. Position arm across chest.	Reduces strain on shoulder and neck muscles.
3. Bring top of binder point over neck on unaffected side.	
4. Bring other binder point over neck on affected side.	
5. Position arm with wrist above elbow. Tie ends behind neck in square knot.	Enhances circulation. Prevents dependent edema of wrist and hand.
6. Place gauze squares between neck and sling knot to pad the area.	Enhances comfort.
7. Fold remaining bandage around elbow for support and fasten with safety pin.	

Nursing Implications: Assess circulation (color, pulses, warmth), mobility, and sensation of extremities. Assess skin daily for signs of pressure or breakdown. Provide padding or readjust sling as necessary.

Procedure: Assisting with a Sitz Bath

Description: A specially designed tub allows the client to sit in warm water without immersing legs or upper trunk.

Purpose: To promote circulation, relaxation, and comfort to incisional areas, wounds, or hemorrhoids.

STEP	RATIONALE
1. Fill sitz tub or bathtub with warm water. Add medications, if ordered.	Excessively warm water can damage tissue and cause burns.
2. Assist client into sitting position in tub. Adjust water temperature if necessary.	Water should feel comfortably warm to client.
3. Place bath blanket around client's shoulders, if desired. Place a call signal next to client.	Prevents chilling. Ensures safety.
4. After 15 minutes, assist client out of tub and dry skin gently.	

Nursing Implications: Instruct client not to attempt to get out of tub alone if he or she is weak or unsteady. For bedridden clients, a plastic sitz basin can be used. Have client notify nurse if symptoms such as dizziness arise. Be prepared to check blood pressure and discontinue sitz bath if hypotension occurs. Properly clean bath basin between uses.

Procedure: Applying Warm Soaks

Description: Affected body part is immersed in warm water or warmed solutions for a prescribed period of time.

Purpose: To debride wounds and improve circulation; to apply medicated solutions that facilitate healing.

STEP	RATIONALE
1. Fill basin with warmed water or solution. Test for proper temperature.	Excessively high temperature may damage tissues or cause burns.

STEP	RATIONALE
2. Place waterproof pad under client if soiling of linen is likely.	
3. Immerse affected body part in basin.	
4. Cover client with a bath blanket to prevent chilling.	Ensures comfort.
5. Allow to soak for 15–20 minutes. Remove and gently pat dry.	

Nursing Implications: If it is not possible to soak a body area in a basin, towels may be soaked in the warmed solution and applied. Wrap toweled area in waterproof pad and leave in place for approximately 15 minutes.

If continuous warm soaks are ordered, wrap a heating pad around the moist towel or sterile saline dressings and waterproof pad; keep on low warming temperature. Wet towel or dressings with solution every 1–2 hours. Check to be sure that temperature is not too warm. Assess skin and wound condition and document.

Procedure: Using a Heat Lamp

Description: An application of dry heat using 40- to 75-watt infrared or regular household bulb situated at a safe distance from the client's skin.

Purpose: To promote circulation and healing without risk of injury from the heat source.

STEP	RATIONALE
1. Provide privacy for client.	
2. Assist client into a comfortable position that exposes the area to be treated. Pad with pillows, if necessary.	Because client will have to maintain position for 15–20 minutes, ensure that position is comfortable.
3. Make sure that skin to be exposed is dry.	Moisture may act as a conductor of heat.
4. Place heat lamp about 24 inches away for 40–60 watts and about 30 inches away for 75 watts. Turn on lamp.	Protects skin from burning.
5. Adjust light for direct effect on area to be treated. Position call bell and instruct client to ring for nurse if experiencing any discomfort.	Ensures that the correct area is treated with heat. Ensures safety.
6. While heat lamp treatment is in progress, check client every 5 minutes. Assess skin and position of lamp.	Some clients may have decreased sensation. Assess any changes in skin condition.
7. After 20 minutes, discontinue the treatment. Assess skin condition and redress wound, if required. Position for comfort.	Some clients may not be able to tolerate the heat treatment for the entire period.

Nursing Implications: Document procedure, including the amount of heat, distance of source from skin, length of treatment, area treated, and client's response.

Procedure: Teaching Controlled Coughing Techniques

Description: When the cough reflex is diminished because of central nervous system depression, anesthesia, pain, or sedation, the potential for atelectasis (collapsed lung) and infection increases.

Purpose: To clear airway of secretions; to prevent pneumonia, atelectasis, and airway infections.

STEP	RATIONALE
1. Identify clients at risk for ineffective cough: those with lung diseases, profound weakness, immobility, postoperative states, central nervous system diseases, depression, lung cancer, or an artificial airway.	Certain conditions predispose client for the nursing diagnosis of ineffective airway clearance.
2. Place client in best position for cough effectiveness. Usually sitting up and leaning forward is most beneficial.	Allows lung expansion and expiratory effort.
3. Deep breathing and coughing: Position client upright. Have client take two or three deep breaths, hold last breath for count of three, then cough twice forcefully while pulling in abdominal muscles.	Taking deep breaths expands the lung, moving air behind mucous secretions. Two consecutive coughs help to remove secretions and dislodge mucus.

STEP	RATIONALE
If client is recovering from surgery, splint incisional area with hands or a pillow.	Splinting reduces the pain of coughing by decreasing incisional pulling.
4. Cascade cough: Have client take slow, deep breaths and hold second breath for count of two. Instruct client to open mouth and cough several times in succession while contracting expiratory muscles. The client should cough until all the air is expelled.	The cascade cough helps to clear large and small airways.
After each cascade cough, have client breathe slowly and quietly, allowing a period of rest.	Rest prevents paroxysms of coughing.
5. Huff cough: Have client take two slow, deep breaths and hold second breath for a count of two. Instead of a series of coughs, have the client say "huff."	Clients with lung disease may not be able to perform cascade cough. Huff cough may be effective in producing natural cough reflex.
6. Quad cough: Have client take two slow, deep breaths and hold second breath for count of two. Have client exhale forcefully while nurse or client presses upward and inward against diaphragm.	External pressure assists the muscular efforts of the cough and assists in expelling secretions.

Nursing Implications: Observe and record effectiveness of coughing techniques. Support and encourage client efforts. For clients with copious or tenacious secretions, coughing techniques may need to be performed every hour. For the routine postoperative client, coughing techniques should be performed every 2 hours.

Procedure: Nasal and Oral Pharyngeal Suctioning

Description: These two procedures involve inserting a plastic suction tube into the nasal or oral pharynx and then applying suction to remove secretions.

Purpose: To remove excess oral and nasal secretions and prevent aspiration of secretions or body fluids; to provide a patent airway.

STEP	RATIONALE
1. Obtain necessary equipment: • Suction source • Suction catheter kit with sterile gloves • Sterile distilled water • Sterile water-soluble lubricant • Connecting tubing • Towel	Organizing necessary equipment allows quick and safe implementation.
2. Have client assume semi-Fowler's position, if allowed, and place towel across the chest.	This position is generally comfortable for the client and accessible for the nurse. The towel protects the client and bed linen from secretions.
3. Turn on suction source and adjust setting. Start with 100–150 mm Hg and increase as necessary.	Excessive suction pressures may cause trauma to tissues. Pressure needed for suctioning may vary depending on catheter size and amount and consistency of secretion.
4. Attach connecting tubing to suction.	
5. Unwrap suction kit package. Open inner suction package and carefully remove sterile basin. Open basin and pour in sterile water. Do not touch inside of sterile basin or any part of the inner suction kit package.	Prevents contamination of equipment.
6. Open lubrication jelly and carefully expel contents onto sterile section of the inner suction package.	Use water-soluble lubricant. Lubrication decreases trauma to tissues and allows easier insertion of suction catheter.
7. Apply sterile gloves.	
8. Pick up suction catheter wrapped in plastic bag with nondominant hand. With dominant hand, remove suction catheter and attach to connecting tubing. Be sure to keep sterile hand and sterile catheter tip from becoming contaminated.	Prepares for suctioning while preventing the spread of microorganisms.
9. Check suction by suctioning a small amount of sterile water from prepared basin.	Checks suction before beginning procedure.

STEP	RATIONALE
10. Coat suction catheter tip with lubricant.	
11. Insert catheter into naris using dominant hand and pass gently into the pharynx using a downward slant. If resistance is met, do not force.	
12. Apply suction by placing nondominant thumb over vent in catheter tubing. Use an intermittent suction rather than continuous suction, pulling back catheter slowly.	Limit suction time to 10 seconds or less. Intermittent suction reduces trauma to tissues.
13. Rinse catheter in sterile water, using continuous suctioning until catheter is clear of secretions.	
14. Repeat steps 12 and 13 until secretions are cleared. Allow rest time between suctioning.	

Nursing Implications: If oxygen is in use, remove before suctioning and replace after suctioning. Observe client's respiratory and cardiac status; suctioning can cause hypoxia, arrhythmias, and bronchospasm.

Document client's response to suctioning, including respiratory status before and after. Note and chart the color, amount, and consistency of secretions. If client requires frequent nasal pharyngeal suctioning, a nasal airway may be required to limit trauma to tissues. In clients with bleeding disorders, nasal pharyngeal suctioning is generally contraindicated.

Procedure: Nasal and Oral Tracheal Suctioning

Description: This procedure involves inserting a suction catheter through the nasal or oral passage into the trachea to clear the airway.

Purpose: To remove secretions and maintain airway clearance; to stimulate deep cough reflex.

STEP	RATIONALE
1. Follow steps 1–9 of the procedure for Nasal and Oral Pharyngeal Suctioning.	
2. Insert lubricated catheter gently into naris with dominant hand. Angle catheter tip downward to pass it through to the pharynx. Do not apply suction. Have client take a breath and pass catheter quickly into trachea. Apply intermittent suction with nondominant thumb over vent in catheter tubing. Limit suction time to 10 seconds. Rotate catheter back and forth while removing slowly. Client usually coughs when trachea entered.	Suctioning during insertion of catheter increases hypoxia. Intermittent suctioning prevents undue trauma to tissues.
3. Rinse catheter in sterile water until catheter is clear of secretions.	
4. Repeat steps 2 and 3, if necessary, allowing a short period of rest between suctioning.	Rest reduces risk of impaired oxygenation.

Nursing Implications: If oxygen is in use, remove before suctioning and replace immediately after. The depth required for proper nasal tracheal suctioning in the adult is approximately 20 cm. To verify correct length, measure from nose to ear and ear to mid-sternum. If resistance is met during suctioning, release suction pressure. If resistance is met passing the catheter, do not force.

Document client response to suctioning, including respiratory status before and after. Note and chart the color, amount, and consistency of secretions. If client requires frequent nasal tracheal suctioning, a nasal airway may be required.

Procedure: Endotracheal or Tracheostomy Tube Suctioning

Description: Involves passing a suction catheter through an endotracheal or tracheostomy tube to remove secretions.

Purpose: To remove secretions and maintain a patent airway; to stimulate cough reflex.

STEP	RATIONALE
1. Collect necessary equipment: • Suction source • Suction catheter kit with sterile gloves • Sterile distilled water • Sterile water-soluble lubricant • Connecting tubing • Ambu bag with reservoir tubing and tracheostomy adaptor • Oxygen supply with appropriate tubing to connect to Ambu bag • Sterile gauze • Sterile saline for suctioning (optional) • Towel	Organizing necessary equipment allows for safe and quick implementation.
2. Connect Ambu bag to oxygen source and turn flowmeter to 15 L. Attach connecting tubing to suction device.	
3. Have client assume semi-Fowler's position, if allowed, and place towel across chest.	This position is generally comfortable for the client and accessible for the nurse. The towel protects the client and bed linen from secretions.
4. Turn on suction source and adjust setting. Start with 100–150 mm Hg and increase as necessary.	Excessive suction pressures may cause trauma to tissues. Pressure needed for suctioning may vary depending on catheter size and/or amount and consistency of secretions.
5. Unwrap suction kit package. Open inner suction package and carefully remove sterile basin. Open basin and pour in sterile water. Do not touch inside of sterile basin or any part of the inner suction kit package.	Avoids contamination of equipment.
6. Apply sterile gloves.	
7. Pick up suction catheter, wrapped in plastic bag, with nondominant hand. With dominant hand, remove suction catheter and attach to connecting tubing. Be sure to keep sterile glove and sterile catheter tip from becoming contaminated.	Prepares for suctioning while preventing the spread of microorganisms.
8. Check suction by aspirating a small amount of sterile water from prepared basin.	
9. Remove oxygen delivery device or humidity source from endotracheal or tracheostomy tube with nondominant hand. Using Ambu bag, deliver two to three hyperinflated breaths.	Preoxygenation reduces risk of altered oxygenation during suctioning procedure.
10. With dominant hand, insert suction catheter into endotracheal or tracheostomy tube and pass gently but quickly into trachea. Do not activate suction during insertion of catheter.	Suctioning during catheter insertion will increase hypoxia.
11. Insert catheter until resistance is met. Recent research indicates that a premeasured depth of insertion decreases trauma. Pull back about 1 cm and activate suction using the nondominant thumb over the vent of the suction tubing. Suction intermittently while pulling back slowly on the catheter, using a rotating movement.	Limit suction time to 10 seconds to prevent hypoxia. Intermittent suctioning reduces trauma to the tissues.
12. Hyperoxygenate client using Ambu bag. Give two to three breaths.	
13. Rinse catheter in sterile water using continuous suctioning until catheter is clear of secretions.	
14. Repeat steps 12 and 13, if necessary. Replace oxygen delivery device after completion of procedure.	

Nursing Implications: Document client response to suctioning, including respiratory status before and after. Note and chart color, amount, and consistency of secretions. Observe respiratory and cardiac status; suctioning can cause hypoxia, arrhythmias, and bronchospasm.

NOTE: If secretions are particularly thick and difficult to remove, sterile saline (about 5–10 ml) may be instilled before hyperoxygenation with Ambu bag. It takes practice to perform endotracheal or tracheostomy tube suctioning alone. The procedure is easier with two nurses, one to operate the Ambu bag and one to suction.

Procedure: Care of the Artificial Eye

Description: Cleansing the artificial eye is performed with soap and water.

Purpose: To provide integrity of the eye socket, prevent infection, and maintain client's self-image.

STEP	RATIONALE
1. Collect necessary equipment: • Washcloth • Wash basin with warm water • Mild soap • Rubber bulb syringe • Saline	Organizing necessary equipment allows safe and quick implementation.
2. Wash hands thoroughly before proceeding with intervention.	Prevents transfer of microorganisms to the eye tissues.
3. To remove prosthesis, gently pull back lower eyelid and press lightly against lower orbital ridge below eyelid.	This breaks the suction within the eye socket and allows the artificial eye to slide out.
4. Clean prosthesis with mild soap and warm water. Handle with care. Rinse well and dry with washcloth or tissue.	Removes microorganisms that may cause infection.
5. Clean eyelid and eye socket with washcloth or gauze moistened with saline. Dry with gauze.	Cleansing without soap is necessary, as soap is difficult to remove and may cause irritation.
6. To replace prosthesis, expose eye socket with thumb and index finger of nondominant hand. Place moistened artificial eye into socket with notched edge toward nose. Depress lower lid to allow artificial eye to slip into place. Make sure eyelashes are turned away from prosthesis.	Careful and correct insertion of prosthesis allows proper fit.
7. Observe the position of the artificial eye and ask the client if proper fit has been achieved.	Ensures proper position of prosthesis.

Nursing Implications: If artificial eye is not replaced in client, store in water in covered plastic case. Observe and report any changes in tissue surrounding the eye, particularly signs of infection. Remove artificial eye and store appropriately before sending client to surgery. Avoid demonstrating any signs of revulsion about the procedure. The procedure for cleansing the artificial eye need not be sterile. Maintain client's dignity and privacy during procedure.

Procedure: Administering Eyedrops and Ointment

Description: Eyedrops and ointment must be instilled correctly.

Purpose: To treat infection and combat irritation; to supply moisture and lubrication to the cornea; to dilate or constrict the pupil.

STEP	RATIONALE
1. Wash hands well before instilling medication.	Prevents transfer of microorganisms.
2. Using forefinger of nondominant hand, pull lower eyelid down by placing finger over cheek bone and pulling down gently. Instruct client to look upward.	Exposes inner surface of lid.
3. Drop eyedrop medication into center of lower lid. If instilling ointment, squeeze tube gently to deposit a ribbon of medication along lower lid.	Medication should not be instilled directly onto cornea. Take care not to touch the eye with the dropper or ointment tube tip. Prevents contamination of medication.
4. Instruct client to slowly close eyes and slowly open.	If medication can cause systemic effects, apply gentle pressure with gloved finger to client's nasolacrimal duct for 30–60 seconds. Allows medication to be distributed evenly. Prevents systemic distribution of drugs, which could cause adverse side effects.
5. Wipe off excess medication with a tissue and instruct client not to rub the eye.	
6. Wash hands after procedure.	Prevents transfer of microorganisms.

Nursing Implications: Observe and record appearance of the eye and response to treatment. If client is to be discharged home with eye medication, teach proper administration to client and family. Medications stored in refrigerator should be warmed to room temperature before use. Provide safety measures if client has blurred vision after instillation of eye medication.

Procedure: Administering Eardrops

Description: Eardrops must be instilled correctly.

Purpose: To treat infection and relieve discomfort; to loosen cerumen for removal.

STEP	RATIONALE
1. Have client lie on side, with affected ear up.	
2. Pull pinna upward and outward to expose ear canal. In children, pull pinna down and back.	Provides easier access to ear canal structures.
3. Instill the prescribed medication. Hold dropper ½ inch above ear canal.	
4. Have client lie on side for several minutes. Apply gentle massage to targus of ear.	Allows even distribution of medication.

Nursing Implications: Do not force eardrops into an occluded ear canal. If cerumen or drainage is present, wipe gently with a cotton-tipped applicator. Do not force cerumen inward. Eardrops should be warmed to room temperature before use.

Record condition of the ear and response to medication. If the client is to be discharged home with eardrops, teach client and family proper procedure.

Procedure: Administering Nasal Medications

Description: Nasal spray and drops must be instilled correctly.

Purpose: To relieve nasal congestion, inflammation, and irritation.

STEP	RATIONALE
Instilling Nasal Spray:	
1. Position client in sitting position and have client tilt head backward.	
2. Ask client to occlude one nostril. Spray required amount in other nostril and ask client to inhale simultaneously.	
3. Repeat step 2 for opposite nostril.	
4. Client may blot nose but should not blow nose for several minutes.	Allows time for medication to be absorbed.
Instilling Nasal Drops:	
1. Place client in supine position.	
2. Tilt head backward. Use a small pillow or rolled towel under neck for support.	This position allows for medication to reach sinus area.
3. Have client breathe through mouth.	Decreases risk of aspiration of medication.
4. Instill nasal drops by holding dropper ½ inch above nares. Instill medication midline toward the ethmoid bone.	Allows proper distribution of medication.
5. Have client remain in same position for 5 minutes.	
6. Client may blot nose but should not blow nose for several minutes.	Allows medication to be absorbed.

Nursing Implications: Nasal decongestants may cause rebound effect and should only be used as directed for 3–5 days. Dropper or applicator need not be sterile; rinse in hot water after each use.

Record effect on breathing. Record color of secretions.

Procedure: Administering Medications Intramuscularly via Z-Track Method

Description: The Z-track method of injection deposits the medication into the muscle without tracking residual medication.

Purpose: To protect the skin and subcutaneous tissues from irritating medications.

STEP	RATIONALE
1. Wash hands thoroughly before preparing medication for injection.	Prevents transfer of microorganisms.
2. Prepare medication for administration as directed. Draw medication into the syringe.	
3. Apply a new needle to the syringe: • 23 gauge 1–1½ inch for adults • 25–27 gauge ½–1 inch for children	Ensures that no solution remains on the needle shaft.
4. Draw up 0.2–0.3 ml of air to create an air lock.	An air lock prevents tracking medication into subcutaneous tissue.
5. Select an intramuscular site, preferably dorsal gluteal or ventrogluteal, and prepare with an antiseptic swab.	
6. Pull the skin and subcutaneous tissues 1–1½ inches laterally.	
7. Holding skin taut with nondominant hand, inject needle at a 90-degree angle deep into muscle tissue.	
8. Aspirate on syringe; then inject medication if no blood return is noted.	Aspirate to ensure that needle is not in blood vessel.
9. After withdrawing needle, release the skin immediately.	This method leaves a zigzag path that seals the medication within the muscle tissue.

Nursing Implications: Medications such as iron should be given via the Z-track method. Record location of injection and method of medication record. Observe site for any signs of tissue irritation.

Procedure: Mixing Medications from Two Vials

Description: Two medications for intramuscular injection are drawn up into one syringe.

Purpose: To reduce the number of injections administered to the client.

STEP	RATIONALE
Mixing Medication from a Single and Multidose Vial:	
1. Check compatibility of medications with pharmacy or their reference. In a syringe, pull back a volume of air equal to the amount of solution needed from the single-dose vial.	
2. Inject the air from the syringe into the single-dose vial.	Creates positive pressure needed to withdraw solution.
3. Using the same syringe, aspirate a volume of air equal to the amount of solution needed from the multidose vial.	
4. Inject air into multidose vial and withdraw desired amount. Withdraw syringe carefully.	
5. Insert needle into single-dose vial and pull back desired dosage.	The positive pressure in single-dose vial allows for easier withdrawal.
6. Discard needle in proper receptacle and place a new needle on syringe.	Decreases potential for transfer of microorganisms. Placing a new needle on the syringe assures that the needle is sharp, especially if injection is to be given intramuscularly. Makes injection less painful.

Nursing Implications: Be certain that medications mixed in the same syringe are compatible. A cloudy appearance noted in the syringe after mixing may indicate incompatibility. Care must be taken not to contaminate the multidose vial. When the volume of the air is injected into the single-dose vial, be careful not to allow the needle to touch the solution.

Some medications may be saved if entire bottle is not used. Other medications should be discarded (e.g., those without a preservative). Narcotics that are wasted must be witnessed by an RN.

Procedure: Administering Blood Products (check with institutional policy and state LPN law)

Description: Procedure involves initiating blood therapy and monitoring client for adverse reactions.

Purpose: To replace blood volume lost as a result of surgery, trauma, or disease process.

STEP	RATIONALE
1. Obtain blood-component consent form, if applicable.	Required by some agencies.
2. Assess IV site for inflammation. Note size of IV catheter. If smaller than 20 gauge, a new IV infusion must be started.	IV catheters smaller than 20 gauge may cause damage to red blood cells and clotting in the catheter. Make sure that IV catheter is patent and of appropriate size before picking up unit from blood bank. The unit must be hung within 20 minutes.
3. According to agency protocol, obtain blood product from blood bank.	
4. Verify blood component with RN. Check and compare the following information: a. Client's name and hospital identification number with the prepared unit b. Client's blood group and Rh type with those of the donor unit c. Crossmatch compatibility of donor unit to client's blood d. Blood expiration date e. Hospital unit number on blood bag and blood slip f. All information, to ensure correctness g. Blood for abnormal appearance (e.g., clots or color changes)	Strict verification procedure must be followed to protect client from incompatible blood.
5. Check client's arm band with blood product information. *Do not* administer if any information (name, hospital number) does not match.	
6. Obtain and record baseline vital signs (including temperature).	Important to note pretransfusion status.
7. Using a Y-tubing blood administration set, spike a 0.9 normal-saline IV administration bag. Flush tubing with normal saline solution and prime the filter chamber. Close all roller clamps after tubing is flushed. Some agencies also require a microaggregate filter.	Normal saline solution is isotonic and reduces hemolysis. Do not administer with dextrose solutions or any medications. Filters remove large aggregates or microaggregates that may form in stored units of whole blood or packed red blood cells.
8. Attach end of flushed Y-tubing to the hub of an 18- or 20-gauge (or larger) IV catheter. Securely tape tubing in place.	A large-bore catheter prevents hemolysis.
9. Spike blood bag with second tubing of blood administration set. Open clamp below blood component bag and regulate flow with roller clamp below filter.	
10. Infuse blood slowly (2–5 ml/min), remaining with client during first 15–20 minutes.	Most blood reactions occur in the first 15–20 minutes.
11. Document client's vital signs according to institutional policy.	Changes in vital signs may be an indication of transfusion reaction.
12. Regulate infusion according to physician's orders. Rotate blood bag periodically.	Infusion rate should be based on age, cardiac status, and rate of blood loss. Rotation mixes and maintains infusion, reducing risk of clotting.
13. Observe client for signs of transfusion reaction such as chills, fever, flushing, rash, dyspnea, chest pain, or itching. Stop infusion and notify physician of any signs of reaction. Start infusion of normal saline at a keep-open rate to maintain IV patency. Follow institutional policy for transfusion reaction, which usually involves sending remaining blood and tubing to the laboratory along with a urine specimen. The physician may order medications such as antihistamines.	
14. After blood is administered, close roller clamp of tubing connected to saline and flush tubing.	Infuses remainder of blood in tubing and filter chamber. Keeps vein open between units.
15. Note and record vital signs 1 hour after infusion.	Blood reactions can occur up to 1 hour after transfusion.

Nursing Implications: If an 18- to 20-gauge or large-bore IV catheter is needed, begin before obtaining the blood from the blood bank. Blood components should not hang for longer than 4–5 hours because of risk for bacterial growth, destruction of red blood cells, and clotting in tubing. Only one unit at a time should be obtained from the blood bank. For rapid infusion, a pressure bag may be used around the unit of blood. Pressure should not exceed 300 mm Hg. *Do not* use infusion machines unless specifically designed for blood; other machines will damage cells. Blood warmers may be required if rapid administration of blood products will be detrimental or if the client has cold agglutinins.

Procedure: Bottle-Feeding an Infant

Description: Nutritional feeding is provided via a nippled bottle.

Purpose: To provide proper nutritional intake for growth and development; to maintain fluid balance; to provide nurturing and bonding.

STEP	RATIONALE
1. Prepare formula according to instructions. Prepare the bottle with sterile nipple.	
2. Check infant's armband to ensure correct identification and correct formula.	Eliminates chance of giving the wrong formula to the infant.
3. Position infant for bottle feeding. Sit comfortably in chair. Cradle infant in one arm, while supporting against chest or lap.	Ensures comfort, safety, and security.
4. Touch corner of mouth with tip of nipple.	Stimulates rooting reflex, causing infant to turn toward nipple.
5. Hold bottle inverted with nipple down and insert filled nipple into infant's mouth.	Holding bottle upright prevents infant from sucking air.
6. Burp infant once during feeding and after feeding is completed. Some infants require more burping than others.	Releases swallowed air. Helps absorption of feeding.
7. Allow baby to feed until satisfied, around 10–25 minutes.	
8. Place infant on back after feeding.	Prevents regurgitation.

Nursing Implications: Assess infant for signs of allergic reaction to formula: rash, flushing, diarrhea, increased crying. Infant should gain weight and demonstrate tolerance to formula. Warm formula to room temperature; do not allow to sit out on counter. Some prepared formulas require refrigeration; others do not.

Procedure: Administering Enteral Nutrition via Nasogastric or Gastrostomy Tube

Description: The procedure involves instilling easily digestible nutrients into the stomach, allowing delivery of partially digested nutrients to the bowel at a slow rate. Enteral feedings are administered via nasogastric or gastrostomy tube.

Purpose: To maintain or promote nutritional status.

STEP	RATIONALE
1. Collect necessary equipment: • Sixty-milliliter syringe • Enteral tube-feeding formula • Enteral feeding bag and tubing • Enteral feeding pump	Organizing necessary equipment allows quick and safe implementation.
2. Connect tubing to bag and add proper formula in ordered strength. Some agencies add blue dye (usually food coloring) to formula to detect aspiration in clients with a tracheostomy.	
3. Prime tubing with formula and set up infusion pump.	An infusion pump helps to regulate continuous feeding.
4. Place client in high-Fowler's position. If client is to receive continuous tube feeding, position client with head elevated at least 30 degrees.	Elevation of head prevents aspiration.
5. Assess for presence of bowel sounds.	Indicates peristalsis.

STEP	RATIONALE
6. Check placement of nasogastric or gastrostomy tube by instilling a small amount of air (10 ml) via 60-ml syringe into tube. Auscultate simultaneously over epigastrium. Air will be heard entering the stomach.	Verifies correct placement of tube, ensuring that tube is not displaced.
7. Aspirate gastric contents to check residual. If greater than 50–100 ml, notify physician and hold feeding.	Indicates delayed gastric emptying.
NOTE: Small, soft feeding tubes usually collapse on aspiration and no residual is obtained. Flush with water after aspirating gastric contents.	
8. Connect tube feeding and begin at prescribed rate. Check for gastric residual at least every 8 hours.	Checking for residual allows assessment of gastric motility and absorption of formula.

Nursing Implications: If client is receiving continuous tube feedings, hang only enough formula to last 3–4 hours. (Some formulas may hang longer at room temperature.) Formulas hanging longer are susceptible to bacterial growth. Change tubing and bag every 24 hours. Check to see if the tape is securely in place.

If pulmonary aspiration occurs, notify physician, suction client to remove gastric contents from lungs, and obtain a chest radiograph. Hold feedings until client is evaluated by physician.

If feeding tube is occluded, remove it and insert a new tube. Follow guidelines for insertion.

If intermittent or bolus feedings are ordered, attach 60-ml syringe, without plunger, to fit the end of tube. Add amount of formula ordered by physician and allow to infuse by gravity. Flush tubing with 30–60 ml of water after bolus feeding. To administer medications, prepare according to hospital policy (crushing tablets or obtaining elixir forms) and give as bolus feedings. Flush tubing with water (30–60 ml) after giving medications.

Check for tube placement at least once every 8 hours and before administering medications.

Note and record residuals every 8 hours. Note and record abdominal assessment, daily weights, electrolytes, and bowel status each day. Clients may develop diarrhea, which requires reducing the strength of the enteral formula or addition of an antidiarrheal agent. To prevent the development of diarrhea, the tube feeding is often started at one-half strength and then increased to full strength over a period of a few days.

If gastrostomy tube is in place, wash area daily with soap and water. A clean gauze dressing may be placed over the site.

Procedure: Administering Enteral Feeding via a Jejunostomy or Nasojejunal Feeding Tube

Description: The procedure involves giving tube feedings via the jejunal route, bypassing the stomach, and is indicated for clients with gastric resection, gastric cancer, or chronic nausea and vomiting.

Purpose: To provide and maintain nutritional status; to reduce risk of aspiration.

STEP	RATIONALE
1. Collect necessary equipment: • Sixty-milliliter syringe • Enteral tube-feeding formula • Enteral feeding bag and tubing • Enteral feeding pump	Organizing necessary equipment ensures quick and safe implementation.
2. Connect tubing to bag containing formula in ordered strength.	Initiation of feeding usually involves administering diluted formula and increasing strength as tolerated.
3. Prime tubing with formula and set up infusion pump.	An infusion pump helps to regulate continuous feeding.
4. Elevate client's head at least 30 degrees.	Elevating the head of bed prevents aspiration, although risk is reduced with the feeding tube in the jejunum.
5. Assess for presence of bowel sounds.	Indicates peristalsis.
6. Check placement of jejunostomy tube by aspirating with syringe. Return of intestinal secretions should be observed.	Indicates proper placement of feeding tube. However, some small or soft tubes collapse during aspiration.
7. Connect feeding tube and begin at prescribed rate. Check for residual at least every 8 hours.	Checking for residual allows for assessment of intestinal motility and absorption of formula.

Nursing Implications: If client is receiving continuous feedings, change formula every 8–12 hours. Formulas hanging longer are susceptible to bacterial growth. Change tubing and bag every 24 hours.

Note and record residuals every 8 hours and abdominal assessment, weight, electrolytes, and bowel status each day. Clients may develop diarrhea, which requires reducing the strength of the enteral formula or feeding rate or addition of an antidiarrheal agent.

The site around the jejunostomy tube should be cleansed with soap and water daily. A gauze dressing may be applied to the site.

If jejunostomy tube is to be clamped intermittently, turn off formula infusion and disconnect tubing. Flush jejunostomy tube with water (30 ml) and place a catheter plug on the end of the tube (a C clamp can be used for this purpose).

If medications are to be administered, prepare according to hospital policy and give via gravity flow through a 60-ml syringe (with appropriate tip to fit jejunostomy tube) with plunger removed. Flush with water to keep tube patent and to deliver all of the medication.

Procedure: Administering Hyperalimentation via Peripheral Vein

Description: This involves infusing total parenteral nutrition (TPN) by way of a peripheral vein. TPN is the infusion of an IV solution and amino acids, glucose, vitamins, electrolytes, minerals, and trace elements.

Purpose: To provide short-term nutritional support.

STEP	RATIONALE
1. Compare peripheral TPN solution prepared by pharmacy with physician's order. Check expiration date and time.	Ensures infusion of proper solution. Peripheral TPN has less glucose than central TPN.
2. Check armband for client's name.	Ensures correct identification.
3. Connect tubing with inline filter. Use macrodrip tubing for rates >100 ml/hr.	Inline filter prevents infusion of microorganisms. TPN solution is a good medium for bacterial growth.
4. Prime tubing and thread it through infusion device.	Tubing is primed to prevent infusion of air.
5. Attach tubing to hub of IV catheter; tape securely.	
6. Set correct rate on infusion device and check once every hour for proper delivery.	The infusion pump regulates flow, but nurse must check to ensure correct delivery.

Nursing Implications: Observe IV site for redness, swelling, or signs of infiltration. Restart IV infusion if necessary. Change tubing and filter every 24 hours. Change IV site every 3 days to prevent infection. Before administering TPN, inspect bag for any particles or signs of contamination. Store TPN in refrigerator; remove 1 hour before hanging to allow solution to warm to room temperature.

Check urine sugars once each shift and report any increase in urine glucose and acetone levels. Assess lung fields at least once each shift for presence of crackles, indicting fluid overload.

If other IV piggyback fluids are needed, consider using a heparin lock at a second IV site to avoid possible compatibility problems.

Procedure: Administering Fat Emulsions

Description: An emulsified fat solution containing linoleic acid is infused simultaneously with hyperalimentation or separately. Linoleic acid is an essential fatty acid that prevents fatty-acid deficiency.

Purpose: To prevent fatty-acid deficiency; to provide a high caloric count and energy supply; to provide and maintain nutritional status.

STEP	RATIONALE
1. Obtain fat emulsion bottle from pharmacy or central supply. Check the order for correct concentration (usually 10–20%). Observe bottle for separation of emulsion. If separated, return to source.	
2. Spike bottle with vented tubing and flush the line. In some cases, special tubing accompanies the solution and should be used for the infusion.	Air vent allows for infusion via IV tubing by allowing air to displace the fat emulsion draining from the bottle.
3. Attach needle to end tubing. Swab primary IV tubing of the TPN solution at an injection site below the filter.	Infusing fat emulsion through filter causes occlusion of tubing.
4. Using an infusion device, set rate appropriately. For the first 30 minutes, infusion should run no faster than 1 ml/min. Check for adverse reactions. Continue at a 4–6 hour rate for 250–500 ml fat emulsion.	Reduces risk of adverse reactions such as chills, fever, flushing, diaphoresis, dyspnea, and chest and back pain.

Nursing Implications: The signs and symptoms of fatty-acid deficiency are dry scaly skin, sparse hair growth, impaired wound healing, decreased resistance to stress, increased susceptibility to respiratory infections, and anemia.

Fat emulsions are contraindicated in clients with abnormal fat metabolism, as in pancreatitis. Inform physician of abnormal liver function tests. Client may not be able to metabolize lipids. Fat emulsion may be piggybacked into peripheral hyperalimentation but should not be mixed with other medications. The emulsion may separate. Phlebitis often occurs when fat emulsions are given.

Procedure: Administering Hyperalimentation via Central Vein

Description: Hyperosmolar TPN is administered into the central circulation.

Purpose: To provide and maintain nutritional support when enteral nutrition is contraindicated, not appropriate, or inadequate to meet needs.

STEP	RATIONALE
1. If refrigerated, remove bag ½–1 hour before use. Check central TPN with physician's orders. Inspect bag for floating particles or signs of contamination. Confirm placement of central line with a chest radiograph if not done previously (if this is the first bag).	Ensures proper solution mixture. If contamination observed, return bag to pharmacy.
2. Check central IV site for redness, swelling, or signs of infiltration. If present, have physician restart line.	Infected central lines can lead to sepsis, a major complication.
3. Compare client armband identification with that on TPN bag.	Correct identification is essential in preventing drug errors.
4. Spike TPN bag with macrodrip tubing with inline filter.	Inline filters help to prevent infusion of microorganisms.
5. Prime tubing and insert in infusion device.	Prevents introduction of air. The infusion device regulates flow rate; it is critical for central TPN because a bolus dose of hyperosmolar glucose solution can produce rapid cellular dehydration.
6. Set desired rate. Check infusion every hour.	The infusion pump regulates flow, but nurse must check to ensure correct delivery.

Nursing Implications: Change tubing and filter every 24 hours. Solution should be changed at least once every 24 hours. Store central TPN in refrigerator; remove 1 hour before hanging to allow solution to warm to room temperature.

Check urine glucose once each shift and report any increase in urine glucose and acetone levels. Assess lung fields at least once each shift for presence of crackles, indicating fluid overload. Notify physician of abnormal electrolyte levels or blood glucose. Client may need to be on insulin while on central TPN.

Initial rate is usually 50 ml/hr, and it is then increased daily as tolerated. The client should be weaned from central TPN gradually. Watch for hypoglycemia at this time. Carefully monitor I&O. Osmotic diuresis can occur.

Do not play "catch-up"—i.e., accelerate administration—if central TPN is behind schedule. Site care should be performed using aseptic technique with masks. If available, use ever-lock connections to prevent air embolus. Do not piggyback other drugs into central TPN, except for lipid emulsions.

Procedure: Catheterizing Bladder Using Indwelling or Intermittent Catheter

Description: A sterile rubber or silicone tube is introduced through the urethra and into the bladder, providing continuous or intermittent outflow of urine.

Purpose: To relieve bladder distention and maintain urinary tract patency; to obtain accurate urine output measures.

STEP	RATIONALE
1. Obtain catheter insertion kit with urine drainage bag or intermittent catheter kit. Bring an extra pair of sterile gloves in case of contamination. If catheterizing a woman, bring an extra catheter.	Kits contain the necessary supplies for quick and safe implementation.
2. Explain procedure and ensure privacy.	Decreases anxiety and embarrassment and increases cooperation.
3. Place bed at comfortable working level.	

STEP	RATIONALE
4. Position client: **Woman:** Supine with knees flexed and thighs relaxed in external rotation **Man:** Supine with legs slightly abducted, with client draped for comfort	Provides proper visualization of urethral opening.
5. Apply clean latex gloves. Wash perineal area with warm water and mild soap; rinse and dry.	Decreases risk of introduction of microorganisms during catheterization.
6. Identify urethral meatus, which in the woman is forward of vagina, and in the man at the tip of the penis.	Identifying structures before proceeding promotes accurate placement of catheter.
7. Using bed or bedside table, open catheter insertion kit. Place moisture-proof pad under the buttocks. Do not touch any part of kit while removing pad.	Protects bed linen and client. Prevents contamination of sterile kit.
8. Put on sterile gloves. Place fenestrated sterile drape with opening over perineal area, exposing structures. Care must be taken to avoid touching contaminated areas. Restless, confused, or weak clients are best draped after setting up the supplies in the kit. If necessary, an assistant can restrain the client.	
9. Open packet containing antiseptic cleaning solution and pour evenly over the cotton balls. (If client is allergic to povidone-iodine [Betadine], use hexachlorophene [Phiso-Hex].)	
10. Examine catheter and check to see that it is securely connected to urine drainage bag. Tip of catheter is surrounded by a balloon. Attach syringe with sterile water to injection port of catheter. Do not inject water into balloon at this point in the procedure.	Equipment should be in good condition and without tears. Prepares catheter for insertion and keeps syringe handy.
11. Open lubricant packet and apply along catheter tip.	Lubrication assists in ease of insertion and promotes client's comfort.
12. Place kit between legs of women or on thighs of men.	
13. Cleanse urethral meatus and surrounding area: a. Woman: With nondominant hand, pull back labia with thumb and forefinger to expose urethral opening. Maintain position with this hand throughout procedure.	Maintains visualization of urethral opening. Assistant's help may be needed to expose if client is contracted, restless, or obese. Additional light source such as flashlight may be needed.
b. With dominant hand, use forceps to grasp a cotton ball soaked in antiseptic solution. Using a downward motion, cleanse the urethral opening by starting above the structure and wiping down past the vaginal area. Drop cotton ball (not on sterile field) and grasp another. Use one cotton ball per wipe. Also cleanse area to the sides of the meatus.	Maintains a sterile dominant hand and avoids contamination. Cleanses area of microorganisms. Reduces chance of bladder contamination.
c. Man: Pull back foreskin, if present, with nondominant hand. Hold penis at shaft below glans and pull upward. Maintain this position throughout procedure.	Exposes meatus for catheterization.
d. With dominant hand using forceps, grasp cotton ball soaked with antiseptic solution. Cleanse in circular motion from meatus to base of glans. Use a new cotton ball for each wipe.	Cleanses area of microorganisms. Reduces chance of bladder contamination.
14. Pick up catheter with dominant hand and insert lubricated tip into urethra. Ask client to take a deep breath and exhale slowly. For men, hold penis perpendicular to body. If resistance is felt, pull back slightly and attempt passage again. Rotating catheter slightly may help. If lubricant in kit is in a syringe, some may be placed directly into the meatus.	Relaxes sphincter muscles and aids in passing catheter. Forcing catheter may damage urethral lining. Some resistance may normally be felt in prostate area.
15. Advance catheter 2–3 inches in women and 7–8 inches in men until urine is noted. Then advance further to ensure that balloon is in bladder.	Ensures placement of catheter in bladder.

STEP	RATIONALE

16. a. Indwelling catheter:
    Inject 10 ml sterile water into injection port of catheter.
    Pull gently until resistance is met.
   b. Intermittent catheterization:
    Drain urine into receptacle provided in the kit. Allow urine to drain until bladder is empty. Remove catheter, cleanse client, and dry well.
	Positions catheter in bladder and prevents dislodging.

17. Place catheter drainage bag below level of bladder. Attach to bed.	Prevents urine from backing up into bladder.
18. Tape catheter to inner side of thigh. Make sure that system drains urine freely without obstruction.	Reduces trauma to meatus and urethra during movement. Maintains patent urine flow.
19. Measure and document amount of urine output. Send urine specimen to laboratory, if ordered. Do not disconnect catheter from tubing to obtain specimens.	
20. Discard used supplies in proper receptacle.	

Nursing Implications: When repositioning client, make sure catheter and tubing are not obstructing flow of urine. Instruct client not to pull on catheter.

In women, if no urine is obtained when inserting catheter, check position: the catheter may be in vagina. If so, insert new sterile catheter into urethra, leaving first catheter in place to avoid repeating error. Remove and discard original catheter. If tube is definitely in bladder but no urine is obtained, notify physician.

Report and record size of catheter placed (use smallest size possible), amount of water used to inflate the balloon, color and character of urine, and amount obtained. Document type of drainage in use.

If intermittent catheterization is ordered, document the amount and character of urine and the time. If client voided before intermittent catheterization, note time and amount.

Procedure: Routine Catheter Care

Description: Perineal hygiene is performed for clients with an indwelling catheter.

Purpose: To reduce risk of bladder infection; to provide complete perineal hygiene.

STEP	RATIONALE
1. Collect necessary supplies: • Clean latex gloves • Mild soap and warm water • Povidone-iodine solution • Povidone-iodine ointment • Sterile swabs • Tape **NOTE:** Some studies have shown soap and water to be as effective as povidone-iodine.	Organizing necessary supplies allows for quick and safe implementation.
2. Ensure privacy. Position client as in catheterization procedure. Drape client with bath blanket.	Provides comfort and lessens embarrassment.
3. Using the gloves, wash perineal area with soap and water. Rinse and dry.	Gloves protect the nurse from transmission of microorganisms. Cleansing reduces possible contaminants.
4. With nondominant hand, pull back labia or foreskin to expose meatus.	Meatus must be visualized for proper cleansing.
5. Cleanse area around meatus with sterile swabs soaked in antiseptic solution. Cleanse along catheter with solution.	Prevents transfer of microorganisms.
6. Apply antiseptic ointment with sterile swab to base of catheter near meatus.	Reduces risk of introduction of microorganisms into urethra.
7. Replace tape anchoring catheter to thigh. Replace drainage bag, if needed, maintaining a sterile connection.	Changing bag when signs of leakage or sediment buildup are noted reduces risk of infection.

Nursing Implications: Document catheter care after performing procedure. Care should be performed daily or more often if area becomes contaminated with stool. Observe and report condition of meatus. Note character of urine and report foul odor or cloudy appearance. Empty catheter drainage bag every 8 hours or when full. Empty bag before transporting client to a diagnostic procedure.

Procedure: Irrigating a Colostomy

Description: This process involves instilling 500–1000 ml of tepid water through colostomy stoma, then allowing the water and stool to drain into a collection bag.

Purpose: To remove stool, prevent continuous oozing of stool; to regulate bowel movements to a routine time; to cleanse the bowel before a diagnostic procedure.

STEP	RATIONALE
1. Collect necessary supplies and equipment: • Irrigator with tubing • Irrigation sleeve with belt • Water-soluble lubricant • Clamps • Irrigation cone	Organizing necessary supplies and equipment allows for quick and safe implementation.
2. If client is ambulatory, position client sitting on toilet. If client is on bedrest, position on side. Provide privacy.	Sitting position is generally comfortable for bowel evacuation.
3. Put on clean gloves. Remove appliance and wash area with soap and water; dry.	
4. Apply irrigation sleeve with belt. Let sleeve hang so that it touches water in toilet.	Allows for direct flow of water and stool into toilet.
5. If client is lying in bed, clamp end of sleeve.	Prevents possibility of spilling contents and controls odor.
6. Fill irrigator with 500–1000 ml of tepid water, and flush tubing.	Sufficient amount of solution to stimulate colon emptying. Flushing tubing prevents air from entering colon.
7. Attach cone to irrigation tubing and apply lubricant to cone tip.	
8. Insert cone into stoma through top of sleeve. Insert carefully without force. May need to dilate stoma before insertion, using gloved lubricated finger. Insert cone in direction of bowel lumen.	Protects stoma from trauma.
9. Begin flow of irrigation solution, clamping tube if cramping occurs. Release clamp as cramping subsides. Hang bag so that bottom is at level of client's shoulder or slightly higher.	If solution enters bowel rapidly, cramping results, reducing ability to hold sufficient volume of solution.
10. Clamp tubing when irrigation completed.	Prevents backflow of irrigation solution.
11. Remove cone carefully so that sleeve covers stoma.	Protects client and area.
12. A gush of fluid return should occur in spurts.	
13. Clamp top of sleeve and allow solution and stool to return.	About 1 hour may be required for complete return. May clamp end of sleeve if client wishes to walk around.
14. When all fecal material has been irrigated from bowel, remove sleeve and belt.	
15. Wash and prepare skin around stoma. Apply new pouch.	Allows pouch to stick firmly without leaks.
16. Wash out sleeve, cone, and irrigator tubing. Store articles in proper place for reuse.	Keeps articles clean for reuse.

Nursing Implications: Avoid frequent irrigation of colostomy with water, which can cause loss of electrolytes and fluid imbalance. To regulate the bowel, irrigation should be performed around the same time each day, preferably an hour after a meal.

Record amount of irrigation instilled and amount returned, if possible. Examine client's abdomen every shift, noting bowel sounds and any areas of tenderness. Record amount and character of returned stool.

Procedure: Collecting a Midstream Urine Specimen

Description: Urine is collected during midstream in a sterile container.

Purpose: To collect urine for culture and sensitivity test in order to determine the presence of bacteria or other organisms.

STEP	RATIONALE
1. Instruct client to wash perineal area with soap and water and rinse well. Provide privacy in bathroom, if possible.	Cleanses perineal area of fecal and other contaminants.
2. Obtain midstream urine kit. Remove antiseptic swab or towelette and have client wipe perineal area front to back in one wipe.	Removes bacteria.
3. Rinse with one wipe of sterile water front to back.	Antiseptic may contaminate specimen and alter results.
4. Instruct client to start to void and stop midstream. Place sterile collection cup under client and instruct to complete voiding.	Initial stream of urine flushes urethra of microorganisms that may give false-positive reading.
5. Screw lid on cup securely. Be careful not to contaminate inside cup.	Ensures an accurate culture test.

Nursing Implications: Label container with name, hospital number, date and time of voiding, and method of collection. Send or take specimen to laboratory as soon as possible. Document procedure in nurse's notes. Obtain culture before administration of antibiotics, if possible. If client is already receiving antibiotics, list drug(s) on laboratory request form.

Procedure: Checking Urine for Glucose and Ketones

Description: This involves measuring glucose and ketones by dipping a chemically prepared strip into clean urine or adding drops of urine to chemically prepared tablets.

Purpose: To identify the presence of glucose and ketones in a urine sample; to quickly assess diabetic status.

STEP	RATIONALE
1. Obtain double voided specimen in clean container. (With children, second voided specimens have not been found to be more accurate.)	Urine that has been in the bladder for a long time does not reflect accurate amount of glucose and ketones.
2. Test urine with glucose reagent tablet: a. With a medicine dropper (supplied with kit) place 10 drops of urine into test tube. b. Rinse dropper; place 10 drops of water into test tube. c. Place test tube in holder and add reagent tablet without touching tablet. d. Allow to "boil." Do not hold tube, which becomes quite hot. e. After 15 seconds, shake test tube and check color against chart provided. Watch for rapid change.	The combination results in a chemical reaction that produces heat. Glucose reagent test tablets measure 0–2% glucose. If solution is allowed to remain in test tube too long, the test results will be inaccurate.
3. Test urine with glucose and ketone reagent strip: a. Insert reagent strip into clean urine and gently shake off excess. b. Follow directions on reagent container for time interval allowed before reading results; use watch to time. c. Compare color change on reagent strip to color chart on container. d. Close reagent-strip bottle tightly.	Each brand of reagent strip requires a specific time for accurate results. Moisture may alter accuracy of test strips.
4. Test urine with acetone tablet. a. Place tablet on paper towel. b. Add one drop of urine to tablet. Wait 30 seconds. c. Compare color change with chart.	Measures presence of ketone bodies.

Nursing Implications: Keep supplies clean and ready for next testing. Discard urine appropriately. Record in nurses' notes or diabetic record and continue with prescribed therapy. Depending on brand of tablet used, be aware of possible false-positive test results that occur with some medications.

Procedure: Collecting a Stool Specimen

Description: A small amount of stool is obtained for laboratory testing.

Purpose: To detect presence of blood, bile, fat, urobilinogen, nitrogen content, ova, parasites, protozoa, or bacteria in the stool.

STEP	RATIONALE
1. Collect stool specimen appropriately for purpose of test.	Stool specimen may have to be collected by a certain method. Check with laboratory if uncertain.
2. Place clean specimen hat in toilet, if client is able to use it.	Prevents stool from falling into toilet water.
3. Explain to client that stool must be free of urine, water, and toilet tissue.	Urine inhibits bacterial growth and may conflict with results.
4. Using clean gloves and tongue blade, place stool specimen in plastic container that has client's label on outside.	Maintains cleanliness and prevents transfer of microorganisms.
5. Place specimen in plastic bag and send to laboratory as soon as possible.	Fresh samples produce more accurate results.

Nursing Implications: Clean all equipment immediately and dispose of tongue blade and gloves in trash receptacle. Document in nurses' notes the color and character of stool and method of collection.

Procedure: Testing for Occult Blood in Stool

Description: This simple laboratory test can quickly assess presence of blood in the stool.

Purpose: To determine presence of GI bleeding.

STEP	RATIONALE
1. Obtain Hemoccult cardboard slide, two wooden sticks, Hemoccult developing agent, and clean stool specimen.	Hemoccult slides are the most commonly used guaiac tests.
2. Put on clean gloves. With wooden stick, obtain small amount of stool. Open flap of cardboard slide and place a smear of stool in circle A. Discard stick.	
3. With second wooden stick, obtain a small smear of stool from a different area of the stool specimen and place on circle B. Close flap.	The results of Hemoccult testing are more conclusive if positive results are obtained from both samples.
4. Turn cardboard slide over and open the other flap. Place 2 drops of Hemoccult developing solution on each circle. Put a drop on monitor circle. Positive one should turn blue and negative one stays white.	Filter paper on slide is prepared with guaiac, which will turn blue if blood loss exceeds 5 ml/day. Ensures that guaiac slide is working properly.
5. Wait 30–60 seconds before reading test results. Bluish color indicates presence of occult blood.	Accurate timing is important for accurate results.
6. Discard cardboard slide, used wooden sticks, and gloves in trash receptacle. Discard stool specimen appropriately.	Prevents transfer of microorganisms.

Nursing Implications: Send to laboratory immediately. Label specimen with name, date, and time. False-positive results may occur if the client has a diet high in meat, bananas, drugs (aspirin), iron preparations, anticoagulants, and corticotropin. Black stools are associated with upper GI bleeding, and bright-red stools with lower GI problems such as hemorrhoids and carcinomas.

Procedure: Collecting Nose and Throat Cultures

Description: A swab of mucosal membranes is performed to be used as a testing specimen for bacterial or fungal growth on a culture medium.

Purpose: To determine the presence of pathogenic organisms and the antibiotics that are effective in treatment.

STEP	RATIONALE

For Throat Culture:
1. Obtain two culturette tubes with sterile swabs. Label each tube with client's name and information.
2. Position client sitting up comfortably with head tilted back.
3. Using tongue blade, visualize the pharynx. Insert swab without touching teeth or gums, and gently swab tonsillar areas and areas of redness or drainage.
4. Carefully withdraw swab without contaminating. Insert swab into culture tube and press tip to crush ampule.

Touching gums or teeth may result in contamination with resident bacteria.

The culture medium maintains the presence of bacteria until testing.

For Nose Culture:
5. Use the second culturette for the nasal specimen. Use penlight to visualize nostrils. Choose nostril with greatest patency. (Client may have to blow nose to open obstruction.)
6. Insert culture swab and swab areas inside nostril that appear red or inflamed. Try not to touch sides of nostril. (A nasal speculum may be used.)
7. Carefully remove swab and place inside culture tube. Press tip of culture tube to break ampule.

Prevents contamination with resident bacteria.

Culture medium maintains the presence of bacteria until testing. Crushing ampule releases medium so that it is in contact with tip of swab.

Nursing Implications: Send to laboratory immediately. Label specimens with name, time, and date. Document procedure in nurses' notes, describing color and character of secretions. Indicate any antibiotics the client is taking.

Procedure: Care of the Client with a T-Tube

Description: During a cholecystectomy, a T-tube is placed in the common bile duct and connected to a drainage bag.

Purpose: To drain bile after a cholecystectomy and bile-duct exploration; to prevent contracture and stenosis of the duct during healing.

STEP	RATIONALE
1. Place client in low-Fowler's to semi-Fowler's position.	Facilitates draining.
2. Check T-tube for kinds of obstruction of drainage.	Prevents possible obstruction of drainage.
3. Measure output and record every 8 hours. With gloved hands, open bottom port of drainage bag and allow bile to drain into graduated container for measuring. Close drainage bag securely.	It is important to record output; record is used to determine when to remove tube.
4. Cleanse and dry area around tube and place sterile dry dressing around insertion site daily.	

Nursing Implications: Assess sclera for yellowish color, which may indicate biliary obstruction. Record stools, noting color and character. The T-tube drain may be removed in 1–2 weeks. Usually, T-tube is clamped at intervals before removing. Be aware of potential for nausea and vomiting or signs of biliary obstruction. Stools will be clay colored if tube is *unclamped.*

CHAPTER 8

Pharmacology Review Tests

Danny Willis, RN, MN

Test 1: Pharmacological Principles

QUESTIONS

1. Meperidine (Demerol) is classified as:
   A. Psychotropic
   B. Antibiotic
   C. Analgesic
   D. Cardiotonic

2. Polycillin is classified as:
   A. Psychotropic
   B. Analgesic
   C. Antibiotic
   D. Diuretic

3. Hydrochlorothiazide (HydroDIURIL) is classified as:
   A. Antibiotic
   B. Analgesic
   C. Cardiotonic
   D. Diuretic

4. Diazepam (Valium) is classified as:
   A. Antibiotic
   B. Psychotropic
   C. Cardiotonic
   D. Diuretic

5. Digoxin (Lanoxin) is classified as:
   A. Antibiotic
   B. Cardiotonic

   C. Diuretic
   D. Psychotropic

6. A drug that is absorbed into the bloodstream and carried to specific organs is said to have:
   A. A systemic effect
   B. A local effect
   C. An untoward effect
   D. An indirect effect

7. A drug has an idiosyncratic effect when:
   A. The drug is absorbed into the body and carried to all cells
   B. Psychological dependence occurs when the drug is injected
   C. Unusual, unpredictable, unexpected reactions occur
   D. All of the drug's intended effects occur

8. A medication that consists of a suspension of fat globules and water is classified as:
   A. An emulsion
   B. An ointment
   C. A tincture
   D. An elixir

9. The action of antibiotics is that:
   A. They allow the body to build up its defenses to fight infection

B. They increase the number of phagocytes to ingest bacteria
C. They break down the bacterial cell wall and inhibit growth of microorganisms
D. They destroy microorganisms

10. The goal of antihypertensive therapy is to:
A. Cure the client of high blood pressure
B. Control the blood pressure and prevent complications
C. Make the client hypotensive and prevent congestive heart failure
D. Prevent the left ventricle from pumping blood

11. The word *antiseptic* means:
A. Increasing body activities
B. Inhibiting the growth of bacteria
C. Slowing down bodily activities
D. Destroying bacteria

12. The most rapid route of administration of a drug is:
A. Subcutaneous (SC)
B. Intramuscular (IM)
C. Intravenous (IV)
D. Oral

13. The single most important organ that detoxifies drugs is the:
A. Lung
B. Stomach
C. Liver
D. Bone marrow

14. Anaphylactic shock can occur as a result of drug allergy. Some of the signs of this reaction are:
A. Flushed skin, dyspnea, hypertension
B. Bradycardia, pallor, edema of the extremities
C. Hypotension, dyspnea, diaphoresis
D. Fever, rash, bradycardia

15. Clients who are receiving antineoplastic agents that depress bone marrow function may require reverse isolation or placement in a pathogen-free environment because:
A. The client has an infection that could be transmitted to others
B. Bacteria normally found in the air could prove fatal
C. Exposure to pathogens might cause hyponatremia
D. Anemia might result

16. Female clients who are receiving androgens for treatment of a neoplasm may develop:
A. Endometrial carcinoma
B. Alopecia
C. Mild to moderate masculinization
D. Ulcerations of the mouth

17. Promethazine (Phenergan), when combined with a narcotic:
A. Causes central nervous system (CNS) stimulation
B. Produces a triple response
C. Potentiates the effect of the narcotic
D. Increases the need for narcotics

18. Chronic use of mineral oil
A. Can cause dysphagia
B. Hinders the absorption of fat-soluble vitamins
C. Chemically interacts with water-soluble vitamins
D. Leads to dumping syndrome

19. Tricyclic drugs are considered to be in which of the following categories of drugs?
A. Antidepressants
B. Antidiarrheals
C. Antiemetics
D. Hypnotics

20. An example of a CNS stimulant is:
A. Thyroxine
B. Diazepam
C. Amphetamine
D. Alcohol

21. Which of the following procedures is recommended if it becomes necessary for a nurse to discard a narcotic?
A. Have another person witness you discarding the drug.
B. Report discarding the narcotic to the physician who prescribed it.
C. Have the pharmacy director issue an identical amount of drug to replace what you had to discard.
D. Save the discarded amount and return it to the pharmacy.

22. A client asks a physician for a specific medication, but the nurse has trouble reading the physician's order. Which of the following persons should the nurse consult in order to clarify the order?
A. The unit clerk who transcribed the order
B. The physician who wrote the order
C. The pharmacist who will fill the order
D. The client, who has been taking the medication on a regular basis over the last 2 years.

23. To verify an alert client's identity, the nurse checks the client's identification band before giving medications. It is also recommended that:
A. The nurse call the client by name
B. The client be asked to state his or her name
C. A relative be asked to verify the client's identification
D. A second nurse be asked to verify the client's identity

24. A nurse notes an error about ½ hour after giving a medication to a client. The nurse's first action in this situation should be to:
A. Prepare an incident report
B. Call the physician
C. Notify the client that an error has been made
D. Check the client's condition

25. The "five rights" for drug administration are:
A. Right time, dose, route, room, client
B. Right dose, route, client, room, medication
C. Right route, dose, client, physician, room
D. Right time, dose, drug, client, route

26. One of the problems encountered in the use of antineo-plastic drugs is that:
    A. Surgery or radiation cannot be used concomitantly to treat the malignancy
    B. The tumor may be too small or too large to treat with drugs
    C. These drugs also affect normal cells
    D. Only a few types of malignancies can be treated with these drugs

27. A client, aged 66 years, had exploratory surgery for possible cancer of the colon. Because the tumor had spread and was inoperable, the physician decided to administer 5-fluorouracil (5-FU) for palliative management of the tumor. The client began to develop adverse drug effects. As a nurse you know that:
    A. Drug therapy will have to be discontinued
    B. This outcome is a sign that the drug is ineffective and another must be tried
    C. There are times when some of these effects must be tolerated in order to obtain optimum therapeutic results
    D. No other type of drug can be given to lessen adverse drug effects

28. After several weeks of chemotherapy treatment, an oncology client begins to develop alopecia and is very upset. What might a nurse suggest to the client or the family about this problem?
    A. Limit visitors to the immediate family, and include only those who are understanding.
    B. Move the client to a private room.
    C. Suggest that client purchase a wig.
    D. Tell the client not to worry because the hair always grows back.

29. An oncology client develops leukopenia, which is manifested by:
    A. Fatigue and shortness of breath
    B. Nausea and vomiting
    C. Easy bruising
    D. Lesions in the buccal cavity

30. A client develops thrombocytopenia, which is manifested by:
    A. Fatigue
    B. Easy bruising
    C. Shortness of breath on exertion
    D. Decreased resistance to infection

31. When a client has a new diagnosis of a convulsive disorder, the nurse should first:
    A. Obtain a thorough history from the client or the family
    B. Explain what epilepsy is to the family
    C. Assure the family that drugs will control the seizures
    D. Never leave the client's bedside

32. Close observation of a client with a convulsive disorder is most important because:
    A. The nurse will ultimately have to describe the seizures to the client's family
    B. Drug therapy cannot begin until the client has another seizure that has been observed by nursing personnel

C. It may help the physician to diagnose the type of convulsive disorder
D. The nurse will be in charge of protecting the client from injury during a seizure

33. Phenytoin has been selected to treat a client with a convulsive disorder. Now that drug therapy has been instituted:
    A. It is no longer necessary to describe the seizures that may occur because the diagnosis has been established.
    B. Ongoing nursing observations often help the physician to evaluate the effectiveness of drug therapy.
    C. The client will have no more seizures.
    D. There is no longer any need to describe the seizure.

34. A client complains of nausea, which appears to be drug related. GI discomfort may be prevented by giving a drug:
    A. Early in the morning
    B. Late in the evening
    C. With two or more glasses of water
    D. With or immediately after meals

35. Ibuprofen (Motrin):
    A. Has only analgesic activity
    B. Provides analgesic and anti-inflammatory activity
    C. Has no known adverse effects
    D. Should always be taken on an empty stomach for best results

36. A tranquilizer that is also used as a muscle relaxant is:
    A. Phenobarbital
    B. Chlorpromazine
    C. Perphenazine
    D. Diazepam

37. You are instructed to give a client 5 ml of an expectorant. The client refuses it. You should:
    A. Leave it by the bedside so that the client can take it later
    B. Discard the medication and report it to the physician
    C. Return the medication to the bottle and report it to the physician
    D. Get somebody to help you force the client to take the medicine

38. A client is taking furosemide (Lasix) 80 mg bid. A nursing action before administering the drug is to check the client's:
    A. History of allergies to penicillins
    B. Red-green discrimination
    C. Optic nerve damage
    D. Potassium level

39. A client is receiving digoxin 0.25 mg PO qd. Before administration of the drug, the nurse would take the client's:
    A. Apical pulse for 30 seconds
    B. Apical pulse for 60 seconds
    C. Radial pulse for 30 seconds
    D. Radial pulse for 60 seconds

40. A client is taking the antacid aluminum hydroxide. The nurse would encourage the client to also:

A. Take milk of magnesia nightly
B. Decrease fluid intake
C. Increase bulk in the diet
D. Decrease bulk in the diet

41. Drugs that initiate a response are called:

    A. Antagonists
    B. Agonists
    C. Depressants
    D. Antiseptics

42. The serum half-life of a drug is:

    A. The time required after absorption for half of the drug to be eliminated
    B. The time required for half of a drug dose to be absorbed
    C. The time required for a drug to exert half of its total effect
    D. Half of the time required for a drug to be completely metabolized

43. Knowledge of drug potency does not enable us to predict whether a potent drug is more or less toxic. The valid indicator that measures the safety of the drug is:

    A. Side effect profile
    B. Therapeutic range
    C. Duration of action
    D. Biological half-life

44. A large initial dose to achieve minimum effective concentration is known as:

    A. Threshold dose
    B. Therapeutic range
    C. Loading dose
    D. Free (unbound) drug

45. A common side effect of many anti-inflammatory agents (e.g., aspirin, indomethacin, ibuprofen) is:

    A. Urinary retention
    B. Increased pulse rate
    C. Behavioral changes
    D. GI disturbances

46. Ibuprofen is one of the newest drugs in the group of NSAIDs. Ibuprofen agents should be administered:

    A. With food or large glass of water
    B. On an empty stomach
    C. Before breakfast, lunch, and dinner, and at bedtime
    D. With aspirin or other NSAIDs

47. The nurse is instructed to give an IM injection in the vastus lateralis. The location of the vastus lateralis for the site for administration is:

    A. At the lateral portion of the thigh with one hand's breadth above the knee and one hand's breadth below the greater trochanter
    B. At the lateral portion of the thigh with one hand's breadth below the knee and one hand's breadth above the greater trochanter
    C. At the lower edge of the acromion to the middle third of the front part of the thigh
    D. At the middle third of the front part of the thigh to above the knee

48. When mixing neutral protamine Hagedorn (NPH) and regular insulin, the best sequence is:

    A. Air into NPH, then air into the regular and draw it up, followed by drawing up the NPH
    B. Air into NPH and draw up, then air into the regular and draw up
    C. Air into regular, then air into NPH and draw up, followed by drawing up regular
    D. Giving two separate injections; do not mix insulin

49. An unconscious client is in shock with metabolic acidosis. The nurse should be sure to have which of the following drugs on hand?

    A. Dobutamine
    B. Sodium nitroprusside
    C. Sodium bicarbonate
    D. Calcium gluconate

50. Drugs can be given IV, intradermally, IM, and SC. Aspiration is contraindicated in which method?

    A. IV
    B. Intradermally
    C. SC
    D. IM

ANSWERS

1. **(C)** Nursing process phase: evaluation; client need: pharmacological and parenteral therapies; content area: pharmacology.

    RATIONALE

    (A) Psychotropics alter the mood. (B) Antibiotics inhibit the growth of bacteria. (C) Analgesics relieve pain. Meperidine is given to relieve pain. (D) Cardiotonics make the heart pump more efficiently.

2. **(C)** Nursing process phase: evaluation; client need: pharmacological and parenteral therapies; content area: pharmacology.

    RATIONALE

    (A) Psychotropics alter the mood. (B) Analgesics relieve pain. (C) Antibiotics inhibit the growth of bacteria. Polycillin is given to inhibit the growth of bacteria. (D) Diuretics promote fluid excretion.

3. **(D)** Nursing process phase: evaluation; client need: pharmacological and parenteral therapies; content area: pharmacology.

    RATIONALE

    (A) Antibiotics inhibit the growth of bacteria. (B) Analgesics relieve pain. (C) Cardiotonics make the heart pump more efficiently. (D) Diuretics promote fluid excretion. Hydrochlorothiazide is given to promote fluid excretion.

4. **(B)** Nursing process phase: evaluation; client need: pharmacological and parenteral therapies; content area: pharmacology.

    RATIONALE

    (A) Antibiotics inhibit the growth of bacteria. (B) Psychotropics alter the mood. Diazepam is given to alter the mood. (C) Cardiotonics make the heart pump more efficiently. (D) Diuretics promote fluid excretion.

5. **(B)** Nursing process phase: evaluation; client need: pharmacological and parenteral therapies; content area: pharmacology.

    RATIONALE

    (A) Antibiotics inhibit the growth of bacteria. (B) Cardiotonics make the heart beat more efficiently. Digoxin is given to make the heart beat more efficiently. (C) Diuretics promote fluid excretion. (D) Psychotropics alter the mood.

6. **(A)** Nursing process phase: evaluation; client need: pharmacological and parenteral therapies; content area: pharmacology.

    RATIONALE

    (A) Drugs that affect the entire body are described as having a systemic effect. (B) A drug with a local effect affects only a targeted local area. (C) An untoward effect is one that is undesirable. (D) An indirect effect occurs as an unplanned consequence and is not the primary effect.

7. **(C)** Nursing process phase: evaluation; client need: pharmacological and parenteral therapies; content area: pharmacology.

    RATIONALE

    (A) A drug that is carried to all cells has a systemic effect. (B) In psychological dependence, the client has an incapacitating need for a drug. (C) An idiosyncratic effect is an unusual, unpredictable, unexpected reaction. (D) An effective drug is one that produces all of its intended effects.

8. **(A)** Nursing process phase: evaluation; client need: pharmacological and parenteral therapies; content area: pharmacology.

    RATIONALE

    (A) An emulsion is a mixture of two insoluble liquids, such as fat and water. (B) An ointment is a topical semisolid. (C) A tincture is an alcohol extract liquid. (D) An elixir is a sweetened, aromatic liquid form of a drug.

9. **(D)** Nursing process phase: evaluation; client need: pharmacological and parenteral therapies; content area: pharmacology.

    RATIONALE

    (A) Building up the body's defenses to fight infection is not the direct action of antibiotics. (B) Antibiotics do not increase the number of phagocytes. (C) Antibiotics do not break down the cell wall. They have no action on growth of new cells. (D) By definition, antibiotics inhibit the growth of or destroy microorganisms.

10. **(B)** Nursing process phase: planning; client need: pharmacological and parenteral therapies; content area: pharmacology.

    RATIONALE

    (A) Antihypertensive drugs help to control high blood pressure, but they do not cure the disease. (B) Hypertension is a chronic disease. The goals are to control the blood pressure and to prevent complications. (C) Hypotension can be a side effect of antihypertensive therapy, but it is not the goal. (D) Antihypertensive drugs allow the heart to pump under reduced pressure. The left ventricle should not be prevented from pumping blood.

11. **(B)** Nursing process phase: evaluation; client need: pharmacological and parenteral therapies; content area: pharmacology.

    RATIONALE

    (A) Catabolic refers to increasing body activities. (B) Antiseptic means inhibiting the growth of bacteria. (C) Anabolic refers to decreasing body activities. (D) Sterilization refers to destroying bacteria.

12. **(C)** Nursing process phase: evaluation; client need: pharmacological and parenteral therapies; content area: pharmacology.

    RATIONALE

    (A) The SC route is faster than oral but slower than IM and IV. (B) The IM route is faster than SC but slower than IV. (C) The IV route is a direct route for administration of a drug that does not require absorption of the drug from the tissues. (D) The slowest route for absorption is the oral form.

13. **(C)** Nursing process phase: evaluation; client need: pharmacological and parenteral therapies; content area: pharmacology.

    RATIONALE

    (A) The lungs help excrete drugs but do not detoxify. (B) The stomach absorbs drugs. (C) The liver is the main organ for detoxification. (D) The bone marrow helps to absorb and store drugs but does not detoxify.

14. **(C)** Nursing process phase: data collection; client need: pharmacological and parenteral therapies; content area: pharmacology.

    RATIONALE

    (A) Shock produces hypotension, not hypertension. (B) Shock produces tachycardia, not bradycardia. (C) Hypotension, dyspnea, and diaphoresis are classic signs of anaphylaxis, which is a life-threatening, acute allergic reaction. (D) Shock produces tachycardia, not bradycardia.

15. **(B)** Nursing process phase: implementation; client need: pharmacological and parenteral therapies; content area: pharmacology.

    RATIONALE

    (A) The client may have an infection that can be transmitted, but reverse isolation is used to protect the compromised client. (B) These clients have decreased reserves to fight normal flora. (C) Exposure to pathogens does not cause hyponatremia. (D) The client may be anemic, but reverse isolation is not used for anemia, a condition with reduced red blood cells (RBCs).

16. **(C)** Nursing process phase: data collection; client need: pharmacological and parenteral therapies; content area: pharmacology.

    RATIONALE

    (A) Androgens do not cause endometrial cancer. **(B)** Alopecia is a side effect of antineoplastic agents. **(C)** Mild to moderate masculinization can result from the administration of male hormones (androgens). **(D)** Ulcerations of the mouth are a side effect of antineoplastic agents.

17. **(C)** Nursing process phase: data collection; client need: pharmacological and parenteral therapies; content area: pharmacology.

    RATIONALE

    (A) Promethazine decreases stimulation of the CNS. **(B)** There is no triple response. **(C)** The action of promethazine is to potentiate the effect of the narcotic. **(D)** Phenergan decreases the need for narcotics.

18. **(B)** Nursing process phase: evaluation; client need: pharmacological and parenteral therapies; content area: pharmacology.

    RATIONALE

    (A) There is no evidence that mineral oil causes dysphagia (difficulty swallowing). **(B)** A side effect of mineral oil is that it hinders the absorption of fat-soluble vitamins. **(C)** Mineral oil does not mix with water-soluble vitamins. **(D)** Dumping syndrome is caused by increased emptying time of the stomach. Mineral oil works on the lower gastrointestinal (GI) tract.

19. **(A)** Nursing process phase: evaluation; client need: pharmacological and parenteral therapies; content area: pharmacology.

    RATIONALE

    (A) Tricyclics affect the mood and are in the category of antidepressants. **(B)** Antidiarrheal drugs help to prevent or reduce diarrhea. **(C)** Antiemetics help to prevent nausea and vomiting. **(D)** Hypnotics induce a clinical state resembling sleep.

20. **(C)** Nursing process phase: evaluation; client need: pharmacological and parenteral therapies; content area: pharmacology.

    RATIONALE

    (A) Thyroxine is a thyroid hormone and increases metabolism, but it is not a CNS stimulant. **(B)** Diazepam is a tranquilizer and decreases CNS stimulation. **(C)** An amphetamine is a CNS stimulant. **(D)** Alcohol is a depressant, not a stimulant.

21. **(A)** Nursing process phase: implementation; client need: pharmacological and parenteral therapies; content area: pharmacology.

    RATIONALE

    (A) Narcotics are included under federal controlled substances regulations. Federal regulations recommend having another person witness you discarding the drug. **(B)** There is no need to notify the physician. **(C)** You may inform the pharmacy about the discard, but not to replace it with an identical amount. **(D)** There is no need to return the discard to the pharmacy; the pharmacy can neither verify the drug nor reissue it.

22. **(B)** Nursing process phase: evaluation; client need: pharmacological and parenteral therapies; content area: pharmacology.

    RATIONALE

    (A) Consulting the unit clerk is not the safest option. The unit clerk did not write the order. **(B)** The only person who really knows the desired order is the physician, and this is the safest option. **(C)** Consulting the pharmacist is not the safest option. The pharmacist did not write the order. **(D)** Consulting the client is not the safest option. The client did not write the order.

23. **(B)** Nursing process phase: planning; client need: pharmacological and parenteral therapies; content area: pharmacology.

    RATIONALE

    (A) A confused client may respond to other than his or her own name, or there may be two persons with the same name. **(B)** The most accurate way is to have the client state his or her name. **(C)** A relative could be asked for verification, but a relative is not the most direct source in this situation. **(D)** A second nurse is not the most direct or accurate way to verify the client's identity in this situation.

24. **(D)** Nursing process phase: implementation; client need: pharmacological and parenteral therapies; content area: pharmacology.

    RATIONALE

    (A) Preparing an incident report is recommended but is not the highest priority in this situation. **(B)** Calling the physician is recommended but is not the highest priority in this situation. **(C)** Notifying the client is a possible action but is not the highest priority in this situation. **(D)** The highest priority is to check the client first to assess the response to the drug.

25. **(D)** Nursing process phase: implementation; client need: pharmacological and parenteral therapies; content area: pharmacology.

    RATIONALE

    (A) Room is not one of the five rights. **(B)** Room is not one of the five rights. **(C)** Room is not one of the five rights. **(D)** These are the five rights. Memorization of them is standard practice.

26. **(C)** Nursing process phase: evaluation; client need: pharmacological and parenteral therapies; content area: pharmacology.

    RATIONALE

    (A) Surgery and radiation are both used to treat malignancy. **(B)** The size of the tumor has no relationship to its treatment with antineoplastic drugs. **(C)** A side effect of antineoplastic agents is that they also affect normal cells. **(D)** Antineoplastic drugs are used to treat a wide variety of malignancies.

27. **(C)** Nursing process phase: planning; client need: pharmacological and parenteral therapies; content area: pharmacology.

    RATIONALE

    (A) Drugs are discontinued for allergic reactions but not necessarily for adverse effects. **(B)** Side effects do not mean that the drug is ineffective; all drugs have some side effects. **(C)** Beneficial effects must be weighed against adverse effects. **(D)** When side effects occur, another drug may be given at the same time to decrease the side effects (e.g., an antiemetic may be given to decrease the side effects of nausea created by an antibiotic).

28. **(C)** Nursing process phase: planning; client need: pharmacological and parenteral therapies; content area: pharmacology.

    RATIONALE

    (A) Limiting visitors will not help with self-esteem and may cause an increased feeling of isolation. **(B)** Moving the client to a private room may create a further feeling of isolation. **(C)** Alopecia is loss of hair. A wig might help this client's self-esteem. **(D)** The hair does not always grow back, so this response may be false reassurance.

29. **(D)** Nursing process phase: evaluation; client need: pharmacological and parenteral therapies; content area: pharmacology.

    RATIONALE

    (A) Anemia may cause fatigue and shortness of breath. **(B)** Nausea and vomiting are side effects of many drugs. **(C)** Easy bruising is not caused by a decreased number of white cells. **(D)** Lesions in the buccal cavity are a side effect of leukopenia.

30. **(B)** Nursing process phase: evaluation; client need: pharmacological and parenteral therapies; content area: pharmacology.

    RATIONALE
    (A) A decrease in RBCs produces fatigue. **(B)** Thrombocytopenia, or a decrease in platelets, affects the clotting of the blood, resulting in easy bruising. **(C)** Shortness of breath results from anemia. **(D)** A reduction in white blood cells (WBCs) decreases resistance to infection.

31. **(A)** Nursing process phase: data collection; client need: pharmacological and parenteral therapies; content area: pharmacology.

    RATIONALE
    (A) The first step in assessment is obtaining a history. **(B)** There is no evidence that the client's specific disorder is epilepsy. **(C)** One cannot assure the family that drugs will control the seizures at this point. **(D)** The client does not require constant attention, only close observation.

32. **(D)** Nursing process phase: planning; client need: pharmacological and parenteral therapies; content area: pharmacology.

    RATIONALE
    (A) Describing the seizures to the family is not as important as protecting the client from injury. **(B)** Drug therapy is important but not the most important reason for close observation of the client. **(C)** Diagnosing the specific type of convulsive disorder is helpful but not the most important reason for close observation of the client. **(D)** It would be most important for the nurse to protect the client from injury.

33. **(B)** Nursing process phase: planning; client need: pharmacological and parenteral therapies; content area: pharmacology.

    RATIONALE
    (A) Describing the seizures is necessary. **(B)** The nurse is still responsible for ongoing assessment. **(C)** Seizures may still occur after treatment is started. **(D)** Describing the seizures is necessary.

34. **(D)** Nursing process phase: implementation; client need: pharmacological and parenteral therapies; content area: pharmacology.

    RATIONALE
    (A) Time of day is less important than food in preventing discomfort. **(B)** Time of day is less important than food in preventing discomfort. **(C)** Water is less important than food in preventing discomfort. **(D)** Manufacturers recommend giving drugs with food to help relieve nausea.

35. **(B)** Nursing process phase: evaluation; client need: pharmacological and parenteral therapies; content area: pharmacology.

    RATIONALE
    (A) Ibuprofen also has an anti-inflammatory effect. **(B)** Ibuprofen is a nonsteroidal anti-inflammatory drug (NSAID) with antipyretic and analgesic properties. **(C)** All drugs have some side effects. **(D)** It is best to take ibuprofen with food to help prevent mucosal irritation.

36. **(D)** Nursing process phase: evaluation; client need: pharmacological and parenteral therapies; content area: pharmacology.

    RATIONALE
    (A) Phenobarbital is not used as a muscle relaxant. **(B)** Chlorpromazine is an antipsychotic. **(C)** Perphenazine is an antiemetic and antipsychotic. **(D)** Diazepam is a muscle relaxant that also has antianxiety effects.

37. **(B)** Nursing process phase: implementation; client need: pharmacological and parenteral therapies; content area: pharmacology.

RATIONALE
(A) The nurse should never leave medicine at the bedside. **(B)** Discarding the medication is safer than risking returning the medication to the wrong bottle. The physician should be notified if the client is not taking medication. **(C)** The nurse should never return the medication to the bottle. **(D)** The nurse should never force a client to take a medicine.

38. **(D)** Nursing process phase: evaluation; client need: pharmacological and parenteral therapies; content area: pharmacology.

    RATIONALE
    (A) Furosemide is a sulfonamide derivative. Check the client for allergies to sulfa drugs. **(B)** Furosemide has no effect on red-green discrimination. **(C)** Furosemide does not cause optic nerve damage, but may cause loss of hearing. **(D)** Furosemide is a potassium-wasting diuretic, so it is important to check potassium levels before its administration. It also increases excretion of chloride and sodium.

39. **(B)** Nursing process phase: implementation; client need: pharmacological and parenteral therapies; content area: pharmacology.

    RATIONALE
    (A) Taking the apical pulse for 30 seconds is not the recommended length of time for the most accurate measurement. **(B)** With all cardiotonics, the only acceptable method to determine pulse rate is to take an apical pulse for a full minute. **(C)** An apical pulse is heard over the apex of the heart and is more accurate than a radial pulse. **(D)** An apical pulse is heard over the apex of the heart and is more accurate than a radial pulse.

40. **(C)** Nursing process phase: implementation; client need: pharmacological and parenteral therapies; content area: pharmacology.

    RATIONALE
    (A) Laxatives are not a first defense. **(B)** Decreasing fluid intake increases the chances of constipation. **(C)** Aluminum hydroxide causes constipation; thus, increasing bulk in the diet will help to prevent constipation. **(D)** Decreasing bulk increases the chances for constipation.

41. **(B)** Nursing process phase: evaluation; client need: pharmacological and parenteral therapies; content area: pharmacology.

    RATIONALE
    (A) An antagonist is a drug that makes another drug less effective. **(B)** By definition, an agonist stimulates receptors to initiate a response. **(C)** A depressant is a drug that slows a vital process. **(D)** Antiseptics inhibit the growth of bacteria.

42. **(A)** Nursing process phase: evaluation; client need: pharmacological and parenteral therapies; content area: pharmacology.

    RATIONALE
    (A) The time it takes for eliminating processes to reduce the blood concentration of the drug by half is called the drug half-life. **(B)** Half-life is measured by elimination, not absorption. **(C)** The time for a drug to exert half of its total effect cannot be measured. **(D)** The time required for a drug to be completely metabolized cannot be measured.

43. **(B)** Nursing process phase: evaluation; client need: pharmacological and parenteral therapies; content area: pharmacology.

    RATIONALE
    (A) All drugs have common side effects. **(B)** By definition, therapeutic range is the ratio between the lethal dose and the mean effective dose. **(C)** Duration of action is how long the drug is circulating in the body. **(D)** Biological half-life is the time it takes for half of the drug to disappear from the serum.

44. **(C)** Nursing process phase: evaluation; client need: pharmacological and parenteral therapies; content area: pharmacology.

    RATIONALE

    (A) The threshold dose of a drug is barely sufficient to produce desired effects. **(B)** Therapeutic range is the ratio between the lethal dose and the mean effective dose. **(C)** A loading dose is a large initial dose to achieve minimum effective concentration. **(D)** Free drug is the amount in the serum that is ineffective in its purpose.

45. **(D)** Nursing process phase: evaluation; client need: pharmacological and parenteral therapies; content area: pharmacology.

    RATIONALE

    (A) Anti-inflammatory drugs do not cause urinary retention. **(B)** Anti-inflammatory drugs do not commonly cause increased pulse rate. **(C)** Anti-inflammatory drugs do not commonly cause behavioral changes. **(D)** Many anti-inflammatory agents irritate the lining of the stomach. These should not be used in clients with a history of ulcers.

46. **(A)** Nursing process phase: planning; client need: pharmacological and parenteral therapies; content area: pharmacology.

    RATIONALE

    (A) Administering ibuprofen with food or a large glass of water helps to prevent gastric irritation. **(B)** Administering NSAIDs on an empty stomach increases the chances for gastric irritation. **(C)** Administering NSAIDs before meals or at bedtime does not provide protection against gastric irritation. **(D)** Administering NSAIDs with aspirin or other NSAIDs increases the chance of gastric irritation.

47. **(A)** Nursing process phase: data collection; client need: pharmacological and parenteral therapies; content area: pharmacology.

    RATIONALE

    (A) These are landmarks for location of the vastus lateralis. The vastus lateralis is the preferred injection site for children because it is well developed and has few major nerves present that could be injured. **(B)** This is not a landmark for an injection of any kind. **(C)** This is not a landmark for an injection of any kind. **(D)** This is not a landmark for an injection of any kind.

48. **(A)** Nursing process phase: implementation; client need: pharmacological and parenteral therapies; content area: pharmacology.

    RATIONALE

    (A) Regular insulin is pure and NPH a mixture; so if contamination does occur, it would be best to contaminate the NPH. **(B)** This sequence may cause contamination of NPH into the pure regular insulin. **(C)** This sequence may cause contamination of NPH into the pure regular insulin. **(D)** You should not give the client two injections if one injection can suffice.

49. **(C)** Nursing process phase: implementation; client need: pharmacological and parenteral therapies; content area: pharmacology.

    RATIONALE

    (A) Dobutamine does not combat metabolic acidosis. **(B)** Sodium nitroprusside does not combat metabolic acidosis. **(C)** Sodium bicarbonate is the only drug listed that helps to reverse acidosis. **(D)** Calcium gluconate does not combat metabolic acidosis.

50. **(B)** Nursing process phase: evaluation; client need: pharmacological and parenteral therapies; content area: pharmacology.

    RATIONALE

    (A) With an IV injection the nurse must aspirate to make sure the needle is in the vein and not in the tissue. **(B)** Intradermal injection is just under the skin; no danger exists of injection into a blood vessel. **(C)** Aspiration is needed in SC injections to make sure that the needle is not in a blood vessel. **(D)** Aspiration is needed in IM injections to make sure that the needle is not in a blood vessel.

Test 2: Calculation of Dosages

 QUESTIONS

51. qid means:
    A. Every 4 days
    B. Every 4 hours
    C. Four times each day
    D. Every day

52. *ac* means:
    A. Before meals
    B. After meals
    C. At mealtime
    D. At once

53. One fluid ounce is equivalent to:
    A. 15 ml
    B. 30 ml
    C. 2 tsp
    D. 3 tsp

54. The physician orders Maalox 15 ml. How many tablespoons would you give?
    A. 3 tsp
    B. 2 tsp
    C. 1 tsp
    D. 1 tbsp

55. One gram is equivalent to:
    A. 10 mg
    B. 100 mg
    C. 1000 mg
    D. 10,000 mg

56. You are instructed to give nitroglycerin 0.4 mg. The drug label reads "1/150-grain tablet." How many tablets would you give?
    A. 1 tablet
    B. ½ tablet
    C. 2 tablets
    D. 1½ tablets

57. You are instructed to give cephalexin monohydrate (Keflex) 0.5 g. The drug comes as 250 mg per capsule. How many capsules would you give?
    A. Five capsules
    B. Four capsules
    C. Two capsules
    D. One capsule

58. You are instructed to give penicillin V potassium (Pen-Vee K suspension) 0.75 g. The drug is available as 250 mg per 5 ml. How many milliliters would you give?
    A. 10 ml
    B. 15 ml

C. 3 ml
D. 20 ml

59. You are instructed to give cyclophosphamide (Cytoxan) 4 mg/kg per day PO. The client weighs 154 lb. How much Cytoxan would you give each day?
    A. 100 mg
    B. 120 mg
    C. 240 mg
    D. 280 mg

60. You are instructed to give cephalexin monohydrate 3 g over the next 24 hours, divided into six equally spaced doses. How much would you give for each dose?
    A. 3000 mg
    B. 500 mg
    C. 1000 mg
    D. 2000 mg

61. Aspirin is available in 5-grain tablet. The physician orders aspirin 300 mg. The amount of drug to be administered is:
    A. One-half tablet
    B. One tablet
    C. Two tablets
    D. One and one-half tablets

62. Vitamin K is available in 1 mg per 0.5 ml. The physician orders vitamin K 0.5 mg. The amount of vitamin K to be administered is:
    A. 2.5 ml
    B. 0.50 ml
    C. 0.25 ml
    D. 1 ml

63. Digoxin is available in 0.125 mg per tablet. The physician orders digoxin 0.25 mg. The amount of drug to be administered is:
    A. One tablet
    B. One-half tablet
    C. Two tablets
    D. One and one-half tablets

64. Meperidine is available in 75 mg/ml. The physician orders Demerol 0.50 mg. The amount of drug to be administered is:
    A. 0.5 ml
    B. 0.6 ml
    C. 0.7 ml
    D. 1.5 ml

65. Codeine is available in 1-grain tablet. The physician orders codeine 30 mg. The amount of drug to be administered is:

A. One tablet
B. One-half tablet
C. One and one-half tablets
D. Three-fourths tablet

66. Hydroxyzine (Vistaril) is available in 25 mg/cc. The physician orders 100 mg q4–6h PRN. How many cc would you give per as-needed dose?

A. 0.25 cc
B. 2.50 cc
C. 4 cc
D. 40 cc

67. The amount of solution and amount of IV aminophylline received by a client each hour when there is 500 mg aminophylline in 250 ml solution given every 24 hours is:

A. 12.5 ml/hr and 0.33 mg/hr
B. 10 ml/hr and 21 mg/hr
C. 21 ml/hr and 20 mg/hr
D. 20 ml/min and 40 ml/hr

68. The amount of solution and amount of IV aminophylline received by the client each minute when there is 250 mg aminophylline in 250 ml solution given over 16 hours is:

A. 0.5 ml/hr and 0.4 mg/ml
B. 10 ml/hr and 5 mg/ml
C. 0.26 ml/min and 0.26 mg/min
D. 1 ml and 1 mg/min

69. The amount of solution and amount of IV aminophylline received by a client each hour when there is 500 mg aminophylline in 500 ml solution over 12 hours is:

A. 21 ml/hr and 20.0 mg/hr
B. 20 ml/min and 40 ml/hr
C. 50 ml/hr and 21 mg/ml
D. 42 ml/hr and 42 mg/hr

70. The amount of solution and amount of IV dopamine received by a client each hour when there is 400 mg dopamine in 500 ml solution over 24 hours is:

A. 21 ml/hr and 17 mg/hr
B. 12.5 ml/hr and 0.33 mg/hr
C. 20 ml/hr and 34 mg/hr
D. 21 ml/hr and 34 mg/min

71. If the client is to receive insulin at 3 units/hr with a solution of 50 units per 100 ml in normal saline (NS), the rate of infusion in milliliters would be:

A. 4 ml/hr
B. 12 gtt/ml
C. 10 ml/hr
D. 6 ml/hr

72. The correct formula for converting total volume and hours of infusion into rate of drops (guttae, abbreviated gtt) per minute using calibration of IV tubing is:

A. $\dfrac{\text{milliliters per gtt} \times \text{set calibration}}{60 \text{ minutes}}$

B. $\dfrac{\text{milliliters per hour} \times \text{gtt per milliliter}}{60 \text{ minutes}}$

C. $\dfrac{\text{milliliters per hour} \times \text{minutes per milliliter}}{60 \text{ minutes}}$

D. $\dfrac{\text{milliliter per hour} \times \text{drop factor}}{10}$

73. You are instructed to give morphine sulfate 10 mg SC. The drug label reads "15 mg/ml." How many milliliters would you give?

A. 0.5 ml
B. 0.6 ml
C. 0.7 ml
D. 1.5 ml

74. Hydroxyzine 25 mg IM has been ordered. Vial reads "100 mg in 2 ml." How many milliliters would you give?

A. 5 ml
B. 4 ml
C. 0.5 ml
D. 1.4 ml

75. The order reads "5000 units heparin SC every 6 hours." Vial reads "20,000 units/ml." How many milliliters would you give?

A. 4 ml
B. 0.4 ml
C. 0.25 ml
D. 2.5 ml

76. The physician orders lactated Ringer's solution 1000 ml to be infused over 8 hours. Drops per milliliter equals 15. How many drops per minute would you give?

A. 30 gtt/min
B. 31 gtt/min
C. 15 gtt/min
D. 16 gtt/min

77. You are instructed to infuse 150 ml of D₅W over 1 hour. Drops per milliliter equals 10. How many drops per minute would you give?

A. 25 ml/min
B. 26 gtt/min
C. 25 gtt/min
D. 50 gtt/min

78. A hypertonic solution of 10% dextrose in water is to be infused over 10 hours via a 16-gauge IV needle. The total amount of fluid is 1000 ml, and the drop factor is 10. How many drops per minute would you give?

A. 16 ml/hr
B. 16 gtt/min
C. 17 gtt/min
D. 17 ml/hr

79. You are instructed to infuse 100 ml of solution in 2 hours. The set calibration is 60 gtt/ml. How many drops per minute would you give?

A. 50 ml/hr
B. 50 gtt/min
C. 60 gtt/min
D. 60 gtt/ml

80. You are instructed to infuse 900 ml of solution in 2 hours. The set calibration is 20 gtt/ml. How many drops per minute would you give?

A. 90 gtt/min
B. 45 gtt/min
C. 150 gtt/min
D. 45 gtt/min

81. You are instructed to infuse 1000 ml of solution in 8 hours. The set calibration is 10 gtt/ml. How many drops per minute would you give?

A. 20 gtt/min
B. 21 gtt/min
C. 125 gtt/min
D. 12.5 gtt/min

82. You are instructed to administer a solution IV at 150 ml/hr. The set calibration is 60 gtt/ml. How many drops per minute would you give?

A. 75 gtt/min
B. 75 ml/min
C. 150 gtt/min
D. 150 ml/min

83. You are instructed to infuse 50 ml of antibiotic in 30 minutes. The set calibration is 60 gtt/ml. How many drops per minute would you give?

A. 100 gtt/min
B. 50 gtt/min
C. 150 gtt/min
D. 10 gtt/min

84. You are instructed to infuse 15 ml of medication over 15 minutes. The set calibration is 60 gtt/ml. How many drops per minute would you give?

A. 15 gtt/min
B. 60 gtt/min
C. 5 gtt/min
D. 6 gtt/min

85. You are instructed to infuse 600 ml of IV fat emulsion (Intralipid) over 8 hours. The set calibration is 10 gtt/ml. How many drops per minute would you give?

A. 10 gtt/min
B. 60 gtt/min
C. 13 gtt/ min
D. 600 gtt/min

86. You are instructed to infuse 150 ml of fluid over 2 hours using minidrip (minidrip equals 60 gtt/ml). How many drops per minute would you give?

A. 150 gtt/min
B. 60 gtt/min
C. 75 gtt/min
D. 7.5 gtt/min

87. A client is to receive 1000 ml D_5 in one-half NS with 20 mEq potassium chloride over 10 hours. Drip factor is 15 gtt/ml. How many drops per minute would you give?

A. 15 gtt/min
B. 25 gtt/min
C. 2.5 gtt/min
D. 25 ml/hour

88. The physician orders 100 ml lactated Ringer's solution to be infused over 2 hours. The set calibration is 10 gtt/ml. How many drops per minute would you give?

A. 8 gtt/min
B. 80 gtt/min
C. 10 gtt/min
D. 20 gtt/min

89. You are instructed to infuse 15 ml of fluid over 30 minutes. The set calibration is 60 gtt/ml. How many drops per minute would you give?

A. 30 gtt/min
B. 30 ml/min
C. 30 ml/hr
D. 3 gtt/min

90. A client is to receive 1800 ml of fluid over 10 hours. The set calibration is 10 gtt/ml. How many drops per minute would you give?

A. 30 gtt/min
B. 10 gtt/min
C. 10 ml/min
D. 30 ml/min

91. The physician orders lactated Ringer's solution 1000 ml to be infused over 6 hours. Drops per milliliter equals 15. How many drops per minute would you give?

A. 4.4 gtt/min
B. 44 gtt/min
C. 42 gtt/min
D. 41 gtt/min

92. You are instructed to infuse D_5W 250 ml over 1 hour. Drops per milliliter equals 15. How many drops per minute would you give?

A. 62 gtt/min
B. 63 gtt/min
C. 52 gtt/min
D. 53 gtt/min

93. A hypertonic solution of 10% dextrose and water is to be infused over 12 hours. The total amount of fluid is 1000 ml and the drop factor 15. How many drops per minute would you give?

A. 20 gtt/min
B. 28 gtt/min
C. 21 gtt/min
D. 208 gtt/min

94. You are instructed to infuse 300 ml of solution in 2 hours. The set calibration is 60 gtt/ml. How many drops per minute would you give?

A. 15 gtt/min
B. 150 gtt/min
C. 75 gtt/min
D. 300 gtt/min

95. You are instructed to infuse 900 ml of fluid in 2 hours. The set calibration is 10 gtt/ml. How many drops per minute would you give?

   A. 450 gtt/min
   B. 750 gtt/min
   C. 75 gtt/min
   D. 7.5 gtt/min

96. You are instructed to infuse 1500 ml of fluid in 8 hours. The set calibration is 10 gtt/ml. How many drops per minute would you give?

   A. 31 gtt/min
   B. 32 gtt/min
   C. 3.2 gtt/min
   D. 3 gtt/min

97. You are instructed to administer an IV infusion of 250 ml of D_5W at 100 ml/hr. The set calibration is 60 gtt/ml. How many drops per minute would you give?

   A. 10 gtt/min
   B. 100 gtt/min
   C. 25 gtt/min
   D. 25 ml/min

98. You are instructed to infuse 60 ml of antibiotic in 15 minutes. The set calibration is 10 gtt/ml. How many drops per minute would you give?

   A. 40 gtt/min
   B. 60 gtt/min
   C. 20 gtt/min
   D. 30 gtt/min

99. You are instructed to infuse 20 ml of medication over 30 minutes. The set calibration is 60 gtt/ml set. How many drops per minute would you give?

   A. 40 gtt/min
   B. 80 gtt/min
   C. 30 gtt/min
   D. 60 gtt/min

100. You are instructed to infuse 800 ml of IV fat emulsion over 6 hours. The set calibration is 20 gtt/ml. How many drops per minute would you give?

A. 44 gtt/min
B. 45 gtt/min
C. 46 gtt/min
D. 47 gtt/min

101. You are instructed to infuse 105 ml of fluid over 2 hours using a minidrip of 60 gtt/min. How many drops per minute would you give?

   A. 53 gtt/min
   B. 50 gtt/min
   C. 60 gtt/min
   D. 62 gtt/min

102. The client is to receive 1000 ml D_5 in one-half NS with 20 mEq potassium chloride over 8 hours. Drip factor is 10 gtt/ml. How many drops per minute would you give?

   A. 20 gtt/min
   B. 21 gtt/min
   C. 22 gtt/min
   D. 60 gtt/min

103. The physician orders 100 ml lactated Ringer's solution to be infused over 2 hours. The set calibration is 10 gtt/ml. How many drops per minute would you give?

   A. 17 gtt/min
   B. 16 gtt/min
   C. 8 gtt/min
   D. 8.5 gtt/min

104. You are instructed to infuse 30 ml over 30 minutes. The set calibration is 60 gtt/ml. How many drops per minute would you give?

   A. 30 gtt/min
   B. 45 gtt/min
   C. 60 gtt/min
   D. 6 gtt/min

105. The client is to receive 1000 ml of fluid over 10 hours. The set calibration is 15 gtt/ml. How many drops per minute would you give?

   A. 100 gtt/min
   B. 115 gtt/min
   C. 25 gtt/min
   D. 125 gtt/min

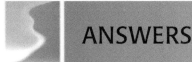
ANSWERS

51. **(C)** Nursing process phase: evaluation; client need: pharmacological and parenteral therapies; content area: pharmacology.
    RATIONALE
    (A) Every 4 days is q4d. **(B)** Every 4 hours is q4h. **(C)** Four times each day is qid. **(D)** Every day is qd.

52. **(A)** Nursing process phase: evaluation; client need: pharmacological and parenteral therapies; content area: pharmacology.
    RATIONALE
    (A) Before meals is ac. **(B)** After meals is pc. **(C)** At meals is cc. **(D)** At once is stat.

53. **(B)** Nursing process phase: evaluation; client need: pharmacological and parenteral therapies; content area: pharmacology.
    RATIONALE
    (A) Fifteen milliliters is ½ oz. **(B)** Thirty milliliters is 1 oz. **(C)** Two teaspoons is 10 ml. **(D)** Three teaspoons is 15 ml.

54. **(D)** Nursing process phase: evaluation; client need: pharmacological and parenteral therapies; content area: pharmacology.
    RATIONALE
    (A) Three teaspoons is 15 ml, but the question asks for tablespoons. **(B)** Two teaspoons is 10 ml, but question asks for tablespoons. **(C)** One teaspoon is 5 ml, but question asks for tablespoons. **(D)** One tablespoon is 15 ml.

55. **(C)** Nursing process phase: evaluation; client need: pharmacological and parenteral therapies; content area: pharmacology.
    RATIONALE
    (A) Ten milligrams is equivalent to 1/100 g. **(B)** One hundred milligrams is equivalent to 1/10 g. **(C)** One thousand milligrams is equivalent to 1 g. **(D)** Ten thousand milligrams is equivalent to 10 g.

56. **(A)** Nursing process phase: evaluation; client need: pharmacological and parenteral therapies; content area: pharmacology.
    RATIONALE
    (A) One tablet would be 0.4 mg − 1 tablet = 1/150 grain = 0.4 mg. **(B)** One-half tablet would be 0.2 mg. **(C)** Two tablets would be 0.8 mg. **(D)** One and one-half tablets would be 0.6 mg.

57. **(C)** Nursing process phase: evaluation; client need: pharmacological and parenteral therapies; content area: pharmacology.
    RATIONALE
    (A) Select another option. **(B)** Select another option. **(C)** 0.5 g = 500 mg, 500 mg : x : 250 mg : 1 capsule, $250x = 500$, $x = 2$ capsules. **(D)** Select another option.

58. **(B)** Nursing process phase: evaluation; client need: pharmacological and parenteral therapies; content area: pharmacology.
    RATIONALE
    (A) Select another option. **(B)** 50 mg : 1 ml : : 750 mg : x, 750 mg : x : : 50 mg : 1 ml, $50x = 750$, $x = 15$ ml. **(C)** Select another option. **(D)** Select another option

59. **(D)** Nursing process phase: evaluation; client need: pharmacological and parenteral therapies; content area: pharmacology.
    RATIONALE
    (A) Select another option. **(B)** Select another option. **(C)** Select another option. **(D)** 1 kg = 2.2 lb, 154 kg ÷ 2.2 lb = 70 kg, 70 kg × 4 mg/kg = 280 mg.

60. **(B)** Nursing process phase: evaluation; client need: pharmacological and parenteral therapies; content area: pharmacology.
    RATIONALE
    (A) Select another option. **(B)** 3 g = 3000 mg in 24 hours, 3000 mg ÷ 6 doses = 500 mg. **(C)** Select another option. **(D)** Select another option.

61. **(B)** Nursing process phase: evaluation; client need: pharmacological and parenteral therapies; content area: pharmacology.
    RATIONALE
    (A) Select another option. **(B)** 1 grain = 60 mg, 60 mg × 5 grains = 1 tablet, 300 mg : 1 tablet : : 300 mg : x, $300x = 300$ mg, $x = 1$ tablet. **(C)** Select another option. **(D)** Select another option.

62. **(C)** Nursing process phase: evaluation; client need: pharmacological and parenteral therapies; content area: pharmacology.
    RATIONALE
    (A) Select another option. **(B)** Select another option. **(C)** 1 mg : 0.5 cc : : 0.5 mg : x, $x = 0.25$ ml. **(D)** Select another option.

63. **(C)** Nursing process phase: evaluation; client need: pharmacological and parenteral therapies; content area: pharmacology.
    RATIONALE
    (A) Select another option. **(B)** Select another option. **(C)** 0.125 mg : 1 tablet : : 0.25 mg : x, $0.125x = 0.25$, $x = 2$. **(D)** Select another option.

64. **(C)** Nursing process phase: evaluation; client need: pharmacological and parenteral therapies; content area: pharmacology.
    RATIONALE
    (A) Select another option. **(B)** Select another option. **(C)** 75 mg : 1 ml : : 50 mg : x, $75x = 50$, $x = 0.66$ or 0.7 ml. **(D)** Select another option.

65. **(B)** Nursing process phase: evaluation; client need: pharmacological and parenteral therapies; content area: pharmacology.
    RATIONALE
    (A) Select another option. **(B)** 1 grain = 60 mg, 60 mg : 1 tablet : : 30 mg : x, $60x = 30$, $x = 0.5$ tablet. **(C)** Select another option. **(D)** Select another option.

66. **(C)** Nursing process phase: evaluation; client need: pharmacological and parenteral therapies; content area: pharmacology.
    RATIONALE
    (A) Select another option. **(B)** Select another option. **(C)** 25 mg : 1 cc : : 100 mg : x, $25x = 100$, $x = 4$ cc. **(D)** Select another option.

67. **(B)** Nursing process phase: evaluation; client need: pharmacological and parenteral therapies; content area: pharmacology.
    RATIONALE
    (A) Select another option. **(B)** 500 mg ÷ 24 hr = 20.8 or 21 mg/hr, 250 ml ÷ 24 hr = 10.4 or 10 ml/hr. **(C)** Select another option. **(D)** Select another option.

68. **(C)** Nursing process phase: evaluation; client need: pharmacological and parenteral therapies; content area: pharmacology.
    RATIONALE
    (A) Select another option. **(B)** Select another option. **(C)** 250 mg ÷ 16 hr = 15.6 mg/hr ÷ 60 min/hr = 0.26 mg/min, 250 ml ÷ 16 hr = 15.6 ml/hr ÷ 60 min/hr = 0.26 ml/min. **(D)** Select another option.

69. **(D)** Nursing process phase: evaluation; client need: pharmacological and parenteral therapies; content area: pharmacology.
    RATIONALE
    (A) Select another option. **(B)** Select another option. **(C)** Select

another option. **(D)** 500 ml ÷ 12 hr = 41.6 or 42 ml/hr, 500 mg ÷ 12 hrs = 41.6 or 42 mg/hr.

70. **(A)** Nursing process phase: evaluation; client need: pharmacological and parenteral therapies; content area: pharmacology.
RATIONALE
(A) 400 mg ÷ 24 hr = 16.6 or 17 mg/hr, 500 ml ÷ 24 hr = 20.8 or 21 ml/hr. **(B)** Select another option. **(C)** Select another option. **(D)** Select another option.

71. **(D)** Nursing process phase: evaluation; client need: pharmacological and parenteral therapies; content area: pharmacology.
RATIONALE
(A) Select another option. **(B)** Select another option. **(C)** Select another option. **(D)** 50 units = 100 ml, 1 unit = 2 ml, 3 unit = 6 ml.

72. **(B)** Nursing process phase: evaluation; client need: pharmacological and parenteral therapies; content area: pharmacology.
RATIONALE
(A) Select another option. **(B)** You must know formula. **(C)** Select another option. **(D)** Select another option.

73. **(C)** Nursing process phase: evaluation; client need: pharmacological and parenteral therapies; content area: pharmacology.
RATIONALE
(A) Select another option. **(B)** Select another option. **(C)** 10 mg : x ml : : 15 mg : 1 ml, $15x$ = 10, x = 0.66 or 0.7 ml. **(D)** Select another option.

74. **(C)** Nursing process phase: evaluation; client need: pharmacological and parenteral therapies; content area: pharmacology.
RATIONALE
(A) Select another option. **(B)** Select another option. **(C)** 25 mg : : x : : 100 mg : : 2 ml, $100x$ = 50, x = 0.5 ml. **(D)** Select another option.

75. **(C)** Nursing process phase: evaluation; client need: pharmacological and parenteral therapies; content area: pharmacology.
RATIONALE
(A) Select another option. **(B)** Select another option. **(C)** 20,000 : 1 ml : : 5000 : : x, 20,000 = 5000x, x = 0.25 ml. **(D)** Select another option.

76. **(B)** Nursing process phase: evaluation; client need: pharmacological and parenteral therapies; content area: pharmacology.
RATIONALE
(A) Select another option. **(B)** 1000 ml × 15 gtt/ml ÷ 60 min/hr × 8 hr = 15,000/480 = 31.2 or 31 gtt/min. **(C)** Select another option. **(D)** Select another option.

77. **(C)** Nursing process phase: evaluation; client need: pharmacological and parenteral therapies; content area: pharmacology.
RATIONALE
(A) Select another option. **(B)** Select another option. **(C)** 150 ml × 10 gtt/ml ÷ 60 min/hr × 1 hr = 1500/60 = 25 gtt/min. **(D)** Select another option.

78. **(C)** Nursing process phase: evaluation; client need: pharmacological and parenteral therapies; content area: pharmacology.
RATIONALE
(A) Select another option. **(B)** Select another option. **(C)** 1000 ml × 10 gtt/ml ÷ 10 hr × 60/min/hr = 10,000/600 = 16.6 or 17 gtt/min. **(D)** Select another option.

79. **(B)** Nursing process phase: evaluation; client need: pharmacological and parenteral therapies; content area: pharmacology.

RATIONALE
(A) Select another option. **(B)** 100 ml × 60 gtt/ml ÷ 60 min/hr × 2 hr = 6000/120 = 50 gtt/min. **(C)** Select another option. **(D)** Select another option.

80. **(C)** Nursing process phase: evaluation; client need: pharmacological and parenteral therapies; content area: pharmacology.
RATIONALE
(A) Select another option. **(B)** Select another option. **(C)** 900 ml × 20 gtt/ml ÷ 60 min/hr × 2 hr = 18,000/120 = 150 gtt/min. **(D)** Select another option.

81. **(B)** Nursing process phase: evaluation; client need: pharmacological and parenteral therapies; content area: pharmacology.
RATIONALE
(A) Select another option. **(B)** 1000 ml × 10 gtt/ml ÷ 8 hr × 60 min/hr = 10,000/480 = 20.8 or 21 gtt/min. **(C)** Select another option. **(D)** Select another option.

82. **(C)** Nursing process phase: evaluation; client need: pharmacological and parenteral therapies; content area: pharmacology.
RATIONALE
(A) Select another option. **(B)** Select another option. **(C)** 150 ml × 60 gtt/ml ÷ 60 ml = 9000/60 = 150 gtt/min. **(D)** Select another option.

83. **(A)** Nursing process phase: evaluation; client need: pharmacological and parenteral therapies; content area: pharmacology.
RATIONALE
(A) 50 ml × 60 gtt/ml ÷ 30 min = 3000/30 = 100 gtt/min. **(B)** Select another option. **(C)** Select another option. **(D)** Select another option.

84. **(B)** Nursing process phase: evaluation; client need: pharmacological and parenteral therapies; content area: pharmacology.
RATIONALE
(A) Select another option. **(B)** 15 ml × 60 gtt/ml ÷ 15 min = 900/15 = 60 gtt/min. **(C)** Select another option. **(D)** Select another option.

85. **(C)** Nursing process phase: evaluation; client need: pharmacological and parenteral therapies; content area: pharmacology.
RATIONALE
(A) Select another option. **(B)** Select another option. **(C)** 600 ml × 10 gtt/ml ÷ 60 min/hr = 6000/480 = 12.5 or 13 gtt/min. **(D)** Select another option.

86. **(C)** Nursing process phase: evaluation; client need: pharmacological and parenteral therapies; content area: pharmacology.
RATIONALE
(A) Select another option. **(B)** Select another option. **(C)** 150 ml × 60 gtt/ml ÷ 60 min/hr × 2 hr = 9000/120 = 75 gtt/min. **(D)** Select another option.

87. **(B)** Nursing process phase: evaluation; client need: pharmacological and parenteral therapies; content area: pharmacology.
RATIONALE
(A) Select another option. **(B)** 1000 ml × 15 gtt/ml ÷ 60 min/hr × 10 hr = 15,000/600 = 25 gtt/min. **(C)** Select another option. **(D)** Select another option.

88. **(A)** Nursing process phase: evaluation; client need: pharmacological and parenteral therapies; content area: pharmacology.
RATIONALE
(A) 100 ml × 10 gtt ÷ 2 hr × 60 min/hr = 1000/120 = 8.3 or 8 gtt/min. **(B)** Select another option. **(C)** Select another option. **(D)** Select another option.

89. **(A)** Nursing process phase: evaluation; client need: pharmacological and parenteral therapies; content area: pharmacology.

    RATIONALE

    (A) 15 ml × 60 gtt/ml ÷ 30 min = 900/30 = 30 gtt/min. **(B)** Select another option. **(C)** Select another option. **(D)** Select another option.

90. **(A)** Nursing process phase: evaluation; client need: pharmacological and parenteral therapies; content area: pharmacology.

    RATIONALE

    (A) 1800 ml × 10 gtt/ml ÷ 60 min/hr × 10 hr = 18,000/600 = 30 gtt/min. **(B)** Select another option. **(C)** Select another option. **(D)** Select another option.

91. **(C)** Nursing process phase: evaluation; client need: pharmacological and parenteral therapies; content area: pharmacology.

    RATIONALE

    (A) Select another option. **(B)** Select another option. **(C)** 1000 ml × 15 gtt/ml ÷ 60 min/hr × 6 hr = 15,000/360 = 41.6 or 42 gtt/min. **(D)** Select another option.

92. **(B)** Nursing process phase: evaluation; client need: pharmacological and parenteral therapies; content area: pharmacology.

    RATIONALE

    (A) Select another option. **(B)** 250 ml × 15 gtt/ml ÷ 60 min/hr × 1 hr = 3750/60 = 62.5 or 63 gtt/min. **(C)** Select another option. **(D)** Select another option.

93. **(C)** Nursing process phase: evaluation; client need: pharmacological and parenteral therapies; content area: pharmacology.

    RATIONALE

    (A) Select another option. **(B)** Select another option. **(C)** 1000 ml × 15 gtt/ml ÷ 12 hr × 60 min/hr = 15,000/720 = 20.8 or 21 gtt/min. **(D)** Select another option.

94. **(B)** Nursing process phase: evaluation; client need: pharmacological and parenteral therapies; content area: pharmacology.

    RATIONALE

    (A) Select another option. **(B)** 300 ml × 60 gtt/ml ÷ 60 min/hr × 2 hr = 18,000/120 = 150 gtt/min. **(C)** Select another option. **(D)** Select another option.

95. **(C)** Nursing process phase: evaluation; client need: pharmacological and parenteral therapies; content area: pharmacology.

    RATIONALE

    (A) Select another option. **(B)** Select another option. **(C)** 900 ml × 10 gtt/ml ÷ 60 min/hr × 2 hr = 9000/120 = 75 gtt/min. **(D)** Select another option.

96. **(A)** Nursing process phase: evaluation; client need: pharmacological and parenteral therapies; content area: pharmacology.

    RATIONALE

    (A) 1500 ml × 10 gtt/ml ÷ 60 min/hr × 8 hr = 15,000/480 = 31.25 or 31 gtt/min. **(B)** Select another option. **(C)** Select another option. **(D)** Select another option.

97. **(B)** Nursing process phase: evaluation; client need: pharmacological and parenteral therapies; content area: pharmacology.

    RATIONALE

    (A) Select another option. **(B)** 100 ml × 60 gtt/ml ÷ 60 min/hr × 1 hr = 6000/60 = 100 gtt/min. **(C)** Select another option. **(D)** Select another option.

98. **(A)** Nursing process phase: evaluation; client need: pharmacological and parenteral therapies; content area: pharmacology.

    RATIONALE

    (A) 60 ml × 10 gtt/ml ÷ 15 min = 600/15 = 40 gtt/min. **(B)** Select another option. **(C)** Select another option. **(D)** Select another option.

99. **(A)** Nursing process phase: evaluation; client need: pharmacological and parenteral therapies; content area: pharmacology.

    RATIONALE

    (A) 20 ml × 60 gtt/ml ÷ 30 min = 1200/30 = 40 gtt/min. **(B)** Select another option. **(C)** Select another option. **(D)** Select another option.

100. **(A)** Nursing process phase: evaluation; client need: pharmacological and parenteral therapies; content area: pharmacology.

     RATIONALE

     (A) 800 ml × 20 gtt/ml ÷ 60 min/hr × hr = 16,000/360 = 44.4 or 44 gtt/min. **(B)** Select another option. **(C)** Select another option. **(D)** Select another option.

101. **(A)** Nursing process phase: evaluation; client need: pharmacological and parenteral therapies; content area: pharmacology.

     RATIONALE

     (A) 105 ml × 60 gtt/ml ÷ 60 min/hr × 2 hr = 6300/120 = 52.5 or 53 gtt/min. **(B)** Select another option. **(C)** Select another option. **(D)** Select another option.

102. **(B)** Nursing process phase: evaluation; client need: pharmacological and parenteral therapies; content area: pharmacology.

     RATIONALE

     (A) Select another option. **(B)** 1000 ml × 10 gtt/ml ÷ 60 min/hr × 8 hr = 10,000/480 = 20.8 or 21 gtt/min. **(C)** Select another option. **(D)** Select another option.

103. **(C)** Nursing process phase: evaluation; client need: pharmacological and parenteral therapies; content area: pharmacology.

     RATIONALE

     (A) Select another option. **(B)** Select another option. **(C)** 100 ml × 10 gtt/ml ÷ 60 min/hr × 2 hr = 1000/120 = 8.3 or 8 gtt/min. **(D)** Select another option.

104. **(C)** Nursing process phase: evaluation; client need: pharmacological and parenteral therapies; content area: pharmacology.

     RATIONALE

     (A) Select another option. **(B)** Select another option. **(C)** 30 ml × 60 gtt/ml ÷ 30 min = 1800/30 = 60 gtt/min. **(D)** Select another option.

105. **(C)** Nursing process phase: evaluation; client need: pharmacological and parenteral therapies; content area: pharmacology.

     RATIONALE

     (A) Select another option. **(B)** Select another option. **(C)** 1000 ml × 15 gtt/ml ÷ 60 min/hr × 10 hr = 15,000/600 = 25 gtt/min. **(D)** Select another option.

CHAPTER 9

Nutrition and Combined Nutrition-Pharmacology Review Tests

Patricia Gauntlett Beare, RN, PhD,
Demetrius J. Porche, RN, CCRN, DNS

Test 1: Nutritional Principles

QUESTIONS

1. After a myocardial infarction, a 52-year-old man has been placed on a 1-g sodium diet. Which of the following choices is considered low sodium?

   A. Canned and dry soups
   B. Ketchup, Worcestershire sauce
   C. Bologna and hot dogs
   D. Fresh or frozen meat, whole-grain bread

2. A 52-year-old male client is 3 weeks post-myocardial infarction. His doctor has ordered a diet to lower his blood cholesterol. Which of the following statements indicates a need for further teaching?

   A. "I ate a grilled cheese sandwich and an avocado salad for lunch yesterday."
   B. "I enjoyed broiled chicken, baked potato, and canned peaches for dinner."
   C. "I fixed a loin lamb chop, macaroni, and an apple-raisin salad for dinner."
   D. "I ate red beans and rice with bread sticks yesterday."

3. A client with a history of strokes has been admitted for evaluation of her dysphagia. Which of the following should the nurse encourage?

   A. Thin, clear liquid foods
   B. Eating in an upright position

C. Using liquids to clear the mouth of food
D. Talking to the client while eating to facilitate the social aspect of eating

4. A client is being evaluated for chronic "heartburn." When teaching the client to avoid gastroesophageal reflux, which of the following client statements indicates a need for further teaching?

   A. "I will limit my lifting of heavy objects."
   B. "I will try to lose some of my extra weight."
   C. "I will lie down for a half hour after meals."
   D. "I will elevate the head of my bed at night."

5. A 42-year-old male client was admitted with peptic ulcer disease. Which of the following decreases gastric acid secretion or increases gastric healing?

   A. Eating at bedtime so that acid can work on food at night
   B. Eating a bland diet
   C. Eliminating only foods that cause discomfort
   D. Drinking caffeinated beverages instead of milk

6. A 19-year-old woman is being treated for ulcerative colitis. After her symptoms are under control, she has been ordered to follow a low-fiber diet. Which of the following statements indicates a need for further teaching?

A. "I can drink coffee, tea, or clear fruit juices."
B. "I can eat pancakes, waffles, Special K, and puffed wheat."
C. "I can eat chicken, eggs, and potatoes."
D. "I can eat peanut butter pie, coconut meringue pie, or cherry pie for dessert."

7. A 76-year-old woman is seen at the clinic with chronic constipation. She has been placed on a high-fiber diet. Which of the following presents good food choices for her?

A. Popcorn, oat bran muffins, brown rice
B. Grits, Cheerios, corn flakes
C. Ripe banana, applesauce, fruit cocktail
D. Well-cooked meat, potatoes, canned vegetables

8. A client with chronic cholecystitis is treated with a fat- and calorie-controlled diet. Which meal is an example for the nurse to help the client choose?

A. English muffin, fresh fruit, Canadian bacon
B. Buttermilk, fried potatoes, pork sausage
C. French toast, chocolate milk, smoked salmon
D. Croissant, corned beef, skim milk

9. A 42-year-old female client underwent a gastrectomy 4 months ago. She has developed pernicious anemia. The nurse anticipates that the physician will order:

A. Vitamin B_{12} in a multivitamin
B. A dietary consultation
C. Parenteral vitamin B_{12}
D. A diet high in vitamin B_{12}

10. The nurse is discussing "old wives' tales" with a group of new mothers. Which of the following statements is actually true about breastfeeding?

A. Limiting nursing time will prevent sore nipples.
B. Limiting breastfeeding will build up a supply of milk.
C. Sore nipples are caused by a tight seal from the baby's lips.
D. A fussy baby should be nursed frequently.

11. A 35-year-old woman is admitted to your unit with nausea and vomiting, cramps, diarrhea, and chills. These symptoms occurred about 30 hours after she ate supper. Which of the following foods is most likely to be the cause?

A. Salad
B. Chicken
C. Gravy
D. Raw seafood or fish

12. The nurse is helping a client with a new diagnosis of diabetes to select his meals. Which of the following statements indicates a need for further teaching?

A. "I will weigh my meat before cooking."
B. "I will trim off visible fat before or after cooking."
C. "I know that meat does not contain fiber."
D. "Many processed meats contain large amounts of carbohydrates."

13. The nurse is helping a client with a new diagnosis of diabetes to select his meals. Which of the following indi-

cates a need for further teaching when selected as a vegetable?

A. Corn
B. Beans
C. Carrots
D. Tomatoes

14. The nurse is helping a client with a new diagnosis of diabetes to select his meals. Which of the following indicates a need for further teaching when selected from the cereal and grain list?

A. Grits
B. Pasta
C. Rice
D. Popcorn

15. A 22-year-old primigravida is 5 ft 5 in tall and weighed 128 lb at the beginning of pregnancy. Her expected weight at term gestation would be:

A. 145 lb
B. 148 lb
C. 155 lb
D. 167 lb

16. A client who is a native of the Middle East normally wears a long robe that covers her arms and body, along with a shawl that covers her head and neck. She is pregnant and the nurse is aware that she will need a supplement of:

A. Vitamin D
B. Calcium
C. Vitamin C
D. Zinc

17. A client experiences morning nausea early in her pregnancy. The nurse advises her to:

A. Eat a small amount of dry, carbohydrate-containing food on awakening
B. Increase her intake of fluids in the early morning
C. Increase her intake of fat to provide enough calories
D. Restrict her intake of fluids throughout the day for a few weeks

18. If an iron supplement is prescribed for a pregnant woman, which point should the nurse emphasize in her teaching?

A. She should take the supplement with food to avoid stomach upsets.
B. She should take the supplement with milk to improve absorption.
C. As long as she takes the supplement, she does not have to worry about including iron sources in her diet.
D. She should include food such as citrus fruits, melons, broccoli, or strawberries in her diet each day.

19. In a teaching plan for a pregnant woman, the nurse would advise her on the need to avoid:

A. Cholesterol
B. Sodium
C. Alcohol
D. Saturated fat

20. A 55-year-old man has liver failure caused by cirrhosis and is in impending hepatic coma. The nurse is assisting him with his diet selection. Which of the following choices indicates a need for further teaching?
    A. Fruit salad
    B. Cooked buttered carrots
    C. Boiled potato
    D. Cream of chicken soup

21. In evaluating a 10-year-old boy's understanding of his diet for celiac disease, the nurse would expect him to order which of these foods for breakfast?
    A. Corn flakes
    B. Buckwheat pancakes
    C. Oat bran muffins
    D. Cereal with wheat germ

22. An 18-year-old female client is admitted to the hospital with acute renal failure. She is oliguric, hypertensive, and hyperkalemic. The nurse would not expect to see which of the following on her meal tray?
    A. Canned, drained pears
    B. Whole-wheat bread
    C. Fresh orange
    D. Unsalted butter

23. A 12-year-old girl has a new diagnosis of insulin-dependent diabetes mellitus. The nurse advises the client that some carbohydrates need to be included in her diet because they:
    A. Insulate the body to prevent heat loss
    B. Furnish the body with energy
    C. Build and repair new tissue
    D. Provide a source of dietary fiber

24. In evaluating a client's understanding of the exchange diet, the nurse would expect the client to state that part-skim-milk mozzarella cheese is:
    A. A milk exchange
    B. A meat exchange
    C. A fat exchange
    D. Either a milk or a meat exchange

25. In teaching the exchange diet to a client with a new diagnosis of diabetes, the nurse would explain that potatoes are:
    A. A vegetable exchange
    B. A starch-bread exchange
    C. A fruit exchange
    D. Either a vegetable or a starch-bread exchange

26. A 57-year-old client has undergone resection of the ileum and much of the jejunum. Postoperatively, the client has experienced diarrhea and steatorrhea. The nurse would expect the diet to be restricted in:
    A. Protein
    B. Fluid
    C. Sodium
    D. Fat

27. A client complains of constipation. The nurse teaches the client to add fiber to the diet. The teaching was effective if the client has:

    A. Carrot-raisin salad
    B. Hamburger on a sesame seed bun
    C. Mashed potatoes with gravy
    D. Canned fruit cocktail

28. A 68-year-old woman is receiving a nasogastric tube feeding. Tube placement is known to be correct if:
    A. A loud "whoosh" can be heard over the left upper quadrant of the abdomen when air is injected through the tube
    B. No air bubbles appear when the free end of the tube is held under water during exhalation
    C. The client experiences no gagging or respiratory distress
    D. An abdominal x-ray shows the tube to be in the body of the stomach

29. A client who undergoes a gastric resection is most likely to require supplementation with:
    A. Magnesium
    B. Folic acid
    C. Chloride
    D. Vitamin B_{12}

30. A 14-year-old boy has third-degree burns over 50% of his body. He is in stable condition. The best snack for him would be:
    A. Peanut butter sandwich and milkshake
    B. Buttered popcorn and soft drink
    C. Orange juice and fresh vegetables with dip
    D. Milk and crackers

31. To promote wound healing in a burn client, the nurse would expect which vitamin or mineral to be supplemented?
    A. Folic acid
    B. Zinc
    C. Iron
    D. Vitamin K

32. The nurse would offer which food to a client on a clear-liquid diet?
    A. Tea
    B. Orange juice
    C. Sherbet
    D. Vegetable soup

33. A client on a full-liquid diet received the following foods on his tray. Which food should be removed?
    A. Chicken noodle soup
    B. Ice cream
    C. Cream of tomato soup
    D. Custard

34. In teaching a client about a low-fat diet, the nurse explains that a food without any limits is:
    A. Avocado
    B. Blueberry muffin
    C. Chocolate bar
    D. Angel food cake

35. A neonate has a diagnosis of phenylketonuria (PKU). Which of the following statements by her mother informs the nurse that more education is needed?

    A. "I must read the ingredient listing on foods before I give them to the baby."
    B. "As the baby grows, her diet will change."
    C. "The baby will need a special infant formula."
    D. "When she becomes a teenager, she won't need a special diet any longer."

36. Which food would the nurse select for a toddler on a low-phenylalanine diet?

    A. Boiled potato
    B. Macaroni
    C. Corn
    D. Applesauce

37. Which food would the nurse select for a child on a galactose-free diet?

    A. Sherbet
    B. Buttered popcorn
    C. Egg noodles
    D. Pancakes

38. A 4-month-old infant is to begin on solid foods. The following are good reasons for starting with infant rice cereal except:

    A. Rice cereal is the most economical infant food.
    B. An infant of this age has developed the ability to digest the carbohydrate provided by the cereal.
    C. Infant cereals are fortified with iron.
    D. Rice cereal is not often associated with allergic reactions.

39. A mother of a 9-month-old infant gave a diet history of feeding the baby the foods listed below. Which food choice indicates that the mother needs further teaching?

    A. Infant formula
    B. Scrambled egg
    C. Toast strips
    D. Cottage cheese

40. A client who has essential hypertension is following a 2-g sodium diet restriction. The nurse would expect the client to avoid:

    A. Fresh flounder
    B. Hard rolls
    C. Peanut butter
    D. Milk

41. When evaluating a client's understanding of a low-sodium diet, the nurse would expect her to state she uses which seasoning?

    A. Worcestershire sauce
    B. Garlic salt
    C. Ketchup
    D. Lemon juice

42. A client has very high blood cholesterol levels. In regard to diet, the nurse implements a teaching plan and encourages the client to reduce intake of:

    A. All types of fats
    B. Saturated fats
    C. Polyunsaturated fats
    D. Monounsaturated fats

43. The nurse would encourage a client on a low-cholesterol diet to drink:

    A. Whole milk
    B. Two percent lowfat milk
    C. Skim milk
    D. Acidophilus milk

44. A client states that she is a strict vegetarian (consuming no animal products). What food could the nurse recommend as a source of calcium?

    A. Strawberries
    B. Raisins
    C. Mustard greens
    D. Corn

45. In teaching a weight-loss class, the nurse emphasizes that the most effective way for people to achieve and maintain weight loss is:

    A. Low-calorie liquid-formula diet
    B. Increased exercise combined with low-calorie diet
    C. Increased exercise
    D. Low-calorie diet selected from common foods

46. The mother of a 7-lb 6-oz newborn is trying to decide whether to breast-feed or bottle-feed. In discussing the decision with her, the nurse can say that:

    A. Growth is better in formula-fed infants
    B. Formula feeding is less expensive than breastfeeding
    C. Breast-fed infants are more likely to have colic than formula-fed ones
    D. Breast-fed infants are less likely to develop allergies

47. A client would like to breast-feed her newborn son. The nurse knows that he will need a supplement to provide:

    A. Zinc
    B. Vitamin E
    C. Fluoride
    D. Thiamine

48. At a baby's 2-week checkup in the clinic, his mother asks whether it is time to start him on solid foods. The nurse can tell her that:

    A. It is best to start solid foods soon because the baby will be more likely to accept them now than when he is older.
    B. Solid foods should not be started until the infant is at least 4 months old, when it will be less likely to cause allergies.
    C. It is a good idea to start solid foods now because doing so will help the baby to sleep through the night at an earlier age.
    D. Solid foods should be started before 2 months of age because doing so will help to prevent the baby from becoming obese.

49. A mother intends to wean her child from breastfeeding at 8 months of age. She asks what he should receive in place of the breast milk. The nurse explains that:

    A. Whole cow's milk is an economical and nutritious substitute for breast milk for an infant of this age.
    B. An infant of this age can be weaned to skim milk because this helps to reduce the risk of his developing heart disease later in life.
    C. Formula without iron is the best choice for a child of this age because it is less likely to cause constipation than a formula with iron.
    D. Iron-fortified formula should be used until the infant is 12 months old.

50. A 3-year-old client comes to the clinic. His mother reports that he drinks several cups of milk daily but dislikes most other foods except peanut butter and french fries. The nurse suspects that the child is most likely to have a deficiency of which nutrient?

    A. Calcium
    B. Phosphorus
    C. Protein
    D. Iron

51. A client with acute pancreatitis is receiving a low-fat diet. The best breakfast for her would be:

    A. Orange juice, corn flakes with skim milk, biscuits with jam, coffee
    B. Grape juice, bran flakes with skim milk, toast with honey, tea
    C. Tomato juice, poached eggs on toast, coffee
    D. Grapefruit sections, blueberry muffins, and tea

52. During a health-care visit, the client states that "sometimes my gums bleed." The nurse in diet teaching explains that bleeding gums are usually a sign of inadequate intake of:

    A. Vitamin C
    B. Vitamin D
    C. Vitamin E
    D. Vitamin A

53. When presenting a class on nutrition, the nurse should emphasize that in the United States, the most likely cause of anemia is deficiency of:

    A. Iron
    B. Folic acid
    C. Vitamin B_{12}
    D. Intrinsic factor

54. A client has an esophageal tumor obstruction. The client has a gastrostomy. Which type of diet would be best for this client?

    A. Full liquid
    B. Soft
    C. Low residue
    D. Tube feeding via gastrostomy

55. A client develops pneumonia. The nurse encourages his wife to select which nutrient to assist in producing adequate antibodies to resist the infection?

    A. Protein
    B. Fat
    C. Thiamine
    D. Riboflavin

56. The nurse might expect the physician to write orders for a low-residue diet for a client 2–3 days before he undergoes:

    A. Oral surgery
    B. GI surgery
    C. Head and neck surgery
    D. Any surgery

57. A client undergoes gastric surgery and experiences postoperative difficulty with symptoms of dumping syndrome. The food that would be most likely to worsen her symptoms is:

    A. Fried fish
    B. Hard-cooked egg
    C. Plain bagel
    D. Fruit gelatin

58. A client is experiencing symptoms of dumping syndrome. The nurse advises the client to drink fluids:

    A. Just before meals
    B. Only with meals
    C. Before and during meals
    D. After meals

59. A client notes that he experiences cramping, bloating, and watery stools when drinking milk. A plan of care for the client would be to encourage a reduction in intake of:

    A. Milk protein
    B. Lactose
    C. Sucrose
    D. Galactose

60. A client reports that the following is typical of his usual daily eating habits: 1 cup oatmeal, 2 slices whole-grain toast, 1 cup orange juice, 1 cup 2% fat milk, 5 oz lasagna, 1 cup orange juice, 1 cup 2% fat milk, 1 cup steamed broccoli, 2 bean tacos, 1 cup tossed salad with olive oil and vinegar, and 30 oz of beer. According to the Food Pyramid and the Dietary Guidelines for Americans, it would be most important for the client to:

    A. Decrease his intake of cholesterol
    B. Decrease his alcohol intake
    C. Increase his fiber intake
    D. Increase his vegetable intake

61. In developing a teaching plan for weight control, the nurse is aware that obesity is usually defined as having a body weight that is at least _____% greater than the desirable body weight.

    A. 5
    B. 20
    C. 40
    D. 55

62. A client is found to be obese. The nurse includes diet teaching and makes the client aware of risk factor(s) for other diseases such as:

A. Peptic ulcer
B. Periodontal disease
C. Scleroderma
D. Hypertension

63. A 6-ft-tall football player who weighs 300 lb has a diagnosis of hiatal hernia and complains of burning chest pain after eating. Which of the following statements by the client indicates a need for further dietary teaching?

A. "I should lie down and rest after eating."
B. "I should not snack before I go to bed."
C. "I should reduce my weight."
D. "I can use an antacid to relieve the burning."

64. A client is placed on a high-fiber diet. Which of the following does the nurse identify as the best source of dietary fiber?

A. Pineapple juice
B. Potatoes au gratin
C. Popcorn
D. Roast beef

65. A 6-month-old formula-fed infant has an acute case of diarrhea. In instructing the mother regarding the infant's care, the nurse needs to know and teach that *lactose* refers to:

A. Fruit sugar
B. Table sugar
C. Milk sugar
D. Corn syrup

66. It is important to observe a 6-month-old admitted with diarrhea for:

A. Dry, sticky mucous membranes
B. Edema
C. Acute weight gain
D. Skin rash

67. When teaching a pregnant client, the nurse knows that iron supplements are recommended:

A. Only during the first trimester of pregnancy
B. Only during the last trimester of pregnancy
C. Throughout pregnancy and lactation
D. Only during lactation

68. If a client's weight before pregnancy was 122 lb, she should aim for a weight of approximately _____ lb at the end of pregnancy.

A. 135
B. 147
C. 159
D. 165

69. When the nurse is teaching a client with insulin-dependent diabetes, a good rule is:

A. All foods in the meal plan should be consumed at the planned time each day.
B. It is safe to omit meat or fat exchanges but not to omit fruits, milk, or breads.
C. Exchanges may be moved from one meal or snack to the next within the same day.

D. Extra exchanges from the diabetic diet may be consumed as long as the client takes extra insulin with the food.

70. If a client develops a complete intestinal obstruction postoperatively, which type of feeding is he or she most likely to receive?

A. Nasogastric tube feeding
B. Full-liquid diet
C. Total parenteral nutrition
D. Low-residue diet

71. A client has been found to have very high blood cholesterol levels. The nurse teaches that, in regard to his diet, he should know that blood cholesterol increases with excessive intake of:

A. All types of fats
B. Saturated fats
C. Polyunsaturated fats
D. Monounsaturated fats

72. A client on a low-cholesterol diet should know that cholesterol is found in:

A. Lean ground beef
B. Avocado
C. Peanuts
D. Palm oil

73. A 60-year-old man with renal failure is not receiving dialysis. If he is hungry between meals, the nurse can offer him:

A. Hard candy
B. Soft drinks
C. Cheddar cheese
D. Fresh fruit

74. The best breakfast food for a person following a low-fat, low-cholesterol diet would be:

A. Biscuits with corn oil margarine
B. Oatmeal with brown sugar
C. Eggs Benedict
D. Bagel with cream cheese

75. The best lunch for someone following a low-sodium diet would be:

A. Cheeseburger, fries, ketchup, soft drink
B. Bologna sandwich, carrot and celery sticks, brownies, iced tea
C. Chicken noodle soup, bran muffins, apple turnover, milk
D. Tossed salad with turkey and hard-cooked egg, vinegar and oil dressing, bread sticks, pineapple rings, iced tea

76. When the nurse is planning the diet for a child with celiac disease, which could be consumed?

A. White sauce made with bleached flour
B. Fried rice
C. Vegetable-barley soup
D. Oatmeal muffins

77. The nurse would be most concerned when finding that a pregnant client took excessive amounts of an over-the-counter vitamin supplement containing which of the following?

    A. Vitamin E
    B. Biotin
    C. Folic acid
    D. Vitamin A

78. A 78-year-old client complains of constipation. Which of the following would be most likely to benefit this client?

    A. Increasing the number of rest periods
    B. Increasing protein intake
    C. Decreasing intake of fluids at mealtime
    D. Increasing intake of complex carbohydrates

Test 2: Nutrition and Pharmacology

Demetrius J. Porche, RN, DNS

 QUESTIONS

79. A 33-year-old client with type I insulin-dependent diabetes is a businessman with a very active lifestyle. He has maintained control of his diabetes until recently. His insulin routine is 5 units of Regular insulin plus 20 units of NPH insulin every morning before breakfast at 7 AM. Because the client takes NPH insulin, he should have a snack at which time of the day?

    A. After breakfast (10 AM)
    B. Midafternoon (2 PM)
    C. Early evening (7 PM)
    D. Before bedtime (9 PM)

80. Which type of insulin can be given intravenously (IV)?

    A Regular
    B. NPH
    C. Lente
    D. Humulin N

81. What would be the correct technique to administer Regular insulin and NPH insulin with one injection?

    A. NPH insulin should never be mixed with any other form of insulin.
    B. Using aseptic technique, first withdraw the proper dose of Regular insulin; then withdraw the proper dose of NPH insulin.
    C. Using aseptic technique, first withdraw the proper dose of NPH insulin; then withdraw the proper dose of Regular insulin.
    D. Regular insulin should never be mixed with any other form of insulin.

82. In the midafternoon, a client with diabetes starts experiencing symptoms of dizziness, weakness, sweating, rapid pulse, and delayed thinking. Which would be the least desirable snack?

    A. Orange juice
    B. Honey
    C. Hard candy
    D. Cheese

83. Which of the following would be the best snack for a client with insulin-dependent diabetes before participating in a 2-hour football game?

    A. Fresh fruit
    B. Orange juice
    C. Cheese and crackers
    D. Soda

84. Intravenous fluids containing potassium are administered slowly and cautiously to prevent:

    A. Metabolic acidosis
    B. Fluid overload
    C. Cardiac arrest
    D. Infiltration

85. A nurse is teaching a client about fat-soluble vitamins. Which statement by the client indicates that further teaching is necessary?

    A. "Vitamin A is fat soluble."
    B. "Vitamin D is fat soluble."
    C. "Vitamin K is fat soluble."
    D. "Vitamin B_{12} is fat soluble."

86. Digoxin (Lanoxin) 0.125 mg IV has been ordered for a cardiac client. The ampule is labeled "digoxin 0.5 mg/2 ml." The nurse should:

    A. Administer ½ ml
    B. Administer ¼ ml
    C. Administer 1 ml
    D. Call the physician to verify the order

87. The physician orders 10 ml of a medication. The medicine is available only to be administered in minims. What is the correct amount to administer?

    A. 30 minims
    B. 35 minims
    C. 80 minims
    D. 160 minims

88. After administration of morphine 10 mg IM for pain relief, which of the following data has lowest priority?
    A. Urine output
    B. Blood pressure
    C. Respiratory status
    D. Pain relief

89. In lactose intolerance, which of the following can be substituted for milk products?
    A. Cheese
    B. Ice cream
    C. Soy milk
    D. Goat milk

90. Lactose intolerance is a deficiency of which enzyme?
    A. Lactase
    B. Maltase
    C. Peptase
    D. Amylase

91. A 22-year-old client verbalizes an understanding of a gluten-free diet. Which statement by the client indicates that further teaching is needed to help the client fully understand the features of a gluten-free diet?
    A. "High protein is a feature of a gluten-free diet."
    B. "Low protein is a feature of a gluten-free diet."
    C. "High calories are a feature of a gluten-free diet."
    D. "High vitamins and minerals are features of a gluten-free diet."

92. There are "five rights" of medication administration to avoid medication errors. Which of the rights is related to reading the armband of a client?
    A. Right client
    B. Right medication
    C. Right dose
    D. Right route

93. Which of the following statements by a client indicates that further teaching is necessary related to a clear-liquid diet?
    A. "Milk is a clear liquid."
    B. "Tea is a clear liquid."
    C. "Broth is a clear liquid."
    D. "Apple juice is a clear liquid."

94. Which of the following is most important before administering any medication?
    A. Check the input and output (I&O) records.
    B. Assess for symptoms.
    C. Check the admitting diagnosis.
    D. Check the client's identification band.

95. A client has experienced third-degree burns on 60–70% of the body. The client is now in stable condition in a private room. The client's diet should consist of:
    A. High protein
    B. Low protein
    C. High carbohydrates
    D. Low carbohydrates

96. Which of the following would be consistent with a burn client's dietary needs?
    A. Hamburger and coleslaw
    B. Peanut butter and milkshake
    C. Orange juice and vegetables
    D. Milk and crackers

97. Celiac disease requires a gluten-free diet. Which of the following should be eliminated from a gluten-free diet?
    A. Milk
    B. Beef
    C. Green vegetables
    D. Wheat bread

98. Which of the following would be a necessary supplemental vitamin for someone with cirrhosis of the liver?
    A. Vitamin B_6
    B. Vitamin B_{12}
    C. Folic acid
    D. Vitamin K

99. An order reads: "Tylenol (acetaminophen) gr X suppository PRN every 4 hours for temperature greater than 100°F." The nurse should administer:
    A. 325 mg
    B. 650 mg
    C. 900 mg
    D. 1200 mg

100. Which finding would indicate a therapeutic response to levodopa therapy?
    A. Increased tremors
    B. Increased rigidity
    C. Decreased tremors
    D. Twitching

101. What is the best instruction a nurse can give for constipation?
    A. "Decrease fluid intake."
    B. "Get bedrest."
    C. "Increase dietary fiber."
    D. "Take Kaopectate."

102. What is the best instruction a nurse can give for diarrhea?
    A. "Decrease fluid intake."
    B. "Increase activity."
    C. "Increase fluid intake with essential electrolytes."
    D. "Encourage extra intake of milk or milk products."

103. A client has a diagnosis of *Pneumocystis carinii* pneumonia. The client is receiving pentamidine in a 300-mg aerosolized treatment every day during the acute illness. What is the correct position for pentamidine aerosolized treatment?
    A. Lying supine
    B. Lying prone
    C. Sitting upright
    D. Turning from side to side every 3–5 minutes

104. Which of the following is considered a full liquid?
    A. Cranberry sauce
    B. Oatmeal
    C. Gelatin
    D. Vegetable soup

105. Mannitol has been administered to a client for cerebral edema. The nurse can evaluate mannitol's effectiveness by assessing:
    A. Increased potassium level
    B. Decreased potassium level
    C. Increased urine output
    D. Increased respiratory rate

106. Which of the following is an indication for a decrease in the dosage of nitroglycerin?
    A. An increase in chest pain
    B. Lightheadedness and dizziness
    C. Increased blood pressure
    D. A pulse rate of 80 bpm

107. Correct heparin administration involves:
    A. Never rotating injection sites
    B. Aspirating to assess for blood vessel entry
    C. Always giving heparin by deep IM injection
    D. Never rubbing the area after the injection

108. A 74-year-old female client with a history of cardiac disease is admitted to the hospital for congestive heart failure (CHF). Her condition is stable. She is receiving furosemide (Lasix) 20 mg bid and digoxin 0.25 mg every morning. Before the digoxin is given, which of the vital signs should be assessed and documented?
    A. Temperature
    B. Apical pulse
    C. Blood pressure
    D. Respiratory rate

109. A client is receiving furosemide therapy. Which of the following foods is a rich source of supplemental potassium?
    A. Squash
    B. Apricots
    C. Oatmeal
    D. Cream of wheat

110. A client is discharged home on a 2-g sodium diet. Which statement made by the client indicates poor understanding of the specified diet?
    A. "Fresh fruit is part of a 2-g sodium diet."
    B. "Potatoes are part of a 2-g sodium diet."
    C. "Eggs are part of a 2-g sodium diet."
    D. "Ice cream is part of a 2-g sodium diet."

111. A client with CHF has a 1000-ml/day fluid restriction with a 2-g sodium diet. Before serving meals to this client, the nurse should:
    A. Check the client's admitting diagnosis
    B. Notify the dietitian about the fluid restriction
    C. Call the physician to clarify the order
    D. Assess the client's total fluid intake up to this meal; then collaboratively decide on the amount of fluid to be consumed with the meal

112. A client in CHF is placed on digoxin and furosemide therapy; the nurse can evaluate the effectiveness of digoxin and furosemide by:
    A. Increased pupillary reaction
    B. Increased respiratory rate
    C. Increased urine output
    D. Increased edema

113. A 35-year-old male client on a telemetry unit begins to have more than 10 unifocal premature ventricular contractions (PVCs) per minute. The nurse should prepare to administer:
    A. Digoxin
    B. Lidocaine
    C. Propranolol (Inderal)
    D. Atropine

114. A postoperative IV fluid order reads: "Lactated Ringer's 1000 ml to be infused over 8 hours." The infusion set delivers 15 gtt/ml. The nurse should regulate the rate of flow at:
    A. 15 gtt/min
    B. 31 gtt/min
    C. 60 gtt/min
    D. 90 gtt/min

115. A client has begun having grand mal seizures. He is now in stable condition. The physician orders 2 g of $MgSO_4$ in 100 ml D_5W over 30 minutes. The infusion set delivers 10 gtt/ml. When this infusion is monitored, the rate of flow should be:
    A. 15 gtt/min
    B. 33 gtt/min
    C. 66 gtt/min
    D. 99 gtt/min

116. During the $MgSO_4$ infusion the nurse should assess for signs of toxicity every 15 minutes. Which of the following is not a sign of $MgSO_4$ toxicity?
    A. Depressed knee jerk
    B. Increased knee jerk
    C. Confusion
    D. Respiratory distress

117. The nurse would expect a 45-year-old male client with renal disease to be placed on a _____ diet.
    A. High-potassium
    B. Potassium-restricted
    C. High-sodium
    D. High-protein

118. In a protein-restricted diet, which of the following should be altered to maintain appropriate caloric intake?
    A. Increase amount of vitamins and minerals.
    B. Increase simple carbohydrates and fats.
    C. Increase protein and decrease carbohydrates.
    D. Decrease amount of vitamins but increase minerals.

119. Which of the following statements made by a client about the potential side effects of aminoglycosides indicates the need for further teaching?

    A. "Ototoxicity can be a side effect."
    B. "Nephrotoxicity can be a side effect."
    C. "Neurotoxicity can be a side effect."
    D. "Photosensitivity can be a side effect."

120. While monitoring a client with histoplasmosis who has been placed on amphotericin B therapy, the nurse identifies:

    A. Afebrile reaction
    B. Hyperkalemia
    C. Hypokalemia
    D. Elevated blood pressure

121. Which statement about antineoplastic medication is incorrect?

    A. Drug combinations increase effectiveness.
    B. Antineoplastic drugs may be used with radiation therapy.
    C. Antineoplastic drugs kill only neoplastic cells.
    D. Common side effects are stomatitis, GI distress, alopecia, and bone marrow suppression.

122. A client is being discharged home on thyroid USP. Which statement made by the client indicates the need for further teaching?

    A. "Weight loss is a potential side effect of thyroid USP."
    B. "Insomnia is a potential side effect of thyroid USP."
    C. "Bradycardia is a potential side effect of thyroid USP."
    D. "Tachycardia is a potential side effect of thyroid USP."

123. Aspirin can be given for the following reasons:

    A. To decrease platelet aggregation
    B. To decrease carbon dioxide retention
    C. To inhibit peptic ulcer disease
    D. To reduce SC emphysema

124. A client has a diagnosis of cholelithiasis and cholecystitis. A fat-restricted diet was ordered. Which food would be allowed?

    A. Chicken
    B. Avocado
    C. Pecan pie
    D. Liver

125. A client's condition has improved with a fat-restricted diet. The diet has been advanced to a controlled-fat–low-fat diet. What food should the nurse remove from the dinner tray?

    A. Liver
    B. Baked potato
    C. Green beans
    D. Chicken

126. Which of the following statements informs the nurse that more education is needed for the mother of a child with PKU?

    A. "As my child grows his diet will change."

    B. "My child has had phenylketonuria and received a special diet since birth."
    C. "I must read the ingredients and nutritional information on foods before I give it to my child."
    D. "My child will be on a special diet only until puberty."

127. When a client is receiving heparin therapy, the nurse should do which of the following?

    A. Shave the client with a straight razor daily.
    B. Assess for irritability.
    C. Assess for ecchymosis or signs of bleeding.
    D. Encourage a full-liquid diet.

128. A new client admitted to the unit has a diagnosis of asthma. Breath sounds exhibit wheezes and rhonchi in all lobes. The client is receiving aminophylline (which contains theophylline) 250 mg q6h. Which of the following indicates that the medication is effective?

    A. Increased wheezes
    B. Decreased wheezes
    C. Increased rhonchi
    D. Decreased rhonchi

129. An 85-year-old client recovering from a cerebrovascular accident (CVA) resides in a skilled nursing facility. There are minimal sequelae from the CVA. The client is able to walk and perform activities of daily living with minimal assistance. However, he is unable to swallow whole pills. Four pills are to be taken at 12 noon. Which of the following would be the most appropriate method of administering the pills?

    A. Give one pill at a time every 5 minutes.
    B. Break pills into pieces, giving one at a time every 5 minutes.
    C. Crush pills and place in applesauce.
    D. Give one pill whole every 15 minutes.

130. The client has received diazepam (Valium) 10 mg PO for anxiety. What would be the most appropriate nursing function?

    A. Encourage client to ambulate independently.
    B. Assist with ambulation.
    C. Counsel client on chemical dependency.
    D. Place in bed with siderail raised and soft restraints on both arms.

131. A client is receiving a fluid-restricted diet of 1000 ml because of CHF. The client's daily intake consists of 3 oz of orange juice, 8 oz of milk, two 8-oz glasses of water, and 6 oz of tea. The client wants to have 8 oz of skim milk for an evening snack. The nurse should:

    A. Ask for a physician's order to increase the fluid restriction to 1500 ml
    B. Permit the client to drink the skim milk
    C. Explain to the client that 8 oz of skim milk would exceed the daily fluid restrictions
    D. Substitute the skim milk with a clear liquid

132. A client is receiving diphenhydramine (Benadryl) 50 mg tid. An appropriate nursing action would be to inform the client that:

A. Drowsiness may occur
B. Tinnitis usually occurs
C. Alcohol has no effect on diphenhydramine
D. Diphenhydramine increases mental alertness

133. Which of the following is important to tell a client receiving phenazopyridine (Pyridium)?

   A. Appetite may increase.
   B. Urine may change color to red-orange.
   C. Urine may change color to blue-purple.
   D. Pain will occur with voiding.

134. Which client statement about rifampin is true?

   A. "Rifampin is usually given with other antituberculosis drugs."
   B. "Rifampin is usually given with other antimalaria drugs."
   C. "My urine and feces may be colored red-orange."
   D. "My saliva, sputum, sweat, and tears may be colored red-orange."

135. A 53-year-old client with a history of coronary artery disease is admitted to the hospital for angina. The physician orders a low-cholesterol diet. The client should decrease the intake of:

   A. Veal
   B. Chicken
   C. Fish
   D. Eggs

136. Which of the following statements by the client about nitroglycerin's administration indicates that further teaching is needed?

   A. "I will need to assess my blood pressure before administration."
   B. "I will need to assess my blood pressure after administration."
   C. "I will need to change positions rapidly."
   D. "The sublingual nitroglycerin may sting when taken."

1. **(D)** Nursing process phase: evaluation; client need: basic care and comfort; content area: nutrition.

   RATIONALE

   (A) Canned and dry soups contain salt. **(B)** Ketchup, sauces, and Worcestershire sauce contain salt. **(C)** Any processed food, such as smoked ham or processed luncheon meat, is high in salt. **(D)** Buttermilk; fresh or frozen meats; whole-grain breads; and fresh, frozen, or canned vegetables without salt are allowed.

2. **(A)** Nursing process phase: evaluation; client need: basic care and comfort; content area: nutrition.

   RATIONALE

   (A) Cheese (American, mozzarella, cheddar) is high in fat. Avocados are also high in fat. **(B)** Lean meats with fat trimmed, potatoes, rice, and canned fruits are low in fat. **(C)** Lean meats, macaroni, and fresh fruits are low in fat. **(D)** Beans, rice, and bread sticks are low in fat.

3. **(B)** Nursing process phase: implementation; client need: basic care and comfort; content area: nutrition.

   RATIONALE

   (A) Thin liquids are more difficult to swallow. **(B)** Eating in an upright position allows gravity to assist the passage of food along the esophagus and helps to prevent choking and aspiration. **(C)** Liquids should be used only after the client has cleared the food from her mouth, to prevent choking and aspiration. **(D)** The client should be supervised, but distractions should be avoided so that the client can focus attention on eating the meal.

4. **(C)** Nursing process phase: evaluation; client need: basic care and comfort; content area: nutrition.

   RATIONALE

   (A) Limiting bending over at the waist and wearing constrictive clothing increase intra-abdominal reflux. **(B)** Obesity increases intra-abdominal pressure. **(C)** The goal of medical treatment is to reduce intra-abdominal pressure and reflux and gastric acid production. The client should not lie down for 2 to 3 hours after meals. **(D)** Elevating the head of the bed at night decreases reflux.

5. **(C)** Nursing process phase: evaluation; client need: basic care and comfort; content area: nutrition.

   RATIONALE

   (A) Eating at bedtime stimulates acid during sleep. **(B)** A bland diet may have adverse effects from ingesting excessive amounts of milk with antacids, causing milk-alkali syndrome and an increase in gastric acid secretion. **(C)** There is little rationale for completely eliminating particular foods unless they cause repeated discomfort. **(D)** Caffeinated and decaffeinated beverages stimulate gastric acid secretions.

6. **(D)** Nursing process phase: evaluation; client need: basic care and comfort; content area: nutrition.

   RATIONALE

   (A) Coffee, tea, carbonated beverages, strained and clear fruits, juices, and milk are allowed. **(B)** Refined breads, rolls, crackers, waffles, and refined dry and cooked cereals are allowed. **(C)** Chicken, well-cooked meats, fish, eggs, white and sweet potatoes are allowed. **(D)** Any dessert made with seeds, nuts, coconuts, or fruit or vegetable pulp is not recommended.

7. **(A)** Nursing process phase: evaluation; client need: basic care and comfort; content area: nutrition.

   RATIONALE

   (A) Foods high in fiber include whole-grain breads, oat bran muffins, brown rice, popcorn, wheat germ, whole-grain cereals, and beans. **(B)** Refined cooked cereals and dry cereals are low in fiber. **(C)** Canned or cooked fruits and vegetables are low in fiber. **(D)** Most well-cooked meats, canned vegetables, white and sweet potatoes are low in fiber.

8. **(A)** Nursing process phase: evaluation; client need: basic care and comfort; content area: nutrition.

   RATIONALE

   (A) English muffins; any whole-grain bread or bagels; fresh, frozen, or dried fruit; and lean pork such as Canadian bacon are low in fat. **(B)** Buttermilk, pork sausage, and fried potatoes are high in fat. **(C)** French toast and chocolate milk are high in fat. The smoked salmon, if canned in water, is acceptable. **(D)** Croissants are very high in fat, as is corned beef. The skim milk is a good choice.

9. **(C)** Nursing process phase: evaluation; client need: basic care and comfort; content area: nutrition.

   RATIONALE

   (A) Pernicious anemia occurs from a deficit in vitamin B_{12}, which cannot be absorbed because of a lack of the intrinsic factor, produced by specialized cells in the stomach. It must be given IM. **(B)** Malabsorption occurs despite adequate dietary intake. **(C)** Because there is no source of intrinsic factor as a result of the gastrectomy, vitamin B_{12} must be given parentally. **(D)** The vitamin cannot be absorbed from food because of the lack of intrinsic factor.

10. **(D)** Nursing process phase: planning; client need: basic care and comfort; content area: nutrition.

    RATIONALE

    (A) Limiting nursing time in the first several days will not prevent sore nipples and may hinder milk production. **(B)** The more a baby nurses, the more milk is produced. **(C)** Sore nipples are usually caused by incorrect nursing position. A tummy-to-tummy position or a football hold is correct. The baby's lips should make a tight seal around the breast. **(D)** A baby undergoes growth spurts at 10 days, 2 weeks, 6 weeks, and 3 months. The baby should nurse frequently. A fussy newborn is probably ready to feed.

11. **(B)** Nursing process phase: evaluation; client need: basic care and comfort; content area: nutrition.

    RATIONALE

    (A) *Staphylococcus aureus* found on skin is transmitted to foods requiring handling in preparation, such as salads. Symptoms occur 2–3 hours after eating the food. **(B)** Eggs, poultry, and other foods containing the organism *Salmonella* can cause symptoms 12–24 hours after eating the contaminated food. **(C)** Meats, gravies, and casseroles can contain *Clostridium perfringens,* which causes cramps or diarrhea from a toxin released by the organism growing in the intestine. **(D)** Raw seafood or fish can cause vibriosis 2–48 hours after eating the contaminated food. Flulike symptoms are exhibited.

12. **(A)** Nursing process phase: evaluation; client need: basic care and comfort; content area: nutrition.

    RATIONALE

    (A) Meat should be weighed after cooking. **(B)** Visible fat should be trimmed off before or after cooking. **(C)** Meat does not contain fiber, but dried beans, peas, and lentils are good sources of fiber. **(D)** Some processed meats, seafood, and soy products contain large amounts of carbohydrates.

13. **(A)** Nursing process phase: evaluation; client need: basic care and comfort; content area: nutrition.

    RATIONALE

    (A) Corn and peas are considered starches. **(B)** One-half cup cooked beans is a vegetable. **(C)** One-half cup carrots is considered a vegetable. **(D)** One-half cup tomatoes is considered a vegetable.

14. **(D)** Nursing process phase: evaluation; client need: basic care and comfort; content area: nutrition.

    RATIONALE

    (A) One-half cup grits counts as a cereal and grain. **(B)** One-half cup pasta counts as a cereal and grain. **(C)** One-third cup rice counts as a cereal and grain. **(D)** Three cups of popcorn counts as one starch and one fat.

15. **(C)** Nursing process phase: planning; client need: basic care and comfort; content area: nutrition.

    RATIONALE

    (A) Her weight before pregnancy was appropriate for her height, and a gain of 15–20 lb would be inadequate; inadequate gains increase the risk of delivering a low-birth-weight infant. **(B)** Her weight before pregnancy was appropriate for her height, and a gain of 15–20 lb would be inadequate; inadequate gains increase the risk of delivering a low-birth-weight infant. **(C)** A gain of 25–30 lb would be associated with the best pregnancy outcome. **(D)** A gain of 39 lb would provide no additional advantage to the infant, and excessive weight gained during pregnancy might be hard for the mother to lose afterward.

16. **(A)** Nursing process phase: evaluation; client need: basic care and comfort; content area: nutrition.

    RATIONALE

    (A) The client receives little sun exposure. Unless her diet history indicates that she consumes a quart of milk or other good sources of vitamin D daily, a supplement is indicated. **(B)** There are no data to indicate the need for a calcium supplement. **(C)** There are no data to indicate the need for a vitamin C supplement. **(D)** There are no data to indicate the need for a zinc supplement.

17. **(A)** Nursing process phase: implementation; client need: basic care and comfort; content area: nutrition.

    RATIONALE

    (A) Plain, dry, carbohydrate-containing foods (e.g., dry toast, crackers) on awakening help to alleviate the nausea experienced by some women. **(B)** Increased intake of fluids during the morning, when nausea is most common, may worsen the symptoms. **(C)** Fatty foods may worsen nausea, and carbohydrates can supply most of her calorie needs. **(D)** Reducing intake of fluids in the early morning may help to reduce nausea, but restricting fluids altogether is inadvisable, because the pregnant woman needs increased fluids for expansion of plasma volume, synthesis of amniotic fluid, excretion of wastes, and other vital bodily processes.

18. **(D)** Nursing process phase: implementation; client need: basic care and comfort; content area: nutrition.

    RATIONALE

    (A) The presence of food in the stomach is likely to inhibit absorption of iron. **(B)** Milk is an inhibitor of iron absorption. **(C)** "Heme" iron from meats is better absorbed than iron from most supplements, and thus enhances iron nutrition. Moreover, during pregnancy, the woman is highly interested in nutrition and

motivated to eat well, and this is a good time to emphasize the principles of a sound diet. **(D)** Vitamin C sources such as these enhance the absorption of iron from the supplement.

19. **(C)** Nursing process phase: implementation; client need: basic care and comfort; content area: nutrition.

    RATIONALE

    (A) Cholesterol intake has no known deleterious effect on the fetus. **(B)** Pregnant women without hypertension have no need to restrict sodium unduly. **(C)** Alcohol consumption during pregnancy may result in congenital malformations and learning disabilities. **(D)** Saturated fat has no deleterious effect on the fetus.

20. **(D)** Nursing process phase: implementation; client need: basic care and comfort; content area: nutrition.

    RATIONALE

    (A) Fruit is low in protein and sodium and thus would not exacerbate liver failure and fluid retention. **(B)** Carrots are low in protein, and butter would help to provide needed calories. **(C)** Boiled potato is low in sodium and protein. **(D)** Unless low-sodium products are used, soup is high in sodium. In addition, the soup could be included in the diet only if the milk products and poultry contained in the soup were included within the daily protein allowance.

21. **(A)** Nursing process phase: evaluation; client need: basic care and comfort; content area: nutrition.

    RATIONALE

    (A) Corn contains no gluten. **(B)** Buckwheat is believed by many authorities to contain gluten. In any event, buckwheat pancakes are normally made with added wheat flour, which would be a gluten source. **(C)** Oats contain gluten. **(D)** Wheat germ contains gluten.

22. **(C)** Nursing process phase: implementation; client need: basic care and comfort; content area: nutrition.

    RATIONALE

    (A) Canned pears, drained of their juice, are almost free of sodium and are low in fluid and potassium. **(B)** Bread is low in water content and potassium. **(C)** Oranges are rich in potassium. **(D)** Unsalted butter is almost free of sodium and provides needed calories.

23. **(B)** Nursing process phase: implementation; client need: basic care and comfort; content area: nutrition.

    RATIONALE

    (A) Fat deposits insulate the body to prevent heat loss. **(B)** The primary role of carbohydrates is to provide energy. Some cells, particularly red blood cells (RBCs) and the central nervous system (CNS) cells, rely primarily on carbohydrates to meet their energy needs. **(C)** Proteins (amino acids) are the primary building blocks for new tissue. **(D)** Some complex carbohydrates do provide fiber, but fiber is not the major reason for consuming dietary carbohydrate.

24. **(B)** Nursing process phase: evaluation; client need: basic care and comfort; content area: nutrition.

    RATIONALE

    (A) Cheese is made from milk, but its protein and fat contents are more similar to those of meat than to the items on the milk exchange list. **(B)** The protein and fat contents of cheese are similar to those of meat. **(C)** Items in the fat exchange list are primarily composed of fat, and cheese is a good source of protein. **(D)** The protein and fat contents of cheese are more similar to those of meat than to the items on the milk exchange list.

25. **(B)** Nursing process phase: implementation; client need: basic care and comfort; content area: nutrition.

RATIONALE

(A) Starchy vegetables such as potatoes are more similar in carbohydrate and protein contents to most foods on the starch-bread exchange list than to other vegetables. (B) Potatoes are similar in carbohydrate and protein contents to foods on the starch-bread exchange list. (C) Potatoes contain more protein than most foods on the fruit exchange list. (D) Starchy vegetables such as potatoes are more similar in their carbohydrate and protein contents to most foods on the starch-bread exchange list than to other vegetables.

26. **(D)** Nursing process phase: planning; client need: basic care and comfort; content area: nutrition.

    RATIONALE

    (A) Protein can be absorbed in the upper portion of the small intestine. Adequate protein is needed to promote healing and hypertrophy (enlargement) of the remaining bowel. (B) Fluid is largely absorbed in the colon. Adequate fluid is needed to replace diarrheal losses. (C) Sodium is lost in diarrhea and needs to be replaced by dietary intake. (D) The ileum is the primary site for fat absorption. After resection of the ileum, fat restriction often reduces the volume of stools and improves client comfort.

27. **(A)** Nursing process phase: evaluation; client need: basic care and comfort; content area: nutrition.

    RATIONALE

    (A) Fresh and dried vegetables and fruits are among the best dietary sources of fiber, which adds bulk to the stools and helps to prevent constipation. (B) Sesame seeds provide some fiber, but the number included on the bun would be inadequate to add bulk to stools. (C) Mashed potatoes contain starch but little fiber. (D) The heating required in the canning process reduces the fiber content of canned fruits and vegetables.

28. **(D)** Nursing process phase: implementation; client need: basic care and comfort; content area: nutrition.

    RATIONALE

    (A) An inrush of air can sometimes be heard over the upper left abdominal quadrant even when the tube is positioned in the bronchus or pleural space. (B) If the tube is in the pleural space or lodged against the wall of the bronchus, air bubbles may not be emitted during exhalation. (C) New "nonreactive" (polyurethane, silicone rubber, and similar substances) tubes are less irritating than the harder tubes previously used and may not cause gagging or respiratory distress even when located in the pulmonary system. In any event, an obtunded client would be unlikely to display these signs. (D) Radiographic evidence is the most certain method of confirming appropriate tube placement.

29. **(D)** Nursing process phase: planning; client need: basic care and comfort; content area: nutrition.

    RATIONALE

    (A) Magnesium absorption is not affected by a gastrectomy. (B) Folic acid absorption can be affected, but vitamin B_{12} is a greater concern because of its neurological and RBC formation effects. (C) Chloride is a principal body anion in the extracellular fluid whose absorption is not affected by a gastrectomy. (D) Hydrochloric acid, produced in the stomach, is required to split vitamin B_{12} away from the proteins to which it is bound in food. Intrinsic factor, produced by the gastric mucosa, must be bound to vitamin B_{12} for the vitamin to be absorbed in the ileum. Adults generally have vitamin B_{12} stores sufficient to last approximately 3 years, but after that time, parenteral vitamin B_{12} will be required.

30. **(A)** Nursing process phase: implementation; client need: basic care and comfort; content area: nutrition.

    RATIONALE

    (A) The client needs a high-protein, high-calorie diet for tissue healing and replacement of blood and tissue proteins lost as a result of the burn. These choices provide the most protein and are also rich in calories. (B) These choices are good sources of calories, which the client needs to meet his energy needs, but they provide little protein. (C) Orange juice and vegetables are low in calories and protein. (D) These choices are lower in protein and calories than a peanut butter sandwich and a milkshake.

31. **(B)** Nursing process phase: planning; client need: basic care and comfort; content area: nutrition.

    RATIONALE

    (A) Folic acid is necessary for forming RBCs, which are lost in burns, but zinc is especially important for increasing the strength of healing wounds. (B) Zinc increases the tensile strength (the force needed to separate the edges) of healing wounds. (C) Iron is needed to replace blood losses, but zinc is especially important for wound healing. (D) Vitamin K is required for formation of clotting factors.

32. **(A)** Nursing process phase: implementation; client need: basic care and comfort; content area: nutrition.

    RATIONALE

    (A) Tea is the only choice that is a clear liquid. (B) This food is not a clear liquid. (C) This food is not a clear liquid. (D) This food is not a clear liquid.

33. **(A)** Nursing process phase: implementation; client need: basic care and comfort; content area: nutrition.

    RATIONALE

    (A) Neither noodles nor chicken chunks would be liquid at room temperature, which is the criterion for including a food in a full-liquid diet. (B) Ice cream is liquid at room temperature. (C) Cream of tomato soup is liquid at room temperature. (D) Custard is liquid at room temperature.

34. **(D)** Nursing process phase: implementation; client need: basic care and comfort; content area: nutrition.

    RATIONALE

    (A) Eighty-eight percent of the kilocalories in avocados are derived from fat. (B) Muffins and other "quick breads" (unless specially prepared) contain oil, butter, or margarine, as well as fat from egg yolk. (C) Chocolate candies contain cocoa butter or other fats. (D) Angel food cake contains no egg yolk or other sources of fat.

35. **(D)** Nursing process phase: implementation; client need: basic care and comfort; content area: nutrition.

    RATIONALE

    (A) It is essential to read labels to determine whether foods contain proteins (because proteins provide phenylalanine) or are sweetened with aspartame. (B) Infants are initially fed a low-phenylalanine formula or breast milk. As children mature, they eat a wider variety of foods, which requires more vigilance by the family. (C) With careful supervision, it is possible for infants with PKU to be breast-fed. If the mother chooses not to breast-feed, the baby will require a special low-phenylalanine formula. (D) Individuals with PKU display improved mental function if they continue the phenylalanine-restricted diet indefinitely. It is especially important that women who wish to have children ensure that their phenylalanine levels are controlled before they conceive and during pregnancy.

36. **(D)** Nursing process phase: implementation; client need: basic care and comfort; content area: nutrition.

    RATIONALE

    (A) Starchy vegetables such as potatoes contain some protein and thus supply phenylalanine. (B) Pasta and other grain products are sources of protein. (C) Corn contains some protein and thus supplies phenylalanine. (**D**) Fruits, which are generally low in protein, provide little phenylalanine.

37. (**C**) Nursing process phase: implementation; client need: basic care and comfort; content area: nutrition.
    RATIONALE
    (**A**) Sherbet generally contains milk and therefore contains galactose. (**B**) Butter contains traces of lactose. (**C**) Noodles are made without milk or lactose and therefore are galactose-free. Food labels or the product manufacturer should be consulted if there is any question about a product's lactose content. (**D**) Unless they are specially prepared, pancakes are made with milk.

38. (**A**) Nursing process phase: implementation; client need: basic care and comfort; content area: nutrition.
    RATIONALE
    (**A**) Infant cereals from all types of grains are usually equivalent in price. (**B**) Pancreatic amylase activity increases from low levels at birth to relatively normal levels at 4 months, and this prepares the infant to digest the starch in cereal grains. (**C**) Infant cereals are a good choice for a first food because they are fortified with iron. Iron stores deposited in utero and in the postnatal period begin to be depleted between 3 and 6 months of age. (**D**) Rice is considered the least allergenic cereal grain for infants; wheat is among the foods that are most likely to cause allergies in infants.

39. (**B**) Nursing process phase: evaluation; client need: basic care and comfort; content area: nutrition.
    RATIONALE
    (**A**) Iron-fortified infant formula, rather than cow's milk, is recommended until 12 months of age because the infant needs good sources of iron and because cow's milk is likely to cause gastrointestinal (GI) blood loss. (**B**) Egg white is not recommended for infants younger than 12 months because it is commonly associated with allergy when started earlier. (**C**) The 9-month-old infant enjoys finger foods such as toast strips. (**D**) Cottage cheese provides high protein.

40. (**C**) Nursing process phase: implementation; client need: basic care and comfort; content area: nutrition.
    RATIONALE
    (**A**) Fish contains some sodium, but unless it is prepared with added salt, there is no need to avoid it on a 2-g sodium diet. (**B**) Hard rolls and most other yeast breads are relatively low in sodium and can be included in a 2-g sodium diet. (**C**) Peanut butter is prepared with salt unless a special salt-free product is used. (**D**) Milk contains sodium, but at this level of sodium restriction, there is no need to limit its intake unduly.

41. (**D**) Nursing process phase: implementation; client need: basic care and comfort; content area: nutrition.
    RATIONALE
    (**A**) Worcestershire sauce, as well as many other seasonings and condiments, is prepared with salt. (**B**) Garlic salt, as well as many other seasonings and condiments, is prepared with salt. (**C**) Ketchup, as well as many other seasonings and condiments, is prepared with salt. (**D**) Lemon juice is virtually sodium-free.

42. (**B**) Nursing process phase: evaluation; client need: basic care and comfort; content area: nutrition.
    RATIONALE
    (**A**) Polyunsaturated and monounsaturated fats do not elevate serum cholesterol. (**B**) Excessive intake of saturated fats is associated with elevations of serum cholesterol. (**C**) Polyunsaturated fats tend to reduce cholesterol levels. (**D**) Monounsaturated fats in the diet tend to reduce serum cholesterol or have a neutral effect on it.

43. (**C**) Nursing process phase: evaluation; client need: basic care and comfort; content area: nutrition.
    RATIONALE
    (**A**) Whole milk is rich in milk fat, which is saturated, and contains cholesterol. (**B**) Two percent milk contains saturated fat and cholesterol. (**C**) Skim milk is virtually devoid of saturated fat. (**D**) Sweet acidophilus milk is usually whole or 2% milk. It contains bacterial cultures, but they do not change the fat content.

44. (**C**) Nursing process phase: evaluation; client need: basic care and comfort; content area: nutrition.
    RATIONALE
    (**A**) Strawberries (and most other fruits) are low in calcium. (**B**) Raisins are low in calcium. (**C**) Deep-green leafy vegetables, with the exceptions of spinach and Swiss chard, are fair sources of calcium. Spinach and chard contain calcium but also contain so much oxalic acid that absorption of their calcium is prevented. (**D**) Corn is a poor calcium source.

45. (**B**) Nursing process phase: planning; client need: basic care and comfort; content area: nutrition.
    RATIONALE
    (**A**) Rapid weight loss often occurs with use of liquid-formula diets, but the weight is usually regained. (**B**) A low-calorie diet, in addition to an increase in activity, is the most effective way to promote lasting weight loss. (**C**) Exercise alone tones the body and increases the muscle mass but rarely results in substantial weight loss. (**D**) A low-calorie diet alone will result in gradual weight loss, but the addition of exercise to the regimen often helps to curb the appetite and to take the dieter's mind off food.

46. (**D**) Nursing process phase: implementation; client need: basic care and comfort; content area: nutrition.
    RATIONALE
    (**A**) Growth in infants receiving breast milk is comparable to growth in those receiving commercial formulas. (**B**) Breastfeeding is often less expensive than formula feeding. The only real cost of breastfeeding (other than a one-time expense for nursing bras) is that resulting from the mother's need for a modest increase in her calorie and protein intake. If she chooses foods wisely, she can meet these increased needs very inexpensively. (**C**) There is no increase in colic in breast-fed infants. (**D**) Young infants are especially prone to development of allergies. Breast milk is much less likely to cause an allergic reaction than cow's milk or soy, the protein sources used in most infant formulas.

47. (**C**) Nursing process phase: planning; client need: basic care and comfort; content area: nutrition.
    RATIONALE
    (**A**) Human milk is adequate in zinc to meet the needs of full-term infants. (**B**) Human milk is adequate in vitamin E to meet the needs of full-term infants. (**C**) Human milk provides little fluoride, so the breast-fed infant usually needs a supplement at an early age to ensure proper tooth formation. (**D**) Human milk has adequate thiamine to meet the infant's needs.

48. (**B**) Nursing process phase: implementation; client need: basic care and comfort; content area: nutrition.
    RATIONALE
    (**A**) Early initiation of solid foods does not improve later acceptance of foods. (**B**) The young infant is prone to development of allergies, and exposure to a wide variety of antigens from foods is apt to result in allergy. (**C**) Research has shown that infants begin to sleep through the night when they reach approximately 11 lb, and introducing solid foods early does not accelerate the process. (**D**) Early introduction of solid foods does not reduce the risk of obesity. Very young infants are less able to communi-

cate their satiety and may be overfed by zealous caregivers. Older infants communicate by turning their heads away, withdrawing eye contact, drooling out food, or refusing to open their lips.

49. **(D)** Nursing process phase: planning; client need: basic care and comfort; content area: nutrition.

    RATIONALE
    (A) Cow's milk is not recommended for infants younger than 12 months because it is a poor source of iron and often causes GI blood loss. **(B)** Infants are rapidly growing and need the kilocalories provided by fat; use of skim milk may impair growth. There is no evidence that use of skim milk in infancy has any beneficial effects on later heart disease. **(C)** A reliable source of iron, such as iron-fortified formula, is needed by rapidly growing infants. Use of formula without iron is likely to result is iron-deficiency anemia. **(D)** Iron-fortified formula is recommended until 12 months of age because it provides a reliable source of iron and helps to prevent iron-deficiency anemia.

50. **(D)** Nursing process phase: evaluation; client need: basic care and comfort; content area: nutrition.

    RATIONALE
    (A) Milk is a good source of calcium, phosphorus, and protein. **(B)** Milk is a good source of calcium, phosphorus, and protein. **(C)** Milk is a good source of calcium, phosphorus, and protein. **(D)** Milk is an extremely poor source of iron. Excessive milk consumption by toddlers results in "milk anemia."

51. **(B)** Nursing process phase: implementation; client need: basic care and comfort; content area: nutrition.

    RATIONALE
    (A) Biscuits are prepared with shortening. **(B)** This meal is almost fat-free. **(C)** Poached eggs contain 5 g of fat each. **(D)** Muffins are prepared with oil or margarine and eggs.

52. **(A)** Nursing process phase: evaluation; client need: basic care and comfort; content area: nutrition.

    RATIONALE
    (A) Vitamin C is necessary for maintaining capillary walls; thus deficiency often results in bleeding. **(B)** Vitamin D is involved primarily in regulation of calcium and phosphorus metabolism. **(C)** Vitamin E is an antioxidant and is important in maintaining red cell membranes and in preventing anemia. **(D)** Vitamin A deficiency is commonly associated with deterioration of vision, roughening of the skin, and atrophy of the mucous membranes.

53. **(A)** Nursing process phase: evaluation; client need: basic care and comfort; content area: nutrition.

    RATIONALE
    (A) Iron-deficiency anemia is the most common nutritional anemia in the United States in virtually all age groups. **(B)** Deficiency of folic acid may occur in malnourished individuals; pregnant women and infants are also at risk, but it is not as widespread as iron deficiency. **(C)** The only individuals at serious risk of dietary deficiency of vitamin B_{12} are strict vegetarians. Also, impaired absorption is likely in individuals with gastric or ileal resection, but this problem affects only a limited number of people. **(D)** Impaired production of intrinsic factor occurs spontaneously in some individuals and also after gastric resection, but this problem affects only a limited number of people.

54. **(D)** Nursing process phase: evaluation; client need: basic care and comfort; content area: nutrition.

    RATIONALE
    (A) If the esophagus is obstructed, no oral feedings would be able to bypass the obstruction. **(B)** If the esophagus is obstructed, no oral feedings would be able to bypass the obstruction. **(C)** If the esophagus is obstructed, no oral feedings would be able to by-

pass the obstruction. **(D)** Gastrostomy feedings would bypass the obstruction.

55. **(A)** Nursing process phase: planning; client need: basic care and comfort; content area: nutrition.

    RATIONALE
    (A) Amino acids derived from proteins are components of antibodies. **(B)** Fat is not a component of antibodies. **(C)** Thiamine is not a component of antibodies. **(D)** Riboflavin is not a component of antibodies.

56. **(B)** Nursing process phase: planning; client need: basic care and comfort; content area: nutrition.

    RATIONALE
    (A) There is no need to prepare the client for oral surgery with a low-residue diet. **(B)** Some physicians use a low-residue diet before GI surgery to decrease the fecal content of the GI tract during surgery. **(C)** There is no need for a low-residue diet before head and neck surgery. **(D)** A low-residue diet is not indicated for any surgery except surgery of the GI tract.

57. **(D)** Nursing process phase: evaluation; client need: basic care and comfort; content area: nutrition.

    RATIONALE
    (A) The fat and protein provided by the fish would be slowly digested and might reduce symptoms of dumping syndrome. **(B)** The fat and protein provided by the egg would be slowly digested and might reduce symptoms of dumping syndrome. **(C)** The starch provided by the bagel would be less likely than simple carbohydrates to cause dumping, because it would be gradually hydrolyzed and would not increase the osmolality of the small bowel as rapidly as simple carbohydrates. **(D)** Simple carbohydrates such as the sucrose in fruit gelatins enter the small bowel quickly after ingestion and rapidly increase the osmolality of the bowel content. Thus, they are the nutrients most likely to cause symptoms in the person with dumping syndrome.

58. **(D)** Nursing process phase: planning; client need: basic care and comfort; content area: nutrition.

    RATIONALE
    (A) Fluids present in the stomach at the same time as food increase the speed of gastric emptying and thus increase the likelihood of dumping syndrome. **(B)** Fluids present in the stomach at the same time as food increase the speed of gastric emptying and thus increase the likelihood of dumping syndrome. **(C)** Fluids present in the stomach at the same time as food increase the speed of gastric emptying and thus increase the likelihood of dumping syndrome. **(D)** Avoiding fluids until at least ½–1 hour after meals reduces the speed with which foods are emptied from the stomach.

59. **(B)** Nursing process phase: evaluation; client need: basic care and comfort; content area: nutrition.

    RATIONALE
    (A) It is unusual to experience maldigestion of milk protein. **(B)** Many adults lack lactase, the enzyme required to digest lactose (milk sugar). The undigested carbohydrate passes into the colon, where it draws fluid into the feces and often causes cramping and diarrhea. **(C)** Select another answer. **(D)** Select another answer.

60. **(B)** Nursing process phase: planning; client need: basic care and comfort; content area: nutrition.

    RATIONALE
    (A) The client's intake of animal products (which are the only sources of cholesterol) is limited to one serving of milk and the meat and cheese contained in the lasagna, so his cholesterol intake should not be excessive. **(B)** The Dietary Guidelines for Americans recommends only a moderate alcohol intake, defined as no more

than 2 drinks per day. A 12-oz glass of beer is equivalent to one drink, so the client's intake is excessive. (C) Whole-grain breads, oatmeal, legumes (beans), and vegetables provide good sources of fiber in the diet. (D) The broccoli and salad are equivalent to three vegetable servings; three to five are recommended.

61. **(B)** Nursing process phase: evaluation; client need: basic care and comfort; content area: nutrition.

    RATIONALE
    (A) Individuals at 5% of desirable weight are usually described as "normal weight." (B) Although there are exceptions, individuals whose weight is ≥20% of the ideal or desirable weight for their height are usually considered obese. (C) Individuals whose weights are at least 20% more than the ideal or desirable weight are usually considered obese. (D) Individuals whose weights are at least 20% more than the ideal or desirable weight are usually considered obese.

62. **(D)** Nursing process phase: evaluation; client need: basic care and comfort; content area: nutrition.

    RATIONALE
    (A) Obesity does not increase the risk of peptic ulcers. (B) Obesity does not increase the risk of periodontal disease. (C) Obesity does not increase the risk of scleroderma. (D) Obesity is a risk factor for development of hypertension.

63. **(A)** Nursing process phase: evaluation; client need: basic care and comfort; content area: nutrition.

    RATIONALE
    (A) Although rest can be important, lying down immediately after eating increases the reflux of acid gastric contents. (B) Snacking at bedtime may cause reflux if the client lies down to sleep shortly afterwards. (C) Obesity is often a precipitating cause of reflux and subsequent pain. (D) Use of antacids may help to control the symptoms.

64. **(C)** Nursing process phase: evaluation; client need: basic care and comfort; content area: nutrition.

    RATIONALE
    (A) One-half cup pineapple has about 2 g of fiber. (B) Potatoes have about 3.8 g of fiber. (C) Popcorn has about 10 g of fiber. (D) Roast beef has about 5 g of fiber.

65. **(C)** Nursing process phase: implementation; client need: basic care and comfort; content area: nutrition.

    RATIONALE
    (A) Fruit sugar is fructose. (B) Table sugar is sucrose. (C) Lactose, or milk sugar, is hydrolyzed or digested by enzymes in the mucosal lining of the GI tract. The concentrations of these enzymes is very low after acute gastroenteritis, and a formula providing carbohydrates other than lactose may be better tolerated than milk-based formulas. (D) Corn syrup is glucose or dextrose.

66. **(A)** Nursing process phase: data collection; client need: basic care and comfort; content area: nutrition.

    RATIONALE
    (A) Dehydration, which can occur relatively rapidly in an infant of this age, is manifested by dry, sticky mucous membranes, poor skin turgor, and an acute weight loss. (B) A fluid does not cause edema or weight gain. The infant may get a "diaper" skin rash if not cleaned properly, but observing for a fluid volume deficit is most critical. (C) The infant has a fluid loss. (D) A fluid does not cause edema or weight gain. The infant may get a diaper skin rash if not cleaned properly, but observing for a fluid volume deficit is most critical.

67. **(C)** Nursing process phase: planning; client need: basic care and comfort; content area: nutrition.

    RATIONALE
    (A) Iron is recommended throughout pregnancy and lactation. (B) Iron is recommended throughout pregnancy and lactation. (C) Iron supplements are recommended throughout pregnancy to allow the marked expansion in RBC production. Although lactation does not require large amounts of iron, because little iron is secreted in milk, an iron supplement is recommended during lactation to replenish stores that may have been depleted during pregnancy. (D) Iron is recommended throughout pregnancy and lactation.

68. **(B)** Nursing process phase: planning; client need: basic care and comfort; content area: nutrition.

    RATIONALE
    (A) A weight of 135 lb is less than the optimal weight gain. (B) Optimal fetal outcome is achieved with a maternal weight gain of approximately 25–30 lb during pregnancy. (C) A weight of 159 lb is over the 25–30 lb weight recommended. (D) A weight of 165 lb is over the 25–30 lb weight recommended.

69. **(A)** Nursing process phase: implementation; client need: basic care and comfort; content area: nutrition.

    RATIONALE
    (A) The diet for the insulin-dependent client is designed to provide carbohydrates at times when insulin is at its peak activity. (B) Exchanges should neither be omitted nor shifted from one time of the day to another. (C) Exchanges should neither be omitted nor shifted from one time of the day to another. (D) Insulin regimens can be adjusted for departures from usual eating and exercise habits, but meal plans are based on an individual's usual food intakes.

70. **(C)** Nursing process phase: implementation; client need: basic care and comfort; content area: nutrition.

    RATIONALE
    (A) When a complete intestinal obstruction develops, particularly one low in the GI tract, enteral feedings are not tolerated. (B) When a complete intestinal obstruction develops, particularly one low in the GI tract, enteral feedings are not tolerated. (C) Only total parenteral nutrition provides nutrients while bypassing the GI obstruction. (D) When a complete intestinal obstruction develops, particularly one low in the GI tract, enteral feedings are not tolerated.

71. **(B)** Nursing process phase: evaluation; client need: basic care and comfort; content area: nutrition.

    RATIONALE
    (A) Different fats have different effects on blood cholesterol levels. (B) Saturated fats tend to increase blood cholesterol. (C) Polyunsaturated fats have a neutral effect on, or lower, blood cholesterol. (D) Monounsaturated fats have a neutral effect on, or lower, blood cholesterol.

72. **(A)** Nursing process phase: evaluation; client need: basic care and comfort; content area: nutrition.

    RATIONALE
    (A) Only animal products contain cholesterol. Even if the visible fat in meats is trimmed away, the tissues contain cholesterol. (B) Avocado is a nonanimal product. (C) Peanuts are a nonanimal product. (D) Palm oil is a nonanimal product.

73. **(A)** Nursing process phase: implementation; client need: basic care and comfort; content area: nutrition.

    RATIONALE
    (A) He is probably receiving a low-protein, low-potassium, low-sodium diet. If the nurse wants to provide him with a snack that has not been figured into his diet plan, then hard candy, a simple carbohydrate, is the safest. (B) Soft drinks provide fluid, and

he probably has a fluid restriction; in addition, they provide phosphorus, which may further reduce kidney function. (C) Cheese is rich in sodium and high in protein. (D) Most fresh fruits are good or excellent sources of potassium.

74. **(B)** Nursing process phase: evaluation; client need: basic care and comfort; content area: nutrition.

    RATIONALE

    (A) Biscuits and other quick breads are high in fat, as is margarine. (B) This choice is the lowest in fat and cholesterol. (C) Eggs are rich in cholesterol. (D) Cream cheese is high in cholesterol.

75. **(D)** Nursing process phase: evaluation; client need: basic care and comfort; content area: nutrition.

    RATIONALE

    (A) Ketchup is high in sodium. (B) Processed meats such as bologna are high in sodium. (C) Soups are high in sodium. (D) All are low-sodium foods.

76. **(B)** Nursing process phase: evaluation; client need: basic care and comfort; content area: nutrition.

    RATIONALE

    (A) Flour contains wheat, which contains gluten. (B) Rice is the only grain listed that does not contain gluten. (C) Barley contains gluten. (D) Oatmeal contains gluten.

77. **(D)** Nursing process phase: data collection; client need: basic care and comfort; content area: nutrition.

    RATIONALE

    (A) Excessive vitamin E may endanger the cardiovascular system but is less harmful than vitamin A. Vitamin A is more dangerous to the liver in both the mother and neonate. (B) Biotin is water soluble and unlikely to be toxic. (C) Folic acid is water soluble. (D) Vitamin A is toxic when taken in excessive amounts.

78. **(D)** Nursing process phase: planning; client need: basic care and comfort; content area: nutrition.

    RATIONALE

    (A) Increasing the number of rest periods decreases GI motility and aggravates constipation. (B) Protein does not affect constipation. (C) Decreasing fluids increases the risk of constipation. (D) The fiber provided by complex carbohydrates increases fecal bulk and reduces constipation.

79. **(B)** Nursing process phase: implementation; client need: pharmacological and parenteral therapies; content area: pharmacology.

    RATIONALE

    (A) After breakfast is too early for action of NPH insulin. (B) The peak action of NPH insulin occurs 6–8 hours after administration. (C) Early evening is too late for the peak action of NPH insulin. (D) Before bedtime is too late for the peak action of NPH insulin.

80. **(A)** Nursing process phase: implementation; client need: pharmacological and parenteral therapies; content area: pharmacology.

    RATIONALE

    (A) Only Regular insulin can be administered IV. (B) NPH insulin is cloudy. Only clear insulin can be given IV. (C) Lente insulin is cloudy. Only clear insulin can be given IV. (D) Humulin N insulin is cloudy. Only clear insulin can be given IV.

81. **(B)** Nursing process phase: implementation; client need: pharmacological and parenteral therapies; content area: pharmacology.

    RATIONALE

    (A) NPH can be mixed with Regular insulin. (B) Regular insulin is drawn first to avoid contaminating it with NPH. NPH cannot be given IV, which could be a problem if the Regular insulin was contaminated with NPH insulin. (C) Do not contaminate Regular insulin with NPH insulin. (D) Regular insulin can be mixed with other types of insulin.

82. **(D)** Nursing process phase: implementation; client need: basic care and comfort; content area: nutrition.

    RATIONALE

    (A) Orange juice is a simple carbohydrate that makes absorption occur rapidly. (B) Honey is a simple carbohydrate that makes absorption occur rapidly. (C) Hard candy is a simple carbohydrate that makes absorption occur rapidly. (D) A simple carbohydrate is needed for fast digestion and absorption; cheese is the most complex carbohydrate listed.

83. **(C)** Nursing process phase: planning; client need: basic care and comfort; content area: nutrition.

    RATIONALE

    (A) Fresh fruit is rapidly absorbed and provides quick energy. This would not help with endurance. (B) Orange juice is rapidly absorbed and provides quick energy. This would not help with endurance. (C) Cheese and crackers are complex carbohydrates that will be digested and absorbed slowly. This will assist in maintaining the blood glucose level at a stable level during the exercise. (D) Soda is rapidly absorbed and provides quick energy. This would not help with endurance.

84. **(C)** Nursing process phase: implementation; client need: pharmacological and parenteral therapies; content area: pharmacology.

    RATIONALE

    (A) Metabolic acidosis can cause hyperkalemia but not the reverse. (B) Rapid infusion of IV fluids can cause fluid overload. Rapid infusion of potassium does not. (C) Potassium chloride should be administered slowly and cautiously to prevent fatal hyperkalemia resulting in cardiac arrest. (D) Infiltration can occur regardless of the type of fluid.

85. **(D)** Nursing process phase: planning; client need: basic care and comfort; content area: nutrition.

    RATIONALE

    (A) Vitamin A is fat soluble. (B) Vitamin D is fat soluble. (C) Vitamin K is fat soluble. (D) Vitamin B_{12} is not fat soluble.

86. **(A)** Nursing process phase: implementation; client need: pharmacological and parenteral therapies; content area: pharmacology.

    RATIONALE

    (A) If 2 ml equals 0.5 mg, then 1 ml equals 0.25 mg, and ½ ml equals 0.125 mg. (B) Math calculation for correct answer explains incorrect answers. (C) Math calculation for correct answer explains incorrect answers. (D) Calling the physician to verify the order is not necessary in this situation.

87. **(D)** Nursing process phase: implementation; client need: pharmacological and parenteral therapies; content area: pharmacology.

    RATIONALE

    (A) Math calculation for correct answer explains incorrect answers. (B) Math calculation for correct answer explains incorrect answers. (C) Math calculation for correct answer explains incorrect answers. (D) 1 ml = 16.2 minims, 10 ml × 16.2 minims/ml = 160 minims.

88. **(A)** Nursing process phase: evaluation; client need: pharmacological and parenteral therapies; content area: pharmacology.

    RATIONALE

    (A) Urine output is not affected by morphine administration. (B)

Morphine may lower the blood pressure. **(C)** Morphine may lower the respiratory rate. **(D)** Pain relief is the desired outcome.

89. **(C)** Nursing process phase: planning; client need: basic care and comfort; content area: nutrition.

    RATIONALE

    (A) Cheese contains lactose. **(B)** Ice cream contains lactose. **(C)** Soybean milk is used as a substitute for milk because it does not contain lactose. **(D)** Goat milk contains lactose.

90. **(A)** Nursing process phase: planning; client need: basic care and comfort; content area: nutrition.

    RATIONALE

    (A) Lactase is the enzyme that digests milk products. Lactase is the deficient enzyme in lactose intolerance. **(B)** Maltase is starch sugar. **(C)** Peptase is not a word. **(D)** Amylase is a pancreatic enzyme.

91. **(B)** Nursing process phase: planning; client need: basic care and comfort; content area: nutrition.

    RATIONALE

    (A) A gluten-free diet should be high in protein, calories, vitamins, and minerals to maintain a balanced nutritional state. **(B)** A low-protein diet does not meet the requirement of a gluten-free diet: high protein, high calories, and high vitamins and minerals. **(C)** A gluten-free diet should be high in protein, calories, vitamins, and minerals to maintain a balanced nutritional state. **(D)** A gluten-free diet should be high in protein, calories, vitamins, and minerals to maintain a balanced nutritional state.

92. **(A)** Nursing process phase: planning; client need: pharmacological and parenteral therapies; content area: pharmacology.

    RATIONALE

    (A) The five rights to correct medication administration are right client, right medication, right dose, right route, and right time. Reading the client's armband allows the nurse to validate the right client. **(B)** The five rights to correct medication administration are right client, right medication, right dose, right route, and right time. Reading the client's armband allows the nurse to validate the right client. **(C)** The five rights to correct medication administration are right client, right medication, right dose, right route, and right time. Reading the client's armband allows the nurse to validate the right client. **(D)** The five rights to correct medication administration are right client, right medication, right dose, right route, and right time. Reading the client's armband allows the nurse to validate the right client.

93. **(A)** Nursing process phase: implementation; client need: basic care and comfort; content area: nutrition.

    RATIONALE

    (A) A clear-liquid diet contains foods that are clear and liquid at room temperature. Milk is not clear at room temperature. **(B)** Tea is a clear liquid at room temperature. **(C)** Broth is a clear liquid at room temperature. **(D)** Apple juice is a clear liquid at room temperature.

94. **(D)** Nursing process phase: data collection; client need: pharmacological and parenteral therapies; content area: pharmacology.

    RATIONALE

    (A) With specific medications, it is necessary to check I&O. **(B)** The nurse would check for symptoms. **(C)** The nurse would be aware of the diagnosis. **(D)** It is most important to check that you are administering the correct medicine to the correct client.

95. **(A)** Nursing process phase: implementation; client need: basic care and comfort; content area: nutrition.

    RATIONALE

    (A) A burn client should be placed on a high-protein diet to assist with tissue repair and restoring a positive nitrogen balance, unless otherwise contraindicated. **(B)** This choice does not meet high-protein requirements. **(C)** This choice does not meet high-protein requirements. **(D)** This choice does not meet high-protein requirements.

96. **(B)** Nursing process phase: implementation; client need: basic care and comfort; content area: nutrition.

    RATIONALE

    (A) Coleslaw is low in protein content. **(B)** Of the foods listed, peanut butter and milkshake have the highest protein and caloric content. **(C)** Vegetables are low in protein content. **(D)** Crackers are low in protein content.

97. **(D)** Nursing process phase: implementation; client need: basic care and comfort; content area: nutrition.

    RATIONALE

    (A) Milk does not contain gluten. **(B)** Beef does not contain gluten. **(C)** Green vegetables do not contain gluten. **(D)** Wheat bread contains glutens, a group of proteins found in grain foods.

98. **(D)** Nursing process phase: planning; client need: basic care and comfort; content area: nutrition.

    RATIONALE

    (A) Vitamin B_6 is not dependent on bile. **(B)** Vitamin B_{12} is not dependent on bile. **(C)** Folic acid is not dependent on bile. **(D)** Vitamin K is dependent on the presence of bile for absorption.

99. **(B)** Nursing process phase: evaluation; client need: pharmacological and parenteral therapies; content area: pharmacology.

    RATIONALE

    (A) Math calculation explains the incorrect answers. **(B)** 1 grain = 64.8 mg, 10 grains $\times$ 64.8 mg/grain = 648 mg. The nurse should administer the 650-mg suppository. **(C)** Math calculation explains the incorrect answers. **(D)** Math calculation explains the incorrect answers.

100. **(C)** Nursing process phase: evaluation; client need: pharmacological and parenteral therapies; content area: pharmacology.

    RATIONALE

    (A) This choice indicates an increase in symptoms. **(B)** This choice indicates an increase in symptoms. **(C)** Levodopa is the drug of choice for parkinsonism. Levodopa relieves the tremors, rigidity, and twitching associated with parkinsonism. **(D)** This choice indicates an increase in symptoms.

101. **(C)** Nursing process phase: implementation; client need: basic care and comfort; content area: nutrition.

    RATIONALE

    (A) Decreasing fluid intake would increase the chance of constipation. **(B)** Bedrest would not stimulate the bowel to empty and would increase the chance of constipation. **(C)** Vegetable fiber provides dietary residue. Increased dietary residue increases the volume of fecal material. The increase in fecal material stimulates the bowel to empty. **(D)** Kaopectate is given for diarrhea.

102. **(C)** Nursing process phase: implementation; client need: basic care and comfort; content area: nutrition.

    RATIONALE

    (A) Decreasing fluid intake could lead to dehydration. **(B)** Increased activity would not decrease the fluidity of the stools or decrease the rapid bowel emptying. **(C)** Diarrhea causes an increase in the fluidity of stool, with a loss of potassium and sodium. Encourage liquids high in potassium and sodium such as Gatorade, soup, broth, water, and apple, orange, and grapefruit juices. (D) Milk and milk products have a laxative effect.

103. **(C)** Nursing process phase: implementation; client need: pharmacological and parenteral therapies; content area: pharmacology.

RATIONALE

(A) Position would not produce this effect. (B) Position would not produce this effect. (C) Lung scans after treatment showed that distribution was most uniform when clients were sitting upright, with more aerosol reaching the upper lung. (D) Position would not produce this effect.

104. **(C)** Nursing process phase: implementation; client need: basic care and comfort; content area: nutrition.

RATIONALE

(A) Cranberry sauce does not liquefy at room temperature. (B) Oatmeal does not liquefy at room temperature. (C) Gelatin liquefies at room temperature. (D) Vegetable soups do not liquefy at room temperature.

105. **(C)** Nursing process phase: evaluation; client need: pharmacological and parenteral therapies; content area: pharmacology.

RATIONALE

(A) Mannitol increases potassium excretion. (B) Mannitol may decrease potassium as a side effect but not as a measure of effectiveness. (C) Mannitol is an osmotic diuretic used to promote diuresis. (D) Mannitol does not increase respirations.

106. **(B)** Nursing process phase: data collection; client need: pharmacological and parenteral therapies; content area: pharmacology.

RATIONALE

(A) Nitroglycerin is a vasodilator that is used to decrease blood pressure and to dilate coronary arteries. (B) Excessive dosage is characterized by headache, lightheadedness and dizziness, syncope, tachycardia, and low blood pressure. (C) Nitroglycerin is a vasodilator that is used to decrease blood pressure and to dilate coronary arteries. (D) A pulse rate of 80 bpm is considered normal.

107. **(D)** Nursing process phase: implementation; client need: pharmacological and parenteral therapies; content area: pharmacology.

RATIONALE

(A) One should always rotate injection sites. (B) One should not aspirate for heparin to decrease possibility of tissue trauma. (C) Heparin is given subcutaneously (SC), not IM. (D) Rubbing the area after heparin administration would increase the likelihood of bleeding.

108. **(B)** Nursing process phase: implementation; client need: pharmacological and parenteral therapies; content area: pharmacology.

RATIONALE

(A) Temperature is not specifically assessed for digitalis administration. (B) A fall in heart rate to 60 bpm in adults is a criterion used for withholding medication and notifying the physician. The apical pulse should be assessed for one full minute, noting rate, rhythm, and quality, before administering digoxin. (C) Blood pressure is not specifically assessed for digitalis administration. (D) Respiration is not specifically assessed for digitalis administration.

109. **(B)** Nursing process phase: implementation; client need: basic care and comfort; content area: nutrition.

RATIONALE

(A) Squash is not high in potassium content. (B) Apricots are high in potassium. (C) Oatmeal is a rich source of iron but not of potassium. (D) Cream of wheat is a refined cereal. Refined foods have very little potassium

110. **(D)** Nursing process phase: implementation; client need: basic care and comfort; content area: nutrition.

RATIONALE

(A) This choice is low in sodium unless sodium is added during cooking. (B) This choice is low in sodium unless sodium is added during cooking. (C) This choice is low in sodium unless sodium is added during cooking. (D) Of the foods listed, ice cream would have the highest sodium content. Ice cream is a processed food.

111. **(D)** Nursing process phase: implementation; client need: basic care and comfort; content area: nutrition.

RATIONALE

(A) Checking the admitting diagnosis will not denote fluid restrictions. (B) The nurse would notify dietary personnel about the fluid restriction before serving the tray. (C) Calling the physician is not necessary for this meal situation. (D) The fluid intake should be evaluated before serving all meals. The client should be allowed to participate in the decision-making process.

112. **(C)** Nursing process phase: evaluation; client need: pharmacological and parenteral therapies; content area: pharmacology.

RATIONALE

(A) These medications have no effect on pupillary responses. (B) These medications do not increase respiratory rate as a therapeutic effect. (C) Furosemide promotes diuresis. The effectiveness of both these drugs in CHF is evident from the increased urine output. (D) Furosemide decreases edema rather than producing it.

113. **(B)** Nursing process phase: planning; client need: pharmacological and parenteral therapies; content area: pharmacology.

RATIONALE

(A) Digoxin may be ordered as a cardiotonic but not as a first choice for PVCs. (B) Lidocaine is the first-line drug of choice for ventricular ectopy. (C) Propranolol may be ordered but not as a first choice for PVCs. (D) Atropine increases the heart rate but has no direct effect on PVCs.

114. **(B)** Nursing process phase: implementation; client need: pharmacological and parenteral therapies; content area: pharmacology.

RATIONALE

(A) Math calculation explains incorrect answers. (B) Amount to be infused × drop factor ÷ Time of infusion in minutes, 1000 ml × 15 gtt/min ÷ 480 min = 31 gtt/min. (C) Math calculation explains incorrect answers. (D) Math calculation explains incorrect answers.

115. **(B)** Nursing process phase: implementation; client need: pharmacological and parenteral therapies; content area: pharmacology.

RATIONALE

(A) Math calculation explains incorrect answers. (B) Amount to be infused × drop factor ÷ Time of infusion in minutes, 100 ml × 10 gtt/ml ÷ 30 min = 33 gtt/min. (C) Math calculation explains incorrect answers. (D) Math calculation explains incorrect answers.

116. **(B)** Nursing process phase: evaluation; client need: pharma-

cological and parenteral therapies; content area: pharmacology.

RATIONALE

(A) Signs of $MgSO_4$ toxicity are flushing, sweating, extreme thirst, hypotension, sedation, confusion, depressed or no reflexes, muscle weakness, depressed cardiac function, and respiratory paralysis. (B) Increased reflexes are not a sign of magnesium toxicity. (C) Signs of $MgSO_4$ toxicity are flushing, sweating, extreme thirst, hypotension, sedation, confusion, depressed or no reflexes, muscle weakness, depressed cardiac function, and respiratory paralysis. (D) Signs of $MgSO_4$ toxicity are flushing, sweating, extreme thirst, hypotension, sedation, confusion, depressed or no reflexes, muscle weakness, depressed cardiac function, and respiratory paralysis.

117. **(B)** Nursing process phase: implementation; client need: basic care and comfort; content area: nutrition.

RATIONALE

(A) A high-potassium diet is contraindicated in treating renal disease. (B) Clients with renal disease are unable to excrete potassium adequately, which causes elevated serum potassium. Therefore, the amount of potassium in the diet must be restricted to prevent complication of hyperkalemia. (C) Sodium is restricted in treating renal disease. (D) Protein is restricted in treating renal disease.

118. **(B)** Nursing process phase: implementation; client need: basic care and comfort; content area: nutrition.

RATIONALE

(A) Vitamins and minerals do not increase calories. (B) Adequate caloric intake must be maintained to prevent catabolism. This is done by increasing the amount of simple carbohydrates and fats in the diet. (C) Decreasing carbohydrates is not recommended. (D) Neither vitamins nor minerals increase calories.

119. **(D)** Nursing process phase: evaluation; client need: pharmacological and parenteral therapies; content area: pharmacology.

RATIONALE

(A) Potential side effects of aminoglycosides include ototoxicity. (B) Potential side effects of aminoglycosides include nephrotoxicity. (C) Potential side effects of aminoglycosides include neurotoxicity. (D) There is no documentation that aminoglycosides cause photosensitivity.

120. **(C)** Nursing process phase: evaluation; client need: pharmacological and parenteral therapies; content area: pharmacology.

RATIONALE

(A) Amphotericin B does not directly cause afebrile reactions, hyperkalemia, or elevated blood pressure. (B) Amphotericin B does not directly cause afebrile reactions, hyperkalemia, or elevated blood pressure. (C) Potential side effects of amphotericin B are anorexia, weight loss, nausea, vomiting, diarrhea, hypokalemia, muscle pain, chills, fever, anemia, and rash. (D) Amphotericin B does not directly cause afebrile reactions, hyperkalemia, or elevated blood pressure.

121. **(C)** Nursing process phase: implementation; client need: pharmacological and parenteral therapies; content area: pharmacology.

RATIONALE

(A) Incorrect option is explained in rationale for correct answer. (B) Incorrect option is explained in rationale for correct answer. (C) The effects of antineoplastic drugs are usually not limited to neoplastic cells. Most antineoplastic drugs are damaging to

dividing cells, thus preventing cell proliferation. (D) Incorrect option is explained in rationale for correct answer.

122. **(C)** Nursing process phase: evaluation; client need: pharmacological and parenteral therapies; content area: pharmacology.

RATIONALE

(A) Potential side effects of thyroid USP are palpitations, arrhythmias, headache, tremors, insomnia, tachycardia, weight loss, nervousness, and anorexia. (B) Potential side effects of thyroid USP are palpitations, arrhythmias, headache, tremors, insomnia, tachycardia, weight loss, nervousness, and anorexia. (C) Bradycardia is not a side effect of thyroid replacement. (D) Potential side effects of thyroid USP are palpitations, arrhythmias, headache, tremors, insomnia, tachycardia, weight loss, nervousness, and anorexia.

123. **(A)** Nursing process phase: planning; client need: pharmacological and parenteral therapies; content area: pharmacology.

RATIONALE

(A) Aspirin may be prescribed to treat headache, arthritis, joint pain, dental pain, and antipyretic effects and to decrease platelet aggregation (clotting). (B) Aspirin has no effect on decreasing carbon dioxide retention. (C) Aspirin does not inhibit peptic ulcer disease and may exacerbate the condition. (D) Aspirin has no effect on SC emphysema.

124. **(A)** Nursing process phase: implementation; client need: basic care and comfort; content area: nutrition.

RATIONALE

(A) Lean meat is low in fat. (B) Hidden sources of fat, such as nuts, avocado, olives, organ meats, chocolate, and coconut, are eliminated from the diet. (C) Hidden sources of fat, such as nuts, avocado, olives, organ meats, chocolate, and coconut, are eliminated from the diet. (D) Hidden sources of fat, such as nuts, avocado, olives, organ meats, chocolate, and coconut, are eliminated from the diet.

125. **(A)** Nursing process phase: implementation; client need: basic care and comfort; content area: nutrition.

RATIONALE

(A) Organ meats are high in fat and cholesterol content. (B) Baked potatoes have no fat. (C) Green beans have no fat. (D) Chicken is low in fat, especially if the skin is removed.

126. **(D)** Nursing process phase: implementation; client need: basic care and comfort; content area: nutrition.

RATIONALE

(A) Incorrect options are explained in rationale for correct answer. (B) Incorrect options are explained in rationale for correct answer. (C) Incorrect options are explained in rationale for correct answer. (D) PKU is a genetic defect affecting the metabolism of phenylalanine. The phenylalanine-restricted diet will change with growth needs but will be necessary throughout the life span.

127. **(C)** Nursing process phase: evaluation; client need: pharmacological and parenteral therapies; content area: pharmacology.

RATIONALE

(A) Shaving with a straight razor increases the chances for nicking the skin and bleeding. (B) Irritability has no effect on heparin administration. (C) Bleeding as evidenced by ecchymosis could be a sign of excessive anticoagulation. (D) A full-liquid diet has no effect on heparin administration.

128. **(B)** Nursing process phase: evaluation; client need: pharmacological and parenteral therapies; content area: pharmacology.

RATIONALE

(A) Aminophylline does not increase wheezing. (B) Aminophylline is prescribed for bronchospasms caused by bronchitis, asthma, and emphysema. Aminophylline should improve the quality and rate of respirations. Aminophylline decreases wheezing. (C) Aminophylline does not increase rhonchi. (D) Aminophylline does not increase rhonchi.

129. **(C)** Nursing process phase: implementation; client need: pharmacological and parenteral therapies; content area: pharmacology.

RATIONALE

(A) Spacing the time when giving the pills will not correct the problem with swallowing the pills. (B) Breaking pills will not correct the problem of not being able to swallow pills. (C) The pills should be crushed and placed in food with good consistency for ease of swallowing. (D) Spacing the time when giving the pills will not correct the problem with swallowing the pills.

130. **(B)** Nursing process phase: implementation; client need: pharmacological and parenteral therapies; content area: pharmacology.

RATIONALE

(A) Ambulation should be supervised. (B) Diazepam may cause CNS reactions such as drowsiness, fatigue, confusion, dizziness, and muscle weakness. Ambulation should be supervised. (C) There is nothing to indicate that the client needs counseling for chemical dependency. (D) There is no need for use of restraints.

131. **(C)** Nursing process phase: implementation; client need: basic care and comfort; content area: nutrition.

RATIONALE

(A) Incorrect options are explained in rationale for correct answer. (B) Incorrect options are explained in rationale for correct answer. (C) The client has consumed a total of 990 ml of fluids. If the client had the evening snack of skim milk, the total intake would be 1230 ml. It should be explained to the client that the skim milk would exceed the fluid restriction. (D) Incorrect options are explained in rationale for correct answer.

132. **(A)** Nursing process phase: implementation; client need: pharmacological and parenteral therapies; content area: pharmacology.

RATIONALE

(A) Drowsiness is the principal side effect of diphenhydramine. (B) There are no data to show that diphenhydramine causes tinnitus. (C) Alcohol potentiates the effects of diphenhydramine. (D) Diphenhydramine decreases alertness; it does not increase alertness.

133. **(B)** Nursing process phase: implementation; client need: pharmacological and parenteral therapies; content area: pharmacology.

RATIONALE

(A) Phenazopyridine has no direct effect on the appetite. (B) Phenazopyridine may color the urine orange-to-red. (C) Phenazopyridine may color the urine orange-to-red, not blue-purple. (D) Phenazopyridine may decrease rather than increase pain on urination.

134. **(A)** Nursing process phase: implementation; client need: pharmacological and parenteral therapies; content area: pharmacalogy.

RATIONALE

(A) Rifampin is an anti-infective and antibiotic active against tuberculosis and some gram-negative and gram-positive organisms. Rifampin is usually prescribed with other antituberculosis drugs for treating tuberculosis. (B) Rifampin has no effect on malaria. (C) Rifampin does not alter the color of body fluids. (D) Rifampin does not alter the color of body fluids.

135. **(D)** Nursing process phase: implementation; client need: basic care and comfort; content area: nutrition.

RATIONALE

(A) Veal is low in cholesterol. (B) Chicken is low in cholesterol. (C) Fish is low in cholesterol. (D) On a low-cholesterol diet, the intake of eggs should be decreased to three egg yolks per week.

136. **(C)** Nursing process phase: implementation; client need: pharmacological and parenteral therapies; content area: pharmacology.

RATIONALE

(A) Assessing blood pressure before administration of nitroglycerin is routine. (B) Assessing blood pressure after administration of nitroglycerin is routine. (C) Dizziness, lightheadedness, and syncope occur because of postural hypotension. Advise the client to change positions slowly. (D) Sublingual nitroglycerin may sting when taken.

Comprehensive Integrated Practice Tests

TEST 1

Patricia Gauntlett Beare, RN, PhD

 ## QUESTIONS

1. The nurse is assessing a 70-year-old man. Normal changes that may increase with age include:

   A. Decrease in blood pressure (BP), decrease in cardiac reserve, increase in coronary artery disease
   B. Prostatic hypertrophy, reduced creatinine clearance, increase in renal blood flow
   C. Diminished peristalsis, constipation, reduced gastric acid secretion
   D. Decrease in bone mineral content, loss of height, decrease in number of taste buds

2. An 80-year-old client is being assessed by the nurse. Which of the following occurs as a result of normal aging?

   A. High-frequency hearing loss
   B. Increased susceptibility to postural hypertension
   C. Increased cardiac reserve
   D. Increased adaptation to dark

3. When assessing clients over 65 years, the nurse would correctly identify which of the following as the most common chronic condition in older Americans?

   A. Arthritis
   B. Hearing impairment
   C. Cataracts
   D. Diabetes

4. The nurse is teaching a group of older people about early signs of aging. Which of the following occurs earliest in most older adults?

   A. Difficulty reading fine print without glasses
   B. Osteoarthritic changes of the cervical spine
   C. Intense awareness that life is limited (midlife crisis)
   D. Difficulty staying up at night and working the next day

5. A 65-year-old client complains of having trouble sleeping at night. The best response by the nurse is:

   A. "Try to drink some warm milk before you go to bed."
   B. "Try staying up and watching television until you fall asleep."
   C. "I will refer you to Dr. Jones for some sleeping pills."
   D. "Most cases of insomnia are normal as you get older."

6. The nurse is assessing a 70-year-old client. Which of the following symptoms is commonly reported by older persons?

   A. Vaginal bleeding
   B. Reduced urinary frequency
   C. Incontinence
   D. Increased weight gain

7. A 65-year-old client has been taking several aspirins daily for her arthritis. It would be most important for the nurse to observe for:

   A. Weight gain
   B. Gastrointestinal (GI) hemorrhage
   C. Oral mucous membrane hypertrophy
   D. Confusion

8. A 68-year-old client is receiving dietary counseling from the nurse. Which of the following statements indicates a need for further teaching?

   A. "I must eat 2–4 servings of fruit per day."
   B. "I must avoid all meats and animal products."
   C. "I should use moderation in my sugar and salt consumption."
   D. "I must eat 6–11 servings of bread, cereal, and pasta per day."

9. The nurse is doing preoperative teaching with a 26-year-old client for a total hysterectomy for severe endometriosis. Which of the following statements indicates a need for further teaching?

   A. "I'm so glad I'm having this surgery. My husband and I want a large family."
   B. "I should lift no more than 10 lb for the next 4 weeks."

C. "I can resume normal sexual relations in about 6 weeks."

D. "I can take Tylenol for pain control."

10. A 50-year-old client is 15 days posthysterectomy. Which of the following symptoms should be immediately reported to the physician?

A. Serosanguinous vaginal drainage

B. A temperature of 99.4°F (37.4°C)

C. Bright-red bleeding from the incisional site or other site

D. Laboratory findings of 12.0 g/dl Hgb and 36 Hct

11. A 48-year-old client has a diagnosis of dumping syndrome after gastric surgery. It would be most important for the client to:

A. Drink concentrated carbohydrates such as milkshakes between meals

B. Lie down after meals

C. Eat large well-balanced meals

D. Drink fluids with meals

12. A 30-year-old woman has just delivered premature twin babies. It is most important for the nurse to inform the parents:

A. That it is in the twins' best interest to stay in the hospital

B. How they (the parents) will be incorporated into the twins' care

C. That they should obtain as much rest as possible in preparation for the twins coming home

D. Not to call the nursery unless it is an emergency

13. The parents of twin baby girls bring them to the pediatrician's office for their first checkup. The parents have numerous questions. The nurse's response should reflect the fact that:

A. Twins are very special and need additional attention

B. Even though they are twins, each baby needs to be viewed as an individual

C. Twins should be treated exactly the same

D. Twins should never be separated during this very early period

14. The nurse is preparing to discharge newborn twins with their parents. It would be most important for the nurse to:

A. Observe the parents feeding, bathing, and dressing the babies

B. Teach the parents what it means when the baby cries

C. Inform the parents when the first immunizations will be given

D. Advise the parents to get help for the first 2 weeks when the twins are at home

15. An 8-year-old child has been hospitalized with a diagnosis of nephrotic syndrome. He has severe edema and proteinuria, and is lethargic. Which of the following nursing measures would be appropriate?

A. Daily measurement of weight and abdominal girth

B. A high-carbohydrate diet

C. Daily exercise and play therapy

D. Promoting adequate fluid intake

16. A 6-month-old child is admitted to the hospital for evaluation of vomiting. Which of the following would the nurse provide as a toy?

A. A large puzzle

B. Push-pull toy

C. Soft, colorful blocks

D. A rocking horse

17. A 20-year-old gravida 2, para 2 vaginally delivered a 7-lb 2-oz girl on April 3 at 10:35 PM. She is rubella immune, has a small right sublabial nick, refused ice application to perineum, is voiding, and has a firm uterus at the level of the umbilicus. She is bottle-feeding her baby. Her blood type is A-negative and her daughter's is A-positive. On the morning of April 4, her lochia is dark red and contains small shreds of tissue. The nurse should describe this discharge as lochia:

A. Alba

B. Leuka

C. Rubra

D. Serosa

18. At 8 AM on the first postpartum day, a client's fundus is 2 cm above the umbilicus and located on the right side of her abdomen. There is a moderate amount of vaginal blood. The nurse should:

A. Ask the client if she had any infections during the last 2 weeks of pregnancy

B. Notify the registered nurse (RN) or midwife immediately

C. Proceed with the data collection and chart the information as noted

D. Provide a way for the client to empty her bladder before proceeding with the data collection

19. A postpartum client asks the nurse how long her vaginal discharge will last. The nurse's best response would be to explain that it will last:

A. About 3 days

B. Longer than if she were breastfeeding

C. Until her checkup in 6 weeks

D. Until the placental site has healed

20. At 10 AM on the first postpartum day, the nurse notes that a client's fundus is firm and that there is a continuous flow of vaginal blood with no clots. As she gets out of bed, the client notices a "gushing" from her vagina and passes a small clot. She becomes frightened. The nurse should explain to her that:

A. She probably got up too soon after delivery and needs to take it a little slower

B. The amount of discharge is increased because she is not breastfeeding

C. The lochia that pools in the vagina while she is lying in bed drains when she stands

D. The vaginal opening is edematous and bruised right after delivery

21. A new mother states that she is afraid to have a bowel movement because she remembers the discomfort she

experienced after delivering her other child. The nurse should encourage her to:

A. Eat a low-roughage diet, drink 8 glasses of water per day, and keep physical activity to a minimum
B. Eat fresh fruits and vegetables, drink 6–8 glasses of water per day, and ambulate frequently
C. Eat small amounts of food for several days so she will be less likely to have a bowel movement until the soreness in her perineum is decreased
D. Eat whatever she wishes, take a mild laxative for several days, and keep up her Kegel exercises

22. A client's Rh antibody titer indicates that she has not been sensitized to the Rh factor. The nurse should anticipate that which of the following will be given after delivery?

A. Bromocriptine mesylate (Parlodel)
B. Oxytocin
C. Rh₀(D) immune globulin (e.g., RhoGAM)
D. Rubella virus vaccine

23. A 22-year-old gravida 1, para 1 delivered a 7-lb 8-oz boy by cesarean birth. She has decided to breast-feed her son. Her abdominal incision is midline and vertical and has a dressing on it. To assess her uterus for position and tone, the nurse should:

A. Ask her how it feels instead of palpating for it
B. Gently palpate above or below the incision
C. Gently palpate on each side of the incision
D. Palpate directly over the incision

24. When a client breast-feeds her baby after a cesarean birth, the nurse can help by suggesting that she:

A. Bottle-feed the baby after each feeding until she is producing milk in sufficient amount
B. Lie on her side with the baby lying beside her and turned toward her
C. Raise the head of her bed and rest the baby high on her abdomen
D. Wash her nipples with soap and water before and after feeding the baby

25. As a client's baby starts to breast-feed, the client begins to experience severe abdominal cramps. The nurse should:

A. Assist her to move the baby off her abdominal incision
B. Explain that breastfeeding does cause discomfort and she should consider bottle feeding instead
C. Explain that when the baby sucks, oxytocin, the hormone that causes the uterus to contract, is released
D. Medicate her for pain and give the baby a bottle for this feeding

26. A new mother complains that her incision hurts when she has to cough, turn, and breathe deeply. The nurse should teach her to:

A. Breathe less deeply, cough gently, and splint her incision to decrease her discomfort
B. Continue with the exercise because she needs to wear off the anesthetic she received during surgery
C. Continue with the exercise while splinting her incision because she needs to fully inflate her lungs to prevent pooling of secretions

D. Discontinue the exercise and inform her physician the next time he or she visits

27. Students were tested on normal fetal circulation and given the following scenario. A baby was born at term by vaginal birth. She was assessed and placed in her mother's arms. Rapid and radical physiological changes occurred at birth as the baby's body established pulmonary ventilation and her circulatory pattern markedly changed. In the neonate, three structures that were necessary for fetal circulation must close as blood supply is increased to the lungs and liver. Which of the following did the students identify incorrectly?

A. Ductus arteriosus
B. Ductus neonatorum
C. Ductus venosus
D. Foramen ovale

28. Data collection of a newborn at 1 minute after birth reveals a heart rate of 98 bpm, good respiratory effort with crying, active motion, vigorous cry, and pink body with blue extremities. Her Apgar score is:

A. 10
B. 9
C. 8
D. 7

29. When the father of a newborn asks why the baby's hands and feet look blue, the nurse should explain that this condition is common and temporary, and is called:

A. Acrocyanosis
B. Acrodermatosis
C. Cyanoacrylate
D. Vernix caseosa

30. By law, a newborn is given eyedrops of a 1% silver nitrate solution or an erythromycin ophthalmic preparation in both eyes. This is done as a prophylactic treatment for:

A. Gonorrheal conjunctivitis
B. Hemorrhagic tendencies
C. Nosocomial infection
D. Staphylococcal infection

31. In the birthing room after the initial data collections are complete, a mother asks to breast-feed her baby. The most appropriate nursing intervention would be to:

A. Ask her to wait until the baby has been thoroughly evaluated in the newborn nursery
B. Ask her to wait until you give the baby glucose water as the initial feeding
C. Assist her to breast-feed the baby
D. Refuse her request

32. A 2-day-old, full-term newborn infant is of normal weight and length and to this point has had an uncomplicated newborn course. His mother is breastfeeding him. He will be in the neonatal period from the time of his birth through his:

A. Fourteenth day of life
B. Twenty-eighth day of life

C. First year of life

D. Time of discharge from the hospital

33. The intraoperative nurse monitoring a client receiving local anesthesia notices an increase in the heart rate. The change may be caused by the release of:

A. Norepinephrine

B. Glucocorticoids

C. Aldosterone

D. Antidiuretic hormone

34. When assessing a newborn's heart rate (preferably when he is asleep), the nurse should:

A. Auscultate the apical pulse for a full minute

B. Auscultate the apical pulse for 30 seconds and double it

C. Auscultate the apical pulse for 15 seconds and multiply by 4

D. Palpate the brachial pulse for 30 seconds and double it

35. While he is awake and quiet, a newborn's pulse, in beats per minute, should average:

A. 80–100

B. 100–120

C. 120–150

D. 150–180

36. Of the following findings on data collection, which is most likely to be normal for a newborn infant?

A. Failure to pass meconium during the first 24 hours of life

B. Failure to void during the first 24 hours of life

C. Inability to pass a rectal thermometer >⅛ inch into the rectum

D. Rust-colored or pink stains on a diaper with voiding

37. A nurse is preparing to obtain a consent for a client preoperatively. Which of the following is correct?

A. The client's decision to have surgery can be revoked at any time.

B. The consent form may be signed by the client if premedication has been given.

C. A spouse, child, or friend may sign the consent form if the client asks him or her to.

D. The perioperative nurse is required to inform the client of all the surgical and anesthetic risks related to the procedure.

38. On the day of birth a newborn was given an intramuscular (IM) injection of a substance because of a transient blood coagulation deficiency. The substance injected was probably:

A. Aquaphor

B. Cyanocobalamin (vitamin B$_{12}$)

C. Erythromycin

D. Phytonadione (vitamin K)

39. A 68-year-old client had bilateral total knee replacements under general anesthesia. The surgical procedure lasted 4 hours. Preoperatively, the client received instructions on deep-breathing exercises to increase lung ventilation and gas exchange postoperatively. The postsurgical nurse observes correct technique when the client is able to:

A. Take quick, shallow breaths through the mouth, hold them, then cough deeply from the chest

B. Take a slow, deep breath through the mouth, hold it, exhale, and cough deeply from the throat

C. Take a slow, deep breath through the nose, hold it, exhale, and cough deeply from the chest

D. Take a quick, deep breath through the nose, hold it, exhale, and cough deeply from the throat

40. While teaching a newborn's mother who is breastfeeding about baby care, the nurse informs her that normal stools for her baby are most likely to be:

A. Brown, well-formed, and up to 2 per day

B. Dark green, loose, and 5–8 per day

C. Pale yellow, formed, pasty, and every other day

D. Yellow, loose, and up to 6–10 per day

41. A newborn's mother asks whether she should feed him foods other than the breast milk. The nurse knows that, according to the American Academy of Pediatrics, breast milk or formula meets all the requirements of growth for the normal infant until the age of:

A. 2 months

B. 6 months

C. 9 months

D. 12 months

42. A 38-year-old woman was hospitalized with a medical diagnosis of cholecystitis. The nurse would expect the history of her present illness to include intolerance to which of the following nutrients?

A. Carbohydrates

B. Fat

C. Protein

D. Vitamin C

43. The preoperative teaching for prevention of postoperative complications includes leg exercises. The nurse teaches leg exercises preoperative to gallbladder surgery to help prevent:

A. Muscle spasms

B. Paralytic ileus

C. Stasis and clot formation

D. Vasogenic shock

44. Before surgery an intravenous (IV) catheter is inserted in a client's forearm. An isotonic solution is administered at a rate sufficient to keep the vein open. The nurse knows that the isotonic solution may be:

A. 0.9% sodium chloride

B. 0.45% sodium chloride

C. 10% dextrose

D. 50% dextrose

45. One hour before surgery is scheduled, the nurse gives a client her preanesthetic (preoperative) medication. Which of the following statements by the nurse is most appropriate after the medication is administered?

A. "Please remain in bed and use this call signal if you need anything. I am leaving the siderails up while no one is in the room with you."
B. "Please remember to empty your bladder before you are taken to the operating room."
C. "You may move about in your room as much as you like, but lie down when you begin to feel sleepy."
D. "While you wait to go to the operating room, I will give you a clear explanation of the surgical procedure so you will know what to expect."

46. Of the following postoperative nursing interventions, the one that will provide the surgical client with the greatest benefits is:
A. Deep-breathing and coughing exercises
B. Early ambulation
C. Leg exercises (calf, quadriceps, and gluteal)
D. Medication for pain

47. On the morning of the second day after surgery, data collection reveals pain, tenderness, and swelling in a client's left calf. She has not taken the as-needed pain medication ordered for her since the previous day. The nurse's next action should be to:
A. Administer the medication ordered every 4 hours as needed for pain, and include the site of the pain as the intervention is recorded
B. Allow the client to be up in her room only and elevate her left leg
C. Immobilize her leg and have her maintain bedrest until the physician examines her leg
D. Massage her leg to relieve pain and swelling, and ask if she would like her pain medication

48. A 78-year-old man has been admitted for total joint replacement of his fractured right hip. In conjunction with the hip surgery, the physician orders aspirin 325 mg every day. The nurse is aware that this medication is probably ordered for which of the following effects?
A. Analgesic
B. Antibiotic
C. Anticoagulant
D. Antipyretic

49. To prevent prosthesis dislocation after a total hip replacement, the nurse teaches a client to maintain which of the following leg positions?
A. Abduction
B. Adduction
C. Flexion
D. Internal rotation

50. While evaluating follow-up teaching, the nurse concludes that a client post–hip replacement surgery is beginning to understand after stating that he will have to learn not to cross his legs and not to flex his hip more than 90 degrees. He says, "but I will gradually get back to doing most of my routine daily activities after_____":
A. 1 week
B. 3 months
C. 9 months
D. 12 months

51. A 73-year-old man is admitted to the cardiac stepdown unit with a diagnosis of congestive heart failure. He has 2+ pitting edema bilaterally up to his calves. The physician has ordered bedrest and the following medications: furosemide (Lasix) 80 mg IV bid, digoxin 0.25 mg orally (PO) every morning, theophylline (Slo-bid) 10 mEq (2 tablets) PO tid, aspirin 325 mg PO every day, and nifedipine (Procardia XL) 10 mg PO bid. During data collection, the nurse notes urine output of 10 cc during the last 4 hours, fatigue, slight lethargy, and complaints of visual disturbances. The next action the nurse should take is to:
A. Administer the next dose of furosemide early to increase urine output
B. Call the physician
C. Chart data collection data and recheck the client in 30 minutes
D. Check laboratory values

52. A client has been placed on furosemide 80 mg IV bid. He has a diagnosis of congestive heart failure. The nurse should be aware that the client's medical diagnosis and treatment put him at risk for potential depletion of which of the following electrolytes?
A. Calcium
B. Chloride
C. Potassium
D. Sodium

53. A 63-year-old woman is admitted to the medical-surgical unit with an exacerbation of symptoms related to ovarian carcinoma. On admission her BP is 122/82 mm Hg, pulse (P) 88 bpm, respirations (R) 20/min, and temperature 98.2°F (36.7°C). She is expected to return home when the symptoms subside. While she is in the hospital, the physician has ordered morphine sulfate 4 mg IV q3–4 h PRN for pain. Her condition worsens. During the nurse's data collection, vital signs include BP 108/64 mm Hg, pulse 63 bpm, and respirations 10/min. Before the nurse leaves the room, tears roll down the client's face as she requests her pain medication. The nurse should:
A. Administer the morphine as ordered
B. Administer the morphine and offer to sit with her for a few minutes
C. Report the vital signs to the charge nurse so that a different narcotic analgesic can be ordered
D. Leave the room to allow her to be alone

54. A 9-month-old child weighs 20 lb and has sustained a fracture of the right femur. The client is admitted and placed in Bryant's traction. The nurse knows that this type of traction is:
A. Continuous, skeletal
B. Continuous, skin
C. Intermittent, skeletal
D. Intermittent, skin

55. For effective traction a 9-year-old boy must be maintained in an appropriate position. The nurse is aware that his buttocks must be:

A. Elevated and clear of the bed
B. Flat on the bed
C. Supported by a well-padded sling
D. Supported by a pillow

56. A 9-month-old infant is hospitalized for a fractured right femur. At this stage in the infant's development, the nurse should:

A. Apply a Band-Aid after injections to give him the security of wholeness
B. Have his mother stay and care for her child, if possible
C. Provide for frequent eye-to-eye contact between parents and child
D. Set limits and allow him to make choices when possible

57. A 10-year-old child has a high fever, headache, vomiting, and scarlatina rash. His throat is sore and dry. Throat culture reveals the presence of group A β-hemolytic streptococcal infection ("strep throat"). When penicillin is prescribed, the nurse should teach the boy or his mother to:

A. Monitor the scarlatina rash to determine when the medication has been effective
B. Take all the medication even if the symptoms subside several days before it is gone
C. Take the medication until his temperature is normal
D. Take the medication until his throat is no longer sore

58. When a 10-year-old child returns for a follow-up examination after a streptococcal infection, his mother asks why a urinalysis is being done. The nurse explains that:

A. Group A β-hemolytic streptococcal infections can be followed by the complication of glomerulonephritis
B. Penicillin has the potential side effect of pyelonephritis
C. The urinalysis will indicate whether a human immunodeficiency virus (HIV) infection is also present
D. Urinary tract infections are common with streptococcal infections and need to receive prompt treatment

59. An 8-year-old boy will miss 4 days of school because of illness. He tells his mother that he does not want to go back after he is well. His mother asks the nurse how to handle this situation. The most helpful intervention would probably be to:

A. Allow him to miss a full week of school to provide for continuity when he returns to school
B. Contact the school counselor for advice
C. Have the boy's teacher send his school work home and see that he completes the assignments before he returns to school
D. Obtain special permission for him to return to school earlier than planned and miss only 2 days

60. A 77-year-old woman has been admitted with occasional urinary incontinence of unknown origin (may be described as functional incontinence). The nurse instructs her on obtaining a clean-catch urine specimen. Which of the following statements related to collection of a clean-catch urine sample from a female client indicates the need for further teaching?

A. "Separate labia to expose urethral opening."
B. "Cleanse from front to back with antiseptic solution."
C. "Collect entire specimen as I void."
D. "Deliver specimen to the nurse immediately."

61. The nurse caring for a client knows that the average quantity of urine produced by "normal" adult kidney function per 24-hour period is approximately:

A. 800–1000 cc
B. 1200–1500 cc
C. 1500–1800 cc
D. 1800–2200 cc

62. A client's orders include keeping a record of her I&O. During lunch she drank 5 oz of iced tea and ate 4 oz of Jell-O and 2 oz of creamed soup. The nurse would record which of the following totals as intake?

A. 150 ml
B. 180 ml
C. 210 ml
D. 330 ml

63. Goals of nursing interventions for clients experiencing temporary incontinence (caused by illness, confusion, or decreased level of consciousness) include (a) prevention of bladder distention and (b) keeping the client dry. Which of the following measures is least likely to help the client to regain voluntary control?

A. Inserting a Foley catheter to keep the client dry
B. Offering the bedpan or commode on arising and at bedtime
C. Scheduling toileting every 2 hours
D. Assisting the client to use the bedpan or toilet about an hour after drinking liquids containing caffeine

64. A 76-year-old client's urinary incontinence causes her to be subject to alterations in skin integrity. Of the following measures, which would be of fundamental importance in prevention of skin breakdown?

A. Wash with soap and water and dry the perineal area after periods of incontinence.
B. Pad the client's clothing or bed with absorbent material.
C. Apply barrier creams to protect skin from contact with urine.
D. Change wet "diaper" frequently on a regular schedule.

65. Inadequate attention to care of a 76-year-old client who is incontinent and immobile can result in a complication known as a:

A. Flexion contracture
B. Pressure ulcer
C. Dermatologic crisis
D. Pressure point

66. Conservative measures have failed to help a 76-year-old client gain voluntary control of voiding. An order has been given for insertion of a Foley catherer. For catheterizing a female client, the preferred body position is:

A. Left Sims'
B. Supine (dorsal)

C. Dorsal recumbent

D. Prone

67. A 76-year-old client's Foley catheter is draining well via a closed system to the drainage bag hanging from the side of the bed. The physician has ordered a urinalysis. While maintaining sterile technique, the nurse will:

A. Allow the urine to flow into the specimen container from the tube at the lower edge of the drainage bag

B. Separate the catheter from the drainage tubing and allow the urine to flow from the catheter into the specimen container

C. Withdraw a quantity of urine from the catheter with a sterile needle and syringe inserted into the catheter above the bifurcation

D. Using a sterile needle, withdraw a specimen from the port located on the urinary drainage tubing

68. The nurse recognizes that the single most effective intervention to limit the spread of nosocomial (hospital-acquired) infections is:

A. Prophylactic anti-infective therapy for susceptible clients

B. Correct handwashing technique faithfully observed

C. Proper disposal of blood and other body fluids

D. Frequent in-service education programs on isolation technique

69. To implement procedures correctly, the nurse must understand the differences among various invasive procedures, that is, which procedures require sterile technique for performance and which can be carried out using clean technique. Which of the following procedures does not require sterility of equipment and solutions used?

A. Urinary catheterization

B. Hyperalimentation

C. Nasogastric feeding

D. Tracheostomy suctioning

70. A 48-year-old client is admitted with fever (temperature 102°F [38.8°C]) and acute severe pain in several joints of the extremities, especially the large toe. Data collection reveals a family history of gout. The nurse anticipates that the physician may initially order which of the following drugs?

A. Allopurinol

B. Colchicine

C. Probenecid

D. Sulfinpyrazone

71. Assessment of a client's large toe with gangrene might reveal which of the following characteristics?

A. Pain

B. Swelling

C. Increased heat

D. Cyanosis

72. Gout results from impaired uric acid production or excretion. The physician has ordered a 24-hour urine collection to begin at 8 AM. The nurse initiating the collection will:

A. Collect and include the urine specimen voided at 8 AM the day the collection is begun

B. Collect all urine voidings after the 8 AM voiding, including the 8 AM specimen 24 hours after the beginning of the collection

C. Maintain the collection in the client's room at room temperature during the 24-hour period

D. Collect as many of the client's voidings as possible during the collection period, using clean-catch technique

73. A client with gout is discharged from the hospital. Which of the following might best describe the dietary regimen on discharge from the hospital?

A. Decreased fluid intake and high-purine diet

B. Fasting, crash diets, or both

C. Shellfish, organ meats, alcohol

D. Potatoes, milk, increased fluids

74. A nursing diagnosis for a client with gout is alteration in comfort as a result of pain, related to the disease process. When talking about what the client can do to provide comfort and relieve pain, the client gives the following measures. Which one indicates a need for further teaching?

A. "Apply pressure to the affected joint as ordered."

B. "Apply cold or heat packs."

C. "Administer analgesics and anti-inflammatory agents."

D. "Provide immobilization for the affected joint."

75. When planning care for a client with gout, the nurse identifies the major goal of drug therapy in arthritis and related conditions as:

A. Providing emotional support

B. Curing the underlying cause

C. Reducing inflammation of joints

D. Preparing the client for surgery

76. A client has an order for a total of 3000 ml of 5% dextrose in water to be infused over 24 hours. What is the approximate infusion rate in drops per minute? Standard drop factor is 10.

A. 21 gtt/min

B. 125 gtt/min

C. 2 gtt/min

D. 60 gtt/min

77. After a client's IV fluids have been infusing for some period, the flow is interrupted. Which of the following measures done by a nurse indicates a need to review the IV procedure for further teaching?

A. Check for swelling at the needle site.

B. Move the client's arm to a new position.

C. Lower the receptacle below the level of the needle.

D. Flush cannula or needle with sterile saline.

78. A 75-year-old client is receiving IV therapy. Later that night the client begins experiencing headache, flushed skin, rapid pulse, increased BP, increased respirations, coughing, and shortness of breath. These symptoms may indicate possible:

A. Circulatory overload

B. Drug overload
C. Superficial thrombophlebitis
D. Air embolism

79. A client has a diagnosis of bronchial asthma. Any of the following drugs may be used in the treatment of asthma. Which of the medications is effective in inhibiting the allergic reaction?

    A. Epinephrine
    B. Terbutaline sulfate
    C. Cromolyn sodium
    D. Theophylline

80. A 57-year-old client has been experiencing anorexia, weight loss, and diarrhea and is admitted for diagnostic purposes. He has an order for enemas in preparation for a barium enema the next day. Which of the following nursing actions represents the best response appropriate to administration of enemas?

    A. Lubricate tip of tubing and insert tubing 2 inches with client lying in the left lateral position with right leg flexed.
    B. Expel air from tubing; lubricate and insert tip of tubing 4 inches with client lying in right lateral position with left leg flexed.
    C. Open clamp and allow solution to flow moderately fast with container at level of 15 inches above anus.
    D. Allow solution to flow slowly until container is empty or until client is unable to take any more; clamp tubing and remove from anus.

81. A 62-year-old client is admitted to the eye unit with a past history of foggy vision, diminished accommodation, nondescript ocular discomfort, and complaint of mild aching in both eyes. Initial data collection is conducted and tonometry (measurement of intraocular pressure) is ordered. Intraocular pressure is 28 mm Hg. The nurse knows that the range for normal intraocular pressure is:

    A. 11–22 mm Hg
    B. 24–32 mm Hg
    C. 34–44 mm Hg
    D. 50–75 mm Hg

82. A client is diagnosed as having chronic (open-angle) glaucoma, the most common form of glaucoma. Medical treatment is used initially, and surgery may be required if medical treatment is not successful. Drugs that either increase the outflow of aqueous humor or decrease the production of aqueous humor may be prescribed. The principal objective of drug treatment of glaucoma is:

    A. Evaluation for diagnostic purposes
    B. Preparation of the client for surgery
    C. Education of the client
    D. Reduction of intraocular pressure

83. The nurse caring for a client with glaucoma knows that a miotic drug:

    A. Dilates the pupil
    B. Constricts the pupil
    C. Cures glaucoma
    D. Anesthetizes the eye

84. Miotic drugs are frequently prescribed for various types of glaucoma. The nurse may administer which of the following drugs to facilitate miosis?

    A. Acetazolamide (Diamox)
    B. Pilocarpine
    C. Mannitol
    D. Phenylbutazone

85. A client's physician has ordered pilocarpine 2%, gtt ii OS qid. To correctly implement the order, the nurse would administer:

    A. 2 drops in left eye four times a day
    B. 11 drops in left eye four times a day
    C. 2 drops in right eye every day
    D. 2 drops in both eyes four times a day

86. Regarding instillation of a client's eyedrops, the nurse should:

    A. Instruct the client to focus gaze straight ahead
    B. Drop the solution gently onto the cornea
    C. Drop medication into the center of the lower lid
    D. Touch the eyedropper gently to the client's lower eyelid

87. While constructing discharge planning with a client with glaucoma and the family, the nurse teaches the client to occlude the nasolacrimal (tear) duct by applying digital pressure at the inner canthus during administration of eyedrops and for 2 minutes afterward. The primary reason for such action is:

    A. To prevent excessive systemic absorption of drugs
    B. To prevent the client from tearing during administration
    C. To prevent blinking of the eyelids during administration
    D. To prevent possible loss of medication

88. The nurse caring for the client should teach the client who has glaucoma not to take:

    A. Beta-blockers
    B. Antiemetics
    C. Mydriatics
    D. Analgesics

89. A 73-year-old client has been admitted to undergo an intraocular lens implant because of a cataract (clouding or opacity of lens) in the right eye. Surgery will be performed under local anesthesia. Plans include the client being discharged home the evening of the day of surgery. Preoperative medication is diazepam (Valium) 10 mg PO. The diazepam supplied consists of scored tablets of 5 mg each. The nurse should administer by mouth:

    A. One-half tablet
    B. One tablet
    C. Two tablets
    D. Two and one-half tablets

90. The nurse is checking a care plan for a client with cataract surgery. Which of the following is an error in nursing care planning for postoperative measures and discharge teaching?

A. Position the client on the operative side with pillows.

B. Patch operative (right) eye and employ protective shield as ordered.

C. Administer prescribed medications for prevention of nausea and constipation.

D. Instruct client not to lift, pull, or push heavy objects.

91. A neighbor asks you, as a nurse, to recommend eyedrops for his mother, who has recently developed an eye irritation. You should recommend:

    A. Visine; it is the most commonly prescribed eye medication

    B. Atropine, as it is inexpensive and very effective

    C. Aspirin to decrease inflammation and provide comfort

    D. Professional assessment to help determine the cause of the problem

92. A 2-year-old child presents holding her ear and rolling her head from side to side. Postauricular and cervical lymph glands are enlarged. Her temperature is 104°F (40°C). Her appetite has been poor, and chewing seems to be painful for her. She has had a cold, and irritability has been characteristic of her temperament for several days. The nurse knows that the client's signs and symptoms may be indicative of which of the following common early childhood health problems?

    A. Conjunctivitis
    B. Tonsillitis
    C. Otitis media
    D. Cystitis

93. The nurse knows that several factors predispose infants and young children to otitis media. Which of the following statements related to susceptibility to otitis media is least accurate?

    A. Eustachian tubes are short, narrow, and lie in a somewhat vertical plane.

    B. Cartilage lining is underdeveloped and may allow eustachian tubes to open inappropriately.

    C. Humoral defense mechanisms are still immature.

    D. Usual lying-down positions favor pharyngeal pooling, which may hinder eustachian tube drainage.

94. To administer a 2-year-old child's ear medication, the nurse must know that there is one fundamental variation in the method employed for adults and the method for infants and children. Which of the following steps for admininistration of otic medications will be altered for the client?

    A. Position the client on the unaffected side.

    B. Pull the pinna (auricle) up and back before administration.

    C. Direct the drops toward the ear canal.

    D. Allow the client to remain positioned for 5–10 minutes (after administration).

95. The nurse is responsible for discharge teaching regarding care of a 2-year-old child with otitis media after the child goes home. To ensure that that the proper technique for administrating otic medication has been learned, the best action the nurse can take is to have the mother or person responsible for administering the eardrops:

A. Repeat the instructions to the nurse verbally

B. Write down the procedure as given by the nurse

C. Take a written test to demonstrate mastery of the technique

D. Perform the procedure in the presence of the nurse

96. A 68-year-old client has experienced a gradual decline in motor function; after a thorough diagnostic workup, a diagnosis of Parkinson's disease has been made. Parkinson's disease is accompanied by brain cell degeneration and dopamine deficiency. Which of the following statements about the disorder is accurate?

    A. Parkinson's disease can be treated with levodopa, which eventually halts the degenerative process.

    B. Parkinson's disease can result in a "parkinsonian crisis," caused by extended use of the drugs used to treat the disorder.

    C. Parkinson's disease is a familial disease.

    D. Parkinson's disease does not usually affect the individual's intellectual faculties.

97. Which of the following drugs used to treat a client's Parkinson's disease may also be used for prevention of lactation and for female infertility?

    A. Levodopa
    B. Bromocriptine mesylate (Parlodel)
    C. Diphenhydramine (Benadryl)
    D. Benztropine mesylate (Cogentin)

98. A client with Parkinson's disease may experience constipation resulting from lack of exercise, medication side effects, or loss of saliva in the GI tract. Which of the following client statements regarding promotion of normal elimination would indicate a need for further teaching?

    A. "I should increase intake of fluid and dietary fiber."

    B. "I should use mild laxatives or stool softeners."

    C. "I should establish a regular time for bowel movements."

    D. "I should take a 2-hour nap each afternoon."

99. Several medications are prescribed for controlling constipation symptoms in a client with Parkinson's disease. Which of the following statements best describes the appropriate nursing action?

    A. When the client needs information about drug therapy, he should be referred to the physician.

    B. When medication information is required, the nurse knows that the pharmacist should provide such information.

    C. When the client requires drug information, the nurse should contact the physician for an order to give the information.

    D. When a drug regimen is begun, the nurse should instruct the client regarding administration, adverse effects, and other fundamental knowledge.

100. A 20-year-old client has a history of epilepsy controlled by medication. Recently the client ceased taking prescribed drugs and subsequently experienced status epilepticus. The condition can best be described as:

A. A period of remission when the client experiences no seizures
B. A time of continuous seizures or seizures in rapid succession
C. A rare degenerative disorder related to epilepsy
D. A term that is synonymous with petit mal seizures

101. An ampule of diazepam contains 5 mg/ml. How many minims are required to administer 2 mg?

    A. 2
    B. 0.4
    C. 10
    D. 6

102. Which of the following actions is least likely to occur within the realm of a practical (vocational) nursing responsibility?

    A. Administering medications
    B. Prescribing drug therapy
    C. Gathering data for research
    D. Evaluating effectiveness of medications

103. Assessment of the gums of a client with epilepsy reveals gingival hyperplasia (hypertrophy). The condition may result from a long-standing use of which of the following drugs?

    A. Phenytoin (Dilantin)
    B. Primidone (Mysoline)
    C. Clonazepam (Klonopin)
    D. Diazepam

104. A client is given the usual medication of choice for status epilepticus. The drug is administered IV, very slowly, until the seizures stop. The drug described is:

    A. Docusate sodium
    B. Digoxin
    C. Diazepam
    D. Dexamethasone

105. A client is seen in the emergency room with an open sucking chest wound. The first action the nurse would take is to:

    A. Administer oxygen
    B. Perform chest physiotherapy and coughing
    C. Administer pain medication
    D. Seal the wound with sterile petroleum gauze

106. A client is being treated with chest tubes because of a pneumothorax. The nurse recognizes that chest tubes may be used to:

    A. Regain positive intrapleural pressure
    B. Prevent pleural irritation
    C. Remove air and fluid from the intrapleural space
    D. Establish negative intra-alveolar pressure

107. Nursing care of the client with closed chest drainage should include:

    A. Clamping chest tube every 2 hours
    B. Elevating chest tube higher than client's chest
    C. Milking chest tube only if obstructed by clots
    D. Clamping chest tube when moving the client

108. While bathing a client with chest tubes, the nurse notices that there is bubbling in the water-seal chamber. This probably means that:

    A. There is a leak in the system
    B. The system is functioning properly
    C. The client is exhaling
    D. The client needs to be turned to the left side

109. A 46-year-old oil company manager is admitted via the emergency room to your unit for observation because of epigastric pain and hematemesis. He has a long history of alcohol use. A tentative diagnosis of gastritis secondary to alcoholism is made. To prevent Wernicke's encephalopathy, a neurological disease manifested by confusion and ataxia, the nurse expects the client to be treated with:

    A. Antabuse
    B. Vitamin C
    C. Chlordiazepoxide (Librium)
    D. Thiamine

110. While assessing a client with alcoholism and related gastritis, it is extremely important for the nurse to try to determine:

    A. How long has the client been sick?
    B. With whom does the client live?
    C. Does the client always have gastric-type pain after he drinks?
    D. When did the client take the last drink?

111. On the second hospital day, the nurse recognizes which signs as impending delirium tremens (DTs) in an alcoholic client?

    A. Elevated BP, visual hallucinations, restlessness
    B. Elevated BP, lowered temperature, seizures
    C. Lowered BP, elevated temperature, restlessness
    D. Lowered BP, elevated temperature, seizures

112. An alcoholic client in DTs becomes belligerent, so the nurse applies four-point leather restraints. It is important to recognize that the nurse needs to do which of the following activities?

    A. Get order for restraints as needed; document every hour; tell him that the restraints are "to put him in his place."
    B. Get as-needed order for restraints; document every half hour; tell him that the restraints are for "disciplinary measures."
    C. Get specific order for restraints; check circulation every 15 minutes and document; tell him that the restraints will be taken off in 1 hour.
    D. Get specific order for restraints; check circulation every 15 minutes and document; tell him that the restraints are to prevent him from hurting himself or others.

113. A 55-year-old plumber suffered a cerebrovascular accident (CVA), or stroke, resulting in right hemiplegia and speech problems. He was admitted to the medical floor of a community hospital, where his wife visits daily. She is very supportive and assists with his care.

Progress is slow for the client, and he has difficulty expressing frustration because of his aphasia. His wife tends to overcompensate for this by pampering him and taking over tasks that he does slowly or clumsily. Physical therapy personnel work daily with him on ambulation; after being fitted with a leg brace, he is able to ambulate with a quadripod cane. The rehabilitation process begins with this client when:

A. He is about to be discharged or transferred to a rehabilitation facility
B. The critical period of illness is passed
C. He is admitted to the hospital
D. He expresses an interest in walking

114. The nurse is using principles of rehabilitation when he or she:

A. Encourages a client to dress in street clothes
B. Bathes a client and combs hair
C. Brushes a client's teeth when the client has trouble or forgets
D. Asks the physician to order a Foley catheter for occasional urinary incontinence

115. The physician orders active and passive range-of-motion (ROM) exercises to all extremities. For the client, passive ROM exercises are:

A. Done by the nurse or therapist without assistance from the client
B. Done by the therapist, who instructs the client which way to move and exercise
C. More effective than active ROM exercises in preventing contractures
D. Done by the client three times a day

116. A nurse is administering the Denver Developmental Screening Test (DDST) and recognizes that the test:

A. Assesses the child from birth to 2 years
B. Cannot be adjusted for prematurity
C. Can be administered to all minority ethnic groups
D. Is not an IQ test

117. The nurse is assessing a 2-year-old child. Which of the following toys is suitable for this child?

A. Squeak toy
B. Pull toy
C. Tricycle, Big Wheel
D. Jungle gym

118. The nurse is assessing a 12-month-old infant. Which of the following is appropriate gross motor development seen for the first time?

A. Sits with support, head steady.
B. Crawls, creeps, or walks holding on to furniture.
C. Walks well, stoops, and recovers.
D. Kicks ball forward, walks up steps, walks backward.

119. A 24-year-old pregnant client comes into the prenatal clinic. She is complaining of severe headaches, vertigo, and blurred vision. The priority nursing action is to:

A. Encourage her to rest more frequently during the day

B. Tell her to take Tylenol or aspirin for the headache pain
C. Immediately notify the physician
D. Refer her for allergy testing

120. The nurse teaches an older client who is undergoing an amniocentesis. Which of the following statements by the client indicates a need for further teaching?

A. "This test will determine if my baby's lungs are mature."
B. "This test will tell me if my baby has Down's syndrome."
C. "This test will tell me if there is a problem with my blood reacting to the baby's blood."
D. "This test will determine the fetal age and position."

121. When preparing a pregnant client for an amniocentesis, the client verbalizes understanding of the procedure to the nurse. Which of the following indicates a need for further teaching?

A. "I will drink lots of water and try not to go to the bathroom."
B. "I will sign a consent form."
C. "I must report any vaginal bleeding or fever afterwards."
D. "I will have my BP, pulse, and respirations taken very frequently before and after the procedure."

122. A 22-year-old client is admitted to the emergency room with vaginal bleeding, low abdominal cramping, and a BP of 80/40 mm Hg, P 130 bpm, R 20/min. The nurse correctly suspects these to be symptoms of:

A. Overdose of aspirin
B. Toxic shock syndrome
C. Endometriosis
D. Spontaneous abortion

123. A 26-year-old woman on a psychiatric unit refuses to sleep in her room because she says that it is "bugged." The most appropriate way in which the nurse might initially handle this situation is to:

A. Simply state that the room is not bugged
B. Change the room
C. Ask her why she believes the room is bugged
D. Ignore her delusion

124. A 31-year-old client is admitted to a psychiatric unit. She thinks that her coworkers are accusing her of indiscretions and spying on her. The initial nursing goal is directed at:

A. Joining in group activities
B. Establishing trust with staff
C. Limiting contacts with other clients
D. Allowing coworkers to visit

125. In teaching a client about the care of a leg brace, the nurse should emphasize:

A. The need to inspect skin daily and to expect some minor irritations
B. The cleaning and maintenance of the brace, which should be done by a professional therapist

C. The importance of keeping brace joints free of lint and oiling them once a week

D. That weight fluctuations have little effect on the fit of the brace

126. A 28-year-old client was injured in a motorcycle accident. The right leg was amputated above the knee. The nurse explains that a temporary prosthesis will be fitted to the leg. The most important use for a temporary prosthesis immediately after surgery is that it:

A. Allows the client to stand with aid within a few days

B. Substitutes for a dressing over the stump

C. Enhances body image

D. Prevents complications of bedrest

127. A client is learning to use crutches for the first time. When planning care for this client, which of the following is most important?

A. Heavy padding of the axillary bar so that it can help support body weight

B. Looking down frequently to see the position of the crutches and feet

C. Having two assistants aid the client

D. Carefully assessing the client's activity level

128. To prepare a client for crutch walking, it would be most important for the nurse to:

A. Refer the client to physical therapy

B. Initiate muscle-strengthening exercises for arms and shoulders

C. Urge the client to conserve strength in other activities to avoid tiring

D. Demonstrate crutch walking: how to sit, stand, and get up from the floor in case of falling

129. When a client receives a permanent prosthesis, the nurse should teach the client to:

A. Wash the prosthesis daily with soap and water

B. Wear it only when going out or having company

C. Inspect the prosthesis daily for loose or worn parts

D. Oil all joints daily

130. In the data collection phase of the nursing process, nurses:

A. Make plans to help the client meet treatment goals

B. Gather, verify, and communicate data about a client's health needs

C. Identify problems and act to eliminate them

D. Communicate with the client and formulate realistic goals to meet his or her health needs

131. An 8-year-old child is admitted to the pediatric unit with a diagnosis of chronic nephrosis. In discussing the plan of care with the client's mother, you share that the purpose of weighing the child is:

A. To measure adequacy of nutritional management

B. To check the accuracy of the fluid intake record

C. To impress on the child the importance of eating well

D. To determine changes in the amount of edema

132. Causing mental distress by name-calling, isolating, ignoring, or ridiculing is an example of:

A. Psychological abuse

B. Physical abuse

C. Active neglect

D. Passive neglect

133. A 90-year-old client is kept locked in a room of a house. The client is diabetic and is fed once a day by relatives. They do not give the client insulin because it is too expensive. The nurse identifies deliberately abandoning an older person or denying health care as an example of:

A. Psychological abuse

B. Physical abuse

C. Passive neglect

D. Active neglect

134. The nurse is observing a physician do a complete examination. Examining by feeling and touching is:

A. Percussion

B. Palpation

C. Inspection

D. Auscultation

135. The nurse identifies the best way to facilitate growth and development in the acutely ill toddler as:

A. Direct efforts at preparing and teaching parents to ensure nonanxious parenting of the child

B. Telling the toddler well in advance of a procedure that is to take place

C. Separating the toddler from parent, especially if there are temper tantrums

D. Encouraging the child to regress to a previous developmental level for familiarity and comfort

136. A 7-year-old child has been hospitalized for dehydration and vomiting. It would be most important for the nurse to remember which of the following?

A. Fear is related to body injury, loss of control, and death, and mutilation fantasies are common.

B. A child may view hospitalization as a punishment for thoughts.

C. Fears are related to body image.

D. A child may exhibit regressive behavior such as whining, tantrums, and thumbsucking.

137. According to Maslow's hierarchy, the first priority in nursing actions must be aimed at:

A. Moving toward satisfaction of creative and emotional needs as early as possible

B. Helping the client gain respect from others to prevent loneliness

C. Doing first things first: meeting the client's physiological needs before moving on to other needs

D. Helping the client to establish close relationships with as many persons as possible

138. The nurse is evaluating a mother's knowledge of steroid therapy because her child is being discharged. It is most important to know whether the mother knows that steroid therapy:

A. Commonly causes hirsutism

B. Aggravates acne
C. Causes cushingoid features to disappear
D. "Masks" infections

139. The first priority of nursing care of the client with a head injury is to:

A. Check level of consciousness
B. Evaluate pupils
C. Protect airway
D. Evaluate motor function

140. An 80-year-old woman is admitted for cataract surgery. When you are first assessing her, she tells you that she used to be several inches taller than she is now. The best response would be to:

A. Tell her she can regain her height by practicing better posture
B. Disregard her statement because she is probably confused owing to her advanced age
C. Acknowledge her statement as being inaccurate because older people do not tend to become shorter with age
D. Ask her how tall she used to be, measure her current height, and include both in your data collection

141. A 64-year-old client frequently complains that the room is too cold. The nurse realizes that the reason for this may be that:

A. A normal decrease in subcutaneous fat predisposes older people to feeling cold
B. Older people often complain because they are lonely
C. Sweat glands diminish in size, number, and activity as they become sclerosed
D. Older persons are more susceptible to heatstroke

142. A nursing home resident has a pressure sore exposing the trochanter of the hip. The nurse identifies this as:

A. Stage I
B. Stage II
C. Stage III
D. Stage IV

143. A chronically debilitated 82-year-old client is admitted to the hospital from a nursing home. The nurse identifies which of the following as risk factors for development of pressure ulcers?

A. Incontinence, immobility, impaired nutrition
B. Immobility, incontinence, agitation
C. Incontinence, impaired nutrition, agitation
D. Agitation, hyperactivity, thin skin

144. An 80-year-old client is hospitalized for cataract surgery. She tells you she sometimes has "palpitations" when she climbs stairs but that she has never had chest pain on exertion. The nurse should know that:

A. The heart of the aging person may respond by temporarily beating faster
B. She is a candidate for myocardial infarction
C. Rapid heartbeat on exertion is a cardinal sign of heart failure
D. She probably has mitral stenosis

145. An 80-year-old client should be encouraged to be up and about during hospitalization for cataract surgery, within prudent limitations imposed by the surgery. This is primarily because:

A. The older person is at high risk for pneumonia
B. The immune system is more efficient in aging persons
C. The intercostal muscles become flabby and dilated
D. Alveolar atrophy is reversed by early ambulation

146. A client has had gallbladder "attacks" in the past and is considered at risk for gallstone formation. The nurse should check that the client's diet is:

A. High in antacids and calcium
B. Low in cholesterol
C. High in protein and carbohydrate
D. Free of electrolytes

147. Antabuse has been ordered for a client to bolster sobriety. In planning discharge teaching sessions, the nurse should include which of the following topics?

A. Importance of reduced smoking
B. Limiting exposure to the sun
C. Medication scheduling and side effects
D. Restricted sexual and physical activity

148. For communicating with the older hearing-impaired person, the nurse issues the following guidelines:

A. "Stand at the person's side, and talk loudly in his or her ear."
B. "Speak at a normal rate."
C. "Speak in short sentences and allow time for a response."
D. "Repeat the message using different words, and raise your voice."

149. When planning the dietary needs of a 68-year-old client, the nurse considers that the older person needs:

A. 800 mg of calcium in the daily diet
B. 1000–1500 mg of calcium in the daily diet
C. 1000–1500 g of calcium in the daily diet
D. 1–1½ g of calcium in the daily diet

150. The nurse is planning fluid intake for a 68-year-old client. The older person should take in the following amount of water daily:

A. 1000 ml
B. 2000 ml
C. 3000 ml
D. 3000 L

151. A 45-year-old client has recently been placed on a low-sodium diet. The nurse is teaching her how to read food labels on food products.

A. "List ingredients contained by amounts, in descending order."
B. "List major ingredients only."
C. "Always give helpful information about sodium content and fiber."
D. "Always list the daily requirements."

152. The nurse recognizes that to communicate with the older person:

A. It should be recognized that silence will create tension
B. Restraints may be necessary to get the older person to listen
C. Ample time must be allowed for questions to be answered and information given
D. Eye contact should be avoided because it may make the older person feel self-conscious

153. When caring for a 68-year-old client, the nurse recognizes that which of the following may contribute to failure to identify the presence of an infection?

A. The cough reflex is less active.
B. The skin is thinner with diminished blood supply.
C. Prostatic hypertrophy reduces the natural ability to flush the bladder.
D. Absence of fever is not unusual.

154. When assessing the home of a 75-year-old home-health client for safety, the nurse identifies that fatal accidents occur most often in the:

A. Bathroom
B. Living room
C. Bedroom
D. Kitchen

155. After assessing the environment of a 70-year-old client, the nurse recognizes the need for further teaching when the client says "I will:

A. Eliminate clutter; ensure a wide pathway."
B. Carpet all stairways, using throw rugs over slippery areas."
C. Keep handles of pans on the stove turned in and away from the pathway."
D. Install and regularly check smoke detectors."

156. A client has a diagnosis of venous thrombosis. The nurse correctly identifies which of the following as a risk factor?

A. Surgical procedures
B. Excessive exercises
C. Decubiti and a diet low in iron
D. Immobility

157. A 24-year-old woman is in active labor with contractions coming every 2 minutes and lasting 60 seconds. Fetal heart rate is 150 bpm. Her BP is 70/50 and the woman's pulse rate 120 bpm. The first nursing action is to:

A. Place the client in lithotomy position
B. Elevate the head of the bed
C. Ask someone else to check the client's pulse
D. Place the client on her left side

158. A 15-year-old girl believes that she is pregnant. Which of the following symptoms does the nurse recognize as one of the earliest indications of pregnancy?

A. Amenorrhea
B. Dysmenorrhea
C. Pica
D. Nausea

159. A 15-year-old girl is 4 months pregnant when she comes to the clinic for her routine checkup. Which of the following symptoms would be abnormal?

A. Urinary frequency
B. Polyphagia
C. Nausea
D. Dysuria

160. A 9-month-old infant is prone to croup. His mother asks what she can do at home to help relieve his symptoms. The nurse suggests:

A. "Give him cough medicine every 4 hours while he is awake."
B. "Give him a warm bath."
C. "Keep the house temperature >80°F (26.6°C)."
D. "Keep the humidity in the house low."

161. A 16-year-old adolescent is 6 hours posttonsillectomy. Which of the following should the nurse include in the care?

A. Position client on her back to promote drainage.
B. Encourage client to cough, clear the throat, or blow the nose frequently.
C. Have the client use a straw to drink cool fluids.
D. Offer a liquid diet and cool fluids first 12–24 hours.

162. A 2-year-old child comes with his mother to the clinic. The child is fussy and irritable, and keeps tugging on his right ear. When assessing the child, the nurse suspects.

A. Ménière's disease
B. Otitis media
C. Otosclerosis
D. Meningitis

163. A 42-year-old client is 5 weeks postileostomy and is beginning to use a permanent appliance. The client is complaining of an odor from the appliance bag. The nurse explains that the best way to prevent odor is to:

A. Use a commercial deodorizer that is sprayed inside the bag
B. Avoid excessive amounts of gas-forming foods
C. Thoroughly clean the bag at regular intervals
D. Refit the bag because of odor leakage

164. The nurse has given the Mantoux tuberculin tests to a family in the clinic. To interpret the results correctly, the nurse would need to know which of the following is a positive reaction at 48 hours?

A. The area of induration
B. The amount of erythema
C. The size of the raised wheal
D. The absence of erythema or induration

165. A 38-year-old client had a cesarean section and delivered premature twins 14 hours ago. She is hungry and wants to start her liquid diet. Before giving a tray to her, the nurse's most important action is to:

A. Check her dressing
B. Check bowel sounds
C. Encourage ambulation
D. Give pain medication

166. A client is unconscious with a head injury from a motor vehicle accident. The nurse is observing him for increased intracranial pressure. Which set of vital signs

would indicate this? His normal vital signs are BP 140/80 mm Hg, P 80 bpm, and R 18/min.

A. R 18, P 100, BP 170/90
B. R 16, P 80, BP 120/76
C. R 12, P 60, BP 180/120
D. R 24, P 120, BP 60/40

167. When giving an enema to a client, the nurse knows that the correct temperature for an enema is:

A. 70–80°F (21.1–26.6°C)
B. 80–90°F (26.6–32.2°C)
C. 102–105°F (38.8–40.5°C)
D. 110–120°F (43.3–48.8°C)

168. A physican asks you to gather equipment so that he can start an (IV) infusion on a client who is to receive blood. The nurse would set up with which IV needle?

A. No. 16 Angiocath
B. No. 22 Angiocath
C. No. 25 butterfly
D. No. 27 butterfly

169. The correct technique for a nurse to use when suctioning is:

A. To occlude the catheter suction port when withdrawing
B. To occlude the catheter suction port when entering
C. To instill 20 ml of normal saline
D. To open the catheter suction port when withdrawing

170. A client is 5 ft 2 in. tall and weighs 100 lb. The nurse is to administer 4.4 ml of gamma globulin IM. The nurse should:

A. Give one injection into the vastus lateralis
B. Give one injection into the gluteus maximus
C. Divide the dosage and give an injection into each deltoid
D. Divide the dosage and give an injection into each buttock in the gluteal muscle

171. The nurse is to administer heparin 5000 units into the abdomen, and should be sure to:

A. Massage the site after the injection
B. Firmly pinch the skin and administer the injection at a 90-degree angle
C. Aspirate before injecting the medicine
D. Give subcutaneously (SC)

172. A 12-year-old boy is in a leg cast for a fractured femur. The most important nursing intervention is to:

A. Palpate for a pedal pulse
B. Palpate for a popliteal pulse
C. Report any drainage on the cast
D. Keep traction on the cast at all time

173. A mother calls the clinic and tells the nurse that her 12-year-old daughter has spilled hot grease on her foot and it has two blisters the size of quarters. The nurse initially advises her to:

A. Break the blisters and cover with a clean dressing
B. Leave the blisters intact and open to air

C. Break the blisters and place ice on the area
D. Leave the blisters intact and apply petrolatum

174. A 3-day-old infant was a healthy newborn. He now has a diagnosis of phenylketonuria (PKU). His mother asks the nurse how the diagnosis was made. Your response is that it was made from which type of specimen?

A. Gastric secretions
B. Arterial blood gases
C. Capillary blood
D. Urine

175. A 14-year-old adolescent is admitted to a behavioral management unit. When planning care, the nurse recognizes that the central task of early adolescence is:

A. Industry versus inferiority
B. Identity versus role confusion
C. Intimacy versus isolation
D. Integrity versus despair

176. While working on a psychiatric unit, the nurse is especially careful to observe depressed clients:

A. In the early morning
B. In the afternoon
C. In the evening
D. At visiting time

177. A 25-year-old client with a diagnosis of schizophrenia is sitting in a corner rocking to and fro, twisting her hands. One of the best initial approaches by the nurse is to:

A. Bring the client some warm milk
B. Hug the client
C. Bring the client a deck of cards
D. Sit quietly by the client

178. Although it is the physician's responsibility to prescribe medication, the nurse should understand the basis for the drug therapy. One of the drugs prescribed is isoniazid for tuberculosis therapy. It would be important for the nurse to know that isoniazid is given with pyridoxine 50–100 mg daily to prevent:

A. Labyrinth damage
B. Peripheral neuritis
C. Renal toxicity
D. GI irritation

179. A client with a diagnosis of tuberculosis has been discharged from the hospital on drug therapy. The most important outcome of the nurse's teaching is for the client to:

A. Take the medications regularly and without interruption
B. Carry extra medication when traveling
C. Learn how to discontinue drugs when symptoms of intolerance occur
D. Wear a Medic Alert bracelet

180. A 40-year-old client is hospitalized with an extensive myocardial infarction. The client is very frustrated with the limitations imposed, such as bedrest. In addition, the client is always complaining about the food. This is an example of:

A. Compensation
B. Denial
C. Displacement
D. Projection

181. The highest-priority nursing intervention for a 39-year-old client with a prolapsed umbilical cord is to:

    A. Leave the room to obtain assistance
    B. Monitor fetal heartbeats
    C. Cover the exposed cord with a sterile dressing
    D. Place in knee-chest or exaggerated Trendelenburg position

182. A 26-year-old client was admitted to the hospital with a diagnosis of appendicitis. Which of the following signs and symptoms are indicative of appendicitis?

    A. Anorexia and high fever
    B. Nausea and vomiting after eating
    C. Tenderness located in the lower right quadrant
    D. Tenderness over McBurney's point

183. Which of the following interventions would be appropriate for a client with suspected appendicitis?

    A. Place a heating pad on the tender area to decrease pain.
    B. Administer an enema preoperatively.
    C. Give the client sips of cool water.
    D. Maintain a semi-Fowler's position.

184. The nurse is sitting with a woman who is in active labor in her home. Because of a hurricane, she cannot be taken to the hospital. What is the most important action for the nurse?

    A. Time contractions for frequency and duration.
    B. Remain calm and support the mother.
    C. Boil water and all the equipment.
    D. Provide the client with a light meal so that she can maintain her strength.

185. A nurse is on a boat where people are eating and drinking. Someone yells "Help! My wife's choking!" The nurse would initially:

    A. Ask the husband, "Can she talk?"
    B. Give a back blow
    C. Give an abdominal thrust
    D. Hit her in the chest

186. The nurse is applying a tourniquet to the upper arm of a client who has sustained a gunshot wound. This is a last resort because:

    A. Tourniquets are difficult to apply
    B. Tourniquets must be released every 20 minutes
    C. Tourniquets may be used below the elbow or knee
    D. Tourniquets cause considerable nerve and tissue damage

187. The nurse is helping to orient a 72-year-old client with organic brain syndrome (OBS) to his room in a nursing home. Which of the following is appropriate?

    A. Give him a complete orientation to the unit and its rules.
    B. Limit the orientation to small, specific amounts of essential information.

C. Show him only his room to avoid further confusion.
D. Ask him questions to determine what he understands.

188. When planning for a 79-year-old client's ADLs, it is essential that the nurse:

    A. Make the client responsible for own care
    B. Encourage the client to do as much of his or her own care as possible
    C. Assign another client to show him or her the routine
    D. Do as much care as possible for the client

189. The physician orders a sputum specimen to be collected on a client suspected of having TB. The specimen is best collected:

    A. At bedtime
    B. In early morning
    C. Before lunch
    D. Time does not matter

190. A client starts having a seizure. It would be most important to:

    A. Protect the head from injury and turn the head to the side
    B. Place a tongue blade or other object between the teeth
    C. Restrain the client to prevent injury
    D. Move the client to the floor and hold her down.

191. A 24-year-old client has been admitted to the emergency room. The physician suspects a head injury and a skull fracture. Cerebrospinal fluid (CSF) leakage may occur. The nurse assesses for:

    A. Watering of the eyes and drainage of mucus from the nose
    B. Clear fluid from the nose or ears
    C. Purulent, thick yellow drainage from the nose or ears
    D. Bleeding from the nose or ears

192. What type of strategy would the nurse teach a 77-year-old client about successful aging?

    A. Eat red meat to keep your protein level up.
    B. Refrain from sexual activity.
    C. Do what makes you happy.
    D. Do not keep any pets.

193. What type of basic nursing intervention is useful in assisting an older person with feelings of self-worth and self-esteem?

    A. Letting the older person decide on his or her food plan
    B. Assisting with hygiene and grooming
    C. Not allowing the older person to take a bath or shower
    D. Refrain from putting cosmetics on the older woman

194. What nursing intervention is appropriate to help maintain mental-health wellness in older adults?

    A. Calling them "honey"
    B. Encouraging dependence
    C. Referring to their diapers used for incontinence
    D. Allowing as much control over care as possible

195. What is the most appropriate response to an older person in teaching about medications?

A. "Take plenty of vitamins."
B. "Use sedatives to help you sleep."
C. "Take daily laxatives."
D. "Take as few medications as possible."

196. What is the responsibility of the hospital nurse in maintaining an older person's mental health?

A. Assess for signs of abuse.
B. Teach instructions for home care to both older person and family.
C. Assess for signs of social isolation.
D. Teach ways to cope with aging.

197. The nurse working in a nursing home identifies which kind of activity that a nursing home resident can have some control over?

A. Administration of routine medications
B. Requesting that certain staff members be assigned to him or her
C. Complete control of the food plan
D. Type and time of bath

198. Which nursing intervention can be used to prevent loneliness in a nursing home resident?

A. Allow clients to wander in other residents' rooms.
B. Provide group learning.
C. Provide individual one-to-one contact.
D. Limit communication for the residents with dementia.

199. What interpersonal impact does humor have on an older person?

A. Humor serves as an outlet for inner tensions and anxieties.
B. Older persons are more likely to be offended when jokes about aging are told by people of their own age group.
C. Humor helps to establish relationships.
D. Humor stimulates alertness.

200. What type of humor intervention can a nurse use in any setting with an older person?

A. Tease the older person even if it is against his or her wishes.
B. Wear scary costumes for effect.
C. Tell grim stories.
D. Use cartoons in teaching materials.

201. How does a nurse develop a culturally appropriate care plan for an older person?

A. By listening to the family's perception of the client's problem
B. By allowing family members time to discuss their perception of the client's problem
C. By acknowledging the older person's viewpoint
D. By recommending a treatment plan based on the physician's recommendation

202. What term is used to describe professional misconduct, negligent care or treatment, or failure to meet the standards of care, resulting in harm to a person?

A. Civil wrongs
B. Torts
C. Malpractice
D. Informed consent

203. Which of the following is not an element of negligence that must be present to substantiate a malpractice claim?

A. Duty
B. Breach of duty
C. Damages
D. Unrelated causal effect

204. Documentation is the best method of defense in a malpractice suit involving an older person. In addition to the malpractice defense, documentation has what other use?

A. Increases the potential areas of legal exposure
B. Describes client education and discharge instructions
C. Relates conversations of nurses among themselves
D. Refrains from recording untoward events such as falls

205. What aspects of documentation about restraints ensures that the nurse acted competently?

A. Failure to document the need for restraints
B. Failure to monitor client's condition properly
C. Documenting client's response to restraints
D. Failure to try alternatives before using restraints

206. What is the nurse's responsibility in obtaining informed consent before surgery?

A. To obtain the informed consent
B. To witness the signature of the client on the informed consent sheet
C. To read the client his or her rights
D. To sign for the client if he or she is unable to do so

207. Clients can exercise their right to refuse treatment in the form of a "do not resuscitate" (DNR) order. How does the nurse ensure that the client's wishes are carried out?

A. Obtain a telephone order from the physician.
B. Request that the physician write a DNR order on the chart.
C. Resuscitate the client on family members' request.
D. Resuscitate the client regardless of the order.

208. To preserve the older person's wishes and protect the health-care providers, the nurse must see that the following is included in the chart:

A. "Slow code" orders
B. Copies of living will and medical power of attorney
C. Telephone order for DNR
D. Physician's request for DNR without family input

209. Which of the following is a common nursing area of legal exposure in caring for older persons?

A. Undermedication
B. Overmedication
C. Reporting complications
D. Assessing the older person's condition every 8 hours

1. **(D)** Nursing process phase: data collection; client need: growth and development through the life span; content area: medical-surgical.

   RATIONALE

   (A) BP increases with age. **(B)** Renal blood flow is nearly halved, renal tubules are less able to concentrate urine, and prostatic hypertrophy is almost universal. Creatinine clearance also steadily decreases with age. **(C)** Peristalsis is decreased, gastric acid is reduced, but constipation rarely arises unless there is poor diet, drug effects, decreased mobility, or disease. **(D)** Average loss in height is 2 inches, the number of taste buds decreases by 70%, and bone mineral content is decreased by 10–15% in men.

2. **(A)** Nursing process phase: data collection; client need: growth and development through the life span; content area: medical-surgical.

   RATIONALE

   (A) High-frequency hearing loss, or presbycusis, occurs with particular problems with high-pitched sounds such as *s, z, sh,* and *ch*. **(B)** Increased susceptibility to postural hypotension occurs because of reduced baroceptor responsiveness. **(C)** Decreased cardiac reserve occurs, making the older person more susceptible to fluid overload. **(D)** Decreased adaptation to dark occurs, making night driving more hazardous.

3. **(A)** Nursing process phase: data collection; client need: growth and development through the life span; content area: medical-surgical.

   RATIONALE

   (A) Arthritis is the most common chronic condition, occurring in 48 of 100 persons over 65 years. **(B)** Hearing impairment occurs in 32 of 100 persons over 65 years. **(C)** Cataracts occur in 17 of 100 persons over 65 years. **(D)** Diabetes occurs in 16 of 100 persons over 65 years.

4. **(D)** Nursing process phase: data collection; client need: growth and development through the life span; content area: medical-surgical.

   RATIONALE

   (A) The gradual loss of lens elasticity, or presbyopia, occurs in the early 40s. **(B)** By age 40, all adults have osteoarthritic changes in the cervical spine. **(C)** Usually in the 40s, a re-examination of the goals and attitudes toward living occurs. **(D)** Difficulty staying up at night and working the next day is the most common early sign of aging.

5. **(D)** Nursing process phase: data collection; client need: growth and development through the life span; content area: medical-surgical.

   RATIONALE

   (A) Although this is a good response because milk helps release hormones and calm the client, it is not the best answer. **(B)** Most older people will not be helped by this. **(C)** Sleep disturbances may occur from nocturia, arthritis, or diabetes. These may require a referral to the doctor; otherwise, sleep disturbance is normal. **(D)** Most older people complain of problems sleeping. A combination of wakefulness, resting, dozing, and sleep is the usual pattern.

6. **(C)** Nursing process phase: data collection; client need: growth and development through the life span; content area: medical-surgical.

   RATIONALE

   (A) Vaginal bleeding is never a normal sign in postmenopausal women. **(B)** Urinary frequency occurs because of decreased bladder capacity and decreased ability of the renal tubules. **(C)** Incontinence may occur because of benign prostatic hypertrophy in men, decreased estrogen in women, and loss of sphincter tone. **(D)** Weight increases until the mid-50s, then declines.

7. **(B)** Nursing process phase: data collection; client need: pharmacological and parenteral therapies; content area: pharmacology.

   RATIONALE

   (A) Weight gain from edema is a common side effect of steroids and nonsteroidal anti-inflammatory drugs (NSAIDs). **(B)** GI hemorrhage occurs when aspirin destroys the lining of the stomach. It can also interfere with platelet functioning. **(C)** Anticonvulsants may cause gingival hypertrophy, but aspirin does not. **(D)** Many drugs, especially histamine H_2 receptor agents, may cause confusion.

8. **(B)** Nursing process phase: data collection; client need: basic care and comfort; content area: medical-surgical.

   RATIONALE

   (A) Fruit and vegetable groups should be increased to 2–4 servings and 3–5 servings per day, respectively. **(B)** Meat, animal products, and dry beans and nuts should be eaten in 2–3 servings per day. **(C)** Sugar and salt intake should be moderate. **(D)** Bread, cereal, and pasta group servings should be 6–11 servings per day.

9. **(A)** Nursing process phase: evaluation; client need: management of care; content area: medical-surgical.

   RATIONALE

   (A) A total hysterectomy involves removal of the uterus. She will no longer be able to have children. **(B)** Lifting of heavy objects and heavy housework should be avoided for 4 weeks. **(C)** Sexual relations can be resumed in 4–6 weeks with physician's approval. **(D)** Mild analgesics can be taken for pain control.

10. **(C)** Nursing process phase: implementation; client need: reduction of risk potential; content area: medical-surgical.

    RATIONALE

    (A) Serosanguinous vaginal drainage is normal for about 2–4 weeks after an abdominal hysterectomy. **(B)** A temperature of 101°F (38.3°C) or more should be immediately reported to the physician. **(C)** Internal hemorrhage from the incision or vagina is a major complication that causes circulating blood volume loss and fluid volume depletion. **(D)** Laboratory findings of 12.0 g/dl Hgb and 36 Hct are normal values.

11. **(B)** Nursing process phase: implementation; client need: reduction of risk potential; content area: medical-surgical.

    RATIONALE

    (A) The client should avoid concentrated carbohydrates because they increase dumping. **(B)** The client should lie down after meals to decrease the effect of gravity. **(C)** The client should eat small, frequent well-balanced meals. **(D)** The client should avoid drinking fluids during and for about 2 hours after eating.

12. **(B)** Nursing process phase: implementation; client need: growth and development through the life span; content area: maternity nursing.

    RATIONALE

    (A) It is important to explain to the parents the necessity of keeping the twins in the hospital, but not of most importance. **(B)** Instructing the parents in how they will be incorporated into the twins' care is most important because it facilitates bonding and identifies expectations. (C) Rest is important, but not of most importance. (D) Parents may call the nursery whenever they need to be reassured or have the need for health teaching.

13. **(B)** Nursing process phase: implementation; client need: growth and development through the life span; content area: pediatrics.
   RATIONALE
   (A) Twins are two individual babies and each needs attention, but not more than usual. (B) Treating the twins as individuals facilitates the future self-identity of each as separate from the other twin. (C) Twins should be treated as individuals, each with his or her own unique personality. (D) New research shows that newborn twins should be kept together to decrease crying, but they may be separated.

14. **(A)** Nursing process phase: implementation; client need: growth and development through the life span; content area: pediatrics.
   RATIONALE
   (A) A return demonstration of parenting skills validates learning. (B) Teaching the parent what to check for when the baby cries is important (i.e., Is the baby wet? Is the baby hungry?). However, safe caregiving is essential. (C) The parents will be taking the babies to the physician's office for follow-up visits. The immunization schedule can be reinforced at that time. (D) Help is not essential for the first few weeks when the babies are brought home.

15. **(A)** Nursing process phase: implementation; client need: physiological adaptation; content area: pediatrics.
   RATIONALE
   (A) Careful monitoring of fluid intake and output (I&O), along with daily measurement of weight and abdominal girth, is essential. (B) A diet high in protein may help to restore the body's normal plasma oncotic pressure. (C) The child with severe edema may be placed on bedrest to promote diuresis. (D) Fluids are restricted based on client's symptoms. Controlling edema is critical.

16. **(C)** Nursing process phase: implementation; client need: growth and development through the life span; content area: pediatrics.
   RATIONALE
   (A) The child does not have the motor skills or intellectual skills to solve a puzzle. (B) The child does not have the motor skills to walk with a push-pull toy. (C) Soft, colorful toys are appropriate for the 6-month-old child. (D) The child does not have the motor skills to ride a rocking horse.

17. **(C)** Nursing process phase: data collection; client need: prevention and early detection of disease; content area: maternity nursing.
   RATIONALE
   (A) Lochia alba (10 days, 6 weeks) is yellowish-white. (B) Leuka is not a valid word. (C) Lochia rubra persists from delivery until about the third day. It is dark red and contains blood, debris from the placenta, and decidua and clots. (D) Lochia serosa is serous, watery pink to brown, occurring from 3 days to 6–10 days.

18. **(D)** Nursing process phase: implementation; client need: physiological adaptation; content area: maternity nursing.
   RATIONALE
   (A) Infections would cause a rise in temperature and are not related to this situation. (B) If it is not an emergency, the midwife or RN does not need to be called. (C) This is a good option, but not the best. (D) A distended bladder can cause uterine relaxation and displace the uterus from its midline position. Emptying the bladder allows the uterus to resume its contracted position.

19. **(D)** Nursing process phase: implementation; client need: basic care and comfort; content area: maternity nursing.
   RATIONALE
   (A) Three days is usually too short. (B) The response that refers to breastfeeding does not address her question appropriately. (C) Although lochia alba may continue normally to the sixth week, it does not always do so. (D) The vaginal discharge will continue until the placental site has healed.

20. **(C)** Nursing process phase: implementation; client need: basic care and comfort; content area: maternity nursing.
   RATIONALE
   (A) Early ambulation is recommended and enhances involution of the uterus. (B) Breastfeeding also enhances involution of the uterus but does not prevent pooling of blood in the vagina. (C) A gush of blood sometimes occurs when the postpartal mother first arises and is caused by pooling of blood in the vagina, which flows out because of gravity when she stands. (D) The vagina does appear edematous and bruised after delivery, but that does not cause the pooling of blood.

21. **(B)** Nursing process phase: implementation; client need: basic care and comfort; content area: maternity nursing.
   RATIONALE
   (A) Limited physical activity, low-roughage diet, and inadequate fluids may postpone the bowel movement and allow it to harden in the rectum, resulting in greater pain at the time of bowel movement. (B) Early ambulation, fluids, and foods with roughage will promote normal evacuation of the bowel, resulting in minimal discomfort as bowel elimination pattern is restored. (C) Encourage foods with roughage to promote normal bowel evacuation. (D) Laxatives may be necessary but should be used as prescribed by the physician. Kegel exercises are important but for reasons other than promoting peristalsis.

22. **(C)** Nursing process phase: planning; client need: reduction of risk potential; content area: maternity nursing.
   RATIONALE
   (A) Bromocriptine mesylate (Parlodel) may be administered after delivery to suppress lactation by preventing the secretion of prolactin. (B) Oxytocin is used to stimulate labor artificially. (C) The mother's blood is Rh-negative while her daughter's is Rh-positive. Injection of $Rh_0(D)$ immune globulin within 72 hours of delivery will prevent her from producing antibodies against the Rh factor, which could harm future pregnancies. (D) Rubella virus vaccine is not related to the Rh factor; it is administered to women who do not already demonstrate immunity.

23. **(C)** Nursing process phase: data collection; client need: prevention and early detection of disease; content area: maternity nursing.
   RATIONALE
   (A) The client should not be asked to provide this information; this could cause the nurse to miss essential data. (B) Above or below the incision is too high or too low. (C) Gentle palpation on the sides of the midline vertical incision should reveal each side of the uterus because the uterus is usually found below the umbilicus and at the midline. (D) To palpate directly over the incision would produce unnecessary pain and trauma to the tissues, and palpation would be hampered by the presence of the dressing material.

24. **(B)** Nursing process phase: implementation; client need: growth and development through the life span; content area: maternity nursing.

RATIONALE
(A) The baby will receive sufficient nutrition from the breast, and giving a bottle after each feeding would prevent successful breastfeeding. (B) A side-lying position, with pillows supporting the mother's head and with baby turned toward mother, provides adequate support for both mother and baby and does not increase incisional pain. (C) Holding the baby high on her abdomen would increase the mother's incisional pain and might not permit the baby adequate access to the nipple. (D) Nipples should be cleansed with water before each feeding; soap may be drying to them.

25. (C) Nursing process phase: implementation; client need: growth and development through the life span; content area: maternity nursing.

RATIONALE
(A) Pain is usually not coming from the abdominal incision. (B) The abdominal discomfort is transitory and will usually be gone in a few days as she continues to breast-feed. (C) The explanation that oxytocin is released and causes the uterus to contract is the response that will promote the mother's understanding, self-care, and breastfeeding success. (D) A mild analgesic may be given 40–60 minutes before the nursing period. Bottle feeding will interfere with the establishment of successful breastfeeding.

26. (C) Nursing process phase: implementation; client need: reduction of risk potential; content area: maternity nursing.

RATIONALE
(A) She needs to breathe deeply to prevent atelectasis and pneumonia. (B) She is not wearing off the anesthetic, and there is no need to contact the physician at this time. (C) She must continue with these measures, which prevent pooling of secretions (hypostatic pneumonia) and collapse of alveoli (atelectasis) during the postanesthesia period. Teach her to splint her incision because the support reduces discomfort. (D) There is no need to call the physician.

27. (B) Nursing process phase: evaluation; client need: growth and development through the life span; content area: maternity nursing.

RATIONALE
(A) The ductus arteriosus connects with the main pulmonary artery and the aorta. These two structures allow most of the fetal blood to bypass the lungs. (B) There is no ductus neonatorum. (C) The ductus venosus is a major blood channel that develops through the embryonic liver from the umbilical vein to the inferior vena cava. (D) The foramen ovale is an opening between the two atria of the heart.

28. (C) Nursing process phase: data collection; client need: growth and development through the life span; content area: maternity nursing.

RATIONALE
(A) Guess again! (B) Recalculate! (C) Apgar scoring allows only one point for a heart rate <100 and one point for pink body with blue extremities. (For each of these to be given two points, the neonate must have a heart rate >100 and a pink body including the extremities.) The other three observations are given two points each, for a total score of eight. (D) Guess again!

29. (A) Nursing process phase: implementation; client need: growth and development through the life span; content area: maternity nursing.

RATIONALE
(A) *Acro* means extremity and *cyanosis* means dark blue. Acrocyanosis of the hands and feet may be normal in an infant within the first few hours after birth. (B) Acrodermatosis is not correct and refers to a skin disease that affects the hands and feet. (C)

Cyanoacrylate adhesives and toxic glues such as "superglue" are not related to description of the infant. (D) Vernix caseosa is a protective sebaceous deposit covering the fetus.

30. (A) Nursing process phase: implementation; client need: reduction of risk potential; content area: maternity nursing.

RATIONALE
(A) Law requires prevention of ophthalmia neonatorum, which is caused by gonococcal organisms, potentially acquired from the mother's birth canal. An erythromycin preparation is preferred over silver nitrate in some institutions. (B) The treatment has no effect on hemorrhagic tendencies. (C) The treatment does not apply to nosocomial infections. (D) The treatment does not apply to staphylococcal infections.

31. (C) Nursing process phase: implementation; client need: growth and development through the life span; content area: maternity nursing.

RATIONALE
(A) There is no reason to wait until the neonatal nursery evaluation is complete or to refuse the request. (B) Even in facilities where sterile water is given as a newborn infant's first feeding, glucose water is not used because, if aspirated, it is dangerous to lung tissue. (C) Putting a baby to the breast after delivery provides both physiological and psychosocial benefits. For example, it stimulates the production of oxytocin, which causes the uterus to contract, assisting with delivery of the placenta and control of bleeding. (D) There is no reason to refuse her request.

32. (B) Nursing process phase: data collection; client need: growth and development through the life span; content area: maternity nursing.

RATIONALE
(A) Select another answer. (B) A neonate is an infant from birth through the first 28 days of life. An infant is a child <1 year of age. (C) Guess again! (D) Guess again!

33. (A) Nursing process phase: implementation; client need: prevention and early detection of disease; content area: medical-surgical.

RATIONALE
(A) Norepinephrine is a stimulant that causes peripheral vasoconstriction and increased blood pressure and heart rate. (B) This hormone causes gluconeogenesis, a negative nitrogen balance, decrease in the immune response, and increased platelet activity. This results in an increase in the amount of available energy fuel, slowing of the tissue repair process, and increased risk of infection and increased clot formation. (C) Release of this hormone causes sodium and water reabsorption, leading to decreased urination and an increased circulatory volume. (D) The release of antidiuretic hormone causes the physiological changes listed in rationale C.

34. (A) Nursing process phase: data collection; client need: prevention and early detection of disease; content area: maternity nursing.

RATIONALE
(A) The apical pulse rate is most accurate. (B) Auscultating for a full minute provides greater opportunity for noting variations and abnormalities. (C) Auscultating for a full minute provides greater opportunity for noting variations and abnormalities. (D) Peripheral pulses should also be evaluated to detect any lags or unusual characteristics.

35. (C) Nursing process phase: data collection; client need: growth and development through the life span; content area: maternity nursing.

RATIONALE
(A) Rates as low as 70–90 during sleep have been reported as nor-

mal. **(B)** Rates of 100–120 are below normal if the baby is awake. **(C)** Rates of 120–150 while the baby is awake are normal. **(D)** Rates may be as high as 180 when the newborn infant is crying.

36. **(D)** Nursing process phase: data collection; client need: prevention and early detection of disease; content area: maternity nursing.

RATIONALE

(A) Normal full-term neonates pass meconium within 24 hours of life, or at least by 48 hours. **(B)** Many newborn infants void immediately after birth, 92% void by 24 hours, and 99% by 48 hours. **(C)** A perforate anus allows passage of a rectal thermometer, so option C is never normal. **(D)** Rust-colored or pink stains on a diaper with voiding are most likely to be normal. Large amounts of uric acid are excreted during the newborn period, and these urates appear as pink stains ("brick dust spots" or "brick dust") on a diaper.

37. **(A)** Nursing process phase: implementation; client need: management of care; content area: medical-surgical.

RATIONALE

(A) This statement is true. If a client should express a lack of understanding of the procedure or an unwillingness to continue with the surgery, this should be reported to the nursing supervisor and to the client's physician immediately. **(B)** No client should receive preoperative medication until the consent form has been signed. Mind-altering medication renders the client mentally incompetent. When the medication has been given, the drug effects should be allowed to wear off before the consent can be obtained. **(C)** Competent adults should sign their own consent forms. Spouses, children, and friends cannot do so legally. **(D)** The surgeon and the anesthesia care provider, not the perioperative nurse, are required to inform the client of the risks of procedures.

38. **(D)** Nursing process phase: implementation; client need: pharmacological and parenteral therapies; content area: maternity nursing.

RATIONALE

(A) Aquaphor is a trade name for petrolatum. **(B)** Cyanocobalamin does not help produce clotting factors. **(C)** Erythromycin is an antibiotic used for prophylaxis of gonorrheal conjunctivitis. **(D)** The absence of normal flora needed to synthesize vitamin K in the newborn infant's gut creates a transient blood coagulation deficiency. There are usually no clinical consequences, but an injection of this substance is given prophylactically on the day of birth to combat the deficiency. Aqua-Mephyton is a trade name for phytonadione (vitamin K).

39. **(C)** Nursing process phase: implementation; client need: reduction of risk potential; content area: medical-surgical.

RATIONALE

(A) A deep breath through the nose is most effective. **(B)** Breathing in through the nose is recommended. **(C)** After surgery there is a decline in lung ventilation and gas exchange that varies with the individual client, length of anesthesia, and surgical site. The client is taught this technique of sustained maximal inspiration to prevent collapse of alveoli and to mobilize secretions after surgery. **(D)** A slow breath through the nose and coughing from the chest is most effective.

40. **(D)** Nursing process phase: data collection; client need: basic care and comfort; content area: maternity nursing.

RATIONALE

(A) Well-formed brown stools are unusual for newborn infants. **(B)** The stools of a breast-fed newborn infant may be pasty green, but dark green is normal only for meconium. **(C)** Normal newborn stools vary in frequency from up to 10 daily to one every 2–3 days. **(D)** Breast-fed infants usually produce stools that are yellow-gold, soft, or mushy. They are more liquid, more frequent, and less pale yellow than those of formula-fed infants.

41. **(B)** Nursing process phase: implementation; client need: basic care and comfort; content area: maternity nursing.

RATIONALE

(A) The American Academy of Pediatrics (1988) recommends breast milk as the optimal food for the first 4–6 months of life. **(B)** The American Academy of Pediatrics (1988) recommends breast milk as the optimal food for the first 4–6 months of life. **(C)** The American Academy of Pediatrics (1988) recommends breast milk as the optimal food for the first 4–6 months of life. **(D)** The American Academy of Pediatrics (1988) recommends breast milk as the optimal food for the first 4–6 months of life.

42. **(B)** Nursing process phase: data collection; client need: prevention and early detection of disease; content area: medical-surgical.

RATIONALE

(A) She should have no difficulty with carbohydrates. Select another option. **(B)** Inflammation of the gallbladder (cholecystitis), presence of gallstones (cholelithiasis), or both interfere with movement of bile from the liver or gallbladder into the small intestine, where it promotes the digestion of fats. **(C)** She should have no difficulty with protein. Select another option. **(D)** She should have no difficulty with vitamin C. Select another option.

43. **(C)** Nursing process phase: implementation; client need: reduction of risk potential; content area: medical-surgical.

RATIONALE

(A) Leg exercises will not help to prevent muscle spasms. **(B)** Paralytic ileus is paralysis of intestines, which may occur after any abdominal surgery but is not prevented by leg exercises. **(C)** Muscle contractions involved in the leg exercise increase venous return and therefore help prevent stasis of blood and clot formation. If a clot forms and becomes dislodged, the resulting embolus can be life threatening. **(D)** Vasogenic shock results from inadequate vascular tone caused by nerve injury, chemicals, or sepsis and is not affected by leg exercises.

44. **(A)** Nursing process phase: implementation; client need: pharmacological and parenteral therapies; content area: medical-surgical.

RATIONALE

(A) Isotonic solutions of the two agents in the question would be 0.9% sodium chloride or 5% dextrose. **(B)** The 0.45% sodium chloride is hypotonic. **(C)** The 10% dextrose is hypertonic. **(D)** The 50% dextrose is hypertonic.

45. **(A)** Nursing process phase: implementation; client need: pharmacological and parenteral therapies; content area: medical-surgical.

RATIONALE

(A) Preoperative medications often cause drowsiness or dizziness. After administration, the bed siderails should be up and the room light dim. The calm, drowsy state should be interrupted only when necessary and then briefly and quietly. **(B)** Her bladder should have been emptied before the medication was administered. **(C)** It is not safe to allow the client to move around in the room. **(D)** The nurse should explain the procedure or answer any questions before the client is premedicated.

46. **(B)** Nursing process phase: implementation; client need: reduction of risk potential; content area: medical-surgical.

RATIONALE

(A) Deep-breathing and coughing mainly affect respiratory function. **(B)** The benefits of early ambulation include improved respiratory, circulatory, and GI function; improved wound healing because of improved circulation; increased comfort and morale; reduced pain; and reduced recovery time, hospital stay, and expenses. **(C)** Leg exercises mainly affect circulatory function. **(D)** Medication for pain increases comfort and rest.

47. **(C)** Nursing process phase: implementation; client need: reduction of risk potential; content area: medical-surgical.

    RATIONALE

    (A) The pain medication may reduce the sensation of pain but would not prevent emboli. **(B)** Pain, tenderness, and swelling in the lower extremity may signal the presence of a clot. She must be placed on bedrest. The physician will decide whether to continue the bedrest. The desired outcome is prevention of an embolism. **(C)** Pain, tenderness, and swelling in the lower extremity after surgery signal the potential presence of phlebothrombosis. Immobilization helps to prevent embolus formation by reducing the chances for thrombi to break loose. **(D)** Massage may cause release of a clot into the bloodstream (i.e., formation of an embolism).

48. **(C)** Nursing process phase: implementation; client need: pharmacological and parenteral therapies; content area: medical-surgical.

    RATIONALE

    (A) Aspirin also reduces pain and fever, but for those effects a higher dosage is usually required. **(B)** Aspirin is not an antibiotic. **(C)** Given in small doses in conjunction with a surgical procedure, aspirin may be used for its prophylactic anticoagulation effect. **(D)** Aspirin also reduces pain and fever, but for those effects a higher dosage is usually required.

49. **(A)** Nursing process phase: implementation; client need: reduction of risk potential; content area: medical-surgical

    RATIONALE

    (A) Postoperative positioning after total hip replacement varies with the type of prosthesis and its method of insertion. However, positioning is usually directed at maintaining abduction and limiting flexion of the hip. **(B)** Leg adduction can cause dislocation. **(C)** Hip flexion >90 degrees can cause dislocation. **(D)** This cannot be done. Select another option.

50. **(B)** Nursing process phase: implementation; client need: reduction of risk potential; content area: medical-surgical.

    RATIONALE

    (A) After total hip replacement it is important not to flex the hip >90 degrees and to avoid extremes of internal rotation, adduction, and flexion of the hip to prevent dislocation. Routine activities of daily living (ADLs) are not possible in 1 week. **(B)** After total hip replacement it is important not to flex the hip >90 degrees and to avoid extremes of internal rotation, adduction, and flexion of the hip to prevent dislocation. Other ADLs are usually possible by 3 months after surgery. **(C)** After total hip replacement it is important not to flex the hip >90 degrees and to avoid extremes of internal rotation, adduction, and flexion of the hip to prevent dislocation. Routine ADLs are possible after 3 months. **(D)** After total hip replacement it is important not to flex the hip >90 degrees and to avoid extremes of internal rotation, adduction, and flexion of the hip to prevent dislocation. Routine ADLs are possible after 3 months.

51. **(D)** Nursing process phase: data collection; client need: pharmacological and parenteral therapies; content area: medical-surgical.

    RATIONALE

    (A) It is inappropriate to simply administer furosemide (Lasix) when urinary output is insufficient. **(B)** Calling the physician is an inappropriate response. The physician will be unable to diag-

nose the problem completely if he or she is not presented with all the facts of the situation. **(C)** The client's symptoms imply a problem requiring immediate attention, not one that may be postponed for 30 minutes. **(D)** Collected data indicate digitalis toxicity; however, additional data regarding blood levels of digoxin are required to determine appropriate action. In this case, the physician would be most likely to hold the digoxin until blood levels return to therapeutic range.

52. **(C)** Nursing process phase: data collection; client need: pharmacological and parenteral therapies; content area: medical-surgical.

    RATIONALE

    (A) Calcium should not be significantly affected. Select another option. **(B)** Chloride should not be significantly affected. Select another option. **(C)** Furosemide is a potassium-depleting diuretic. **(D)** Sodium should not be significantly affected. Select another option.

53. **(C)** Nursing process phase: implementation; client need: pharmacological and parenteral therapies; content area: medical-surgical.

    RATIONALE

    (A) Administration of additional morphine may result in respiratory arrest. **(B)** Administration of additional morphine may result in respiratory arrest. **(C)** Decreased respiratory rate is an early sign of morphine toxicity. If the client's respiratory rate is 8–10 or less, withhold a repeated dose and consult the physician. Another narcotic may relieve the pain without depression of respiration. **(D)** Leaving the room to allow the client to be alone does not address her current need.

54. **(B)** Nursing process phase: implementation; client need: reduction of risk potential; content area: medical-surgical.

    RATIONALE

    (A) Bryant's traction is continuous skin traction. **(B)** Bryant's traction is skin traction applied to both legs to minimize potential trauma to the affected leg while maintaining appropriate position of the bone fragments. It involves bilateral vertical extension of the legs and is continuously applied. **(C)** Bryant's traction is continuous skin traction. **(D)** Bryant's traction is continuous skin traction.

55. **(A)** Nursing process phase: implementation; client need: reduction of risk potential; content area: medical-surgical.

    RATIONALE

    (A) With Bryant's traction, the child's weight serves as counter-traction to the vertical pull of the weights. It is necessary, then, for his buttocks to be elevated and clear of the bed to allow his weight to pull against the force of the weights. An abdominal restraint is usually necessary to keep him from turning from side to side. **(B)** The buttocks must be elevated to allow countertraction to the vertical pull of the weights. An abdominal restraint is usually necessary to keep him from turning side to side. **(C)** A sling is not appropriate. **(D)** A pillow is not appropriate.

56. **(B)** Nursing process phase: implementation; client need: growth and development through the life span; content area: medical-surgical.

    RATIONALE

    (A) The Band-Aid applies to toddlers, not infants. **(B)** One of the primary developmental concerns at 8–12 months of age is separation anxiety. The infant becomes more possessive of his mother, clings to her to avoid separation, and fears strangers. **(C)** Eye contact and touch are especially important during the first month of life when bonding between mother and child is beginning. **(D)** The limits and choices apply to toddlers, not infants.

57. **(B)** Nursing process phase: implementation; client need: pharmacological and parenteral therapies; content area: pediatrics.

RATIONALE

(A) The medication is ordered for a set number of days and is given whether or not a rash is present. **(B)** Penicillin G is given for 7–10 days to eradicate the streptococcal infection completely and prevent its complications, although symptoms will usually subside within the first couple of days. **(C)** The medication is ordered for a set number of days whether or not the temperature is normal. **(D)** The medication is ordered for a set number of days whether or not the throat is sore.

58. **(A)** Nursing process phase: implementation; client need: reduction of risk potential; content area: pediatrics.

RATIONALE

(A) Urinalysis allows early diagnosis and treatment of acute glomerulonephritis. Some of the serious complications that can follow infections with group A β-hemolytic streptococci include acute glomerulonephritis, rheumatic fever, peritonsillar abscess, pneumonia, and meningitis. **(B)** Urinalysis is not usually associated directly with pyelonephritis. Select another option. **(C)** Urinalysis is not usually associated with HIV (AIDS). Select another option. **(D)** Urinalysis is not usually associated with urinary tract infections. Select another option.

59. **(C)** Nursing process phase: implementation; client need: coping and adaptation; content area: pediatrics.

RATIONALE

(A) Missing a full week would only add to this problem. **(B)** The school counselor is not needed. **(C)** Because he is an 8-year-old school-age child, the boy's problem is probably concern about falling behind in school, resulting in the loss of his role or position at school. He may fear loss of recently mastered skills, and keeping up with his work could prevent this fear. **(D)** Returning to school early may interfere with his physical recovery.

60. **(C)** Nursing process phase: implementation; client need: reduction of risk potential; content area: medical-surgical.

RATIONALE

(A) Labia must remain separated during collection. **(B)** Cleansing is from least contaminated area to most contaminated area, or front to back. **(C)** The initial stream of urine is allowed to flow into the bedpan or toilet, the midstream portion is collected, and the sterile specimen container is removed from the stream while the client is still voiding. **(D)** Examination of urine is most reliable if examined within the hour after voiding.

61. **(B)** Nursing process phase: data collection; client need: physiological adaptation; content area: medical-surgical.

RATIONALE

(A) Select another option. **(B)** Urine volume varies depending on fluid intake, cardiac and renal condition of the client, hormonal influences, and loss of fluid in perspiration or exhaled air. **(C)** Select another option. **(D)** Select another option.

62. **(D)** Nursing process phase: data collection; client need: physiological adaptation; content area: medical-surgical.

RATIONALE

(A) Select another option. **(B)** Select another option. **(C)** Select another option. **(D)** Jell-O and creamed soup are considered liquids along with the tea. Eleven ounces multiplied by 30 ml/oz yields a total of 330 ml.

63. **(A)** Nursing process phase: planning; client need: basic care and comfort; content area: medical-surgical.

RATIONALE

(A) Inserting a Foley catheter will not help the client to regain voluntary control of bladder function. **(B)** Nursing interventions are appropriate to goals sought. **(C)** Nursing interventions are appropriate to goals sought. **(D)** Nursing interventions are appropriate to goals sought.

64. **(A)** Nursing process phase: implementation; client need: basic care and comfort; content area: medical-surgical.

RATIONALE

(A) Proper cleansing and drying are basic to maintenance of skin integrity. **(B)** Padding clothing or bed linen and applying barrier creams may be important but secondary to providing a clean, dry skin surface. **(C)** Padding clothing or bed linen and applying barrier creams may be important but are secondary to providing a clean, dry skin surface. **(D)** Use of diapers should be discouraged because they are demeaning and may convey the impression that incontinence is permissible.

65. **(B)** Nursing process phase: planning; client need: physiological adaptation; content area: medical-surgical.

RATIONALE

(A) A flexion contracture is a permanent contraction of a muscle resulting from spasm or paralysis. **(B)** A pressure ulcer results from continued pressure, usually over a bony prominence. Skin breakdown can be hastened by improper cleansing or infrequent alteration of position. Massage can promote circulation in the areas of concern, helping to decrease the possibility of skin breakdown. **(C)** A pressure ulcer may be considered a "dermatologic crisis," but this is not the appropriate answer to the question. **(D)** Any pressure point is not itself a "complication."

66. **(C)** Nursing process phase: planning; client need: reduction of risk potential; content area: medical-surgical.

RATIONALE

(A) The left Sims' position is between a lateral and a prone position and is suitable for vaginal and rectal access. **(B)** In the supine or dorsal position, the client is in a back-lying position with legs extended. **(C)** In the dorsal recumbent position, the client lies on her back with knees flexed and hips rotated eternally, a position that allows access to the urinary meatus in the female client. **(D)** In the prone position, the client is lying flat on her abdomen.

67. **(D)** Nursing process phase: implementation; client need: reduction of risk potential; content area: medical-surgical.

RATIONALE

(A) Option A is incorrect because a specimen of urine that has been standing in the bag should never be used for examination. Urine changes on standing, and sterility cannot be ensured at the drainage port. **(B)** Option B also is incorrect: a system designed to remain closed should never be opened; again, sterility cannot be ensured. **(C)** As suggested in option C, puncture above the bifurcation may damage the channel used to inflate the balloon and may lead to deflation; also, some materials used in the manufacture of catheters do not close completely after puncture. **(D)** The port is designed to allow penetration with a sterile system and closure on withdrawal of a needle.

68. **(B)** Nursing process phase: implementation; client need: reduction of risk potential; content area: medical-surgical.

RATIONALE

(A) Prophylactic therapy is used in some instances. **(B)** Proper handwashing by all personnel and clients is fundamental to the control of all infections. No other measures surpass handwashing in importance for controlling the spread of infection. **(C)** Proper disposal of potentially infective materials is essential. No other measures surpass handwashing in importance for controlling the spread of infection. **(D)** Educational programs may be helpful, but such knowledge is most valuable when applied in practice.

69. **(C)** Nursing process phase: implementation; client need: safety and infection control; content area: medical-surgical.

    RATIONALE

    (A) To minimize the possibility for infection, no unsterile solutions or equipment should be introduced into the urethra, urinary bladder, or trachea. **(B)** Hyperalimentation is a means of providing nutrients IV. Clients receiving total parenteral nutrition (TPN) are particularly susceptible to catheter-related infections. Strict aseptic technique must be maintained during the TPN procedure and in regard to the dressings at the site. **(C)** The alimentary canal is not sterile; therefore, unsterile (but clean) equipment and solutions can be introduced to that body system. Other procedures carried out using clean technique include gastrostomy feedings, colostomy care, and enemas. **(D)** To minimize the possibility for infection, no unsterile solutions or equipment should be introduced into the urethra, urinary bladder, or trachea.

70. **(B)** Nursing process phase: data collection; client need: pharmacological and parenteral therapies; content area: medical-surgical.

    RATIONALE

    (A) Allopurinol, probenecid, and sulfinpyrazone are maintenance drugs used for chronic gout. The choice among these drugs depends on the physiological mechanism underlying the disorder. **(B)** Decrease in client symptoms on administration of colchicine is useful in establishing a diagnosis of gout or gouty arthritis. **(C)** Allopurinol, probenecid, and sulfinpyrazone are maintenance drugs used for chronic gout. The choice among these drugs depends on the physiological mechanism underlying the disorder. **(D)** Allopurinol, probenecid, and sulfinpyrazone are maintenance drugs used for chronic gout. The choice among these drugs depends on the physiological mechanism underlying the disorder.

71. **(D)** Nursing process phase: data collection; client need: prevention and early detection of disease; content area: medical-surgical.

    RATIONALE

    (A) Pain, swelling, increased heat, and redness are classic manifestations of inflammation such as gout. **(B)** Pain, swelling, increased heat, and redness are classic manifestations of inflammation such as gout. **(C)** Pain, swelling, increased heat, and redness are classic manifestations of inflammation such as gout. **(D)** The toe would exhibit cyanosis.

72. **(B)** Nursing process phase: implementation; client need: reduction of risk potential; content area: medical-surgical.

    RATIONALE

    (A) The first voided specimen at 8 AM on the day of collection is discarded. **(B)** All other voidings after the 8 AM voiding, including the final voiding at 8 AM on the day the collection ends, must be included in the sample. **(C)** The sample must be kept refrigerated or cooled in the room during collection. **(D)** All urine is saved for 24-hour collections.

73. **(D)** Nursing process phase: planning; client need: physiological integrity; content area: medical-surgical.

    RATIONALE

    (A) Clients with gout should increase fluids to 3000 ml/day unless contraindicated. **(B)** Fasting and crash diets increase the serum uric acid level and should be avoided. **(C)** High-purine diet (shellfish, liver, organ meats, sardines, anchovies) and excessive alcohol intake should be avoided to avoid precipitation of an acute attack of gout. **(D)** Increased fluids and alkaline foods such as potatoes or milk increase the urine pH and decrease formation of uric acid crystals, which may lead to formation of kidney stones.

74. **(A)** Nursing process phase: implementation; client need: basic care and comfort; content area: medical-surgical.

    RATIONALE

    (A) Gout is one of the most excruciatingly painful conditions that the nurse may see. Often a cradle is required to keep the pressure of a sheet from the affected joint. Any or all of the additional measures may be appropriate nursing interventions. Pressure will not relieve pain in the affected joint. **(B)** Cold or heat may relieve pain. **(C)** Analgesics or anti-inflammatory agents may relieve pain. **(D)** Immobilization may decrease pain.

75. **(C)** Nursing process phase: planning; client need: pharmacological and parenteral therapies; content area: medical-surgical.

    RATIONALE

    (A) Administration of drugs for emotional support is not viable. **(B)** There is no known cure for arthritis. **(C)** Reduction of pain and inflammation is the major purpose of drug therapy. **(D)** Drugs may be given in preparation for surgery, but option D is inappropriate for the question asked.

76. **(A)** Nursing process phase: planning; client need: pharmacological and parenteral therapies; content area: medical-surgical.

    RATIONALE

    (A) The standard drop factor indicates the number of drops per milliliter that the tubing will deliver. Multiplying the drop factor of 10 by the total milliliters gives 30,000, the number of drops to be given in 24 hours. Multiplying 60 minutes by 24 hours calculates the total number of minutes in 24 hours (1440). Dividing 30,000 drops by 1440 minutes comes to 21.5 drops/min. The nurse should set the infusion to administer approximately 21 drops/min to administer 3000 ml in 24 hours. **(B)** Recalculate. **(C)** Recalculate. **(D)** Recalculate.

77. **(D)** Nursing process phase: data collection; client need: pharmacological and parenteral therapies; content area: medical-surgical.

    RATIONALE

    (A) Option A is appropriate because swelling may demonstrate the presence of edema, suggesting infiltration. **(B)** Option B is appropriate because the client may have moved an arm, which may have caused the bevel of the needle to lie against the side of the vein, thereby obstructing the flow of solution. **(C)** Option C may be appropriate because patency of the tubing may be assessed by observing return of blood from the client into the IV tubing when the receptacle is lowered. **(D)** Never flush the needle or cannula by injecting saline with a syringe and needle directly into the tubing because such action may force a blood clot into circulation.

78. **(A)** Nursing process phase: data collection; client need: pharmacological and parenteral therapies; content area: medical-surgical.

    RATIONALE

    (A) In addition to the aforementioned symptoms, a client experiencing circulatory overload may exhibit venous distention, syncope, shock, dyspnea, and cyanosis resulting from pulmonary edema. **(B)** Drug overload may occur from receiving an excessive amount of fluid containing drugs; and symptoms may include dizziness, fainting leading to shock, and symptoms specific to the offending drug. **(C)** Superficial thrombophlebitis may produce tenderness at first with subsequent pain along the course of the vein, edema and redness at injection site, and excessive warmth in the affected arm as compared with the other arm. These signs are characteristic of inflammation. **(D)** An air embolism results when air gets into the circulatory system. Symptoms may include hypotension, cyanosis, tachycardia, increased venous pressure, and loss of consciousness.

79. **(C)** Nursing process phase: planning; client need: pharmacological and parenteral therapies; content area: medical-surgical.

RATIONALE

(A) Epinephrine, terbutaline sulfate, and theophylline each act to relieve bronchospasm. **(B)** Epinephrine, terbutaline sulfate, and theophylline each act to relieve bronchospasm. **(C)** Cromolyn sodium has no bronchodilator, anti-inflammatory, or antihistamine action. Cromolyn is not effective for acute bronchial asthmatic attacks. Cromolyn inhibits the allergic reaction if inhaled before the challenge by the antigen. **(D)** Epinephrine, terbutaline sulfate, and theophylline each act to relieve bronchospasm.

80. **(D)** Nursing process phase: implementation; client need: reduction of risk potential; content area: medical-surgical.

RATIONALE

(A) Tubing should be inserted 3–4 inches for an adult (1–2 inches for a child). **(B)** For some radiologic procedures (relating to the transverse colon), the client may need to receive the enema while lying on the right side, but unless specified, the left side is the position of choice. **(C)** Solution should not flow moderately fast. **(D)** Fluid should flow slowly, the client should take as much as possible of amount ordered, and tubing should be clamped before removing from anus to prevent leakage. Tip is lubricated and left lateral position is the preferred position for administration of an enema, because it facilitates flow of solution by gravity into the sigmoid and descending colon, which are on the left side.

81. **(A)** Nursing process phase: data collection; client need: prevention and early detection of disease; content area: medical-surgical.

RATIONALE

(A) The tonometer is placed directly on the anesthetized cornea. A reading of 11–22 mm Hg indicates intraocular pressure that is within normal limits. **(B)** A reading of 24–32 mm Hg suggests glaucoma. **(C)** A reading of 35–44 mm Hg suggests glaucoma. **(D)** Readings of 50–75 mm Hg can occur with acute attacks in clients with acute (angle-closure) glaucoma.

82. **(D)** Nursing process phase: planning; client need: pharmacological and parenteral therapies; content area: medical-surgical.

RATIONALE

(A) Diagnosis has already been made if treatment has begun. **(B)** Control of intraocular pressure may be desired before surgery, but the primary objective of treatment for glaucoma is reduction of intraocular pressure, which may damage the optic nerve and result in blindness. **(C)** Option C has no relationship to the question. **(D)** Reduction of intraocular pressure is the ultimate goal in drug treatment of glaucoma.

83. **(B)** Nursing process phase: planning; client need: pharmacological and parenteral therapies; content area: medical-surgical.

RATIONALE

(A) Dilation of the pupil could obstruct the flow of aqueous humor and thereby increase intraocular pressure. **(B)** A miotic drug causes the pupil to contract, allowing the iris to draw away from the cornea, thus facilitating the drainage of aqueous humor through lymph spaces in the canal of Schlemm. **(C)** Glaucoma is a disorder that can be controlled rather than cured. **(D)** Anesthetic action is needed during tonometry but not for treatment of glaucoma.

84. **(B)** Nursing process phase: implementation; client need: pharmacological and parenteral therapies; content area: medical-surgical.

RATIONALE

(A) Acetazolamide is a carbonic anhydrase inhibitor that decreases production of aqueous humor. **(B)** Pilocarpine constricts the pupil (miosis) and contracts ciliary musculature, facilitating aqueous outflow. **(C)** Mannitol reduces intraocular pressure by increasing blood osmolality. **(D)** Phenylbutazone is an anti-inflammatory agent not associated with ocular therapy.

85. **(A)** Nursing process phase: implementation; client need: pharmacological and parenteral therapies; content area: medical-surgical.

RATIONALE

(A) The symbol for the number 2 in the apothecary system of measurement is two lowercase "i's." The abbreviation for left eye is OS. The abbreviation for four times a day is qid. **(B)** Eleven drops is incorrect. **(C)** The right eye would be designated OD, and every day is qd. **(D)** Both eyes would be designated OU.

86. **(C)** Nursing process phase: implementation; client need: pharmacological and parenteral therapies; content area: medical-surgical.

RATIONALE

(A) The client should focus gaze upward toward the forehead. **(B)** The medication should not hit the sensitive cornea. **(C)** The nurse pulls the lower lid down gently and drops medication into the center of the lower lid as the client focuses gaze upward toward the forehead. **(D)** The eyedropper should remain sterile. An eyedropper that touches the lower lid will be contaminated. Bacterial contamination of the solution may result.

87. **(A)** Nursing process phase: planning; client need: pharmacological and parenteral therapies; content area: medical-surgical.

RATIONALE

(A) Excessive absorption of strong drugs (e.g., epinephrine) may occur through the nasolacrimal duct, leading to undesirable effects. **(B)** This option is not a priority reason. **(C)** This option does not prevent blinking. **(D)** Option D is also a correct reason for occlusion of the nasolacrimal duct but may be secondary in importance to prevention of systemic absorption of the drug.

88. **(C)** Nursing process phase: planning; client need: pharmacological and parenteral therapies; content area: medical-surgical.

RATIONALE

(A) Beta-blockers may be used to achieve miosis. **(B)** Antiemetics may be employed to help prevent vomiting in a client with acute glaucoma (which could increase intraocular pressure). **(C)** Mydriatics (e.g., atropine) in a glaucomatous eye may precipitate an acute glaucoma attack that may result in blindness. (Mydriatics cause pupillary dilation.) It is important also that the client be cautioned against using over-the-counter drugs such as antihistamines, as these may contain mydriatics. **(D)** Analgesics may be prescribed to alleviate pain of acute glaucoma.

89. **(C)** Nursing process phase: implementation; client need: pharmacological and parenteral therapies; content area: medical-surgical.

RATIONALE

(A) Recalculate. **(B)** Recalculate. **(C)** The ratio and proportion method helps ensure accurate calculation of drug dosages. In this problem, 5 mg is to 1 tablet as 10 mg is to x tablets. Cross-multiplying gives $5x = 10$ mg. Then $x = 10$ mg $\div$ 5 mg. Finally, $x = 2$ tablets. **(D)** Recalculate.

90. **(A)** Nursing process phase: implementation; client need: reduction of risk potential; content area: medical-surgical.

RATIONALE

(A) The client is positioned on the unoperative side to eliminate pressure on the suture line. **(B)** The patch and shield protect the eye from accidental injury. **(C)** Antiemetics and laxatives should be administered as ordered. **(D)** The client should not lift, pull, or push heavy objects.

91. **(D)** Nursing process phase: planning; client need: management of care; content area: medical-surgical.

    RATIONALE
    (A) The cause of a problem should be determined before treatment is instituted. **(B)** The cause of a problem should be determined before treatment is instituted. **(C)** The cause of a problem should be determined before treatment is instituted. **(D)** Vocational nurses are not licensed to prescribe medications.

92. **(C)** Nursing process phase: data collection; client need: prevention and early detection of disease; content area: pediatrics.

    RATIONALE
    (A) Conjunctivitis is inflammation of the conjunctiva (lines the eyelids and is reflected onto the eyeball). **(B)** Otitis media may result from tonsillitis, but the listed characteristics better described otitis media than tonsillitis. **(C)** The presenting signs and symptoms are characteristic of otitis media. The client may also exhibit signs of vomiting and diarrhea. **(D)** Cystitis is inflammation of the urinary bladder.

93. **(A)** Nursing process phase: evaluation; client need: growth and development through the life span; content area: pediatrics.

    RATIONALE
    (A) In infants and young children, the eustachian tubes are short, wide, and straight and lie in a somewhat horizontal plane. **(B)** This statement is accurate. **(C)** This statement is accurate. **(D)** This statement is accurate.

94. **(B)** Nursing process phase: implementation; client need: pharmacological and parenteral therapies; content area: pediatrics.

    RATIONALE
    (A) This intervention is part of the correct procedure. **(B)** For infants and children <3 years of age, the nurse pulls the pinna down and back to administer eardrops. Because the external auditory canal is cartilaginous and straight, downward action separates the walls of the canal for instillation. The adult ear canal has more ossification and angles slightly, so a gentle pull upward straightens the canal. Positioning the client on the unaffected side allows medication to flow inward by gravity. Allowing the client to remain in the same position keeps the medication from running out of the canal. The drops are directed toward the ear canal because drops that hit the tympanic membrane directly may cause pain. Two additional measures associated with instillation of eardrops are (1) warm the medication by rolling the bottle in the hands for a few minutes (cold medication may induce nausea or vertigo), and (2) the nurse's hand should rest on the client's head for stabilization to help prevent injury if the client moves. **(C)** This intervention is part of the correct procedure. **(D)** This intervention is part of the correct procedure.

95. **(D)** Nursing process phase: evaluation; client need: pharmacological and parenteral therapies; content area: pediatrics.

    RATIONALE
    (A) Theoretical knowledge of a procedure or memorization of factual information concerning the process may not ensure ability to apply the knowledge in practice. **(B)** Theoretical knowledge of a procedure or memorization of factual information concerning the process may not ensure ability to apply the knowledge in practice. **(C)** Theoretical knowledge of a procedure or memorization of factual information concerning the process may not ensure ability to apply the knowledge in practice. **(D)** Demonstration of the procedure in the presence of the nurse allows the nurse to evaluate the person's ability to apply as well as to comprehend the information. Successful performance of the procedure may also enhance the person's self-confidence to perform the task properly.

96. **(D)** Nursing process phase: data collection; client need: physiological adaptation; content area: medical-surgical.

    RATIONALE
    (A) Currently, no treatment stops the degenerative process of Parkinson's disease. **(B)** Parkinsonian crisis occurs on abrupt withdrawal of prescribed medications or with emotional trauma—and this is a medical emergency. **(C)** Parkinson's disease is not familial. **(D)** Intellectual capacity is not lost, although mood disturbances often occur.

97. **(B)** Nursing process phase: planning; client need: pharmacological and parenteral therapies; content area: medical-surgical.

    RATIONALE
    (A) Select another option. **(B)** All the aforementioned drugs are antiparkinsonian agents. Bromocriptine mesylate is used also for amenorrhea, galactorrhea, prevention of lactation, and female infertility. **(C)** Select another option. **(D)** Select another option.

98. **(D)** Nursing process phase: planning; client need: basic care and comfort; content area: medical-surgical.

    RATIONALE
    (A) This response is correct. **(B)** This response is correct. **(C)** This response is correct. **(D)** An afternoon nap will not help to facilitate bowel function. Any of the other three choices may help to prevent constipation.

99. **(D)** Nursing process phase: implementation; client need: pharmacological and parenteral therapies; content area: medical-surgical.

    RATIONALE
    (A) The nurse may be instructed by the physician on specific knowledge required by the client. **(B)** The pharmacist is not usually contacted to give drug information to the client (although he or she may provide information when the client purchases the drugs). **(C)** The nurse does not need a physician's order to provide information related to the drug regimen. **(D)** The nurse is the person closest to the client. The nurse has knowledge (or can find out) about the medications, and he or she has the responsibility for independent nursing action in discharge teaching.

100. **(B)** Nursing process phase: data collection; client need: pharmacological and parenteral therapies; content area: medical-surgical.

    RATIONALE
    (A) This answer is not true; select another option. **(B)** Status epilepticus is a medical emergency in which the client has continuous seizures or seizures in rapid succession lasting at least 30 minutes. There are many kinds of status epilepticus. **(C)** This answer is not true; select another option. **(D)** This is not true; select another option.

101. **(D)** Nursing process phase: planning; client need: pharmacological and parenteral therapies; content area: medical-surgical.

    RATIONALE
    (A) Recalculate. **(B)** Recalculate. **(C)** Recalculate. **(D)** This problem requires conversion of milliliters to minims first. The nurse must know that 1 ml is equivalent to 15–16 minims. The correct dosage can be ascertained by ratio and proportion calculation as follows: 2 mg is to x minims as 5 mg is to 15 minims. Cross-multiplying gives $5x = 30$; then $x = 30 \div 5$. Finally, $x = 6$ minims.

102. **(B)** Nursing process phase: evaluation; client need: management of care; content area: medical-surgical.

    RATIONALE
    (A) This action is within the standard practice of nursing. **(B)** Only physicians are licensed to prescribe medications. **(C)** This

action is within the standard practice of nursing. **(D)** This action is within the standard practice of nursing.

103. **(A)** Nursing process phase: data collection; client need: pharmacological and parenteral therapies; content area: medical-surgical.

    RATIONALE

    (A) All of the drugs listed are anticonvulsant medications with various side effects. Long-term use of phenytoin has been known to result in hypertrophy of gingival tissue. Special attention to meticulous oral care is important for clients receiving this drug. **(B)** Primidone does not cause gingival hypertrophy. **(C)** Clonazepam does not cause gingival hypertrophy. **(D)** Diazepam does not cause gingival hypertrophy.

104. **(C)** Nursing process phase: implementation; client need: pharmacological and parenteral therapies; content area: medical-surgical.

    RATIONALE

    (A) Docusate sodium is a stool softener. **(B)** Digoxin is a cardiac glycoside. **(C)** Diazepam is the usual medication of choice. **(D)** Dexamethasone is a synthetic adrenocorticosteroid.

105. **(D)** Nursing process phase: implementation; client need: reduction of risk potential; content area: medical-surgical.

    RATIONALE

    (A) Although oxygen therapy is given to maintain adequate ventilation and oxygenation, it is not the priority action. **(B)** Chest physiotherapy and coughing with support to the chest wall are used primarily for pulmonary contusions to maintain airway clearance, but are not the priority action. **(C)** Pain medication may be administered, but it is not the priority. **(D)** The wound must be sealed immediately to prevent the development of a tension pneumothorax.

106. **(C)** Nursing process phase: evaluation; client need: reduction of risk potential; content area: medical-surgical.

    RATIONALE

    (A) The purpose is to regain normally negative intrapleural pressure. **(B)** Chest tubes have no effect on plural irritation. **(C)** Chest tubes are used because the normally negative pressure that causes inspiration has been interrupted. To regain negative intrapleural pressure, a tube is inserted and negative pressure applied with the aid of a water seal and/or negative-pressure pump to remove both air and fluid. **(D)** The purpose is to establish normal negative intrapleural pressure.

107. **(C)** Nursing process phase: planning; client need: reduction of risk potential; content area: medical-surgical.

    RATIONALE

    (A) The chest tube may be clamped temporarily to determine whether there is an air leak (bubbling in the water-seal chamber). **(B)** The chest drainage devices should always be kept lower than the client to prevent reflux into the chest. **(C)** Gentle milking should be instituted only if a flow becomes obstructed because of clot formation. **(D)** The chest tube should not be clamped for client transport. When transporting a client, the suction may be disconnected, but the water seal must be maintained.

108. **(A)** Nursing process phase: evaluation; client need: reduction of risk potential; content area: medical-surgical.

    RATIONALE

    (A) Bubbling means that there is a leak from the pleural cavity or drainage system. **(B)** Bubbling indicates a leak in the system and that the system is not functioning properly. **(C)** The water level in the water-seal chamber will rise and fall with inspiration and expiration. **(D)** Turning on the side does not cause bubbling; a leak in the system does.

109. **(D)** Nursing process phase: planning; client need: basic care and comfort; content area: medical-surgical.

    RATIONALE

    (A) Antabuse is a drug used to treat alcohol abuse. **(B)** Vitamin C is not used to prevent encephalopathy. **(C)** Chlordiazepoxide may be used to treat delirium tremens. **(D)** Thiamine deficiency may occur with alcoholism because of damaged GI tract and lack of absorption or malnutrition. Wernicke's encephalopathy is caused by thiamine deficiency.

110. **(D)** Nursing process phase: planning; client need: prevention and early detection of disease; content area: medical-surgical.

    RATIONALE

    (A) Asking this question is not the most important priority. **(B)** Asking this question is not the most important priority but will become more important at discharge. **(C)** Asking this question is not the most important priority. **(D)** Alcoholics may have seizures or delirium tremens related to withdrawal. Usually, the seizures occur from 12 to 48 hours after the last drink. Some seizures have been reported up to 2 weeks after the last drink.

111. **(A)** Nursing process phase: planning; client need: prevention and early detection of disease; content area: medical-surgical.

    RATIONALE

    (A) Alcoholic withdrawal may include visual and tactile hallucinations; auditory hallucinations are more likely to occur in psychosis. The BP is elevated because of an outpouring of norepinephrine-epinephrine. **(B)** Temperature is usually not affected. **(C)** The BP is elevated because of an outpouring of norepinephrine-epinephrine; temperature is not affected. **(D)** Temperature is usually not affected.

112. **(D)** Nursing process phase: implementation; client need: safety and infection control; content area: medical-surgical.

    RATIONALE

    (A) Restraints are applied to prevent the client from hurting himself or others, not for punitive measures. **(B)** Physicians should write a specific order for restraints, not an as-needed order. **(C)** The restraints may not necessarily be taken off in 1 hour. **(D)** Because the client is severely immobilized, his circulation should be checked frequently, and documentation should occur every 15 minutes. (A flowsheet is appropriate for this.)

113. **(C)** Nursing process phase: implementation; client need: prevention and early detection of disease; content area: medical-surgical.

    RATIONALE

    (A) At discharge, it is too late to encourage the client to become as independent as possible. **(B)** His needs should be assessed on admission and re-evaluated as he progresses. **(C)** Rehabilitation is best when started at the time of admission. **(D)** He must be encouraged to exercise and walk as soon as possible.

114. **(A)** Nursing process phase: implementation; client need: basic care and comfort; content area: medical-surgical.

    RATIONALE

    (A) The nurse should promote activity that allows a client to function and look as normal as possible. **(B)** Bathing the client and combing hair does not promote independence. **(C)** The nurse may remind client to brush teeth, but not do it. **(D)** Foley catheter can introduce bacteria into the urinary tract system. Instituting Kegel exercises would be more appropriate.

115. **(A)** Nursing process phase: implementation; client need: reduction of risk potential; content area: medical-surgical.

    RATIONALE

    (A) Passive ROM is the range of movement at a particular joint that is accomplished by the use of a machine or an assistant. **(B)**

Active ROM is the range of movement at a particular joint that a client is able to accomplish without assistance. (**C**) Active ROM exercises are more effective than passive ROM. (**D**) With passive ROM, there is no assistance from the client.

116. (**D**) Nursing process phase: data collection; client need: prevention and early detection of disease; content area: pediatrics.

    RATIONALE

    (**A**) The DDST assesses the child from birth to 6 years. (**B**) The DDST adjusts for premature birth by subtracting the number of weeks of prematurity from the chronological age. (**C**) The value of the DDST is questionable in minority ethnic groups. (**D**) The DDST is not an intelligence test but measures four skill areas: gross motor, fine motor, language, and personal-social skills.

117. (**C**) Nursing process phase: evaluation; client need: growth and development through the life span; content area: pediatrics.

    RATIONALE

    (**A**) Squeak toys are appropriate for the 6–12-month-old child. (**B**) Pull toys are appropriate for the 12–18-month-old child who walks well. (**C**) By 2–4 years the child can pedal a tricycle. (**D**) A 4–6-year-old child has the dexterity and motor skills to play on a jungle gym.

118. (**B**) Nursing process phase: data collection; client need: growth and development through the life span; content area: pediatrics.

    RATIONALE

    (**A**) By 0–6 months, the infant can sit with support and roll over from side to back. (**B**) At 6–12 months, the infant can crawl, creep, or walk holding on to furniture. (**C**) At 12–18 months, the child can walk well, stoop, and recover. (**D**) At 18–24 months, the child can kick a ball forward, walk up steps, walk backwards, and throw a ball overhand.

119. (**C**) Nursing process phase: evaluation; client need: growth and development through the life span; content area: maternity nursing.

    RATIONALE

    (**A**) Although this may be true, these symptoms need to be evaluated by a physician. (**B**) Tylenol or aspirin may relieve the pain, but these symptoms may indicate serious complications and must be evaluated by the physician. (**C**) These signs require immediate notification of the physician, because the pregnancy may be in jeopardy. (**D**) The nurse cannot make a judgment as to whether or not these symptoms are a result of the allergy.

120. (**D**) Nursing process phase: evaluation; client need: growth and development through the life span; content area: maternity nursing.

    RATIONALE

    (**A**) The amniocentesis determines the fetal lung maturity with lecithin:sphingomyelin ratio. (**B**) The amniocentesis ascertains the presence of chromosomal aberrations. (**C**) The extent of ABO, RH can be determined by amniocentesis. (**D**) A sonogram, not an amniocentesis, allows visualization of the fetus, uterus, and placenta.

121. (**A**) Nursing process phase: evaluation; client need: reduction of risk potential; content area: maternity nursing.

    RATIONALE

    (**A**) Encouraging bladder fullness is appropriate for a sonogram. Bladder fullness could result in puncture of the bladder in an amniocentesis. (**B**) The client will sign an informal consent. (**C**) Vaginal bleeding and elevated temperature should be observed for and reported. (**D**) Vital signs are taken every 5 minutes during the procedure and every 15 minutes after the procedure.

122. (**D**) Nursing process phase: evaluation; client need: growth and development through the life span; content area: maternity nursing.

    RATIONALE

    (**A**) Aspirin may cause decreased platelet aggregation, GI bleeding, and abdominal pain. It is not likely to cause vaginal bleeding. (**B**) Toxic shock syndrome is caused by certain strains of *Staphylococcus aureus*. The fever is 102°F (38.9°C) or greater; hypotension, GI vomiting, severe myalgia, alterations in consciousness are some of the symptoms. (**C**) Endometriosis may cause abdominal cramping but not shock symptoms. (**D**) A spontaneous abortion occurs naturally during the second or third month. Symptoms include vaginal bleeding, spotting or hemorrhaging, low abdominal cramping, passing of tissue through the vagina, or shock.

123. (**A**) Nursing process phase: implementation; client need: psychosocial adaptation; content area: psychiatric nursing.

    RATIONALE

    (**A**) Psychiatric clients cannot be reasoned with or argued with because they believe a delusion to be true. The best approach is a simple statement of reality. (**B**) Changing her room would feed her delusion. (**C**) Psychiatric clients cannot identify why, but they accept a delusion as being true. (**D**) This option does not point out the reality.

124. (**B**) Nursing process phase: planning; client need: coping and adaptation; content area: psychiatric nursing.

    RATIONALE

    (**A**) Joining in group activities initially is inappropriate until she is less delusional. (**B**) Establishing trust is of primary importance because she is so paranoid and lacks trust in others. (**C**) Limiting contacts with other clients is important, but developing a sense of trust with staff is the priority. (**D**) Coworkers should not visit until she becomes less delusional.

125. (**A**) Nursing process phase: implementation; client need: basic care and comfort; content area: medical-surgical.

    RATIONALE

    (**A**) Inspect skin to monitor for irritation and breakdown. (**B**) This is not a relevant option for care of a brace. (**C**) This is not a relevant option for care of a brace. (**D**) Weight fluctuations may cause the brace to become loose or tight.

126. (**A**) Nursing process phase: implementation; client need: basic care and comfort; content area: medical-surgical.

    RATIONALE

    (**A**) Allowing the client to stand with aid helps to prevent complications resulting from immobility. (**B**) A prosthesis does not substitute for a dressing. (**C**) A prosthesis does not enhance body image. (**D**) A prosthesis does prevent complications of immobility, but does so because it allows the client to stand.

127. (**D**) Nursing process phase: data collection; client need: basic care and comfort; content area: medical-surgical.

    RATIONALE

    (**A**) Leaning on an axillary bar may cause nerve damage. (**B**) The client should be taught to walk upright, looking straight ahead. (**C**) Although making sure that adequate help is available to support the client initially, option C is not as important as option D. (**D**) If the client cannot tolerate the physical activity, he or she will not adjust to crutch walking.

128. (**B**) Nursing process phase: implementation; client need: basic care and comfort; content area: medical-surgical.

    RATIONALE

    (**A**) The nurse cannot order physical therapy. (**B**) The client will need strength before using crutches. (**C**) It is most important for the client to do muscle-strengthening exercises. **(D)** Although option D is also correct, it is a physical priority for the client to have the necessary strength to perform crutch walking.

129. **(C)** Nursing process phase: evaluation; client need: basic care and comfort; content area: medical-surgical.

RATIONALE

(A) The prosthesis must be kept in working order, and water can cause rusting. **(B)** The client needs to wear the prosthesis all the time. **(C)** The prosthesis should be maintained in good working order. **(D)** The joints should not be oiled.

130. **(B)** Nursing process phase: data collection; client need: prevention and early detection of disease; content area: medical-surgical.

RATIONALE

(A) This action occurs during the planning phase. **(B)** Data collection is the first phase of the nursing process in which nurses establish a database about the client's problems and needs, level of wellness, health practices, and past illnesses. **(C)** This action occurs during the problem identification stage. **(D)** This action occurs during the planning stage.

131. **(D)** Nursing process phase: planning; client need: basic care and comfort; content area: pediatrics.

RATIONALE

(A) Although weighing a client is a factor in determining nutritional management, it is not the primary reason for daily weights. **(B)** Weight does not accurately reflect fluid intake, but rather fluid balances. **(C)** This response is not a viable option. **(D)** Measurement of daily weight is the primary way of evaluating edema and fluid shifts.

132. **(A)** Nursing process phase: evaluation; client need: coping and adaptation; content area: psychiatric nursing.

RATIONALE

(A) Psychological abuse is causing mental distress by name-calling, isolating, ignoring, or ridiculing an individual. **(B)** Excessive or improper use of physical force on an individual is physical abuse. **(C)** Active neglect is deliberately denying ordered health care to an individual. **(D)** Passive neglect is the unintentional abuse in which the caregiver does not do something that is required because of a lack of skills, knowledge, or ability.

133. **(D)** Nursing process phase: evaluation; client need: psychosocial adaptation; content area: medical-surgical.

RATIONALE

(A) Psychological abuse is causing mental distress by name-calling, isolating, ignoring, or ridiculing an individual. **(B)** Physical abuse is the excessive or improper use of physical force on an individual. **(C)** Unintentional abuse in which the caregiver does not do that which is required because of a lack of skills, knowledge, or ability is called passive neglect. **(D)** Active neglect is deliberately denying ordered health care to an individual.

134. **(B)** Nursing process phase: data collection; client need: prevention and early detection of disease; content area: medical-surgical.

RATIONALE

(A) Percussion is the use of the fingertips to tap the body lightly but sharply to determine position, size, and consistency of an underlying structure. **(B)** Palpation is the process of examining by application of the hands or fingers to the external surface of the body to detect evidence of disease or abnormalities in the various organs. **(C)** Inspection is the visual examination of the external surface of the body as well as its movements and posture. **(D)** Auscultation is the process of listening for sounds within the body—usually to sounds of the thoracic or abdominal viscera—to detect some abnormal condition.

135. **(A)** Nursing process phase: planning; client need: growth and development through the life span; content area: pediatrics.

RATIONALE

(A) Toddlers benefit most from having parents who are not overtly anxious and trust the hospital personnel. **(B)** The toddler will not remember well in advance of the procedure. **(C)** Separation anxiety is strongest during the toddler years. Promote care by parents. **(D)** Providing objects such as a blanket or toys from home for familiarity and comfort encourages regression.

136. **(A)** Nursing process phase: evaluation; client need: growth and development through the life span; content area: psychiatric nursing.

RATIONALE

(A) In the 7-year-old child, fears are related to body injury; allow the child to participate in procedures and prepare the child in advance. **(B)** For the 4–6-year-old child, the child's magical thoughts and fantasies may distort the hospital experience. The nurse should explain simply the relationship between cause, illness, and treatment. **(C)** For the 12–18-year-old adolescent, fears are related to body image. The nurse should promote privacy, provide detailed information, and promote self-care. **(D)** The 16-month-old to 4-year-old toddler is resistive and exhibits regressive behaviors such as tantrums. Provide for routines and promote care by parents.

137. **(C)** Nursing process phase: planning; client need: basic care and comfort; content area: psychiatric nursing.

RATIONALE

(A) Physiological needs are first priority. **(B)** This action relates to love and belonging, which come after physiological needs. **(C)** If physiological needs are not met, psychological needs cannot be met. Maslow's hierarchy goes from physical needs to safety and security, to love and belonging, and to self-esteem and self-actualization. **(D)** This action relates to love and belonging and is a lower priority than physiological and safety and security needs.

138. **(D)** Nursing process phase: evaluation; client need: pharmacological and parenteral therapies; content area: pediatrics.

RATIONALE

(A) All options are true, but infections are life threatening and therefore are most important to recognize. **(B)** All options are true, but infections are life threatening and therefore are most important to recognize. **(C)** All options are true, but infections are life threatening and therefore are most important to recognize. **(D)** All options are true, but infections are life threatening and therefore are most important to recognize.

139. **(C)** Nursing process phase: evaluation; client need: physiological adaptation; content area: medical-surgical.

RATIONALE

(A) The nurse should assess the level of consciousness after the airway is established. **(B)** Pupils are evaluated after an open airway is established. **(C)** The first priority of nursing care is to ensure protection of the airway and to stabilize cervical injuries. **(D)** Motor function is evaluated after the airway is evaluated.

140. **(D)** Nursing process phase: data collection; client need: prevention and early detection of disease; content area: medical-surgical.

RATIONALE

(A) Option A is not a true statement. **(B)** Option B makes the client seem foolish. **(C)** Option C is not true because vertebral column spacing decreases with aging. **(D)** Option D is correct and is necessary for a baseline data collection.

141. **(A)** Nursing process phase: evaluation; client need: growth and development through the life span; content area: medical-surgical.

    RATIONALE
    (A) Subcutaneous fat works as an insulator against cold. **(B)** This statement may be true, but there is a physical reason. **(C)** There is no change in sweat glands. **(D)** This option does not respond to the question.

142. **(D)** Nursing process phase: evaluation; client need: physiological adaptation; content area: medical-surgical.

    RATIONALE
    (A) A stage-I pressure sore consists of an area of redness that does not blanch or fade. **(B)** A stage-II pressure sore consists of partial-thickness skin loss involving the epidermis or dermis. **(C)** A stage-III pressure sore consists of full-thickness loss involving necrosis of subcutaneous tissue. **(D)** A stage-IV pressure sore consists of full-thickness loss involving damage to bone, muscle, or supporting structures.

143. **(A)** Nursing process phase: evaluation; client need: prevention and early detection of disease; content area: medical-surgical.

    RATIONALE
    (A) The primary risk factors for pressure ulcers are immobility and limited activity. Other risk factors include altered level of consciousness, incontinence, and impaired nutritional status. **(B)** Immobility and incontinence are risk factors for pressure ulcers; agitation is not. **(C)** Incontinence and impaired nutrition are risk factors; agitation is not. **(D)** Loss of subcutaneous fat support in the skin is a normal process of aging; agitation and hyperactivity are not risk factors.

144. **(A)** Nursing process phase: data collection; client need: growth and development through the life span; content area: medical-surgical.

    RATIONALE
    (A) Increased exercise causes BP to increase and the person can feel his or her own heartbeat. **(B)** There is no indication that she is a candidate for myocardial infarction. **(C)** This is not a cardinal sign of heart failure. Dyspnea and edema of the extremities are more likely symptoms. **(D)** There is no indication of mitral stenosis.

145. **(A)** Nursing process phase: evaluation; client need: reduction of risk potential; content area: medical-surgical.

    RATIONALE
    (A) Older persons have decreased lung expansion because of rib cage inelasticity, and a decreased immune response, which predisposes older persons to pneumonia. **(B)** There is a decrease in the immune response with aging. **(C)** Aging has little effect on the pulmonary system; respiratory muscle strength remains unchanged. **(D)** Immobile clients are at increased risk for pneumonia postoperatively because of decreased functional reserve and a decreased cough reflex.

146. **(B)** Nursing process phase: planning; client need: basic care and comfort; content area: medical-surgical.

    RATIONALE
    (A) A diet high in antacids and calcium has no effect on formation of biliary calculi. **(B)** Biliary calculi are high in cholesterol; therefore, the cholesterol intake of this client needs to be limited. **(C)** A diet high in protein and carbohydrate has no effect on formation of biliary calculi. **(D)** An electrolyte-free diet has no effect on formation of biliary calculi.

147. **(C)** Nursing process phase: implementation; client need: pharmacological and parenteral therapies; content area: medical-surgical.

RATIONALE
(A) Reduced smoking may be healthy, but Antabuse has no effect. **(B)** Antabuse has no effects connected to the sun. **(C)** In a person taking Antabuse, the general physical symptoms experienced after ingesting even a small amount of alcohol may be severe. The drug remains in the body for several days after being discontinued. **(D)** There would be no restricted sexual or physical activity.

148. **(C)** Nursing process phase: implementation; client need: growth and development through the life span; content area: medical-surgical.

    RATIONALE
    (A) Talking loudly distorts sounds. High-frequency-hearing sound loss causes older people to have problems discriminating certain high-pitched sounds. Speak in front of the person so that he or she can see your lip movement. **(B)** Speaking more slowly and distinctly will help the older person to process the information. **(C)** The best communication is face to face, using short sentences and talking in a normal voice tone. **(D)** Repeating the message may confuse the client, and raising your voice distorts the sound.

149. **(D)** Nursing process phase: evaluation; client need: basic care and comfort; content area: medical-surgical.

    RATIONALE
    (A) The Food and Drug Administration (FDA) recommendation to delay bone degeneration is to include 1–1½ g of calcium in the daily diet. **(B)** The FDA recommendation to delay bone degeneration is to include 1–1½ g of calcium in the daily diet. **(C)** The FDA recommendation to delay bone degeneration is to include 1–1½ g of calcium in the daily diet. **(D)** The FDA recommendation to delay bone degeneration is to include 1–1½ g of calcium in the daily diet.

150. **(C)** Nursing process phase: planning; client need: basic care and comfort; content area: medical-surgical.

    RATIONALE
    (A) A 1000-ml intake is inadequate for daily fluid needs. **(B)** A 2000-ml intake is inadequate for daily fluid needs. **(C)** The need for fluid intake does not decrease with age. Three thousand milliliters is about 3 quarts of fluid. **(D)** Three thousand liters is appproximately 3000 quarts of fluid.

151. **(A)** Nursing process phase: evaluation; client need: basic care and comfort; content area: medical-surgical.

    RATIONALE
    (A) The FDA requirement is to list ingredients by amounts in descending order. **(B)** This statement is not true; select another option. **(C)** This statement is not true; select another option. **(D)** This statement is not true; select another option.

152. **(C)** Nursing process phase: planning; client need: coping and adaptation; content area: medical-surgical.

    RATIONALE
    (A) Silence allows the person to think and add information. **(B)** Neither chemical nor physical restraints should be used as a punitive measure. **(C)** This is a tenet for good communication with all persons, but it is especially true for the older person, who may take more time to process material. **(D)** Eye contact may aid in the communication process.

153. **(D)** Nursing process phase: evaluation; client need: prevention and early detection of disease; content area: medical-surgical.

    RATIONALE
    (A) The cough reflex is less active and may contribute to development of an infection, but this is not the question. **(B)** The skin

is the body's primary barrier against infection, but this is not the question. (C) Prostatic hypertrophy, with increased residual urine, reduces the natural process of flushing the bladder, but this is not the question. (D) Absence of fever in the face of bacterial infection is not unusual in older persons.

154. (A) Nursing process phase: evaluation; client need: safety and infection control; content area: medical-surgical.

RATIONALE

(A) Although falls can occur anywhere, most occur in the bathroom because of slippery floors and bath fixtures, as well as inadequate support fixtures such as rails. (B) In the living room, many falls occur from throw rugs or from unstable chairs or furniture. (C) Many falls occur in the bedroom when the older person gets up during the night to go to the bathroom. (D) Burns occur in the kitchen from stoves or hot pots or pans left on the stove.

155. (B) Nursing process phase: evaluation; client need: safety and infection control; content area: medical-surgical.

RATIONALE

(A) Elimination of clutter promotes safety by decreasing the chances of falling or tripping. (B) Carpets, especially throw rugs, increase the chance for tripping or sliding. (C) Handles of pans should be turned inward so the client does not accidentally reach for them or knock them off the stove. (D) Smoke detector batteries need to be changed regularly. A good method is to change them twice a year when standard time and daylight saving time change.

156. (D) Nursing process phase: evaluation; client need: reduction of risk potential; content area: medical-surgical.

RATIONALE

(A) Some surgical procedures may cause immobility, but not all. (B) Immobility, rather than excessive exercise, is more likely to cause venous thrombosis. (C) A low-iron diet or decubiti will not affect the formation of venous thrombosis. (D) Prolonged immobility promotes stasis of blood and subsequent venous thrombosis.

157. (D) Nursing process phase: evaluation; client need: growth and development through the life span; content area: maternity nursing.

RATIONALE

(A) This action will not help; select another option. (B) Elevating the head of the bed may actually decrease her BP; select another option. (C) The pulse will not change if another person takes it; reassess the situation. (D) Placing the client on her left side relieves pressure on the vena cava to increase venous return and thereby increase BP.

158. (A) Nursing process phase: evaluation; client need: growth and development through the life span; content area: maternity nursing.

RATIONALE

(A) Amenorrhea is an early sign of pregnancy. (B) Dysmenorrhea, or painful menses, is not a sign of pregnancy and may occur at any time during a menstrual period. (C) Pica occurs when a pregnant woman has a desire for claylike substances. (D) Nausea is a later sign that can occur.

159. (D) Nursing process phase: evaluation; client need: growth and development through the life span; content area: maternity nursing.

RATIONALE

(A) Urinary frequency is normal and occurs because of pressure on the bladder. (B) Polyphagia, or increased appetite, is common. (C) Nausea is common until after the 16th week of preg-

nancy. (D) Dysuria, or painful urination, could indicate a bladder infection.

160. (B) Nursing process phase: data collection; client need: basic care and comfort; content area: pediatrics.

RATIONALE

(A) Croup is an inflammation of the larynx, trachea, and bronchi causing narrowing of the air passages from edema. Cough medicine is inappropriate. (B) Warm, moist air is required to decrease epiglottal edema. (C) Warm, dry heat will make the symptoms worse. (D) Warm, dry heat will make the symptoms worse.

161. (D) Nursing process phase: implementation; client need: basic care and comfort; content area: pediatrics.

RATIONALE

(A) The client should be positioned on her side or stomach to promote drainage. (B) Coughing, clearing the throat, or blowing his nose will increase bleeding. (C) Using a straw will increase the chance of bleeding. (D) Cool fluid and a liquid diet promote fluid intake and healing.

162. (B) Nursing process phase: data collection; client need: prevention and early detection of disease; content area: pediatrics.

RATIONALE

(A) Ménière's disease is a chronic disease of adulthood characterized by sudden attacks of vertigo, tinnitus, and hearing loss. (B) Otitis media is an infection of the middle ear, primarily the result of a blocked eustachian tube. In infants, there is a tendency to rub, hold, or pull the affected ear. (C) Otosclerosis is a disorder of the middle ear characterized by slow formation of spongy bone around the stapes, which causes progressive hearing loss. (D) Meningitis is an inflammation of the lining of the brain. Irritability is a symptom, but usually it is accompanied by nuchal pain, fever, vomiting, or headache.

163. (C) Nursing process phase: implementation; client need: basic care and comfort; content area: medical-surgical.

RATIONALE

(A) A commercial deodorizer can be used, but there is a better option. (B) Gas-forming foods can cause odor, but there is a better option. (C) Cleaning the bag frequently gets rid of the basis of the odor problem—fecal residue. (D) The bag may need to be refitted, but there is a better option.

164. (A) Nursing process phase: evaluation; client need: prevention and early detection of disease; content area: medical-surgical.

RATIONALE

(A) The area of induration is 10 mm but may vary with HIV infection and close contact with active tuberculosis (TB) cases or persons with a chest x-ray consistent with healed TB. Tuberculin reactions should be measured and recorded in millimeters after 48 hours at the largest diameter of the induration. (B) A normal response to the purified protein derivative (PPD) is erythema; select another option. (C) An intradermal injection of PPD causes a wheal to form; select another option. (D) Absence of erythema or induration is a negative response to the test.

165. (B) Nursing process phase: data collection; client need: basic care and comfort; content area: maternity nursing.

RATIONALE

(A) It is important to check her dressing, but this question is related to feeding. (B) You might do all the listed interventions, but the correct answer to the question is option B. Make sure bowel sounds have returned before providing nourishment after surgery. (C) It is important to encourage ambulation, but the question is related to feeding. **(D)** It is important to give pain medication, but this question is related to feeding.

166. **(C)** Nursing process phase: data collection; client need: prevention and early detection of disease; content area: medical-surgical.

    RATIONALE

    (A) Increased BP may not necessarily be a sign of increased intracranial pressure. **(B)** The vital signs are all normal. **(C)** Classic signs of increased intracranial pressure are a decrease in respirations, a decrease in pulse rate, and an increase in BP. **(D)** This information indicates impending shock.

167. **(C)** Nursing process phase: evaluation; client need: basic care and comfort; content area: medical-surgical.

    RATIONALE

    (A) A temperature range of 70–90°F (21.1–32.2°C) can cause spasm because it is too cold. **(B)** A temperature range of 80–90°F (26.6–32.2°C) can cause spasm because it is too cold. **(C)** The temperature should be just greater than body temperature. **(D)** A temperature of 110°F (43.3°C) will burn.

168. **(A)** Nursing process phase: evaluation; client need: pharmacological and parenteral therapies; content area: medical-surgical.

    RATIONALE

    (A) To administer blood, you need a large-bore needle. The only needle listed that can deliver blood is the No. 16 Angiocath. **(B)** This Angiocath is too small; select another size. **(C)** This butterfly is too small; select another size. **(D)** This butterfly is too small; select another size.

169. **(A)** Nursing process phase: implementation; client need: reduction of risk potential; content area: medical-surgical.

    RATIONALE

    (A) When suctioning, the nurse should occlude the suction port on withdrawal. Other options would either deprive the client of oxygen or provide an inadequate vacuum. **(B)** This technique will deprive the client of oxygen. **(C)** Instilling 20 ml of normal saline may cause a fluid overload if this is instilled each time. **(D)** Opening the catheter suction port when withdrawing will cause an inadequate vacuum.

170. **(D)** Nursing process phase: implementation; client need: pharmacological and parenteral therapies; content area: medical-surgical.

    RATIONALE

    (A) A volume of 4.4 ml is too great for one injection. **(B)** A volume of 4.4 ml is too great for one injection. **(C)** A volume of 2.2 ml is too great for administration in the deltoid muscle. **(D)** Because a volume of 4.4 ml is too great for one injection, the dosage must be divided.

171. **(D)** Nursing process phase: implementation; client need: pharmacological and parenteral therapies; content area: medical-surgical.

    RATIONALE

    (A) The skin should not be massaged after the injection. **(B)** Heparin should be given as an SC injection, not IM. **(C)** Heparin should not be aspirated because of the possibility of causing bruising or bleeding. **(D)** Heparin should be given SC.

172. **(A)** Nursing process phase: data collection; client need: reduction of risk potential; content area: pediatrics.

    RATIONALE

    (A) Absence of a pedal pulse is of the utmost importance because it indicates circulatory compromise. **(B)** You cannot palpate for a popliteal pulse through a cast. **(C)** Some drainage is expected. **(D)** There is no mention that the client is in traction.

173. **(B)** Nursing process phase: evaluation; client need: basic care and comfort; content area: pediatrics.

    RATIONALE

    (A) The blisters should be kept intact to prevent infection. **(B)** Skin should be kept intact to prevent infection. **(C)** Ice or cool water helps to disperse heat and prevent further damage, but skin should be kept intact. **(D)** Petrolatum only makes the blister worse by containing the heat and limiting air exposure.

174. **(C)** Nursing process phase: evaluation; client need: prevention and early detection of disease; content area: pediatrics.

    RATIONALE

    (A) Analysis of gastric secretions does not detect PKU. **(B)** PKU is not detected in arterial blood gases. **(C)** This test is performed on capillary blood, although the phenylpyruvic acid is excreted in the urine. Phenylketonuria is a hereditary disease caused by the body's failure to oxidize an amino acid because of a defective enzyme. This is called the *Guthrie test*. **(D)** Serum phenylalanine levels of 12–15 mg per 100 ml will begin to appear in the urine. By this time, some degree of irreversible mental damage may have occurred.

175. **(B)** Nursing process phase: planning; client need: growth and development through the life span; content area: psychiatric nursing.

    RATIONALE

    (A) Industry versus inferiority is characteristic of the school-age child. **(B)** Erikson's stages of development indicate that the early adolescent is achieving role identity. **(C)** Intimacy versus isolation is characteristic of the young adult. **(D)** Integrity versus despair is characteristic of the older adult.

176. **(A)** Nursing process phase: evaluation; client need: psychosocial adaptation; content area: psychiatric nursing.

    RATIONALE

    (A) Morning-evening variation in symptoms occurs with psychotic depression. The client is most depressed in the morning and experiences a slight elevation of mood as the day progresses. **(B)** Mood is usually better in the afternoon; select another option. **(C)** Mood is usually elevated toward evening; select another answer. **(D)** Visiting time may either increase or decrease mood, depending on the client's relationship with the visitors.

177. **(A)** Nursing process phase: implementation; client need: psychosocial adaptation; content area: psychiatric nursing.

    RATIONALE

    (A) Because the basic trauma in schizophrenia is a disturbed parent-infant relationship, giving the client some milk will promote trust. **(B)** Hugging is very intrusive; select another option. **(C)** Bringing the client a deck of cards is an option, but there are better ones. **(D)** This is an excellent option; sitting quietly with the client may help to decrease agitation and promotes sharing of feelings. However, there is a better option.

178. **(B)** Nursing process phase: evaluation; client need: pharmacological and parenteral therapies; content area: medical-surgical.

    RATIONALE

    (A) Streptomycin (not isoniazid) can cause eighth cranial nerve damage, is nephrotoxic, and causes labyrinth damage and hepatitis. **(B)** Isoniazid can cause peripheral neuritis; pyridoxine is given prophylactically. **(C)** Streptomycin and ethambutol (not isoniazid) are rarely used with people with renal disease. **(D)** Para-aminosalicylic acid (PAS) and ethionamide (not isoniazid) can cause gastric disturbance.

179. **(A)** Nursing process phase: evaluation; client need: pharmacological and parenteral therapies; content area: medical-surgical.

RATIONALE

(A) Discontinuance of even one drug may cause organisms to become drug resistant. **(B)** This outcome is important, but not the most important. **(C)** Drugs should never be discontinued by the client, only by the physician. **(D)** It is important to wear a Medic Alert bracelet, but not of highest importance.

180. **(C)** Nursing process phase: evaluation; client need: coping and adaptation; content area: medical-surgical.

    RATIONALE

    (A) Compensation is covering up a weakness by emphasizing a desirable trait. An example is a physically handicapped individual who is an outstanding scholar. **(B)** Denial is the refusal to accept reality. **(C)** Displacement is the discharging of pent-up feelings to a less dangerous object or area. He is displacing his anger about his medical restrictions to a less dangerous one such as diet. **(D)** Projection is the attribution of one's own undesirable traits to someone else.

181. **(D)** Nursing process phase: evaluation; client need: growth and development through the life span; content area: maternity nursing.

    RATIONALE

    (A) The nurse should not leave the room. Relieving the pressure is the highest priority. Use the call light to obtain help. **(B)** Fetal heart rate should be monitored, but this is not the highest priority. **(C)** This is not an appropriate answer. **(D)** Cord prolapse is an extremely serious complication that calls for immediate action because pressure on the cord deprives the baby of oxygen. The highest priority is to relieve the pressure of the fetal body or head from the cord.

182. **(C)** Nursing process phase: data collection; client need: prevention and early detection of disease; content area: medical-surgical.

    RATIONALE

    (A) Clients usually present with a low-grade fever. **(B)** Nausea and vomiting may occur, but they are not related to eating. **(C)** Tenderness in the lower right quadrant is a classic sign. It is usually located over McBurney's point. **(D)** The area of tenderness is McBurney's point.

183. **(D)** Nursing process phase: implementation; client need: basic care and comfort; content area: medical-surgical.

    RATIONALE

    (A) A heating pad may cause the appendix to rupture. **(B)** An enema is never given preoperatively in appendicitis because it could cause the appendix to rupture, and peritonitis could result. **(C)** Keep client NPO to decrease peristalsis. **(D)** A semi-Fowler's position relieves abdominal pain and tension.

184. **(B)** Nursing process phase: implementation; client need: growth and development through the life span; content area: maternity nursing.

    RATIONALE

    (A) Timing contractions is only important to determine when the baby will be delivered. **(B)** Remaining calm will let nature take its course. **(C)** Boiling water works in the cinema and gives nervous people something to do. **(D)** She should be NPO because digestion stops when labor begins.

185. **(A)** Nursing process phase: implementation; client need: prevention and early detection of disease; content area: medical-surgical.

    RATIONALE

    (A) Asking the man if his wife can talk establishes whether she has something in her airway. A victim is unable to talk if she is choking. **(B)** Giving a blow to the back if the person is choking

will cause the food to move further down in the airway. **(C)** An abdominal thrust is done after the rescuer knows the airway is blocked. **(D)** Hitting the person on the chest is done after establishing an airway, if cardiopulmonary resuscitation (CPR) is being done. This is not appropriate for this situation.

186. **(D)** Nursing process phase: evaluation; client need: physiological adaptation; content area: medical-surgical.

    RATIONALE

    (A) Tourniquets are not difficult to apply. **(B)** If a tourniquet is applied, it should be released only by the physician. **(C)** Direct pressure and elevation usually control bleeding in these areas. **(D)** Tourniquets can cause a considerable amount of damage, which may be permanent.

187. **(B)** Nursing process phase: evaluation; client need: growth and development through the life span; content area: medical-surgical.

    RATIONALE

    (A) Give only essential information because he will not be able to remember a lot of information. **(B)** The orientation should be limited to small, specific amounts of essential information. He will not be able to remember a lot of facts or details. **(C)** This is too specific, and will not provide visual clues for him. **(D)** Questions will further confuse him and add to his anxiety.

188. **(B)** Nursing process phase: planning; client need: basic care and comfort; content area: medical-surgical.

    RATIONALE

    (A) Making the client responsible for his or her own care may not be appropriate based on the client's physiological and psychological functioning. **(B)** The plan needs to be based on the client's level of functioning with self-care and independence, reinforced as much as possible. **(C)** Assigning another client is not appropriate. **(D)** The client should be encouraged to be independent and care for himself or herself as much as possible.

189. **(B)** Nursing process phase: implementation; client need: prevention and early detection of disease; content area: medical-surgical.

    RATIONALE

    (A) An early morning specimen contains the most cells and bacteria. **(B)** The best time to collect a sputum specimen is the first thing in the morning. These specimens are more likely to contain cells and bacteria. **(C)** Before or after lunch is not conducive to the appetite or digestion and, most important, does not contain the cells or bacteria that an early morning specimen would. **(D)** Time does matter; select another option.

190. **(A)** Nursing process phase: implementation; client need: prevention and early detection of disease; content area: medical-surgical.

    RATIONALE

    (A) Protecting the client from injury and decreasing the risk of aspiration are the priorities for client safety. **(B)** A tongue blade or other object might cause injury to the client's teeth or jaw, but aspiration is the major danger. **(C)** Restraints during a seizure might cause injury to the client. **(D)** Trying to move the client to the floor and holding the client down might cause injury.

191. **(B)** Nursing process phase: data collection; client need: prevention and early detection of disease; content area: medical-surgical.

    RATIONALE

    (A) Clear fluid from the nose or ears is the correct answer. **(B)** CSF is clear fluid from the nose or ears. The nurse should test the drainage for the presence of glucose. **(C)** CSF is clear, thin fluid from the nose or ears. **(D)** Bleeding would indicate intracranial bleeding or skull fracture.

192. **(C)** Nursing process phase: implementation; client need: growth and development through the life span; content area: medical-surgical.

    RATIONALE

    (A) People who live a long time generally have a modest caloric intake, do not eat a lot of meat or processed foods, and eat fresh vegetables, fruits, and grains. **(B)** Sexual activity does not have to decline with age, and continued activity may extend life. **(C)** A little "enlightened selfishness" will make the older person and his or her friends feel better and live longer. **(D)** Having friends, relatives, or pets increases survival.

193. **(B)** Nursing process phase: implementation; client need: growth and development through the life span; content area: medical-surgical.

    RATIONALE

    (A) Letting the person decide on a food plan may be contrary to physician's orders. **(B)** Appearance often affects the way people feel. Basic nursing interventions related to cleanliness, hygiene, and grooming are important in helping older people maintain feelings of self-worth and self-esteem. **(C)** Providing hygiene maintains an older person's feelings of self-worth and self-esteem. **(D)** Older women often like cosmetics but prefer those that are appropriate for older skin.

194. **(D)** Nursing process phase: implementation; client need: coping and adaptation; content area: medical-surgical.

    RATIONALE

    (A) Call the client by his or her last name preceded by "Mr.," "Mrs.," or "Miss," not by an endearing term such as "honey." **(B)** Encourage independence. **(C)** Avoid comments or actions that reflect ageism, such as reference to diapers. **(D)** Allowing as much control of care and environment as possible is a general nursing intervention that can be used to help maintain mental-health wellness in older adults.

195. **(D)** Nursing process phase: implementation; client need: pharmacological and parenteral therapies; content area: medical-surgical.

    RATIONALE

    (A) Encourage nutritional diet instead of vitamin pills. **(B)** Encourage exercise and activities with others instead of sedatives, hypnotics, antianxiety agents, and alcohol. **(C)** Advise exercise and high-bulk foods instead of laxatives. **(D)** Discourage misuse of medications by teaching the client to administer as few medications as possible, to prevent possible delirium and other complications such as falls.

196. **(B)** Nursing process phase: implementation; client need: coping and adaptation; content area: psychiatric nursing.

    RATIONALE

    (A) Hospital nurses are not able to view the family dynamics that may indicate abuse during the short stay in the hospital. **(B)** Hospital nurses have the responsibility in the discharge planning and teaching of older clients and their families to reduce anxiety and promote mental health. **(C)** Hospital nurses may not be able to assess social isolation during the short stay in the hospital. **(D)** Because of the short stay in the hospital, the nurse will not be able to teach effective ways to cope with aging.

197. **(D)** Nursing process phase: implementation; client need: basic care and comfort; content area: psychiatric nursing.

    RATIONALE

    (A) Whether to take medications ordered "as needed" is not an example of the kind of activity that a nursing home resident can

have some control over. **(B)** Assignment of staff members is not the responsibility of a nursing home resident. **(C)** Participating in a partial choice of food plan is an example of the kind of activity that a nursing home resident can have some control over, but the control is not complete. **(D)** Type and time of bath is an example of the kind of activity that a nursing home resident can have some control over.

198. **(C)** Nursing process phase: implementation; client need: coping and adaptation; content area: psychiatric nursing.

    RATIONALE

    (A) Allowing a resident to wander into another resident's room is inappropriate and does not prevent loneliness. **(B)** Group activities may be helpful, but one-to-one contact is most beneficial. **(C)** Group activities may be helpful, but people can feel lonely even in a group without some one-to-one contact and communication. **(D)** Effective communication, even with patients with dementia, should be a primary goal of all nursing home staff members.

199. **(C)** Nursing process phase: evaluation; client need: coping and adaptation; content area: psychiatric nursing.

    RATIONALE

    (A) Humor serving as an outlet for inner tensions and anxieties is a psychological effect. **(B)** Older persons are less offended when people of their own age group joke about aging than when younger persons joke about aging. **(C)** Interpersonally, humor has been referred to as a "social lubricant" because it helps to establish relationships and promote group cohesion. **(D)** Stimulating awareness is a physiological effect of humor.

200. **(D)** Nursing process phase: implementation; client need: coping and adaptation; content area: psychiatric nursing.

    RATIONALE

    (A) Teasing an older person without his or her consent is a violation of the person's boundaries. **(B)** Funny costumes, false noses, and hats, not scary costumes, can be worn for visual impact. **(C)** Funny stories or jokes should be told rather than grim or frightening stories. **(D)** Post or otherwise share cartoons with clients and their families. Use cartoons as teaching materials.

201. **(C)** Nursing process phase: implementation; client need: management of care; content area: psychiatric nursing.

    RATIONALE

    (A) The nurse should listen with understanding to the older person's own perception of the problem, not the family's. **(B)** The nurse needs to explain his or her own perception of the problem. **(C)** The nurse should acknowledge and discuss the differences and similarities between the older person's and the nurse's viewpoint. **(D)** The nurse should recommend a treatment plan within the constraints of his or her own ideas and those of the client.

202. **(C)** Nursing process phase: evaluation; client need: management of care; content area: medical-surgical.

    RATIONALE

    (A) Civil wrongs are the same as torts. **(B)** Torts are civil wrongs that cause harm or damage to a person or party. **(C)** Malpractice is defined as professional misconduct, negligent care or treatment, or failure to meet the standards of care, resulting in harm to a person. **(D)** Informed consent is not an area of legal action of negligence.

203. **(A)** Nursing process phase: evaluation; client need: management of care; content area: medical-surgical.

    RATIONALE

    (A) Duty is not an element of negligence. **(B)** Breach of duty is an element of negligence. **(C)** Damage is an element of negligence. **(D)** The court must find a causal connection between the breach and the damages, if any, to substantiate the claim.

204. **(B)** Nursing process phase: evaluation; client need: management of care; content area: medical-surgical.

RATIONALE

(A) Documentation decreases the potential areas of legal exposure. **(B)** Documentation describes client education and discharge instructions. **(C)** Documentation relates physicians' conversations, family comments, and client's concerns and feelings. **(D)** Documentation records untoward events such as falls.

205. **(C)** Nursing process phase: implementation; client need: management of care; content area: medical-surgical.

RATIONALE

(A) Document the need for restraints (describe the client's specific behavior and the type of restraints used). **(B)** For a client check, document skin integrity, circulation, respiratory status, client's verbal response, reasons based on client behavior for continued restraints, and physician's orders. **(C)** Documenting client's response to restraints ensures that a nurse is operating from a standard of care. **(D)** Document alternatives used before restraints.

206. **(B)** Nursing process phase: implementation; client need: management of care; content area: medical-surgical.

RATIONALE

(A) The physician usually has the duty to obtain the informed consent. **(B)** The nurse's responsibility is to witness the signature of the client on the informed consent sheet. **(C)** Clients are read their rights on entering the hospital, not when an informed consent is obtained before surgery. **(D)** If the client is confused, is mentally incompetent, or cannot give informed consent, the

next person who is legally permitted to consent must be given the elements of informed consent.

207. **(B)** Nursing process phase: implementation; client need: management of care; content area: medical-surgical.

RATIONALE

(A) The physician may refuse to sign the telephone order, thus exposing the nurse to liability. **(B)** The attending physician must write a DNR order on the chart to protect the health-care providers legally. **(C)** Competent clients have the right to refuse resuscitation even if family members request it. **(D)** If there is a signed physician's order not to resuscitate, the nurses are covered legally.

208. **(B)** Nursing process phase: implementation; client need: management of care; content area: medical-surgical.

RATIONALE

(A) "Slow code" orders must not be accepted because they are not legal and have ethical implications. **(B)** Copies of the living will and medical durable power of attorney should be included in the client's chart. **(C)** DNR orders must be written as an order in the client's chart. **(D)** Discussions with the client and family should be documented.

209. **(B)** Nursing process phase: implementation; client need: management of care; content area: medical-surgical.

RATIONALE

(A) Overmedication, not undermedication, is an area of legal exposure. **(B)** Areas of legal exposure include decubitus ulcers, overmedication, falls, and restraints. **(C)** Reporting complications is not an area of legal exposure. **(D)** Assessing an older person's condition every 8 hours is not an area of legal exposure.

TEST 2

Patricia Gauntlett Beare, RN, PhD
Larry P. Purnell, RN, PhD

QUESTIONS

1. The focus and purpose of health teaching are to:

   A. Resolve the problem
   B. Facilitate teaching methods
   C. Facilitate client's mastery
   D. Facilitate teacher's control

2. When should the nurse begin teaching of an older client?

   A. At the time of admission
   B. At the time of discharge
   C. At home
   D. When the older client is physically capable

3. In teaching an older person administration of medications, the nurse's best response would be:

   A. "Take your medications tid."
   B. "The doctor wants you to take your medicine every 6 hours."
   C. "Take your medicine when you go to bed at night."
   D. "Take your medicine ac and hs."

4. The presenting signs and symptoms of disease in the older person are frequently atypical and nonspecific, such as:

   A. An elevated white blood cell (WBC) count and fever in sepsis
   B. Chest pain in myocardial infarction
   C. Apathy in thyrotoxicosis.
   D. Polyuria and polydipsia in diabetic emergencies

5. Which of the following does the nurse need to consider first before setting goals with an older adult?

   A. What does the nurse expect the older person to accomplish?
   B. What kind of relaxation time does the older person have?
   C. What kind of social support does the older person have?
   D. Does the older person enjoy being alone?

6. A 72-year-old client leaving rehabilitation still requires assistance with walking. The physician orders her to relocate to a center that will permit daily assistance in walking. Concerned about leaving her husband, who is in poor health, she tells the nurse that she would rather give up walking than leave her husband. The nurse's response is:

   A. "Your needs come first."
   B. "Your husband would want what is best for you."
   C. "I understand that staying with your husband is more important than walking."
   D. "Are you sure you want to throw all of your success away?"

7. The nurse is orienting a 78-year-old client to her new room in the long-term care facility. The nurse instructs the client to:

   A. Stay away from the men's hall
   B. Refrain from socializing in the lounge
   C. Personalize her living space with personal possessions
   D. Be aware that she will be treated as if she were "sick"

8. How can the nurse intervene to make the dining area and mealtime pleasant in a long-term care facility?

   A. Serve the food quickly and remove the trays on time.
   B. Seat residents alphabetically.
   C. Seat residents according to social preferences.
   D. Have residents eat alone in their rooms.

9. A client is to receive 30 units of neutral protamine Hagedorn (NPH) insulin and 4 units of Regular insulin at 8 AM. The nurse would:

   A. Inject air into the Regular insulin first
   B. Draw up the insulins in separate syringes
   C. Inject air into the NPH insulin first
   D. Ask the pharmacy for the desired mixture

10. The physician orders norethindrone (Norlutin) 7.5 mg PO for a young woman experiencing breakthrough

bleeding. The pharmacist dispenses 5-mg tablets and instructs the client to take _____ tablet(s).

A. 0.5
B. 1.0
C. 1.5
D. 2.0

11. The nurse is doing a physical data collection on a 6-month-old infant. The baby is sitting quietly on the mother's lap. Which of the following parts of the data collection should the nurse do first?

A. Auscultate heart and lungs.
B. Examine eyes, ears, and mouth.
C. Examine head and move toward the feet.
D. Palpate peripheral pulses.

12. A client who is in mechanical restraints asks the nurse when they can be removed. Which one of the following is the best response by the nurse?

A. "Please tell me why you were physically violent."
B. "When apologies are made for creating such a disturbance."
C. "When your behavior is under control and you are no longer a danger to yourself or others."
D. "When the medication has calmed your violent behavior."

13. The nurse caring for a 4-year-old child after a tonsillectomy and adenoidectomy monitors for signs and symptoms of hemorrhage. Which of the following would be an early indication of hemorrhage?

A. Swallowing infrequently
B. Dark-brown emesis of approximately 25 ml
C. Pulse rate of 95 bpm
D. Drooling of bright-red secretions

14. A pregnant client is started on an iron supplement. What information can the nurse give the client to aid in absorption of the supplement?

A. "Take your iron with milk."
B. "Take your supplement with your prenatal vitamins."
C. "Take your iron with orange juice."
D. "Take your iron in the morning with breakfast."

15. During an otoscopic examination on a 9-month-old infant, the nurse pulls the pinna in which direction?

A. Down and back
B. Down and forward
C. Up and back
D. Up and forward

16. After reviewing danger signs during pregnancy that should be reported immediately to the health-care provider, which of the following responses would indicate to the nurse that the client understands?

A. "Intermittent vomiting."
B. "Vaginal bleeding."
C. "Leukorrhea."
D. "Urinary frequency."

17. A nurse is teaching a 27-year-old, first-time mother of a healthy full-term girl. Which of the following statements by the newborn's mother indicates a need for further teaching?

A. "I need to place my daughter on her side to sleep."
B. "I need to place my daughter on her back to sleep."
C. "I need to place my daughter on her abdomen to sleep."
D. "I need to place my daughter upright to burp her before I put her to sleep after her bottle."

18. The nurse, in planning program activities for clients in a day treatment setting, should:

A. Facilitate diversional activities for the lower-functioning clients
B. Focus on pathology
C. Provide for meaningful social interaction
D. Provide for multifaceted needs

19. A client arrives in the clinic for her first prenatal visit. She states that her last menstrual period was May 12 to 16. Using Naegele's rule, determine her expected date of confinement:

A. February 23
B. August 15
C. February 19
D. March 3

20. Which of the following statements indicates to the nurse the best understanding of placental functioning?

A. "The placenta filters out harmful substances."
B. "The placenta is where my blood circulates through my baby."
C. "The umbilical cord has one vein and one artery."
D. "The placenta gives my baby oxygen and nutrients."

21. A 58-year-old client is 4 days postoperative status for a coronary bypass graft surgery. The nurse encourages him to cough and deep-breathe to clear the thick secretions from his lungs. The client states that it hurts too much to breathe. Which of the following nursing actions would be appropriate to help this client minimize the pain from his chest incision?

A. Administer morphine sulfate as ordered.
B. Use incentive spirometer every hour.
C. Use a pillow to splint the chest.
D. Teach diaphragmatic breathing to the client.

22. A 33-year-old client is experiencing severe irritability secondary to acute alcohol withdrawal. The physician orders lorazepam (Ativan) mg IV tid. Using a 4-mg/ml vial, how many milliliters does the nurse administer?

A. 0.5
B. 1.0
C. 1.5
D. 2.0

23. A 38-year-old client is admitted with fever and dyspnea and is intubated and placed on a ventilator for respiratory distress. After the endotracheal tube has been placed in the client, the nurse would immediately do which of the following?

A. Check for bilateral breath sounds.
B. Call for a chest x-ray.
C. Obtain stat arterial blood gases.
D. Check the client's vital signs.

24. A 49-year-old client is admitted with signs and symptoms of pulmonary embolism. The nurse is aware that which of the following is a risk factor associated with pulmonary embolism?

    A. Hypervolemia
    B. Arthritis
    C. Long-bone fracture
    D. Osteoporosis

25. A child with neutropenia has just been admitted to the pediatric unit. Which of the following actions by the nurse would take highest priority?

    A. Encourage eating raw vegetables and fruits for their vitamin C content.
    B. Prohibit any activity and maintain strict bedrest.
    C. Report immediately any temperature elevation.
    D. Screen visitors.

26. A 46-year-old client is 3 days postoperative status from a craniotomy. The client develops diabetes insipidus. The nurse realizes that which of the following causes diabetes insipidus?

    A. Increased antidiuretic hormone (ADH) production
    B. Decreased ADH production
    C. Hypovolemia
    D. Renal failure

27. A 78-year-old male client is admitted for shortness for breath on exertion and extreme fatigue. Some time after lunch, he asks the nurse if there are any large-print magazines or books in the hospital to read. He tells the nurse that it is the only type of print he can read. The nurse would identify which of the following conditions as the reason for the client's visual problem?

    A. Cataracts
    B. Presbyopia
    C. Xerostomia
    D. Arcus senilis

28. Which of the following statements by a 23-weeks-pregnant client indicates to the nurse the need for further instruction on improving circulation?

    A. "I should avoid crossing my legs while sitting."
    B. "I should put on my support pantyhose after I have walked to the bathroom."
    C. "I should elevate my legs whenever I sit at work."
    D. "I should dorsiflex my feet if I have been standing for a long period of time."

29. What is the single most effective mechanism to prevent and control the spread of hepatitis A in any setting?

    A. Education
    B. Handwashing
    C. Avoidance of illicit drug use
    D. Immunization to prevent hepatitis B virus infection

30. The second stage of labor is complete when:

    A. The cervix is completely dilated
    B. The client begins the pushing process
    C. The infant is delivered
    D. The placenta has been delivered

31. A 28-year-old client is admitted with Cushing's syndrome. Which of the following physical changes would the nurse expect to observe in a client with this disorder?

    A. Bronzing of the skin, weight loss, and alopecia
    B. Hyperactivity, acne, and ecchymosis
    C. Moon face, hirsutism, and thin extremities
    D. Buffalo hump, thin extremities, and girdle obesity

32. Which of the following information is most important in teaching parents about the hygiene of a preschooler?

    A. The parent should assist with or supervise all of his or her hygienic needs, especially bathing, until age 5 years.
    B. The preschooler is fearful of being pulled down the drain because of the inability to judge size.
    C. The child cannot dress himself or herself completely until age 4 years.
    D. Specific instructions and directions with no options are best to ensure proper bathing and dressing.

33. A client is 4 days after delivery by cesarean section. Which of the following is true regarding uterine involution after a cesarean section?

    A. The uterus involutes 1 cm/day.
    B. Lochia increases about day 5.
    C. Lochia decreases about day 5.
    D. There is less risk for endometritis.

34. A 6-year-old boy has asthma. His mother asks the nurse if he can participate in any sports. The nurse would recommend which of the following?

    A. Basketball
    B. Long-distance running
    C. Swimming
    D. Soccer

35. A mother has her 12-year-old daughter in the arthritis clinic. The physician prescribes naproxen (Naprosyn)—first dose 500 mg, then 250 mg every 8 hours—for signs and complaints of inflamed joints and pain. The mother asks how long it will take for the naproxen to be effective. Which of the following is the most accurate response by the nurse?

    A. "It is a long-acting drug and will take several months for therapeutic effect."
    B. "Therapeutic effects may not be noticed for 3 to 4 weeks."
    C. "The medicine works rapidly, so she will be moving her joints better in 24 hours."
    D. "She will have relief of pain after the first dose, but the inflammation will not decrease for several days."

36. A client gave birth 10 minutes ago. The placenta has still not delivered. The nurse should:

    A. Inform the primary health-care provider

B. Apply traction to the umbilical cord
C. Prepare the client for surgery
D. Reassure the client that this is normal

37. The nurse is caring for a 4-year-old child admitted with a history of spontaneous pneumothorax. The child has a closed-chest drainage system. The purpose of the water in the closed-chest drainage chamber is to:

A. Decrease the danger of sudden change in pressure in the tube
B. Prevent entrance of air into the pleural cavity
C. Provide faster removal of chest secretions by capillary action
D. Facilitate emptying bloody drainage from the chest

38. Discharge instructions for a client recovering from severe iron-deficiency anemia should emphasize the need for:

A. Planned rest periods
B. Fluid intake of 3000 ml daily
C. A diet high in vatamin B_{12}
D. A diet high in folic acid

39. A 2-year-old girl has a diagnosis of urinary tract infection (UTI). While teaching the mother, the nurse identifies the following factor as having predisposed her daughter to a UTI:

A. Increased fluid intake
B. Frequent emptying of the bladder
C. Ingestion of highly acidic juices
D. Short urethra in young girls

40. For many women, one of the first signs of pregnancy is a fullness or tingling of the breasts. These changes are a result of:

A. The presence of breast milk
B. An enhanced sexual drive
C. A decreased blood supply
D. Hormonal changes

41. An 8-year-old child was admitted to the hospital with an acute illness. During the admission assessment, the nurse notes the child's religious affiliation as Mormon. What beliefs about diet and food practices are common to this religion?

A. Members may not have blood transfusions.
B. Members may eat meat from animals that are vegetable eaters, have cloven hooves, and chew their cud.
C. Members should avoid tea, coffee, chocolate, and other products containing caffeine.
D. Members must fast for 6 hours before receiving Holy Communion.

42. A 15-year-old female client is seen at the clinic and is given a diagnosis of a UTI infection. In preparing to teach her, the nurse would include which of the following in the plan of care?

A. Inform her that the cause of such infection in adolescents is usually sexual activity.
B. Tell her that drinking large amounts of carbonated beverages can help to dilute the urine.

C. Tell her that douching will help to rid the vagina of bacteria.
D. Tell her that it is best to take showers because baths may contribute to bacterial growth that may predispose a female to a UTI.

43. A 4-year-old boy is admitted to the children's surgical unit for first stage repair of hypospadias. In considering the level of development of the preschool-age child, which of the following statements accurately describes this stage of development?

A. He is experiencing the Electra complex.
B. He is beginning to question his sexuality.
C. He is anxious about penile size.
D. He is afraid of mutilation.

44. An alcoholic client is discharged from the inpatient treatment setting on disulfiram (Antabuse). The nurse should instruct the client to avoid the use of:

A. Vinegar-based dressings, cough elixirs, and cologne
B. Cough elixirs, cologne, and acetaminophen
C. Cologne, acetaminophen, and penicillin
D. Acetaminophen, penicillin, and vinegar-based dressings

45. A nurse is teaching a 65-year-old client about closed-angle glaucoma. Which of the following statements indicates a clear understanding of closed-angle glaucoma?

A. "I should never take over-the-counter medications without consulting my doctor."
B. "If I forget to take my eyedrops, I just wait for the next dose."
C. "I can stop taking my eyedrops when my vision improves."
D. "I will return to my eye doctor for a checkup every 2 years."

46. A 17-year-old female client suspects that she is 10 days pregnant. Because she cannot come to the clinic this week, the client tells the nurse that she will use a home pregnancy test. The nurse should emphasize the fact that:

A. Consumer tests have a high rate of false-positive results.
B. Consumer tests are easy to use.
C. A test with a negative result should be repeated in a week if amenorrhea continues.
D. The results of clinic tests are kept private.

47. Which of the following is expected behavior in a 4-year-old child?

A. The child may tell "tall tales" and have imaginary playmates.
B. The child may make extra demands for attention because fear of loss of love is common.
C. The child still clings to the security blanket.
D. The child will be more tranquil than at 3 years old.

48. An 8-year-old child is admitted to the pediatric unit with a diagnosis of acute glomerulonephritis (AGN). A nursing care plan would include which of the following?

A. Forcing fluids
B. Increasing sodium in the diet

C. Weighing daily

D. Taking vital signs once per shift

49. When the client's membranes spontaneously rupture, the nurse's first action is to:

A. Change the client's linen

B. Notify the primary health-care provider

C. Assess fetal heart tones

D. Document the client's response to the event

50. On the second-day postpartum cesarean section, the nurse notes that a breastfeeding client's uterus is 3 cm below her umbilicus. The nurse would expect this finding to be:

A. Abnormal because her baby weighed >7 lb

B. Abnormal because this is her first baby

C. Normal because she has had a cesarean birth

D. Normal because she is breastfeeding

51. A 45-year-old client performs the repetitive act of checking the front door of her house to make certain that it is locked. The client feels out of control and requests admission to the hospital. During the initial interview, the nurse observes that the client is restless and has difficulty focusing on a topic. The nurse is aware that the client's behavior represents an effort to:

A. Relieve tension

B. Control her thoughts

C. Seek attention

D. Control a phobia

52. A 20-year-old client has third-degree burns on 9% of the body. The nurse explains to the family that one leg has been burned and that third degree means that:

A. Subcutaneous (SC) tissues and possibly underlying tissues are involved

B. Destruction of epidermis and dermis has occurred

C. Only the epidermis has been lost

D. The leg is covered by erythema and blisters

53. A 16-year-old girl developed macrocytic anemia secondary to pregnancy. The physician orders 1 mg of folic acid intramuscularly (IM) for 4–5 days. Using a 5-mg/ml vial, the nurse administers how many milliliters?

A. 0.1

B. 0.2

C. 0.3

D. 1.0

54. Which finding indicates that a client who takes nitroglycerin (NTG) needs further teaching to prevent complications?

A. Client took six NTGs before notifying the physician.

B. Client places the tablet under the tongue until dissolved.

C. Client stores the medication in an airtight, dark bottle.

D. Client reports that he premedicates before sexual intercourse.

55. A client with diabetes had 30 units of NPH insulin SC at 8 AM. The nurse might plan for this client to have a snack between:

A. 10 AM and 2 PM

B. 12 noon and 4 PM

C. 2 PM and 8 PM

D. 4 PM and 7 PM

56. The descent of the fetal head into the pelvis before delivery is called:

A. Quickening

B. Effacement

C. Lightening

D. Station

57. Which of the following approaches by the nurse is best when administering an IM injection of an antibiotic to a 2-year-old child?

A. Tell the child it will not hurt, secure the child, and administer the antibiotic IM.

B. Tell the child there will be a little stick in the arm and explain that it will hurt a little.

C. Allow the child to assist in drawing up the medication beforehand.

D. Enter the room with medication prepared, briefly state that he or she is giving the child a shot, administer it, and comfort the child.

58. When planning nursing care for a 5-year-old child, which nursing action is most appropriate for the child placed under an oxygen mist tent?

A. Encourage the child to keep stuffed animals in bed with him or her.

B. Encourage the use of a battery-operated tape player for music.

C. Use only synthetic-material blankets under the tent.

D. Use a plastic or vinyl doll for play.

59. A client with newly diagnosed diabetes is being discharged; the client is to give himself insulin when he goes home. Before discharging the client, the nurse ensures that he:

A. Explains all of the details about how to give the insulin

B. Administers the injection into an orange

C. Administers the injection to a significant other

D. Administers the insulin to himself

60. On afternoon rounds, the nurse sees the mother of a terminal cancer client weeping silently. What would be the most appropriate nursing intervention?

A. Tell her that you (the nurse) know how she feels.

B. Tell her she must not cry and that everything is going to be all right.

C. Go immediately to her and ask her what she is crying about.

D. Sit in the chair beside her, put your hand on her hand, and wait for her to speak.

61. The nursing process is a systematic, rational method of planning and providing nursing care based on a client's actual or potential health-care needs. The step in which the nurse carries out planned nursing interventions is called:

A. Planning

B. Evaluation

C. Implementation

D. Data collection

62. A 4-year-old child is seen in the clinic. She is pulling on her ear and says, "My ear hurts." This statement is an example of:

A. Secondary data

B. Constant data

C. Objective data

D. Subjective data

63. According to Maslow's hierarchy of needs, a client having respiratory distress would fit under the category with the highest priority, called:

A. Safety and security needs

B. Physiological needs

C. Self-actualization

D. Psychosocial needs

64. An 85-year-old client in a skilled nursing care facility is complaining of chest pain. Essential nursing data collection includes:

A. The location, intensity, and duration of the pain

B. How well the client slept last night

C. Whether the pain increases on movement

D. The client's body temperature

65. A 67-year-old client is admitted with pulmonary emphysema. Signs and symptoms that the nurse might expect to note in data collection may include:

A. Severe chest pain, hot dry skin, minimal breath sounds, inspiratory wheezing

B. Exertional dyspnea, cough with copious amounts of mucopurulent sputum, barrel-shaped chest

C. Anxiety, cyanosis, hypotension, dysphagia, chronic respiratory alkalosis

D. Orthopnea, inspiratory wheezing, lack of chest movement on the left side, severe knifelike chest pain

66. Medications often used in the treatment of chronic obstructive pulmonary disease (COPD) include bronchodilators to relax smooth muscle and to increase vital capacity. An example of a bronchodilator is:

A. Spironolactone (Aldactone)

B. Nifedipine (Procardia)

C. Aminophylline

D. Digoxin

67. The nurse needs to monitor clients receiving bronchodilators for side effects or toxic effects of these drugs, which include:

A. Seeing halos around lights and having blurred vision, tachycardia, hypotension, anorexia

B. Dehydration, hypokalemia, urticaria, abdominal or epigastric pain

C. Tachycardia, cardiac arrhythmias, photosensitivity, headache, confusion

D. Restlessness, tachycardia, insomnia, nausea, vomiting, palpitations, seizures

68. A client with pulmonary emphysema has severe difficulty breathing and orthopnea. Orthopnea means that the client:

A. Has respiratory distress

B. Has blood gases that show respiratory acidosis

C. Has periods of apnea

D. Can breathe more easily when sitting upright

69. The flow rate for O_2 administration to a client with severe emphysema (i.e., COPD) will be in low concentrations, 1–2 L/min, because:

A. High levels of O_2 will cause tachypnea and hypoxemia

B. The respiratory center in the brain has adapted to low levels of O_2 as the main stimulus for respiration, and administration of high concentrations of O_2 will depress respirations

C. COPD clients often need to receive long-term oxygen therapy, and high levels of O_2 could create a dependency

D. Higher levels of O_2 should be administered only as a last resort to prevent carbon dioxide retention and respiratory alkalosis

70. Safety precautions in the use of oxygen therapy include:

A. Posting "No smoking" signs on the door of the room

B. Not using any electrical equipment near the oxygen flow meter

C. Instructing the client that smoking is permitted only when the oxygen is not on

D. Avoiding use of medications that might interact with oxygen

71. A client's oral temperature is 102°F (38.8°C). This is:

A. Within the normal range for an oral temperature

B. Afebrile

C. Febrile and higher than normal

D. An indication that the electronic thermometer needs to be recharged

72. Factors that can affect normal body temperature include:

A. Diet, blood pressure, time of day

B. Medications taken, mood, health status, exercise

C. Smoking, environment, weight, medications

D. Age, diurnal variations, environment, exercise

73. A 44-year-old client has type I, or insulin-dependent, diabetes mellitus and is receiving 30 units of Humulin neutral protamine Hagedorn (NPH) insulin every morning. The nurse will observe him for signs and symptoms of hypoglycemia:

A. 30–60 minutes after administration

B. 8–12 hours after administration

C. 18 hours after administration

D. 2–4 hours after administration

74. Symptoms of hypoglycemia include:

A. Hunger, inability to concentrate, tremors, tachycardia, diaphoresis, diplopia, blurred vision

B. Hypothermia, anorexia, lethargy, increased thirst, nausea, vomiting

C. Irritability; loss of appetite; dry, hot flushed skin; diplopia

D. Inability to concentrate, air hunger, headaches, blood glucose level of 140

75. A client is to receive Regular and NPH insulin. The nurse will:

   A. Draw up the amount of Regular insulin into the syringe first
   B. Draw up the NPH insulin first because this will enhance mixing of the two insulins
   C. Inject a volume of air equal to that of medication into the NPH insulin vial first and withdraw the NPH insulin before withdrawing the amount of Regular insulin
   D. Draw up the Regular insulin into the syringe first

76. The normal route of administration of insulin is:

   A. IM
   B. Intradermal
   C. SC
   D. Oral

77. The nurse is assigned to care for a 47-year-old female client who is first-day postoperative cholecystectomy. She will be kept on nothing by mouth (NPO) postoperatively until:

   A. She no longer has nausea and her appetite returns
   B. She is fully awake and the effects of the anesthesia have worn off
   C. Her physician writes an order for clear liquids as tolerated
   D. Peristalsis has returned, as evidenced by auscultation of bowel sounds and the ability to pass flatus

78. A postoperative cholecystectomy client is receiving a clear liquid diet. Which of the following foods is allowed?

   A. Jell-O, cream of chicken soup, milk
   B. Oatmeal, orange juice, vanilla pudding
   C. Water, coffee or tea, sherbet, pureed bananas
   D. A grape popsicle, plain gelatin, apple juice, water

79. Medications that may be given to a postoperative client experiencing nausea and vomiting include:

   A. Trimethobenzamide (Tigan) or promethazine (Phenergan)
   B. Glycopyrrolate (Robinul) or diphenhydramine (Benadryl)
   C. Merperidine (Demerol) or pentazocine (Talwin)
   D. Atropine or morphine

80. A most important nursing intervention in which the nurse instructs the client to prevent postoperative respiratory complications is:

   A. To perform range-of-motion and leg exercises as soon as the anesthetic has worn off
   B. To stop smoking and to cough and deep-breathe at least every 2 hours
   C. To elevate the feet when sitting up and to wear antiembolic stockings during postoperative ambulation
   D. To provide low-flow oxygen and to increase vitamin C intake

81. The nursing intervention that will quickly alert the nurse to any changes in a postoperative client's condition is:

   A. Measuring and recording intake and output (I&O)
   B. Assessing pain quality and intensity
   C. Monitoring vital signs
   D. Inspecting the dressing or drainage tubes, or both, for bleeding

82. The nurse has just administered digoxin (Lanoxin) 0.25 mg to a client, and the client asks, "How does this medicine help my heart beat?" The nurse's best response is:

   A. "It helps to dilate the blood vessels, which increases your heart rate."
   B. "It increases the force of the contraction of the heart muscle and also strengthens the heartbeat."
   C. "It constricts the coronary arteries, which helps to supply more blood to your heart."
   D. "It lengthens the number of impulses generated, which in turn slows down your heart rate."

83. The nurse instructs a client in the cardiac unit to take his radial and apical heart rate, and the client asks, "Why is this important?" The nurse's best response is:

   A. "It is important for you to know how to take your own pulse."
   B. "You will know what your normal pulse rate is."
   C. "The physician will want you to call him or her and perhaps omit your digoxin if your pulse rate falls below a certain level."
   D. "Knowing your normal pulse rate will alert you to changes, which may require omitting or even increasing the amount of your medication."

84. A 67-year-old executive is hospitalized with a cerebrovascular accident (CVA), or stroke. Blood pressure on admission is 170/110 mm Hg. The executive has some weakness in the left arm and leg. The cause of this left-sided weakness is:

   A. A hemorrhage or clot on the left side of the brain, which has cut off the blood supply to the spinal cord
   B. Hypertension, and it is a temporary condition
   C. A hemorrhage or clot on the right side of the brain
   D. A thrombosis of the spinal cord, which has decreased the blood supply to the extremities

85. A 66-year-old male client's blood pressure of 170/110 mm Hg is:

   A. Within the normal range for a man of his age
   B. Serious hypertension
   C. Slightly higher than normal
   D. Slightly high but probably a result of his hospitalization and diagnosis

86. Some clients with CVAs experience expressive aphasia, which is:

   A. Inability to speak because of intellectual impairment related to brain damage
   B. Inability to read and understand
   C. Difficulty in speaking and swallowing related to neuromuscular impairment and brain damage
   D. Inability to speak, understand, or write because of impairment of the blood supply to the speech center

87. Maintenance of body function and prevention of complications is crucial in the nursing management of a

client who has suffered a CVA. Nursing interventions that will aid in recovery and prevent contractures include:

A. Turning and repositioning client every 2 hours, using a footboard and pillows, and encouraging range-of-motion exercises to all extremities.
B. Elevating the head of the bed 40 degrees; instructing client to turn, cough, and deep-breathe every 2–4 hours.
C. Performing neurological assessment every 2 hours, turning and repositioning client, using flotation mattress, and auscultating lung sounds.
D. Changing client's position from side to side every 2 hours, monitoring vital signs, and observing for signs of dehydration and electrolyte imbalance.

88. Discharge instructions to give a client with a CVA to aid in preventing a recurrence include:

A. "Use community resources, keep appointments for speech and physical therapy, take medication as ordered, and maintain a diet high in protein and vitamin E."
B. "Lose weight and stop smoking (if applicable), follow dietary instructions (low salt, low cholesterol, and low fat), keep blood pressure under control, and report any changes in your condition to your physician."
C. "Keep blood pressure under control, perform aerobic exercises three times a week, and maintain 1500-kcal American Diabetes Association (ADA) diet."
D. "Stop smoking (if applicable), avoid overexposure to very cold weather, continue speech and physical rehabilitation, and monitor daily I&O."

89. A 34-year-old woman is first day postappendectomy. The nurse assists her in coughing and deep-breathing every 2 hours to:

A. Prevent pulmonary complications
B. Help to remove secretions from the lungs and bronchi
C. Prevent postoperative thrombophlebitis
D. Mobilize secretions and prevent paralytic ileus

90. Nursing interventions that help to prevent circulatory problems in postoperative clients include:

A. Performing leg exercises and early ambulation
B. Checking vital signs every 4 hours
C. Decreasing fluid intake and assessing for edema
D. Administering oxygen via nasal cannula

91. The appearance of a second postoperative day surgical wound should have:

A. A slight erythema at the distal portion and slight sanguineous drainage
B. Absence of redness or swelling and edges well approximated
C. Minimal to moderate swelling and slight purulent discharge
D. Slight scar tissue and minimal serous drainage

92. A 36-year-old male client is experiencing dyspnea and chest pain. This assessment is an alteration in which of his basic needs?

A. The need for love and belonging
B. Physiological needs (i.e., oxygen)
C. Self-esteem
D. Safety and security (i.e., comfort)

93. Surgical wound infections are the second most frequent type of nosocomial infection found in hospitals. Health personnel could best reduce these infections by:

A. Leaving incisions open to air to promote healing
B. Using strict surgical asepsis when changing all dressings
C. Strictly adhering to the principles of effective handwashing
D. Always cleansing incisions from bottom to top—from the least contaminated to the most contaminated area

94. An 85-year-old client in a skilled care facility has an infected leg ulcer. Hot moist packs are ordered. The nurse will use extreme caution in applying these packs because many older clients have:

A. Reduced sensitivity to pain
B. Reduced sensation to temperature stimuli
C. Thickened integumentary areas
D. Increased sensation of nerve pathways

95. The nurse is applying an elastic bandage to the sprained ankle of a client in an outpatient clinic. The nurse leaves the toes exposed to:

A. Allow range-of-motion exercises and prevent potential complications
B. Decrease discomfort and potential edema
C. Allow the skin to breathe
D. Check for circulation and sensation of the extremity

96. A 72-year-old client has nausea and vomiting, arrhythmias, diarrhea, and changes in color vision. The client has been taking digoxin 0.25 mg daily for the last 6 months. These symptoms are:

A. Probably a result of something that the client ate
B. A toxic effect of digoxin
C. A side effect of digoxin
D. A result of a dose of digoxin too high for client's age

97. Nursing interventions for a client receiving SC heparin include:

A. Monitoring apical pulse and blood pressure before each administration
B. Strictly monitoring the client's I&O
C. Assessing skin, mucous membranes, urine, and other body secretions for possible bleeding
D. Assessing the client for an electrolyte imbalance

98. A teenage girl is very angry about a test she failed in school today and accuses the teacher of wanting to make her feel "stupid." This is an example of:

A. Anger
B. Repression
C. Projection
D. Denial

99. A client with pancreatitis has a history of alcohol abuse. The nurse will observe the client for agitation; nausea and vomiting; delirium tremens; and visual, auditory, and tactile hallucinations. These are indications of:

   A. Possible cirrhosis of the liver
   B. Alcohol withdrawal
   C. Depression
   D. Suicidal thoughts

100. The nurse is assisting a third-day postoperative client in selecting a dinner menu. Vitamin C is essential in tissue healing. Which of the following menus will best aid in providing vitamin C?

   A. Roast chicken, corn on the cob, mashed potatoes, butterscotch pudding
   B. Fish fillet, brown rice, green beans, tomato juice, Jell-O with sliced fruit
   C. Chicken breast fillet in tomato sauce, potatoes, broccoli, cantaloupe with sliced strawberries
   D. Veal parmesan, white rice, carrots, tossed salad, custard pudding

101. The nurse is to administer iron dextran IM to a client with iron-deficiency anemia. Because this drug is irritating to tissues, the nurse will:

   A. Carefully inject it into the ventrogluteal site, which has a large muscle mass
   B. Administer it into the ventrogluteal site using the Z-track technique and a 2- to 3-inch long needle
   C. Administer it into a large muscle and massage the area thoroughly for absorption into the muscle
   D. Administer it IV because the nurse knows that it will cause less irritation by this route

102. The nurse is to administer 500 mg of amoxicillin PO to a client with pneumonia. The medication on hand is labeled in grams. The nurse will give:

   A. 0.5 g
   B. 5 g
   C. 1.5 g
   D. 50 g

103. A 4-year-old child has varicella (chickenpox). In the future, the child should have what type of immunity?

   A. Artificially acquired immunity
   B. Natural passive immunity
   C. Actively acquired immunity
   D. Naturally acquired active immunity

104. Handwashing is crucial in preventing the spread of infection. This practice breaks the chain of infection during which phase of the cycle?

   A. Portal of entry to host
   B. Reservoir
   C. Method of transmission
   D. Portal of exit from source

105. The data collection phase of the nursing process is best described as:

   A. Evaluating whether the problem has been resolved
   B. Putting planned nursing strategies into action
   C. Setting priorities with the client that will resolve the identified problem
   D. Gathering, communicating, and verifying data about health needs of the client

106. An 86-year-old client is admitted with a diagnosis of hypernatremia. The nurse should expect the blood plasma level to be:

   A. High in sodium ions
   B. High in calcium levels
   C. Low in sodium ions
   D. Low in chlorides

107. A 16 year-old adolescent admitted with sickle cell crisis has complaints of dyspnea and leg pain. The pain of sickle cell anemia is caused by:

   A. The disturbance in cellular metabolism
   B. Enlargement of the bone marrow and a decrease in the number of circulating RBCs
   C. The sickling (clumping) of the cells, which obstructs the capillary blood flow and causes occlusion and thrombosis
   D. Bleeding into the joints because of the rapid destruction of RBCs by the bone marrow

108. Genetic counseling is very important in sickle cell anemia because it is:

   A. A nonserious condition with a very poor prognosis
   B. A hereditary chronic form of anemia that results in a shortened life span
   C. An acquired immunosuppressive condition resulting in little resistance to infection
   D. A sex-linked inherited coagulation disorder causing spontaneous bleeding

109. A 20-month-old baby is admitted to the pediatric unit with injuries that could possibly have resulted from child abuse. The mother states that the child "fell down the stairs." Which of the following will provide the nurse with additional information when assessing the baby?

   A. Ask the mother why such a young child was left unattended.
   B. Talk to the child and ask what happened.
   C. Observe the interaction between mother and child.
   D. Pick up and examine the child more carefully.

110. A nurse comes upon the scene of an automobile accident. On further investigation, the driver does not appear to be conscious. What is the nurse's first priority?

   A. Establish a patent airway.
   B. Assess for pulselessness.
   C. Assess for unresponsiveness.
   D. Call for help.

111. A 52-year-old male client is admitted with a possible myocardial infarction. His wife is very frightened and asks the nurse, "Is he going to die?" Which would be the most appropriate response by the nurse?

   A. "I really can't tell you that; you'll have to talk to his doctor."

B. "You have to be brave for your husband now; let's not talk like that."

C. "I know you're scared; would you like to sit and talk for a while?"

D. "Perhaps your husband is not really as sick as he appears. Most people don't die from a heart attack."

112. An adult client's pulse is rapid and irregular; this would be referred to as:

A. Weak and thready
B. Tachycardia and arrhythmia
C. Tachycardia and bounding
D. Tachycardia and hypotension

113. A 4-year-old child is admitted with acute lymphocytic leukemia. Which of the following symptoms are typical of this type of leukemia?

A. Pallor, weakness, fatigue, lymphadenopathy
B. Hypotension, anorexia, thrombosis, alopecia
C. Thrombocytopenia, enlarged cervical lymph nodes, chest pain
D. Anemia, spontaneous bleeding, decreased urinary output

114. The nurse must be extremely careful in protecting a client with leukemia from any source of infection primarily because:

A. If these clients acquire an infection and antibiotics are ordered, they would suffer very serious side effects from such drugs
B. They might contact pneumonia and become even more ill
C. Leukemia seriously affects the blood-forming system (WBCs) and its ability to ward off infection
D. An infection could precipitate spontaneous bleeding and hemorrhage

115. A 47-year-old client is having surgery to remove gallstones. This surgery is called:

A. Cholelithotomy
B. Cholelithiasis
C. Lithotripsy
D. Cholecystostomy

116. Nurses are responsible for assessing urinary function in their clients. A *urinometer* is:

A. An instrument used to measure a client's output accurately
B. A device used to obtain a urine specimen from a client
C. An instrument used to measure the specific gravity of urine
D. A device used to test the urine for sugar and acetone

117. When measuring the specific gravity of the urine of a client who is dehydrated, the nurse would expect:

A. A specific gravity below the norm because of decreased urinary output
B. An increase in specific gravity because of the concentration of the urine and excess sodium
C. An increased specific gravity because of increased urinary output

D. A specific gravity within the normal range, unless the client's output is higher than usual

118. When doing preoperative and postoperative teaching with a client who is very anxious, the nurse must remember that:

A. The client's stress level is only temporary
B. The client may not be able to follow directions or explanations given at this time
C. The client may have a lot of misplaced hostility and may be noncompliant
D. The client's anxiety is probably not related to fear of the unknown

119. Nurses can experience anxiety, especially in a new or an unknown situation, such as performing a procedure for the first time. Which of the following will help to decrease the nurse's anxiety in such a situation?

A. Ask another team member to do the procedure.
B. Relax and remain confident, and performance will be effective.
C. Ask questions and review the procedure, because knowledge and competence help to allay anxiety.
D. Assume that anxiety often releases hormones that improve effectiveness and performance.

120. A client has just been told by the physician that his condition is extremely grave and the prognosis very poor. When the nurse enters his room, he says, "The doctor said I am just fine and can go home today." What is the probable rationale for his statement?

A. He refuses to believe what the doctor has said and is using denial as a means of coping.
B. He probably misunderstood the doctor's explanation.
C. He is bargaining in an attempt to be discharged and postpone facing his prognosis.
D. He is depressed and just wants to go home and pretend he didn't hear what the doctor said.

121. Which of the following is the nurse's first intervention in the treatment of an adult client in respiratory arrest?

A. Pinch the victim's nose and administer two quick breaths into the mouth.
B. Administer 100% O_2 with an Ambu bag.
C. Open the victim's airway using the head-tilt–chin-lift maneuver.
D. Begin chest compressions at a ratio of 15 compressions:2 ventilations.

122. When a nurse is performing cardiopulmonary resuscitation (CPR) on an adult and is the only rescuer, the compression:ventilation ratio is:

A. 5 compressions:2 ventilations
B. 15 compressions:2 ventilations
C. 5 compressions:1 ventilation
D. 15 compressions:1 ventilation

123. A client with cancer of the lung is receiving chemotherapy. The nurse will monitor blood values, specifically the WBC count, because:

A. These drugs cause proliferation of red blood cells

(RBCs) and the nurse needs to be aware of any pertinent changes

B. These drugs cause polycythemia and could precipitate thrombosis

C. These drugs depress the bone marrow, inhibiting the production of blood cells, and a serious decrease in WBCs increases susceptibility to infection

D. A serious decrease in WBCs could alter the effects of the drug and even cause bleeding tendencies

124. Nurses encounter many ethical dilemmas in their practice. Which of the following could be considered an ethical dilemma?

A. A client refuses to take digoxin as ordered.

B. A terminally ill client's pain is not being properly managed.

C. A child is admitted with signs and symptoms of physical abuse.

D. The nurse observes another nurse on the unit taking a controlled substance that was meant for a client.

125. A licensed practical nurse (LPN) working in a health-care agency is expected to practice:

A. Within the same standards as other LPNs in a similar setting

B. According to the guidelines of the nurse or physician under whose supervision the LPN is practicing

C. Within the scope of his or her knowledge and experience

D. To the best of his or her ability and experience

126. Which lunch menu should the nurse recommend for a child with celiac disease?

A. Hot dog, french fries, milk, and cake

B. Spaghetti, garlic bread, salad, and pudding

C. Pizza, cookies, and malt

D. Baked fish, corn on the cob, and apple

127. A client complains of nausea and headache. This is an example of:

A. Objective data

B. Variable data

C. Constant data

D. Subjective data

128. When taking an oral temperature with a glass thermometer, to obtain an accurate reading the nurse must leave it in place for:

A. Five to 10 minutes

B. Approximately 2–4 minutes

C. Thirty to 60 seconds

D. Approximately 1–1½ minutes

129. Before administering digoxin, the nurse checks:

A. The client's blood pressure

B. The apical pulse for 60 seconds

C. The radial pulse

D. The client for pitting edema

130. When discharging a client with a prescription for warfarin (Coumadin), the nurse instructs the client not to take aspirin because aspirin:

A. Can cause irritation to the lining of the stomach

B. Frequently has delayed effects and is not readily absorbed in the body

C. Interferes with clot formation and could precipitate bleeding

D. Is not very effective and causes more side effects than most medications

131. In giving dietary discharge instruction to a client with a recent myocardial infarction, the nurse instructs him to avoid foods that:

A. Are high in potassium, because this could seriously alter his serum electrolytes

B. Contain caffeine, such as chocolate and tomato juice

C. Are high in saturated fats

D. Are high in sugar and vitamin B

132. A 53-year-old client with a recent stroke is very frustrated because he will not be able to return to his occupation as an airline pilot. He is very angry today and refuses his medication. What should the nurse understand?

A. Clients who can no longer be as independent as in the past experience a great deal of frustration.

B. His feelings are temporary, and he will soon learn to adapt.

C. He is using his anger and noncompliance to get attention.

D. He is denying his illness and displaying immature behavior.

133. A 24-year-old woman is pregnant for the first time. The term for a first pregnancy is:

A. *Primipara*

B. *Multigravida*

C. *Primigravida*

D. *Para*

134. A 19-year-old primigravida is admitted with preeclampsia. The nurse will monitor her very closely for:

A. Hypotension

B. Nausea

C. Bleeding

D. Evidence of seizure activity

135. A 4-year-old child is admitted with a fever of 105°F (40.5°C) and a potential diagnosis of infectious meningitis. The physician has ordered a lumbar puncture. The purpose of this test is:

A. To decrease the pressure on the brain

B. To bring down fever

C. To examine the cerebrospinal fluid (CSF) for evidence of bacteria indicative of meningitis

D. To examine the spinal column for evidence of bleeding

136. After a lumbar puncture, the nurse will position the client:

A. In semi-Fowler's position to allow for drainage of CSF

B. Flat for about 6 hours to prevent a possible spinal headache

C. In a prone position to prevent post-test meningeal irritation

D. On the side with the head of the bed slightly elevated to prevent aspiration

137. A neighbor, who is working in the yard burning leaves, suddenly begins screaming for help. His clothing is on fire and he is screaming uncontrollably. The nurse's first action is to:

A. Grab a garden hose and try to put out the fire
B. Throw dirt on the victim to smother the flames
C. Place him in a horizontal position and roll him in a blanket or coat to smother the flames
D. Call the fire department for assistance

138. On arrival at the hospital, the primary focus for a client with a thermal injury is:

A. Attention to respiratory and emotional problems
B. Maintaining a patent airway, determining respiratory status, assessing the extent of the injury, and meeting fluid needs
C. Determining the cause of the accident
D. Inserting an endotracheal tube and determining potential need for skin grafting

139. The nurse is to make an entry on a client's chart at 4 PM using military time. The time the nurse enters is:

A. 0400
B. 400
C. 1400
D. 1600

140. Which of the following most accurately exemplifies documentation of objective data?

A. Respirations appear shallow and noisy.
B. The client seems to be depressed today.
C. Dressing was changed, and incision is clean and healing, with 2 cm of serosanguineous drainage.
D. The client has complaints of pain in her left lower quadrant (LLQ), not relieved by medication.

141. Erik Erikson defines the developmental stage of late adulthood (age 60 or older) as:

A. Generativity versus stagnation
B. Ego integrity versus despair
C. Intimacy versus isolation
D. Retirement versus depression

142. An 18 year-old client sustained a compound fracture of the left tibia while skiing and is admitted to the emergency room (ER). The rationale for cleaning the wound from the area of least contamination to the area of greatest contamination is to:

A. Help to promote wound healing by removing any drainage
B. Remove any moisture that harbors organisms that may have collected
C. Prevent introduction of organisms into the wound
D. Prevent contaminating areas previously cleaned

143. The Apgar scale is an assessment tool that rates the

physiological characteristics of the newborn infant. The maximum total score is:

A. 10
B. 12
C. 5
D. 4

144. An infant whose respirations are slow and irregular at 1 and 5 minutes after birth will receive an Apgar respiratory score of:

A. 3
B. 10
C. 1
D. 2

145. The most appropriate position for giving a client a back rub at the hour of sleep is:

A. Supine
B. Prone
C. Lateral
D. Semi-Fowler's

146. A frequent site and cause of nosocomial infection is the:

A. Urinary tract, related to placing the drainage bag above the bladder
B. Incision, related to use of aseptic technique when changing the dressing
C. Bloodstream, related to self-administration of insulin
D. Respiratory system, related to clients coughing without covering their mouths

147. A second-day postoperative client is having incisional pain. The client was medicated an hour ago. Which of the following noninvasive nursing interventions will best aid in decreasing pain at this time?

A. Change position and give a back rub.
B. Assist in range-of-motion exercises.
C. Give an injection of meperidine (Demerol) as ordered.
D. Explain to the client that medication has just been given and to try to relax.

148. A nurse is working in the ER and receives a frantic phone call from a mother whose 2-year-old child has swallowed a bottle of aspirin (about 20 tablets). The nurse instructs her to:

A. Call the poison control center
B. Induce vomiting if the child is conscious and bring her to the ER
C. Give the child an antiemetic and observe closely for the next 24 hours
D. Dilute the aspirin by having the child drink a glass of milk

149. When positioning a postoperative client who has had a total hip replacement, the nurse is careful to keep the operative leg:

A. Flexed
B. Abducted
C. Adducted
D. Supported by pillows under the knee and foot

150. An adult client with angina has a radial pulse of 58 bpm. This slow rate is considered below normal and is called:

    A. Tachycardia
    B. Arrhythmia
    C. Sinus rhythm
    D. Bradycardia

151. A 23-year-old client is 3 months pregnant and has hypertension as a complication of pregnancy. Which food would the nurse encourage her to avoid?

    A. Peanut butter
    B. Smoked ham
    C. Broccoli
    D. Chicken

152. A pregnant client who has hypertension is given a prescription for furosemide (Lasix), a potassium-wasting diuretic. The nurse would encourage her to eat:

    A. Bananas
    B. Apples
    C. Rice
    D. Grapefruit

153. A client has delivered a healthy 6-lb 2-oz baby. She does not want to breast-feed. The nurse explains to her that she should:

    A. Restrict fluids to 1000 ml daily
    B. Increase fluids to 3500 ml daily
    C. Wear a tight bra or binder on her breasts
    D. Apply warm compresses to her breasts

154. The nursing assistant on a nurse's unit is 8 months pregnant. While in the cafeteria at lunch time, she begins choking on roast turkey. The nurse's first intervention is to:

    A. Ask, "Can you talk?"
    B. Give her three back blows
    C. Give her three chest thrusts
    D. Perform the Heimlich maneuver

155. A 22-year-old client prematurely delivered a 5-lb 1-oz baby. She has Rh-negative blood and is to receive $Rh_0(D)$ immune globulin (RhoGAM). She asks the nurse why. The nurse explains to her that:

    A. $Rh_0(D)$ immune globulin is given to all mothers
    B. $Rh_0(D)$ immune globulin is given to Rh-negative mothers with Rh-positive babies
    C. $Rh_0(D)$ immune globulin is given to Rh-negative mothers with Rh-negative babies
    D. $Rh_0(D)$ immune globulin is given to all Rh-negative mothers

156. A client does not want to breast-feed her baby. To suppress milk production, the nurse administers:

    A. Acetazolimide (Diamox)
    B. Hydromorphone (Dilaudid)
    C. Dexamethasone (Decadron)
    D. Estradiol valerate (Deladumone)

157. A 42-year-old client has had a full-term pregnancy. Her labor is not progressing, and oxytocin (Pitocin) is started. During induction, the nurse observes her to make sure her resting phase is adequate. Her resting phase should be at least:

    A. 15 seconds
    B. 20 seconds
    C. 30 seconds
    D. 60 seconds

158. A primigravida who is 3 months pregnant is experiencing nausea. She asks the nurse why she has nausea. The nurse explains that:

    A. It is caused by her anxiety over having her first child
    B. It is caused by a change in hormonal levels
    C. A change in diet will relieve the nausea
    D. Adequate rest will relieve the nausea

159. A 15-year-old client thinks that she is pregnant and wants an abortion. She does not want her parents to know. The nurse's best advice is to:

    A. Tell her parents anyway
    B. Encourage her to talk with the father of her child
    C. Encourage her not to have an abortion
    D. Help her to make an appointment with the local clinic

160. A 30-year-old pregnant client has insulin-dependent diabetes. Her insulin requirements will:

    A. Decrease during her pregnancy
    B. Not change during her pregnancy
    C. Vary during her pregnancy
    D. Change the requirement for the type of insulin needed during her pregnancy

161. Which of the following drains is considered an open drain?

    A. Penrose
    B. Jackson-Pratt
    C. Hemovac
    D. Surgivac

162. The nurse is to apply an Ace bandage to a sprained ankle. The nurse would wrap it beginning at the _____ aspect.

    A. Medial
    B. Distal
    C. Lateral
    D. Proximal

163. A nurse is going to remove an indwelling catheter from an 80-year-old client. The nurse's first action is to:

    A. Deflate the balloon
    B. Disconnect the bag and tubing
    C. Clamp off the tubing
    D. Explain the procedure to the client

164. One method of determining the IM injection site in the gluteal muscle is to imagine that it is divided into four equal quadrants. The injection site is in which quadrant?

    A. Inner upper quadrant
    B. Upper outer quadrant

C. Lower outer quadrant
D. Lower inner quadrant

165. The angle of the needle for an intradermal injection is:

A. 10 degrees
B. 30 degrees
C. 45 degrees
D. 90 degrees

166. A nurse is going to give an SC injection. An appropriate needle length and size is:

A. 1 inch, 25 gauge
B. 1 inch, 20 gauge
C. 1½ inches, 18 gauge
D. ⅝ inch, 26 gauge

167. Which of the following is not a purpose of a nasogastric tube?

A. For gastric decompression
B. For gastric feeding
C. To remove flatus from the colon
D. To administer medications

168. Which of the following is not an acceptable position for a client when receiving a tube feeding?

A. Semi-Fowler's on the back
B. Flat or supine
C. Semi-Fowler's on the right side
D. Semi-Fowler's on the left side

169. A client is receiving an IV infusion using a volume-controlled pump. To check to see if it is infusing at the proper rate, the nurse's first step is to:

A. Check the rate on the pump
B. Count the drops with the door open
C. Count the drops with the door closed
D. Position the pump at least 18 inches above the bed

170. Which of the following is used for urinary diversion?

A. Colostomy
B. Ileostomy
C. Ureterostomy
D. Gastrostomy

171. The preferred IM injection site for a 1-year-old infant is the:

A. Deltoid
B. Gluteus
C. Rectus femoris
D. Triceps

172. A 9-year-old child has a short-leg cast for a fractured ankle. Instruction to the child and mother on discharge from the ER includes:

A. Dry the cast thoroughly with a hair dryer.
B. Use a coat hanger to scratch under the cast.
C. Keep the leg flat for 24 hours.
D. Avoid lifting the cast with the fingertips.

173. Toys to be avoided by a 5-year-old child who has hemophilia include:

A. Tricycle
B. Swings
C. Plastic toys with sharp edges
D. Large Lincoln logs

174. A 7-year-old child has a diagnosis of hypothyroidism. The nurse would suggest that the mother keep the room temperature at:

A. 60°F (15.5°C)
B. 70°F (21.1°C)
C. 75°F (23.8°C)
D. 85°F (29.4°C)

175. An infant client was born with a cleft lip and palate. What method would the nurse use to feed the client?

A. Medicine dropper
B. Metal spoon
C. Soft long nipple
D. Gastrostomy tube

176. A 3-year-old client has just been given a diagnosis of a volvulus. The child's father asks the nurse what it is. The nurse explains that it is:

A. A twisted bowel
B. The bowel telescoping into itself
C. The presence of adhesions
D. A very short large intestine

177. A 12-year-old client has had surgical correction of a ruptured appendix. Postoperatively the client should be positioned:

A. Flat and side-lying
B. Supine
C. Prone
D. In semi-Fowler's position

178. A 2-year-old child fell from a bicycle and hit her head. On her discharge from the ER, the nurse explains to her parents that they should immediately return her to the ER if she:

A. Has a headache
B. Changes her level of consciousness
C. Does not eat
D. Begins crying

179. A neighbor rushes to a nurse's house because her 6-month-old baby has stopped breathing. The nurse's first response is to establish an airway. Next the nurse tries breathing for the baby. How many breaths does the nurse give initially?

A. 1
B. 2
C. 3
D. 4

180. Which of the following congenital disorders is a genetic defect?

A. Congenital hip dysplasia
B. Sickle cell anemia
C. Fetal alcohol syndrome
D. Cerebral palsy

181. The physician has ordered Tylenol 650 mg PO. The nurse has available Tylenol 5 grains. How many tablets would the nurse give?

    A. ½
    B. 1
    C. 1½
    D. 2

182. The physician has ordered 1000 ml D$_5$W plus 80 mEq potassium chloride to run over 12 hours via IV volume-controlled pump. At what hourly rate would the nurse set the pump?

    A. 83 ml/hr
    B. 84 ml/hr
    C. 100 ml/hr
    D. 183 ml/hr

183. The physician has ordered neutral protamine Hagedorn (NPH) insulin 35 units plus Regular insulin 10 units. The nurse's first step in drawing up these two insulins into the same syringe is:

    A. Injecting air into the Regular insulin
    B. Injecting air into the NPH insulin
    C. Drawing up the Regular insulin
    D. Drawing up the NPH insulin

184. The physician has ordered gentamicin 1 mg/kg body weight IM×1. The client weighs 176 lb. How much would the nurse administer?

    A. 17.6 mg
    B. 35.2 mg
    C. 70 mg
    D. 80 mg

185. The physician has ordered cephalexin (Keflex) 1 g PO. Cephalexin 250-mg capsules are available. How many capsules would the nurse give?

    A. 1
    B. 2
    C. 3
    D. 4

186. The physician has ordered renal dopamine 1 g/kg body weight. In evaluating the response to dopamine, the nurse would expect the following:

    A. Increase in blood pressure
    B. Decrease in blood pressure
    C. Increase in urine output
    D. Decrease in urine output

187. A 38-year-old client received her 20 units of Regular insulin at 7:30 AM. She refuses to eat breakfast. The nurse would be sure to observe her for:

    A. Diaphoresis
    B. Polyuria
    C. Polydipsia
    D. Polyphagia

188. A 7-year-old child is receiving insulin. He is going to camp tomorrow. He asks the nurse if he should take his insulin before he goes. The nurse suggests that:

    A. He increase his daily dose by 5 units
    B. He increase his daily dose by 10 units
    C. He take the same dose as usual
    D. He not take any insulin until after he arrives at camp

189. Which of the following statements reflects a value conflict that may influence interpersonal relationships?

    A. The client says, "My pain is worse today."
    B. The nurse says, "All alcoholics are manipulative."
    C. The nurse's aide says, "Not all drug users are worthless."
    D. The client says, "Not all nurses are unfeeling."

190. Unacceptable manipulative behavior is best controlled by:

    A. Prevention
    B. Controlling
    C. Limit setting
    D. Firmness

191. A 22-year-old client is admitted to the psychiatric unit with a diagnosis of schizophrenia, which was first diagnosed 2 years ago. The client is disheveled and has not bathed recently. The parents inform you that the client has not left her room for 10 days. On admission, the client tells the nurse, "They lied, I didn't kill my mother. You're the killers." This response is an example of:

    A. Grandiose delusions
    B. Auditory hallucinations
    C. Persecutory hallucinations
    D. Paranoid delusions

192. A schizophrenic client tells the nurse, "They lied; I did not kill my mother." The nurse's best response to the client about the mother is:

    A. "I just saw your mother; she's fine."
    B. "Tell me more about your mother."
    C. "I'll put you in an isolation room."
    D. "I'll have your mother come to see you now."

193. A client is actively hallucinating and withdrawn. The nurse wants to engage the client in a reality-oriented activity. The best approach is:

    A. To state, "I'd like you to be my partner in this game."
    B. To insist that the client join a group activity.
    C. To explain the benefits of a group activity.
    D. To ask, "Would you like to play checkers?"

194. An 80-year-old client had an ileostomy 3 days ago. He is asking the nurse about his ileostomy and wants to know whether he will have to irrigate it as his brother, who has a colostomy, has to. Based on knowledge of the GI tract, the nurse can tell him that:

    A. He will need to irrigate it daily.
    B. He should ask his physician.
    C. Ileostomies do not need irrigating.
    D. He could have his brother demonstrate an irrigation.

195. A 57-year-old client is recovering from a peptic ulcer and asks about foods. The nurse's directions include:

A. "Drink lots of milk."
B. "Eat anything that does not seem to bother you."
C. "Drink orange juice for breakfast."
D. "Limit calories to 1500 kcal daily."

196. A 77-year-old client seeks the nurse's advice on constipation. Which of the following is not good advice?

A. "Take a mild laxative daily at bedtime."
B. "Increase fluids."
C. "Eat bran on a daily basis."
D. "Eat more fruits and vegetables."

197. A female client has an indwelling urinary catheter. The nurse notices that the urine has a strong odor and is cloudy. The nurse's next action is to:

A. Send a urine specimen to the laboratory for routine urinalysis
B. Send a urine specimen to the laboratory for cultures
C. Irrigate the catheter
D. Measure the specific gravity

198. Classic subjective complaints of a UTI are:

A. Polyuria and frequency
B. Oliguria and pressure
C. Discharge and pressure
D. Frequency and dysuria

199. A 32-year-old client had a cholecystectomy 2 hours ago. The client weighs 250 lb and had general anesthesia. The client is complaining of pain. Priority nursing diagnosis at this time is:

A. Alteration in comfort
B. High risk for airway impairment
C. Alteration in fluid volume
D. Knowledge deficit

200. A 66-year-old client is seen at the clinic. She has had nausea and vomiting for 2 days and is complaining of dizziness. She thinks she has food poisoning. Evaluating her vital signs, the nurse would also include:

A. Taking blood pressure in both arms and legs
B. Simultaneously taking apical and radial pulses
C. Assessing orthostatic vital signs
D. Palpating the bladder

201. Which of the following is not a risk factor for the development of cardiovascular disease?

A. Being underweight
B. Smoking
C. Having hypertension
D. Maintaining a sedentary lifestyle

202. When administering transdermal NTG, it is most important to:

A. Check blood pressure before each dose
B. Check pulse after administration
C. Have the client in the sitting position
D. Check the client's potassium level

203. A 53-year-old client is following a low-sodium diet. A dinner tray arrives. Which food would the nurse remove?

A. Pears
B. Baked chicken
C. Olives
D. Baked potato

204. A 76-year-old client has left-sided congestive heart failure (CHF). Physical assessment findings to be expected include:

A. Dependent edema
B. Distended neck veins
C. LLQ pain
D. Dyspnea on exertion

205. A 46-year-old construction worker has arterial insufficiency of the lower extremities. Expected physical findings include:

A. Lymphedema
B. Pedal edema
C. Absence of pedal pulses
D. Bluish cast to extremities

206. The master endocrine gland is controlled by the:

A. Pineal gland
B. Sympathetic nervous system
C. Hypothalamus
D. Pituitary gland

207. A 44-year-old client has had a thyroidectomy. Planning for return from the recovery room, which item would the nurse have ready?

A. Jackson-Pratt drain
B. Tracheostomy tray
C. Salem sump tube
D. IV potassium infusion

208. A term used to describe an infection that develops as a result of a hospital stay is:

A. Pathogenic
B. Synergistic
C. Diagnostic
D. Nosocomial

1. **(C)** Nursing process phase: implementation; client need: prevention and early detection of disease; content area: medical-surgical.

   RATIONALE
   (A) The purpose of health teaching is to define the problem. **(B)** The purpose of health teaching is to facilitate client's mastery. **(C)** The focus and purpose of health teaching are to define the problem, suggest coping behaviors, and facilitate client's mastery and control. **(D)** The purpose of health teaching is to facilitate client's control.

2. **(D)** Nursing process phase: implementation; client need: prevention and early detection of disease; content area: medical-surgical.

   RATIONALE
   (A) Teaching should begin when the older client is physically capable. **(B)** Teaching should begin when the older client is physically capable. **(C)** Teaching should begin when the older client is physically capable. **(D)** Client teaching should not be done at the time of discharge, but as soon as the older person is physically capable, has the energy and stamina, and has minimal anxiety over the illness or control over the anxiety.

3. **(C)** Nursing process phase: implementation; client need: pharmacological and parenteral therapies; content area: medical-surgical.

   RATIONALE
   (A) Clients do not understand medical jargon "tid." **(B)** Clients may not be able to read a clock and know the time. **(C)** Asking when the client goes to bed at night and gets up in the morning and specifically planning medication to be taken around those times has meaning for the client. **(D)** Clients do not understand medical jargon "ac" and "hs."

4. **(C)** Nursing process phase: data collection; client need: reduction of risk potential; content area: medical-surgical.

   RATIONALE
   (A) An older person with sepsis does not have a febrile response. **(B)** An older person with myocardial infarction would present with fatigue and shortness of breath, not chest pains. **(C)** An older person with thyrotoxicosis presents with apathy rather than the hypermetabolic picture typically found in young adults. **(D)** An older person with a diabetic emergency presents with a change in level of consciousness.

5. **(A)** Nursing process phase: planning; client need: management of care; content area: medical-surgical.

   RATIONALE
   (A) The nurse needs to consider what the older person desires from the health-care system, both now and in the future. **(B)** The nurse needs to consider the older person's leisure-time activities. **(C)** The nurse needs to consider the nature of the older person's relationships and social support system. **(D)** The nurse needs to consider the nature of the older person's relationships and social support system.

6. **(C)** Nursing process phase: implementation; client need: coping and adaptation; content area: medical-surgical.

   RATIONALE
   (A) Validating an older person's concern is important in the rehabilitation process. **(B)** Validating an older person's concern is important in the rehabilitation process. **(C)** Rehabilitation concepts in a geriatric population help individuals to determine what physical activities have inherent meaning and what choices an older person may make to meet his or her own priorities. **(D)** Validating an older person's concern is important in the rehabilitation process.

7. **(C)** Nursing process phase: implementation; client need: coping and adaptation; content area: psychiatric nursing.

   RATIONALE
   (A) This response is not appropriate. **(B)** The lounge is to be used for socializing. **(C)** Residents and their families should be encouraged to personalize the living space by placing personal possessions. **(D)** The resident is less likely to be labeled as "sick" if she personalizes the living space.

8. **(C)** Nursing process phase: implementation; client need: basic care and comfort; content area: psychiatric nursing.

   RATIONALE
   (A) Serve the food to give the resident ample time to eat. **(B)** Meal service times for residents with behavioral problems should be staggered. **(C)** Having to eat with others who behave disruptively during meals is a very unpleasant experience; nurses should seat the residents according to social preference. **(D)** Mealtime can be a time for socializing.

9. **(C)** Nursing process phase: implementation; client need: pharmacological and parenteral therapies; content area: medical-surgical.

   RATIONALE
   (A) If NPH is drawn up first, this intermediate-acting insulin could be mixed with Regular insulin. **(B)** The client would receive two injections, and this is not necessary. **(C)** After air is injected into the NPH, the Regular insulin is drawn into the syringe first. If some Regular insulin should get into the vial of NPH, the action of the NPH would not be greatly affected. **(D)** The nurse can mix the two insulins without the assistance of the pharmacy.

10. **(C)** Nursing process phase: implementation; client need: prevention and early detection of disease; content area: maternity nursing.

    RATIONALE
    (A) Select another answer. **(B)** Select another answer. **(C)** 5 mg : 1 tablet = 7.5 : x = 1.5 tablets. **(D)** Select another answer.

11. **(A)** Nursing process phase: implementation; client need: basic care and comfort; content area: maternity nursing.

    RATIONALE
    (A) If an infant is quiet, begin with auscultating the heart, lungs, and abdomen. This is difficult to do if the child is fussing. **(B)** Traumatic data collections, such as from eyes, ears, and mouth, should be completed last or while the infant is crying. **(C)** The head-to-toe data collection should be altered to meet the developmental needs of the infant. **(D)** Percussion and palpation of areas should follow auscultation.

12. **(C)** Nursing process phase: planning; client need: safety and infection control; content area: psychiatric nursing.

    RATIONALE
    (A) "Why" questions may put the client on the defensive and increase the agitated state. **(B)** Apologies are no assurance that the client has the ability to control behavior. **(C)** The decision to release the client from mechanical restraints is based on assessment data that indicate the client's ability to control his violent behavior. **(D)** Current medication practice involves a combination of

neuroleptics and antianxiety medications. However, there is no assurance that the medication will calm violent behavior.

13. **(D)** Nursing process phase: assessment; client need: physiological adaptation; content area: pediatrics.

    RATIONALE

    (A) Swallowing frequently, not infrequently, would be a sign or symptom of hemorrhage. **(B)** Dark-brown emesis is old blood and is usually present in the emesis after tonsillectomy and adenoidectomy. **(C)** A pulse rate of 95 bpm is normal for a 4-year-old child. **(D)** Drooling of bright-red secretions may be an early indication of hemorrhage after tonsillectomy and adenoidectomy.

14. **(C)** Nursing process phase: implementation; client need: pharmacological and parenteral therapies; content area: maternity nursing.

    RATIONALE

    (A) Milk and calcium supplements decrease absorption of iron. **(B)** Milk and calcium supplements decrease absorption of iron. **(C)** Research has shown that iron is absorbed best if taken at bedtime with citrus juice. **(D)** Iron is absorbed best at bedtime and on an essentially empty stomach.

15. **(A)** Nursing process phase: data collection; client need: prevention and early detection of disease; content area: pediatrics.

    RATIONALE

    (A) To straighten the ear canal in an infant, the pinna is pulled down and back. **(B)** The pinna is not pulled forward to straighten the ear canal. **(C)** With older children, usually over the age of 3 years, the pinna is pulled up and back to allow visualization of the tympanic membrane. **(D)** The pinna is not pulled forward to straighten the ear canal.

16. **(B)** Nursing process phase: evaluation; client need: growth and development through the life span; content area: maternity nursing.

    RATIONALE

    (A) Intermittent vomiting is not a danger sign; continuous vomiting is. **(B)** Vaginal bleeding is the number one danger sign to be reported because of the high risk of injury to the mother and the fetus. The client should seek health care immediately. **(C)** Leukorrhea, or vaginal discharge, is not a threat to the mother's life or that of her fetus. Vaginal discharge is a common occurrence during pregnancy. **(D)** Urinary frequency is a common discomfort of pregnancy because of the increased pressure on the maternal bladder.

17. **(C)** Nursing process phase: evaluation; client need: basic care and comfort; content area: pediatrics.

    RATIONALE

    (A) The mother is correct to place the infant on the side as recommended by the American Academy of Pediatrics (AAP). **(B)** The mother is correct to place the infant in a supine position to sleep as recommended by the AAP. **(C)** The mother needs further teaching because the abdomen is no longer recommended as a sleeping position for healthy newborns. Only infants with breathing problems or excessive vomiting should sleep prone. **(D)** The upright position is appropriate for burping, which is indicated after feedings.

18. **(C)** Nursing process phase: planning; client need: psychosocial adaptation; content area: psychiatric nursing.

    RATIONALE

    (A) Diversional activities for lower-functioning clients may precipitate anxiety and regression. **(B)** Program activities should focus on strengths rather than on pathology. This approach may help the client to relinquish the sick role and to demonstrate more adaptive behavior. **(C)** Day treatment centers provide social interaction and recreational and learning activities for persons who might otherwise be isolated. **(D)** Day treatment centers provide social-skills training, opportunities for socialization, structure, and support for the client. The remaining needs are provided by significant others.

19. **(C)** Nursing process phase: data collection; client need: growth and development through the life span; content area: maternity nursing.

    RATIONALE

    (A) The correct answer is C. **(B)** The correct answer is C. **(C)** Naegele's rule, the most common method of determining a delivery date, is obtained by subtracting 3 months from the first day of the last menstrual period and then adding 1 year and seven days to that date. The correct answer is determined by: May minus 3 months is February. Adding 1 year and 7 days to the 12th results in an EDC of February 19. **(D)** The correct answer is C.

20. **(D)** Nursing process phase: evaluation; client need: growth and development through the life span; content area: maternity nursing.

    RATIONALE

    (A) The placenta does not filter out harmful substances. Whatever the mother takes in, the fetus eventually gets. **(B)** The maternal blood and fetal blood do not directly mix. Maternal nutrients and fetal wastes permeate the capillary walls of the placental villi. **(C)** The umbilical cord has two arteries and one vein. **(D)** The placenta is the connection between maternal nutrition and fetal waste.

21. **(D)** Nursing process phase: implementation; client need: reduction of risk potential; content area: medical-surgical.

    RATIONALE

    (A) This would not help the client clear the thick secretions from his lungs. Morphine sulfate can decrease deep breathing and increase the client's chance of developing pneumonia. **(B)** An incentive spirometer is used to help the client improve tidal volume and deep breathing. It does not help to alleviate pain and is uncomfortable with a fresh chest incision. **(C)** Using a pillow as a splint helps the client to cough after abdominal or thoracic surgery. It does not alleviate pain with breathing. **(D)** This answer is correct. The client can benefit from diaphragmatic breathing by using accessory muscles. The client can deep-breathe without placing pressure on the incision.

22. **(B)** Nursing process phase: implementation; client need: pharmacological and parenteral therapies; content area: psychiatric nursing.

    RATIONALE

    (A) Select another answer. **(B)** 4 mg : 1 ml = 4 mg : x = 1 ml. **(C)** Select another answer. **(D)** Select another answer.

23. **(A)** Nursing process phase: implementation; client need: prevention and early detection of disease; content area: medical-surgical.

    RATIONALE

    (A) The first action a nurse should do after the placement of an endotracheal tube is check the breath sounds of the client to ensure correct tube placement and bilateral expansion of the lungs. **(B)** A chest x-ray would be done after the nurse has assessed the client and after the physician has written the order. **(C)** Obtaining arterial blood gases is a respiratory therapist's function and also needs a physician's orders. However, the nurse is responsible for making sure the physician's orders have been carried out. **(D)** The nurse would check the client's vital signs only after having assessed the breath sounds and tube placement.

24. **(C)** Nursing process phase: planning; client need: prevention and early detection of disease; content area: medical-surgical.

RATIONALE

(A) Hypovolemia, not hypervolemia, can predispose an individual to pulmonary embolus and can produce hypercoagulability of the blood. **(B)** Arthritis is an inflammation of the joints and would not predispose a client to pulmonary embolus. **(C)** A long-bone fracture can predispose a client to pulmonary embolus by causing trauma and a change in the peripheral blood flow. **(D)** Osteoporosis is the thinning of the density of the bone and does not predispose a client to pulmonary embolus.

25. **(C)** Nursing process phase: implementation; client need: safety and infection control; content area: pediatrics.

RATIONALE

(A) Raw vegetables, fruit, and fish should be prohibited because they can introduce bacteria. **(B)** Total restriction of activity is not necessary. Games or toys that can be disinfected and watching TV are appropriate activities. **(C)** Any temperature elevation is significant, and temperature elevations of 100.4°F (38°C) or greater are reported to the physician. **(D)** Persons with colds, sore throats, or infections should be prohibited from visiting, but reporting temperature elevation is more important.

26. **(B)** Nursing process phase: planning; client need: physiological adaptation; content area: medical-surgical.

RATIONALE

(A) An increase in the production of ADH would cause fluid retention, leading to syndrome of inappropriate antidiuretic hormone (SIADH) and not diabetes insipidus, which is marked by dehydration. **(B)** This answer is correct. There is a decrease in the amount of ADH produced by the pituitary. The syndrome is marked by excessive urination, dehydration, and fluid and electrolyte imbalances. **(C)** Hypovolemia would be a result of diabetes insipidus and not a cause for the disorder. **(D)** Renal failure would not be a cause of diabetes insipidus.

27. **(B)** Nursing process phase: data collection; client need: growth and development through the life span; content area: geriatrics.

RATIONALE

(A) Cataracts cause an opacity of the lens and lead to a gradual loss of vision. Images are usually hazy and the client is bothered by glare. **(B)** This answer is correct. This condition is marked by the inability to read objects up close and is caused by the loss of elasticity of the lens of the eye. This is a common result of the aging of the eye lens. **(C)** Xerostomia is a condition seen in older persons in which they suffer from frequent dry mouth. **(D)** Arcus senilis is the deposition of lipids in the iris of the eye. It is usually seen as a slight yellow ring around the iris and is associated with aging.

28. **(B)** Nursing process phase: implementation; client need: growth and development through the life span; content area: maternity nursing.

RATIONALE

(A) Dependent edema of the lower extremities may occur because of poor venous return related to crossing the legs. **(B)** To prevent dependent edema, support pantyhose should be put on in the morning before putting the lower extremities in a dependent position such as walking. **(C)** Sitting with feet elevated facilitates venous return. **(D)** Dorsiflexion improves circulation and prevents venous stasis.

29. **(B)** Nursing process phase: implementation; client need: safety and infection control; content area: pediatrics.

RATIONALE

(A) Education of children and parents is important, but action is needed to prevent and control hepatitis. **(B)** The single most effective method of prevention is the use of handwashing. **(C)** Illicit drug use places individuals at risk for the development of hepatitis B. **(D)** The current vaccine is effective only against the hepatitis B organism.

30. **(C)** Nursing process phase: data collection; client need: growth and development through the life span; content area: maternity nursing.

RATIONALE

(A) Stage 1 is completed when the cervix is completely dilated. **(B)** Pushing occurs at the end of stage 1 and beginning of stage 2. **(C)** Stage 2 begins when the client is fully dilated and is complete on delivery of the infant. **(D)** From the time the infant delivers until delivery of the placenta is stage 3. The delivery of the placenta is the beginning of the recovery stage, stage 4.

31. **(C)** Nursing process phase: data collection; client need: prevention and early detection of disease; content area: medical-surgical.

RATIONALE

(A) These are physical changes associated with Addison's disease, which is caused by a decrease in glucocorticoid production. **(B)** Acne and ecchymosis are physical changes seen in Cushing's syndrome; however, hyperactivity is not associated with this disorder. **(C)** This answer is correct. Cushing's syndrome is a disease in which there is an excessive amount of glucocorticoid and hyperplasia of the adrenal cortex. Other physical symptoms associated with this disease include purplish striae, delayed wound healing, and a buffalo hump noted in the upper back. **(D)** These are normal physical changes associated with aging.

32. **(A)** Nursing process phase: data collection; client need: basic care and comfort; content area: pediatrics.

RATIONALE

(A) The parent should supervise or assist with hygiene, especially bathing, until the age of 5 years to prevent injury or drowning and to ensure proper technique. **(B)** The preschooler is fearful about the drain, but physiological safety takes priority over psychological safety. **(C)** Usually the 3-year-old child can dress himself or herself, except for back buttons, and should be allowed to do so. **(D)** Options can be allowed if they exist. The option to bathe and dress should not be allowed.

33. **(B)** Nursing process phase: data collection; client need: growth and development through the life span; content area: maternity nursing.

RATIONALE

(A) After a cesarean birth, there is about a 5-day delay in involution. **(B)** Lochia increases when the uterus begins to involute, around day 5. **(C)** Lochia is scant the first few days. Then, as involution occurs, the lochia increases. **(D)** Because of delayed involution, there is an increased risk of an infection, endometritis.

34. **(C)** Nursing process phase: implementation; client need: physiological adaptation; content area: pediatrics.

RATIONALE

(A) Exercise-induced asthma is common to all persons with asthma. This condition is rare in activities that require only short bursts of energy (e.g., baseball, gymnastics, skiing) compared with those that involve endurance exercise (e.g., soccer, basketball, and distance running). **(B)** Exercise-induced asthma is common to all persons with asthma. This condition is rare in activities that require only short bursts of energy (e.g., baseball, gymnastics, skiing) compared with those that involve endurance exercise (e.g., soccer, basketball, and distance running). **(C)** Swimming, even long-distance swimming, is recommended because the child breathes air saturated with moisture, and exhaling under water prolongs expiration and increases end-expiratory pressure. **(D)** Exercise-induced asthma is common to all persons with asthma. This is rare in activities that require only short bursts of energy (e.g., baseball, gymnastics, skiing) compared with those that involve endurance exercise (e.g., soccer, basketball, and distance running).

35. **(B)** Nursing process phase: implementation; client need: pharmacological and parenteral therapies; content area: pediatrics.

    RATIONALE
    (A) The therapeutic effects may not be seen immediately but are apparent in 2–4 weeks. **(B)** The normal time for the effects to be apparent is anywhere from 2–4 weeks. **(C)** The naproxen does not work that quickly for the inflammatory response from arthritis. **(D)** Beneficial effects for arthritis take longer than for other conditions, such as menstrual cramps.

36. **(D)** Nursing process phase: implementation; client need: growth and development through the life span; content area: maternity nursing.

    RATIONALE
    (A) The primary health-care provider should be present until after the delivery of the placenta. If the physician or midwife is not there at this time, this is a normal finding and would not be an indication to call him or her. **(B)** The primary health-care provider may sometimes apply tension to the cord to facilitate delivery of the placenta. This is not the role of the nurse, and traction on the cord increases the risk of complications such as uterine inversion. **(C)** Ten minutes is still within the acceptable time frame for the third stage of labor. If the client does not deliver the placenta within 30 minutes, the physician will explore the uterus and may determine that the client has a placenta accreta, which would require surgical intervention. **(D)** The normal time frame for delivery of the placenta is 5–30 minutes. Most placentas are delivered within 5 minutes, but 10 minutes is certainly within the expected time frame for this stage.

37. **(B)** Nursing process phase: planning; client need: reduction of risk potential; content area: pediatrics.

    RATIONALE
    (A) The purpose of the water in the closed-chest drainage system is to prevent entrance of air into the pleural cavity. It is not to decrease the danger of sudden change in pressure in the tube. **(B)** The purpose of the water in the closed-chest drainage system is to prevent entrance of air into the pleural cavity. **(C)** The purpose of the water in the closed-chest drainage system is to prevent entrance of air into the pleural cavity. It is not the faster removal of chest secretion by capillary action. **(D)** The purpose of the water in the closed-chest drainage system is to prevent entrance of air into the pleural cavity. It is not to facilitate emptying bloody drainage from the chest.

38. **(A)** Nursing process phase: implementation; client need: basic care and comfort; content area: medical-surgical.

    RATIONALE
    (A) The client may feel weak and fatigue easily because of tissue hypoxia caused by diminished red blood cells (RBCs) with oxygen-carrying capacity. Rest is indicated. **(B)** A high fluid intake is desirable, but it is not the priority intervention for a client recovering from iron deficiency. **(C)** A diet rich in vitamin B_{12} will not necessarily prevent iron-deficiency anemia. **(D)** A diet high in folic acid is indicated for anemia caused by folate deficiency, not iron-deficiency anemia.

39. **(D)** Nursing process phase: implementation; client need: prevention and early detection of disease; content area: pediatrics.

    RATIONALE
    (A) Increased fluid intake leads to diuresis. Diuresis enhances the antibacterial properties of the renal medulla. **(B)** The single most important factor influencing the occurrence of UTI is urinary stasis. The act of frequently emptying the bladder flushes away organisms causing UTI. **(C)** Concentrated and alkaline urine predisposes a client to UTI. Ingestion of highly acidic juices, such as cranberry juice, acidify the urine. **(D)** The short urethra, which measures ¾ inch in young girls, provides a ready pathway for the invasion of organisms.

40. **(D)** Nursing process phase: planning; client need: growth and development through the life span; content area: maternity nursing.

    RATIONALE
    (A) Breast milk does not develop in the breast early in pregnancy. **(B)** Although some women do experience an increase in sexual drive early in pregnancy, the changes in the breast are not a result of this. **(C)** The tender breasts that occur with early pregnancy result from an increased blood supply. **(D)** The hormones of pregnancy, particularly estrogen and progesterone, prepare the body for breastfeeding. Estrogen has an influence on the development of the ducts, and progesterone causes alveolar and lobule development. Blood vessels enlarge and become prominent, and the darkening and enlargement of the tubercles of Montgomery are related to the action of estrogen.

41. **(C)** Nursing process phase: data collection; client need: basic care and comfort; content area: pediatrics.

    RATIONALE
    (A) This is a belief of the Jehovah Witness faith. **(B)** Particular types of meat are not forbidden. **(C)** The Mormon faith encourages the avoidance of such stimulants as tea, coffee, chocolate, and other products containing caffeine. **(D)** Mormons fast for 24 hours on the first Sunday of each month.

42. **(D)** Nursing process phase: planning; client need: prevention and early detection of disease; content area: pediatrics.

    RATIONALE
    (A) Sexual intercourse may produce transient bacteriuria in female adolescents and is associated with increased risk of UTI, but it would not be appropriate to teach that it is usually the cause of UTI in adolescents. **(B)** Drinking large amounts of carbonated beverages would be contraindicated with UTI because this may be a contributing factor to UTI. **(C)** Douching may contribute to bacteriuria in females and is not recommended. **(D)** UTIs have been related to the use of hot tubs or whirlpool baths, and thus, if one is predisposed to UTIs, it is best to avoid tub baths.

43. **(D)** Nursing process phase: planning; client need: growth and development through the life span; content area: pediatrics.

    RATIONALE
    (A) The Electra complex is a phenomenon of female development in which the girl wishes to kill her mother and marry her father. **(B)** Adolescence, not the preschool years, is a period during which individuals commonly question their sexual orientation. **(C)** Penile size is not a concern of a 4-year-old boy. **(D)** Mutilation and castration anxiety are normal according to Freud's oedipal or phallic stage for the preschool child.

44. **(A)** Nursing process phase: implementation; client need: pharmacological and parenteral therapies; content area: psychiatric nursing.

    RATIONALE
    (A) Vinegar-based salad dressing, cough elixirs, and cologne all contain alcohol and could cause a severe reaction in the presence of disulfirum. **(B)** Cough elixirs and cologne contain alcohol; acetaminophen does not. **(C)** Cologne contains alcohol; acetaminophen and penicillin do not. **(D)** Acetaminophen and penicillin do not contain alcohol; vinegar-based salad dressing does.

45. **(A)** Nursing process phase: implementation; client need: physiological adaptation; content area: medical-surgical.

RATIONALE

(A) Medications that dilate the pupil could further increase intraocular pressure by blocking drainage from the eye through the canal of Schlemm. **(B)** Doses of eyedrops should not be missed. **(C)** Eyedrops will probably be given over the client's lifetime. **(D)** Clients with glaucoma should see their ophthalmologist at least yearly.

46. **(C)** Nursing process phase: implementation; client need: growth and development through the life span; content area: maternity nursing.

RATIONALE

(A) Consumer tests actually have higher rates of false-negative results. This is related to the test being performed too soon after a missed period. **(B)** There are many variables that must be controlled for, such as specimen contamination, timing, or movement of sample. The ease of testing is relative. **(C)** Because of the increased chance of false-negative results, it is important to determine pregnancy at the earliest time to provide prenatal care and to minimize fetal risk. **(D)** Home testing does ensure privacy, so the client is the only one who will know the result.

47. **(A)** Nursing process phase: data collection; client need: growth and development through the life span; content area: pediatrics.

RATIONALE

(A) Tall tales and imaginary playmates are normal for the 4-year-old child. **(B)** The 3-year-old child is more likely to have a security blanket or other object and to fear loss of love. **(C)** The 3-year-old child is more likely to have a security blanket or other object and to fear loss of love. **(D)** The 4-year-old child is typically more aggressive than the 3-year-old child and will become more tranquil at 5 years old.

48. **(C)** Nursing process phase: planning; client need: physiological adaptation; content area: pediatrics.

RATIONALE

(A) Fluid restriction is seldom necessary in the treatment of AGN. Forcing fluids would be contraindicated because of the edema associated with AGN. **(B)** Sodium may be restricted during the edematous phase. Increasing sodium in the diet would be contraindicated. **(C)** A record of daily weight is the most useful means to assess fluid balance in a child with AGN. **(D)** Regular measurements of vital signs, not once a shift, are essential to identify the acute hypertension associated with AGN.

49. **(C)** Nursing process phase: implementation; client need: growth and development through the life span; content area: maternity nursing.

RATIONALE

(A) Because of the risk of cord prolapse with the rupture of membranes, the nurse must first ensure fetal well-being before performing comfort measures. **(B)** Because of the risk of cord prolapse with the rupture of membranes, the nurse must first ensure fetal well-being before notifying the physician or midwife. **(C)** The nurse should first evaluate fetal well-being by assessing the fetal heart tones. There is a high risk of cord prolapse with the rupture of the amniotic membranes. **(D)** Because of the risk of cord prolapse with the rupture of membranes, the nurse must first ensure fetal well-being before documenting the client's response.

50. **(D)** Nursing process phase: data collection; client need: growth and development through the life span; content area: maternity nursing.

RATIONALE

(A) This finding is not abnormal. **(B)** This finding is not abnormal. **(C)** Cesarean section does not affect uterine contraction. **(D)** Stimulation of the nipple with breastfeeding causes the release of oxytocin, the hormone that causes the uterus to contract. This results in greater uterine muscle tone; consequently, smaller uterine size is possible earlier than if the mother were not breastfeeding. It is not abnormal, nor is it the result of cesarean birth.

51. **(A)** Nursing process phase: planning; client need: psychosocial adaptation; content area: psychiatric nursing.

RATIONALE

(A) Compulsions are attempts to relieve tension. **(B)** Obsessions are recurring thoughts that cannot be dismissed from the consciousness. **(C)** Compulsive behavior is a defense against anxiety. It is not an attention-seeking behavior. **(D)** The client is suffering from a compulsive disorder, not a phobia.

52. **(A)** Nursing process phase: planning; client need: prevention and early detection of disease; content area: medical-surgical.

RATIONALE

(A) Third-degree burns may extend into SC tissue, muscle, and nerves. **(B)** Loss of the dermis and epidermis are characteristic of second-degree burns. **(C)** Loss of only the epidermis would mean that the burns were first degree. **(D)** Blisters and erythema are seen in second-degree burns.

53. **(B)** Nursing process phase: implementation; client need: pharmacological and parenteral therapies; content area: maternity nursing.

RATIONALE

(A) Select another option. **(B)** 5 mg : 1 ml = 1 mg : x = 0.2 ml. **(C)** Select another option. **(D)** Select another option.

54. **(A)** Nursing process phase: evaluation; client need: pharmacological and parenteral therapies; content area: medical-surgical.

RATIONALE

(A) This behavior would indicate a need for further teaching. The client should notify the physician if original pain is unrelieved by three doses of NTG. **(B)** This action should be taken by the client receiving NTG. It does not indicate a need for further teaching. **(C)** This action should be taken by the client receiving NTG. It does not indicate a need for further teaching. **(D)** This action should be taken by the client receiving NTG. It does not indicate a need for further teaching.

55. **(C)** Nursing process phase: planning; client need: pharmacological and parenteral therapies; content area: medical-surgical.

RATIONALE

(A) NPH insulin SC peaks in 6–12 hours; this is too soon. **(B)** NPH insulin SC peaks in 6–12 hours; this is too soon. **(C)** NPH insulin SC peaks in 6–12 hours; this is appropriate. **(D)** NPH insulin SC peaks in 6–12 hours; this is too late.

56. **(C)** Nursing process phase: data collection; client need: growth and development through the life span; content area: maternity nursing.

RATIONALE

(A) Quickening refers to the first movements of the growing fetus that are felt by the mother. **(B)** Effacement refers to the shortening and thinning of the cervix that occurs before delivery. **(C)** Lightening refers to the tilting or dropping of the fetal head forward and downward into the true pelvis. This usually occurs 2–3 weeks before labor in the primigravida but frequently does not occur until the beginning of labor in many multigravidas. **(D)** Station is defined as the location of the presenting part of the fetus in relation to the ischial spines of the birth canal.

57. **(D)** Nursing process phase: implementation; client need: pharmacological and parenteral therapies; content area: pediatrics.

    RATIONALE

    (A) Honesty is preferred. An IM antibiotic will probably hurt. (B) Children take things literally and will assume that the nurse is putting a real stick in the arm. (C) Although seeing and holding supplies may be beneficial in some instances, the child is not able to properly prepare an IM. (D) Brief explanations presented positively and immediately before a procedure are best.

58. **(D)** Nursing process phase: implementation; client need: reduction of risk potential; content area: pediatrics.

    RATIONALE

    (A) Stuffed animals are not suitable toys because moisture will dampen the toys and make it difficult to keep them dry. (B) The toy may be a source of sparks and a potential fire hazard. (C) Synthetic blankets can initiate sparks, which may cause a fire. (D) Vinyl or plastic items do not absorb moisture and can be easily wiped dry.

59. **(D)** Nursing process phase: evaluation; client need: pharmacological and parenteral therapies; content area: medical-surgical.

    RATIONALE

    (A) Knowledge of a psychomotor skill is evaluated best by demonstration. (B) The nurse must see a demonstration of the procedure as it will be done in the home. (C) The client needs to show that fear of sticking one's self, not another, with a needle can be overcome. (D) This is the exact procedure that will be carried out at home.

60. **(D)** Nursing process phase: implementation; client need: coping and adaptation; content area: psychiatric nursing.

    RATIONALE

    (A) Telling her that you understand how she feels is not an appropriate response. It is a closed statement and does not invite a response. (B) Telling her not to cry and that everything is going to be all right is not an appropriate response. It is a nontherapeutic statement. (C) Going immediately to her and asking her what is she crying about does invite a response; however, it is not as therapeutic as being attentive and letting her know you care by your touch and waiting for her to speak. (D) Sitting in the chair beside her and letting her feel your presence and waiting for her to speak is a therapeutic response.

61. **(C)** Nursing process phase: implementation; client need: management of care; content area: medical-surgical.

    RATIONALE

    (A) Planning is the phase that comes before implementation. (B) Evaluation is determining whether needs have been met. (C) Implementation is carrying out the goals and plans. (D) Data collection identifies the need for which implementation strategies are planned.

62. **(D)** Nursing process phase: data collection; client need: prevention and early detection of disease; content area: medical-surgical.

    RATIONALE

    (A) Secondary data come from someone other than the client. (B) Constant is not a classification for client data. (C) Objective data are data that are visible or obtained from laboratory or diagnostic tests. (D) Subjective data come from the client.

63. **(B)** Nursing process phase: data collection; client need: physiological adaptation; content area: medical-surgical.

    RATIONALE

    (A) Safety and security needs come after physiological needs. (B) A client with respiratory distress has a need for adequate oxygen, which is the most essential physiological need. Physiological needs are given the highest priority in Maslow's hierarchy because they are necessary for survival. (C) Self-actualization is a need that is not reached until later in one's life. (D) Psychosocial needs are not higher than physiological needs.

64. **(A)** Nursing process phase: data collection; client need: prevention and early detection of disease; content area: medical-surgical.

    RATIONALE

    (A) The location, intensity, and duration of the pain indicate how life-threatening the pain might be. (B) The nurse may collect this information, but it is not as important as the location, intensity, and duration. (C) The nurse may collect this information, but it is not as important as the location, intensity, and duration. (D) The nurse may collect this information, but it is not as important as the location, intensity, and duration.

65. **(B)** Nursing process phase: data collection; client need: prevention and early detection of disease; content area: medical-surgical.

    RATIONALE

    (A) Severe chest pain and hot dry skin are not signs and symptoms of pulmonary emphysema. (B) Pulmonary emphysema (i.e., chronic obstructive pulmonary disease) has specific symptoms related to permanent lung changes and chronic acidosis. Exertional dyspnea is the predominant one because of air trapping and loss of lung elasticity; the swelling and overdistention of the alveoli sacs result in a cough producing copious amounts of mucopurulent sputum. Chronic hyperinflation and use of accessory muscles in breathing causes an increase in anteroposterior chest diameter, commonly referred to as "barrel chest." (C) Dysphagia and alkalosis are not signs and symptoms of pulmonary emphysema. Acidosis is a characteristic, not alkalosis. (D) Lack of chest movement on one side and knifelike chest pain are not signs and symptoms of pulmonary emphysema.

66. **(C)** Nursing process phase: data collection; client need: pharmacological and parenteral therapies; content area: medical-surgical.

    RATIONALE

    (A) Spironolactone is a potassium-sparing diuretic. (B) Nifedipine is an antihypertensive drug. (C) Aminophylline is a theophylline salt, a common bronchodilator to relax the smooth muscle of the respiratory tract and frequently used in the treatment of COPD. (D) Digoxin is a cardiotonic. Clients with COPD who also have cardiovascular complications frequently receive this medication, but it is not specific for treating the COPD.

67. **(D)** Nursing process phase: data collection; client need: pharmacological and parenteral therapies; content area: medical-surgical.

    RATIONALE

    (A) These are not typical side effects of bronchodilators. (B) These are not typical side effects of bronchodilators. (C) These are not typical side effects of bronchodilators. (D) The aim of bronchodilator therapy is to keep the client's theophylline level within the normal range (10–20 g/ml). Minor side effects usually decrease after a few days of therapy; serious side effects or toxic effects are generally related to theophylline serum levels >20 g/ml.

68. **(D)** Nursing process phase: planning; client need: basic care and comfort; content area: medical-surgical.

    RATIONALE

    (A) This is not a definition of orthopnea. (B) This is not a definition of orthopnea. (C) This is not a definition of orthopnea. (D) Orthopnea is a respiratory condition in which there is discomfort in breathing in any position except sitting or standing. It is seen in heart failure, pulmonary edema, and severe emphysema. The client may be in respiratory distress, be acidotic, and have periods of apnea as well; but the question asks for a definition of orthopnea.

69. **(B)** Nursing process phase: evaluation; client need: physiological adaptation; content area: medical-surgical.

    RATIONALE
    (A) High levels of O_2 will not cause tachycardia or hypoxemia. **(B)** Chronic pulmonary emphysema causes permanent lung damage to the alveolar walls and capillaries, resulting in air trapping, loss of elasticity, and chronic respiratory acidosis. The constant high levels of CO_2 in the blood, tissues, and brain (respiratory center) cause the emphysema client to rely on low levels of O_2 as the stimulus for respiration. Administering high levels of O_2 (>2 L/min) could decrease the hypoxic drive and result in respiratory depression or arrest. **(C)** Although some clients on long-term oxygen therapy may become psychologically dependent, this does not answer the question. **(D)** This may be a true statement, but it does not answer the question.

70. **(A)** Nursing process phase: implementation; client need: physiological adaptation; content area: medical-surgical.

    RATIONALE
    (A) Oxygen supports combustion, and even the tiniest spark could cause a fire or explosion if it came in contact with the oxygen. "No smoking" signs should be posted, and the clients and visitors must be told that smoking is not permitted in the room where oxygen is present. **(B)** Well-grounded electrical equipment can be safely used near the flow meter. **(C)** Turning off the oxygen does not eliminate the possibility of a spark causing a fire to occur. **(D)** Medications usually do not interact with oxygen.

71. **(C)** Nursing process phase: data collection; client need: prevention and early detection of disease; content area: medical-surgical.

    RATIONALE
    (A) This is above the normal range for a temperature. **(B)** Afebrile means that there is no temperature elevation. This is a temperature elevation. **(C)** The temperature of the body taken orally in a healthy individual is 98.6°F (37°C). A higher temperature than that is considered fever. **(D)** If an electronic thermometer needed to be recharged, it would not register a temperature.

72. **(D)** Nursing process phase: data collection; client need: prevention and early detection of disease; content area: medical-surgical.

    RATIONALE
    (A) Diet does not affect the body temperature. **(B)** Medications and mood do not affect the body temperature. **(C)** Weight and medications do not affect the body temperature. **(D)** Factors that can affect the client's body temperature include:
    Age: The temperature of the very young is labile because of immature physiological control mechanisms; and that of older persons is labile because of deteriorating control mechanisms.
    Diurnal variations: Body temperature is lowest at 1–4 AM and peaks at 4–6 PM.
    Environmental extremes: These can lower or raise body temperature accordingly.
    Exercise: This raises the basal metabolic rate and can also increase body temperature.

73. **(B)** Nursing process phase: data collection; client need: pharmacological and parenteral therapies; content area: medical-surgical.

    RATIONALE
    (A) NPH insulin does not start acting this quickly. Regular insulin starts acting within this time. **(B)** Humulin NPH insulin is an intermediate-acting insulin that peaks at 8–12 hours after administration, which would be a potential time for a hypoglycemic reaction to occur. **(C)** This is too long a period for an insulin reaction to occur. **(D)** This is too soon for an insulin action to occur for NPH insulin.

74. **(A)** Nursing process phase: data collection; client need: prevention and early detection of disease; content area: medical-surgical.

    RATIONALE
    (A) Hypoglycemia occurs when there is too much insulin in the bloodstream in relation to the available glucose; it can occur during peak insulin administration times, causing symptoms such as hunger, inability to concentrate, tremors, increased pulse rate, diaphoresis, and visual disturbances. **(B)** Hot dry skin, nausea, and vomiting are not signs of hypoglycemia. **(C)** These are not signs of hypoglycemia. **(D)** Hypoglycemia does not occur until the blood glucose is <80 mg/dl.

75. **(A)** Nursing process phase: implementation; client need: pharmacological and parenteral therapies; content area: medical-surgical.

    RATIONALE
    (A) Regular insulin does not contain a modifying protein to slow absorption and is the only type of insulin that can be given IV. For that reason, the nurse always draws up the Regular insulin first when mixing two types, to prevent possible contamination of the Regular insulin with the added protein, which could slow absorption. **(B)** This answer is incorrect; see rationale A. **(C)** This answer is incorrect; see rationale A. **(D)** This answer is incorrect; see rationale A.

76. **(C)** Nursing process phase: implementation; client need: pharmacological and parenteral therapies; content area: medical-surgical.

    RATIONALE
    (A) Insulin is not given IM. **(B)** Insulin is not given intradermally. **(C)** Insulin is normally given SC 15–30 minutes before breakfast to maintain postprandial blood sugar 80–140 mg/dl. Insulin is never given IM because it would be absorbed too rapidly. Regular insulin can be given IV in acute situation. **(D)** Insulin is destroyed by gastric juices if taken orally.

77. **(D)** Nursing process phase: implementation; client need: reduction of risk potential; content area: medical-surgical.

    RATIONALE
    (A) Having an appetite and no nausea does not mean that bowel sounds have returned. **(B)** She may be awake, but this does not mean that bowel sounds have returned. **(C)** Even though the nurse has an order for clear liquids, this does not ensure that bowel sounds have returned. **(D)** Most general anesthetics and preoperative medications decrease gastric motility. Trauma and manipulation of gastric organs also disturb normal digestion and elimination. Food and fluids are withheld in postoperative clients until bowel sounds and the ability to pass flatus have returned and nausea and vomiting have subsided.

78. **(D)** Nursing process phase: planning; client need: basic care and comfort; content area: medical-surgical.

    RATIONALE
    (A) These items are not on a clear liquid diet. **(B)** These items are not on a clear liquid diet. **(C)** Pureed bananas are not on a clear liquid diet. **(D)** A clear liquid diet includes foods that are clear; it is often limited to water, tea, broth, ginger ale, and plain

gelatin. The major objective is to relieve thirst and to prevent dehydration.

79. **(A)** Nursing process phase: implementation; client need: pharmacological and parenteral therapies; content area: medical-surgical.

    RATIONALE

    (A) Trimethobenzamide is an antiemetic that acts by blocking the chemoreceptor trigger zone, which in turn acts on the vomiting center. Promethazine is an antihistamine that acts on the gastrointestinal (GI) system by blocking histamine to provide sedation and decrease nausea. **(B)** Glycopyrrolate is not an antiemetic; diphenhydramine is an antihistamine that does not decrease nausea. **(C)** Merperidine and pentazocine are analgesics and may cause nausea. **(D)** Morphine is an analgesic, and atropine decreases peristalsis, which does not decrease nausea.

80. **(B)** Nursing process phase: implementation; client need: reduction of risk potential; content area: medical-surgical.

    RATIONALE

    (A) These exercises may increase activity but are not primary interventions for decreasing respiratory complications. **(B)** Prevention of postoperative respiratory complications begins with teaching coughing and deep breathing and encouraging clients to stop smoking, which immobilizes cilia and impairs oxygenation. **(C)** These activities will not prevent respiratory complications. **(D)** These interventions are not specific to preventing respiratory complications.

81. **(C)** Nursing process phase: implementation; client need: prevention and early detection of disease; content area: medical-surgical.

    RATIONALE

    (A) Although the nurse may perform these activities on a postoperative client, they will not alert the nurse to an acute problem. **(B)** These symptoms are expected after surgery. **(C)** Vital signs (temperature, pulse, respirations, and blood pressure) are indicators of a person's health status. They are a quick and efficient way of monitoring a client's condition or identifying the presence of problems (especially potential bleeding or shock in a postoperative client). **(D)** These options are appropriate interventions but will not provide an overall health status.

82. **(B)** Nursing process phase: evaluation; client need: pharmacological and parenteral therapies; content area: medical-surgical.

    RATIONALE

    (A) Except in toxic doses, digoxin decreases the heart rate. **(B)** Digoxin is a cardiotonic drug that increases the force of contraction of the myocardium, thereby increasing cardiac output. Cardiotonics also depress the sinoatrial node and slow conduction of the electrical impulses to the atrioventricular node, decreasing the number of ventricular contractions per minute. **(C)** Digoxin does not constrict the arteries. **(D)** Digoxin does not lengthen the number of impulses generated.

83. **(C)** Nursing process phase: evaluation; client need: prevention and early detection of disease; content area: medical-surgical.

    RATIONALE

    (A) This statement is true, but it is not the best response. **(B)** This statement is true, but it is not the best response. **(C)** Digoxin can cause serious side effects or toxic effects, and many physicians want the client to monitor the pulse rate and be given instructions to notify the physician if it falls below or exceeds a certain rate. **(D)** This is a true statement, but it is not the best response.

84. **(C)** Nursing process phase: evaluation; client need: physiological adaptation; content area: medical-surgical.

    RATIONALE

    (A) A hemorrhage in the brain does not cut off blood supply to the spinal cord. **(B)** Hypertension may have precipitated the stroke but does not cause the symptoms; the symptoms are brought on by the stroke. **(C)** When a client suffers a stroke, the hemorrhage or clot causes weakness or hemiplegia on the opposite side of the brain, because there is a crossover of nerves in the pyramidal tract as they lead from the brain down the spinal column. **(D)** There is no thrombosis of the spinal cord in a stroke.

85. **(B)** Nursing process phase: data collection; client need: prevention and early detection of disease; content area: medical-surgical.

    RATIONALE

    (A) This blood pressure is not in normal range. **(B)** Normal blood pressure for adults ranges from about 100/60–140/90 mm Hg. A sustained systolic pressure of 150 mm Hg or higher and a sustained diastolic blood pressure of 90 mm Hg or higher is usually considered hypertension. Blood pressure of 170/110 is considered serious hypertension and may be directly related to a CVA. **(C)** This blood pressure is more than slightly elevated. **(D)** This blood pressure is more than "slightly high."

86. **(D)** Nursing process phase: data collection; client need: physiological adaptation; content area: medical-surgical.

    RATIONALE

    (A) This response meets the criteria for aphasia but is not complete. **(B)** This response meets the criteria for aphasia but is not complete. **(C)** This response does not meet the criteria for aphasia. **(D)** A hemorrhage or clot to the brain often affects the blood supply to the speech center located in the brain, causing various types of aphasia.

87. **(A)** Nursing process phase: implementation; client need: basic care and comfort; content area: medical-surgical.

    RATIONALE

    (A) A contracture is a permanent tightening or shortening of a muscle because of a paralysis. Range-of-motion exercises increase circulation, strengthen muscles, and prevent contractures. Position changes, as well as use of footboards and pillows, also help to keep the body in good alignment, prevent footdrop, and hasten recovery by preventing other complications (respiratory, circulatory, and skin breakdown). **(B)** These interventions are appropriate but will not prevent contractures. **(C)** These interventions are appropriate but will not prevent contractures. **(D)** These interventions will not prevent contractures.

88. **(B)** Nursing process phase: planning; client need: reduction of risk potential; content area: medical-surgical.

    RATIONALE

    (A) This is good advice but will not prevent recurrence of a stroke. **(B)** Being overweight and smoking cigarettes decrease blood supply to vital organs and contribute to arteriosclerosis and atherosclerosis, which are etiological factors in stroke. A diet that is too high in salt, fat, or cholesterol also can contribute to another stroke, by causing fluid retention and narrowing of arteries. Alerting the doctor to any changes in physical condition will also help to maintain health and to prevent further complications. **(C)** This is good advice but will not prevent recurrence of a stroke. **(D)** This is good advice but will not prevent recurrence of a stroke.

89. **(B)** Nursing process phase: evaluation; client need: reduction of risk potential; content area: medical-surgical.

    RATIONALE

    (A) These exercises will not prevent pulmonary complications. **(B)** Anesthetics impair respiratory function. Coughing and deep breathing postoperatively help to remove secretions from the lungs and bronchi and to prevent respiratory complications of pneumonia and atelectasis. **(C)** Coughing and deep breathing will not prevent thrombophlebitis. **(D)** Coughing and deep breathing will not prevent a paralytic ileus.

90. **(A)** Nursing process phase: implementation; client need: reduction of risk potential; content area: medical-surgical.

    RATIONALE

    (A) The decreased mobility after surgery, side effects of anesthesia, and possible electrolyte imbalances all increase the risk of circulatory complications such as thrombophlebitis and pulmonary embolus. Leg exercises aid in preventing the formation of a thrombus. Ambulation stimulates circulation in the lower extremities, preventing venous stasis, thrombophlebitis, and possible pulmonary embolus. **(B)** Checking vital signs will not prevent complications. **(C)** Decreasing fluids may increase complications. Assessing for edema will not prevent complications. **(D)** Oxygen is important but will not prevent circulatory problems.

91. **(B)** Nursing process phase: data collection; client need: prevention and early detection of disease; content area: medical-surgical.

    RATIONALE

    (A) There should be no redness or swelling on a second-day postoperative wound. **(B)** A surgical wound heals by primary intention. Wound edges should be well approximated with no evidence of redness or swelling and with a scant to moderate amount of serosanguineous drainage on the second day after surgery. **(C)** There should not be purulent drainage, indicating that an infection has started on the second day postoperatively. **(D)** Scar tissue would not occur until much later after healing has taken place.

92. **(B)** Nursing process phase: data collection; client need: safety and infection control; content area: medical-surgical.

    RATIONALE

    (A) The need for love and belonging involves physical and emotional relationships. **(B)** Abraham Maslow's hierarchy of human needs is a theory nurses use to understand the relationships of basic human needs. Physiological needs (of which oxygen is the most essential) have the highest priority. The client's chest pain and dyspnea are interfering with basic need for oxygen. **(C)** Self-actualization and self-esteem are higher on the hierarchy (i.e., less important) than physiological needs. **(D)** Safety and security needs include thirst, hunger, sleep, and rest.

93. **(C)** Nursing process phase: implementation; client need: safety and infection control; content area: medical-surgical.

    RATIONALE

    (A) This option is appropriate, but the best response is handwashing. **(B)** This option is appropriate, but the best response is handwashing. **(C)** Research shows that 70% of all nosocomial infections occur in postoperative clients. In a hospital study of 541 nosocomial infections over 7 months, 21% were caused by the same species as that found on hands. Handwashing is considered one of the best ways to prevent the spread of infection. **(D)** This option is appropriate, but the best response is handwashing.

94. **(B)** Nursing process phase: evaluation; client need: reduction of risk potential; content area: medical-surgical.

    RATIONALE

    (A) Older clients frequently have decreased sensitivity to pain, but the question refers to the application of heat. **(B)** Older persons often have sensory impairment and are unable to perceive that heat is damaging the tissues; they are therefore at risk for burns. They also have a low heat tolerance, which puts them at risk for burns, as well as impaired circulation, which puts them

at risk for tissue damage. **(C)** Older persons do not have thickened skin. **(D)** Older persons have decreased sensation of nerve pathways.

95. **(D)** Nursing process phase: implementation; client need: basic care and comfort; content area: medical-surgical.

    RATIONALE

    (A) This is not the rationale for leaving the toes exposed. **(B)** Leaving the toes exposed will not decrease discomfort. **(C)** This is not the rationale for leaving the toes exposed. **(D)** When bandaging an extremity, the end of the body part should be exposed whenever possible so that the nurse (or the client) will be able to determine the adequacy of blood circulation to the extremity.

96. **(B)** Nursing process phase: evaluation; client need: pharmacological and parenteral therapies; content area: medical-surgical.

    RATIONALE

    (A) Change in color vision would not be caused by something the client ate. **(B)** These are symptoms of digitalis toxicity. There is a narrow margin of safety between the full therapeutic effects and the toxic effects of cardiotonics. Clients taking digitalis preparations must be instructed in these adverse effects and in how to monitor their pulse rate, and keep all appointments for laboratory (serum levels) or diagnostic tests. **(C)** These symptoms are a result of toxicity, not side effects. **(D)** These symptoms are caused by a high dose of digoxin, but they have nothing to do with the client's age. This is not the best answer.

97. **(C)** Nursing process phase: data collection; client need: pharmacological and parenteral therapies; content area: medical-surgical.

    RATIONALE

    (A) Heparin per se is not an indication to monitor vital signs. **(B)** Heparin per se is not an indication to monitor I&O. **(C)** The principal adverse reaction to heparin, an anticoagulant, is bleeding. The nurse will monitor the client for any evidence of bleeding and take precautions to prevent it. **(D)** Heparin will not cause an electrolyte imbalance.

98. **(C)** Nursing process phase: evaluation; client need: coping and adaptation; content area: psychiatric nursing.

    RATIONALE

    (A) An expression of anger would be stating feelings about the self without blaming others. **(B)** Repression is excluding memories from awareness. **(C)** Projection, an adaptive mechanism for dealing with inner stress, is the attribution of one's own feelings, ideas, or characteristics (usually undesirable ones) to another person. **(D)** Denial is ignoring or refusing to accept disagreeable realities.

99. **(B)** Nursing process phase: data collection; client need: prevention and early detection of disease; content area: medical-surgical.

    RATIONALE

    (A) Alcoholics may have cirrhosis of the liver, but the symptoms listed are not those of cirrhosis. **(B)** Alcohol is a central nervous system depressant; when alcohol is withdrawn abruptly, the alcoholic may develop alcohol withdrawal syndrome. Alcohol withdrawal symptoms (as listed) are considered a hyperexcitable state or a rebound phenomenon and have been called a "sympathetic storm." Recognition of early signs and symptoms is crucial: delirium tremens is fatal in 15% of clients. **(C)** There is no indication that the client is depressed, nor are these symptoms of that condition. **(D)** There is no indication that the client is suicidal, nor are these symptoms of that condition.

100. **(C)** Nursing process phase: planning; client need: basic care and comfort; content area: medical-surgical.

    RATIONALE

    (A) These foods do not contain any significant amounts of vitamin C. **(B)** These foods do not contain any significant amounts of vitamin C. **(C)** Vitamin C is essential in tissue healing. Tomato sauce, potatoes, broccoli, cantaloupe, and strawberries are all excellent sources of vitamin C. **(D)** These foods do not contain any significant amounts of vitamin C.

101. **(B)** Nursing process phase: planning; client need: pharmacological and parenteral therapies; content area: medical-surgical.

    RATIONALE

    (A) This site is acceptable but does not indicate that the nurse is using a Z-track technique. **(B)** Iron dextran, often used in the treatment of iron-deficiency anemia, is very irritating to SC tissue. The nurse should therefore give it deep IM into a large muscle, with a 2–3-inch long needle, using the Z-track technique. This prevents oozing of the drug back into subcutaneous tissue. **(C)** This answer does not include the Z-track technique. **(D)** Iron dextran cannot be given IV.

102. **(A)** Nursing process phase: planning; client need: pharmacological and parenteral therapies; content area: medical-surgical.

    RATIONALE

    (A) There are 1000 mg in a gram. Therefore, if the nurse is to administer 500 mg, the nurse will give 0.5 g or ½ g. **(B)** Math calculation explains incorrect options. **(C)** Math calculation explains incorrect options. **(D)** Math calculation explains incorrect options.

103. **(D)** Nursing process phase: evaluation; client need: prevention and early detection of disease; content area: pediatrics.

    RATIONALE

    (A) Artificially acquired immunity occurs with immunizations. **(B)** Natural passive immunity occurs with placental transfer. **(C)** Active acquired immunity occurs with an injection of human or animal serum. **(D)** When a person contracts chickenpox, antibodies are formed in the presence of active infection in the body. This is a naturally acquired type of active immunity, which should produce a lifelong immunity to that disease.

104. **(C)** Nursing process phase: planning; client need: safety and infection control; content area: medical-surgical.

    RATIONALE

    (A) Intact skin is the main mechanism in the portal of entry. **(B)** The reservoir will not prevent the spread of infection. **(C)** The aim of most hospital precautions is breaking the chain during the mode (method) of transmission phase of the cycle. Handwashing (especially between client contacts), which prevents the spread of infection during the mode of transmission, is the most effective means of controlling and preventing the spread of microorganisms. **(D)** Careful isolation and disposal of waste and waste products (portal of exit) will decrease the spread of infection but will not break the chain.

105. **(D)** Nursing process phase: evaluation; client need: management of care; content area: medical-surgical.

    RATIONALE

    (A) This choice describes the evaluation phase. **(B)** This choice describes the implementation phase. **(C)** This choice describes the planning phase. **(D)** Data collection is the first phase of the nursing process. The nurse gathers, verifies, and communicates data about a client to establish a database about the client's level of wellness, health practices, past illnesses, and related experiences and health-care goals.

106. **(A)** Nursing process phase: data collection; client need: physiological adaptation; content area: medical-surgical.

    RATIONALE

    (A) Hypernatremia means sodium excess in the blood plasma. The nurse would therefore expect a sodium level higher than the norm of 135–145 mEq/L (plasma). **(B)** Hypercalcemia is a high blood level of calcium. **(C)** Hyponatremia is a low blood level of sodium. **(D)** Hypochloremia is a low blood level of chlorides.

107. **(C)** Nursing process phase: data collection; client need: physiological adaptation; content area: medical-surgical.

    RATIONALE

    (A) Cellular metabolism may be affected, but it does not cause the pain. **(B)** The number of circulating RBCs decreases, but this decrease is not the cause of the pain in sickle cell anemia. **(C)** In sickle cell anemia, the RBCs that contain the sickle cell hemoglobin are deoxygenated, causing them to elongate and become crescent-shaped. They are then unable to pass through the bloodstream, causing thrombosis, pain, and infarction because of the decreased blood supply. **(D)** There is no bleeding in the joints with sickle cell anemia.

108. **(B)** Nursing process phase: implementation; client need: prevention and early detection of disease; content area: maternity nursing.

    RATIONALE

    (A) Sickle cell anemia is a serious condition. **(B)** Sickle cell anemia is an inherited severe multisystem disease for which there is no known cure. Genetic counseling is important because the disease can be transmitted to offspring. **(C)** Sickle cell anemia is not an acquired immunosuppressive condition. **(D)** Sickle cell anemia is not sex linked.

109. **(C)** Nursing process phase: implementation; client need: psychosocial adaptation; content area: pediatrics.

    RATIONALE

    (A) Asking the mother why the child was left unattended will put her on the defensive. **(B)** A 20-month-old child cannot describe what happened. **(C)** In a suspected case of child abuse, some additional information may be obtained by observing the parent-child interaction. How does the parent talk to the child? Is verbalization negative or positive? How does the parent respond to the child? Does the child seek comfort from the parent? **(D)** Examining the child will give the nurse more assessment data on physical injuries, but it will not help to determine the interaction between mother and child. This is not the best response.

110. **(C)** Nursing process phase: implementation; client need: physiological adaptation; content area: medical-surgical.

    RATIONALE

    (A) This is not the first step in CPR. **(B)** This is not the first step in CPR. **(C)** Before beginning CPR, the nurse should first assess for unresponsiveness and should then look, listen, and feel for any signs of spontaneous respirations. These are the standard steps in CPR. **(D)** This is not the first step in CPR.

111. **(C)** Nursing process phase: implementation; client need: coping and adaptation; content area: psychiatric nursing.

    RATIONALE

    (A) This response will not decrease her anxiety. **(B)** This response will not decrease her anxiety. **(C)** Therapeutic communication is crucial at this time. Listen to the client's wife and allow her to ventilate her feelings. Provide the opportunity for her to express her feelings and fears; to ask further questions; and to seek comfort, support, and understanding. This is the best response for the circumstances. **(D)** This response will not decrease her anxiety.

112. **(B)** Nursing process phase: data collection; client need: prevention and early detection of disease; content area: medical-surgical.

 RATIONALE

 (A) Thready means a very weak pulse. **(B)** By definition, "tachy" is derived from the Greek *tachys*, meaning swift. "Cardia" is from the Greek *kardia*, meaning heart. The Greek word *rhythmos* means rhythm (measured time or movement; regular occurrence of an impulse). *Arhythmos* means without rhythm or lacking rhythm, or not regular. **(C)** There is no indication that the pulse is bounding. **(D)** There is no indication that there is hypotension. It does not fit the definition of rapid and irregular.

113. **(A)** Nursing process phase: data collection; client need: prevention and early detection of disease; content area: pediatrics.

 RATIONALE

 (A) Early signs and symptoms of acute lymphocytic leukemia include pallor, weakness, fatigue, and lymphadenopathy. Leukemia, a malignant disorder of the bone marrow and lymph nodes, leads to an increase in uncontrollable WBCs, which enlarges lymph tissue (lymphadenopathy) and causes a decrease in other blood cells (RBCs and platelets), resulting in pallor, weakness, and fatigue. **(B)** The symptoms listed are not characteristic of acute lymphocytic leukemia. **(C)** The symptoms listed are not characteristic of acute lymphocytic leukemia. **(D)** The symptoms listed are not characteristic of acute lymphocytic leukemia.

114. **(C)** Nursing process phase: implementation; client need: safety and infection control; content area: medical-surgical.

 RATIONALE

 (A) Side effects of antibiotics are not more serious in these clients than in other clients. This is not the best response. **(B)** Correct, but with the explanation given in option C. **(C)** Clients with acute leukemia have an increased potential for infection because they have many immature WBCs that are incapable of fighting infection. **(D)** An infection will not precipitate bleeding.

115. **(A)** Nursing process phase: implementation; client need: physiological adaptation; content area: medical-surgical.

 RATIONALE

 (A) Cholelithotomy is the removal of gallstones through an incision. **(B)** Cholelithiasis means the formation or presence of calculi or bile stones in the gallbladder. **(C)** Lithotripsy is the process of crushing stones through shock waves. **(D)** Cholecystectomy is removal of the gallbladder.

116. **(C)** Nursing process phase: planning; client need: basic care and comfort; content area: medical-surgical.

 RATIONALE

 (A) A urinometer does not measure output. **(B)** A urinometer is not used to take a specimen. **(C)** A urinometer is an instrument that measures specific gravity of urine, comparing its weight with that of water. **(D)** This is not a device for measuring glucose (sugar) and acetone.

117. **(B)** Nursing process phase: evaluation; client need: prevention and early detection of disease; content area: medical-surgical.

 RATIONALE

 (A) A dehydrated client will have an increased specific gravity. **(B)** When a client is dehydrated or hypovolemic, sodium and other electrolytes are lost through excretion along with water, resulting in urine that is more concentrated. The more concentrated the urine, the higher its specific gravity (and weight) will be. A dehydrated client would have decreased urinary output. **(C)** Dehydrated clients have a decreased urine output. **(D)** Dehydrated clients have a decreased urine output.

118. **(B)** Nursing process phase: planning; client need: psychosocial adaptation; content area: psychiatric nursing.

 RATIONALE

 (A) The anxiety may not be temporary. **(B)** Anxiety is an emotional response to a threat to one's self-esteem or well-being. Clients undergoing a surgical procedure are often highly stressed and unable to follow directions or explanations given. The nurse first needs to listen, allow the client to express any fears, and answer questions before giving teaching or explanation. **(C)** This statement may or may not be true, but it does not address anxiety. **(D)** Anxiety may or may not be related to fear of the unknown. This is not the best response.

119. **(C)** Nursing process phase: planning; client need: psychosocial adaptation; content area: psychiatric nursing.

 RATIONALE

 (A) This strategy might help to reduce the nurse's anxiety, but it is not the best response. **(B)** The nurse may have confidence, but the anxiety will still remain. **(C)** Anxiety often impairs functioning and can also lead to errors in judgment and performance. Nurses unfamiliar with a procedure need to take time to review it, to ask questions, and to remember that knowledge and competence guard against anxiety and that as knowledge and competence increase, anxiety lessens. **(D)** This statement may be true, depending on the level of anxiety. This is not the best response.

120. **(A)** Nursing process phase: data collection; client need: coping and adaptation; content area: psychiatric nursing.

 RATIONALE

 (A) Clients often at first deny the seriousness of their illness and go through elaborate mental "gymnastics" (such as denial) to prove to themselves that this is not really happening to them. This mental mechanism is a means of helping them to cope, until they are able to begin to deal with the reality of their illness. **(B)** It is more likely that he is in denial rather than not hearing the physician. **(C)** Bargaining is a later stage of coping with a grave prognosis. **(D)** Depression is a later stage of coping with a grave prognosis.

121. **(C)** Nursing process phase: implementation; client need: physiological adaptation; content area: medical-surgical.

 RATIONALE

 (A) This is not the first intervention in CPR. **(B)** This is not the first intervention in CPR. **(C)** Of the foregoing choices, in a client with respiratory arrest the nurse must first open the airway before proceeding with other interventions. Opening the airway often will aid in spontaneous respirations. This is standard protocol for CPR. **(D)** This is not the first intervention in CPR.

122. **(B)** Nursing process phase: implementation; client need: physiological adaptation; content area: medical-surgical.

 RATIONALE

 (A) This ratio does not meet the standards of CPR. **(B)** The American Medical Association and American Health Association guidelines for CPR are 15 chest compressions:2 ventilations in a one-person rescue. **(C)** This ratio does not meet the standards of CPR. **(D)** This ratio does not meet the standards of CPR.

123. **(C)** Nursing process phase: data collection; client need: pharmacological and parenteral therapies; content area: medical-surgical.

RATIONALE
(A) These drugs do not cause proliferation of RBCs. (B) These drugs do not cause polycythemia. (C) Chemotherapy is aimed at destroying cancer cells, which are rapidly dividing cells. In the process, chemotherapy also destroys other rapidly dividing cells (e.g., bone marrow), which could cause a profound decrease in WBCs, putting the client at risk for infection, which he or she may not be able to fight off. (D) Chemotherapy does not cause bleeding tendencies.

124. **(D)** Nursing process phase: implementation; client need: management of care; content area: psychiatric nursing.

RATIONALE
(A) A client's refusal to take medication is not an ethical dilemma. (B) This choice does not meet the definition of an ethical dilemma. (C) Physical abuse is reportable by law; thus there is no ethical dilemma. (D) An ethical dilemma occurs when there is a conflict of values. Ethics concerns what is right or wrong; values influence how one perceives others and how one acts. In option D, the nurse's values come into conflict, because the nurse does not want to report the colleague but knows that he or she needs help and that the behavior could endanger clients. As a professional, the nurse is accountable to maintain standards of practice and assumes an ethical responsibility to clients.

125. **(A)** Nursing process phase: implementation; client need: management of care; content area: medical-surgical.

RATIONALE
(A) Nurses are responsible for practicing within the standards of care developed by their licensing agencies and profession. These standards are guidelines for determining whether a nurse has acted as any reasonable prudent nurse with the same level of education and experience would have acted. (B) The Board of Nursing sets guidelines for LPNs, not individual nurses or physicians. (C) This choice does not meet the criteria for the Board of Nursing. (D) This choice does not meet the requirements for the Board of Nursing.

126. **(D)** Nursing process phase: implementation; client need: basic care and comfort; content area: pediatrics.

RATIONALE
(A) Hot dogs, bread, and cake contain gluten. This child needs a gluten-free diet. (B) All these foods (except salad) contain gluten. (C) All these foods contain gluten. (D) These foods are gluten-free and should be recommended for this child's diet.

127. **(D)** Nursing process phase: data collection; client need: prevention and early detection of disease; content area: medical-surgical.

RATIONALE
(A) Complaints of nausea and headache are not objective data. (B) Variable data are used in research. (C) Constant data are used in research. (D) Complaints of nausea and headache are subjective data information only—the client's perceptions or feelings about a health problem. Objective data are concrete data that can be palpated, observed, or auscultated.

128. **(B)** Nursing process phase: implementation; client need: prevention and early detection of disease; content area: medical-surgical.

RATIONALE
(A) Five minutes is longer than necessary. (B) The nurse must allow sufficient time for the temperature to register. The recommended time is 2 minutes or 3 minutes for a glass thermometer. (C) Thirty to 60 seconds is not long enough to register a temperature on a glass thermometer. (D) One to 1½ minutes is not long enough to register a temperature on a glass thermometer.

129. **(B)** Nursing process phase: evaluation; client need: pharmacological and parenteral therapies; content area: medical-surgical.

RATIONALE
(A) It is not necessary to take the blood pressure before giving digoxin. (B) It is necessary to take an apical pulse for a full minute before administering digoxin, a cardiotonic. Changes in pulse quality, rate, and rhythm cannot always be easily assessed by a radial pulse. The physician may want the nurse to hold the drug and notify him or her if the apical pulse rate falls below 60 bpm or the client displays any symptoms of digitalis toxicity (arrhythmias or changes in pulse rhythm). (C) Before giving digoxin, the apical pulse is taken, not the radial pulse. (D) One does not need to check for pitting edema before giving digoxin.

130. **(C)** Nursing process phase: implementation; client need: pharmacological and parenteral therapies; content area: medical-surgical.

RATIONALE
(A) This statement is true, but it is not the reason for not taking aspirin with warfarin. (B) This statement is true, but it is not the reason for not taking aspirin with warfarin. (C) Aspirin interferes with clot formation and potentiates the action of anticoagulants (warfarin) and could cause bleeding or hemorrhage. Clients taking warfarin should be instructed to use acetaminophen instead of aspirin. (D) This statement is true, but it is not the reason for not taking aspirin with warfarin.

131. **(C)** Nursing process phase: planning; client need: prevention and early detection of disease; content area: medical-surgical.

RATIONALE
(A) There is no reason to restrict potassium in the diet of a client who has had a myocardial infarction unless he is on a special medication that can cause a retention of potassium. (B) Tomato juice is not high in caffeine. (C) Following a diet that is high in saturated fats constitutes a risk factor for myocardial infarction and the development of coronary artery disease. (D) The client with myocardial infarction does not normally need to be concerned about vitamin B in the diet.

132. **(A)** Nursing process phase: evaluation; client need: coping and adaptation; content area: medical-surgical.

RATIONALE
(A) This client's frustration is a natural reaction, especially because his illness interferes with his occupation and his means of earning a living. A change in occupation may be more difficult because of his age and condition. (B) His behavior may not be temporary. (C) His behavior is not related to a desire for attention. (D) His behavior is not related to immaturity.

133. **(C)** Nursing process phase: data collection; client need: growth and development through the life span; content area: maternity nursing.

RATIONALE
(A) *Primipara* means having given birth once. (B) *Multigravida* means having had more than one pregnancy. (C) *Primigravida* is the term used for a woman during her first pregnancy: *primi* meaning first or one and *gravida* meaning pregnant or heavy with child. (D) *Para* means past pregnancies.

134. **(D)** Nursing process phase: data collection; client need: growth and development through the life span; content area: maternity nursing.

RATIONALE
(A) Clients with preeclampsia have hypertension. (B) The client may have nausea, but this does not require frequent monitoring. (C) Preeclampsia is not associated with bleeding. (D) Preeclampsia, or toxemia of pregnancy, if not monitored and

treated promptly, can lead to eclampsia. Symptoms of eclampsia include convulsive seizures and coma—a very grave condition of pregnancy. The nurse may monitor this client for the other conditions, as well, but they do not characterize preeclampsia, which is what the question is about.

135. **(C)** Nursing process phase: data collection; client need: prevention and early detection of disease; content area: medical-surgical.

RATIONALE

(A) The purpose of a lumbar puncture is diagnostic, not to relieve pressure on the brain. **(B)** Performing a lumbar puncture will not bring down the temperature. **(C)** In meningitis, an inflammation of the meninges of the brain, CSF surrounds the brain and spinal cord. A lumbar puncture is performed in this instance to examine the CSF for evidence of bacteria (which causes meningitis) or increased WBCs resulting from inflammation or infection. **(D)** The spinal fluid can be examined for blood, but the primary reason for a lumbar puncture in this case is diagnostic in nature.

136. **(B)** Nursing process phase: implementation; client need: reduction of risk potential; content area: medical-surgical.

RATIONALE

(A) Maintaining the client in a semi-Fowler's position would increase the likelihood of headache. **(B)** Keeping the room dark and the bed flat, as well as increasing hydration, will relieve discomfort and help to prevent headache. **(C)** Keeping the client prone would not prevent meningeal irritation. **(D)** Some clients experience a "spinal" headache after the removal of CSF, and lying on the side would not relieve it.

137. **(C)** Nursing process phase: implementation; client need: physiological adaptation; content area: medical-surgical.

RATIONALE

(A) This may be a later activity, but it is not the first action. **(B)** This may be a later activity, but it is not the first action. **(C)** At the scene of a fire, the first priority is to prevent further injury to the victim. Laying the victim flat prevents the fire, hot air, and smoke from rising toward the head and respiratory passages. Rolling the victim in a blanket or article of clothing will help to smother the fire. **(D)** This may be a later activity, but it is not a first priority.

138. **(B)** Nursing process phase: planning; client need: prevention and early detection of disease; content area: medical-surgical.

RATIONALE

(A) Paying attention to emotional needs will come later. **(B)** Maintaining a patent airway should always be the nurse's primary focus. Primary areas of assessment and intervention also include determining the extent of the burn and fluid and electrolyte needs. The extent and depth of injury control the physiological response and the type of treatment required. Fluid replacement is the cornerstone to successful treatment and early survival of the burn client because of massive fluid shifts and potential hemodynamic shock. **(C)** Determining the cause of the accident will come later. **(D)** Assessing the need for skin grafting will occur later.

139. **(D)** Nursing process phase: implementation; client need: management of care; content area: medical-surgical.

RATIONALE

(A) This time is 4 AM. **(B)** This is not a military time. **(C)** This time is 2 PM. **(D)** To provide continuity and less chance of error in documentation of time, many agencies use military time in their documentation. After 12 noon, time is recorded as 1300 for 1 PM; thus, 4 PM would be recorded as 1600.

140. **(C)** Nursing process phase: data collection; client need: prevention and early detection of disease; content area: medical-surgical.

RATIONALE

(A) This choice is objective data but not descriptive or measurable ("appear" is a vague description). **(B)** This choice is subjective data. **(C)** Objective data are the results of direct observation by the nurse. **(D)** This choice is subjective data.

141. **(B)** Nursing process phase: planning; client need: growth and development through the life span; content area: medical-surgical.

RATIONALE

(A) Generativity versus stagnation occurs in the middle years. **(B)** Erikson views life development as a continuous struggle for emotional and social equilibrium. The conflict of late adulthood (age 65 or older) is ego integrity versus despair. During this stage, the older adult struggles to feel a sense of worth about life and achievements. **(C)** Intimacy versus isolation occurs in young adulthood. **(D)** Retirement versus depression is not a stage of Erikson.

142. **(C)** Nursing process phase: implementation; client need: safety and infection control; content area: medical-surgical.

RATIONALE

(A) This is not the rationale for cleaning the wound in this fashion. **(B)** This is not the rationale for cleaning the wound in this fashion. **(C)** Wounds are cleaned from the least contaminated to the most contaminated area to prevent introduction of organisms back into the wound. **(D)** This is not the rationale for cleaning the wound in this fashion.

143. **(A)** Nursing process phase: data collection; client need: growth and development through the life span; content area: maternity nursing.

RATIONALE

(A) The Apgar score is a system of assessing the newborn infant's physical condition at 1 minute after birth (and again at 1, 2, or 5 minutes after birth). A score of 0, 1, or 2 is given for the heart rate, respiratory effort, muscle tone, response to stimuli, and color, for a maximum score of 10. **(B)** This is above the maximum score possible. **(C)** The maximum score is 10. **(D)** The maximum score is 10.

144. **(C)** Nursing process phase: data collection; client need: growth and development through the life span; content area: maternity nursing.

RATIONALE

(A) This score is too high. **(B)** This score is too high. **(C)** In Apgar scoring of the newborn infant, respiratory effort is given a normal score of 2 for good respirations and in an infant who is crying. A score of 1 is given for slow and irregular respirations, and 0 is given for absence of respirations. **(D)** This score is too high.

145. **(B)** Nursing process phase: planning; client need: basic care and comfort; content area: medical-surgical.

RATIONALE

(A) The nurse cannot give a back rub in this position. **(B)** Having the client in the prone position when giving a back rub makes it easier to apply necessary pressure to back muscles, to promote relaxation and to relieve muscle tension. **(C)** Prone position is better than lateral. **(D)** This is a difficult position to give a back rub.

146. **(A)** Nursing process phase: evaluation; client need: safety and infection control; content area: medical-surgical.

RATIONALE

(A) A nosocomial infection is one that results from the delivery of health services in a health-care facility. The urinary tract is a prime site; placing the urinary drainage bag above the level of the bladder allows reflux of urine in the catheter or bag (which could be contaminated) to reenter the bladder and become a source of infection. **(B)** Aseptic technique would help to prevent nosocomial infections. **(C)** Self-administration of insulin would not cause a nosocomial infection. **(D)** Spreading germs by not covering the mouth is not an example of a nosocomial infection.

147. **(A)** Nursing process phase: implementation; client need: basic care and comfort; content area: medical-surgical.

RATIONALE

(A) Changing position and giving a back rub are simple noninvasive ways to reduce pain perception and to promote relaxation when it is too soon to administer another pain medication. **(B)** Range-of-motion exercises would increase pain. **(C)** Giving another injection of meperidine is an invasive action. **(D)** Explaining to this client that medication has just been given will not decrease pain.

148. **(B)** Nursing process phase: implementation; client need: pharmacological and parenteral therapies; content area: pediatrics.

RATIONALE

(A) It is not appropriate to have the mother call the poison control center. **(B)** The procedure for accidental aspirin poisoning in a conscious client is to induce vomiting and to bring the client to the ER for gastric lavage. Inducing vomiting may not ensure complete emptying of stomach contents, and absorption could cause serious complications. Immediate gastric lavage will clear the stomach of the drug and prevent further absorption. **(C)** The antiemetic should be given in the ER rather than at home. **(D)** Diluting the medicine will not prevent further absorption.

149. **(B)** Nursing process phase: implementation; client need: reduction of risk potential; content area: medical-surgical.

RATIONALE

(A) Flexion is not the correct position for this client. **(B)** The leg of a client who has had a total hip replacement must be maintained in a position of abduction in the early postoperative period to prevent adduction and flexion and potential dislocation. **(C)** Adduction is not the correct position for this client. **(D)** This positioning alone will not prevent adduction.

150. **(D)** Nursing process phase: data collection; client need: prevention and early detection of disease; content area: medical-surgical.

RATIONALE

(A) Tachycardia is a pulse rate above 100. **(B)** Arrhythmia means an irregular heartbeat. **(C)** Sinus rhythm means the heartbeat is initiated from the sinoatrial node. The normal adult pulse rate is 60–100. **(D)** A pulse rate <60 is called bradycardia, derived from the Greek *bradys,* meaning slow, and *kardia,* meaning heart: slow heart rate.

151. **(B)** Nursing process phase: planning; client need: growth and development through the life span; content area: maternity nursing.

RATIONALE

(A) There is nothing in peanut butter that would aggravate hypertension. **(B)** Smoked ham is high in sodium, which increases fluid retention, which in turn increases blood pressure. **(C)** There is nothing in broccoli that would contraindicate it during pregnancy. **(D)** Chicken is allowed for a client with hypertension as long as it is not prepared high in salt.

152. **(A)** Nursing process phase: planning; client need: pharmacological and parenteral therapies; content area: maternity nursing.

RATIONALE

(A) Bananas are high in potassium. **(B)** Apples are healthy but they will not supply the needed potassium. **(C)** Rice is healthy but it will not supply the needed potassium. **(D)** Grapefruit is healthy but it will not supply the needed potassium.

153. **(C)** Nursing process phase: implementation; client need: growth and development through the life span; content area: maternity nursing.

RATIONALE

(A) Do not restrict fluids to 1000 ml/day; the client needs more than this. **(B)** Increasing fluids will increase milk production. **(C)** A tight bra or binder will decrease milk production. **(D)** Applying warm compresses will increase milk production.

154. **(A)** Nursing process phase: implementation; client need: physiological adaptation; content area: maternity nursing.

RATIONALE

(A) The first step is to determine how serious the situation is. If she can talk, the choking is not serious. **(B)** Back blows are a later action. **(C)** In the late stages of pregnancy, chest thrusts should be performed with the victim standing or sitting; however, this is not the first action. **(D)** The Heimlich maneuver is contraindicated in pregnancy.

155. **(B)** Nursing process phase: evaluation; client need: pharmacological and parenteral therapies; content area: maternity nursing.

RATIONALE

(A) $Rh_o(D)$ immune globulin is not given to all mothers. **(B)** $Rh_o(D)$ immune globulin is given only to Rh-negative mothers who have Rh-positive babies. **(C)** $Rh_o(D)$ immune globulin is not given in this situation. **(D)** $Rh_o(D)$ immune globulin is not given in this situation.

156. **(D)** Nursing process phase: implementation; client need: pharmacological and parenteral therapies; content area: maternity nursing.

RATIONALE

(A) Acetazolamide is a diuretic and is not given to suppress milk production. **(B)** Hydromorphone is an analgesic and is not given to suppress milk production. **(C)** Dexamethasone is a steroid and is not given to suppress milk production. **(D)** Estradiol valerate is the only drug listed that suppresses milk production.

157. **(C)** Nursing process phase: data collection; client need: pharmacological and parenteral therapies; content area: maternity nursing.

RATIONALE

(A) To be adequate, a resting phase must be at least 30 seconds long. **(B)** To be adequate, a resting phase must be at least 30 seconds long. **(C)** To be adequate, a resting phase must be at least 30 seconds long. This meets the criteria. **(D)** To be adequate, the resting phase must be at least 30 seconds long. Sixty seconds is more than required.

158. **(B)** Nursing process phase: implementation; client need: growth and development through the life span; content area: maternity nursing.

RATIONALE

(A) Nausea during pregnancy is not caused by anxiety. **(B)** Nausea during pregnancy has a physiological basis because of hormone levels and is independent of rest, anxiety, or foods. **(C)** A change in diet will not stop her nausea. **(D)** Adequate rest will not relieve her nausea.

159. **(D)** Nursing process phase: data collection; client need: growth and development through the life span; content area: psychiatric nursing.

RATIONALE

(A) Telling her parents would not be respecting her privacy or confidentiality. (B) The nurse might suggest this, but the nurse does not know whether the client knows who the father is or whether she has an ongoing relationship with him. (C) The nurse remains nonjudgmental regarding a client's abortion. (D) The clinic staff will help her with counseling and explore reasons for the abortion. The nurse respects the confidentiality of the client.

160. **(C)** Nursing process phase: data collection; client need: pharmacological and parenteral therapies; content area: medical-surgical.

RATIONALE

(A) Insulin needs will increase during certain phases of pregnancy. (B) Insulin requirements change during pregnancy. (C) Insulin requirements change during pregnancy during each trimester and with weight gain. (D) Pregnancy does not alter the type of insulin needed.

161. **(A)** Nursing process phase: implementation; client need: reduction of risk potential; content area: medical-surgical.

RATIONALE

(A) A Penrose drain is an open drain. (B) A Jackson-Pratt is a closed drain. (C) A Hemovac is a closed drain. (D) A Surgivac is a closed drain.

162. **(B)** Nursing process phase: implementation; client need: basic care and comfort; content area: medical-surgical.

RATIONALE

(A) An Ace bandage cannot be wrapped medially. (B) Ace bandages are wrapped from distal to proximal to increase venous return. (C) An Ace bandage cannot be wrapped laterally. (D) Wrapping a bandage beginning at the proximal site decreases venous return.

163. **(D)** Nursing process phase: implementation; client need: basic care and comfort; content area: medical-surgical.

RATIONALE

(A) The nurse would deflate the balloon, but this is not the first step. (B) The nurse does not have to disconnect the bag and tubing. (C) The nurse might clamp off the tubing, but this is not the first step. (D) The first step of any procedure is to explain it to the client even if he or she is confused.

164. **(B)** Nursing process phase: data collection; client need: pharmacological and parenteral therapies; content area: medical-surgical.

RATIONALE

(A) In this area the nurse might hit the sciatic nerve. (B) This is the quadrant without major blood vessels or nerves. (C) This quadrant is painful and has many blood vessels. (D) This quadrant has major nerves and blood vessels.

165. **(A)** Nursing process phase: implementation; client need: pharmacological and parenteral therapies; content area: medical-surgical.

RATIONALE

(A) An intradermal injection is just under the skin. (B) This angle would go too deep. (C) This angle would go too deep. (D) This angle would go too deep.

166. **(D)** Nursing process phase: implementation; client need: pharmacological and parenteral therapies; content area: medical-surgical.

RATIONALE

(A) This needle is too long for an SC injection. (B) This needle is too long and has too large a gauge for an SC injection. (C) This needle is too long and has too large a gauge for an SC injection. (D) SC needle length is ½–⅝ inch. Acceptable gauges are 25, 26, or 27.

167. **(C)** Nursing process phase: evaluation; client need: reduction of risk potential; content area: medical-surgical.

RATIONALE

(A) A nasogastric tube can be used for decompression of the stomach. (B) A nasogastric tube can be used for gastric feeding. (C) A nasogastric tube can remove air from the stomach but not from the colon. (D) A nasogastric tube can be used for administering medications.

168. **(B)** Nursing process phase: evaluation; client need: reduction of risk potential; content area: medical-surgical.

RATIONALE

(A) This is an acceptable position to help prevent regurgitation in most clients. (B) This position increases chances for regurgitation and aspiration. (C) This is an acceptable position to help prevent regurgitation in most clients. (D) This is an acceptable position to help prevent regurgitation in most clients.

169. **(A)** Nursing process phase: implementation; client need: pharmacological and parenteral therapies; content area: medical-surgical.

RATIONALE

(A) The first step is to look at the pump. (B) Counting drops will not give an accurate rate with a pump. (C) Counting drops will not give an accurate rate with a pump. (D) The height of the pump will not affect volume-controlled pumps.

170. **(C)** Nursing process phase: implementation; client need: reduction of risk potential; content area: medical-surgical.

RATIONALE

(A) A colostomy is a fecal diversion. (B) An ileostomy is a fecal diversion. (C) A utereostomy is used for urinary diversion. (D) A gastrostomy tube is used for gastric feeding.

171. **(C)** Nursing process phase: implementation; client need: pharmacological and parenteral therapies; content area: medical-surgical.

RATIONALE

(A) Only the leg is used for children this age. (B) Only the leg is used for children this age. (C) Only the leg is used for IM injections in children <2 years old. Other muscles are not fully developed. (D) Only the leg is used for children this age.

172. **(D)** Nursing process phase: implementation; client need: prevention and early detection of disease; content area: medical-surgical.

RATIONALE

(A) It is preferable for casts to air dry. (B) One should not put anything down a cast. (C) The leg should be elevated to prevent edema. (D) To prevent pressure on the underlying tissue, the cast should be lifted with the flat part of the hand.

173. **(C)** Nursing process phase: evaluation; client need: growth and development through the life span; content area: pediatrics.

RATIONALE

(A) Preventing cuts is important because hemophilia is a disorder that leads to easy bleeding. A tricycle is a relatively safe toy. (B) Preventing cuts is important because hemophilia is a disorder that leads to easy bleeding. Swings are relatively safe toys. (C) Preventing cuts is important because hemophilia is a disorder that leads to easy bleeding. This is an unsafe toy for a child with hemophilia. The sharp edges can cause cuts leading to bleeding. (D) Lincoln logs are a relatively safe toy.

174. **(C)** Nursing process phase: implementation; client need: basic care and comfort; content area: pediatrics.

   RATIONALE

   (A) A client with hypothyroidism gets cold easily. This room temperature is too cold. **(B)** A client with hypothyroidism gets cold easily. This room temperature is too cold. **(C)** Persons with hypothyroidism have a tendency to be cold. A temperature of 75°F (23.8°C) is warmer than usual and is a good temperature for a child with hypothyroidism. **(D)** A temperature of 85°F (29.4°C) is too warm.

175. **(C)** Nursing process phase: implementation; client need: basic care and comfort; content area: pediatrics.

   RATIONALE

   (A) A medicine dropper is inappropriate; the child needs a nipple to stimulate the sucking reflex. **(B)** The child with a cleft lip and palate cannot use a metal spoon. **(C)** This child cannot drink fluids normally. She needs a long soft nipple for best results to prevent injury and to promote oral feeding. **(D)** A gastrostomy tube is not a good choice if food can be provided orally.

176. **(A)** Nursing process phase: implementation; client need: physiological adaptation; content area: pediatrics.

   RATIONALE

   (A) A twisted bowel is the pathology of volvulus. **(B)** Telescoping is known as intussusception. **(C)** Adhesions are scar tissue formations. **(D)** A volvulus does not affect the length of the intestine.

177. **(D)** Nursing process phase: implementation; client need: reduction of risk potential; content area: medical-surgical.

   RATIONALE

   (A) Lying flat will pull on the incision and increase pain. **(B)** A supine position would increase the pain. **(C)** A prone position would increase the pain. **(D)** A semi-Fowler's position would prevent contaminated abdominal contents from ascending above the diaphragm

178. **(B)** Nursing process phase: evaluation; client need: prevention and early detection of disease; content area: medical-surgical.

   RATIONALE

   (A) A headache is to be expected. **(B)** The most significant serious finding in head injury is an alteration in consciousness that would signify increased intracranial pressure. **(C)** Not eating is not of great concern at this time. **(D)** It is normal for a 2-year-old child to cry.

179. **(D)** Nursing process phase: implementation; client need: physiological adaptation; content area: maternity nursing.

   RATIONALE

   (A) The recommendation of the American Heart Association is 4 initial breaths. **(B)** The recommendation of the American Heart Association is 4 initial breaths. **(C)** The recommendation of the American Heart Association is 4 initial breaths. **(D)** This is the American Heart Association guideline.

180. **(B)** Nursing process phase: evaluation; client need: physiological adaptation; content area: maternity nursing.

   RATIONALE

   (A) This is a nongenetic congenital disorder. It is not passed on genetically. **(B)** Sickle cell anemia B is an inherited chronic form of anemia in which abnormal sickle or crescent-shaped RBCs are present. **(C)** Fetal alcohol syndrome is a nongenetic congenital disorder. It is not passed on genetically. **(D)** Cerebral palsy is a nongenetic congenital disorder. It is not passed on genetically.

181. **(D)** Nursing process phase: implementation; client need: pharmacological and parenteral therapies; content area: medical-surgical.

   RATIONALE

   (A) This amount is not enough; see calculations in rationale D. **(B)** This amount is not enough; see calculations in rationale D. **(C)** This amount is not enough; see calculations in rationale D. **(D)** 1 grain = 65 mg. 5 grains = 325 mg, or 1 tablet : 325 mg :: x : 650 mg. x = 650 mg/325 mg, or 2 tablets.

182. **(A)** Nursing process phase: implementation; client need: pharmacological and parenteral therapies; content area: medical-surgical.

   RATIONALE

   (A) 1000 ml/12 hr = 83.3 or 83 ml/hr. **(B)** This amount is too much; see math calculation in rationale A. **(C)** This amount is too much; see math calculation in rationale A. **(D)** This amount is too much; see math calculation in rationale A.

183. **(B)** Nursing process phase: implementation; client need: pharmacological and parenteral therapies; content area: medical-surgical.

   RATIONALE

   (A) Air is drawn into the NPH insulin to prevent contamination of the Regular insulin, as it is pure insulin. See correct steps in rationale B. **(B)** The correct steps to complete mixing are to (1) draw air into the NPH vial, (2) draw air into the Regular insulin vial and draw up the insulin, and (3) reenter NPH vial and draw up required amount. **(C)** See correct steps in rationale B. **(D)** See correct steps in rationale B.

184. **(D)** Nursing process phase: implementation; client need: pharmacological and parenteral therapies; content area: medical-surgical.

   RATIONALE

   (A) See math calculations in rationale D. **(B)** See math calculations in rationale D. **(C)** See math calculations in rationale D. **(D)** 1 lb = 2.2 kg. 176 lb ÷ 2.2 kg = 80 kg = 1 mg/kg = 80 mg. Math calculation explains incorrect options.

185. **(D)** Nursing process phase: implementation; client need: pharmacological and parenteral therapies; content area: medical-surgical.

   RATIONALE

   (A) See math calculations in rationale D. **(B)** See math calculations in rationale D. **(C)** See math calculations in rationale D. **(D)** 1 g = 1000 mg. 1000 mg ÷ 250 = 4 capsules. Math calculation explains incorrect options.

186. **(C)** Nursing process phase: evaluation; client need: pharmacological and parenteral therapies; content area: medical-surgical.

   RATIONALE

   (A) Low-dose renal dopamine does not affect blood pressure. **(B)** Low-dose renal dopamine does not affect blood pressure. **(C)** Vasodilation will increase urine output. **(D)** Low-dose dopamine will increase urine output, not decrease it.

187. **(A)** Nursing process phase: data collection; client need: pharmacological and parenteral therapies; content area: medical-surgical.

   RATIONALE

   (A) Diaphoresis is a symptom of hypoglycemia, which can result from taking insulin without eating. **(B)** Polyuria results from a high blood glucose level. **(C)** Polydipsia results from a high blood glucose level. **(D)** Polyphagia results from a high blood glucose level.

188. **(C)** Nursing process phase: evaluation; client need: pharmacological and parenteral therapies; content area: pediatrics.

RATIONALE

(A) He will not go to camp until tomorrow; therefore, he should take the same dose today. **(B)** He will not go to camp until tomorrow; therefore, he should take the same dose today. **(C)** Because of increased exercise at camp, the need for insulin will be decreased. **(D)** He should take his insulin when he eats breakfast and before leaving for camp.

189. **(B)** Nursing process phase: implementation; client need: psychosocial adaptation; content area: psychiatric nursing.

RATIONALE

(A) There is no value statement here. The client is making a subjective comment. **(B)** The nurse is being judgmental when he or she classifies people into groups and assumes that all people are the same. **(C)** There is no value conflict in this statement. The aide is being respectful of people. **(D)** There is not a value conflict in this statement.

190. **(C)** Nursing process phase: implementation; client need: coping and adaptation; content area: psychiatric nursing.

RATIONALE

(A) The nurse cannot prevent manipulative behavior. **(B)** The nurse cannot control manipulative behavior. **(C)** It is essential that the nurse enforce limit setting to help control manipulative behavior. **(D)** Firmness is not as successful in controlling manipulative behavior as limit setting.

191. **(C)** Nursing process phase: evaluation; client need: psychosocial adaptation; content area: psychiatric nursing.

RATIONALE

(A) This is an example of persecutory hallucinations, not grandiose delusions, such as thinking that the person is a superior being. **(B)** This is an example of persecutory hallucinations, not auditory hallucinations, such as hearing voices that do not exist. **(C)** Persecutory hallucinations occur when people think that someone is after them for something they did not do or that is not reality based. **(D)** Paranoid delusions occur when the individual thinks that someone is blaming him or her incorrectly.

192. **(B)** Nursing process phase: evaluation; client need: psychosocial adaptation; content area: psychiatric nursing.

RATIONALE

(A) The client may not believe this statement by the nurse. **(B)** The best intervention is to get the client to talk about her mother and her feelings. **(C)** Isolation will not be beneficial in this situation. **(D)** If the client is hallucinating, the presence of the mother may encourage more erratic behavior.

193. **(A)** Nursing process phase: implementation; client need: psychosocial adaptation; content area: psychiatric nursing.

RATIONALE

(A) The client needs simple, straightforward directions. **(B)** Insisting on the client's joining may aggravate the condition. **(C)** Explaining the benefits will not be successful. The client is too ill at this time. **(D)** The client is not ready to make decisions at this time.

194. **(C)** Nursing process phase: implementation; client need: reduction of risk potential; content area: medical-surgical.

RATIONALE

(A) Ileostomies have continuous liquid to semiliquid drainage and normally do not need irrigating. **(B)** The nurse can answer the question; it does not need to be referred to the physician. **(C)** Because ileostomies do not need irrigation, the client does not need anyone to show him the irrigation procedure. **(D)** There is no need for demonstrating the irrigation procedure. Ileostomies do not need irrigating.

195. **(B)** Nursing process phase: implementation; client need: prevention and early detection of disease; content area: medical-surgical.

RATIONALE

(A) Milk may irritate ulcers and may increase acid production. **(B)** Clients with ulcers can eat anything that does not bother them. **(C)** Juice may irritate ulcers. **(D)** There is no need to reduce calories according to this scenario.

196. **(A)** Nursing process phase: implementation; client need: basic care and comfort; content area: medical-surgical.

RATIONALE

(A) This is not good advice. Diet control should be tried first before depending on laxatives. **(B)** Increasing fluids will help to prevent constipation. **(C)** Including bran (bulk) on a daily basis will help to prevent constipation. **(D)** Eating more fruits and vegetables will help to prevent constipation.

197. **(B)** Nursing process phase: data collection; client need: prevention and early detection of disease; content area: medical-surgical.

RATIONALE

(A) The client has symptoms of a bladder infection. Sending a routine urinalysis to the laboratory will not help to diagnose a bladder infection. **(B)** Client has symptoms of a UTI, so the specimen must be cultured. **(C)** Irrigating the catheter will not help a bladder infection. **(D)** Measuring the specific gravity will not help the client's bladder infection.

198. **(D)** Nursing process phase: data collection; client need: prevention and early detection of disease; content area: medical-surgical.

RATIONALE

(A) Polyuria and frequency may be caused by increased fluid intake. **(B)** Oliguria and pressure may be caused by decreased fluid intake. **(C)** Discharge and pressure are more diagnostic of a vaginal infection. **(D)** Classic symptoms of a UTI are frequency and dysuria.

199. **(B)** Nursing process phase: data collection; client need: reduction of risk potential; content area: medical-surgical.

RATIONALE

(A) Airway problems have priority over comfort. **(B)** The airway is of highest priority in postoperative clients after general anesthesia. **(C)** There is a potential for fluid volume alteration, but airway management takes priority. **(D)** The client may have a knowledge deficit, but airway problems have the highest priority.

200. **(C)** Nursing process phase: data collection; client need: prevention and early detection of disease; content area: medical-surgical.

RATIONALE

(A) The nurse may take blood pressure in both arms for comparison, but the essential need here is for orthostatic vital signs. **(B)** There is no indication that the priority is for taking both the apical and radial pulse simultaneously. **(C)** Change in orthostatic vital signs (e.g., blood pressure) will indicate severity of dehydration. **(D)** Palpating the bladder will not help assess for fluid volume deficit.

201. **(A)** Nursing process phase: data collection; client need: prevention and early detection of disease; content area: medical-surgical.

RATIONALE
(A) Being underweight is not a risk factor. (B) Smoking is a risk factor for the development of cardiovascular disease. (C) Having hypertension is a risk factor for the development of cardiovascular disease. (D) Maintaining a sedentary lifestyle is a risk factor for the development of cardiovascular disease.

202. **(A)** Nursing process phase: implementation; client need: pharmacological and parenteral therapies; content area: medical-surgical.

RATIONALE
(A) NTG causes vasodilation, which can cause significant hypotension. (B) The nurse may also check the pulse, but it is most important to check the blood pressure. (C) The client does not have to be in a sitting position. (D) NTG does not directly affect blood potassium level.

203. **(C)** Nursing process phase: implementation; client need: basic care and comfort; content area: medical-surgical.

RATIONALE
(A) Pears are not high in sodium. (B) Baked chicken is not high in sodium, unless specifically prepared with salt. (C) Olives are high in sodium. (D) Baked potatoes are not high in sodium unless salt is added by the client.

204. **(D)** Nursing process phase: data collection; client need: prevention and early detection of disease; content area: medical-surgical.

RATIONALE
(A) This is an expected finding in right-sided heart failure. (B) This is an expected finding in right-sided heart failure. (C) LLQ pain is not a sign of CHF. (D) Dyspnea is a classic symptom of congestive failure resulting from fluid backup into the lungs.

205. **(C)** Nursing process phase: data collection; client need: prevention and early detection of disease; content area: medical-surgical.

RATIONALE
(A) Lymphedema is a sign of venous insufficiency. (B) Pedal edema is a sign of venous insufficiency. (C) The absence of pedal pulses indicates arterial insufficiency. (D) A bluish cast to the extremities is suggestive of venous insufficiency.

206. **(C)** Nursing process phase: evaluation; client need: physiological adaptation; content area: medical-surgical.

RATIONALE
(A) The pineal gland does not control the pituitary gland. (B) The sympathetic nervous system does not control the pituitary gland. (C) The master endocrine gland is the pituitary gland and is controlled by the hypothalamus. The pituitary gland has sympathetic nervous system innervation but does not control it. (D) The master endocrine gland *is* the pituitary gland.

207. **(B)** Nursing process phase: implementation; client need: reduction of risk potential; content area: medical-surgical.

RATIONALE
(A) A Jackson-Pratt drain would be placed in surgery, if needed. (B) Edema in the neck can lead to respiratory distress. A tracheostomy set should be available for this emergency. (C) There is no indication for a Salem sump tube. (D) There is no reason to have an IV potassium infusion at the bedside.

208. **(D)** Nursing process phase: evaluation; client need: safety and infection control; content area: medical-surgical.

RATIONALE
(A) Pathogenic means having organisms capable of causing disease. (B) Synergistic means working together. (C) Diagnostic means pertaining to a disease. (D) Nosocomial pertains to a hospital- or infirmary-acquired infection.

TEST 3

Larry D. Purnell, RN, PhD

QUESTIONS

1. The most common cause of myocardial infarction is:
   A. Atherosclerosis
   B. Synergistic effects
   C. Pulmonary embolism
   D. Blows to the chest

2. An 80-year-old client is recovering from cardiogenic shock. She has a urinary catheter for continuous drainage. Urinary output in this stage should be:
   A. <20 cc/hr
   B. >30 cc/hr
   C. >100 cc/hr
   D. <150 cc/hr

3. The mother of a 5-year-old child calls the emergency room and tells the nurse that her husband is bringing the child in because of a wasp sting, to which the child is allergic. What is the first medicine the nurse would have available?
   A. Diphenhydramine (Benadryl)
   B. Methylprednisolone (Solu-Medrol)
   C. Epinephrine
   D. Sodium bicarbonate

4. Objective signs that a client is in shock are:
   A. An increase in blood pressure and a decrease in pulse
   B. An increase in blood pressure and an increase in pulse
   C. A decrease in blood pressure and a decrease in pulse
   D. A decrease in blood pressure and an increase in pulse

5. An 80-year-old client has third-degree burns on 25% of the body. The priority nursing diagnosis is:
   A. Alteration in comfort
   B. Fluid volume deficit
   C. Alteration in nutrition
   D. Circulation, altered

6. A 47-year-old client had a supratentorial craniotomy after a motorcycle accident. Positioning after surgery is:
   A. Semi-Fowler's
   B. Flat
   C. Prone
   D. Lateral

7. A client is experiencing an increase in intracranial pressure. The nurse would expect his blood pressure to be:
   A. Systolic up, diastolic down
   B. Systolic down, diastolic down
   C. Systolic up, diastolic up
   D. Systolic down, diastolic up

8. A 77-year-old client who is taking Lanoxin (digoxin) has a low blood potassium level. The nurse would be especially sure to monitor:
   A. Pulse
   B. Blood pressure
   C. Urinary output
   D. Specific gravity

9. A client has acute pancreatitis. To determine its severity, the nurse would look at which laboratory test?
   A. Serum transaminase
   B. Serum amylase
   C. Serum sodium
   D. Serum magnesium

10. A 59-year-old client has a nasogastric tube for suction. Which of the following would be contraindicated for this client?
    A. Ice chips
    B. Glycerine swabs
    C. Hard candies
    D. Peroxide gargles

11. An 80-year-old client with unconsciousness of unknown

etiology has just been admitted. The priority nursing diagnosis is:

  A. Airway maintenance
  B. Alteration in nutrition
  C. Alteration in consciousness
  D. Alteration in elimination

12. A client with acute renal failure now has an hourly urine output of 150 cc. The client is in what stage of renal failure?

  A. Oliguria phase
  B. Initial phase
  C. Diuretic phase
  D. Recovery phase

13. The most serious electrolyte abnormality for a client in chronic renal failure is:

  A. Hypokalemia
  B. Hyperkalemia
  C. Hyponatremia
  D. Hypernatremia

14. A 38-year-old client has chronic cirrhosis and is jaundiced. To decrease pruritus from the jaundice, the nurse would:

  A. Use wool blankets
  B. Keep the room temperature above 75°F (23.8°C)
  C. Keep the room temperature below 70°F (21.1°C)
  D. Use lots of soap in the bath water

15. The most likely side effect of chemotherapy is:

  A. Fatigue
  B. Nausea
  C. Dehydration
  D. Skin ulceration

16. A 77-year-old client with thrombocytopenia and dementia likes to talk about her younger days and occasionally confabulates. This behavior:

  A. Prevents aggression
  B. Gains attention
  C. Indicates acute psychosis
  D. Maintains self-esteem

17. For which condition must the nurse notify the state health department?

  A. Chlamydia
  B. Syphilis
  C. Nonspecific urethritis
  D. Herpes

18. Oxygen is transported in which component of the blood?

  A. Serum
  B. Plasma
  C. Red blood cells (RBCs)
  D. White blood cells (WBCs)

19. The charge nurse asks the nurse to bring a 1000-ml intravenous (IV) bag of D_5 and normal saline (NS). The nurse selects:

  A. D_5/0.33 NS
  B. D_5/0.45 NS
  C. D_5/0.9 NS
  D. D_5/0.2 NS

20. Which of the following is not a complication of IV therapy?

  A. Extravasation
  B. Phlebitis
  C. Infiltration
  D. Renal shutdown

21. Uses of a tracheostomy tube include:

  A. Promotion of nutrition
  B. Relief of flatus
  C. Achievement of an artificial airway
  D. Increasing dead space

22. A 32-year-old client has a thoracotomy tube in place. To best promote drainage, the nurse should:

  A. Keep the client on the unaffected side
  B. Keep water seal at chest level
  C. Reposition the client every 2 hours
  D. Turn him on his affected side

23. A complication that can occur during the insertion of a subclavian catheter is:

  A. Arterial spasm
  B. Pulmonary infection
  C. Phlebitis
  D. Air embolism

24. A 22-year-old client just had a leg cast applied. Which symptom would be of most concern to the nurse?

  A. Swelling of the toes
  B. Blood drainage on the cast
  C. Toes cool to the touch
  D. Loss of sensation in the toes

25. Hypertension is called a "silent health problem." Which of the following is not a symptom of hypertension?

  A. Headache
  B. Nausea
  C. Vertigo
  D. Epistaxis

26. Collection of fluid in the pleural cavity is called:

  A. Hemothorax
  B. Pneumothorax
  C. Atelectasis
  D. Pleural effusion

27. Generalized edema is called:

  A. Anasarca
  B. Pitting
  C. Ascites
  D. Lymphedema

28. What is the name of the hormonal dysfunction that causes increased growth in the hands, feet, and facial bones?

  A. Myxedema

B. Acromegaly
C. Gigantism
D. Addison's disease

29. A 43-year-old client has a hormonal disturbance characterized by hirsutism, truncal obesity, and a buffalo hump. These are symptoms of the disease called:

A. Acromegaly
B. Myxedema
C. Cushing's disease
D. Graves' disease

30. In which of the following situations is reading the temperature orally contraindicated?

A. A 45-year-old client with a duodenal ulcer
B. A client who has recently suffered a heart attack
C. An adult client with an elevated temperature
D. A confused older client

31. Which of the following groups is most susceptible to extreme changes in environmental temperature?

A. Toddlers
B. Newborn infants
C. Young adults
D. Adolescents

32. Which of the following pulse sites is most frequently used in measuring blood pressure in adults?

A. Brachial
B. Femoral
C. Carotid
D. Radial

33. Which of the following terms means an irregular pulse?

A. Tachycardia
B. Diastole
C. Arrhythmia
D. Bradycardia

34. What is the appropriate site for taking the pulse of an infant?

A. Apical
B. Radial
C. Femoral
D. Temporal

35. The difference in pressure during relaxation of the left ventricles and that which remains constant is called:

A. Pulse pressure
B. Maximal pressure
C. Systolic pressure
D. Diastolic pressure

36. A 35-year-old client is hospitalized with a fractured right femur. Which of the following blood pressures would be considered within the normal range for him?

A. 88/50 mm Hg
B. 124/80 mm Hg
C. 180/110 mm Hg
D. 144/92 mm Hg

37. A 45-year-old auto accident victim has fractures of both

arms. The client is in bilateral (both sides) casts from the shoulders to the hands. Appropriate sites to take the client's pulse include:

A. Temporal or brachial
B. Brachial or femoral
C. Radial or carotid
D. Carotid or femoral

38. A 15-year-old client is admitted with a fever of 103°F (39.4°C). The client is flushed and complains of a headache. The nurse also notes that the skin is warm and dry and the lips and oral membranes are parched. This represents which part of the nursing process?

A. Planning
B. Implementation
C. Data collection
D. Evaluation

39. A client has a fever that is possibly the result of a throat infection. This would be which part of the nursing diagnosis statement?

A. P—the problem
B. E—the etiology or cause
C. E—the evaluation of the problem
D. S—the signs and symptoms manifested

40. The nurse administers acetaminophen (Tylenol), 10 grains, for a client's fever, as ordered by the physician. The administration of acetaminophen represents which phase of the nursing process?

A. Implementation
B. Evaluation
C. Planning
D. Reassessment

41. Twenty minutes after giving acetaminophen to a client with an elevated temperature, the nurse notes her response to the medication (decreased temperature). This represents which phase of the nursing process?

A. Planning
B. Data collection
C. Analysis
D. Evaluation

42. Assessment of a client's dry skin and parched oral mucous membranes is an example of what type of data?

A. Constant
B. Objective
C. Subjective
D. Modifiable

43. Which of the following is considered a client strength?

A. Shallow respirations
B. Irregular pulse rate
C. History of bronchial asthma
D. Weight within normal range

44. Which of the following conditions could cause a decrease in blood pressure?

A. Fever
B. Hemorrhage

C. Stress

D. Obesity

45. When measuring a client's blood pressure, the first faint clear tapping sounds the nurse hears on release of the hand valve indicate:

A. Diastolic pressure

B. Venous pressure

C. Pulse pressure

D. Systolic pressure

46. When a nurse makes an error in charting, which of the following nursing actions should be taken?

A. Draw a line through the error, and begin again.

B. Use white correction fluid, rewrite the data, and initial the corrections.

C. Draw a line through the error, initial above it, and write "error."

D. Draw a line through the error and write the correct data above.

47. Using a "source-oriented" medical record, the nurse will find a client's age, address, and other biographical data on the:

A. Graphic sheet

B. Admission sheet

C. Progress notes

D. Nurses' notes

48. One of the orders written on a client's chart is abbreviated NPO. This means:

A. Normal physical observations

B. Normal preoperative orders

C. Nothing by mouth

D. No physician orders written

49. When a new client is admitted to the hospital, which of the following actions should the nurse take first?

A. Collect a urine specimen.

B. Assist the client to undress and record items on a clothing list.

C. Take and record vital signs.

D. Greet the client, identify himself or herself, explain hospital routine, and identify reason for admission.

50. An 87-year-old client with pneumonia is assigned to a nurse's care. Which of the following assessments takes first priority?

A. Rapid, irregular respirations of 32/min

B. Skin warm, flushed, and dry

C. Temperature of 99.4°F (37.4°C)

D. Dry unproductive cough

51. The data collection on a client with pneumonia identifies dyspnea. This means:

A. Respirations are shallow

B. The client is breathing very rapidly

C. The client cannot breathe in a supine position

D. Breathing has become difficult and labored

52. The optimal position to enhance optimal ventilation for a client with pneumonia is:

A. In Fowler's position

B. Lying on the unaffected side

C. In Sims' position

D. In the dorsal recumbent position

53. The physician has ordered O_2 via nasal cannula at 3 L/min. Safety precautions when oxygen is in use include:

A. Avoiding use of all types of lotions for skin care

B. Placing "No smoking" signs in prominent places in the client's room

C. Keeping the flow rate <4 L/min to prevent toxicity

D. Making sure that the room is well ventilated

54. When teaching health care to an older client with osteoporosis, the nurse would:

A. Remind the client to take her anti-inflammatory medication to prevent joint stiffness

B. Remind the client of the importance of a yearly physical examination

C. Instruct the client to eat foods rich in calcium and to increase physical activity

D. Encourage the client to avoid long walks and becoming fatigued

55. Constipation is frequently a problem among older persons. Which of the following is a means of prevention?

A. Good attention to nutrition and avoidance of enriched foods

B. Increased exercise; a low-bulk and low-fat diet

C. A diet high in calcium and carbohydrates

D. Increased fluid intake, increased exercise, and adequate bulk in the diet

56. The nurse is to administer an injection of vitamin B_{12} to an adult client. Which of the following nursing interventions will decrease irritation to subcutaneous (SC) tissue?

A. Injecting the medication into the deltoid muscle

B. Using the Z-track method of intramuscular (IM) injection into the ventrogluteal muscle

C. Changing the needle before injection into the gluteus maximus

D. Injecting the medication into the gluteus medius and firmly massaging the area after the injection

57. The nurse enters a client's room to administer her oral medications and the client states that one of the medications is different from what she has taken in the past. Which of the following nursing interventions will prevent a medication error?

A. Recheck the medication in question against the physician's order before proceeding.

B. Tell the client that it must be a new medication that her physician has ordered.

C. Leave her medications at the bedside and tell her that they are what her physician has ordered.

D. Omit the medication and record the fact that it was refused.

58. Symptoms that the nurse would expect to find in collecting data on a client with pulmonary emphysema include:

A. Hemoptysis, unproductive cough, cardiac arrhythmias, and pedal edema
B. Exertional dyspnea, cough, increased mucous production, and wheezing
C. Chronic cough, diminished breath sounds, bradycardia, and epistaxis
D. Chest pain, hemoptysis, inspiratory wheezing, and right-sided atelectasis

59. The nurse would expect the blood gases of a client with emphysema to show:

A. Hypoxia, respiratory alkalosis, elevated PaO_2
B. Hypoxemia, hypercapnia, respiratory acidosis
C. Elevated SaO_2, hypocapnia, respiratory acidosis
D. Increased SaO_2, hypocapnia, respiratory acidosis

60. A 75-year-old male client is admitted with a diagnosis of left-sided cerebrovascular accident (CVA). A nursing priority in caring for this client is:

A. Assessing level of consciousness and neurological functioning at frequent intervals
B. Passive range-of-motion exercises to prevent contractures
C. Administration of laxatives to prevent constipation
D. Minimal neurological stimulation to prevent a change in condition

61. When communicating with a post-CVA client with expressive aphasia, the nurse would understand that:

A. The client may have difficulty in understanding what is being said
B. Communication in writing might be necessary
C. It might be difficult to understand the client
D. The client will have difficulty in speaking and in writing

62. In collecting data on a client with a urinary tract infection, the nurse would expect symptoms to include:

A. Abdominal pain, nocturia, elevated temperature
B. Frequency, urgency, dysuria, suprapubic pressure
C. Flank pain, hematuria, abdominal distention
D. Urinary retention, elevated pulse rate, crystalluria

63. Nursing interventions and teaching in caring for a client with a urinary tract infection include:

A. Increasing fluid intake, cleansing the perineal area from front to back after elimination, administering medications ordered to acidify the urine
B. Administering anti-inflammatory drugs, measuring intake and output (I&O) and specific gravity of urine
C. Monitoring blood pressure, assessing for fluid retention, measuring I&O
D. Increasing fluid intake, administering diuretics, monitoring electrolytes

64. A high-risk factor in a potential suicide client is:

A. Increased physical activity
B. A recent change in mood
C. Hypersomnia
D. Crying; increased verbal activity

65. A gravida 2 obstetric client is Rh-negative. There could be a complication to the fetus if:

A. The mother received $Rh_o(D)$ immune globulin (RhoGAM) after her first delivery
B. The father is Rh-negative
C. The father is Rh-positive
D. The baby is Rh-negative

66. The best source of dietary calcium to recommend to a pregnant client is:

A. Milk
B. Bananas
C. Salad greens
D. Orange juice

67. In which client care situation on a general care unit should surgical asepsis be used?

A. Before removing a dressing
B. When inserting a urinary catheter
C. When administering a saline enema
D. When giving perineal care

68. The single most important means of preventing the spread of infection is:

A. Effective handwashing
B. Use of clean gloves in performing client care
C. Isolation precautions
D. Disinfectants

69. After assessing a client's pulse and finding it to be 124 bpm and rapid, the nurse would chart this as:

A. Bradycardia
B. Pulse paradox
C. Arrhythmia
D. Tachycardia

70. Nursing interventions for hyperthermia should increase heat loss and decrease heat production, such as:

A. Increasing fluids and increasing physical activity
B. Providing extra blankets and offering acetaminophen as ordered
C. Increasing fluids and administering tepid sponge baths
D. Offering warm fluids and reducing physical activity

71. In collecting data on a client and documenting subjective data, the nurse charts data that:

A. The nurse assessed and observed, including interpretations and conclusions drawn
B. The client perceives, and the way he or she expresses it
C. The nurse observed, including responses to treatment
D. The nurse perceived and gathered in the client assessment

72. The nursing process should be integrated into the documentation because:

A. It includes observations made and problems identified
B. It is the best means of communicating with other members of the health-care team and is the foundation of nursing practice
C. It includes the nurse's assessment and information that should be charted
D. It is pertinent data and should be charted on the Kardex and kept updated

73. A client is terminally ill. When the nurse enters the room, it is evident that the client has been crying. A statement to enhance communication would be:

    A. "You seem sad and depressed today; what is the problem?"
    B. "How are you feeling today?"
    C. "Come on, cheer up, I'm sure things will look brighter tomorrow."
    D. "I see that you have been crying. Would you like to talk about it?"

74. To listen attentively to a client, the nurse needs to:

    A. Respond quickly to statements made and questions asked so the client knows that the nurse is interested
    B. Listen to what the client says and ask why he or she feels that way
    C. Listen with all of the senses and maintain eye contact with the client
    D. Sit down, lean back in the chair, and cross the arms

75. What is the nurse's first action when discovering a hospitalized client who appears to have ceased breathing?

    A. Determine unresponsiveness.
    B. Begin cardiac compression.
    C. Give two quick breaths.
    D. Call for help.

76. Which is the best indicator to use to determine that external cardiac compressions should be started?

    A. Unresponsiveness
    B. Absence of carotid pulse
    C. Cessation of respirations
    D. Fixed and dilated pupils

77. The steps of the nursing process, in the correct order, are:

    A. Data collection, discrimination, planning, evaluation, reevaluation
    B. Data collection, analysis, intervention, planning, diagnosis
    C. Data collection, discovering, evaluation, planning, reassessment
    D. Data collection, planning, implementation, and evaluation

78. The basic four food groups are:

    A. Fruits and vegetables, milk and cheese, breads and cereals, vitamins and minerals
    B. Fruits and vegetables, milk and milk products, breads and cereals, meats and poultry and alternates
    C. Milk and milk products, breads and cereals, carbohydrates and protein, vitamins and minerals
    D. Milk and milk products, fruits, vegetables, cheese and poultry

79. The "five rights" for safe administration of medications are:

    A. Right drug, right dose, right client, right amount, right route
    B. Right drug, right client, right order, right route, right time

C. Right drug, right dose, right time, right route, right client
    D. Right client, right drug, right strength, right time, right documentation

80. A 66-year-old client is admitted with dehydration and hypernatremia. Clinical signs and symptoms for which the nurse will observe the client include:

    A. Cool moist skin, hypotension, elevated serum sodium, hypothermia
    B. Extreme thirst; dry, sticky mucous membranes; flushed skin; elevated temperature; elevated sodium serum
    C. Agitated behavior, hyperpyrexia, decreased specific gravity of urine, hypotension
    D. Anorexia, cool moist skin, fatigue, elevated serum sodium, personality changes

81. Normal serum potassium concentration levels range from:

    A. 3.2–4.5 mEq/L
    B. 2.5–4.5 mEq/L
    C. 3.5–5.5 mEq/L
    D. 3.5–4.0 mEq/L

82. A client with dehydration and hypokalemia is to receive an IV infusion of 1000 ml of D5/0.33 sodium chloride with 20 mEq of potassium chloride. It is to be administered over an 8-hour period. The administration set has a drop factor of 20 gtt/ml. The nurse will set the flow rate at:

    A. 20 gtt/min
    B. 42 gtt/min
    C. 60 gtt/min
    D. 32 gtt/min

83. A 27-year-old client is scheduled for an appendectomy. The nurse will be certain that the client has emptied the bladder before surgery primarily because:

    A. A full bladder preoperatively could cause postoperative urinary retention
    B. A full bladder could very easily be injured during the surgical procedure (surgical trauma)
    C. A full bladder could cause urinary stasis and a potential postoperative urinary tract infection
    D. The nurse will need to obtain a urinalysis before surgery

84. The nurse will be certain that a surgical client has been given informed consent. Informed consent means that:

    A. The client has given full consent for the surgical procedure
    B. A properly informed and fully competent client has given full consent to the surgical procedure
    C. The client has been prepared for surgery and given full consent to the procedure
    D. The physician has fully explained the surgical procedure to the client

85. Food and fluids are withheld before a surgical procedure primarily:

    A. Because the client may experience nausea and vomiting because of anxiety

B. To reduce postoperative nausea and vomiting

C. To reduce preoperative and postoperative discomfort

D. Because food or fluids in the stomach increase the possibility of aspiration of stomach contents while the client is anesthetized

86. In some instances, the surgical area is shaved of hair before surgery. The primary rationale for this is:

A. To prevent postoperative discomfort

B. To destroy microorganisms and to reduce the chance of infection

C. To prevent pain and discomfort during postoperative dressing changes

D. To provide a better view of the surgical area

87. The physician orders 5000 units of heparin every 12 hours SC for the first 48 hours postoperatively. The rationale for this medication is:

A. To decrease the risk of postoperative emboli

B. To prevent the risk of postoperative hemorrhage

C. To increase blood coagulation

D. To prevent possible postoperative paralytic ileus

88. Which of the following signs could indicate a possible wound infection?

A. Elevated body temperature, erythema, swelling surrounding the suture line, increased abdominal pain

B. Diaphoresis, anorexia, serosanguineous drainage, diminished bowel sounds

C. Swelling around the incision, serosanguineous drainage, skin edges well approximated

D. Elevated body temperature, bright-red drainage, increased urine output

89. A nurse arrives on the scene of an automobile accident and finds the driver unconscious and bleeding from a head laceration. The first action the nurse will take is:

A. Ensure that the victim has a patent airway

B. Try to stop the bleeding by applying pressure to the nearest artery and by elevating the extremity above the heart

C. Go to the nearest telephone and activate the emergency medical system

D. Elevate the victim's head, and begin cardiopulmonary resuscitation (CPR)

90. A client is to undergo ionizing radiation treatment for breast cancer. To explain this to the client, the nurse understands that radiation attempts to kill cancer cells by:

A. Dissolving the cell nucleus via heat and destroying cancer cells

B. Altering the normal pattern of normal cells which in turn will kill off the cancer cells

C. Radiation passing through living tissues and inhibiting cell division protein

D. Disrupting cancer cells via magnetic resuscitation

91. A nurse is caring for a client with a radioactive uterine implant. Nursing interventions will focus on:

A. Observing the principles of time, distance, and shielding

B. Keeping at least 12 ft away from the source of radiation

C. Keeping the client on protective isolation and allowing the client to do as much self-care as possible

D. Wearing a radiation film badge and spending only 10 minutes at a time at the bedside

92. A nurse and community health educator can teach prevention of chest injuries by:

A. Teaching clients that both passive and active smoking contribute to chest injuries

B. Encouraging the use of passenger seat belts in motor vehicles

C. Teaching clients to drive at or below the speed limit to prevent potential automobile accidents and resultant chest injuries

D. Teaching that children must be placed in the back seat of moving vehicles to prevent chest injury in the event of an accident

93. A 68-year-old client is admitted to the hospital with increased breathlessness, a productive cough, and fever and chills. His arterial blood gas values are PaO_2 58 mm Hg, $PaCO_2$ 55 mm Hg, and pH 7.0. These are indicative of:

A. Hypoventilation and respiratory alkalosis

B. Metabolic alkalosis resulting from uncompensated respiratory alkalosis

C. Respiratory acidosis resulting from hypoventilation

D. Respiratory alkalosis resulting from pulmonary disease

94. With early signs of hypoxia, the nurse would expect to assess a chronic obstructive pulmonary disease client for:

A. Dyspnea, neurological changes, hypertension, diminished breath sounds

B. Increased rate and depth of respirations, headache, changes in behavior, decreased judgment, drowsiness

C. Orthopnea, use of accessory muscles to breathe, cyanosis of nailbeds

D. Labored breathing, crowing respirations, inspiratory wheezing

95. A 45-year-old client is post–myocardial infarction. The client is placed on a low-salt, low-cholesterol diet. Some foods that the nurse will instruct the client to decrease in amounts include:

A. Green leafy vegetables, citrus fruits

B. Bananas, whole-grain breads, nuts

C. Potatoes, cruciferous vegetables, raisins

D. Organ meats, whole milk, egg yolks, shellfish

96. A 66-year-old client takes a potassium-depleting diuretic. Foods that will help to keep the client's potassium level within normal limits include:

A. Dairy products, whole-grain cereals, starchy vegetables

B. Citrus fruits, liver and organ meats, dark-green vegetables

C. Bananas, oranges, cantaloupe, fish, spinach, whole-grain cereals

D. Nuts, dairy products, citrus fruits, enriched bread

97. Medications usually used in the treatment of rheumatoid arthritis include:

A. Anti-inflammatory agents
B. Antilipemic agents
C. Antibiotics
D. Sympatholytic agents

98. A 24-year-old woman is admitted in labor at 39 weeks' gestation. The nurse will position her in the Sims' position because:

A. It increases fetal activity
B. It facilitates descent of the presenting part through the birth canal
C. It enhances maternal and placental circulation and promotes relaxation
D. It decreases the intensity of the labor pains, especially in back labor

99. A fetal heart rate of 132 bpm in a client who is in labor should be interpreted as:

A. Abnormal
B. Fetal distress
C. Within the normal limits
D. Slightly above the norm

100. The nurse times the frequency of a client's labor contractions from the:

A. Beginning of one contraction until relaxation of the uterus
B. Beginning of one contraction until the beginning of the next
C. Peak of one contraction until the beginning of the next
D. Contraction of the uterus until its relaxation

101. The third stage of labor is defined as:

A. The stage when the placenta and membranes are delivered
B. The beginning of the first contraction, ending with the birth of the baby
C. The time when the cervix is fully dilated, lasting until the delivery of the baby
D. The period when the baby is delivered, ending with the delivery of the placenta and membranes

102. A 3-month-old infant is admitted with possible pyloric stenosis. A classic sign of this condition is:

A. Anemia
B. Projectile vomiting
C. Diarrhea
D. Anorexia

103. While caring for a client with acute glomerulonephritis, an important nursing intervention would be:

A. Monitoring and assessing I&O
B. Monitoring pulse and respirations
C. Forcing fluids
D. Increasing ambulation

104. Which of the following would be the best food choice to select for a post-tonsillectomy 4-year-old child?

A. Ice slush
B. A glass of milk
C. Orange juice
D. Decaffeinated soda pop

105. The primary purposes of changing a postoperative client's dressing are:

A. To inspect the dressing
B. To inspect the incisional area for healing and for evidence of infection
C. To inspect the dressing and to provide comfort for the client
D. To chart the type and amount of drainage

106. A client will be ambulatory on the first day after surgery. The primary benefits of early ambulation are:

A. To improve circulation, stimulate elimination, and prevent dependence
B. To facilitate the normal functioning of all body organs and systems, and reduce the danger of potential postoperative complications
C. To improve appetite, prevent nausea and vomiting, and prevent potential evisceration
D. To prevent formation of emboli, promote ventilation, and stimulate diaphoresis

107. A client, aged 75 years, is admitted to the hospital with a diagnosis of congestive heart failure (CHF). This condition develops as a result of:

A. Increased cardiac output resulting from hypovolemia
B. Increased metabolic needs of the body
C. Accumulation of serous fluid in the pleural space
D. The heart's inability to pump effectively to meet the demands of the body

108. A client is receiving chemotherapy for treatment of breast cancer. She has begun to experience alopecia (loss of hair). It is important to inform her that the alopecia is:

A. Temporary and that hair will grow again soon after chemotherapy is discontinued
B. Permanent but that wearing a wig will help her overall self-concept and cosmetic appearance
C. Not life threatening and the hair may even begin to grow again when she is in remission
D. Never permanent and that it will aid her in finding ways to improve her appearance

109. A client, aged 52 years, has a diagnosis of hypertension. Admission blood pressure is 200/110 mm Hg, and the client is complaining of a severe headache and dizziness. The licensed practical nurse's (LPN's) first priority is to:

A. Document the blood pressure in the admission notes
B. Report this immediately to the registered nurse (RN)
C. Give the client acetaminophen as prescribed for headache
D. Ask the client if there is a history of hypertension in the family

110. A client who is a two-pack-per-day cigarette smoker changes the topic of conversation whenever her smok-

ing is brought up. This psychological defense mechanism is called:

A. Sublimation
B. Repression
C. Denial
D. Compensation

111. A 22-month-old infant is admitted with gastroenteritis, hyperthermia, and dehydration. Which nursing intervention will most effectively aid in reducing fever?

A. Giving 5 grains of aspirin
B. Sponging the client with alcohol
C. Applying extra blankets
D. Giving the client a tepid sponge bath

112. When instilling eardrops in the left ear of a 3-year-old child, the nurse will:

A. Ask the child to sit in an upright position
B. Pull the auricle upward and forward during instillation
C. Pull the pinna upward and backward during instillation
D. Straighten the ear canal by grasping the pinna and gently pulling it down and backward

113. Which of the following side effects are commonly seen during initial treatment with nitrates (vasodilators)?

A. Flushing, hypotension, bradycardia
B. Headache, postural hypotension, flushing
C. Drowsiness, anorexia, hypertension
D. Tachycardia, hypertension, hypokalemia

114. Two days after her cholecystectomy, a client has been experiencing nausea and vomiting. The client has a T-tube in place. For what electrolyte imbalance will the nurse monitor?

A. Hypernatremia
B. Hyperkalemia
C. Hypervolemia
D. Hypokalemia

115. Before administering an antihypertensive agent, the nurse will:

A. Check all extremities for any pitting edema
B. Measure and record the client's blood pressure
C. Weigh the client
D. Take an apical pulse reading

116. A client is receiving Regular insulin according to 6-hour fasting blood sugar levels. The nurse will observe her for side effects within:

A. 2–4 hours
B. 30–60 minutes
C. 15–20 minutes
D. 2–3 hours

117. The nurse is caring for a client with thrombophlebitis. A medication that may be administered in the treatment of this condition is:

A. Ampicillin
B. Heparin
C. Propranolol (Inderal)
D. Nitroglycerin

118. A 22-year-old primipara has had a cesarean delivery. The nurse will observe her for possible postpartum hemorrhage by:

A. Monitoring her pulse rate and checking her dressing
B. Monitoring her vital signs and palpating the level of the fundus
C. Checking her blood pressure and the color of her nailbeds
D. Monitoring the color and amount of her flow

119. Pulmonary tuberculosis is on the increase. Signs and symptoms of this condition for which the nurse will assess a client include:

A. Elevated WBC count, diaphoresis, hypertension, anorexia
B. Anorexia, fatigue, low-grade afternoon fever, weight loss, cough, possible hemoptysis
C. Chest pain, tachycardia, enlarged cervical lymph nodes, joint pain, fatigue
D. Bradycardia, weight gain, subnormal temperature, general malaise, elevated sedimentation rate

120. A 34-year-old client has been recently admitted to the hospital for the third time this past month with anxiety, nausea and vomiting, and a tentative diagnosis of hypochondriasis. Which of the following statements correctly defines this disorder?

A. The outward manifestation of anger that the client is not able to express directly and that is manifested in physical symptoms
B. The inability to acknowledge thoughts or feelings in oneself and attributing them to another
C. A defense used by the ego when it does not wish to remember a painful feeling or emotion
D. A defense by the ego when it feels severely threatened or during periods of internal psychic stress

121. A nurse in a long-term psychiatric unit finds that a client with depression has not showered for a week and is very unkempt in appearance. The nurse would:

A. Do nothing and wait until the client is ready to shower on his or her own
B. Tell the client to go and shower now
C. Assist the client in gathering the necessary items to bathe
D. Obtain physical help and carry the client to the shower

122. A 22-year-old computer programmer was admitted last night with schizophrenia. He is watching television in the day room. As the nurse approaches him, he says, "Leave me alone, don't bother me." The nurse would:

A. Introduce himself or herself and stay with him for a while
B. Stay at his side for an hour to let him know that he is not in control
C. Leave with plans to return in 1 hour
D. Gently touch his hand and offer help

123. A 34-year-old client is scheduled for major surgery. Since admission, the client has been very demanding, continuously calling the nurse to straighten a pillow

and pour a glass of water. The nurse identifies this as an example of which defense mechanism?

A. Regression
B. Conversion
C. Denial
D. Projection

124. A single father brings his 17-year-old daughter to the clinic because she refuses to leave the house for fear of meeting someone she does not know. He wants to know what this condition is called. The nurse explains that it is called:

A. Acrophobia
B. Xenophobia
C. Claustrophobia
D. Agoraphobia

125. During change of shift report, the nurse reports that a new admission has bulimia. The nurse recognizes that bulimia is

A. A phobia of obesity
B. A disorder associated with starvation
C. A disorder associated with vomiting
D. A disorder associated with bingeing and vomiting

126. A 78-year-old client with senile dementia is wandering the halls in a long-term care facility. He is looking for his 5-year-old son. The nurse would:

A. Ask him when he last saw his son
B. Remind him that his son is now a grown man
C. Ask him to describe his son
D. Help him back to his room

127. A home health nurse is caring for a client with a colostomy. Her family asks the nurse for advice on coping with their father, who has organic brain syndrome. He is very forgetful and gets angry when the family reminds him that he should remember. The nurse's best advice for the family is that they should:

A. Place him in a long-term care facility because he is potentially dangerous to himself
B. Give detailed instructions to him when he does something wrong
C. Reorient him when he loses contact with reality
D. Provide flexibility in his daily activities

128. A 22-year-old client with an antisocial personality refuses to participate in group activities and makes fun of other clients, calling them "nut cases." Which of the following nursing plans would be most effective for the staff to follow?

A. Isolate the client from the other clients to avoid disturbing them with the name calling.
B. Set ground rules.
C. Call a team meeting to discuss the treatment plan.
D. Require the client's participation in all group activities.

129. A 44-year-old paranoid client is admitted for corrective orthopedic surgery. He refuses oral medication, saying that the nurse is trying to poison him. The nurse would:

A. Insist that he take the medicine because it is not poison

B. Skip the medicine and report the behavior to the physician
C. Give him the choice of taking it orally or IM
D. Ask him why he thinks it is poison

130. A 24-year-old female client has refused to get out of bed for 3 days. Her mother brings her to the hospital. The client is given a diagnosis of depression. After 4 days on the unit, she refuses to take her oral medicine because she says it is causing her to have difficulty seeing. The nurse would:

A. Administer it IM
B. Hold the medicine until the client is evaluated further
C. Insist that she take the medicine orally
D. Confine her to her room until she is ready to take her medicine

131. A home health nurse gives the mother of a 9-month-old child instructions for recurrent attacks of croup. The nurse recommends to the mother that when the child begins to cough, she should:

A. Give an additional dose of the prescribed expectorant
B. Keep the child warm
C. Turn the child upside down and give gentle back blows
D. Turn the shower on and create a warm mist

132. A 45-year-old client has just had electroconvulsive therapy. The nurse would:

A. Take his vital signs every 5 to 10 minutes
B. Observe the client for nausea and vomiting
C. Reorient the client to time and place
D. Place the client on bedrest for the next 24 hours

133. A woman who is 8 months pregnant is at the clinic for her regular appointment. She confides in the nurse that her husband wants her to bottle-feed the baby. He thinks that breast-feeding will distort her breasts. She asks the nurse's opinion. The nurse's response is:

A. "To please your husband, you should bottle-feed."
B. "Have you tried talking with your mother about the problem?"
C. "You should discuss this with your doctor."
D. "What would you like to do?"

134. An 18-year-old mother delivers a healthy full-term baby boy. Three days later he is given a diagnosis of phenylketonuria (PKU). The mother asks the nurse if this condition will affect the child's eating habits when he gets older. The nurse tells her that the child will have to avoid eating:

A. Foods high in protein
B. Fruit juices
C. Leafy green vegetables
D. Foods with caffeine

135. It is apparent that a 24-year-old client is going to abort. She is very apprehensive. Which of the following statements is best to give the client support?

A. "Just try to stay calm; everything will be all right."
B. "Is this your first spontaneous abortion?"

C. "It is best to abort now rather than later on in your pregnancy."
D. "I will stay with you to help you through this."

136. A 19-year-old female client is admitted to the psychiatric unit because she talks to herself, is suspicious of other people, laughs inappropriately, and hears voices telling her to kill herself. She is sitting in the lounge quietly talking to a card table. The nurse would:

A. Ignore the behavior; she is not bothering anyone
B. Try to engage her in some physical activity
C. Tell her to stop talking
D. Ask her with whom is she talking

137. A 48-year-old male client is in restraints for severe agitation. The best way to assess whether he is ready to have the restraints removed is:

A. Give him a sedative, wait 30 minutes, and then remove the restraints.
B. Check his pupils for dilation.
C. Observe him for tense muscles.
D. Ask him if he is in control now.

138. A 34-year-old primipara has just had her water break. The nurse's next action is to:

A. Complete a vaginal exam.
B. Ask her husband to leave the room.
C. Take her vital signs.
D. Check the fetal heart rate.

139. A newborn has an elevated bilirubin and phototherapy is ordered. The nurse would:

A. Cover the baby with a blanket to prevent chilling
B. Keep the baby NPO during the therapy
C. Cover the baby's eyes to prevent retinal damage
D. Prepare for an IV infusion

140. To evaluate the effects of phototherapy for an infant with increased bilirubin, the nurse would expect that the:

A. Infant's appetite will increase
B. Infant will become less irritable
C. Skin color will become less jaundiced
D. Photophobia will decrease

141. In an automobile manufacturing plant, coworkers bring a woman who is about to deliver a baby to the nurse's office. The nurse has the secretary call for help and assists with the impending delivery. The nurse would:

A. Apply gentle pressure to the delivering head
B. Have her cross her legs to delay the delivery until help arrives
C. Discourage the mother from pushing
D. Encourage the mother to hold her breath

142. The nurse in the delivery room has just been handed a newborn baby. The nurse's first action is to:

A. Gently slap the baby's bottom to stimulate breathing
B. Hold the baby's head down to help the mucus drain
C. Place the baby on the mother's abdomen
D. Take the baby's vital signs

143. A 54-year-old client is having delusions. It is important that the nurse:

A. Correct the delusions
B. Not talk about the delusions
C. Tell the client to think about something else
D. Not disagree with the client about the delusions

144. A 62-year-old client with glaucoma is reluctant to have surgery. He asks the nurse what will happen if he does not have the surgery. The nurse explains that he:

A. Could get a detached retina
B. Will become nearsighted
C. Will become farsighted
D. May become blind

145. A 2-year-old is admitted with bacterial meningitis. The priority nursing intervention is to:

A. Complete neurological checks
B. Take vital signs
C. Administer antibiotics
D. Encourage good nutrition

146. A nurse enters the room of a 36-year-old client who is speaking as if someone else is in the room. He wants to introduce the nurse to his friend. The nurse's best response is to:

A. Offer to give him some medication.
B. Tell him that no one is there except the client and nurse
C. Ask him what the person's name is
D. Ask him to describe his friend

147. A delusional client thinks the rest of the clients are "out to take his things." The best nursing response to this behavior is:

A. Ignore it because it is not hurting anyone.
B. Correct the thinking each time the client says it.
C. Involve the client in a physical activity.
D. Ask the client to clarify what he means.

148. A 22-year-old client is admitted for emergency surgery because of an ectopic pregnancy. Priority nursing intervention for this client is:

A. Getting a signed consent for sterilization
B. Obtaining a type and crossmatch for blood replacement
C. Giving her postoperative instructions
D. Obtaining a thorough obstetric history

149. A 42-year-old client has just delivered a stillborn infant. She is rather upset and quietly crying. The nurse's best response to comfort her is:

A. Assure her that everything will be okay
B. Ask her if she would like to talk about why she is crying
C. Tell her to not worry, she can have another baby
D. Tell her that this is best because the baby would have had other problems

150. A 10-year-old child is admitted to the pediatric unit with glomerulonephritis. The first nursing priority is:

A. Checking blood pressure
B. Checking stool for occult blood

C. Preparing for a urinary catheterization

D. Preparing for insertion of a GI tube

151. A 6-month-old client is brought to the pediatric clinic with diarrhea. The nurse would be sure to check:

A. Blood pressure

B. Skin turgor

C. For decreased respirations

D. For decreased pulse

152. A nurse is visiting the home of a 4-year-old client with hemophilia. A priority area to check for bleeding is the:

A. Thorax

B. Abdomen

C. Skull

D. Joints

153. A 3-month-old client has congenital hip dysplasia. The nurse would teach the parents to:

A. Keep the child's hips wrapped in blankets

B. Keep the child's hips aligned with the feet

C. Carry the child straddling the hip

D. Carry the child in a manner that keeps the legs straight

154. A 2-year-old has had diarrhea for 2 days. Which of the following would the nurse instruct the parents to avoid?

A. Apple juice

B. Cooked carrots

C. Creamed soup

D. Applesauce

155. The nurse is teaching the parents of a 1-year-old child to administer eardrops for otitis media. The nurse instructs them to:

A. Pull the pinna up and back before giving the drops

B. Pull the pinna down and back before giving the drops

C. Pull the pinna forward and down after giving the drops

D. Pull the pinna straight toward them before giving the drops

156. The 19-year-old parents of a 3-week-old newborn bring their child to the clinic because he is vomiting every time he eats. The physician determines that this is normal newborn regurgitation. The nurse reassures the parents by explaining that this is normal because the:

A. Formula is richer than breast milk

B. Stomach is very small

C. Cardiac sphincter is not fully mature

D. Stomach lining is easily irritated

157. A 2-month-old client has had surgical repair of a cleft lip. The nurse teaches the parents to feed the baby using a

A. Teaspoon

B. Small plastic cup

C. Bottle with a soft nipple

D. Syringe with a soft catheter

158. A 15-month-old child has tetrology of Fallot and will have surgery in 2 months. What toy does the nurse recommend for the child?

A. Stacking blocks

B. A pull toy

C. A horn

D. Bouncing balls

159. A 7-year-old client has a diagnosis of hypothyroidism and is placed on levothyroxine. The nurse instructs the parents to give the medicine:

A. Until symptoms disappear

B. Daily in the morning

C. Until constipation develops

D. Until weight is stabilized

160. A mother brings her 9-year-old daughter to the clinic because she is overweight. What is the best advice to give the mother to help her child lose weight?

A. As she progresses in school, she will become more active and lose weight naturally.

B. Eliminate all sweets from the diet.

C. Give her large doses of supplemental vitamins to suppress the appetite.

D. Begin a program of activity and exercise.

161. The nurse is monitoring the blood pressure of a 23-year-old client in active labor. The nurse takes her blood pressure:

A. During contractions

B. Between contractions

C. Immediately after contractions

D. At the peak of contractions

162. A newborn with meningomyelocele is delivered to the nursery. In what position would the nurse place the child?

A. Side-lying

B. Prone

C. Dorsal

D. Fowler's

163. A 28-year-old woman who has been raped presents herself in the emergency room. The nurse's first action is to:

A. Report it to the police

B. Report it to the supervisor

C. Determine her most immediate needs

D. Call her family for support

164. Three hours after delivery, a 22-year-old client complains of severe perineal pain. Which nursing strategy has priority?

A. Give her an ordered pain medicine.

B. Check her fundus.

C. Inspect her perineum.

D. Give a sitz bath.

165. Percussion and postural drainage are ordered for a 6-month-old child with tracheobronchitis When is the best time to schedule this intervention?

A. Immediately after meals

B. Immediately before meals

C. Just before play time

D. Midway between meals

166. A 6-year-old child being seen at the school clinic has a diagnosis of lead poisoning. Lead poisoning can lead to:

    A. Increased urination
    B. Decreased urination
    C. Malnutrition
    D. Anemia

167. A nurse's 17-year-old neighbor admits to having sexual activity and is now having a thick white discharge. The nurse tells her to:

    A. Drink lots of water and if it does not go away in 2 days, go to the clinic
    B. Not to worry about it just yet; this is a natural occurrence and will go away on its own
    C. Suggest that she be seen as soon as possible in the clinic; she may have a sexually transmitted disease
    D. Tell her mother

168. As part of the school health clinic staff, a nurse notices that a 12-year-old child has illegible handwriting and continuously transposes figures. The nurse refers him for further testing because she suspects:

    A. Aphasia
    B. A learning disability
    C. Visual problems
    D. A neurological disorder

169. An 8-year-old client has a seizure disorder. In preparing the environment to protect the child from injury during a seizure, the nurse would:

    A. Place a wooden tongue blade near the bedside
    B. Place a plastic bite block near the bedside
    C. Keep restraints near the bedside to be used in case of a seizure
    D. Keep a syringe of antiseizure medication at the bedside

170. The nurse is giving medication instructions to a 45-year-old client with minimal English skills. The best way to ensure compliance is to:

    A. Speak slowly
    B. Exaggerate the words
    C. Speak loudly
    D. Provide written instructions

171. A 12-year-old client needs a leg operation. Who should sign the consent form?

    A. The mother.
    B. The father.
    C. Both the mother and father.
    D. Let the parents decide.

172. A 68-year-old Islamic male client needs to have a urinary catheter inserted. Who is the best person to do the procedure?

    A. A female registered nurse
    B. A male orderly
    C. The client's wife
    D. A male LPN

173. An 82-year-old traditional Native American female client does not maintain eye contact with the nurse when the nurse is giving discharge instructions. The nurse should interpret this behavior to mean that:

    A. She does not understand the instructions
    B. She is not interested in the instructions
    C. This is probably normal in her culture
    D. She prefers a physician to give the instructions

174. The father of a Vietnamese child with bronchitis is rubbing the child's back with a coin. The coin leaves red marks. The nurse should:

    A. Suspect the possibility of child abuse
    B. Recognize this as a traditional healing method among Vietnamese
    C. Not allow the father to be alone with his child
    D. Forbid this practice while the child is in the hospital

175. A 45-year-old client is scheduled for knee surgery. Because he does not like the hospital food, his wife brings food from home. He is on a regular diet. The nurse's first response is to:

    A. Ask her to not do this. It is against hospital policy.
    B. Make a referral to the dietitian.
    C. Allow the client to eat the food.
    D. Take the food away.

176. A 67-year-old Japanese client has been given a diagnosis of cancer of the liver. The family does not want the client to know. Which of the following is the most appropriate initial action?

    A. Tell him anyway; it is his right to know.
    B. Respect the family's wishes.
    C. Refer the situation to the ethics committee.
    D. Insist that the family tell the client.

177. A 57-year-old Mexican client with a myocardial infarction has been transferred to the cardiac step-down unit. The extended family comes to visit. The most appropriate action is to:

    A. Restrict visitors to two at a time.
    B. Ask for a family member to help control visitors on a rotational basis.
    C. Ask the physician to speak with the family.
    D. Act as the control person.

178. A 35-year-old client in a long-term care facility has terminal breast cancer. She is taking herbal tea for her indigestion. The nurse's first action is to:

    A. Carefully explain that herbal teas are not permitted
    B. Report the situation to her physician
    C. Report the situation to the pharmacist
    D. Allow her to take the herbal teas

179. A 34-year-old client with a new diagnosis of insulin-dependent diabetes refuses to take insulin when she goes home. She tells the nurse that God will take care of her. The nurse's most appropriate action is to:

    A. Ask her physician to prescribe an oral hypoglycemic agent.
    B. Have the chaplain talk with her.
    C. Ask her physician to talk with her about this "nonsense."
    D. Explain to her that God cannot heal diabetes.

180. A 72-year-old Filipino client is in the long-term care fa-

cility for cancer of the lung. The client is reluctant to cough and deep-breathe, maintains a rigid position in bed, and refuses needed pain medication. The best initial approach is to:

A. Give the pain medication
B. Ask the physician to order the medicine around the clock instead of on an as-needed basis
C. Explore the reasons for not taking the pain medication
D. Report the situation to the nursing supervisor

181. A 63-year-old client being prepared for surgery becomes visibly upset when the nurse tries to remove a beaded bracelet from the client's wrist. The nurse should:

A. Tape the bracelet in place
B. Encourage the family to remove the bracelet
C. Delay the surgery until the bracelet is removed
D. Enclose the hand and wrist in a mitten

182. A 42-year-old laminectomy client is discharged home. He tells the nurse that he still has pain and is going to see an acupuncturist when he gets home. What is the nurse's best response?

A. "The acupuncturist may ruin the surgery."
B. "Be sure to tell your physician that you are seeing an acupuncturist, and be sure to tell the acupuncturist that you have had a laminectomy."
C. "The acupuncture cannot do as much good as the surgery."
D. "I do not think that is a good idea."

183. A 45-year-old home-care client on crutches is demonstrating her crutch walking for the nurse. The nurse knows that she is using the crutches correctly if she:

A. Has both feet far apart
B. Places her weight on the axilla
C. Places her weight on the palms of her hands
D. Does not swing her weight through the crutches

184. During a home visit to a client, her husband tells the nurse that he is experiencing urinary frequency, extreme thirst, and blurred vision. What is the nurse's best advice?

A. Encourage him to make an appointment with his physician as soon as possible; he may have diabetes mellitus.
B. Instruct him to go to the emergency room immediately.
C. Tell him it is probably nothing to worry about, but if it continues, he should make an appointment with his physician.
D. Call the supervisor and ask for advice.

185. A 22-year-old client had an allergic reaction to a home permanent. She is being discharged from the emergency room with a prescription for methylprednisolone tablets. The nurse stresses the importance of:

A. Taking the pills as long as her symptoms continue
B. Completing the medication exactly as instructed or some serious complications can develop
C. Taking the medicine at bedtime
D. Taking the medicine before breakfast

186. A 60-year-old client has a 15-year history of heavy alcohol abuse. The nurse's priority intervention is to:

A. Increase nutritional status
B. Increase fluid intake
C. Monitor neurological status
D. Monitor vital signs

187. The nurse is giving discharge instructions in the emergency room to a client with cholecystitis. What foods are important for the client to avoid?

A. Meats
B. Fruits high in sugar
C. Fatty foods
D. Vegetables high in fiber

188. As part of a community health fair, a nurse is teaching residents to do breast self-examinations. The best time to conduct a breast self-examination is:

A. The first of the month
B. The end of the month
C. Three days before the menses begins
D. Three days after the menses begins

189. A 56-year-old client with cirrhosis and renal failure has pruritus. To help decrease the itching, the nurse suggests:

A. Taking a bath with very warm water
B. Keeping his bedroom temperature between 80 and 85°F (26.6 and 29.4°C)
C. Avoiding soap in the bath water as much as possible
D. Using perfumed lotion after bathing

190. The nurse is evaluating the hemodialysis shunt on a 54-year-old client. A functioning shunt would:

A. Be cool to touch
B. Have a visible pulsation
C. Have a palpable rush of blood
D. Be outlined with erythematous skin

191. A 42-year-old ambulatory client who has had abdominal surgery just had the wound edges separate. What is the nurse's priority action?

A. Put the client back to bed.
B. Place moist saline gauze over the wound.
C. Call the physician.
D. Medicate the client for pain.

192. A 76-year-old client with CHF has just expired. Several family members are at the bedside. One of the daughters sits on the floor and begins to wail. The nurse would:

A. Tell her that everything will be okay
B. Help her to sit in a chair
C. Call the physician for a tranquilizer
D. Stay close to her and ask if she needs anything

193. An 87-year-old client in the long-term care facility has chronic constipation. The first priority is dietary control. Which of the following foods will help to decrease constipation?

A. Lean meat and meat by-products

B. Fruits and vegetables
C. Poultry and fish
D. Rice and potatoes

194. A 76-year-old home-care client has angina pectoris. When he has an attack, he should first:

A. Take a nitroglycerin tablet
B. Call the rescue squad
C. Stop all activity
D. Ignore the pain for at least 3 minutes before taking nitroglycerin

195. A 24-year-old client is in hypovolemic shock secondary to hemorrhage. The most significant change in vital signs that indicates worsening of the condition includes:

A. A decrease in pulse rate
B. An increase in respirations
C. A decrease in respirations
D. An increase in pulse rate

196. A 54-year-old client who has had major abdominal surgery has been returned to the nursing unit from the recovery room. The best position for comfort is:

A. High-Fowler's position
B. Semi-Fowler's position
C. Prone
D. Supine

197. A 52-year-old home-care client is 3 days' postprostatectomy. Priority teaching includes:

A. Drinking at least 3000 ml of fluid each day
B. Avoiding citrus drinks
C. Avoiding milk and milk products
D. Drinking only cranberry and apple juices

198. A 53-year-old mastectomy client has a HemoVac in place. After emptying the HemoVac, the nurse would:

A. Place it in a dependent position to improve drainage
B. Completely collapse the HemoVac before reinserting the air plug
C. Milk the tubing every 2 hours to prevent clotting
D. Reattach it to the wall suctioning unit

199. A 33-year-old client is recovering from an endoscopy. Before giving fluids, the most important assessment is determining:

A. A gag reflex
B. Thirst
C. Bowel sounds
D. Degree of alertness

200. The nurse in an endocrine referral clinic is reviewing the records for the day's appointments. One of the clients has Cushing's syndrome. The nurse would expect this client to have the following appearance:

A. Truncal obesity and hirsutism
B. Enlarged hands and feet
C. A large jaw and large feet
D. A buffalo hump and large hands

201. A 32-year-old female client is receiving dexamethasone (Decadron). While planning nursing care, the nurse would be sure to include the client's predisposition to:

A. Renal calculi
B. Infection
C. Gallstones
D. Hypotension

202. A 37-year-old client has been returned to her room after a thyroidectomy. In what position would the nurse place the client?

A. Right side
B. Left side
C. Semi-Fowler's
D. Low-Fowler's

203. A 57-year-old client with a parathyroidectomy is being returned to the room postoperatively. What tray would the nurse be sure to have at the bedside?

A. Thoracotomy
B. Tracheostomy
C. Paracentesis
D. Pericardiocentesis

204. A 27-year-old client enters the emergency room and has a screwdriver protruding from the right flank. The nurse would:

A. Remove the screwdriver and apply manual pressure
B. Leave it in place and help the client to a stretcher
C. Tether the screwdriver in place
D. Remove the screwdriver and put on a sterile dressing

205. A 16-year-old adolescent with a deep, bleeding laceration on the leg enters the clinic. The nurse's first action is to:

A. Clean the wound of debris
B. Apply a tourniquet above the bleeding site
C. Apply a tourniquet below the bleeding site
D. Apply direct pressure to the wound

206. An 87-year-old client is scheduled for an above-the-knee amputation. To best prepare the client for postoperative therapy, the nurse would:

A. Explain phantom limb pain
B. Demonstrate dressing changes
C. Teach crutch walking
D. Teach leg exercises on the unaffected leg

207. A 53-year-old anxious client with arthritis is having difficulty sleeping because of anxiety. The most appropriate activity to promote sleep is:

A. Administer a tranquilizer
B. Administer a sleeping pill
C. Help the client to explore feelings
D. Provide a snack with warm milk

208. A 36-year-old client with hemorrhoids will be having surgery in 3 days. Before surgery, the nurse would instruct the client to follow what kind of diet?

A. High fiber
B. Low fiber
C. High fat
D. High carbohydrate

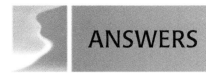

ANSWERS

1. **(A)** Nursing process phase: evaluation; client need: physiological adaptation; content area: medical-surgical.
   RATIONALE
   (A) Although other factors may rarely cause myocardial infarction, the most common cause is atherosclerosis. **(B)** The primary cause of myocardial infarction is atherosclerosis. **(C)** The primary cause of myocardial infarction is atherosclerosis. **(D)** The primary cause of myocardial infarction is atherosclerosis.

2. **(B)** Nursing process phase: assessment; client need: physiological adaptation; content area: medical-surgical.
   RATIONALE
   (A) Less than 20 cc/hr is not enough to keep renal perfusion within normal parameters. **(B)** The minimum expected hourly urine output in shock is 30 cc/hr. **(C)** This amount is too great to expect from a client recovering from cardiogenic shock. **(D)** This amount is too great to expect from a client recovering from cardiogenic shock.

3. **(C)** Nursing process phase: evaluation; client need: pharmacological and parenteral therapies; content area: medical-surgical.
   RATIONALE
   (A) Diphenhydramine is the second medicine to have available. **(B)** Methlyprednisolone may or may not be given, determined by the allergic reaction. **(C)** The first emergency drug in an allergic reaction is epinephrine. **(D)** Sodium bicarbonate is not used as a first-line drug in anaphylaxis.

4. **(D)** Nursing process phase: data collection; client need: prevention and early detection of disease; content area: medical-surgical.
   RATIONALE
   (A) In shock the blood pressure drops and the pulse increases to compensate. **(B)** In shock the blood pressure drops and the pulse increases to compensate. **(C)** In shock the blood pressure drops and the pulse increases to compensate. **(D)** In shock the blood pressure drops and the pulse increases to compensate.

5. **(B)** Nursing process phase: data collection; client need: physiological adaptation; content area: medical-surgical.
   RATIONALE
   (A) There is no pain in third-degree burns. **(B)** As large areas of skin are burned, large amounts of fluids are lost. **(C)** Nutrition is important but not the highest priority. **(D)** Circulation, altered is not an acceptable nursing diagnosis.

6. **(A)** Nursing process phase: implementation; client need: physiological adaptation; content area: medical-surgical.
   RATIONALE
   (A) The physician should order the client's positioning; however, the semi-Fowler's is used to decrease intracranial pressure. **(B)** This position will not decrease intracranial pressure. **(C)** This position will not decrease intracranial pressure. **(D)** This position will not decrease intracranial pressure.

7. **(A)** Nursing process phase: evaluation; client need: prevention and early detection of disease; content area: medical-surgical.
   RATIONALE
   (A) Widened pulse pressure is indicative of increased intracranial pressure. **(B)** This pattern is not a widened pulse pressure. **(C)** This pattern is not a widened pulse pressure. **(D)** This pattern is not a widened pulse pressure; it is a narrowed pulse pressure, which occurs in shock.

8. **(A)** Nursing process phase: implementation; client need: pharmacological and parenteral therapies; content area: medical-surgical.
   RATIONALE
   (A) Electrolyte imbalance of potassium affects the conduction system of the heart, causing abnormal rates or rhythm. **(B)** Potassium does not have a direct effect on the blood pressure. **(C)** Potassium does not have an effect on urinary output. **(D)** Potassium does not have a primary effect on the urine specific gravity.

9. **(B)** Nursing process phase: evaluation; client need: reduction of risk potential; content area: medical-surgical.
   RATIONALE
   (A) Serum transaminase is not diagnostic of pancreatitis. **(B)** Severity of pancreatitis is directly correlated to level of amylase, a pancreatic enzyme. **(C)** Serum sodium is not diagnostic of pancreatitis. **(D)** Serum magnesium levels are not diagnostic of pancreatitis, although clients with pancreatitis frequently have low magnesium levels.

10. **(A)** Nursing process phase: evaluation; client need: reduction of risk potential; content area: medical-surgical.
    RATIONALE
    (A) Ice chips deplete electrolytes by washing out stomach fluid contents. **(B)** Glycerine can be comforting to the client. **(C)** Hard candies can be comforting to the client, although they should be limited in quantity. **(D)** Peroxide gargles can be comforting to the client without depleting electrolytes.

11. **(A)** Nursing process phase: data collection; client need: reduction of risk potential; content area: medical-surgical.
    RATIONALE
    (A) Establishing an airway always has highest priority. **(B)** This option is appropriate but does not have the highest priority. **(C)** This option is appropriate but does not have the highest priority. **(D)** This option is appropriate but does not have the highest priority.

12. **(C)** Nursing process phase: evaluation; client need: physiological adaptation; content area: medical-surgical.
    RATIONALE
    (A) In the oliguric stage, the client does not put out much urine. **(B)** In the initial phase, the client is usually oliguric. **(C)** The abnormally large amount of urine output indicates the diuretic phase. **(D)** The recovery phase is not a recognized term for urinary output for clients in renal failure.

13. **(B)** Nursing process phase: data collection; client need: physiological adaptation; content area: medical-surgical.
    RATIONALE
    (A) Renal failure clients have problems with hyperkalemia, not hypokalemia. Hypokalemia does not occur with renal failure. **(B)** Hyperkalemia causes cardiac rhythm problems because of retention of potassium. **(C)** Hyponatremia is not a common problem with renal failure. **(D)** Hypernatremia is not as serious as hyperkalemia.

14. **(C)** Nursing process phase: implementation; client need: reduction of risk potential; content area: medical-surgical.
    RATIONALE
    (A) Wool blankets increase pruritis. **(B)** Keeping a room at this temperature increases perspiring and increases pruritis. **(C)** A decrease in sweating decreases pruritus. **(D)** Soap residue can increase sweating or cause further skin irritation and pruritis.

15. **(B)** Nursing process phase: data collection; client need: pharmacological and parenteral therapies; content area: medical-surgical.

    RATIONALE

    (A) Fatigue may be a side effect of chemotherapy, but the most common side effect is nausea. **(B)** Nausea is the most common side effect of chemotherapy. **(C)** Dehydration may be a side effect of chemotherapy, but the most common side effect is nausea. **(D)** Skin ulceration may be a side effect of chemotherapy, but the most common side effect is nausea..

16. **(D)** Nursing process phase: evaluation; client need: coping and adaptation; content area: psychiatric nursing.

    RATIONALE

    (A) Confabulation does not prevent aggression. **(B)** The person does not confabulate to get attention but confabulates for self-esteem. **(C)** Confabulation does not denote acute psychosis. **(D)** Confabulation increases self-esteem.

17. **(B)** Nursing process phase: implementation; client need: safety and infection control; content area: medical-surgical.

    RATIONALE

    (A) Chlamydia is not reportable to the health department. **(B)** Syphilis is federally mandated to be reported in all states. **(C)** Nonspecific urethritis is not reportable to the health department. **(D)** Herpes is not reportable to the health department.

18. **(C)** Nursing process phase: evaluation; client need: physiological adaptation; content area: medical-surgical.

    RATIONALE

    (A) The majority of oxygen is carried in the RBCs, not the serum. **(B)** The majority of oxygen is carried in the RBCs, not the plasma. **(C)** RBCs carry oxygen to the tissues in the body and give up carbon dioxide when passing through the lungs. **(D)** WBCs do not carry oxygen.

19. **(C)** Nursing process phase: evaluation; client need: pharmacological and parenteral therapies; content area: medical-surgical.

    RATIONALE

    (A) NS is 0.9. **(B)** NS is 0.9. **(C)** NS is 0.9. **(D)** NS is 0.9.

20. **(D)** Nursing process phase: evaluation; client need: pharmacological and parenteral therapies; content area: medical-surgical.

    RATIONALE

    (A) Extravasation is a common complication of IV therapy. **(B)** Phlebitis is a common complication of IV therapy. **(C)** Infiltration is a common complication of IV therapy. **(D)** Renal shutdown is a result of hypovolemic states; it is not a complication of IV therapy.

21. **(C)** Nursing process phase: implementation; client need: basic care and comfort; content area: medical-surgical.

    RATIONALE

    (A) A tracheostomy tube cannot be used for nutrition. **(B)** A tracheostomy tube cannot be used to relieve flatus. **(C)** A tracheostomy is defined as creation of an artificial airway. **(D)** Tracheostomy decreases dead space.

22. **(D)** Nursing process phase: implementation; client need: reduction of risk potential; content area: medical-surgical.

    RATIONALE

    (A) Keeping the client on the unaffected side deters drainage. **(B)** Keeping a water seal is a function of the drainage system, not the level of the system. **(C)** Repositioning will help drainage only when the client is on the affected side. This is not the best response. **(D)** Turning the client on the affected side is the best way to promote drainage.

23. **(D)** Nursing process phase: evaluation; client need: reduction of risk potential; content area: medical-surgical.

    RATIONALE

    (A) A subclavian catheter goes into a vein; therefore, it cannot cause an arterial spasm. **(B)** A subclavian catheter cannot cause a pulmonary infection. **(C)** Phlebitis is a later complication, not one that can occur on insertion. **(D)** Air embolism can occur on insertion of a subclavian catheter if the entry port is not occluded.

24. **(D)** Nursing process phase: evaluation; client need: reduction of risk potential; content area: medical-surgical.

    RATIONALE

    (A) Some swelling of the toes is expected. **(B)** Depending on the reason for the cast, some blood drainage is expected. **(C)** Toes may be cool (not cold) from inactivity. **(D)** Loss of sensation in the toes may indicate that the cast is too tight and should be reported to the physician.

25. **(B)** Nursing process phase: data collection; client need: prevention and early detection of disease; content area: medical-surgical.

    RATIONALE

    (A) Headache is a common symptom of hypertension. **(B)** Nausea is not a symptom of hypertension. **(C)** Vertigo is a common symptom of hypertension. **(D)** Epistaxis is a common symptom of hypertension.

26. **(D)** Nursing process phase: data collection; client need: physiological adaptation; content area: medical-surgical.

    RATIONALE

    (A) *Hemothorax* is blood in the chest cavity. **(B)** *Pneumothorax* is air in the pleural space. **(C)** *Atelectasis* is a collapse of part of the lung. **(D)** *Pleural effusion* is defined as fluid in the pleural cavity between the visceral and parietal pleura.

27. **(A)** Nursing process phase: data collection; client need: physiological adaptation; content area: medical-surgical.

    RATIONALE

    (A) *Anasarca* is defined as severe, generalized edema. **(B)** *Pitting* is a term to describe the degree of edema. **(C)** *Ascites* is fluid in the abdomen. **(D)** *Lymphedema* describes fluid in the lymphatic drainage system but is not generalized.

28. **(B)** Nursing process phase: evaluation; client need: physiological adaptation; content area: medical-surgical.

    RATIONALE

    (A) Myxedema is a thyroid disorder. **(B)** Acromegaly is the disorder that causes these symptoms in adults. **(C)** Gigantism is a disease of children that causes abnormal long bone growth. **(D)** Addison's disease is a disease of the adrenal glands that causes mineralocorticoid abnormalities.

29. **(C)** Nursing process phase: evaluation; client need: prevention and early detection of disease; content area: medical-surgical.

    RATIONALE

    (A) Acromegaly is a disorder that causes enlargement of the hands, feet, and facial bones. **(B)** Myxedema is a hypothyroid disorder. **(C)** In Cushing's disease, a hypersecretion of the adrenal cortex occurs with an excessive production of glucocorticoids, resulting in these symptoms. **(D)** Graves' disease is a hyperthyroid condition.

30. **(D)** Nursing process phase: implementation; client need: reduction of risk potential; content area: medical-surgical.

    RATIONALE

    (A) There are no contraindications to taking an oral temperature in this client. **(B)** There are no contraindications to taking an oral temperature in this client. **(C)** There are no contraindications to taking an oral temperature in this client. **(D)** Taking an oral temperature reading is contraindicated in older, confused clients because of potential injury.

31. **(B)** Nursing process phase: implementation; client need: prevention and early detection of disease; content area: maternity nursing.

    RATIONALE

    (A) These clients have well-developed temperature-regulating mechanisms. **(B)** A newborn infant's body temperature-regulating mechanism is immature, and infants are greatly influenced by environmental temperatures and must be protected from extreme changes. **(C)** These clients have well-developed temperature-regulating mechanisms. **(D)** These clients have well-developed temperature-regulating mechanisms.

32. **(A)** Nursing process phase: implementation; client need: prevention and early detection of disease; content area: medical-surgical.

    RATIONALE

    (A) The upper arm (site of brachial artery) is usually used for measuring blood pressure. **(B)** The femoral artery cannot be used for measuring blood pressure. The radial artery is sometimes used to measure the blood pressure—especially in hypotensive clients. **(C)** The carotid artery is not usually used for measuring the blood pressure. **(D)** The brachial artery is larger than the radial and therefore is preferred for measuring the blood pressure.

33. **(C)** Nursing process phase: implementation; client need: physiological adaptation; content area: medical-surgical.

    RATIONALE

    (A) Tachycardia is a term meaning a fast heart rate. **(B)** Diastole is the period of time that the heart is at rest. **(C)** Pulse rhythm is the pattern of the beats and the intervals between beats. An irregular rhythm is called an arrhythmia, taken from the Latin word for "without rhythm." **(D)** Bradycardia is a term meaning a slow heart rate.

34. **(A)** Nursing process phase: implementation; client need: prevention and early detection of disease; content area: medical-surgical.

    RATIONALE

    (A) The apical site is routinely used to assess the pulse of infants and children up to 3 years of age. The average pulse of an infant is 125 bpm or more, and a rapid rate is more accurately determined when the pulse is taken apically. **(B)** The radial pulse is not the preferred site for taking a pulse in an infant. **(C)** The femoral pulse is not the preferred site for taking a pulse in an infant. **(D)** The temporal pulse is not the preferred site for taking a pulse in an infant.

35. **(D)** Nursing process phase: implementation; client need: physiological adaptation; content area: medical-surgical.

    RATIONALE

    (A) Pulse pressure is the difference between the systolic and diastolic pressures. **(B)** Maximal pressure is not an acceptable term. **(C)** Systolic pressure is the pressure exerted on the vessel wall at the end of ventricular contraction. **(D)** Blood moves in waves, and the *diastolic pressure* is the pressure when the ventricles are at rest—the lower pressure, present at all times within the arteries.

36. **(B)** Nursing process phase: implementation; client need: prevention and early detection of disease; content area: medical-surgical.

    RATIONALE

    (A) This blood pressure is considered low. **(B)** The average blood pressure of a healthy young adult is 120/80 mm Hg. **(C)** This

blood pressure indicates hypertension. **(D)** This blood pressure indicates hypertension.

37. **(D)** Nursing process phase: implementation; client need: prevention and early detection of disease; content area: medical-surgical.

    RATIONALE

    (A) Both arms are in long casts; the nurse cannot take a brachial pulse. **(B)** Both arms are in long casts; the nurse cannot take a brachial pulse. **(C)** Both arms are in long casts; the nurse cannot take a radial pulse. **(D)** There are nine common peripheral pulse sites. Because of the bilateral casts in this situation, only the carotid or femoral arteries are accessible for palpation.

38. **(C)** Nursing process phase: data collection; client need: physiological adaptation; content area: medical-surgical.

    RATIONALE

    (A) Planning is the second stage of the nursing process. **(B)** Implementation is the third stage of the nursing process. **(C)** Data collection is the first stage of the nursing process; it includes gathering objective and subjective data and verification. **(D)** Evaluation is the last stage of the nursing process.

39. **(B)** Nursing process phase: implementation; client need: physiological adaptation; content area: medical-surgical.

    RATIONALE

    (A) The problem is the stem. **(B)** The etiology of the problem or contributing factors are the second part of a nursing diagnosis statement. **(C)** Evaluation occurs as the result of nursing interventions. **(D)** Signs and symptoms are the contributing factors.

40. **(A)** Nursing process phase: implementation; client need: pharmacological and parenteral therapies; content area: medical-surgical.

    RATIONALE

    (A) Implementation is putting nursing strategies into action in this situation, a dependent nursing action (physician's order). **(B)** Evaluation occurs after the acetaminophen has been given and is based on a reassessment of the contributing factors. **(C)** Planning occurs after a nursing diagnosis is formulated. **(D)** Reassessment occurs as a result of evaluation findings.

41. **(B)** Nursing process phase: implementation; client need: physiological adaption; content area: medical-surgical.

    RATIONALE

    (A) Planning occurs after the nursing diagnosis is formulated. **(B)** Data collection is collecting objective and subjective data and verification. **(C)** Analysis occurs to formulate the diagnosis. **(D)** To evaluate is to judge or appraise; in this case, the client's response to the medication given.

42. **(B)** Nursing process phase: data collection; client need: prevention and early detection of disease; content area: medical-surgical.

    RATIONALE

    (A) Constant data do not change. **(B)** Objective data are data that are detectable by the observer, in this case, dry skin and parched oral mucous membranes. Objective data can be seen, heard, felt, or smelled. **(C)** Subjective data are data that the client tells the nurse about. **(D)** Modifiable data are data that can be changed. This is not a commonly used term in nursing data collection.

43. **(D)** Nursing process phase: implementation; client need: prevention and early detection of disease; content area: medical-surgical.

    RATIONALE

    (A) Shallow respirations are a client weakness. **(B)** Irregular pulse is a client weakness. (**C**) A history of bronchial asthma is a client weakness. (**D**) Normal weight is a client strength. Nurses need to assess strengths as well as weaknesses.

44. (**B**) Nursing process phase: implementation; client need: physiological adaptation; content area: medical-surgical.

    RATIONALE
    (**A**) Fever is likely to cause an increase in blood pressure. (**B**) Hypotension may be caused by excessive blood loss (hemorrhage), as a result of the decreased blood volume. When circulating blood volume falls, as in hemorrhage, the blood pressure falls. (**C**) Stress is likely to increase blood pressure. (**D**) Obesity is likely to cause an increase in blood pressure.

45. (**D**) Nursing process phase: implementation; client need: prevention and early detection of disease; content area: medical-surgical.

    RATIONALE
    (**A**) The diastolic pressure is the last sound heard on release of pressure. (**B**) Venous pressure is not a term used in measuring blood pressure. (**C**) Pulse pressure is the difference between the systolic and diastolic readings. (**D**) The point on the manometer when the first clear Korotkoff sound is heard (contraction of the ventricles) indicates systolic blood pressure.

46. (**C**) Nursing process phase: implementation; client need: management of care; content area: medical-surgical.

    RATIONALE
    (**A**) There is no acceptable method of making a correction in a medical record as stated other than option C. (**B**) There is no acceptable method of making a correction in a medical record other than option C. (**C**) If an error is made in charting, the nurse should not erase it or scratch it out but should draw a line through the error, write the word "error," and sign or initial it above. (**D**) There is no acceptable method of making a correction in a medical record other than option C.

47. (**B**) Nursing process phase: implementation; client need: management of care; content area: medical-surgical.

    RATIONALE
    (**A**) The graphic sheet is a record of vital signs. (**B**) Information is grouped according to the source or the health-care department in this type of record. (**C**) Progress notes contain the physician's recording. (**D**) Nurses' notes contain nurses' documentations.

48. (**C**) Nursing process phase: implementation; client need: basic care and comfort; content area: medical-surgical.

    RATIONALE
    (**A**) There is no standard abbreviation for this phrase. (**B**) There is no standard abbreviation for this phrase. (**C**) WPO is a universal abbreviation. Many abbreviations are taken from root Latin or Greek words (*per ora*). (**D**) There is no standard abbreviation for this phrase.

49. (**D**) Nursing process phase: implementation; client need: basic care and comfort; content area: medical-surgical.

    RATIONALE
    (**A**) Collecting a urine specimen would come later. (**B**) Assisting the client to undress is a later priority. (**C**) Taking and recording vital signs would be a second priority. (**D**) One of the most important steps in the admission procedure is to make the client feel welcome, orient him or her to the new surroundings, and allay any anxieties.

50. (**A**) Nursing process phase: implementation; client need: reduction of risk potential; content area: medical-surgical.

    RATIONALE
    (**A**) The ABCs (*a*irway, *b*reathing, *c*irculation) are always the first priority. Rapid, irregular respirations of 32/min need immediate intervention. (**B**) Skin warm, flushed, and dry does not take as high a priority as increased respirations. (**C**) This slight temperature elevation is not a priority. (**D**) Dry, unproductive cough is not a priority.

51. (**D**) Nursing process phase: implementation; client need: prevention and early detection of disease; content area: medical-surgical.

    RATIONALE
    (**A**) Shallow respirations do not necessarily mean that the client is compromised. (**B**) Rapid breathing is called tachypnea and could be a physiological compensatory mechanism. (**C**) Fowler's position enhances breathing by promoting lung expansion. (**D**) Dyspnea means difficult breathing (taken from the Latin *dys* for "difficult" and *pnea* for "breath").

52. (**A**) Nursing process phase: implementation; client need: reduction of risk potential; content area: medical-surgical.

    RATIONALE
    (**A**) In Fowler's position the head and knees are elevated, facilitating breathing. (**B**) Lying on the side is not as effective as the semi-Fowler's or Fowler's position and may aggravate the client's dyspnea. (**C**) Sims' position will aggravate the client's dyspnea. (**D**) The dorsal recumbent position will aggravate the client's dyspnea.

53. (**B**) Nursing process phase: implementation; client need: basic care and comfort; content area: medical-surgical.

    RATIONALE
    (**A**) Skin lotions do not interfere with oxygen. (**B**) Oxygen is a highly combustible gas that can easily ignite on contact with a spark. The nurse should promote the client's safety by posting "No smoking" signs and by explaining that smoking is not permitted when oxygen is in use. (**C**) The flow rate is 3 L, not 4 L. (**D**) All rooms should be well ventilated.

54. (**C**) Nursing process phase: implementation; client need: prevention and early detection of disease; content area: medical-surgical.

    RATIONALE
    (**A**) A client who takes anti-inflammatory medications may be increasing his or her chance of developing osteoporosis. (**B**) All clients should have a yearly checkup, but this does not answer the question in relation to osteoporosis. (**C**) Adequate calcium intake and exercise have been found to delay some of the bone mineral loss associated with osteoporosis and aging. (**D**) Encouraging walking would help calcium absorption.

55. (**D**) Nursing process phase: implementation; client need: basic care and comfort; content area: medical-surgical.

    RATIONALE
    (**A**) Avoidance of enriched foods may not meet the requirements for decreasing constipation. (**B**) A low-bulk diet increases the chances for constipation. (**C**) A diet high in calcium and carbohydrates will increase constipation. (**D**) Increased daily fluid intake, extra bulk in the diet, and regular exercise help to stimulate normal motility of the intestines.

56. (**B**) Nursing process phase: implementation; client need: pharmacological and parenteral therapies; content area: medical-surgical.

    RATIONALE
    (**A**) The deltoid muscle should not be used for administering irritating medications. (**B**) Z-track injection of IM medications is recommended for medications that could be irritating to tissues. Retracting the skin and SC tissue to one side and maintaining that traction for 10 seconds after injection interrupts the needle track, preventing the medication from seeping into the needle

track or SC tissue and causing irritation. **(C)** Changing the needle will not help to prevent irritating SC tissue. **(D)** Do not massage the injection site after injecting irritating medications; it increases the irritation.

57. **(A)** Nursing process phase: implementation; client need: pharmacological and parenteral therapies; content area: medical-surgical.

RATIONALE

(A) Always recheck the medication against the physician's order when the client notes a discrepancy. Most often the client is correct, and this will avoid a medication error. **(B)** It may not be a new medication; check to make sure. **(C)** Never leave the medication at the client's bedside. **(D)** Do not omit the medication; the client did not refuse it but has questioned it.

58. **(B)** Nursing process phase: implementation; client need: prevention and early detection of disease; content area: medical-surgical.

RATIONALE

(A) Hemoptysis occurs in clients with pulmonary edema. **(B)** Exertional dyspnea, chronic cough, wheezing, and increased mucus production are symptoms of pulmonary emphysema as a result of specific morphologic changes in lung tissue: distention of the alveolar sacs, rupture of the alveolar walls, and destruction of the alveolar capillary bed. **(C)** Epistaxis is not a symptom of pulmonary emphysema. **(D)** Not all of these are symptoms of emphysema.

59. **(B)** Nursing process phase: implementation; client need: reduction of risk potential; content area: medical-surgical.

RATIONALE

(A) Alkalosis is not consistent with pulmonary emphysema. **(B)** The chronic damage to the alveolar walls and capillaries and their decreased elasticity result in a decrease in the exchange of gases between the bloodstream and the air and a retention of carbon dioxide (hypercapnia). **(C)** Elevated SaO_2 and hypocapnia are not associated with pulmonary emphysema. **(D)** Hypocapnia is not a symptom of emphysema.

60. **(A)** Nursing process phase: implementation; client need: reduction of risk potential; content area: medical-surgical.

RATIONALE

(A) During the initial stages of a CVA, it is imperative to maintain cerebral circulation. This can best be done by frequent monitoring of neurological functioning and level of consciousness. **(B)** Range-of-motion exercise could be done but would not have first priority. **(C)** Laxatives may be administered if listed therapy did not control constipation, but this is not the priority. **(D)** Some neurological stimulation is encouraged.

61. **(D)** Nursing process phase: implementation; client need: reduction of risk potential; content area: medical-surgical.

RATIONALE

(A) Aphasic clients do not have difficulty in understanding. **(B)** Writing is not an option with aphasia. **(C)** The nurse may have difficulty understanding the client but will be able to communicate using alternative methods, depending on the client. **(D)** When a CVA affects the left hemisphere of the brain, damage to the speech center may occur. In expressive aphasia, the client has difficulty speaking and writing.

62. **(B)** Nursing process phase: implementation; client need: prevention and early detection of disease; content area: medical-surgical.

RATIONALE

(A) There is suprapubic pressure in urinary tract infections, but not abdominal pain. **(B)** When pathogens invade the urinary tract,

the bladder loses its elasticity. Its filling capacity becomes ineffective, and a moderate stretching of the bladder results in symptoms mentioned in option B. **(C)** There is not usually distention. **(D)** Elevated pulse rate is not a symptom of urinary tract infection.

63. **(A)** Nursing process phase: implementation; client need: physiological adaptation; content area: medical-surgical.

RATIONALE

(A) Practicing good perineal care can prevent contamination from the vagina and rectum. Acidifying the urine via medication or drinking cranberry or prune juice is believed to discourage bacterial multiplication. Increased fluid intake helps to flush out the bacteria present. **(B)** These would not be taught to a client with a urinary tract infection. **(C)** These would not be taught to a client with a urinary tract infection. **(D)** These would not be taught to a client with a urinary tract infection.

64. **(B)** Nursing process phase: implementation; client need: physiological adaptation; content area: psychiatric nursing.

RATIONALE

(A) Increased physical activity is not specific for suicide. **(B)** Most suicidal persons give verbal or behavioral (mood change) warnings before committing suicide. They feel and act less depressed because they have come to terms with a decision to end their lives. **(C)** Hypersomnia is not specific for suicide. **(D)** Increased verbal activity is not specific for suicide.

65. **(C)** Nursing process phase: implementation; client need: reduction of risk potential; content area: maternity nursing.

RATIONALE

(A) If the mother received $Rh_o(D)$ immune globulin after her first pregnancy, there would be no complication. **(B)** If the father is Rh-negative, there would be no complication. **(C)** In a second pregnancy, an Rh-negative mother may produce antibodies against the Rh factor (Rh-positive baby), which cross the placenta and attack the fetus's RBCs if she has not been given $Rh_o(D)$ immune globulin within 72 hours after delivery of her first baby. The possibility exists that if the father is Rh-positive, the infant may also be Rh-positive. **(D)** The baby being Rh-negative is not a complication.

66. **(A)** Nursing process phase: implementation; client need: growth and development through the life span; content area: maternity nursing.

RATIONALE

(A) Pregnancy increases calcium requirements by nearly 50%. Milk is the single most important source of this nutrient. **(B)** Bananas are high in potassium but not in calcium. **(C)** Salad greens also contain calcium but not as much as milk contains. **(D)** Orange juice does not contain any significant amount of calcium.

67. **(B)** Nursing process phase: implementation; client need: safety and infection control; content area: medical-surgical.

RATIONALE

(A) Surgical aseptic technique is not required to remove a dressing. **(B)** Urinary catheterization is an invasive procedure, and surgical asepsis is crucial to prevent introduction of bacteria and a subsequent urinary infection. **(C)** Administering an enema does not require surgical aseptic technique. **(D)** Giving perineal care does not require surgical aseptic technique.

68. **(A)** Nursing process phase: implementation; client need: physiological integrity; content area: medical-surgical.

RATIONALE

(A) Research has proved that most microorganisms are transferred by direct contact and that effective handwashing is considered one of the most effective infection-control measures. **(B)** This option will help to reduce the spread of infection, but the single most important measure is handwashing. **(C)** This option will help to reduce the spread of infection, but the single most important measure is handwashing. **(D)** This option will help to reduce the spread of infection, but the single most important measure is handwashing.

69. **(D)** Nursing process phase: implementation; client need: management of care; content area: medical-surgical.

    RATIONALE

    (A) Bradycardia is a slow pulse rate. **(B)** Pulse paradox is reduction of amplitude of the pulse during inspiration. **(C)** Arrhythmia is an irregular pulse. **(D)** A pulse rate >100 bpm is called tachycardia (taken from the Greek *tachys,* meaning "swift" or "rapid," and *kardia,* meaning "heart").

70. **(C)** Nursing process phase: implementation; client need: reduction of risk potential; content area: medical-surgical.

    RATIONALE

    (A) Increasing physical activity will increase heat production. **(B)** Providing extra blankets will increase heat production. **(C)** Increasing fluid intake will counteract potential dehydration, and giving tepid sponge baths will increase heat loss through conduction. **(D)** Offering warm fluids will not increase heat loss.

71. **(B)** Nursing process phase: implementation; client need: management of care; content area: medical-surgical.

    RATIONALE

    (A) This option is objective data. **(B)** Subjective data are data resulting from the feelings or temperament of the subject (client)—data apparent only to the person affected, which can be described or verified only by that person. **(C)** This option is objective data. **(D)** This option is objective data.

72. **(B)** Nursing process phase: implementation; client need: management of care; content area: medical-surgical.

    RATIONALE

    (A) This is only part of the reason for using the nursing process. **(B)** The nursing process provides a framework of accountability, and the client's record serves as the vehicle by which different members of the health-care team communicate assessments, interventions, and evaluations. **(C)** This is only part of the reason for using the nursing process. **(D)** This is only part of the reason for using the nursing process.

73. **(D)** Nursing process phase: implementation; client need: psychosocial adaptation; content area: psychiatric nursing.

    RATIONALE

    (A) This option does not display an open communication system. **(B)** This option does not display an open communication system. **(C)** This option does not display an open communication system. **(D)** This is an open-ended statement that shows that the nurse has observed the client's distress and allows verbalization of feelings.

74. **(C)** Nursing process phase: implementation; client need: psychosocial adaptation; content area: medical-surgical.

    RATIONALE

    (A) This behavior does not display open attentive listening. **(B)** This behavior does not display open attentive listening. **(C)** Attentive listening requires all the senses and skills; maintaining eye contact helps the nurse to interpret the nonverbal as well as the verbal message and lets the client know the nurse is listening and involved. **(D)** This behavior does not display open attentive listening.

75. **(A)** Nursing process phase: implementation; client need: physiological adaptation; content area: medical-surgical.

    RATIONALE

    (A) The first intervention when the nurse arrives on the scene if the client appears to have "ceased breathing" is to determine whether he or she is responsive. This is the first step of basic CPR. **(B)** This is not the first step of CPR. **(C)** This is not the first step of CPR. **(D)** This is not the first step of CPR.

76. **(A)** Nursing process phase: implementation; client need: physiological adaptation; content area: medical-surgical.

    RATIONALE

    (A) The first step of CPR is to establish unresponsiveness. **(B)** Absence of the carotid pulse determines pulselessness and cardiac arrest. It is essential to assess the carotid pulse accurately because performing external chest percussions on a client with a pulse can lead to serious medical complications. **(C)** The second step of CPR is to determine cessation of respirations. **(D)** Fixed and dilated pupils are not an indication to start or stop breathing or compressions.

77. **(D)** Nursing process phase: implementation; client need: basic care and comfort; content area: medical-surgical.

    RATIONALE

    (A) This is not the correct order for the nursing process. **(B)** This is not the correct order for the nursing process. **(C)** This is not the correct order for the nursing process. **(D)** The nursing process consists of a four-step process of data collection, analysis or planning, implementation, and evaluation. The nursing process uses a systematic, rational, and logical manner to plan, provide, and evaluate nursing care.

78. **(B)** Nursing process phase: implementation; client need: basic care and comfort; content area: medical-surgical.

    RATIONALE

    (A) Vitamins and minerals are essential in the diet, but they are not one of the four basic food groups. **(B)** The "basic four" food guide was introduced by the U.S. Department of Agriculture (USDA) in 1956. This plan is based on four basic groups for sound nutrition: milk and milk products, meats and alternates, breads and cereals, and fruits and vegetables. **(C)** Vitamins and minerals are not one of the four basic food groups. **(D)** Poultry by itself is not one of the four basic food groups.

79. **(C)** Nursing process phase: implementation; client need: pharmacological and parenteral therapies; content area: medical-surgical.

    RATIONALE

    (A) Right amount and right dose are the same thing. **(B)** Right order is not one of the five rights. **(C)** The five rights are the essential guidelines for safe administration of medications. **(D)** Right documentation is important, but it is not one of the five rights.

80. **(B)** Nursing process phase: implementation; client need: prevention and early detection of disease; content area: medical-surgical.

    RATIONALE

    (A) Cool moist skin and hypothermia are not indicative of dehydration. **(B)** Sodium excess can occur with dehydration when water loss exceeds sodium loss, manifesting these symptoms because of hyperosmolarity of the extracellular fluid. **(C)** Decreased specific gravity of urine is not a symptom of dehydration. **(D)** Anorexia and cool moist skin are not symptoms of dehydration.

81. **(C)** Nursing process phase: implementation; client need: reduction of risk potential; content area: medical-surgical.

    RATIONALE

    (A) A potassium level of 3.2 is too low. **(B)** A potassium level of 2.5 is too low. **(C)** Potassium is a major cation of intracellular fluid, in which 98% of this electrolyte is found. Serum potassium levels, however, are based on the portion of potassium in the extracellular fluid, where the normal range is 3.5–5.5 mEq/L. **(D)** A potassium level of 4.0 is not the upper range of normal.

82. **(B)** Nursing process phase: implementation; client need: pharmacological and parenteral therapies; content area: medical-surgical.

    RATIONALE

    (A) See rationale B for correct math calculation. **(B)** The formula for calculating drops per minute of an IV infusion is: Total infusion volume $\times$ df $\div$ Number of hours $\times$ 60 = drops per minute. 1000 ml $\times$ 20 gtt/ml $\div$ 8 hr $\times$ 60 min = 20,000/480 = 41.66 or 42 gtt/min. **(C)** See rationale B for correct math calculation. **(D)** See rationale B for correct math calculation.

83. **(B)** Nursing process phase: implementation; client need: reduction of risk potential; content area: medical-surgical.

    RATIONALE

    (A) This may be correct, but it is not the primary purpose for emptying the bladder before surgery. **(B)** The primary purpose of emptying the bladder before surgery is to prevent inadvertent injury to the bladder during the surgical procedure. **(C)** This may be correct, but it is not the primary purpose for emptying the bladder before surgery. **(D)** This option may be correct, but it is not the primary reason for emptying the bladder before surgery.

84. **(B)** Nursing process phase: implementation; client need: management of care; content area: medical-surgical.

    RATIONALE

    (A) This option does not cover the entire extent of informed consent. **(B)** Informed consent is an agreement by a client to accept a course of treatment or a procedure after complete information, including the risks of treatment and facts relating to it, has been provided by the physician. It is a part of the Patient's Bill of Rights. This protects clients from having any surgical procedure they do not want or do not know about, and it also protects the hospital and health personnel from a claim by a client or family that permission was not granted. **(C)** This option does not cover the entire extent of informed consent. **(D)** This option does not cover the entire extent of informed consent.

85. **(D)** Nursing process phase: implementation; client need: reduction of risk potential; content area: medical-surgical.

    RATIONALE

    (A) This may be a true statement for some clients but is not the reason why food and fluids are withheld before surgery. **(B)** This may be a true statement for some clients but is not the reason why food and fluids are withheld before surgery. **(C)** This may be a true statement for some clients but is not the reason why food and fluids are withheld before surgery. **(D)** Anesthesia depresses gastrointestinal (GI) functioning, and because of the danger that the client may vomit during induction of anesthesia, the client should be NPO for at least 6–8 hours before surgery to prevent possible aspiration of food or fluids.

86. **(B)** Nursing process phase: implementation; client need: reduction of risk potential; content area: medical-surgical.

    RATIONALE

    (A) Shaving before a surgical procedure does not prevent postoperative discomfort. **(B)** The primary purpose of removing hair from the surgical area is to destroy microorganisms and thus to reduce the chance of infection. **(C)** Shaving before a surgical procedure does not prevent pain. **(D)** Shaving before a surgical procedure does not provide a better view of the surgical area.

87. **(A)** Nursing process phase: implementation; client need: pharmacological and parenteral therapies; content area: medical-surgical.

    RATIONALE

    (A) Heparin (an anticoagulant) is often used postoperatively to prevent thromboembolic complications arising from surgery. **(B)** Heparin use would increase the risk of postoperative hemorrhage. **(C)** Heparin would decrease blood coagulation. **(D)** Heparin does not prevent postoperative paralytic ileus.

88. **(A)** Nursing process phase: implementation; client need: prevention and early detection of disease; content area: medical-surgical.

    RATIONALE

    (A) The clinical signs of wound infection include redness, swelling, pain, induration, fever, and leukocytosis. **(B)** Anorexia, diminished bowel sounds, and serosanguineous drainage are not symptoms of a wound infection. **(C)** Well-approximated edges and serosanguineous drainage are not signs of a wound infection. **(D)** Bright-red drainage is abnormal but not indicative of wound infection.

89. **(A)** Nursing process phase: implementation; client need: reduction of risk potential; content area: medical-surgical.

    RATIONALE

    (A) The ABCs of CPR are airway, breathing, and circulation. **(B)** Airway and circulation need to first be assessed before definitive treatment is implemented. **(C)** This is not the first action in this scenario. **(D)** The nurse would not elevate the client's head to begin CPR.

90. **(C)** Nursing process phase: implementation; client need: pharmacological and parenteral therapies; content area: medical-surgical.

    RATIONALE

    (A) Radiation does not kill by heat. **(B)** This is not how radiation works. See rationale C. **(C)** Ionizing radiation is energy in the form of waves or particles transmitted to rapidly dividing cancer cells, which are radiosensitive. Radiation chemically alters tissue protein and disrupts the cancer cells by inhibiting their division. **(D)** There is no such thing as magnetic resuscitation.

91. **(A)** Nursing process phase: implementation; client need: pharmacological and parenteral therapies; content area: medical-surgical.

    RATIONALE

    (A) To prevent overexposure to radiation when caring for clients with radioactive implants, close-contact time should not exceed 15 minutes daily. As the distance from the source of radiation is increased, exposure is decreased. Shielding is necessary for safe protection, especially when the principles of time and distance cannot always be adhered to. **(B)** One does not have to stay 12 ft away. **(C)** The client does not have to be on protective isolation. **(D)** One does not have to wear a film badge, and one can stay in the room for 15 minutes.

92. **(B)** Nursing process phase: implementation; client need: prevention and early detection of disease; content area: medical-surgical.

    RATIONALE

    (A) Passive and active smoking do not cause chest injuries. **(B)** A significant number of chest injuries result from passengers being unrestrained (without seat belts) in automobile accidents and are caused by the forces of acceleration and deceleration. **(C)** Driving below the speed limit may increase the opportunity for accidents. **(D)** Placing children in the back seat does not decrease chest injury unless they are also restrained in seat belts.

93. **(C)** Nursing process phase: implementation; client need: physiological adaptation; content area: medical-surgical.

    RATIONALE

    (A) Hypoventilation causes acidosis. **(B)** The client is acidotic, not alkalotic. **(C)** The client's PaO_2 is far less than the norm of

80–95 mm Hg; his $PaCO_2$ is elevated from the norm of 35–45 mm Hg; and his pH is well below the norm of 7.35–7.45. These indicate respiratory acidosis, and hypoventilation is the primary factor. (D) This is acidosis, not alkalosis.

94. (B) Nursing process phase: implementation; client need: prevention and early detection of disease; content area: medical-surgical.

RATIONALE

(A) Hypertension is a late sign of hypoxia. (B) Hypoxia is a diminished oxygen supply to the cells of the body, resulting in the symptoms listed. The respiratory control center is located in the brain; therefore, judgment can also be impaired. (C) Cyanosis is a late sign of hypoxia. (D) Crowing respirations are characteristic of obstruction.

95. (D) Nursing process phase: implementation; client need: prevention and early detection of disease; content area: medical-surgical.

RATIONALE

(A) There is no need to decrease these foods in the diet. (B) There is no need to decrease these foods in the diet. (C) There is no need to decrease these foods in the diet. (D) Foods high in cholesterol, especially in low-density lipoproteins such as those mentioned in option D, are believed to contribute to the occurrence of myocardial infarction and other coronary and vascular disorders. The other foods listed are not high in cholesterol.

96. (C) Nursing process phase: implementation; client need: reduction of risk potential; content area: medical-surgical.

RATIONALE

(A) These foods are not high in potassium. (B) These foods are not high in potassium. (C) These are potassium-rich foods that will help to keep potassium levels within normal limits when clients are receiving potassium-depleting diuretics. (D) These foods and nuts are not high in potassium.

97. (A) Nursing process phase: implementation; client need: pharmacological and parenteral therapies; content area: medical-surgical.

RATIONALE

(A) Anti-inflammatory agents are used to treat arthritis because they counteract inflammation. (B) Antilipemic drugs are not beneficial in treating arthritis. (C) Antibiotics are not useful in treating arthritis, especially on a long-term basis. (D) Sympatholytic agents are not beneficial in treating arthritis.

98. (C) Nursing process phase: implementation; client need: growth and development through the life span; content area: medical-surgical.

RATIONALE

(A) This position does not increase fetal activity. (B) This position does not facilitate the descent into the birth canal. (C) The Sims' position promotes conscious relaxation, facilitates focusing and breathing techniques, and enhances fetal and maternal circulation, as well as preventing supine hypotension (which can occur in the supine position). (D) This position does not decrease the intensity of labor pains.

99. (C) Nursing process phase: implementation; client need: growth and development through the life span; content area: maternity nursing.

RATIONALE

(A) This is not an abnormal heart rate for an infant. (B) This heart rate does not indicate distress. (C) A normal fetal heart rate is 120–160 bpm. (D) This heart rate is not above the norm.

100. (B) Nursing process phase: implementation; client need: growth and development through the life span; content area: maternity nursing.

RATIONALE

(A) This response defines duration. (B) The frequency of contractions refers to the time interval from the beginning of one contraction to the beginning of the next. (C) This is not a method for measuring the frequency of contractions. (D) This is not a method for measuring the frequency of contractions.

101. (D) Nursing process phase: implementation; client need: growth and development through the life span; content area: maternity nursing.

RATIONALE

(A) This is a part of stage 3 but not the entire stage. (B) This is part of stage 1. (C) This is a part of stage 2. (D) The process of labor is traditionally divided into three stages. The third stage begins when the baby is delivered and ends with the delivery of the placenta and membranes. Currently, a fourth stage has been added to allow for full evaluation of the newly delivered mother.

102. (B) Nursing process phase: data collection; client need: prevention and early detection of disease; content area: pediatrics.

RATIONALE

(A) Anemia may occur as a result of poor nutrition but is not a classic sign. (B) Pyloric stenosis (narrowing) is a disorder of the digestive tract caused by an overgrowth of the circular muscles of the pylorus. This narrowing causes partial blockage that prevents food from properly emptying into the duodenum, resulting in forceful (projectile) vomiting. (C) Diarrhea is not a classic symptom of pyloric stenosis. (D) Anorexia is not a classic symptom of pyloric stenosis.

103. (A) Nursing process phase: implementation; client need: physiological adaptation; content area: medical-surgical.

RATIONALE

(A) In acute glomerulonephritis, urinary output is decreased, specific gravity is high, and fluid restriction may be necessary (because of possible impaired renal function); therefore, keeping I&O in balance and assessing color and character of the urine is important. (B) Monitoring pulse and respirations is important but is not the most important intervention. (C) Fluids are to be restricted rather than encouraged. (D) Ambulation does not affect glomerulonephritis.

104. (A) Nursing process phase: implementation; client need: basic care and comfort; content area: medical-surgical.

RATIONALE

(A) Clear liquids are given to a postoperative tonsillectomy client. An ice slush may be more appealing to a 4-year-old child. Many ice slushes contain synthetic fruit juices, which are not as irritating as natural juices. (B) Milk is not a clear liquid. (C) Orange juice is not a clear liquid. (D) Decaffeinated soda pop still has carbonation.

105. (B) Nursing process phase: implementation; client need: safety and infection control; content area: medical-surgical.

RATIONALE

(A) The nurse would perform this intervention, but it is not the primary reason for changing the dressing. (B) Inspection and assessment of the incisional area and prevention of potential problems (infection, dehiscence, bleeding) are the main reasons why a client's dressing is changed. (C) Dressings do not necessarily prevent an infection or provide comfort. (D) Charting is important but is not the reason for changing a dressing.

106. **(B)** Nursing process phase: implementation; client need: reduction of risk potential; content area: medical-surgical.

RATIONALE

(A) Early ambulation does not prevent dependence. **(B)** Research has shown that early postoperative ambulation helps to restore all body systems to normal and prevents potential postoperative complications. **(C)** Early ambulation does not prevent nausea and vomiting. **(D)** Diaphoresis is not a desirable outcome.

107. **(D)** Nursing process phase: implementation; client need: physiological adaptation; content area: medical-surgical.

RATIONALE

(A) Increased cardiac output does not usually result from hypovolemia. **(B)** Increased metabolic needs do not cause CHF. **(C)** Accumulation of serous fluid in the pleural space does not lead to CHF. **(D)** In CHF the heart fails, becomes filled with fluid, and no longer can adequately pump blood throughout the body.

108. **(A)** Nursing process phase: implementation; client need: pharmacological and parenteral therapies; content area: medical-surgical.

RATIONALE

(A) Hair cells (like other rapidly dividing cells) are very sensitive to chemotherapeutic drugs. Clients should be assured that hair loss is temporary but that the texture and color of the regrowth may differ from the original. **(B)** Alopecia from chemotherapy is rarely permanent. **(C)** This statement about alopecia being "not life threatening" will not help the client's self-esteem. **(D)** One should not tell the client that alopecia is never permanent; the rest of this statement will not help the client's self-esteem.

109. **(B)** Nursing process phase: implementation; client need: management of care; content area: medical-surgical.

RATIONALE

(A) The nurse would document the blood pressure in the chart, but this is not the priority action. **(B)** An LPN always reports to the RN significant changes in vital signs as well as subjective or objective symptoms that indicate a change in the client's condition. A blood pressure reading of 200/110 and the accompanying symptoms bear immediate reporting. **(C)** Giving acetaminophen is the next action after notifying the registered nurse. **(D)** The LPN would inquire about family history of hypertension, but this is not of the highest priority.

110. **(C)** Nursing process phase: data collection; client need: coping and adaptation; content area: psychiatric nursing.

RATIONALE

(A) *Sublimation* is acceptance of a socially approved substitute. **(B)** *Repression* is involuntary exclusion of an undesirable thought from the memory. **(C)** *Denial* is a refusal to admit the reality of or to acknowledge the presence of something painful. **(D)** *Compensation* is the process by which a person makes up for a deficiency by emphasizing an asset.

111. **(D)** Nursing process phase: implementation; client need: physiological adaptation; content area: medical-surgical.

RATIONALE

(A) Giving aspirin is not the first priority. **(B)** Sponging with alcohol would be done if the tepid bath did not work. **(C)** Applying blankets would increase the child's temperature. **(D)** A tepid sponge bath increases heat loss through conduction and is the first measure used to reduce fever in a young child.

112. **(D)** Nursing process phase: implementation; client need: pharmacological and parenteral therapies; content area: pediatrics.

RATIONALE

(A) Having the child sit upright would make it more difficult to instill eardrops. **(B)** This is not the correct technique for instilling eardrops in a child. **(C)** This is not the correct technique for instilling eardrops in a child. **(D)** To straighten the auditory canal of an infant or toddler (which is shorter than that of an adult), gently pull the pinna down and backward.

113. **(B)** Nursing process phase: data collection; client need: pharmacological and parenteral therapies; content area: medical-surgical.

RATIONALE

(A) Bradycardia is not commonly seen in vasodilator therapy. **(B)** Vasodilators (antihypertensives) lower the blood pressure by dilating arterial blood vessels. These agents stimulate central adrenergic receptors, resulting in the adverse effects listed. **(C)** Hypertension is not commonly seen in vasodilator therapy. **(D)** Hypokalemia is not commonly seen in vasodilator therapy.

114. **(D)** Nursing process phase: implementation; client need: physiological adaptation; content area: medical-surgical.

RATIONALE

(A) Gastric suction may cause hyponatremia, not hypernatremia. **(B)** Gastric suction would cause hypokalemia, not hyperkalemia. **(C)** Gastric suctioning would not cause hypervolemia; fluid is being lost. **(D)** Gastric secretions are high in potassium.

115. **(B)** Nursing process phase: implementation; client need: pharmacological and parenteral therapies; content area: medical-surgical.

RATIONALE

(A) This option constitutes assessment data collected in patients with cardiac disease but is not of first priority when administering antihypertensive medications. **(B)** Because the purpose of giving an antihypertensive agent is to lower arterial blood pressure, it is always crucial first to measure the client's blood pressure to establish a baseline and also to be certain the blood pressure is not too low, in which case the administration of an antihypertensive agent would result in serious adverse effects. **(C)** This option constitutes assessment data collected in patients with cardiac disease but is not of first priority when administering antihypertensive medications. **(D)** This option constitutes assessment data collected in patients with cardiac disease but is not of first priority when administering antihypertensive medications.

116. **(B)** Nursing process phase: data collection; client need: pharmacological and parenteral therapies; content area: medical-surgical.

RATIONALE

(A) This is too late for a Regular insulin reaction. **(B)** Regular insulin is a rapid-acting insulin, reaching its onset within 30–60 minutes, which might precipitate adverse effects (hypoglycemia) because of too much insulin in the bloodstream. **(C)** This is too soon for Regular insulin to peak. **(D)** This is past the peak of Regular insulin.

117. **(B)** Nursing process phase: implementation; client need: pharmacological and parenteral therapies; content area: medical-surgical.

RATIONALE

(A) Ampicillin is an antibiotic. **(B)** Heparin is an anticoagulant and inactivates several of the factors necessary for the clotting of blood. It is often ordered to treat thrombophlebitis (inflammation of a vein with formation of a thrombus) to prevent a potential embolus that could lodge in the lungs, heart, or brain, causing serious complications or death or both. **(C)** Propranolol is used for cardiac conditions, not phlebitis. **(D)** Nitroglycerin is used for cardiac conditions.

118. **(B)** Nursing process phase: implementation; client need: growth and development through the life span; content area: medical-surgical.

    RATIONALE

    (A) This is an activity the nurse would do, but it is not the best answer because the signs may not be detected before significant bleeding occurs. **(B)** Significant changes in vital signs will quickly alert the nurse to potential hemorrhage. Assessment and palpation of the fundus is one way to check for height and tone, presence of clots, and possible uterine atony to prevent a potential hemorrhage. **(C)** Nailbed color change is a late sign of hemorrhage. **(D)** Monitoring color and amount of flow will not necessarily indicate hemorrhage.

119. **(B)** Nursing process phase: implementation; client need: prevention and early detection of disease; content area: medical-surgical.

    RATIONALE

    (A) Mycobacterium does not cause hypertension or anorexia. **(B)** Presence of the mycobacterium acid-fast gram-positive bacillus causes symptoms as listed. Initial symptoms are related to the infectious process. Cough and hemoptysis occur if there is pulmonary involvement. **(C)** Mycobacterium does not cause enlarged lymph nodes. **(D)** Mycobacterium does not cause bradycardia or weight gain.

120. **(A)** Nursing process phase: implementation; client need: psychosocial adaptation; content area: psychiatric nursing.

    RATIONALE

    (A) Hypochondriasis is a defense used by the ego when it has real or imagined aggressive, critical feelings toward others. The critical feelings are turned back on the ego and are experienced as guilt, often transformed into physical complaints. **(B)** This is projection. **(C)** This is suppression. **(D)** This is repression.

121. **(C)** Nursing process phase: implementation; client need: psychosocial adaptation; content area: psychiatric nursing.

    RATIONALE

    (A) Doing nothing will not meet the client's basic grooming needs. **(B)** Telling the client to bathe may not accomplish the task. **(C)** Clients with depression frequently do not have the energy to take care of their personal grooming needs. The nurse assists with these needs without fostering dependence. **(D)** This option will not promote independence.

122. **(A)** Nursing process phase: implementation; client need: psychosocial adaptation; content area: psychiatric nursing.

    RATIONALE

    (A) The nurse will stay with the client initially for a short period to begin developing trust. **(B)** It is not necessary to stay for an hour; besides, this is not a matter of control. **(C)** The best plan is to stay a short while and then return later. **(D)** Therapeutic touch is not appropriate until trust is established.

123. **(A)** Nursing process phase: planning; client need: psychosocial adaptation; content area: psychiatric nursing.

    RATIONALE

    (A) Regression is adopting behavioral patterns characteristic of an earlier stage to reduce stress. **(B)** Conversion is channeling psychological stress into physical symptoms. **(C)** Denial occurs when the anxiety-producing situations are rejected as they actually are. **(D)** Projection is attributing undesirable symptoms to other people or objects.

124. **(B)** Nursing process phase: planning; client need: coping and adaptation; content area: psychiatric nursing.

RATIONALE

(A) Acrophobia is fear of height. **(B)** Xenophobia is fear of strangers. **(C)** Claustrophobia is fear of enclosed spaces. **(D)** Agoraphobia is fear of open spaces.

125. **(D)** Nursing process phase: planning; client need: coping and adaptation; content area: psychiatric nursing.

    RATIONALE

    (A) Bulimia is not a phobia. **(B)** Anorexia is a disorder involving starving oneself. **(C)** Bulimia is more than just vomiting. **(D)** Bulimia is eating massive amounts of food and then purging by either vomiting or taking laxatives.

126. **(D)** Nursing process phase: planning; client need: psychosocial adaptation; content area: psychiatric nursing.

    RATIONALE

    (A) This action will only reinforce his confusion. **(B)** This is a short-term solution and may initiate a defense mechanism. **(C)** If he can describe his son, this reinforces his confusion. He does not have a 5-year old son. **(D)** This action will help to orient him to his surroundings.

127. **(C)** Nursing process phase: implementation; client need: psychosocial adaptation; content area: psychiatric nursing.

    RATIONALE

    (A) He may be potentially dangerous to himself, but the family is not asking to have him placed in a long-term care facility. **(B)** Giving detailed instructions to clients with organic brain syndrome will only increase their confusion. **(C)** Organic brain syndrome clients need frequent reality orientation. **(D)** This will only increase his anxiety and confusion.

128. **(C)** Nursing process phase: planning; client need: psychosocial adaptation; content area: psychiatric nursing.

    RATIONALE

    (A) This approach will reinforce the antisocial behavior. **(B)** Setting ground rules does not mean the client will follow them. **(C)** This approach ensures that all team members are engaged in the treatment plan. **(D)** Requiring participation does not mean that the client will participate.

129. **(C)** Nursing process phase: implementation; client need: pharmacological and parenteral therapies; content area: psychiatric nursing.

    RATIONALE

    (A) The nurse is pitting himself or herself against the client. **(B)** This is not an option; he needs his medication or his behavior will get worse. **(C)** Giving him a choice allows him to have some control. **(D)** The client is paranoid; he does not know why he thinks this. This approach will only reinforce his paranoid thoughts.

130. **(B)** Nursing process phase: data collection; client need: pharmacological and parenteral therapies; content area: psychiatric nursing.

    RATIONALE

    (A) The client needs her symptoms evaluated; giving the medicine IM is inappropriate at this time. **(B)** Holding the medicine until the client's symptoms can be evaluated is the correct choice. **(C)** Insisting that she takes her medicine will not control her visual problems. **(D)** The client needs to be evaluated, not confined to her room.

131. **(D)** Nursing process phase: implementation; client need: physiological adaptation; content area: pediatrics.

    RATIONALE

    (A) This action could potentially overdose the child. **(B)** Keeping the child warm would increase the cough. **(C)** Turning the child upside down might increase epiglottal edema and make the child worse. (D) This is the best choice because a warm mist reduces epiglottal edema and relieves coughing.

132. **(C)** Nursing process phase: implementation; client need: reduction of risk potential; content area: psychiatric nursing.

RATIONALE

(A) It is not necessary to take vital signs every 5 to 10 minutes after electroconvulsive therapy. (B) Nausea and vomiting are not usual side effects of electroconvulsive therapy. (C) Clients undergoing electroconvulsive therapy are usually confused after therapy and need reorientation. (D) Bedrest is not required after electroconvulsive therapy.

133. **(D)** Nursing process phase: planning; client need: growth and development through the life span; content area: psychiatric nursing.

RATIONALE

(A) The nurse should be a client advocate. This statement is the nurse's opinion. (B) The problem is between the husband and wife, not the woman's mother. (C) The woman is asking the nurse for help. This is not the best response. (D) This statement will help the client to discuss her feelings before any decision is made.

134. **(A)** Nursing process phase: planning; client need: prevention and early detection of disease; content area: pediatric nursing.

RATIONALE

(A) Children with PKU must restrict the amount of protein in their diet because accumulation of phenylalanine is toxic to the brain. (B) Juices are not restricted in children with PKU. (C) Leafy green vegetables do not have to be restricted in children with PKU. (D) Caffeine does not have to be restricted in children with PKU.

135. **(D)** Nursing process phase: implementation; client need: growth and development through the life span; content area: psychiatric nursing.

RATIONALE

(A) The nurse does not know that everything will be all right. This is false reassurance. (B) This statement will not help to ease the client's apprehension. (C) This statement may increase the client's apprehension. (D) Remaining with the client will help to provide support through the aborting process.

136. **(B)** Nursing process phase: implementation; client need: psychosocial adaptation; content area: psychiatric nursing.

RATIONALE

(A) Ignoring the behavior reinforces the hallucinations. (B) Engaging her in physical activity helps to decrease hallucinations. (C) Telling her to stop talking may increase her agitation. (D) She probably does not know with whom she is talking, and this response reinforces the hallucinations.

137. **(C)** Nursing process phase: data collection; client need: safety and infection control; content area: psychiatric nursing.

RATIONALE

(A) Giving a sedative may be an unnecessary intervention. (B) Dilated pupils will not tell the nurse if the client is agitated. (C) A client with relaxed muscles is not agitated. (D) He may say yes, but he is not in control and may then hurt himself or someone else.

138. **(A)** Nursing process phase: implementation; client need: growth and development through the life span; content area: maternity nursing.

RATIONALE

(A) Completing a vaginal examination to check for a prolapsed

cord is the next action. (B) The husband does not need to leave the room; he is a support. (C) This may be a nursing action, but it is not the first action. (D) This may be a nursing action, but it is not the first action.

139. **(C)** Nursing process phase: implementation; client need: reduction of risk potential; content area: maternity nursing.

RATIONALE

(A) The baby should not be covered in order to get maximum exposure to the light. (B) The baby needs fluids to eliminate the bilirubin. (C) The baby's eyes should be covered to prevent retinal damage. (D) An IV infusion is not necessary. The baby can take fluids orally.

140. **(C)** Nursing process phase: evaluation; client need: reduction of risk potential; content area: maternity nursing.

RATIONALE

(A) Phototherapy does not usually affect the infant's appetite. (B) Phototherapy does not increase an infant's irritability. (C) The phototherapy light should decrease the jaundice in the infant, thereby allowing the nurse to know that it is effective. (D) Phototherapy does not cause photophobia.

141. **(A)** Nursing process phase: implementation; client need: growth and development through the life span; content area: maternity nursing.

RATIONALE

(A) Applying gentle pressure to the head prevents tearing of the perineum. (B) The nurse should not encourage the mother to cross the legs to impede the delivery. (C) The nurse should not discourage the delivery. (D) The nurse should do nothing that will impede the delivery.

142. **(B)** Nursing process phase: implementation; client need: growth and development through the life span; content area: maternity nursing.

RATIONALE

(A) The nurse should not slap the baby's bottom; this could cause cardiac problems. (B) Holding the head in a dependent position helps the mucus to drain and stimulates breathing. (C) The first action is to clear the baby's airway. (D) Vital signs will be taken later.

143. **(D)** Nursing process phase: implementation; client need: psychosocial adaptation; content area: psychiatric nursing.

RATIONALE

(A) Correcting the delusions will make them more fixed. (B) Avoiding talking about the delusions is not therapeutic. (C) This response is not therapeutic. (D) If the nurse disagrees with the client, the delusions become more fixed.

144. **(D)** Nursing process phase: implementation; client need: reduction of risk potential; content area: medical-surgical.

RATIONALE

(A) Glaucoma does not cause a detached retina. (B) Glaucoma does not affect nearsightedness. (C) Glaucoma does not affect farsightedness. (D) If left untreated, glaucoma can lead to blindness.

145. **(C)** Nursing process phase: implementation; client need: physiological adaptation; content area: medical-surgical.

RATIONALE

(A) This is an appropriate nursing strategy but not the first priority. (B) This is an appropriate nursing strategy but not the first priority. (C) The first priority is administering antibiotics. (D) This is an appropriate nursing strategy but not the first priority.

146. **(B)** Nursing process phase: implementation; client need: psychosocial adaptation; content area: psychiatric nursing.

    RATIONALE

    (A) Giving him medication right now will not stop his delusions. (B) This is therapeutic without reinforcing his delusions. (C) This response would reinforce his delusions. (D) This response would reinforce his delusions.

147. **(C)** Nursing process phase: implementation; client need: psychosocial adaptation; content area: psychiatric nursing.

    RATIONALE

    (A) Ignoring the behavior reinforces the delusions. (B) Correcting the behavior may lead to an argument and reinforce the delusions. (C) Physical activity may help the delusions to diminish. (D) This approach reinforces the delusion.

148. **(B)** Nursing process phase: implementation; client need: growth and development through the life span; content area: maternity nursing.

    RATIONALE

    (A) A sterilization consent is not always necessary for an ectopic pregnancy. (B) Blood replacement is crucial in case of hemorrhage. (C) This is a nursing action but not the priority. (D) This is appropriate but not the first priority.

149. **(B)** Nursing process phase: implementation; client need: psychosocial adaptation; content area: psychiatric nursing.

    RATIONALE

    (A) This response is false reassurance. (B) Asking the client if she wishes to talk about the event is therapeutic. (C) This is not a therapeutic response, and the nurse does not know the client's wishes at this time. (D) This is not a therapeutic response.

150. **(A)** Nursing process phase: implementation; client need: physiological adaptation; content area: pediatrics.

    RATIONALE

    (A) Acute hypertension may occur in children with glomerulonephritis. The nurse must check the blood pressure to prevent complications. (B) Clients with glomerulonephritis do not usually have occult bleeding. (C) A urinary catheterization may be ordered, but this is not the priority nursing action. (D) There is no indication for GI intubation.

151. **(B)** Nursing process phase: data collection; client need: prevention and early detection of disease; content area: pediatrics.

    RATIONALE

    (A) Blood pressure is not a reliable measure of dehydration in small children. (B) Skin turgor is decreased in clients with dehydration. (C) Clients with dehydration have increased respirations. (D) Clients with dehydration have an increased pulse rate.

152. **(D)** Nursing process phase: data collection; client need: prevention and early detection of disease; content area: pediatrics.

    RATIONALE

    (A) Although bleeding can occur in the thorax, this is not the most common site for bleeding in children with hemophilia. (B) Although bleeding can occur in the abdomen, this is not the most common site for bleeding in children with hemophilia. (C) Although bleeding can occur in the skull, this is not the most common site for bleeding in children with hemophilia. (D) The most common site of bleeding in children with hemophilia is the joints.

153. **(C)** Nursing process phase: implementation; client need: prevention and early detection of disease; content area: pediatrics.

RATIONALE

(A) This practice limits hip abduction. (B) This practice limits hip abduction. (C) This position promotes hip abduction. (D) This position limits hip abduction.

154. **(C)** Nursing process phase: implementation; client need: prevention and early detection of disease; content area: pediatrics.

    RATIONALE

    (A) Apple juice is permitted in children with diarrhea. (B) Cooked carrots are permitted in children with diarrhea. (C) Milk and milk products should be avoided because they aggravate diarrhea. (D) Applesauce is permitted in children with diarrhea.

155. **(A)** Nursing process phase: implementation; content area: pharmacological and parenteral therapies; content area: pediatrics.

    RATIONALE

    (A) To straighten the ear canal in a child, the pinna is pulled up and back. (B) This method is used to straighten the ear canal in an adult. (C) This method will not straighten the ear canal. (D) This method will not straighten the ear canal.

156. **(C)** Nursing process phase: implementation; client need: basic care and comfort; content area: pediatrics.

    RATIONALE

    (A) This is not the reason for normal regurgitation in the newborn. (B) Although the stomach is small, this is not the reason for normal newborn regurgitation. (C) Because the cardiac sphincter is not fully mature, newborns have frequent regurgitation. (D) There is no scientific evidence to support this statement.

157. **(D)** Nursing process phase: implementation; client need: reduction of risk potential; content area: pediatrics.

    RATIONALE

    (A) A teaspoon is too hard and may injure the surgical repair. (B) The child is too young to drink from a cup. (C) A soft nipple may stimulate the sucking reflex and injure the surgery. (D) A syringe with a soft catheter allows feedings to be given to the side and back of the mouth without injuring the surgery.

158. **(A)** Nursing process phase: implementation; client need: growth and development through the life span; content area: pediatrics.

    RATIONALE

    (A) Stacking blocks is a quiet activity that does not increase oxygen needs. (B) A pull toy is a physical activity that increases oxygen demands. (C) A horn increases oxygen demands. (D) Bouncing balls increase physical activity and therefore increase oxygen demands.

159. **(B)** Nursing process phase: implementation; client need: pharmacological and parenteral therapies; content area: pediatrics.

    RATIONALE

    (A) The medicine will need to be continued for the rest of the child's life. (B) This medicine should be given daily in the morning. (C) A symptom of toxicity from this medicine includes diarrhea, not constipation. (D) The child should continue to gain weight; otherwise, toxicity may be present.

160. **(D)** Nursing process phase: implementation; client need: prevention and early detection of disease; content area: pediatrics.

    RATIONALE

    (A) Progressing in school does not automatically mean that she will lose weight. **(B)** Not all sweets have to be eliminated from the diet. **(C)** Large doses of vitamins are inappropriate and will not suppress her appetite. **(D)** A planned program of activity and physical exercise will help her to lose weight.

161. **(B)** Nursing process phase: implementation; client need: growth and development through the life span; content area: maternity nursing.
   RATIONALE
   (A) Taking the blood pressure during a contraction will give an inaccurate reading. **(B)** Taking blood pressure between contractions will give the most accurate blood pressure. **(C)** Taking the blood pressure immediately after a contraction will give an inaccurate blood pressure. **(D)** Taking the blood pressure at the peak of a contraction will give an inaccurate blood pressure.

162. **(B)** Nursing process phase: implementation; client need: physiological adaptation; content area: pediatrics.
   RATIONALE
   (A) The side-lying position is a difficult position to maintain in an infant. **(B)** The prone position will prevent injury to the affected area. **(C)** The dorsal position will harm the affected area. **(D)** The Fowler's position will harm the affected area.

163. **(C)** Nursing process phase: implementation; client need: psychosocial adaptation; content area: psychiatric nursing.
   RATIONALE
   (A) Although the nurse would notify the police, this is not the first priority. **(B)** Although the nurse may report it to the supervisor, this is not the first priority. **(C)** The first priority is to determine the client's immediate needs so she can establish a sense of control. **(D)** The nurse would not call her family until she has agreed to their being called.

164. **(C)** Nursing process phase: data collection; client need: growth and development through the life span; content area: maternity nursing.
   RATIONALE
   (A) Although the nurse may administer a pain medicine, the first priority is assessment. **(B)** Although the nurse may check her fundus, the first priority is to inspect the perineum. She may have a hematoma. **(C)** Assessment of the perineum is the first priority. She may have a hematoma. **(D)** A sitz bath may be given later, but assessment of the perineum has priority.

165. **(B)** Nursing process phase: planning; client need: reduction of risk potential; content area: pediatrics.
   RATIONALE
   (A) Percussion and postural drainage after meals may cause the child to vomit. **(B)** Percussion and drainage immediately before meals will decrease congestion and improve the appetite. **(C)** It is too difficult to schedule this activity between unpredictable playtimes. **(D)** Midway between meals will not improve her appetite.

166. **(D)** Nursing process phase: planning; client need: physiological adaptation; content area: pediatrics.
   RATIONALE
   (A) Lead poisoning does not cause increased urination. **(B)** Lead poisoning does not cause decreased urination. **(C)** Lead poisoning does not usually cause malnutrition. **(D)** One of the initial signs of lead poisoning is anemia.

167. **(C)** Nursing process phase: implementation; client need: prevention and early detection of disease; content area: medical-surgical.
   RATIONALE
   (A) Drinking lots of water will not help the discharge. She needs

antibiotics. **(B)** Thick white discharge is not a normal occurrence. She needs to see a health provider at the clinic or her private physician. **(C)** She needs treatment as soon as possible to prevent long-range damage to the urinary and reproductive systems. **(D)** Do not tell her mother. She may not want her mother to know.

168. **(B)** Nursing process phase: implementation; client need: growth and development through the life span; content area: pediatrics.
   RATIONALE
   (A) This is not aphasia. Aphasia is having difficulty expressing oneself. **(B)** Transposing figures is one of the symptoms that the child has a learning disability. **(C)** Transposing figures is not consistent with visual problems. **(D)** There are no indications that there is a neurological disorder. Many 12-year-olds have illegible handwriting.

169. **(B)** Nursing process phase: planning; client need: physiological adaptation; content area: medical-surgical.
   RATIONALE
   (A) Do not use wooden tongue blades during a seizure; they can splinter and cause damage. **(B)** Hard plastic bite blocks are preferred to prevent biting the tongue. **(C)** Restraining a person during a seizure can cause more harm. **(D)** It is an unsafe practice to keep a syringe of medicine near the bedside.

170. **(A)** Nursing process phase: implementation; client need: prevention and early detection of disease; content area: medical-surgical.
   RATIONALE
   (A) Speak slowly so that the client has a better chance of understanding. **(B)** Exaggerating the words causes increased confusion. **(C)** The client is not hard of hearing; she does not understand the language. **(D)** Written instructions do not ensure understanding. She may not be able to read the language either.

171. **(D)** Nursing process phase: implementation; client need: management of care; content area: medical-surgical.
   RATIONALE
   (A) Although the mother may sign, it is best to let both parents decide. **(B)** Although the father may sign, it is best to let both parents decide. **(C)** There is no need for both parents to sign the consent form. **(D)** Letting both parents decide avoids cultural imposition.

172. **(D)** Nursing process phase: implementation; client need: coping and adaptation; content area: medical-surgical.
   RATIONALE
   (A) It is usually unacceptable for a woman to touch a male's body in the Islamic culture. **(B)** Although the orderly is a male, he may not be permitted to insert a catheter. The male nurse is the best person to insert the catheter. **(C)** It is preferable to have a trained person do the procedure. **(D)** The male LPN is the best person to do the procedure.

173. **(C)** Nursing process phase: implementation; client need: coping and adaptation; content area: medical-surgical.
   RATIONALE
   (A) Just because someone does not maintain eye contact does not mean that he or she does not understand. **(B)** Just because someone does not maintain eye contact does not mean that he or she is not interested in the conversation. **(C)** Not maintaining eye contact with superiors (the nurse in this case) is common among some Native Americans. **(D)** Not maintaining eye contact does not mean that the client prefers a physician to give the instructions.

174. **(B)** Nursing process phase: planning; client need: coping and adaptation; content area: medical-surgical.

    RATIONALE
    (A) This is not child abuse; coining is a traditional Vietnamese treatment. **(B)** Coining is a traditional Vietnamese treatment that is used for respiratory conditions. **(C)** The practice is not harmful; the father can stay with his child. **(D)** There is no reason to discontinue this practice while the child is in the hospital; it does not interfere with other therapies.

175. **(C)** Nursing process phase: implementation; client need: basic care and comfort; content area: psychiatric nursing.

    RATIONALE
    (A) Although it may be against hospital policy, it should not be and the client should be allowed to eat the food. **(B)** A dietitian should be consulted at a later time. The immediate priority is to let the client eat the food. **(C)** The client is on a regular diet; he can eat the food. **(D)** Do not take the food away.

176. **(B)** Nursing process phase: planning; client need: psychosocial adaptation; content area: medical-surgical.

    RATIONALE
    (A) The client may eventually be told, but initially the nurse should respect the family's wishes. **(B)** Respect the family's wishes initially. In the Japanese culture, to give the client a terminal diagnosis means to give up hope. **(C)** This may be a later action. **(D)** Insisting that the family tell the client about the terminal diagnosis is cultural imposition.

177. **(B)** Nursing process phase: planning; client need: psychosocial adaptation; content area: psychiatric nursing.

    RATIONALE
    (A) Restricting visitors in this cultural group may not help the situation. **(B)** Eliciting the help of family members will give the client and family some autonomy. In the Mexican culture, it is a family obligation for all family members to visit the hospitalized family member. **(C)** Control of visitors is a nursing function, not a physician function. **(D)** Acting as the control person will not give the family autonomy.

178. **(D)** Nursing process phase: implementation; client need: basic care and comfort; content area: psychiatric nursing.

    RATIONALE
    (A) There is no reason why the client cannot take herbal teas. They do not interfere with other treatments. **(B)** The nurse may report the situation to the physician later, but the first action is to let her drink her herbal tea. **(C)** The nurse may report the situation to the pharmacist later so it can be added to her profile, but the initial action is to let the client drink her herbal tea. **(D)** Herbal tea gives the client some relief and autonomy.

179. **(B)** Nursing process phase: planning; client need: psychosocial adaptation; content area: psychiatric nursing.

    RATIONALE
    (A) Oral hypoglycemic medications do not work for insulin-dependent diabetes mellitus. **(B)** Because this is a spiritual and religious issue, the chaplain may have more influence with the client. **(C)** Clients' beliefs should never be labeled as nonsense. **(D)** This statement is an example of cultural imposition.

180. **(C)** Nursing process phase: planning; client need: psychosocial adaptation; content area: psychiatric nursing.

    RATIONALE
    (A) This action negates client autonomy and rights. **(B)** The physician may eventually order the medicine around the clock, but this is not the first action. **(C)** Exploring the reason for not taking the medicine is the first action. Many Filipino clients are stoical about pain because "it is God's will." **(D)** Although the

nurse may report the situation to the nursing supervisor, the first action is to explore the client's reasons for not taking the pain medication.

181. **(A)** Nursing process phase: implementation; client need: psychological adaptation; content area: psychiatric nursing.

    RATIONALE
    (A) Tape the bracelet in place. The bracelet provides for spiritual needs. **(B)** It is not necessary to have the family remove the bracelet. **(C)** It is not necessary to delay the surgery. **(D)** Do not enclose the hand in a mitten. The nailbeds will be used in surgery to help determine oxygenation.

182. **(B)** Nursing process phase: implementation; client need: reduction of risk potential; content area: medical-surgical.

    RATIONALE
    (A) It is unlikely that the acupuncturist will ruin the surgery. **(B)** Both the physician and the acupuncturist should be made aware of each other's involvement. **(C)** In some cases, the acupuncture may be as effective as the surgery. **(D)** This statement is judgmental and does not promote client autonomy.

183. **(C)** Nursing process phase: evaluation; client need: reduction of risk potential; content area: medical-surgical.

    RATIONALE
    (A) The feet should not be far apart; this increases the chances of catching her feet on the crutches. **(B)** Placing weight on the axilla can cause damage to the nerves in the axilla. **(C)** Proper crutch walking is placing the weight on the palms of the hands. **(D)** Proper crutch walking includes a swing-through gait.

184. **(A)** Nursing process phase: implementation; client need: prevention and early detection of disease; content area: medical-surgical.

    RATIONALE
    (A) The nurse should recognize these symptoms as being consistent with diabetes. She should encourage him to make an appointment with his physician as soon as possible. **(B)** The nurse would encourage him to go to the emergency room only if he gets significantly worse or is unable to obtain an appointment with his physician. **(C)** These symptoms, consistent with diabetes, should not be taken lightly. **(D)** The nurse does not need to notify the supervisor at this time.

185. **(B)** Nursing process phase: implementation; client need: pharmacological and parenteral therapies; content area: medical-surgical.

    RATIONALE
    (A) She will continue the medicine even after the symptoms have disappeared. **(B)** The methylprednisolone prescription will include instructions for taking a different number of tablets each day on a decreasing basis. Serious adrenal complications may occur if she does not take the medication exactly as instructed. **(C)** The client will be taking the medication several times each day in the beginning. **(D)** The client will be taking the medication several times each day in the beginning.

186. **(D)** Nursing process phase: implementation; client need: prevention and early detection of disease; content area: medical-surgical.

    RATIONALE
    (A) Although increasing nutritional status is important, the first priority is to monitor vital signs. **(B)** Although increasing fluid intake is important, the first priority is to monitor vital signs. **(C)** Although monitoring neurological status is important, the first priority is to monitor vital signs. **(D)** A change in vital signs is the most sensitive indicator of a change in status of the client with alcohol abuse.

187. **(C)** Nursing process phase: implementation; client need: prevention and early detection of disease; content area: medical-surgical.

RATIONALE

(A) Meats are allowed as long as they are not fatty. **(B)** Fruits of all kinds are permitted. **(C)** Fatty foods will increase the pain associated with cholecystitis. **(D)** Vegetables of all kinds are permitted.

188. **(D)** Nursing process phase: implementation; client need: prevention and early detection of disease; content area: medical-surgical.

RATIONALE

(A) Accurate assessments cannot be made on this schedule. **(B)** Accurate assessments cannot be made on this schedule. **(C)** Three days before the menses begins is not the preferred timing for breast self-examinations. **(D)** The preferred timing for breast self-examinations is 3 days after the menses begin because this is the time with the least amount of breast engorgement.

189. **(C)** Nursing process phase: implementation; client need: basic care and comfort; content area: medical-surgical.

RATIONALE

(A) Taking a bath in very warm water will increase perspiration and increase itching. **(B)** Keeping the room this warm will increase perspiration and increase itching. **(C)** Avoiding soap whenever possible will decrease itching. The residue left by soaps will increase itching. **(D)** Perfumed lotions can irritate the skin and increase itching.

190. **(C)** Nursing process phase: implementation; client need: prevention and early detection of disease; content area: medical-surgical.

RATIONALE

(A) The shunt should be warm to the touch. **(B)** It is unlikely that a visible pulsation would be seen. **(C)** A normally functioning shunt has a palpable rush of blood. **(D)** An outline of erythematous skin would denote a possible infection.

191. **(A)** Nursing process phase: implementation; client need: reduction of risk potential; content area: medical-surgical.

RATIONALE

(A) The priority action is to place the client back in bed to prevent evisceration. **(B)** There is no need for a moist dressing. **(C)** Calling the physician is the next priority. **(D)** The client may need pain medication, but the first priority is to put the client back to bed.

192. **(D)** Nursing process phase: implementation; client need: psychosocial adaptation; content area: psychiatric nursing.

RATIONALE

(A) This statement is an attempt to console the client but is inappropriate. **(B)** She may not want to sit in a chair. **(C)** Calling the physician is not a first priority. **(D)** This behavior may be culture-bound, and the most appropriate action at this time is to remain close to her and offer support.

193. **(B)** Nursing process phase: implementation; client need: basic care and comfort; content area: medical-surgical.

RATIONALE

(A) Lean meats and meat by-products will not help to alleviate constipation. **(B)** Fruits and vegetables provide fiber and help to alleviate constipation. **(C)** Poultry and fish will not help to alleviate constipation. **(D)** Rice and potatoes will make the constipation worse.

194. **(C)** Nursing process phase: implementation; client need: physiological adaptation; content area: medical-surgical.

RATIONALE

(A) Taking nitroglycerin is the second priority. **(B)** He would call the rescue squad only if he does not get relief after repeated doses of nitroglycerin. **(C)** His first priority is to stop all activity to reduce oxygen needs to the myocardium. **(D)** He should not ignore the pain; he could be having a myocardial infarction.

195. **(D)** Nursing process phase: planning; client need: prevention and early detection of disease; content area: medical-surgical.

RATIONALE

(A) The pulse rate would increase if the condition worsens. **(B)** Although respirations may increase, the most sensitive indicator that the condition is worsening would be indicated by an increase in pulse rate. **(C)** Respirations would increase if his condition is worsening. **(D)** The most sensitive indicator of shock is an increase in pulse rate.

196. **(B)** Nursing process phase: implementation; client need: reduction of risk potential; content area: medical-surgical.

RATIONALE

(A) High Fowler's position may impede the airway in clients immediately postoperatively. **(B)** Semi-Fowler's position will help to decrease pull on the incision and to improve ventilation. **(C)** This position would increase pain and impede ventilation immediately postoperatively. **(D)** The supine position would cause pull on the incision.

197. **(A)** Nursing process phase: implementation; client need: reduction of risk potential; content area: medical-surgical.

RATIONALE

(A) The priority is to drink at least 3000 ml of fluid each day to prevent clotting. **(B)** There is no need to eliminate citrus drinks. **(C)** There is no need to eliminate milk and milk products from the diet. **(D)** Although cranberry and apple juices are recommended postoperatively, any liquid is okay to drink.

198. **(B)** Nursing process phase: implementation; client need: reduction of risk potential; content area: medical-surgical.

RATIONALE

(A) The position of the HemoVac is not important; drainage is maintained by negative pressure within the unit. **(B)** Completely collapsing the unit before the air plug is inserted will ensure a proper negative pressure within the unit. **(C)** There is no need to milk the tubing. **(D)** Negative pressure in a HemoVac is maintained within the unit; it should not be attached to the wall unit.

199. **(C)** Nursing process phase: implementation; client need: reduction of risk potential; content area: medical-surgical.

RATIONALE

(A) The presence of a gag reflex does not ensure that the client can take fluids. **(B)** The client's thirst is not an indicator of ability to tolerate fluids. **(C)** The presence of bowel sounds is the most reliable indicator that the client can tolerate fluids without aspirating. **(D)** Degree of alertness does not ensure the presence of bowel sounds.

200. **(A)** Nursing process phase: planning; client need: prevention and early detection of disease; content area: medical-surgical.

RATIONALE

(A) Clients with Cushing's syndrome have truncal obesity and hirsutism. **(B)** Enlarged hands and feet are consistent with acromegaly. **(C)** A large jaw and large feet are consistent with acromegaly. **(D)** Clients with Cushing's syndrome have a buffalo hump, but they do not have large hands.

201. **(B)** Nursing process phase: planning; client need: pharmacological and parenteral therapies; content area: medical-surgical.

RATIONALE

(A) Clients on dexamethasone are not prone to renal calculi. (B) Clients on dexamethasone are prone to infection. (C) Clients on dexamethasone are not prone to gallstones. (D) Clients on dexamethasone are not prone to hypotension.

202. **(C)** Nursing process phase: implementation; client need: reduction of risk potential; content area: medical-surgical.

RATIONALE

(A) This position will not facilitate breathing. (B) This position will not facilitate breathing. (C) This is the best position to maintain adequate breathing postoperatively. (D) Semi-Fowler's is better than low-Fowler's.

203. **(B)** Nursing process phase: planning; client need: reduction of risk potential; content area: medical-surgical.

RATIONALE

(A) A thoracotomy tray is used for the insertion of a chest tube. (B) A tracheostomy tray is needed in case of breathing difficulties. (C) A paracentesis tray is used for an abdominal tap. (D) A pericardiocentesis tray is used for draining fluid from the pericardium.

204. **(B)** Nursing process phase: implementation; client need: physiological adaptation; content area: medical-surgical.

RATIONALE

(A) Do not remove the screwdriver; it may be tamponading a bleeding site. (B) Leave the screwdriver in place until adequate medical help is in place. (C) This is a later action. (D) Do not remove the screwdriver; it may be tamponading a bleeding site.

205. **(D)** Nursing process phase: implementation; client need: physiological adaptation; content area: medical-surgical.

RATIONALE

(A) Cleaning the wound is a second priority. (B) Using a tourniquet is a last resort. (C) If a tourniquet is needed, it would be applied above the laceration. (D) Apply direct pressure first to control the bleeding.

206. **(C)** Nursing process phase: implementation; client need: reduction of risk potential; content area: medical-surgical.

RATIONALE

(A) Not all clients have phantom limb pain. (B) Demonstrating dressing changes is a later activity. (C) Teaching crutch walking is the best activity to prepare him for postoperative therapy. (D) Teaching leg exercises has a lower priority than teaching crutch walking.

207. **(C)** Nursing process phase: implementation; client need: psychosocial adaptation; content area: psychiatric nursing.

RATIONALE

(A) This intervention does not help the client to understand the anxiety. (B) This intervention does not help the client to understand the anxiety. (C) The most appropriate initial intervention is to help the client to understand the anxiety. (D) This activity may help the client to sleep, but it does not help the client to understand the anxiety.

208. **(A)** Nursing process phase: implementation; client need: reduction of risk potential; content area: medical-surgical.

RATIONALE

(A) A high-fiber diet will help to ensure a soft stool and to decrease the chance for bleeding and pain postoperatively. (B) A low-fiber diet will cause bowel irritation. (C) A high-fat diet may cause diarrhea postoperatively. (D) A high-carbohydrate diet may cause constipation postoperatively.

APPENDIX

State Boards of Nursing

Alabama Board of Nursing
PO Box 303900
Montgomery, AL 36130
Phone: (334) 242-4060
FAX: (334) 242-4360

Alaska Board of Nursing
Dept of Comm and Econ Develop
Div of Occupational Licensing
3601 C St, Ste 722
Anchorage, AK 99503
Phone: (907) 269-8161
FAX: (907) 269-8156

American Samoa Health Services
    Regulatory Board
LBJ Tropical Medical Ctr
Pago Pago, AS 96799
Phone: (684) 633-1222
FAX: (684) 633-1869

Arizona State Board of Nursing
1651 E Morten Ave, Ste 150
Phoenix, AZ 85020
Phone: (602) 255-5092
FAX: (602) 906-9365

Arkansas State Board of Nursing
University Tower Building
1123 S University, Ste 800
Little Rock, AR 72204
Phone: (501) 686-2700
FAX: (501) 686-2714

California Board of Vocational Nurse and
    Psychiatric Technician Examiners
2535 Capitol Oaks Dr, Ste 205
Sacramento, CA 95833
Phone: (916) 263-7800
FAX: (916) 263-7859

Colorado Board of Nursing
1560 Broadway, Ste 670
Denver, CO 80202
Phone: (303) 894-2430
FAX: (303) 894-2821

Connecticut Board of Examiners for Nursing
    Div of Health Systems Regulation
410 Capitol Ave, MS# 12HSR #340308
Hartford, CT 06134
Phone: (860) 509-7624
FAX: (860) 509-7286

Delaware Board of Nursing
Cannon Building, Ste 203
PO Box 1401
Dover, DE 19903
Phone: (302) 739-4522
FAX: (302) 739-2711

District of Columbia Board of Nursing
614 H St, NW
Washington, DC 20001
Phone: (202) 727-7468
FAX: (202) 727-7662

Florida Board of Nursing
4080 Woodcock Dr, Ste 202
Jacksonville, FL 32207
Phone: (904) 858-6940
FAX: (904) 858-6964

Georgia State Board of Licensed Practical
    Nurses
166 Pryor St, SW
Atlanta, GA 30303
Phone: (404) 656-3921
FAX: (404) 651-9532

Guam Board of Nurse Examiners
PO Box 2816
Agana, GU 96910
Phone: (671) 475-0251
FAX: (671) 477-4733

Hawaii Board of Nursing
Professional and Vocational Licensing Div
PO Box 3469
Honolulu, HI 96801
Phone: (808) 586-2695
FAX: (808) 586-2689

Idaho Board of Nursing
PO Box 83720
Boise, ID 83720
Phone: (208) 334-3110
FAX: (208) 334-3262

Illinois Department of Professional
    Regulation
James R. Thompson Ctr
100 W Randolph, Ste 9-300
Chicago, IL 60601
Phone: (312) 814-2715
FAX: (312) 814-3145

Indiana State Board of Nursing
Health Professions Bureau
402 W Washington St, Ste 041
Indianapolis, IN 46204
Phone: (317) 232-2960
FAX: (317) 233-4236

Iowa Board of Nursing
State Capitol Complex
1223 E Court Ave
Des Moines, IA 50319
Phone: (515) 281-3255
FAX: (515) 281-4825

Kansas State Board of Nursing
Landon State Office Bldg
900 SW Jackson, Ste 551-S
Topeka, KS 66612
Phone: (913) 296-4929
FAX: (913) 296-3929

Kentucky Board of Nursing
312 Whittington Pkwy, Ste 300
Lousiville, KY 40222
Phone: (502) 329-7006
FAX: (502) 329-7011

Louisiana State Board of Practical Nurse
    Examiners
3421 N Causeway Blvd, Ste 203
Metairie, LA 70002
Phone: (504) 838-5791
FAX: (504) 838-5279

Maine State Board of Nursing
158 State House Station
Augusta, ME 04333
Phone: (207) 287-1133
FAX: (207) 287-1149

Maryland Board of Nursing
4140 Patterson Ave
Baltimore, MD 21215
Phone: (410) 764-5124
FAX: (410) 358-3530

Massachusetts Board of Registration in
    Nursing
Leverett Saltonstall Bldg
100 Cambridge St, Rm 1519
Boston, MA 02202
Phone: (617) 727-9961
FAX: (617) 727-2197

State of Michigan
 CIS/Office of Health Services
Ottawa Towers North
611 W Ottawa, 4th Fl
Lansing, MI 48933
Phone: (517) 373-9102
FAX: (517) 373-2179

Minnesota Board of Nursing
2829 University Ave SE, Ste 500
Minneapolis, MN 55414
Phone: (612) 617-2270
FAX: (612) 617-2190

Mississippi Board of Nursing
239 N Lamar St, Ste 401
Jackson, MS 39201
Phone: (601) 359-6170
FAX: (601) 359-6185

Missouri State Board of Nursing
PO Box 656
Jefferson City, MO 65102
Phone: (573) 751-0681
FAX: (573) 751-0075

Montana State Board of Nursing
111 N Jackson
Helena, MT 59620
Phone: (406) 444-2071
FAX: (406) 444-7759

Dept of Health and Human Services
 Regulation and Licensure Credentialing
 Div—Nursing/Nursing Support Section
PO Box 94986
Lincoln, NE 68509
Phone: (402) 471-4376
FAX: (402) 471-3577

Nevada State Board of Nursing
1755 E Plumb Ln, Ste 260
Reno, NV 89502
Phone: (702) 786-2778
FAX: (702) 322-6993

New Hampshire Board of Nursing
Health & Welfare Bldg
6 Hazen Dr
Concord, NH 03301
Phone: (603) 271-2323
FAX: (603) 271-6605

New Jersey Board of Nursing
PO Box 45010
Newark, NJ 07101
Phone: (201) 504-6586
FAX: (201) 648-3481

New Mexico Board of Nursing
4206 Louisiana Blvd, NE, Ste A
Albuquerque, NM 87109
Phone: (505) 841-8340
FAX: (505) 841-8347

New York State Board of Nursing
State Education Dept
Cultural Education Ctr, Rm 3023
Albany, NY 12230
Phone: (518) 474-3845
FAX: (518) 473-0578

North Carolina Board of Nursing
3724 National Dr
Raleigh, NC 27602
Phone: (919) 782-3211
FAX: (919) 781-9461

North Dakota Board of Nursing
919 S 7th St, Ste 504
Bismarck, ND 58504
Phone: (701) 328-9777
FAX: (701) 328-9785

Ohio Board of Nursing
77 S High St, 17th Fl
Columbus, OH 43215
Phone: (614) 466-3947
FAX: (614) 466-0388

Oklahoma Board of Nursing
2915 N Classen Blvd, Ste 524
Oklahoma City, OK 73106
Phone: (405) 525-2076
FAX: (405) 521-6089

Oregon State Board of Nursing
800 NE Oregon St, Box 25
Ste 465
Portland, OR 97232
Phone: (503) 731-4745
FAX: (503) 731-4755

Pennsylvania State Board of Nursing
PO Box 2649
Harrisburg, PA 17105
Phone: (717) 783-7142
FAX: (717) 783-0822

Commonwealth of Puerto Rico
 Board of Nurse Examiners
Call Box 10200
Santurce, PR 00908
Phone: (787) 725-8161
FAX: (787) 725-7903

Rhode Island Board of Nurse Registration
 and Nursing Education
Cannon Health Bldg
Three Capitol Hill, Rm 104
Providence, RI 02908
Phone: (401) 277-2827
FAX: (401) 277-1272

Commonwealth Board of Nurse Examiners
Public Health Ctr
PO Box 1458
Saipan, Marianas 96950
Phone: (670) 234-8950
FAX: (670) 234-8930

South Carolina State Board of Nursing
110 Centerview Dr, Ste 202
Columbia, SC 29210
Phone: (803) 896-4550
FAX: (803) 896-4525

South Dakota Board of Nursing
3307 South Lincoln Ave
Sioux Falls, SD 57105
Phone: (605) 367-5940
FAX: (605) 367-5945

Tennessee State Board of Nursing
426 Fifth Ave N
Cordell Hull Building, 1st Fl
Nashville, TN 37247
Phone: (615) 532-5166
FAX: (615) 741-7899

Texas Board of Vocational Nurse
 Examiners
William P. Hobby Building, Tower 3
333 Guadalupe St, Ste 3-400
Austin, TX 78701
Phone: (512) 305-8100
FAX: (512) 305-8101

Utah State Board of Nursing
Div of Occupational and
 Professional Licensing
Salt Lake City, UT 84145
Phone: (801) 530-6628
FAX: (801) 530-6511

Vermont State Board of Nursing
109 State St
Montpelier, VT 05609
Phone: (802) 828-2396
FAX: (802) 828-2484

Virgin Islands Board of Nurse
 Licensure
Veterans Drive Station
St Thomas, VI 00803
Phone: (340) 776-7397
FAX: (340) 777-4003

Virginia Board of Nursing
6606 W Broad St, 4th Fl
Richmond, VA 23230
Phone: (804) 662-9909
FAX: (804) 662-9943

Washington State Nursing Care
 Quality Assurance Commission
Dept of Health
Olympia, WA 98504
Phone: (360) 753-2686
FAX: (360) 586-2165

West Virginia State Board of Examiners
 for Practical Nurses
101 Dee Dr
Charleston, WV 25311
Phone: (304) 558-3572
FAX: (304) 558-4367

Wisconsin Department of Regulation and
 Licensing
1400 E Washington Ave
Madison, WI 53708
Phone: (608) 266-2112
FAX: (608) 267-0644

Wyoming State Board of Nursing
2020 Carey Ave, Ste 110
Cheyenne, WY 82002
Phone: (307) 777-7601
FAX: (307) 777-3519

Index

Numbers followed by a "t" indicate tabular material.